Progress in Allergy and Clinical Immunology

Progress in Allergy and Clinical Immunology

Proceedings of the 13th International Congress of Allergology and Clinical Immunology

Edited by

Werner J. Pichler, Beda M. Stadler, Clemens Dahinden,
Alain R. Pécoud, Philippe C. Frei, Conrad Schneider,
Alain L. de Weck

Institute of Clinical Immunology, Inselspital, Bern
and
Centre Hospitalier Universitaire Vaudoise, Dept. Immuno-allergie, Lausanne

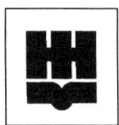

Hogrefe & Huber Publishers
Toronto • Lewiston, NY • Bern • Göttingen • Stuttgart

Library of Congress Cataloging-in-Publication Data

International Congress of Allergology and Clinical Immunology (13th : 1988: Montreux, Switzerland)
Progress in allergy and clinical immunology : proceedings of the XIIIth International Congress of Allergology and
Clinical Immunology / Werner J. Pichler ... [et al.]. (editors).
p. cm.
Congress held Oct. 16–21, 1988, in Montreux, Switzerland.
Includes bibliographies
1. Allergies—Congresses. 2. Immunologic diseases—Congresses. I. Pichler, Werner J., 1949–   . II. Title.
[DNLM: 1. Allergy and Immunology—congresses. QW 504 I5918p]
RC583.2I57   1989   616.97—dc19

Canadian Cataloguing in Publication Data

International Congress of Allergology and Clinical Immunology (13th : 1988: Montreux, Switzerland)
Progress in allergy and clinical immunology

Bibliography: p.

1. Allergy—Congresses. 2. Immunopathology—Congresses. I. Pichler, Werner J., 1949–   . II. Title.
RC583.2I67   1989   61697'079   C89-093285-9

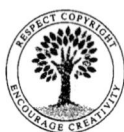

P. O. Box 51
Lewiston, NY   14092

12–14 Bruce Park Ave.
Toronto, Ontario M4P 2S3

Printed in Germany

ISBN 0-920887-45-7
Hans Huber Publishers • Toronto • Lewiston, NY • Bern • Stuttgart
ISBN 3-456-81780-0
Hans Huber Publishers • Bern • Stuttgart • Toronto • Lewiston, NY

Foreword

When you hold this book in your hands, the 13th International Congress of Allergology and Clinical Immunology will have taken place in Montreux a few months ago. Every three years, the world community of allergologists and clinical immunologists gathers to exchange information on the latest research developments and clinical experiences. The value of such large congresses is sometimes questioned: Is the effort in time and money devoted by the concerned—from participants to organizers and exhibitors—worth it?

The presence of over 3400 delegates was in itself an answer to this question. Despite all the problems associated with large congresses, they still represent a major opportunity to assess the state of the art, to establish the uniqueness of our discipline in an increasingly complex world, and to form or renew old friendships with colleagues from around the world.

Allergy and Clinical Immunology have experienced considerable progress in diagnosis and therapy over the past decade. This con-

gress demonstrated that the momentum is continuing. However, we are facing new challenges. The increasing impact of a changing environment on allergic diseases, both in the industrialized and in the third world, was a central theme of the congress. The emergence of new immunological diseases, like AIDS, also poses a global challenge to the world community.

Besides recalling pleasant memories in the minds of the participants (and also of the organizers!), the Proceedings volume represents a concrete way to determine our state of knowledge and also to disseminate the information to those who could not attend.

At this point I would like to thank the contributors to the volume, the editors who put it together, and also the publishers for their excellent cooperation.

Prof. Dr. Alain L. de Weck
President IAACI
President Organization Committee
XIIIth ICACI

Table of Contents

Human Mast Cell Neutral Proteases: Markers of Mast Cell Heterogeneity and Function

Lawrence B. Schwartz*

Tryptase, chymase, and carboxypeptidase are three neutral proteases uniquely concentrated in the secretory granules of mast cells in human tissues. Although their biologic functions have not been convincingly demonstrated, their abundance in mast cells and their secretion with other granule components suggest a purposeful presence for each protease. Tryptase levels, measured by immunoassay, in complex biologic fluids such as serum, nasal and bronchoalveolar lavage fluids, and skin chamber fluid serve as an indicator of mast cell activation and may be useful in the diagnosis and monitoring of allergic diseases. Tryptase and chymase have been used as markers of distinct subpopulations of human mast cells, tryptase$^+$, chymase$^-$ (MC$_T$ cells) and tryptase$^+$, chymase$^+$ (MC$_{TC}$ cells). MC$_T$ and MC$_{TC}$ cells are further distinguished by ultrastructure, tissue distribution, and apparent dependence on functional T lymphocytes. They appear to develop along separate pathways, at least from the time at which granule formation begins. Determination of the functional properties of these mast cell subpopulations along with those of the mast cell proteases should prove critical to our understanding of allergic disease.

Two types of mast cells have been defined in humans on the basis of their protease compositions [1], ultrastructural features [2], and apparent dependence on T lymphocytes [3]. The characteristic tissue distribution for each mast cell type defines, in part, the target tissue and consequent physiologic response to release of mediators. Purposeful yet distinct functions for each mast cell type are likely. This article reviews data concerning the neutral proteases and subpopulations of human mast cells.

Tryptase, Chymase, and Carboxypeptidase

Neutral proteases are the major protein components of human mast cells secretory granules and serve as specific markers for mast cells relative to other cell types and for mast cell subpopulations (Table 1).

Tryptase is a tetramer of 134,000 m.w. with subunits of 31,000 to 35,000 m.w., each with an active site for the cleavage of proteins on the carboxyl side of basic (lys, arg) amino acids ([4–7]. Tryptase is biochemically, antigenically, and genetically distinct from pancreatic trypsin. Based on a specific immunoassay, the mean level of tryptase in a mast cell from adult lung was calculated to be 12 pg and from adult foreskin 35 pg [8]. Negligible amounts were found in normal basophils (0.04 pg/cell) [9],

Table 1. Neutral proteases of human mast cells.

Characteristic	Tryptase	Chymase	Carboxypeptidase
Size (daltons)	134,000	30,000	34,000
Subunit composition	tetramer	monomer	monomer
pH optimum	neutral	neutral	neutral
Specificity	lys, arg (internal)	tyr, phe (internal)	leu, ala (external)
pg/cell			
T mast cell	10	0.04	
TC mast cell	35	4.5	10–25
Basophil	0.04	0.04	

*   Section of Allergy and Immunology, Department of Medicine, Medical College of Virginia, Virginia Commonwealth University, Richmond, Virginia, USA.
This work was supported in part by NIH grant AI-210487 and the Charles W. Thomas Arthritis Fund.

foreskin 35 pg [8]. Negligible amounts were found in normal basophils (0.04 pg/cell) [9], but none has been detected in other cell types. Tryptase is released from secretory granules in parallel with histamine [10], but has a half-life in the circulation of about 2 hours (compared to 1–3 min for histamine). Tryptase levels in complex biologic fluids, including plasma or serum [11] and nasal lavage [12], skin chamber [13, 14], and bronchoalveolar lavage [15] fluids have been used as a specific indicator of mast cell- mediated activity in conditions such as systemic anaphylaxis and mastocytosis, asthma, and allergic rhinitis.

Chymase is a monomer of 30,000 m.w. which cleaves proteins on the carboxyl side of aromatic (tyr, phe) amino acids [16–19]. Chymase is immunologically and biochemically distinct from pancreatic chymotrypsin and neutrophil cathepsin G. The mean level of immunoreactive chymase in mast cells obtained from adult foreskin is 4.5 pg/cell. Both immunoreactive and enzymatic levels of chymase are approximately 10-fold greater in mast cells derived from skin compared to those from lung [8]. In the foreskin preparations 99% of the mast cells were of the MCTC (connective tissue) types, whereas those from lung were composed of about 90% MCT (mucosal) and 10% MCTC cells, the latter cell type most likely accounting for the chymase found in lung mast cells.

Carboxypeptidase is a monomer of about 34,000 m.w. which catalytically removes carboxyterminal leu or val residues from proteins [20, 21]. This mast cell enzyme is distinct from carboxypeptidases A and B and from keratinocyte carboxypeptidase. Approximately 10–25 pg/adult foreskin mast cell have been detected; 5- to 10-fold lower levels are found in mast cells obtained from human lung.

Tryptase, chymase, and carboxypeptidase are stored in mast cell secretory granules as fully active enzymes, probably kept under control by the acid pH within these granules [22]. After release into the extracellular space, these enzymes are maximally active near their neutral pH optima. Tryptase is not susceptible to inhibition by the classical protease inhibitors that reside in tissues and in the circulation; rather, tryptase is stabilized by its ionic association with heparin proteoglycan and destabilized after dissociation of this complex [23, 24]. On the other hand, chymase is inhibited by classical protease inhibitors such as α1-antitrypsin, which should limit expression of chymase activity after its release.

The biologic functions of these proteases are not clearly understood. Of potential interest is the ability of tryptase to generate C3a from C3 [25], destroy high molecular weight kininogen [26] and fibrinogen [27], and activate synovial latent collagenase [28]; of chymase to generate angiotensin II from I [29] and weaken the integrity of the dermal/epidermal basement membrane [30]; and of carboxypeptidase to convert angiotensin to des-leu10 angiotensin I, an inhibitor of angiotensin converting enzyme [28]. These activities may be important components of various mast cell-mediated inflammatory reactions.

T and TC Types of Human Mast Cells

Mast cells containing tryptase together with chymase (TC or MCTC type) and other mast cells containing tryptase alone (T or MCT type) have been detected with immunohistochemical techniques by light [1] and electron [2] microscopy (Table 2). These compositions were confirmed with enzymatic and immunologic assays on material extracted from foreskin- and lung-derived dispersed mast cells [8]. In tissue sections MCT cells were found to be the predominant type in lung and bowel mucosa,

Table 2. Selected characteristics of different types of human mast cells.

Characteristic	MCT (mucosal, atypical)	MCTC (connective tissue, typical)
Neutral protease	tryptase	tryptase chymase
Tissue distribution	lung, bowel mucosa	skin, bowel submucosa
Granule ultrastructure	discrete scrolls	gratings/lattices
T lymphocyte-dependence	+	−

stantial numbers of both mast cell types, making it nearly impossible to define mast cell type based on tissue location alone.

Ultrastructural features of MC_T and MC_{TC} cells were determined by electron microscopy after the mast cell types was first determined with an immunogold technique using antitryptase and antichymase antibodies [2]. All granules of MC_T cells stained strongly for tryptase; all granules of MC_{TC} cells stained strongly for tryptase and chymase. Small amounts of chymase in MC_T cells could not be excluded by this technique.

Morphologic differences between MC_T and MC_{TC} cells were found predominantly within granules. The most common pattern observed for MC_T cells included granules with characteristic discrete scrolls; these were not observed in MC_{TC} cells. Occasional MC_T cells (less than 10%) had a majority of granules with particulate or beaded substructures. Discrete scroll and particulate patterns sometimes appeared together, suggesting a close relationship between MC_T cells with these features, possibly representing different activation states.

At high magnification a portion of the granules of MC_{TC} cells contained characteristic grating and lattice substructures. A single cell containing granules with features characteristic for both mast cell types has not been observed in the author's lab, indicating that direct interconversions between mature human mast cells—if they occur at all—are either very rare or occur very rapidly in normal tissues.

Alternative interpretations of the ultrastructural data to being representative of different cell types involve differences in state of activation, stage of maturation, plane of section or tissue processing. However, both cell types appear mature without evidence of ongoing or recent activation. Different planes of section through the same granule do not produce both discrete scroll and grating/lattice patterns. Finally MC_T and MC_{TC} cell types sometimes reside close enough to one another (particularly in bronchial tissue) to be in the same section, thereby being subjected to identical processing conditions and clearly exhibit the characteristic and distinguishing ultrastructural features described above. Thus, mast cells may be classified as MC_T or MC_{TC} on the basis of characteristic ultrastructural features as well as on the basis of compositional differences.

The question of lineage for MC_T and MC_{TC} cells has not been completely resolved. However, two pieces of experimental data indicate that they mature along distinct developmental pathways. First, patients with combined immunodeficiency diseases as well as those with the acquired immunodeficiency syndrome (AIDS) showed a marked and selective reduction of MC_T cells in the mucosa and submucosa of otherwise normal appearing bowel [3]. MC_{TC} cell numbers were not significantly different from normal values, which suggests that T lymphocyte function affects the development of MC_T cells, but not of MC_{TC} cells.

Additional insight concerning the lineage of MC_T and MC_{TC} mast cells was obtained by examination in situ of immature mast cells using electron microscopic techniques [31]. Immature mast cells were identified by concomitant criteria, including a small cell size, high nuclear:cytoplasmic ratio, and low number and small size of secretory granules in the absence of features of ongoing or recent coupled activation-secretion. Like mature mast cells, immature MC_{TC} cells could be distinguished from MC_T cells by their markedly higher content of chymase, as determined by the immunogold technique. Immature MC_{TC} cells accounted for virtually all mast cells in newborn foreskin, 5% in adult foreskin, and 15% in adult bowel submucosa. Immature MC_T cells accounted for about 10% of the mast cells in adult lung and bowel mucosa. Granules of immature MC_T cells usually showed characteristic discrete scrolls and occasionally a particulate pattern, similar to the larger granules of mature MC_T cells. In contrast, granules of immature MC_{TC} cells contained one or more round, amorphous electron dense core surrounded by a less electron-dense region. The occasional presence of dense core granules within a single TC mast cell suggested that dense core granules develop into those found in mature MC_{TC} cells. These compositional and ultrastructural differences between immature MC_T and MC_{TC} types of cells indicate that there are distinct developmental pathways for each cell type at or before the stage of granule formation.

Assuming a common precursor for T and TC types of human mast cells, analogous to rodent mast cells [32], a divergent pathway of maturation whereby T lymphocytes facilitate the development of MC_T but not MC_{TC} cells is likely. Granule formation appears to begin after a tissue site of residence has been established, but commitment to a particular lineage may occur prior to this event, particularly in light of the close proximity of these mast cells to one another in selected tissues. Whether or not transdifferentiation [33] or direct [34] pathways of interconversion, as postulated for rodent mast cells, occur in humans needs to be clarified. However, direct interconversions appear to be a rare to nonexistent event in normal human tissues. The mechanisms and factors involved with the selective differentiation and tissue distributions as well as the functional compositional differences of distinct mast cell subpopulations will prove to be critical for a better understanding of allergy-related disease.

References

1. Irani, A. A., N. M. Schechter, S. S. Craig, G. De-Blois, and L. B. Schwartz. 1986. Two human mast cell subsets with distinct neutral protease compositions. Proc. Natl. Acad. Sci. USA 83: 4464.

2. Craig, S. S., N. M. Schechter, and L. B. Schwartz. 1988. Ultrastructural analyses of human T and TC mast cells identified by immunoelectron microscopy. Lab. Invest. 68: 682.

3. Irani, A. A., G. DeBlois, S. S. Craig, C. O. Elson, and N. M. Schechter. 1987. Deficiency of the T mast cell type in gastrointestinal mucosa of patients with defective T lymphocyte function. J. Immun. 138: 4381.

4. Schwartz, L. B., R. A. Lewis, and K. F. Austen. 1981. Tryptase from human pulmonary mast cells: Purification and characterization. J. Biol. Chem. 256: 11939.

5. Smith, T. J., M. W. Hougland, and D. A. Johnson. 1984. Human lung tryptase purification and characterization. J. Biol. Chem. 259: 11046.

6. Cromlish, J. A., N. G. Seidah, M. Marcinkiewics, J. Hamelin, D. A. Johnson, and M. Chretein. 1987. Human pituitary tryptase: Molecular forms, NH2-terminal sequence, immunocytochemical localization, and specificity with prohormone and fluorogenic substrates. J. Biol. chem. 262: 1363.

7. Schwartz, L. B. 1985. Monoclonal antibodies against human mast cell tryptase demonstrate shared antigenic sites on subunits of tryptase and selective localization of the enzyme to mast cells. J. Immunol. 134: 526.

8. Schwartz, L. B., A. A. Irani, K. Roller, M. C. Castells, and N. M. Schechter. 1987. Quantitation of histamine, tryptase and chymase in dispersed human T and TC mast cells. J .Immunol. 138: 2611.

9. Castells, M. C., A. A. Irani, and L.B. Schwartz.

10. Schwartz, L. B., R. A. Lewis, D. Selden, and K. F. Austen. 1981. Acid hydrolases and tryptase from secretory granules of dispersed human lung mast cells. J. Immunol. 129: 1290.

11. Schwartz, L. B. 1987. Tryptase levels as an indicator of mast cell activation in systemic anaphylaxis and mastocytosis. New Engl. J. Med. 316: 1622.

12. Castells, M., and L. B. Schwartz. 1987. Tryptase levels in nasal lavage fluid as an indicator of the immediate allergic response. J. Allergy Clin. Immunol., in press.

13. Schwartz, L. B., P. C. Atkins, T. R. Bradford, P. Fleekop, M. Shalit, and B. Zweiman. 1987. Release of tryptase together with histamine during the immediate cutaneous response to allergen. J. Allergy Clin. Immunol. 80: 850.

14. Shalit, M., L. B. Schwartz, C. VonAllman, M. Valenzano, P. Fleekop, P. C. Atkins, and B. Zweiman. 1988. Release of histamine and tryptase in vivo after prolonged cutaneous challenge with allergen in humans. J. Immunol. 141: 821.

15. Wenzel, S. E., A. A. Fowler, and L. B. Schwartz. 1988. Activation of pulmonary mast cells by bronchoalveolar allergen challenge: In vivo release of histamine and tryptase in atopic subjects with and without asthma. Amer. Rev. Res. Dis. 137: 1002.

16. Schechter, N. M., J. E. Fraki, J. C. Gersin, and G. S. Lazarus. 1983. Human skin chymotryptic protease. Isolation and relation to cathepsin G and rat mast cell proteinase I. J. Biol. Chem. 258: 2973.

17. Johnson, L. A., K. E. Moon, and M. Eisenberg. 1986. Purification to homogeneity of the human skin chymotryptic proteinase "chymase". Analyt. Biochem. 155: 358.

18. Sayama, S., R. V. Iozzo, G. S. Lazarus, and N. M. Schechter. 1987. Human skin chymotrypsin-like proteinase chymase: subcellular localization to mast cell granules and interaction with heparin and other glycosaminoglycans. J. Bio. Chem. 262: 6808.

19. Wintroub, B. U., C. E. Kaempfer, N. M. Schechter, and D. Proud. 1986. A human lung mast cell chymotryptic-like enzyme: identification and partial characterization. J. Clin. Invest. 77: 196.

20. Goldstein, S. M., Kaempfer, C. E., Proud, D., L. B. Schwartz, A. A. Irani, and B. U. Wintroub. 1987. Detection and partial characterization of a human mast cell carboxypeptidase. J. Immunol. 139: 2724.

21. Goldstein, S. M., Kaempfer, C. E., and B. U. Wintroub. 1988. Purification of human mast cell carboxypeptidase. Fed. Proc. 2: A1234.

22. Lagunoff, D., and A. Richard. 1983. Evidence for control of mast cell granule protease in situ by low pH. Exp. Cell Res. 144: 353.
23. Schwartz, L. B., and T. M. Bradford. 1986. Regulation of tryptase from human lung mast cells by heparin: stabilization of the active tetramer. J. Biol. Chem. 261: 7372.
24. Alter, S. C., D. D. Metcaradford, and L. B. Schwartz. 1987. Stabilization of human mast cell tryptase: effects of enzyme concentration, ionic strength and the structure and negative charge density of polysaccharides. Biochem. J. 248: 821.
25. Schwartz, L. B., M. D. Kawahara, T. E. Hugli, D. Vik, D. T. Fearon, and K. F. Austen. 1983. Generation of C3a anaphylatoxin from human C3 by human mast cell tryptase. J. Immunol. 130: 1891.
26. Maier, M., J. Spragg, and L. B. Schwartz. 1984. Inactivation of human high molecular weight kininogen by human mast cell tryptase. J. Immunol. 130: 2571.
27. Schwartz, L. B., T. M. Bradford, B. L. Littman, and B. U. Wintroub. 1985. The fibrinolytic activity of purified tryptase from human lung mast cells. J. Immunol. 135: 2762.
28. Gruber, B. L., L. B. Schwartz, N. S. Ramamurthy, A. M. Irani, and M. J. Marchese. 1988. Activation of latent rheumatoid synovial collegenase by human mast cell tryptase. J. Immunol. 139: 2724.
29. Wintroub, B. U., N. B. Schechter, G. S. Lazarus, C. E. Kaempfer, and L. B. Schwartz. 1984. Angiotensin I conversion of human and rat chymotryptic proteinases. J. Invest. Derm. 83: 336.
30. Briggaman, R. A., N. M. Schechter, J. Fraki, and G. S. Lazarus. 1984. Degradation of the epidermal-dermal junction by a proteolytic enzyme from human skin and human plymerphonuclear leukocytes. J. Exp. Med. 160: 1027.
31. Craig, S. S., N. M. Schechter, and L. B. Schwartz. Ultrastructural analysis of maturing human T and TC mast cells in situ. Labs in situ. Lab. Invest., in press.
32. Kobayashi, T., T. Nakano, T. Nakahata, H. Asai, Y. Yagi, K. Tsuji, A. Komiyama, T. Akabane, S. Kojima, and Y. Kitamura. 1986. Formation of mast cell colonies in methylcellulose by mouse peritoneal cells and differentiation of these cloned cells in both skin and the gastric mucosa of W/WV mice: evidence that a common precursor can give rise to both "connective tissue-type" and "mucosal" mast cells. J. Immunol. 136: 1378.
33. Kitamura, Y., Nokano, and Y. Kanayama. 1986. Probable dedifferentiation of mast cells in mouse connective tissues. Curr. Top. Dev. Biol. 20: 325.
34. Levi-Schaffer, F., K. F. Austen, P. M. Gravellese, and R. L. Stevens. 1986. Coculture of interleukin 3-dependent mouse mast cells with fibroblasts results in aphenotypic change of the mast cells. Proc. Natl. Acad. Sci. USA. 83: 6485.

Eosinophils in Diseases: Receptors and Mediators

*Monique Capron**

Through membrane receptors for immunoglobulins (IgG, IgE, IgA) and for complement (CR1, CR3) eosinophils interact with immunoglobulins, antigens, and immune complexes. Eosinophils are incriminated in diseases by releasing preformed mediators such as the cationic proteins (MBP, ECP, EDN-EPX, or EPO) as well as newly formed ones (PGE2, LTC4, PAF-acether). The comparison of IgE receptors present on human eosinophils to CD23 present on B cells reveals the existence of a common structure between the two receptors. Pharmacologically active mediators (EPO, MBP, PAF-acether) are released after IgE-dependent stimulation, whereas IgA-dependent activation leads to the release of EPO. A differential release of eosinophil mediators in response to a given stimulus of activation is confirmed by electron microscopy and immunogold staining. The pathological potential of eosinophils is illustrated in a parasitic infection (eosinophilic meningitis due to *A. cantonensis*) and in eosinophilic gastroenteritis. Finally, a possible involvement of HTLV1 in the malignant form of the hypereosino-philic syndrome (HES) is discussed.

Identified at the end of the past century, eosinophils have long been considered as "inflammatory cells," able to be mobilized at the sites of inflammation by various chemotactic factors. Increased blood eosinophilia has been associated mainly to parasitic and allergic diseases, whereas Gordon, inducing a neurotoxic syndrome in experimental animals after injection of lymph nodes rich in infiltrating eosinophils from Hodgkin's patients, suggested the pathological potential of eosinophils. In recent decades, some functions of eosinophils have been elucidated, and their role in diseases has been partially defined. Evidence [1] indicates the "dual" function of eosino-phils: Eosinophils are involved in *protection*, both by their down-regulatory effect of immediate-type hypersensitivity reactions and by their cytotoxic role against parasite larvae. However, the identification of eosinophil cytolytic molecules and their involvement in damage of normal mammalian cells conferred to eosinophils a role in *path-

ology*. Finally, the demonstration of membrane receptors for IgE and their participation in the release of mediators suggested the essential role of eosinophils in hypersensitivity reactions.

After a brief survey of some general aspects concerning eosinophil membrane receptors with a particular emphasis on IgE and IgA receptors, the release of pharmacologically active mediators will be discussed in response to immunoglobulin-dependent activation. Some recent data related to the involvement of eosinophils in pathology will then be considered.

General Aspects (Figure 1)

Similar to other leukocytes, eosinophils possess membrane receptors for IgG (Fc$_\gamma$R) for IgE (Fc$_\varepsilon$R) and, more recently described, for IgA (Fc$_\alpha$R), whereas the existence of receptors for IgM has not been confirmed. Besides these Fc receptors, eosinophils have receptors for C3b (CR1) and for C3bi (CR3) allowing them to interact with immunoglobulins, antigens and immune complexes. The presence of pharmacological receptors has also been demonstrated, for oestradiol, histamine, glucocorticoïds and more recently PAF-acether.

Eosinophils can be incriminated in diseases by releasing various preformed mediators, among which specific components such as the granule cationic proteins, Major Basic Protein (MBP) present in the crystalloïd, eosinophil cationic protein or ECP, eosinophil-derived neurotoxin or EDN, eosinophil peroxidase or EPO, present in the matrix (Figure 1). Eosinophils can also generate newly formed mediators such as Prostaglandins (PGE2), Leukotrienes (LTC4, 5 or 15 HETE) or PAF-acether. Eosinophils from hypereosinophilic patients (with helminth infections, allergic diseases, with the hypereosinophilic syndrome, HES, or with some myeloproliferative disorders) are very heterogeneous with respect to their mor-

* Centre d'Immunologie et de Biologie Parasitaire, Institut Pasteur, 1, rue du Professeur Calmette, B.P. 245, 59019 Lille, France.
This work was supported by the Unité Mixte INSERM U167-CNRS 624, Institut Pasteur, Lille, France.

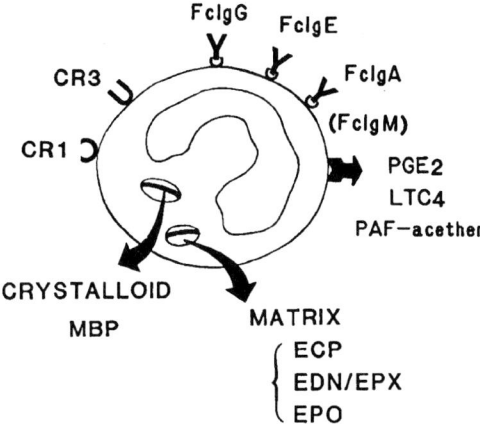

FcIgG FcIgE

CR3

FcIgA

CR1

(FcIgM)

PGE2
LTC4
PAF−acether

CRYSTALLOID
MBP

MATRIX
ECP
EDN/EPX
EPO

Figure 1. Schematic illustration of an human eosinophil representing membrane immunological receptors, main granule proteins, and newly formed mediators.

phology, their membrane receptors or their oxidative metabolism. By centrifugation upon discontinuous density gradients, two subpopulations of human eosinophils differing by their cell density ("normodense" or "hypodense") and by their morphology (inversion of the electron density of the crystalloïd and reduced size of the granules in the case of hypodense eosinophils) were identified. Hypodense eosinophils represent not only the activated state but also the cells in contact to the target tissues, directly involved in pathology. Eosinophil mediators participate to the dual function of eosinophils: in *protection* by a cytotoxic effect against parasites (MBP, ECP, EDN, EPO) or tumor cells (EPO); but also in *damage* against normal mammalian cells with a particular tropism of MBP for tracheal epithelial cells, of EPO for lung cells, of ECP and EDN (neurotoxins) for nervous cells and cardiac cells. However, a large variety of target cells (epidermic, endothelial, intestinal cells) are susceptible to the effect of eosinophil cationic proteins (reviewed in [1]). In addition, the newly generated mediators (LTC4, PAF-acether) are also involved in various pathological processes, as emphasized in numerous studies.

Receptors

IgE Receptors

IgE receptors have been demonstrated on human eosinophils and they participate directly in the effector function of eosinophils against parasite larvae (reviewed in [2]). The production of a monoclonal antibody (BB10) raised against human $Fc_\varepsilon R$-positive eosinophils and able to inhibit the IgE-dependent cytotoxicity of eosinophils, platelets and monocytes, has confirmed the common antigenicity of these $Fc_\varepsilon R$, now referred to as $Fc_\varepsilon RII$ [3].

A common feature of these $Fc_\varepsilon RII$ is their increased expression on activated cells. In the particular situation of human eosinophils, IgE-dependent effector function seems to be restricted to a subpopulation of eosinophils with low density (hypodense), suggesting that the presence of a functional $Fc_\varepsilon R$ could be considered as one marker of eosinophil heterogeneity. Another membrane receptor (CR3) which acts in synergy with $Fc_\varepsilon RII$ has also an increased expression on hypodense eosinophils [4]. Eosinophil heterogeneity was confirmed by using the monoclonal antibody (mAb) BB10, which selectively stains hypodense and not normodense eosinophils [3]. In addition, this mAb allowed us to biochemically characterize the eosinophil receptor for IgE, by using immunosorbent chromatography of eosinophil detergent extracts, passed over either IgE or BB10 immunosorbents [5]. Under reducing conditions, three polypeptide fragments were obtained with apparent molecular weights of 45–50, 23 and 15 kDa. Similar results were recently obtained by immunoprecipitation, and moreover eosinophil $Fc_\varepsilon RII$ was compared to CD23. Whereas BB10 precipitated 3 polypeptides of apparent MW 45–50, 20–25 and 15 kDa on eosinophils and on a B cell line (WIL-2WT), an mAb anti-CD23 (mAb135 kindly provided by Dr G. Delespesse, University of Montreal, Canada) bound to a major 45–50 kDa component both on eosinophils and on WIL-2WT cells. This study, together with previous results, confirms the existence of a common structure between $Fc_\varepsilon RII$ present on eosinophils, platelets, macrophages, and B lymphocytes [2]. On occasion, it has been argued that the low affinity of this second receptor could lessen its real biological significance in IgE-dependent reactions. In fact, the affinity observed for monomeric IgE is comparable with or even higher than the affinity generally reported for the IgG receptors. On the other hand, the increased extrinsic affinity of FcεRII for IgE dimers or complexes gives this class of receptors a particular significance in all situations where IgE complexes are produced, such as parasitic infections and allergic diseases (reviewed in [2]). In this respect, our demonstration of surface-bound IgE to rat and human eosinophils indicates that in spite of the low affinity of FcεRII for monomeric IgE in vitro, IgE immunoglobulins are able to bind to eosinophil FcεRII in vivo.

IgA Receptors

Whereas receptors for IgA have been detected on various leukocyte populations, their presence has not been reported on normal human eosinophils. The recent demonstration of surface IgE and IgA on intestinal eosinophils from parasite infected mice [6] or on blood eosinophils from patients with filariasis [7] suggested the existence of receptors for IgA on activated eosinophils. The binding of monomeric IgA to purified human eosinophils (> 95% purity) was evaluated by flow cytofluorometry analysis after staining with fluorescein-labelled anti-human IgA. Between 5% and 60% of eosinophils were able to bind IgA. Moreover, the proportion of surface IgA bearing eosinophils increased in the case of allergic patients [8]. These results very interestingly showed similarities between the percentages of eosinophils able to bind IgE and IgA. The association between the two receptors at the level of individual cells is presently under investigation.

Receptor for glucocorticoïds

In the context of eosinophil heterogeneity, recent findings suggest a variability between normodense and hypodense eosinophils, in the expression of another receptor, the glucocorticoïd (G.C.) receptor [9]. Whereas normodense eosinophils bear high affinity and saturable G.C. receptors, hypodense eosinophils show absence or loss of G.C. binding. This is correlated with the eosinophil sensitivity to G.C., since hypodense eosinophils appear less sensi-

tive to G.C. than normodense eosinophils. The exact mechanisms modulating G.C. receptor expression on eosinophils require additional investigations. Bearing in mind the inhibitory effects of G.C. on FcεRI, it would probably be of interest to explore the interactions between G.C. receptors and FcεRII.

Release of Mediators

IgE-Dependent Activation

The demonstration of surface IgE on eosinophils from patients with increased IgE levels and particularly on lung eosinophils confirmed the biological relevance of the interaction between eosinophils and IgE antibodies. In order to investigate the role of these cytophilic IgE in eosinophil function and to evaluate their specificity, further experiments measuring the release of various mediators were then performed.

Eosinophil peroxydase (EPO) was detected in the supernatants of eosinophils from hypereosinophilic patients after incubation either with the specific antigen or with anti-IgE antibodies. This was obtained not only in the case

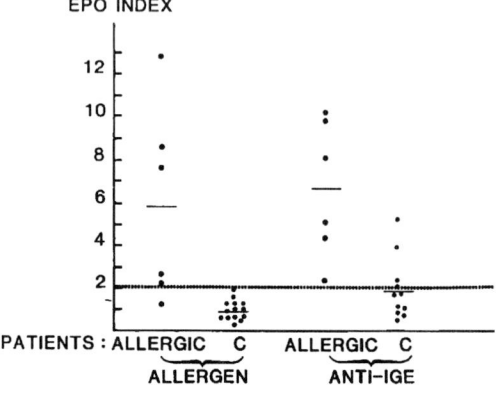

Figure 2. Release of eosinophil peroxydase (EPO) from allergic patients. Purified eosinophils from allergic or nonallergic (control) patients are incubated with the specific allergen or with antihuman IgE mAb. EPO is measured in the supernatants by chemiluminescence and results are expressed as EPO index [10].

of patients with filarial infections [10] but recently confirmed in the case of allergic patients [7]. As shown in Figure 2, only allergens related to the patient allergy and giving positivity in the skin tests induced extracellular release of EPO. However, no release of EPO was obtained when the same allergens were added to eosinophils from nonallergic patients. Not only EPO, but also Major Basic Protein (MBP) was released after addition of anti-IgE antibodies [7]. These results suggest that cell-bound IgE with very restricted antibody specificity could play a role in the activation of hypodense eosinophils in inducing the release of granule proteins with potent cytolytic functions.

Selectivity of Mediator Release

Eosinophil peroxydase (EPO) and Major Basic Protein (MBP) were released after addition of anti-IgE but not anti-IgG antibodies. In contrast, ECP measured by a radioimmunoassay using monoclonal antibodies (EG1, kindly performed by Dr P.C. Tai, London) was only detected after the addition of anti-IgG antibodies. These results, showing no correlation between EPO and ECP release, suggested a variability in the response of eosinophils to different stimuli (IgE versus IgG). Similar results have been recently reported concerning a differential release of EPO and ECP in response to activation by opsonized zymosan (11).

They were more recently confirmed by studies on a factor named HRF (histamine releasing factor) able to induce histamine release after addition to IgE-bearing basophils [12]. When surface IgE bearing eosinophils were incubated with partly purified HRF factor, EPO was detected in the supernatants but not ECP, similarly to the IgE dependent activation. These results show that the release of eosinophil mediators can be induced not only by antigens or anti-IgE, but as well by soluble factors such as HRF. HRF, which is present in nasal lavage fluids and blister fluids during the late cutaneous reaction, has a MW of 15–30 kDa, and can be considered in some aspects as an "IgE binding factor." It is produced in vitro by lung macrophages and platelets, both cell populations bearing in common the second receptor for IgE ($Fc_\varepsilon RII$). However, no similar studies have been related with the production of such IgE binding factors by eosinophils. In prelimi-

nary experiments we have recently shown that $Fc_\varepsilon R$ + hypodense eosinophils are able to release soluble factors of a molecular weight comparable to the previously described IgE binding factors, and able to bind IgE [2].

Finally, the production of a newly formed mediator such as PAF-acether in response to IgE-dependent triggering of hypodense eosinophils confirm the selectivity in the mediators produced by eosinophils according to the stimulus of activation. These findings have to be considered in relation to human eosinophil heterogeneity. Indeed, it has been recently shown that lung eosinophils produced 1000-fold more PAF-acether in response to anti-IgE antibodies than corresponding blood eosinophils from the same patients [13]. Moreover, normodense eosino-phils seemed to produce significant although limited amounts of PAF, in response to IgG triggering and not to IgE triggering [14].

IgA-Dependent Activation

The existence of surface IgA bound to eosinophils from allergic or parasite-infected patients led us to investigate the IgA-dependent release of mediators. Eosinophil peroxydase was evaluated after addition of anti-IgA antibodies to highly purified eosinophils. A significant release of EPO (between 2.5 and 6 times more than in controls) were obtained after addition of anti-IgA. These results suggested that, similar to IgE, surface IgA could participate to eosinophil activation, by inducing the release of mediators [8]. Further experiments are in progress to determine the respective role of IgA and IgE receptors in the effector function of eosinophils.

Implications in Pathology

Much of our knowledge on eosinophil functions in human pathology derives from studies performed in parasitic infections or in allergic diseases. In addition to previous studies suggesting the role of eosinophils in such situations (increased numbers of eosinophils in the biological fluids or detection of specific eosinophil mediators in the lavage or on tissue sections), our results show that eosinophils, through their surface immunoglobulins, are able to interact with antigens and release their various mediators. Among the various immunoglobulin isotypes, surface IgE and IgA seem particularly involved in mediator release, and these findings may have in vivo implications in the context of tissue reactions, especially in the lungs and in the intestine.

In a very recent study concerning experimental infections with a nematode parasite, *Angiostrongylus cantonensis*, responsible for eosino-philic meningitis in nonpermissive hosts including man, we could show the functional duality of eosinophils [15]. Whereas eosinophils are effector cells able to damage helminth larvae in vitro and in vivo, cytolytic mediators can be generated by eosinophils as the consequence of the interaction with antibody-coated parasites, leading to damage of bystanding host cells. In nonpermissive hosts for *A. cantonensis*, neurological alterations are associated to an eosino-philic response and to the presence of eosinophil granule proteins in the cerebrospinal fluid [15].

Our results suggesting a differential release of eosinophil granule mediators, in response to a given stimulus of activation, seem incompatible with the hypothesis of exocytosis of the whole granules. Preliminary studies using electron microscopy and immunogold staining are in favor of a release process of the individual components from the granules through the cytoplasm, suggesting that eosinophil degranulation occurs by a mechanism similar to the "piece-meal" degranulation of basophils observed during certain cell-mediated immune reactions and involving a vesicular transport mechanism [16]. Such an attractive hypothesis was recently confirmed by studies on tissue eosinophils from a patient suffering from eosinophilic gastroenteritis, with a story of milk allergy [17]. Immunogold staining with the appropriate specific antibodies directed against MBP (kindly donated by Dr. Gleich), EPO (kindly donated by Dr. Venge, Uppsala, Sweden), or ECP (EG2, kindly provided by Dr. Tai, London), showed that in ulcerated areas, MBP was virtually absent from the crystalloïd, but detected in the matrix and out of the granules, whereas EPO and ECP were still present in the matrix of the granules [17]. These findings bring morphologic evidence consistent with the hypothesis of a selective release of granule constituents from activated eosinophils. They suggest that the inversion of the electron density of the granule cristalloïd, reported by several authors is due to a loss of MBP. The precise mechanisms for the induction of eosinophil degranulation are unknown and further in vitro studies are now being undertaken to follow the kinetics of eosinophil degranulation in response to given stimuli.

Besides parasitic infections and allergic diseases, commonly associated with increased IgE levels, the precise role of eosinophils remains obscure in some clinical circumstances such as systemic diseases, hematologic malignancies or disorders affecting lung skin or the gastrointestinal tract. The hypereosinophilic syndrome (HES), characterized by a dramatic increase of blood and tissue eosinophils, is associated to multi-organ system lesions, often affecting the heart and the central nervous system. In a recent publication, we suggested that a human T-lymphotropic retrovirus (HTLV1) might be associated with a subset of HES [18]. Both HTLV1 specific antibodies and the proviral sequence of HTLV1 were found in patients with HES prior to the apparition of a T-cell lymphoma and without any evidence of HTLV1 risk factors [18]. Much work remains to be done on the incidence of HTLV1 infection in malignant HES.

Conclusion

In conclusion, our studies appear to have opened a new cellular pathway in the mechanisms of hypersensitivity reactions. The demonstration of receptors for IgE on inflammatory cells has certainly broadened our current view on the cellular mechanisms of allergic reactions. The further demonstration that the activation of these receptors is associated with the selectivity and the dynamics of pharmacological mediator release might have significant implications for our understanding of the physiopathology of allergic and inflammatory reactions, but also for the definition of novel therapeutic strategies. More generally, our studies have now clearly established that eosinophils, for years ambiguous cells for immunologists, are essential cellular components of protective mechanism against parasites as well as effectors of hypersensitivity reactions.

References

1. Gleich, G. J., and C. R. Adolphson. 1986. The eosinophilic leukocyte. Adv. Immunol. 39: 77.
2. Capron, M., C. Leprevost, G. Torpier, and A. Capron. 1989. The second receptor for IgE in eosinophil effector function. Progr. in Allergy, in press.
3. Capron, M., T. Jouault, L. Prin, M. Joseph, J. C. Ameisen, A. E. Butterworth, J. P. Papin, J. P. Kusnierz, and A. Capron. 1986. Functional study of a monoclonal antibody to IgE Fc receptor (FcεRII) of eosinophils, platelets and macrophages. J. Exp. Med. 164: 72.
4. Capron, M., M. D. Kazatchkine, E. Fischer, M. Joseph, A. E. Butterworth, J. P. Kusnierz, L. Prin, J. P. Papin, and A. Capron. 1987. Functional role of the chain of complement receptor type 3 in human eosinophil-dependent antibody-mediated cytotoxicity against schistosomes. J. Immunol. 139: 2059.
5. Jouault, T., M. Capron, J. M. Balloul, J. C. Ameisen, and A. Capron. 1988. Quantitative and qualitative analysis of the Fc receptor for IgE (FcεRII) on human eosinophils. Eur. J. Immunol. 18: 237.
6. Van der Vorst, E., H. Dhont, J. Y. Cesbron, M. Capron, J. P. Dessaint, and A. Capron. 1988. The influence of an *Hymenolepis diminuta* infection on the IgE and IgA bound to mouse intestinal eosinophils. Int. Archs Allergy Appl. Immunol., in press.
7. Capron, M., C. Leprevost, L. Prin, M. Tomassini, G. Torpier, S. MacDonald, and A. Capron. 1988. Immunoglobulin-mediated activation of eosinophils. In Eosinophils in Asthma, J. Morley, ed. Academic Press, London, in press.
8. Capron, M., M. Tomassini, E. Van der Vorst, J. P. Kusnierz, J. P. Papin, and A. Capron. 1988. Existence et fonctions d'un récepteur pour l'IgA sur les éosinophiles humains. C.R. Acad. Sci. 307 (série III): 397.
9. Prin, L., P. Lefebvre, V. Gruart, M. Capron, A. B. Tonnel, D. Formstecher, S. Loiseau, and A. Capron. 1988. Variability in the expression of eosinophil glucocorticoïd receptors: Correlation with corticoresistance in hypereosinophilic patients. J. Clin. Invest., in press.
10. Khalife, J., M. Capron, J. Y. Cesbron, P. C. Tai, H. Taelman, L. Prin, and A. Capron. 1986. Role of specific IgE antibodies in peroxidase (EPO) release from human eosinophils. J. Immunol. 137: 1659.
11. Venge, P. 1988. Eosinophil biochemistry and killing mechanisms. In Eosinophils in Asthma, J. Morley, ed. Academic Press, London, in press.
12. Liu, M. C., D. Proud, L. M. Lichtenstein, D. W. MacGlashan Jr., R. P. Schleimer, N. F. Adkinson Jr., A. Kagey-Sobotka, E. S. Schulman, and M. Plaut. 1986. Human lung macrophage-derived histamine-releasing activity is due to IgE dependent factors. J. Immunol. 136: 2588.
13. Bruynzeel, P. L. B., and J. Verhagen. 1988. Lipid metabolism by eosinophils. In Eosinophils in Asthma. J. Morley, ed. Academic Press, London, in press.
14. Kay, A. B., A. J. Frew, R. Moqbel, G. M. Walsh, K. Kurihara, O. Cromwell, A. Champion, A. Hartnell, and A. J. Wardlaw. 1988. The activated eosinophil in allergy and asthma. In Biochemistry of the Acute Allergic Reactions. Vth Int. Symp. Alan R. Liss, Inc., N.Y., in press.
15. Perez, O., M. Capron, M. Lastre, P. Venge, J. Khalife, and A. Capron. 1988. Angiostrongylus cantonensis: Role of eosinophils in the neurotoxic syndrome (Gordon-like phenomenon). Exp. Parasit., in press.
16. Galli, S. J., A. M. Dvorak, and H. F. Dvorak. 1984. Basophils and mast cells: Morphologic insights into their biology secretory patterns and function. Progr. Allergy 34: 1.
17. Torpier, G., J. F. Colombel, C. Mathieu-Chandelier, M. Capron, J. P. Dessaint, A. Cortot, J. C. Paris, and A. Capron. 1988. Eosinophilic gastroenteritis: Ultrastructural evidence for a selective release of eosinophil Major Basic Protein. Clin. Exp. Immunol., in press.
18. Prin, L., M. Leguern, J. C. Ameisen, S. Saragosti, O. B. Letry, P. Fenaux, J. P. Levy, and A. Capron. 1988. HTLV1 and malignant hypereosinophilic syndrome. Lancet II: 569.

Basophil Activation and Recruitment in Allergic Disease

*Bruce S. Bochner, Robert P. Schleimer, Ernest N. Charlesworth, Ana M. Lamas, and Lawrence M. Lichtenstein**

Pathogenetically significant numbers of basophils and their mediators accumulate in several inflammatory reactions in humans. In allergic disease, for example, it has become appreciated that, during the experimental late phase allergic response induced by intranasal or intradermal allergen provocation, basophils appear along with eosinophils and neutrophils [1, 2]; the same phenomenon appears to occur in the lower airways after antigen challenge in allergic subjects. While basophils represent a minority of the cells that accumulate at the antigen challenge sites and do not account for all of the clinical manifestations of allergic disease, several lines of evidence indicate that these cells release histamine, leukotrienes, and other mediators, and thus play an important role in the late phase response. This report summarizes these in vivo findings and presents data that bear on the possible mechanisms by which activation and recruitment of basophils may influence chronic allergic disease.

Involvement of Basophils in Allergic Reactions

It has been known for over a decade that increased numbers of basophils are seen in individuals with atopic diseases. For example, elevated numbers of basophils and basophil progenitors are found in peripheral blood of atopic subjects, including those with allergic rhinitis and asthma, and basophil numbers increase prior to exacerbations of asthma [3, 4]. They are increased in nasal secretions of individuals with allergic rhinitis, and accumulate in nasal secretions, skin windows, and skin test sites several hours after allergen challenge in allergic subjects (reviewed in [5]). Furthermore, increased numbers of basophils in nasal secretions appear concomitantly with a decrease in the number of peripheral blood basophils, sug-

gesting their recruitment from the circulation [6]. More recently, it was demonstrated that intranasal antigen challenge resulted in a dramatic increase in both the proportion and total number of basophils recovered from nasal lavage fluids during the late phase [7]. The severity of nasal symptoms during natural exposure to allergen correlated with the number of peripheral blood basophils; similarly, the influx of basophils into nasal secretions correlated with the severity of experimental antigen-induced nasal late phase symptoms [7, 8].

A link between the appearance of basophils and their role in late phase allergic reactions was initially suggested by the studies of Naclerio et al. Using the nasal allergen challenge model, they observed that during the acute allergic response levels of histamine, LTC_4 and PGD_2 were increased in lavage fluid [9]. In contrast, mediators detected during the late response included histamine and LTC_4, but not PGD_2. Since human mast cells, but not basophils, are capable of PGD_2 production, this led to the hypothesis that basophils recruited during the late phase were responsible for the observed pattern of symptoms and mediator release. This was confirmed by blinded morphometric analysis of these cells, and functional studies of the cells obtained from late phase lavage fluid also revealed them to be basophils. This hypothesis was supported by observations made using the skin blister, antigen challenge model. In these studies, antigen provocation resulted in both acute and late phase increases in histamine levels [10]. While an acute rise in mast cell-derived tryptase and PGD_2 levels was observed, there was no subsequent rise in either of these two mediators during the late phase cutaneous response. Interestingly, the rise in late phase histamine levels in these fluids correlated closely with an

* Division of Clinical Immunology, The Johns Hopkins University School of Medicine at The Good Samaritan Hospital, 5601 Loch Raven Boulevard, Baltimore, Maryland 21239.
Supported by Grants AR31891, AI7290, and AI8270 from the National Institutes of Health.

influx of basophils into the blister. In this model it was also clear that there was a marked increase in the number of basophils in the dermis itself, a finding not appreciated in previous studies of the cutaneous late response to antigen.

Basophil Activation and Recruitment

The fact that basophils and basophil-derived mediators appear during certain inflammatory responses such as the allergic late phase suggests that mechanisms exist which favor the activation and recruitment of these cells to extravascular inflammatory sites. Activation events for other leukocytes such as the neutrophil have been defined by several criteria including releasability of preformed and newly generated mediators. Information regarding the release of certain basophil-derived mediators such as histamine has begun to emerge. For example, data exist suggesting that basophil releasability is enhanced in allergic individuals. Basophils from children with food allergies reportedly have increased spontaneous histamine release [11], and deuterium oxide (D$_2$O) enhances spontaneous histamine release from basophils of atopic individuals [12]. In addition, culture of basophils with cytokines such as IFN-γ and IL-3, which may be generated in tissue sites of allergic inflammation, leads to enhanced histamine release [13]. Perhaps more importantly, however, are the series of observations establishing that the type of IgE molecule present on the surface of the basophil determines whether the cell can be activated by a family of so-called histamine-releasing factors (HRFs). These HRFs, isolated from a variety of cell types and biological fluids, distinguish atopic from non-atopic individuals in that basophils from the former but not the latter degranulate when exposed to HRFs [14, 15]. The reason for this is due to the presence on the basophil of a subset of IgE antibody (termed IgE+) which is only found in the serum of atopic subjects [16]. In addition to the observation that passive sensitization with IgE+ of basophils from non-allergic subjects confers responsiveness to HRFs [16] and IL-3 [17], it also confers releasability to D$_2$ [18], a response, as mentioned above, characteristic of basophils isolated from atopic donors. Since at least one

such HRF has been detected at the site of the cutaneous late phase response [19], the presence of IgE+ on basophils may be responsible for basophil activation and mediator release during the late phase. Other indicators of leukocyte activation include increased adhesiveness for biological surfaces and augmented cell surface adherence glycoprotein expression. Leukocyte adherence to endothelium and other substrates is mediated through a family of adherence molecules including Mo1 (the C3bi receptor, also referred to as CR3), p150,95, and LFA-1. These molecules share a common beta subunit termed CD18 and are recognized by a variety of monoclonal antibodies which can be used in vitro to inhibit many leukocyte functions including cell adherence and chemotaxis. The importance of these cell surface glycoproteins in vivo is highlighted by studies in which infusion of monoclonal antibodies against Mo1 molecules into laboratory animals prior to initiation of an inflammatory event (e.g., myocardial ischemia) drastically reduces subsequent inflammatory damage [20]. Recently, investigators have begun to study the expression of these cell surface glycoproteins on leukocytes isolated from sites of ongoing allergic reactions. Using a skin chamber model, it has been demonstrated that neutrophils accumulating in skin blister fluids five hours after antigen challenge appear activated compared to peripheral blood granulocytes on the basis of both morphologic changes (e.g., polarization) and increased expression of Mo1 [21, 22]. Incubation of these neutrophils in vitro with several chemotactic factors led to an additional 2- to 3-fold increase in Mo1 expression, suggesting that leukocytes from these sites are capable of further activation [22]. While we plan to study adherence glycoprotein expression on basophils isolated from these and other sites, other experiments similar to those mentioned above have already been performed. Agents with chemotactic and/or secretagogue activity such as the complement fragment C5a, formyl-methionyl-leucyl-phenylalanine (FMLP), and platelet-activating factor (PAF) have been shown to directly stimulate basophil adhesiveness, and while basophils apparently lack p150,95, their adherence to endothelium can be blocked in vitro with antibodies to the common CD18 antigen [23, 24]. The traditional approach to the study of leukocyte recruitment has been to identify and characterize chemotactic responses. Several previous studies of basophil recruitment have identified stimuli such as C5a, IFN-γ and other lymphokines, and sera from atopic donors which were chemotactic for human basophils (reviewed in [5]). While chemotaxis is certainly an important aspect of basophil recruitment, chemotactic factors that would preferentially promote migration of basophils have not yet been identified. Other investigators have identified increased numbers of circulating basophil/mast cell progenitors in the blood of atopic individuals [4]. They also have identified growth factors from culture supernatants of human nasal polyp epithelium or T lymphocytes which are apparently specific for basophils [25, 26]. These investigators have therefore hypothesized that homing of progenitor cells to the sites of allergic respiratory disease, with subsequent proliferation and differentiation to mature cells under the influence of growth factors produced in situ, may in part explain the accumulation of metachromatic cells that is seen at sites of allergic disease [4].

Regardless of these details, the critical step in the development of a basophil-rich infiltrate involves the margination and adherence of circulating cells, either mature or progenitors, to the vascular endothelium adjacent to the inflammatory site. Once removed from the circulation, subsequent diapedesis and chemotaxis would ultimately result in their appearance in the inflammatory infiltration. Thus, agents capable of activating basophils (including those mentioned above) or endothelium might be critical for the regulation of basophil recruitment. It now appears that local recruitment of leukocytes in vivo is the result of specific interactions between cell surface structures on both the endothelial cell and the leukocyte. As seen with the neutrophil, eosinophil, and other leukocytes, agents such as IL-1 and TNF-α promote the adherence of basophils by inducing the transient de novo expression of adherence glycoproteins such as endothelial leukocyte adherence molecule-1 (ELAM-1) on the surface of the endothelial cells [24, 27]. Adhesiveness induced in endothelial cells by these stimuli in vitro is maximal by 4 to 6 hours and gradually declines over 24 hours, kinetics reminiscent of the influx of granulocytes during the late phase response [24]. One group of investigators has been successful in raising monoclonal antibodies which recognize at least one of these cytokine-induced endothelial cell surface proteins,

which can block the adherence of leukocytes to activated endothelial cells in vitro [27]. Interestingly, endothelial cells at sites of human dermatologic conditions including delayed hypersensitivity reactions and chronic dermatitis of various etiologies display these cell surface antigens, while normal endothelium does not, suggesting that endothelial cell activation occurs in vivo in association with these inflammatory skin conditions [28].

Since none of the above stimuli or events are specific for basophils, we hypothesized that there must exist certain basophil-specific stimuli of adhesion which would promote basophil influx during the late phase responses, and we reasoned that it might be a basophil-specific secretagogue. Experiments have now shown that in vitro treatment of human basophils with either anti-IgE or antigen induces dose-dependent increases in their adherence to endothelial cells [29]. Activation of basophil adhesiveness was seen at extremely low concentrations of anti-IgE or antigen that do not cause histamine release; similar treatment of neutrophils (which lack receptors for IgE) or eosinophils (which possess low affinity IgE receptors) did not effect their adhesiveness [29; Lamas, A.M. & R.P. Schleimer, unpublished observations]. Antigen treatment of basophils from nonallergic subjects had no effect on basophil adherence [29]; passive sensitization of these basophils with sera from appropriate allergic donors resulted in transfer of antigen-induced adherence responses to these cells. Furthermore, IgE-dependent increases in basophil adherence to endothelial cells involved CD18 antigens, since treatment of basophils with a monoclonal antibody to CD18 resulted in greater than 80% inhibition of adhesion induced by anti-IgE [29]. IL-3, a cytokine known to promote basophil differentiation and degranulation, is unique among other cytokines in its ability to induce adhesiveness of basophils, but not neutrophils or eosinophils [17, 30]. Whether HRFs are also capable of promoting adherence of basophils to endothelium is currently under investigation. These data suggest that in vivo exposure to exceedingly low doses of appropriate cytokines and/or antigen in the airways or skin may result in rapid localized basophil recruitment by promoting their adherence to endothelium. Subsequent migration, under the influence of chemotactic factors, would then result in basophil accumulation in the tissues. Eventually, after an appropriate period of time and upon exposure to higher antigen concentrations in situ, basophil degranulation would occur.

Pharmacologic Regulation of Basophil Activation and Recruitment

The importance of cell recruitment in chronic allergic diseases such as rhinitis and asthma is supported by the fact that the treatment modalities most effective for these conditions are those that prevent the late phase accumulation of inflammatory cells. Glucocorticoids are perhaps the most effective anti-allergic drugs available, due in large part to inhibition of late phase reactions [31]; they have little or no effect upon the immediate response, except in the case of prolonged topical application [32]. Systemic glucocorticoid administration has profound effects on circulating numbers of leukocytes including suppression of circulating basophil numbers [31]. In addition, glucocorticoids are known to inhibit IgE-dependent histamine release from human basophils but not from human mast cells [33]. This is important, because nasal and cutaneous antigen challenge studies have demonstrated that treatment of allergic subjects with glucocorticoids inhibited the clinical late phase response and the influx of basophils and eosinophils (but not neutrophils] into these sites [7]. Glucocorticoids have no effect on the ability of activated endothelial cells to acquire adhesiveness for basophils, nor do they affect leukocyte chemotaxis [24, 31]. Therefore, the ability of glucocorticoids to inhibit basophil accumulation during the late phase response may be due to their ability to block production of factors responsible for cell activation and recruitment.

Cromolyn sodium, another less potent pharmacologic agent often used in the treatment of allergic diseases, also inhibits late phase reactions, but it differs from oral glucocorticoids in its ability to inhibit the immediate allergic response [34]. While studies with basophils are lacking, it has been shown that pretreatment with cromolyn sodium reduces the number of eosinophils accumulating in bronchoalveolar lavage fluid of asthmatics after antigen challenge [35]. Treatment of neutrophils, eosinophils, and monocytes in vitro with cromolyn sodium inhibits a wide range of leukocyte activation events including rosetting to C3b-coated red blood cells [36]. Thus, these drugs may block the accumulation of basophils and other leukocytes during late phase allergic reactions by inhibiting leukocyte activation and recruitment.

Histamine H_1 antagonists are among the most frequently prescribed medications for the treatment of allergic diseases. These agents are thought to be therapeutic as a result of their ability to competitively inhibit the binding of histamine to H_1 receptors. It was quite intriguing, then, when it was reported that cetirizine, the major metabolite of hydroxyzine, effectively blocked the accumulation of eosinophils at skin window sites [37]. Subsequent experiments have confirmed and extended these observations, demonstrating that while cetirizine had no effect on either histamine release (as measured in skin blisters) or the clinical manifestations of the dermal late phase response, it did inhibit PGD_2 production and the accumulation of basophils, eosinophils and neutrophils during the late phase by approximately 70% [38]. This effect does not appear to be directed against the interaction of granulocytes with endothelium, since cetirizine treatment of neutrophils, eosino-phils, basophils, or umbilical vein endothelial cells did not alter their adherence responses in vitro. Thus, drugs including cetirizine may be capable of inhibiting leukocyte activation and recruitment by as yet undefined pharmacologic effects; the significance of these findings in terms of the pathophysiology of allergic late phase reactions remains to be determined.

Summary

The activation and recruitment of circulating basophils, along with other leukocytes including eosinophils and neutrophils, is a crucial and characteristic event of the late phase allergic response, with the eventual release of preformed and newly synthesized mediators from basophils and other cells present at these inflammatory sites. Mechanisms for the activation and localized recruitment of circulating basophils to sites of allergic inflammation, including the initial step of margination and adherence to the vascular endothelium adjacent to the inflammatory response, may be under the influence of a variety of factors including cytokines and perhaps even the antigens themselves. Among the medications most effective for the treatment of allergic disease, several share the ability to inhibit the late phase recruitment of leukocytes to the inflammatory site. By improving our knowledge of how basophils are activated and recruited from the circulation to target organs of allergic reactions, future studies may suggest new ways of blocking the influx of basophils so as to alleviate the clinical manifestations of chronic allergic diseases such as rhinitis and asthma.

References

1. Solley, G. O., G. J. Gleich, R. E. Jordan, and A. L. Schroeter. 1976. The late phase of the immediate wheal and flare skin reaction. J. Clin. Invest. 58: 408.

2. deShazo, R. D., A. I. Levinson, H. F. Dvorak, and R. W. Davis. 1979. The late phase skin reaction: evidence for activation of the coagulation system in an IgE dependent reaction in man. J. Immunol. 122: 692.

3. Kimura, I., Y. Moritani, and Y. Tanizaki. 1973. Basophils in bronchial asthma with reference to reagin-type allergy. Clin. Allergy 3: 195.

4. Denburg, J. A., S. Telizyn, A. Belda, J. Dolovich, and J. Bienenstock. 1985. Increased numbers of circulating basophil progenitors in atopic patients. J. Allergy Clin. Immunol. 76: 466.

5. Mitchell, E. B., and P. W. Askenase. 1983. Basophils in human disease. Clin. Rev. Allergy 1: 427.

6. Ohtsuka, H., M. Okuda, and Y. Sakaguchi. 1984. Study of basophilic cells in nasal allergy. Part VI. Relationship between basophils and mast cells. Jpn. J. Otolaryngol. 87: 141.

7. Bascom, R., M. Wachs, R. M. Naclerio, U. Pipkorn, S. J. Galli, and L. M. Lichtenstein. 1988. Basophil influx occurs after nasal antigen challenge: Effects of topical corticosteroid pretreatment. J. Allergy Clin. Immunol. 81: 580.

8. Otsuka, H., J. Dolovich, D. Befus, J. Bienenstock, and J. Denburg. 1986. Peripheral blood basophils, basophil progenitors, and nasal metachromatic cells in allergic rhinitis. Am. Rev. Respir. Dis. 133: 757.

9. Naclerio, R. M., D. Proud, A. G. Togias, N. F. Adkinson Jr., D. A. Meyers, A. Kagey-Sobotka, M. Plaut, P. S. Norman, and L. M. Lichtenstein. 1985. Inflammatory mediators in late antigen-induced rhinitis. N. Engl. J. Med. 313: 65.

10. Shalit, M., L. B. Schwartz, N. Golzar, C. von Allman, M. Valenzano, P. Fleekop, P. C. Atkins, and B. Zweiman. 1988. Release of histamine and tryptase in vivo after prolonged cutaneous challenge with allergen in humans. J. Immunol. 141: 821.

11. May, C. D., and L. Remigio. 1982. Observations on high spontaneous release of histamine from leukocytes in vitro. Clin. Allergy. 12: 229.

12. Tung, R., and L. M. Lichtenstein. 1982. In vitro histamine release from basophils of asthmatic and atopic individuals in D_2O. J. Immunol. 128: 2067.

13. Schleimer, R. P., D. A. Davidson, C. Derse, S. Gillis, M. Plaut, and L. M. Lichtenstein. 1988. The effect of cytokines on human basophils. J. Allergy Clin. Immunol. 81: 301 (Abstract).

14. MacDonald, S. M., A. Kagey-Sobotka, D. Proud, R. M. Naclerio, and L. M. Lichtenstein. 1987. Histamine releasing factor: Release mechanism and responding population. J. Allergy Clin. Immunol. 79: 248 (Abstract).

15. Fisher, R. H., A. Kagey-Sobotka, D. Proud, M. A. Orchard, and L. M. Lichtenstein. 1987. Platelet-basophil interactions: Clinical correlates. J. Allergy Clin. Immunol. 79: 196 (Abstract).

16. MacDonald, S. M., L. M. Lichtenstein, D. Proud, M. Plaut, R. M. Naclerio, and A. Kagey-Sobotka. 1987. Studies of IgE-dependent histamine releasing factors: Heterogeneity of IgE. J. Immunol. 139: 506.

17. MacDonald, S. M., A. Kagey-Sobotka, S. Gillis, and L. M. Lichtenstein. 1988. Human recombinant interleukin 3 (IL3) induces histamine release from human basophils. J. Allergy Clin. Immunol. 81: 301 (Abstract).

18. MacDonald, S. M., J. M. White, A. Kagey-Sobotka, D. W. MacGlashan Jr., D. Proud, and L. M. Lichtenstein. 1987. Heterogeneity of IgE: Transfer of D_2O sensitivity. Clin. Res. 35: 641A (Abstract).

19. Warner, J. A., M. M. Pienkowski, M. Plaut, P. S. Norman, and L. M. Lichtenstein. 1986. Identification of histamine releasing factor(s) in the late phase of cutaneous IgE-mediated reactions. J. Immunol. 136: 2583.

20. Simpson, P. J., R. F. Todd III, J. C. Fantone, J. K. Mickelson, J. D. Griffin, and B. R. Lucchesi. 1988. Reduction of experimental canine myocardial reperfusion injury by a monoclonal antibody (Anti-Mo1, anti-CD11b) that inhibits leukocyte adhesion. J. Clin. Invest. 81: 624.

21. Shalit, M., D. E. Campbell, C. Von Allmen, P. C. Atkins, S. D. Douglas, and B. Zweiman. 1987. Neutrophil activation in human inflammatory skin reactions. J. Allergy Clin. Immunol. 80: 87.

22. Shalit, M., C. Von Allman, P. C. Atkins, and B. Zweiman. 1987. Increased expression of CR3 (C3bi receptor) on neutrophils in human inflammatory skin reactions. J. Clin. Immunol. 7: 456.

23. deBoer, M., and D. Roos. 1986. Metabolic comparison between basophils and other leukocytes from human blood. J. Immunol. 136: 3447.

24. Bochner, B. S., P. T. Peachell, K. E. Brown, and R. P. Schleimer. 1988. Adherence of human basophils to cultured umbilical vein endothelial cells. J. Clin. Invest. 81: 1355.

25. Otsuka, H., J. Dolovich, M. Richardson, J. Bienenstock, and J. A. Denburg. 1987. Metachromatic cell progenitors and specific growth and differentiation factors in human nasal mucosa and polyps. Am. Rev. Respir. Dis. 136: 710.

26. Denburg, J. A., S. Hutt-Taylor, M. Haak-Frendscho, A. Kaplan, T. Ishizaka, and D. Harnish. 1988. A possible unique basophil differentiation factor derived from T-cells and nasal polyp epithelium. J. Allergy Clin. Immunol. 81: 281 (Abstract).

27. Bevilaqua, M. P., J. S. Pober, D. L. Mendrick, R. S. Cotran, and M. A. Gimbrone Jr. 1987. Identification of an inducible endothelial leukocyte adhesion molecule. Proc. Natl. Acad. Sci. USA 84: 9238.

28. Cotran, R. S., M. A. Gimbrone Jr., M. P. Bevilaqua, D. L. Mendrick, and J. S. Pober. 1986. Induction and detection of a human endothelial activation antigen in vivo. J. Exp. Med. 164: 661.

29. Bochner, B. S., G. V. Marcotte, D. W. MacGlashan Jr., and R. P. Schleimer. 1988. IgE-dependent and independent regulation of human basophil adhesiveness. J. Allergy Clin. Immunol. 81: 301 (Abstract).

30. Haak-Frendscho, M., N. Arai, K. Arai, M. L. Baeza, A. Finn, and A. P. Kaplan. 1988. Human recombinant granulocyte-macrophage colony-stimulating factor and interleukin 3 cause basophil histamine release. J. Clin. Invest. 81: 17.

31. Schleimer, R. P. 1988. Glucocorticosteroids: Their mechanism of action and use in allergic diseases. In: Allergy Principles and Practice (3rd edition). E. Middleton, C. E. Reed, E. F. Ellis, N. F. Adkinson, Jr., and J. W. Yunginger, eds. Mosby, Washington, DC, pp. 739–765.

32. Pipkorn, U., D. Proud, L. M. Lichtenstein, A. Kagey-Sobotka, P.S. Norman, and R. P. Naclerio. 1987. Inhibition of mediator release in allergic rhinitis by pretreatment with topical glucocorticosteroids. N. Engl. J. Med. 316: 1506.

33. Schleimer, R. P., L. M. Lichtenstein, and E. Gillespie. 1981. Inhibition of basophil histamine release by antiinflammatory steroids. Nature 292: 454.

34. Howarth, P. H., S. R. Durham, T. H. Lee, A. B. Kay, M. K. Church, and S. T. Holgate. 1985. Influence of albuterol, cromolyn sodium, and ipratropium bromide on the airway and circulating mediator responses to allergen bronchial provocation in asthma. Am. Rev. Respir. Dis. 132: 986.

35. DeMonchy, J. G. R., H. F. Kauffman, P. Venge, G. H. Koeter, H. M. Jansen, H. J. Sluiter, and K. DeVries. 1985. Bronchoalveolar eosinophilia during allergen-induced late asthmatic reactions. Am. Rev. Respir. Dis. 131: 373.

36. Kay, A. B., G. M. Walsh, R. Moqbel, A. J. MacDonald, T. Nagakura, M. P. Carroll, and H. B. Richerson. 1987. Disodium cromoglycate inhibits activation of human inflammatory cells in vitro. J. Allergy Clin. Immunol. 80: 1.

37. Fadel, R., N. Herpin-Richard, J. P. Rihoux, and E. Henolg. 1987. Inhibitory effect of cetirizine 2HCl on eosinophilia in vivo. Clin. Allergy 17: 373.

38. Charlesworth, E. N., A. Kagey-Sobotka, P. S. Norman, and L. M. Lichtenstein. 1988. Effect of cetirizine on mast cell mediator release and cellular traffic during the cutaneous late phase reaction. J. Allergy Clin. Immunol., in press.

Lymphocytes and Lymphokines in Immediate Type Hypersensitivity

Beda M. Stadler, Jean-François Gauchat, Kazunori Nakajima, Dominique Gauchat, Claudia Vassella, Stefan Brantschen, Qiu Gang, Xiaodong Yang, Michèle Mandallaz, Alain L. de Weck*

Accumulating in vitro data suggest that cytokines may play a crucial role in the development of allergies. They regulate in an antigen and isotype non-specific manner the formation of IgE. Furthermore, many cytokines promote growth and differentiation and also alter the function of effector cells involved in allergic reactions. Although there are no known hierarchies in the biological activity of these cytokines, it seems that interleukin 3 and 4 as well as γ-interferon play a crucial role in the ontogeny of allergies. One of the consequences of this nonspecific regulation might be the production of isotype-specific IgG anti-IgE antibodies that are capable of interfering with the sensitization process during an allergic reaction.

Cytokines are very promising mediators that may help to understand the cellular networks leading to allergic responses. The difficulty in fully understanding the bioactivities of cytokines lies in their pleiotropy. One cytokine may act either as a growth factor or else as a differentiation or activation factor on a whole variety of different cell types, and many cytokines act also on cells outside the immune system.

It is well known that allergic responses are under direct T cell control [1]. However, no one can yet propose a clear hierarchy of cytokines, and it would therefore be appealing if certain T cell subpopulations were to produce only a certain and limited number of cytokines. Indeed, in the mouse such a system has been described [2]. Murine cloned T helper cell lines may be classified according to their cytokine production and not according to their surface markers. Th1 cells produce γ-interferon, IL-3 and GM-CSF as well as IL-2, while the Th2 cells produce IL-3, IL-4, IL-5, and GM-CSF. As we will see later, the implication of this diversity of cytokine production might be that the Th1 cell is a kind of suppressor cell for the IgE response as well as for many effector cells in allergy. On the other hand, the Th2 cell could be an inducer cell for IgE synthesis and for growth and differentiation of mast cells, basophils and eosinophils.

The question remains whether such a system also exists in the human. The first problem is that presently no antigens are known that would exclusively stimulate either Th1 or Th2 cells. We analyzed human mononuclear cells for their cytokine gene expression and found a distinct pattern of cytokines that was dependent on the applied type of stimulation [3]. Perhaps the most interesting cytokine pattern resulted after anti CD3 antibody stimulation, yielding, for example, very low interleukin 2 mRNA levels. All polyclonal stimuli induced—even though to a variable extent—IL-1 to IL-5 as well as the CSF mRNAs. However, polyclonal stimuli only mimic a "physiological" stimulation. We therefore used antigens such as tetanus toxoid or candida albicans to stimulate human mononuclear cells. Again, antigens induced a different pattern of cytokines than polyclonal stimuli. This opens new and exciting possibilities to explain the sensibilization against allergens. Consequently, we might speculate that allergens stimulate preferentially certain T cell subpopulations resulting in a special "cocktail" of cytokines favoring allergic responses.

Of course, antigens do not only stimulate T helper cells. This complicates even further a potential regulation by a given subpopulation. We have analyzed human mononuclear cells

*   Institute of Clinical Immunology, Inselspital, CH-3010 Bern, Switzerland.
     This work was supported in part by the Swiss National Science Foundation, Grant Nos. 3.249-0.85, 3.885-0.88 and 3.887-1.87.
     Acknowledgements: We would like to thank Drs. Max Schreier, Barbara Fagg, and Franco Di Padova from Sandoz AG, Basel for their generous gifts of recombinant IL-3 and IL-4.

stimulated by polyclonal agents using in situ hybridization techniques [4]. We found that even though a majority of T cells are activated (within the G1 phase of the cell cycle), there seem to be only very few cells that produced a certain cytokine at a given time [4]. We found, for example, approximately 20% of the cells producing γ-interferon, while only approximately 10% of the cells were producing GM-CSF. Thus, this pattern completely contradicts the pattern found in Th1 and Th2 cells in the mouse, where both Th1 and Th2 produce GM-CSF and only Th1 produce γ-IFN [2].

Cytokines and Effector Cells in Allergy

Interleukin 3 was the first cloned cytokine that was clearly relevant to allergic responses. In the mouse it was even called mast cell growth factor in the beginning because this factor induced abundant in vitro growth of mast cell-like cells. While being a pan-specific growth factor for hemopoietic cells in the mouse, it still remains interesting that this factor maintains long-time growth of a cell type, denominated "mast cell" by many authors (for review of topic, see [5]). In the human we searched for a mast cell growth factor, which could be the potential analogue for murine interleukin-3. Then, we described the basophil-promoting activity (BaPA), which promoted growth of a cell type that resembled rather basophils than mast cells [6]. Recently, by using monoclonal antibodies against human recombinant interleukin-3, we have been able to show that BaPA is indeed human interleukin-3 [7]. Most likely, the cell types which are grown by mouse IL-3 or human IL-3 only differ by nomenclature but not by nature and still belong to a rather immature basophil/mast cell phenotype [8, 9].

Interleukin-4 is an additional factor which plays a crucial role in allergic responses. For cultured basophil/mast cell like cells, IL-4 is a differentiation factor [10]. IL-4 changes their morphology and increases their intracellular mediator content. But besides IL-3 and IL-4 there might be still additional factors that may induce the typical phenotype of a basophil or a mast cell as encountered in vivo [11].

Cytokines not only play a role as growth factors for effector cells in allergy, they also act on differentiated effector cells of allergy. For example, interleukin-3 is capable of priming basophils for an enhanced releasability of pharmacologically active mediators. This fact again complicates the hierarchy of cytokine activity. The future will tell whether in atopic patients a certain "cocktail" of cytokines is actually important for the generation of effector cells or their responsiveness toward allergens.

Cytokines and IgE Regulation

Many different factors have been described phenomenologically to play a role for the synthesis of IgE immunoglobulins [1]. According to our present knowledge, many of these crude supernatants or semipurified factors contained one dominant cytokine, namely, interleukin-4. This factor induces IgE synthesis in murine and human systems [12, 13]. All polyclonal stimuli and antigens that we have tested so far induced interleukin-4 mRNA in human mononuclear cells. Thus, one factor is always present that, when added exogenously, induces IgE synthesis in normals and atopics. Even though IL-4 does not mediate isotype specificity in the regulation, it seems that the IgE response is percent wise more affected than IgG1 synthesis [14].

Nevertheless, we never found an induction of IgE synthesis when using polyclonal stimuli in the human [15]. As we know now, this may be in part because of an antagonistic cytokine, namely, γ-interferon. In vitro, γ-interferon clearly inhibits ongoing IgE synthesis or IgE synthesis induced by interleukin-4 [14]. Thus, it has become clear that IgE regulation depends on the ratio of these two cytokines. Already 0.1 unit γ-interferon clearly inhibits IgE synthesis, which suggests that γ-interferon by itself might even be more decisive for IgE production than IL-4, which is the prerequisite.

IgE binding factors, which are most likely the secreted form of the low affinity IgE receptor [16] (CD23) have also been postulated to be involved in the regulation of IgE. How this lectin-like, shed surface receptor might influence IgE synthesis is presently not known. What remains interesting is that IL-4 also induces CD23, while γ-interferon inhibits its expression [17]. Thus, again a cocktail of cytokines together with shed surface receptors may form a microenvironment that either favors or disfavors an allergic response. For future treatment it will be important to know the composition and ratios of certain cytokines that might inhibit in vivo IgE synthesis.

We have analyzed gene expression for interleukin-4 and γ-interferon in normal subjects and atopic patients. Mononuclear cells expressed enhanced IL-4 mRNA levels together with decreased levels of γ-interferon in atopics. IL-4 levels correlated positively and γ-IFN negatively with the patients serum IgE levels which is in agreement with what one would predict from the in vitro data as discussed above.

Cytokines and IgG Anti-IgE Autoantibodies

Auto antibodies against IgE have been described [18–22]. Because cytokines, such as interleukin-4 or γ-interferon lack antigen specificity, we investigated whether a polyclonal induction of IgE synthesis (as it is induced by IL-4) might also result in the production of IgG anti-IgE antibodies. Indeed, polyclonal stimuli induced in vitro IgG anti-IgE antibodies, which resulted in the formation of IgG anti-IgE complexes. IgE within these complexes are hidden for many PRIST-like IgE determination assays which might have also contributed to the past controversy on the human in vitro IgE synthesis. Thus, it might be that in vivo an IgE synthesis may be accompanied by the formation of IgG anti-IgE auto antibodies.

Next, we investigated the functional role of such anti isotype antibodies. By means of defined murine monoclonal anti human IgE antibodies we were able to demonstrate that there exist two types of naturally occurring IgG anti-IgE antibodies. One type, which we called the "anaphylactogenic naturally occurring" anti-IgE antibody, is capable of directly triggering mediator release from human basophils. The so-called non-anaphylactogenic IgG anti-IgE antibody is still capable of recognizing cytophilic IgE, though it does not trigger histamine release [23]. Both types are capable, if complexed with IgE, of inhibiting the binding of IgE to basophils or the CD23 receptor, for example, on human B-cells. Furthermore, both types of IgG anti-IgE antibodies are capable of removing IgE bound to the low affinity IgE receptor [24].

Conclusion

Cytokines form a complex network of cellular mediators which clearly regulate the allergic response. Interestingly, cytokines such as IL-4 or γ-interferon, which are mainly or exclusively produced by T cells, play a central role in the regulation of IgE synthesis and the growth of the effector cells of allergy. Other cytokines, such as the colony-stimulating factors, IL-5, and potentially many others are not exclusively or mainly produced by T lymphocytes and seem to play a less decisive role than those produced by T cells. The example of IL-4 and γ-interferon clearly illustrates that it is not so much an individual cytokine that dominates the allergic response, but rather the ratio within the cocktail which might lead to a normal or an allergic response in a microenvironment. These two cytokines also demonstrate that it is eventually not necessary to postulate a strict isotype-specific regulation for the formation of IgE. The products of this regulation, namely, the immunoglobulins, might not be important only during the sensitization and triggering process, but also during the ontogeny of allergies. Auto anti-IgE antibodies, induced by these polyclonally active cytokines, may by themselves be physiological regulators, since they are capable of inhibiting sensitization. On the other hand, by being capable of directly triggering mediator release, such antibodies might even mimic some of the functions of the cytokines itself. Again, not the absolute quantity of IgE might be of importance, but the quantity of complexed, free IgE or free IgG anti-IgE antibodies might contribute much to the known clinical symptoms of allergies.

References

1. Ishisaka, K. 1985. Twenty years with IgE: From the identification of IgE to regulatory factors for the IgE response. J. Immunol. 135: 1.
2. Coffman, R. L., B. W. P. Seymour, D. A. Lebman, D. D. Hiraki, J. A. Christiansen, B. Shrader, H. M. Cherwinski, H. F. J. Savelkoul, F. D. Finkelman, M. W. Bond, and T. R. Mosmann. 1988. The role of helper T cell products in mouse B cell differentiation and isotype regulation. Immunological Reviews 102: 5.
3. Gauchat, J.-F., C. Walker, A. L. de Weck, and B. M. Stadler. 1988. Stimulation dependent lymphokines mRNA levels in human mononuclear cells. Eur. J. Immunol. 18: 1441.

4. Gang, Q., J. F. Gauchat, U. Wirthmüller, A. L. de Weck, and B. M. Stadler. 1988. Lymphokine production by human peripheral blood lymphocytes: Analysis by in situ hybridization. Lymphokine Research, in press.

5. Bienenstock, J., A. D. Befus, J. Denburg, R. Goodacre, F. Pearce, and F. Shanahan. 1983. Mast cell heterogeneity. Monogr. Allergy 18: 124.

6. Tadokoro, K., B. M. Stadler, and A. L. de Weck. 1983 Factor-dependent in vitro growth of human normal bone marrow-derived basophil-like cells. J. Exp. Med. 158: 857.

7. Fagg, B., K. Hirai, K. Nakajima, and B. M. Stadler. 1988. Human recombinant IL-3 promotes the growth of human basophils/mast cells.In: UCLA Symposia on Molecular and Cellular Biology, New series, Volume 100, J. Groopman, C. Evans, and D. Golde, eds. New York: Alan R. Liss.

8. Hirai, K., A. L. De Weck, and B. M. Stadler. 1988. Characterization of a human basophil-like cell promoting activity. J. Immunol. 140: 221.

9. Stadler, B. M., and K. Hirai. 1988. Human growth factors for metachromatically staining cells. Lymphokines 15: 341.

10. Hamaguchi, Y., Y. Kanakura, J. Fujita, S. Takeda, T. Nakano, S. Tarui, T. Honjo, and Y. Kitamura. 1987. Interleukin-4 as an essential factor for in vitro growth of murine connective tissue-type mast cells. J. Exp. Med. 165: 268.

11. Levi-Schaffer, F., K. F. Austen, P. M. Gravallese, and R. L. Stevens. 1986. Coculture of interleukin 3-dependent mouse mast cells with fibroblasts results in a phenotypic change of the mast cells. Proc. Natl. Acad. Sci. 83: 6485.

12. Snapper, C. M., and W. E. Paul. 1987. Interferon γ and B-cell stimulatory factors 1 reciprocally regulate Ig isotype production. Science 236: 944.

13. Yokota, T., T. Otsuka, T. Mosmann, J. Banchereau, T. DeFrance, D. Blanchard, J. E. De Vries, F. Lee, and D. Arai. 1986. Isolation and characterization of a human interleukin cDNA clone, homologous to mouse B-cell stimulatory factor 1, that expresses B-cell and T-cell-stimulating activities. Proc. Natl. Acad. Sci. 83: 5894.

14. Yang, X. D., A. L. de Weck, B. M. Stadler. 1988. Induction of human IgE synthesis via stimulation by anti-CD3 antibody. Eur. J. Immunol. 18: 436.

15. Yang, X. D., A. L. de Weck, and B. M. Stadler. 1988. Effect of recombinant human interleukin 4 on spontaneous in vitro IgE synthesis. Eur. J. Immunol., in press.

16. Meinke, G. C., A. M. Magro, D. A. Lawrence, and H. L. Spiegelberg. 1978. Characterization of an IgE receptor isolated from cultured B-type lymphoblastoid cells. J. Immunol. 121: 1321

17. Defrance, T., J. F. Aubry, F. Rousset, B. Vanbervliet, J. Y. Bonnefoy, N. Aray. Y. Takebe, T. Yokata, F. Lee, K. Arai, J. de Vries, and J. Banchereau. 1987. Human recombinant interleukin 4 induces Fc ε receptor (CD23) on normal human B lymphocytes. J. Exp. Med. 165: 1459.

18. Williams, R. C. Jr., R. W. Griffiths, J. D. Emmons, and R. C. Field. 1972. Naturally occurring human antiglobulins with specificity for γ-E. J. Clin. Inves. 51: 955.

19. Inganäs, M., S. G. O. Johansson, and H. Bennich. 1981. Anti-IgE antibodies in human serum: Occurrence and specificity. Int. Archs Allergy Appl. Immunol. 65: 51.

20. Stevens, W. J., and C. H. Bridts. 1984. IgG-containing and IgE-containing circulating immune complexes in patients with asthma and rhinitis. J. Allergy Clin. Immunol. 73: 276.

21. Nawata, Y., T. Koike, H. Hosokawa, H. Tomioka, and S. Yoshida. 1985. Anti-IgE autoantibody in patients with atopic dermatitis. J. Immunol. 135: 478.

22. Quinti, I., C. Brozek, N. Wood, R. S. Geha, and D. Y. M. Leung. 1986. Circulating IgG autoantibodies to IgE in atopic syndromes. J. Allergy Clin. Immunol. 77: 586.

23. Stadler, B. M., K. Nakajima, X. Yang, and A. L. de Weck. 1988. Potential role of anti-IgE antibodies in vivo. Progress in allergy, CIA meeting A. Sehon, ed. Basel: S. Karger, in press.

24. Nakajima, K., A. L. de Weck, and B. M. Stadler. 1988. Effect of anti IgE antibodies on IgE binding to CD23. Allergy, in press.

Platelets in Allergy

*André Capron, Claude Auriault, Jean-Yves Cesbron, Véronique Pancré,
André-Bernard Tonnel, Anne Tsicopoulos, Michel Joseph**

Allergy has long been viewed as a classical tragedy involving two partners: a special type of antibody, IgE and possibly an anaphylactic subclass of IgG, and particular cells i.e., basophils and mast cells. Extensive studies initiated in parasitic diseases have now unequivocally established that IgE antibodies can trigger mononuclear phagocytes, eosinophils and platelets directly through specific surface IgE receptors now identified as $Fc_\varepsilon R_{II}$ [1]. Genes encoding for this class of receptors have been cloned, and although studies on molecular structure indicate a close homology between $Fc_\varepsilon R_{II}$ on inflammatory cells and on B cells, there are now emerging indications of some degree of post-transcriptional heterogeneity among the second receptor for IgE. Whilst the evidence for the direct participation of other inflammatory cells, such as eosinophils, in allergic reactions is now widely recognized, the role of platelets as effector cells remains a matter of controversy, and the concept that platelets might be active cellular partners in allergy is still debatable.

In this review, the attempt is made to discuss, in the light of recent information, the experimental evidences pleading for such an active participation.

Mechanisms of Platelet Activation

In allergic disorders, platelet activation was for long believed to occur indirectly through the effects of platelet activating factor (PAF or PA-acether). PAF is released by a variety of IgE sensitized cells that express either $Fc_\varepsilon R_I$ (mast cells, basophils) or $Fc_\varepsilon R_{II}$ (macrophages, eosinophils). PAF is also released by stimulated endothelial cells and by activated platelets themselves [2]. That platelets can participate directly in some IgE-mediated processes has arisen from the demonstration of the involvement of this cell population in IgE-dependent killing of parasites [3].

These studies, confirmed by others [4], indicated that human platelets can bind IgE in vitro, and that cross-linking of surface bound IgE with anti-IgE or antigen-induced platelet activation and secretion. Further experiments led to the demonstration of a specific receptor for the Fc fragment of IgE on the platelet membrane. Scatchard analysis showed that there were between 600 and 1000 binding sites for IgE per platelet with an affinity constant of $3 \times 10^7 M^{-1}$ [5].

Several lines of evidence pointed to similarities between the platelet IgE receptor and the $Fc_\varepsilon R$ on monocytes, macrophages, and eosinophils. In particular a unique monoclonal antibody BB10, raised against the eosinophil IgE receptor, inhibited IgE-binding and IgE-dependent platelet activation. It should be stressed that the platelet IgE receptor clearly appears as distinct from the previously described IgG-binding sites and, that cross-linking of surface bound IgE can also be achieved with "so-called" IgE-binding factor, known as histamine-releasing factor (HRF), released by macrophages and platelets themselves.

Purification and subsequent gel analysis of the platelet IgE receptor has provided evidence of two subunits of 43 kD and 30 kD, the latter differing from the smaller subunit in eosinophils and monocytes generally identified as a 23–25 kD molecule [6]. An interesting feature of the platelet $Fc_\varepsilon R_{II}$ is its association with a platelet membrane glycoprotein, which plays an essential role in haemostasis, the GPIIb/IIIa complex. Platelets from patients with Glanzman thrombasthenia selectively lacked both the GPIIb/IIIa complex and the IgE receptor, and monoclonal antibodies to GPIIb and IIIa inhibited the binding of IgE and the IgE-mediated cytotoxicity in normal platelets, indicating that the binding of IgE to human platelets required the presence of the GPIIb/IIIa complex [7]. Recent studies performed in parallel on

* Centre d'Immunologie et de Biologie Parasitaire, Institut Pasteur, B.P. 245, 1 rue du Prof. Calmette, 59019 Lille Cédex, France.
This work was supported by the Unité Mixte INSERM U167-CNRS 624.

eosinophils and platelets indicated that $Fc_\varepsilon R_{II}$ and GPIIb/IIIa share common characters of adhesiotopes and, more precisely, the RGD sequence commonly involved in the primary structure of adhesion proteins.

In the framework of allergic or inflammatory disorders other biological mediators of platelet triggering have also been demonstrated. C reactive protein, for instance, appeared as a potent inducer of platelet activation. Platelets collected during the acute phase of experimental infection of rodents by schistosomes were highly cytotoxic for schistosome larvae, and normal platelets could be triggered into effector cells by highly purified C reactive protein [8]. More recently, it has been shown that the neuropeptide substance P could directly trigger platelet activation [9]. Interestingly, the amino acid sequence of substance P actively involved in platelet activation is confined to the N-terminal region of the molecule, as for stimulation of T lymphocyte proliferation, whereas amino acids of the C-terminal portion induces histamine release from mast cells. The construction of various synthetic peptides derived from the sequence of substance P has allowed the demonstration that the AA sequence 5-11 corresponded to the most active site of the molecule. In competition experiments, it has been also demonstrated that platelet activation by substance P can be inhibited by IgE itself and that the competitive inhibition observed might be related to the existence of limited but significant conformational homology between the primary structure of substance P and the domain of the ε chain.

Taken together, these examples, which do not represent an exhaustive list of the molecules potentially involved in platelet activation, provide evidence, in the framework of allergic disorders, that relevant stimuli such as IgE, IgE-binding factors, C reactive protein, or substance P can directly participate to platelet activation and to secretion of platelet derived mediators.

Expression of Platelet Activation

Both in animal and in humans, allergic challenge or asthmatic shock—but not the nonallergic bronchoconstriction mediated by methacholine—has been shown to induce the release into plasma of platelet-specific proteins, such as platelet factor 4 (PF4) [10] and a-thromboglobulin (aTG) [11]. These increases however varied widely from patients to patients and were not observed by all investigators [12–13]. In the bronchoalveolar lavage of asthmatics, significant elevations of aTG and fibrinopeptide-A from fibrinogen were measured during early and late phase response to allergen challenge [14].

A Scenario for Free Radicals In IgE-Mediated Platelet Activation

In the framework of our studies, platelets isolated from patients with allergic asthma or with *Hymenoptera* venom hypersensitivity reacted in vitro to specific allergen or to anti-IgE by releasing cytotoxic mediators and oxygen-derived free radicals evidenced respectively by the death of parasitic larvae and by chemiluminescence [15].

How can platelets affect cellular targets ? Our challenging opinion sees the cytotoxicity of platelets as involving the participation of (OX)-type radical species. Four sets of arguments appear in support of this working hypothesis:

1. Free radical scavengers and oxidoreductases (superoxide dismutase, catalase, glutathione peroxidase) removing O^-_2, H_2O_2 and lipid peroxides strongly inhibit cytocidal effects of IgE- dependent platelet activation. The data obtained are consistent with a lipid peroxidation process in platelets [16].

2. Mobilized pools of metal ions, particularly iron, are important in accelerating damaging free radical reactions, and conversely chelating agents can be used as protective compounds. We have, in this context, shown an increased IgE-dependent activation by Fe^{++} down to 10^{-11} M. In addition, the presence of 10^{-6} M of the iron chelator o-phenanthroline abolished the action of Fe^{++} [16].

3. IgE-stimulated platelets induce significant catalase- inhibitable chemiluminescence, reaching its maximum between 3 and 5 minutes after the stimulus and decaying slowly.

4. Spin trapping of hydroxyl radicals by reaction with stable nitroxyl radicals and the generation of electron paramagnetic reso-

nance (EPR) spectra have allowed the identification of °OH radicals after IgE-dependent activation. As a whole the data gathered render highly probable the participation of free radical reactions as a result of IgE- dependent platelet activation. The possibility that oxygen free radicals contribute directly to tissue damage seems unlikely considering the short life span of these molecules. Whatever the primary radical event occurring within cells, it is reasonable to think that it sets off radical chain reactions, leading to lipoperoxidation of lipids in membranes. Lipid peroxides can fragment to give a wide range of more stable products, such as aldehydes. No relationship between the arachidonic acid metabolism of platelets and their cytocidal properties after IgE-dependent activation has been evidenced in our hands. We have been in particular unable to correlate significant changes in arachidonate products with platelet activation, although the cytotoxicity was abolished with various lipoxygenase and cycloxygenase inhibitors. Evidence that Phospholipase A2, which preferentially hydrolyzes peroxidized fatty acids rather than arachidonic acid, might play a crucial role in platelet cytotoxicity is consistent with the above observations. One must admit, however, that we are still left with a working hypothesis in our understanding of molecular mechanisms governing cytocidal properties of platelets following IgE-dependent activation, so that much work in this area is still needed. It might be reassuring to keep in mind that almost 20 years after the discovery of cytotoxic T cells and NK cells our understanding of their killing mechanism is still very fragmentary.

Regulatory Mechanisms

The demonstration of effector functions of platelets in parasitic diseases raised the question of their possible regulation by T-cells. Normal human platelets treated with culture supernatants from mitogen- or antigen-stimulated CD4$^+$/CD8$^-$ T-cells developed the capacity to kill the larvae of *S. mansoni* in the absence of IgE antibodies. The physicochemical properties of the factors involved, strongly suggested that IFNγ was likely one of the lymphokine stimulating platelet cytotoxicity. The neutrali-

zation by monoclonal and polyclonal anti-IFNγ antibodies of the induction of the platelet killer effect, the presence of IFNγ in the CD4$^+$/CD8$^-$ lymphocyte supernatants and finally the direct inducer effect of recombinant IFNγ clearly demonstrated that this lymphokine was one of the factors responsible for the induction of platelet cytotoxic functions [17]. The in vivo relevance of this effect was studied in the rat model: the passive transfer of normal rat platelets treated with rat recombinant IFNγ to normal syngenetic recipients on the day of challenge infection led to a high degree of protection. Moreover, IFNγ could also act on the IgE-dependent platelet cytotoxicity by enhancing the IgE receptor expression on the platelet membrane [18].

The demonstration of interrelationship between IFNγ and platelet function has to be related to the work of Molinas et al. [19], who demonstrated that human IFNγ was able to bind to an estimate of 150–200 high-affinity specific receptors on human platelets with an apparent equilibrium dissociation constant (Kd) of 2×10^{-10} M.

A second inducing factor of platelet cytotoxicity exhibiting a neutral pI was also previously evidenced in CD4$^+$/CD8$^-$ stimulated T lymphocyte supernatant. This factor was identified as tumor necrosis factor (TNF). Indeed, recombinant TNF-β and to a lesser extend TNFα-induced normal platelets into cytotoxic effectors for *S. mansoni* larvae [20]. An additive effect of TNF and IFNγ has been also observed. The characterization of TNF receptor(s) onto the platelet membrane is presently underway.

We have demonstrated that ConA- and antigen-stimulated CD4$^-$/CD8$^+$ T lymphocytes released a factor able to inhibit the IgE-, IFN-, and TNF β-dependent platelet cytotoxicity toward the parasitic larvae. The production of oxygen metabolites by platelets in an IgE-anti-IgE reaction was likewise strongly inhibited by the lymphokine [21]. This platelet activity suppressive lymphokine (PASL) was identified as an acid- and heat-stable polypeptide of 15–20 Kd with a pI of 4.6. The factor was specifically absorbed by platelet membrane suggesting its action through the binding to a receptor. The in vivo relevance of PASL could be established by a complete abolition of the protection normally conferred toward a challenge infection by the intravenous passive transfer of platelets from immune to normal rats, after PASL-treatment of transferred platelets [22]. The molecular cloning of PASL is presently underway.

Taken together, these results demonstrated that in addition to IgE, antigen-specific CD4$^+$/CD8$^-$ T lymphocytes could activate platelets through IFNγ and TNF production while a feedback regulation of the platelet immune functions should be under the control of CD4$^-$/CD8$^+$-stimulated T-cells through PASL generation.

Of possible interest is the observation that whereas IL4 has been shown to induce FcϵR$_{II}$ expression on B cells, monocytes and eosinophils, IL4 did not increase, in our studies, IgE-dependent platelet activation. Conversely, γ-IFN, which enhances the expression of FcϵR$_{II}$ on the platelet membrane, does not exhibit such an effect on eosinophils. These differences in the activity of this interleukin on FcϵR$_{II}$, together with the observation mentioned above of differences in the structure of one of the subunit of IgE platelet receptor, might be an indication of some heterogeneity among IgE receptors on inflammatory cells.

Platelets and Allergic Disorders

While the participation of inflammatory cells expressing the low affinity receptor for IgE, like mononuclear phagocytes or eosinophils, is now largely accepted, the exact role of platelets in allergic diseases certainly remains to be more clearly established [23].

Signs of Platelet Activation in Allergic Disorders

Three different situations were explored in this context. Platelets isolated from asthmatic patients with mite or grass pollen sensitivity reacted in vitro to specific allergens or to anti-IgE by releasing cytocidal mediators and oxygen free radicals. Anti-IgG was unable to produce such an activation. Normal platelets could be passively sensitized by the serum of allergic patients and induced into effectors by the addition of specific ligands. IgE but not IgG depletion abrogated the ability of allergic patient sera to passively sensitize normal platelets to allergens [5]. The involvement of IgE receptors was further confirmed by the total inhibition of both parameters of activation

after preincubation with anti-FcϵR$_{II}$ monoclonal antibody. Similarly, in patients with *Hymenoptera* venom sensitivity, platelets could also be specifically triggered by venom allergen. This platelet activation was allergen specific allowing to differentiate honey-bee and *Vespula* sensitivity.

Finally, platelets isolated from patients with aspirin-sensitive asthma exhibited in vitro an abnormal response to aspirin- generating oxygen metabolites in the presence of acetylsalicylic acid or non-steroidal anti-inflammatory drugs [24].

Changes in the Behavior of Platelets from Allergic Patients

In aspirin-induced asthma, platelets lost their property to generate cytocidal factors after induction of a refractory period obtained by daily ingestion of high doses of aspirin. In this syndrome, platelets were deactivated at the very period when patients were insensitive to the drug, and they recovered full reactivity as soon as the treatment with aspirin has been discontinued and patients were sensitive again [24].

Similarly, in *Hymenoptera* venom hypersensitivity, platelets from patients undergoing specific immunotherapy by rush desensitization lost their specific reactivity to allergens in vitro, becoming unable to generate free radicals and cytotoxic mediators, in contrast with the properties they exhibited before desensitization [25]. The in vitro sensitivity of platelets exactly correlated the sensitivity of patients to venom. Recent experiments favor the possible intervention of lymphokines in the observed modification of platelet reactivity. Indeed, lymphocyte supernatants obtained from patients after rush desensitization were able to down regulate platelet reactivity. Similarly, sera obtained from desensitized patients were able to suppress IgE- dependent platelet activation. Physiochemical characterization of the suppressive factor present in lymphocyte supernatants and in serum showed properties very similar to those previously described for PASL, indicating that this lymphocyte factor might be preferentially expressed during the course of desensitization.

Platelet Dependence of Bronchoconstriction

Beyond the events reported above, the exposure of airways to allergen challenge induces, in asthmatic patients or in sensitized rabbits and guinea-pigs, bronchoconstriction as a primary effect. Platelet depletion of experimental animals suppressed the allergic respiratory syndrome [26]. In this context, the role of PAF-acether in immediate response, although well documented [2], is far from being fully understood. Nonetheless PAF-acether was shown to induce acute airway response after intravenous injection or intratracheal instillation [27]. Platelets seem to play a crucial role in this effect of PAF- acether. Thrombocytopenia has been associated with PAF-induced bronchoconstriction [28]. Platelet depletion, or platelet inhibition by prostacyclin, in rabbit or guinea-pig, suppressed the effects induced by PAF-acether on the lungs [29]. In vitro PAF-acether contracted strongly surgical specimens of human bronchi, but only in the presence of platelets: Neither PAF- acether nor platelets alone could induce bronchospasm [30]. Platelet activation mediated by PAF-acether is expressed by granule exocytosis. Compounds able to inhibit the platelet release also impaired the bronchoconstriction induced by antigen or PAF-acether [29]. In the rat, whose platelets have no PAF-acether receptors, the intravenous injection of this phospholipid was unable to provoke bronchoconstriction [29].

Another approach has recently been developed which has led to the identification of anti-platelet antibodies in some patients with non-allergic, so-called intrinsic asthma. Such antibodies can induce in vitro platelet activation and secretion, similarly to what is observed after IgE-dependent activation.

Conclusion

In the light of the observations reported here, it appears that if the definitive demonstration of a platelet involvement in the immediate response of type I hypersensitive reactions and in their associated inflammatory effects is not acquired, the participation of these blood constituents in the cellular network leading to the physiopathological process of allergic reactions is largely documented and can be considered now as more than a hypothesis. The suggestion that platelets could be generated mainly in the lung vasculature [31] may strengthen the implication of thrombocytes in the asthmatic pathology, and it opens new perspective to their involvement in various allergic and inflammatory disorders. Furthermore, as far as the cellular network is concerned, it should be unrealistic to stress on the only platelets as responsible for such pathologies. Their reactivity has to be reconsidered in the general concept of intercellular communications, with the recruitment of a large variety of active cell populations, among which especially eosinophils, and with the implication of endothelial cells and, possibly, cells from the peripheral nervous system. In the context of the eosinophil participation to bronchial hyperreactivity and tissue damage, it has been reported that platelet depletion reduced PAF-acether- and allergen-mediated eosinophil infiltration into the lungs of normal and allergic animals respectively [32]. Such observations also focus to new therapeutical approaches in the control of allergic diseases and associated inflammatory disorders.

References

1. Capron, A., J. P. Dessaint, M. Capron, M. Joseph, J. C. Ameisen, and A.B. Tonnel. 1986. From parasites to allergy: A second receptor for IgE. Immunology Today 7: 15.
2. Barnes, P. J., K. F. Chung, and C. P. Page. 1988. Platelet-activating factor as a mediator of allergic disease. J. Allergy Clin. Immunol. 81: 919.
3. Joseph, M., C. Auriault, A. Capron, H. Vorng, and P. Viens. 1983. A new function for platelets: IgE-dependent killing of schistosomes. Nature 303: 810.
4. Cines, D. B., H. van der Keyl, and A.I. Levinson. 1986. In vitro binding of an IgE protein to human platelets. J. Immunol. 136: 3433.
5. Joseph, M., A. Capron, J. C. Ameisen, M. Capron, H. Vorng, V. Pancré, J. P. Kusnierz, and C. Auriault. 1986. The receptor for IgE on blood platelets. Eur. J. Immunol. 16: 306.
6. Capron, M., T. Jouault, L. Prin, M. Joseph, J. C. Ameisen, A. E. Butterworth, J. P. Papin, J. P. Kusnierz, and A. Capron. 1986. Functional study of a monoclonal antibody to IgE Fc receptor ($Fc_\varepsilon R_2$) of eosinophils, platelets, and macrophages. J. Exp. Med. 164: 72.
7. Ameisen, J. C., M. Joseph, J. P. Caen, J. P. Kusnierz, M. Capron, B. Boizard, J.L. Wautier, S. Levy-Toledano, H. Vorng, and A. Capron. 1986.

A role for glycoprotein IIb-IIIa complex in the binding of IgE to human platelets and platelet IgE-dependent cytotoxic functions. Br. J. Haematol. 64: 21.

8. Bout, D., M. Joseph, M. Pontet, H. Vorng, D. Deslée and A. Capron. 1986. Rat resistance to schistosomiasis: Platelet- mediated cytotoxicity induced by C-reactive protein. Science, 231: 153.

9. Damonneville, M., M. Joseph, C. Auriault, H. Gras-Masse, A. Tartar, M. Joseph, and A. Capron. 1988. The neuropeptide substance P stimulates the effector functions of platelets. Ninth European Immunology Meeting, Rome, September 14–17, 1988.

10. Knauer, K. A., L. M. Lichtenstein, N. F. Adkinson, and J. E. Fish. 1981. Platelet activation during antigen-induced airway reactions in asthmatic subjects. N. Engl. J. Med. 304: 1404.

11. Gresele, P., T. Todisco, F. Merante, and G. G. Nenci. 1982. Platelet activation and allergic asthma. N. Engl. J. Med. 306: 549.

12. Greer, I. A., J. H. Winter, D. Gaffney, K. McLoughlin, J. J. F. Belch, G. Boyd, and C. D. Forbes. 1984. Platelets in asthma. Lancet, ii: 1479.

13. Durham, S. R., J. Dawes, and A. B. Kay. 1985. Platelets in asthma. Lancet, ii: 36.

14. Metzger, W. J., G. W. Hunninghake, and H. B. Richerson. 1985. Late asthmatic response: Inquiry into mechanisms and significance. Clin. Rev. Allergy 3: 145.

15. Capron, A., M. Joseph, J. C. Ameisen, M. Capron, V. Pancré, and C. Auriault. 1987. Platelets as effectors in immune and hypersensitivity reactions. Int. Arch. Allergy appl. Immunol. 82: 307.

16. Cesbron, J. Y., A. Capron, B. B. Vargaftig, M. Lagarde, J. Pincemail, P. Braquet, H. Taelman, and M. Joseph. 1987. Platelets mediate the action of diethylcarbamazine on microfilariae. Nature, 325: 533.

17. Pancré, V., M. Joseph, C. Mazingue, J. Wietzerbin, A. Capron, and C. Auriault. 1987. Induction of platelet cytotoxic functions by lymphokine: Role of gamma interferon. J. Immunol. 138: 4490.

18. Pancré, V., M. Joseph, A. Capron, J. Wietzerbin, J. P. Kusnierz, H. Vorng, and C. Auriault. 1988. Recombinant human immune interferon induces increased IgE receptor expression on human platelets. Eur. J. Immunol. 18: 829.

19. Molinas, F. C., J. Wietzerbin, and E. Falcoff. 1987. Human platelets possess receptors for a lymphokine: Demonstration of high specific receptors for Hu IFNγ. J. Immunol. 138: 802.

20. Damonneville, M., J. Wietzerbin, V. Pancré, M. Joseph, A. Capron, and C. Auriault. 1988. Recombinant Tumor Necrosis factor mediate plate-

let cytotoxicity to Schistosoma mansoni larvae. J. Immunol. 140: 3962.

21. Pancré, V., C. Auriault, M. Joseph, J. Y. Cesbron, J. P. Kusnierz, and A. Capron. 1986. A suppressive lymphokine of platelet cytotoxic functions. J. Immunol. 137: 591.

22. Pancré, V., M. Joseph, A. Capron, A. Delanoye, H. Vorng, and C. Auriault. A suppressive factor of platelet cytotoxic functions in human and rat Schistosomiasis mansoni (submitted).

23. Joseph, M. 1988. Platelets in Allergy: Assays and interpretation. Clin. Rev. Allergy, 6: 191.

24. Ameisen, J. C., A. Capron, M. Joseph, J. Maclouf, H. Vorng, V. Pancré, E. Fournier, B. Wallaert, and A. B. Tonnel. 1985. Aspirin-sensitive asthma: Abnormal platelet response to drugs inducing asthmatic attacks. Int. Arch. Allergy appl. Immunol. 78: 438.

25. Tsicopoulos, A., A. B. Tonnel, B. Wallaert, M. Joseph, J. C. Ameisen, P. H. Ramon, J. P. Dessaint, and A. Capron. 1988. Decrease of IgE-dependent platelet activation in *Hymenoptera* hypersensitivity after specific rush desensitization. Clin. exp. Immunol. 71: 433.

26. Pinckard, R. N., M. Halonen, J. D. Palmer, C. Butler, J. O. Shaw, and P. M. Henson. 1977. Intravascular aggregation and pulmonary sequestration of platelets during IgE-induced systemic anaphylaxis in the rabbit: Abrogation of lethal anaphylactic shock by platelet depletion. J. Immunol. 119: 2185.

27. Denjean, A., B. Arnoux, R. Masse, A. Lockart, and J. Benveniste. 1983. Acute effects of intratracheal administration of platelet-activating factor in baboons. J. Appl. Physiol. 55: 799.

28. Gateau, O., B. Arnoux, H. Deriaz, P. Viars, and J. Benveniste. 1984. Acute effects of intratracheal administration of PAF-acether in humans. Am. Rev. Resp. Dis. 129: 3.

29. Vargaftig, B. B., and J. Benveniste. 1983. Platelet-activating factor today. Trends Pharmacol. Sci. 4: 341.

30. Schellenberg, R. R., B. Walker, and F. Snyder. 1983. Platelet-dependent contraction of human bronchi by platelet- activating factor. J. All. Clin. Immunol. 71: 145.

31. Trowbridge, E. A., J. F. Martin, and D. N. Slater. 1982. Evidence for a theory of physical fragmentation of megakaryocytes, implying that all platelets are produced in the pulmonary circulation. Thromb. Res. 28: 461.

32. Lellouch-Tubiana, A., J. Lefort, M. T. Simon, A. Pfister, and B. B. Vargaftig. 1988. Eosinophil recruitment into guinea pig lungs after PAF-acether and allergen administration. Modulation by prostacyclin, platelet depletion, and selective antagonists. Am. Rev. Respir. Dis. 137: 948.

Leukotrienes and Other Arachidonic Acid Metabolites

*Charles W. Parker**

As the leukotrienes have continued to be studied, the spectrum of their known actions has expanded from the originally described effects on smooth muscle contraction and the microvasculature to include effects on secretion, cell proliferation, lipid storage, neuronal activity, and ciliary function. Of particular importance is the ability of leukotrienes to potentiate the production or actions of other allergic mediators including PAF, thromboxane A_2 and C5a. The stimulation of PAF production by endothelial cells and leukocytes by leukotrienes taken together with their effects on vascular permeability and chemotaxis appear to be of particular interest for leukocytic migration into inflamed tissues.

One of the key proteins in the production of biologically active arachidonic acid (AA) metabolites is the enzyme 5-lipoxygenase (5-LO). This enzyme catalyzes the first two steps in the production of leukotrienes from AA, the formation of the 5-hydroperoxide and its 5,6 epoxy derivative, LTA_4 [1]. The 5-LO is an unusual lipoxygenase in that it is inactive until activated by Ca^{2+} [2]. Activation normally occurs when cells are treated with an inflammatory or immunologic stimulus and an influx of Ca^{2+} occurs. The partially purified enzyme is unstable, probably due in part to the removal of several nondialysable constituents that contribute to its enzymatic activity. The 5-LO gene from a cDNA library of the human HL60 leukocytic cell line has recently been isolated and sequenced [3]. The cDNA clone encodes a 674 amino acid sequence with areas of homology for interface binding domains of human lipoprotein lipase and rat hepatic lipase, for rabbit reticulocyte and soybean lipoxygenase, and with weak homologies for consensus Ca^{2+} binding sites for lipocortin and calmodulin. The new information on 5-LO structure should lead to a better understanding of its mechanism of action and inactivation and more rapid progress in the area.

The major known sources of leukotrienes in vivo are mast cells, basophils, neutrophils, monocytes, and perhaps lymphocytes, with maximal production normally occurring within the first 5 to 10 min after cell activation [4, 5]. Major initial 5-LO products include LTA_4, LTB_4, LTC_4, and 5-HETE. In neutrophils, much of the LTB_4 produced early remains associated with the cells, but ultimately the bulk of the LTB_4 appears in the medium either as LTB_4 itself or one of its metabolites. At $37\,^{\circ}C$ human neutrophils rapidly metabolize LTB_4 to its 20-OH and 20-COOH derivatives [6], both of which are significantly less active in aggregation, chemotaxis, and granule enzyme release than LTB_4 itself. LTC_4 production occurs primarily in monocytes, mast cells, eosinophils, and basophils. Neutrophils normally make only small amounts of LTC_4. However, LTA_4 can be transferred from neutrophils to endothelial cells, which in turn convert it to LTC_4 [7, 8]. Mast cells, and to a variable extent the other cell types, convert LTC_4 to LTD_4, which is actually more potent biologically than LTC_4 in some systems. Normally, leukotriene production is transient. More sustained responses can be induced in monocytes and presumably in other leukotrine-producing cells by bacterial lipopolysaccharides and interleukins such as IL-1 and tumor necrosis factor from monocytes [9].

A recent study of macrophages from animals infected with *Leishmania donovani* indicates that exposure to the organism for 24 hours in vitro is associated with a marked increase in the ability of the cells to produce LTC_4 when they are additionally stimulated by LPS or zymogen [10]. Under certain circumstances it appears that an infectious agent itself may produce leukotrienes. A study with Cercaria from Schisto-

---

*   Howard Hughes Medical Institutes, Washington University School of Medicine, Dept. of Medicine/Div. Immunology, St. Louis, MO 63110, USA.

soma mansoni, the form of the organism which traverses the skin and leads to human infection, indicates that they are capable of producing substantial quantities of leukotrienes in the skin [11].

Biologic Actions

LTB4 appears to be a major mediator of leukocyte inflammation since low concentrations are capable of stimulating cell aggregation, increased oxidative metabolism, lysosomal enzyme release, chemokinesis and chemotaxis and complement receptor expression [12]. LTB4 has also been suspected to be an important regulator of T cell function, but the evidence is inconclusive at present. LTB4 is a particularly potent stimulator of leukocyte aggregation producing responses at concentrations in the high picomolar range, making it among the most potent known activators of leukocytes [13–18]. There are marked similarities in these responses to those produced by other activators of leukocyte function such as C5a, F-met-leu-phe (F-MLP), LTB4, PAF, and ATP, which all enhance cell aggregation, migration, and the release of granule enzymes extracellularly. When the cell-agglutinating activity of LTB4 for leukocytes from various species is compared with that of its diasteroisomers and metabolites hydroxylated or carboxylated at the C20 position, LTB4 is considerably more potent than the other agents, indicating that LTB4 is acting on cells through specific receptors [12, 18]. Direct binding studies with radiolabeled LTB4 with human and animal leukocytes have confirmed the existence of saturable and reversible binding inhibited by excess unlabeled ligand [13, 14, 17, 18]. Because LTB4 is rapidly metabolized at 37°C, the results of the binding studies are more easily interpreted at lower temperatures, particularly at 4°C. Detailed inhibition studies with a wider range of analogues of LTB4 than previously have recently been reported. This study indicates the C-12 hydroxyl group plays a more important role in binding activation at the receptor than the C-5 OH group [16]. A detailed analysis of the binding curves with human polymorphonuclear leukocytes by several laboratories indicates the existence of at least two classes of binding sites of differing affinities [13, 14, 17]. The high affinity receptor on human polymorphonuclear leukocytes is active at concentrations of <1 nM, in the concentration range where LTB4 produces cell aggregation. Chemokinetic and chemotactic responses occur at considerably higher LTB4 concentrations and may involve the lower affinity receptor. At least one antagonist of the LTB4 receptor, dimethylamide LTB4, has been reported [16], but a wider range of antagonists is needed.

The work of Goetzl and his colleagues has led to a partial characterization of the structure of the receptor for LTB4 in human leukocytes [18]. In broken cell preparations, the receptor is primarily in membrane-rich fractions, suggesting a plasma membrane localization. Cross-linking experiments indicate that the LTB4 binding protein has an apparent molecular weight of about 60 Kd in SDS polyacrylamide gels.

Studies of the mechanism of LTB4 action in human leukocytes suggest that LTB4 induces a rapid increase in Ca^{2+} uptake by cells and an initial decrease, followed by an increase in intracellular pH. Other evidence indicates that the receptor may interact with a GTP-dependent regulatory protein thought to be important in transducing extracellular stimuli to the cell interior [18]. F-MLP, which acts on leukocytes through a different receptor than LTB4, also enhances Ca^{2+} uptake in these cells, and both F-MLP and LTB4 produce an increase in Na influx during stimulation. These observations suggest a possible common activation mechanism.

Not much is known about the factors controlling the number of LTB4 receptors on cells or their possible variation in various disease states [12, 18]. LTB4 receptors can be induced in vitro when the immature leukocyte precursor cell lines such as HL60 and U937 are induced to differentiate. This induction parallels that of a number of other cell surface markers and receptors that increase during cell maturation. Because their protein synthesizing activity is limited, it is doubtful that mature polymorphonuclear leukocytes can upregulate LTB4 receptor levels by synthesizing new LTB4 receptors during stimulation but redistribution of pre-existing receptors is not excluded. Down regulation of high affinity receptors after extended incubation of leukocytes with high concentrations of LTB4 has been demonstrated.

Slow-Reacting Substances (LTC$_4$, LTD$_4$, LTE$_4$)

The biologic activity of slow-reacting substances (SRS) that has received most attention is its spasmogenic action on smooth muscle [2, 4]. Concentrations of LTD$_4$ as low as 0.1 pmole/ml produce easily detectable contractile responses on guinea pig ileal and tracheal smooth muscle preparations. In addition to its high potency, SRS produces an exceptionally sustained contractile response without tachyphylaxis, raising the possibility of an unusually prolonged action in vivo [19]. In the lung SRS interacts both central and peripheral airways and has long been suspected to be an important mediator in bronchial asthma. Slow-reacting substances are more selective in the spectrum of smooth muscle preparations they affect than the primary prostaglandins. LTC$_4$ and LTD$_4$ also have been reported to act at low concentrations on cutaneous blood vessels producing increases in vascular permeability and potentiating the action of other vasoactive agents [20], indicating that they could act as mediators in urticarial reactions as well.

Other biological actions of LTC$_4$ and LTD$_4$ [12] have also been demonstrated. These substances stimulate Purkinje nerve cell function [21], chemotaxis and granule enzyme release in leukocytes [4], and secretion of luteinizing hormone [22]. 5-LO products such as LTC$_4$ also have a possible role in cholesterol ester accumulation in macrophages, which may be of relevance for the development of atherosclerosis [23]. Cholesterol ester accumulation in cultured human macrophages is suppressed by lipyxygenase inhibitors such as nordihydroguaretic acid. Cholesterol-rich macrophages have a considerable increase in 12-plus 15-lipoxygenase activity with a small increase in 5-LO. LTC$_4$ effects on mucin production [24, 25] and ciliary action are also reported, suggesting additional effects in asthma other than airway muscle contraction per se.

There is increasing evidence for close collaborations between platelets, neutrophils, monocytes, lymphocytes, and endothelial cells during the early phases of inflammatory and immunologic responses. Through their effects on the production and action of other mediators, leukotrienes appear to play an important role in these interactions. Lipoxygenase products can affect the production of both platelet activating factor (PAF) and thromboxane A$_2$ (TxA$_2$). In human neutrophils stimulated with A-23187, the production of PAF was greatly augmented by 5-HETE, 5-HPETE, and LTB$_4$ [26]. LTC$_4$ and LTD$_4$ stimulate PGI$_2$ and PAF production and neutrophil binding in endothelial cells [27], reinforcing the effects of other pro-inflammatory agents such as IL-1. Another reported and potentially important action of LTC$_4$ in the vascular system is in the promotion of proliferation in glomerular epithelial cells [28]. Proliferative effects of LTC$_4$ on the vasculature have recently been confirmed in aortic endothelial cells, although the magnitude of the response is rather small. Whether or not leukotrienes regulate MHC antigen expression in endothelial cells as described for severe monokines and lymphokines [27] remains to be fully evaluated. This question is being investigated in our laboratory. Another question that requires careful study is the variation within the vascular system in mediator availability and responsiveness. In perfused lungs, leukotrienes also increase thromboxane formation [29]. Since PAF and TxA$_2$ are highly active autocoids, the potentiation of their formation by lipoxygenase products could markedly amplify the local tissue response. Like histamine and bradykinin LTC$_4$ and LTD$_4$ have little direct effect on neutrophil emigation into tissue. However, if a potent chemotactic stimulator such as C5a or F-met-leu-phe is present, these vasoactive stimulators can markedly potentiate the response [30]. Other mediators may also increase leukotriene production. Lipoxygenase products appear to serve as amplifiers of C5a-induced smooth muscle contraction in the isolated guinea pig trachea [31]. FPL-55712, a selective antagonist of SRS, almost completely inhibits the response to C5a. This indicates that the C5a-induced tracheal contraction is mediated by lipoxygenase products, most likely LTC$_4$ or LTD$_4$.

Thromboxane A$_2$ and the prostaglandin endoperoxides have received relatively little emphasis in recent years, in part because of their instability. However, evidence is emerging that platelets and vascular smooth muscle have specific distinct receptors for these biologically potent AA metabolites [32]. Hopefully, new information will soon be emerging on the mechanism of their effects on tissues and possible role in inflammation.

References

1. Rouzer, C. A., and B. Samuelsson. 1985. On the nature of the 5-lipoxygenase reaction in human leukocytes: Enzyme purification and requirement for multiple stimulatory factors. Proc. Natl. Acad. Sci. USA. 80: 4175.
2. Parker, C. W. 1982. The chemical nature of slow-reacting substances. In: Advances and inflammation research. G. Weissman, ed. New York: Raven Press, p. 1.
3. Dixon, R. A. F., R. E. Jones, R. E. Diehl, C. D. Bennett, S. Kargman, and C. A. Rouzer. 1988. Cloning of the cDNA for human 5-lipoxygenase. Proc. Natl. Acad. Sci. USA. 85: 416.
4. Parker, C. W. 1984. Mediators: Release and function. In: Fudamental immunology. W. E. Paul, ed. New York: Raven Press, p. 697.
5. Samuelsson, B. 1983. Leukotrienes: Mediators of immediate hypersensitivity reactions and inflammation. Science 220: 568.
6. Samuelsson, B. 1982. The leukotrienes: An introduction. Adv. Prost. Thromb. Leuk. Res. 9: 1.
7. Claesson, H.-E., and J. Haeggstrom. 1988. Human endothelial cell stimulate leukotriene synthesis and convert granulocyte released leukotriene A_4 into leukotrienes B_4, C_4, D_4, and E_4. Eur. J. Biochem. 173: 93.
8. Feinmark, S. J., and P. J. Cannon. 1986. Endothelial cell leukotriene C_4 synthesis results from intercellular transfer of leukotriene A_4 synthesized by polymorphonuclear leukocytes. J. Biol. Chem. 261: 16466.
9. Roubin, R., P. P. Elsas, W. Fiers, and A. J. Dessein. 1987. Recombinant human tomour necrosis factor (rTNF) enhances leukotriene biosyntehsis in neutrophils and eosinophils stimulated with Ca^{2+} ionophore A23187. Clin. exp. Immuno. 70: 484.
10. Reiner, N. E., and C. J. Malemund. 1985. Arachidonic acid metabolism by murine perioneal macrophages infected with *Leishmania donovani*: Evidence for parasite-induced alterations in cyclooxygenase and lipxygenase pathways. J. Immunol. 134: 556.
11. Fusco, A. C., B. Salafsky, and M. B. Kevin. 1985. Schistosoma mansoni: Eicosanoid production by cercyriae. Exp. Parasitol. 59: 44.
12. Parker, C. W. 1986. Lipid mediators and inflammation. In: New trends in Allergy II. J. Ring and G. Burg, eds. Berlin: Springer-Verlag, p, 78.
13. Goldman, D. W., and E. J. Goetzl. 1984. Heterogeneity of human polymorphonuclear leukocyte receptors for leukotriene B_4. J. Exp. Med. 159: 1027.
14. Kreisle, R., C. W. Parker, G. L. Griffin, R. M. Senior, and W. F. Stenson. 1985. Studies of leukotriene B_4-specific binding and function in rat

15. Kreisle, R., and C. W. Parker. 1983. Specific binding of leukotriene B_4 to a receptor on human polynorphonuclear leukocytes. J. Exp. Med. 157: 628.
16. Rokach, J., and B. J. Fitzsimmons. 1988. Lipoxygenase metabolites. Chemistry and Biochemistry. In: Cellular and molecular aspects of inflammation. G. Poste and S. T. Crooke, eds. New York: Plenum Press, p. 171.
17. Lin, A. H., P. L. Ruppel, and R. R. Gorman. 1984. Leukotriene B_4 binding to human neutrophils. Prostaglandins 28: 837.
18. Koo, C. H., L. Baud, J. W. Sherman, J. P. Harvey, D. W. Goldman, and E. J. Goetzl. 1988. Molecular properties of leukocyte receptors for leukotrienes. In G. Poste and S. T. Crooke, eds. Cellular and molecular aspects of inflammation. New York: Plenum Press, p. 305.
19. Kellaway, H. C., and E. R. Trethewie. 1940. The liberation of a slow-reacting smooth muscle-stimulating substance in anaphylaxis. Q. J. Exp. Physiol. 30: 122.
20. Drazen, J. M., K. F. Austen, R. A. LÖewis, D. A. Clark, G. Goto, A. Marfat, and E. J. Corey. 1980. Comparative airway and vascular activities of leukotrienes C-1 and D in vivo and in vitro. Proc. Natl. Acad. Sci. USA. 77: 4354.
21. Palmer, M. P., R. Mathews, R. C. Murphy, and B. Hoffer. 1980. Leukotriene C elicits a prolonged excitation of cerebellar Purkinje neurons. Neurosci. Ltt. 18: 173.
22. Hulting, A.-L., J. A. Lindgren, T. Hokfelt, P. Eneroth, S. Werner, C. Patrono, and B. Samulsson. 1985. Leukotriene C4 as a mediator of luteinizing hormone release from rat anterior pituitary cells. Proc. Natl. Acad. Sci. USA. 82: 3834.
23. Van der Schroeff, J. G., L. Havekes, A. M. Weerheim, J. J. Emeis, and B. J. Vermeis. 1985. Suppression of cholesteryl ester accumulation in cultured human monocyte-derived macrophages by lipoxygenase inhibitors. Biochem. Biophys. Res. Comm. 127: 366.
24. Marom, Z., J. H. Shelhamer, and M. Kaliner. 1981. Effects of arachidonic acid, monohydroxy-eicosatetraenoic acid and prostaglandins on the release of mucous glycoproteins from human airways in vitro. J. Clin. Invest. 67: 1695.
25. Richardson, P. S., A. C. Peatfield, D. M. Jackson, and P. J. Piper. 1982. The effect of leukotrienes on the output of mucins from the cat trachea. In: Leukotrienes and other lipxygenase products. P. J. Piper, ed. New York: Raven Press, p. 178.
26. Billah, M. M., R. W. Bryant, and M. I. Siegel. 1985. Lipoxygenase products of arachidonic acid modulate biosynthesis of platelet-activating factor. J. Biol. Chem. 260: 6899.

27. Harlan, J. M. 1985. Leukocyte-endothelial interactions. Blood. 65: 513.

28. Baud, L., J. Sraer, J. Perez, M.-P. Nivez, and R. Ardaillou. 1985. Leukotriene C4 binds to human glomerular epithelial cells and promotes their proliferation in vitro. J. Clin. Invest. 76: 374.

29. Engineer, D. M., H. R. Morris, P. J. Piper, and P. Sirois. 1978. The release of prostaglandins and thromboxanes from guinea-pig lung by slow reacting substance of anaphylaxis, and its inhibition. Br. J. Pharmacol. 64: 211.

30. Issekutz, A. C. 1981. Effect of vasoactive agents on polymorphonuclear leukocyte emigration in vivo. Lab. Invest. 45: 234.

31. Regal, J. F., and R. J. Pickering. 1981. C5a-induced tracheal contraction: Effect of an SRS-A antagonist and inhibitors of arachidonate metabolism. J. Immunol. 126: 313.

32. Halushka, P. V., D. E. Mais, and D. L. Saussy, Jr. 1988. Characterization of thromboxane A_2/prostaglandin H_2 receptors. In: Cellular and molecular aspects of inflammation. G. Poste and S. T. Crooke, eds. New York: Plenum Press, p. 355.

Leukotrienes and Other Lipoxygenase Metabolites: Mediators, Autocoids or Second Messengers?

Clemens A. Dahinden, Urs Wirthmüller, Urs Müller, Yoshiyuki Kurimoto, Alain L. de Weck*

The metabolism of arachidonic acid by the different lipoxygenases generates a large number of oxygenated products, including leukotrienes, potent lipid mediators. The physiological role of most metabolites remains to be determined, but there is some indirect evidence that lipid hydroperoxides (or derivatives) may have a role in signal transduction. On the other hand, lipid mediators do not have an obligatory autocoid role in signal transduction of neutrophils. No leukotrienes are formed after triggering with soluble peptide agonists alone. We found that preexposure of neutrophils with a cytokine, i.e., GM-CSF, is absolutely required for the induction of LTB4 and PAF synthesis by a soluble agonist, C5a, or fMLP. Lipid mediator synthesis occurs very rapidly after triggering with the second signal, and under identical conditions O_2-release is enhanced. IL-3, another hemopoietic growth factor, enhances granule release and, more profoundly, LTC4 synthesis in basophils stimulated by different agonists. Sequential stimulation with IL-3 and C5a results in the production of large quantities of LTC4, while neither factor alone induces the release of lipid mediators. We conclude that a major function of these cytokines is to allow lipid mediator synthesis in effector cells after triggering with agonists which are by themselves not stimulatory. We also propose that lipid mediators represent an autocrine amplification pathway in effector cells.

Lipid mediators are cell derived products with potent biological activities. In the recent years three novel classes of lipid mediators have been characterized and the biochemistry and biology of these compounds has been extensively reviewed [1]. Sulfidoleukotrienes (sLT), LTC4, LTD4, LTE4, formerly called SRS-A, which are produced mainly by mast cells, basophils, eosinophils, and monocytes, increase vascular permeability and induce smooth muscle contraction (i.e., bronchoconstriction), and participate in the vascular phase of inflammation. Leukotriene B4 (LTB4) and its metabolites, produced by neutrophils and monocytes, are potent chemotactic factors that participate in the cellular component of the inflammatory response. Platelet-activating factor (PAF) [2, 3] has even a broader range of activities and mediates both, the vascular and cellular component of inflammation. Figure 1 schematically presents the biosynthetic pathways for the synthesis of these factors. Note that the activation of a single enzyme, phospholipase A2 (PLA2), provides the precursor molecules for all the lipid mediators [4, 5]. The 5-lipoxygenase (5-LOX) generates LTA4, an unstable epoxide, which is converted to LTB4 or LTC4, depending on which enzyme is present in a certain effector cell type. There are two major differences between the cyclooxigenase and the LOX pathway. First, the activity of the 5-LOX depends on a high calcium concentration [6], and the LOX is therefore inactive in resting cells [7]. Thus, the generation of leukotrienes does not solely depend on the availability of free arachidonic acid, as with prostanoids. And the different precursor molecules in each step of the LT-synthesis pathway are also released in relatively large amounts and can be taken up by other cells to be further metabolized [8],which leads to generation of a large variety of hydroperoxides, HETEs, DiHETES (LTB4-isomers), Tri-HETEs, lipoxins and epoxides through the cellular interaction of different types of inflammatory effector cells. The biological function of most of these lipids is still unknown.

*   Institute of Clinical Immunology, Inselspital, CH-3010 Bern, Switzerland.
Supported by the Swiss National Science Foundation, Grant Nr. 3.278.085, 3.058.087.

33

Lipoxygenase Products as Second Messengers

Second messengers are intracellular chemicals necessary for signal transduction, linking occupation of a receptor to the cellular response. The role of G-protein-dependent activation of phospholipase C resulting in the generation of inositolphosphates and diacylglycerol has been well documented in many cells including inflammatory effector cells [9]. However, there are still arguments for the existence of yet undefined chemicals necessary for signal transduction. Lipoxygenase products may be such second messengers, because a) AA can directly activate cells, and b) nordihydroguaiaretic acid, an inhibitor of AA oxygenation, blocks agonist-induced responses in many cell types, including cells that are not able to produce leukotrienes [10, 11]. It is, therefore, possible that a lipid hydroperoxid or -derivative is necessary for signal transduction, though this hypothesis has not been proven. A reason for the very slow progress in this field lies in technical difficulties in detecting small amounts of these products, and in the large number of potential candidates for a second messenger. (see Figure 1).

Lipid Mediators as Autocoids

LTB4 is a potent chemotactic factor for neutrophils (PMN), but PMN triggered with calcium ionophore are also the major source of these mediators. In general, cells that are able to produce LTB4 and/or PAF also respond to these factors. A major role of the lipids may therefore be to attract more effector cells to an inflammatory site. Alternatively, LTB4 might also mediate as an autocoid the PMN response induced by other agonists like C5a or fMLP, in analogy to the function of interleukin 2 in T-helper cells. However, we—and others—did not find a neutrophil agonist capable of inducing LTB4 synthesis [7, 12]. Also, fMLP and C5a induces a transient increase in intracellular calcium concentration even in cells pretreated with LTB4, which are desensitized to a second response to same factor [unpublished data]. Finally LTB4 does not induce a respiratory burst comparable to C5a and fMLP. These findings argue against a necessary autocoid function of LTB4 in the PMN response to other agonists.

Effector Response-Modification by Cytokines

Neutrophils

PMN produce large amounts of LTB4 upon stimulation with Ca-ionophore. However, as pointed out above, soluble agonists do not induce the synthesis of appreciable amounts of lipid mediators. This intriguing observation, that PMN possess the machinery to produce leukotrienes, but do not release LTB4 upon receptor mediated activation, has been called the "leukotriene paradox" by G. Weissmann's group [12]. The solution to this problem came from our observation that PMN generate relatively large quantities of LOX-metabolites upon appropriately timed sequential stimulation with granulocyte-macrophage colony-stimulating factor (GM-CSF) and fMLP or C5a, while neither factor alone induces leukotriene synthesis [13]. Recent studies also showed that PAF synthesis by the phospholipase A2 diacylglycerollipase pathway is regulated in an identical manner [20]. These observations suggest that in GM-CSF-primed cells the signal transduction of PMN-agonists becomes coupled to the phospholipase A2 pathway, by a yet unknown mechanism. LTB4 and PAF produced under these conditions might be important in amplifying inflammatory reactions by attracting more leukocytes to an inflammatory site. The altered mediator profile of GM-CSF-primed PMN might even change the pathology of an inflammatory reaction.

Basophils

Basophils are important effector cells of hypersensitivity reactions and inflammation. Cross-linking of the IgE-receptors triggers the release of preformed mediators, histamine, and proteases, as well as the generation of lipid mediators, in particular leukotriene C4 (also called SRS-A) [14]. The anaphylatoxin C5a is a potent IgE-independent agonist of basophil degranulation, but is unable to stimulate the release of newly formed lipid mediators. Interleukin 3, a product of antigen-activated T-cells, is a pluripotent growth factor for leukocyte precursors [15]. We now demonstrate that IL-3 strongly affects the function of mature basophils [21]. IL-3 alone does not directly induce basophil mediator release, but primes these cells to release larger amounts of histamine and even more profoundly LTC4 after challenge with different IgE-dependent and -independent agonists. Most interestingly, basophils sequentially exposed to IL-3 and C5a produce very large quantities of LTC4, while neither factor alone triggers the generation of lipid mediators (Figure 2). This establishes a novel function of IL-3 and shows that basophil releasability and, more importantly, even the mediator profile can be modulated by a cytokine. We propose that a major function of hematopoietic growth factors is to allow lipid media-

Figure 1. Lipid mediators.

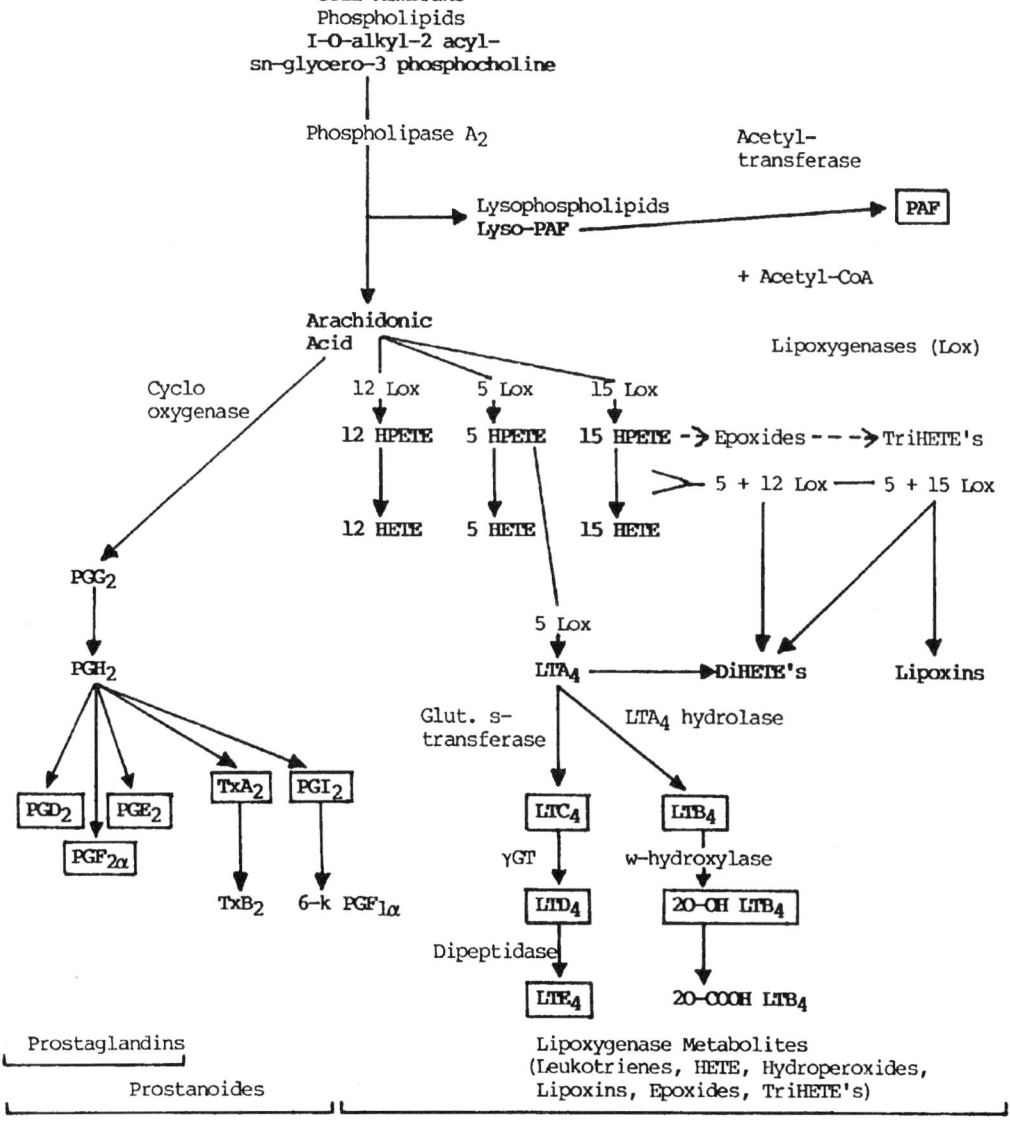

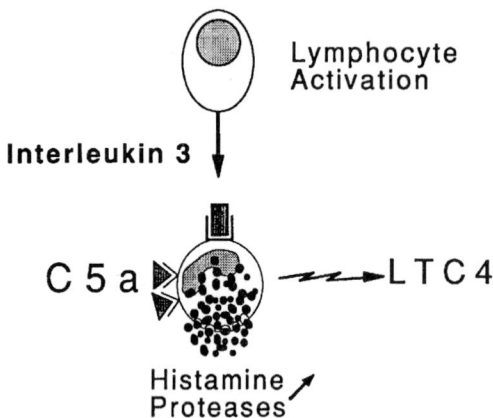

Figure 2. Interaction between specific immune system and basophil effector function.

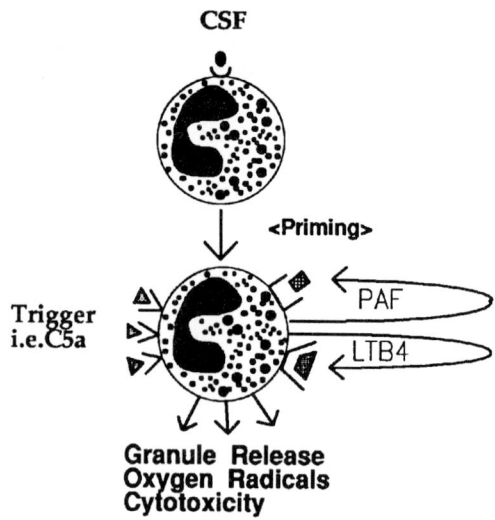

Figure 3. Lipid mediators as autocrine response amplifiers.

tor synthesis upon activation with agonists, which by themselves are not stimulatory. Our data demonstrate that a product of the specific immune system strongly affects the effector response of allergic reactions and inflammation. Such phenomena might also explain how (non-specific) cofactors, like viral infections, can precipitate symptoms of IgE-dependent and -independent hypersensitivity reactions.

The Concept of Autocrine Response Amplification by Lipid Mediators

As pointed out above, LTB4 and PAF are generally produced by the same cell types that also respond to these factors. Furthermore, PAF tends to remain cell-associated, particularly in PMN. Although these lipids do not seem to be necessary for signal transduction, they might represent an autocrine response amplification loop and be responsible for the known enhancement of effector cell function (superoxide production, granule release, cytotoxicity) induced by certain cytokines [16, 17]. Indeed, lipid mediators are formed very rapidly after triggering with a second signal, at the same time superoxide is produced. Also, low levels of PAF, LTB4(18) and 5-HETE [19], at concentrations that do not directly stimulate cell functions, enhance the response to an agonist, even when these lipids are added shortly before or simultaneously with the triggering agent.

In conclusion, we propose that lipid mediators formed by effector cells preexposed to

cytokines are not only important in the pathogenesis of inflammatory reactions, but may even change the function of the effector cell producing it (Figure 3).

References

1. Lewis, R. A., and K. F. Austen. 1984. The biologically active leukotrienes. Biosynthesis, metabolism, receptors, functions, and pharmacology. J. Clin. Invest. 73: 889–897.
2. Demopoulos, C. A., R. N. Pinckard, and D. J. Hanahan. 1979. Platelet-activating factor. Evidence for 1-O-alkyl-2-acetyl-*sn*-glyceryl-3-phosphorylcholine as the active component. J. Biol. Chem. 254: 9355–9358.
3. Benveniste, J., M. Tence, P. Varenne, J. Bidault, C. Boullet, and J. Polonski. 1979. Semi-synthesis and proposed structure of platelet-activating factor (PAF): PAF-acether, an alkyl ether analog of lysphosphatidylcholine. C. R. Seances Acad. Sci. 289:1037–1040.
4. Chilton, F. H., J. M. Ellis, S. C. Olson, and R. L. Wylke. 1984. 1-O-Alkyl-2-arachidonoyl-*sn*-glycero-3-phosphocholine: A common source of platelet-activating factor and arachidonate in human polymorphonuclear leukocytes. J. Biol. Chem. 259: 12014–12019.
5. Snyder, F., T.-C. Lee, and R. L. Wylke. 1985. Ether-linked glycero-lipids and their bioactive species: enzymes and metabolic regulation. In The Enzymes of Biological Membranes, Vol. 2. A. N. Maronosi, ed. New York: Plenum Press, pp. 1–58.

6. Rouzer, C. A., T. Matsumoto, and B. Samuelsson. 1986. Single protein from human leukocytes possesses 5-lipoxygenase and leukotriene A4 synthase activities. Proc. Natl. Acad. Sci. USA. 80: 857.

7. Clancy, R. M., C. A. Dahinden, and T. E. Hugli. 1983. Arachidonate metabolism by human polymorphonuclear leukocytes stimulated by N-formyl-Met-Leu-Phe or complement component C5a is independent of phospholipase activation. Proc. Natl. Acad. Sci. USA. 80:7200–7204.

8. Dahinden, C. A., R. M. Clancy, M. Gross, J. M. Chiller, and T.E. Hugli. 1985. Leukotriene C4 production by murine mast cells: Evidence of a role for extracellular leukotriene A4. Proc. Natl. Acad. Sci. USA. 82:6632–6636.

9. Smith, C. D., B. C. Lane, I. Kusaka, M. W. Verghese, and R. Snyderman. 1985. Chemoattractant receptor-induced hydrolysis of phosphatidylinositol 4,5-bisphosphate in human polymorphonuclear leukocyte membranes: Requirement for a guanine nucleotide regulatory protein. J. Biol. Chem. 260: 5875–5878.

10. Metz, S., M. v. Rollins, R. Strife, W. Fujimoto, R. P. Robertson. 1983. Lipoxygenase pathway in islet endocrine cells: Oxidative metabolism of arachidonic acid promotes insulin release. J. Clin. Invest. 72: 1191–1205.

11. Sasakawa N., S. Yamamoto, and R. Kato. 1984. Effects of inhibitors of arachidonic acid metabolism on calcium uptake and catecholamine release in cultured adrenal chromaffin cells. Biochem. Pharmacol. 33: 2733–2738.

12. Haines K. A., K. N. Giedd, A. M. Rich, H. M. Korchak, and G. Weissmann. 1987. The leukotriene B4 paradox: Neutrophils can, but will not, respond to ligand-receptor interactions by forming leukotriene B4 or its omega-metabolites. Biochem J. 241: 55.

13. Dahinden, C. A., J. Zingg, F. E. Maly, and A. L. de Weck. 1988. Leukotriene production in human neutrophils primed by recombinant human granulocyte-macrophage colony-stimulating factor and stimulated with the complement component C5a and FMLP as second signals. J. Exp. Med. 167: 1281–1295.

14. Grant, J. A., M. A. Lett-Brown, J. A. Warner, M. Plaut, L. M. Lichtenstein, M. Hask-Frendscho, and A. P. Kaplan. 1986. Activation of basophils. Fed. Proc. 45: 2653.

15. Interleukin 3: The panspecific hemopoietin. 1988. In: Lymphokines, Vol. 15. J. W. Schrader, ed. Orlando, FL: Academic Press.

16. Weisbart, R. H., D. W. Golde, S. C. Clark, G. G. Wong, and J. C. Gasson. 1985. Human granulocyte-macrophage colony-stimulating factor is a neutrophil activator. Nature. 314: 361–373.

17. Lopez, A. F., D. J. Williamson, J. R. Gamble, C. G. Begley, J. M. Harlan, S. J. Klebanoff, A. Waltersdorpf, G. Wong, S. C. Clark, and M. A. Vadas. 1986. Recombinant human granulocyte-macrophage colony-stimulating factor stimulates in vitro mature human neutrophil and eosinophil function, surface receptor expression, and survival. J. Clin. Invest. 78: 1220–1228.

18. Dewald, B., and M. Baggiolini. 1985. Activation of NADPH oxidase in human neutrophils. Synergism between FMLP and the neutrophil products PAF and LTB4. Biochem. Biophys. Res. Commun. 128: 297–304.

19. O'Flaherty, J.T. 1985. Neutrophil degranulation: Evidence pertaining to its mediation by the combined effect of leukotriene B4, platelet-activating factor, and 5-HETE. J. Cell. Physiol. 122: 229–239.

20. Wirthmüller U., A. L. de Weck, and C. A. Dahinden. 1988. PAF production in human neutrophils by sequential stimulation with granulocyte-macrophage colony-stimulating factor and the chemotactic factors C5a or fMLP. Submitted.

21. Kurimoto Y., A. L. de Weck, and C. A. Dahinden. 1988. Human interleukin 3 is a basophil response modifier. Submitted.

Eosinophil and Neutrophil Chemotactic Factors in Allergy and Asthma

*A. B. Kay**

During the past few years there have been a number of advances in our knowledge of the scope and nature of allergy- and asthma-associated eosinophil and neutrophil chemotactic factors, the most potent factors described so far being PAF. In this study, C5a and LTB4 proved to be somewhat less active compared with PAF. T-cell products including IL-5 and other recombinant cytokines had negligible activity. On the other hand, T-cells produce appreciable neutrophil chemotactic activity. Of particular interest is a 10 kD NCA from allergen-stimulated T-cell lines and clones as well as a slightly higher (approx. 20 kD) NCA released spontaneously from cultured blood mononuclear cells from severe asthmatics. The relationship of these to the 600 kD HMW-NCA detected in the serum during provoked asthma is at present unclear.

Eosinophil Chemotactic Factors

Eosinophils are associated with a wide variety of disease states including bronchial asthma, atopic allergy, infection with helminthic parasites, and a number of malignant disorders. However, it is still unclear as to which mediators are responsible for attracting and localizing eosinophils to the site of allergic inflammation and other eosinophil- associated pathological reactions. A number of agents are known to have weak eosinophil chemotactic properties. These include mast cell-derived products such as histamine [1], histamine catabolites [2] and the acidic tetrapeptides (Val-Gly-Ser-Glu and Ala-Gly-Ser-Glu) [3], which represents a very small part of the activity originally termed "eosinophil chemotactic factor of anaphylaxis (ECF-A)" [4]. Leukotriene B4 activates granulocytes, particularly neutrophils, and has some eosinophil chemotactic activity [5] and is released from antigen-challenged sensitized lung fragments [6]. Platelet activating factor (PAF) was shown to be the most potent chemically characterized eosinophil chemotactic factor so far described, being much more effective than LTB4, histamine, and ECF-A tetrapeptide [7]. Several lymphocyte-derived factors have also been shown to influence eosinophil locomotion. These include eosinophil chemotactic factor precursor substance [8], eosinophil stimulation promotor [9], specific eosinophil chemotactic factor [10], delayed eosinophil chemotactic factor (a and b) and eosinophil chemotactic inhibitory factor [11]. However, their biological significance is unclear, and they are, for the large part, chemically uncharacterized. Nevertheless, there is clearly an important biological relationship between eosinophils and lymphocytes, and in rodents eosinophilopoiesis is under T-cell control.

Recently, a novel lymphokine (eosinophil differentiating factor or IL-5) was shown to induce the production and differentiation of eosinophils from bone marrow cultures in mouse [12]. In addition, IL-5 was also able to enhance a number of biological functions of mature murine [12] and human eosinophils [13]. Very recently, murine IL-5 was shown to be modestly chemotactic for mouse peritoneal eosinophils [14]. Thus, IL-5 plays a role at several stages in eosinophil development, both from maturation, to activation of the fully differentiated cells. Whether this or other lymphokines play a role in preferentially attracting eosinophils to the site of inflammation has not yet been determined.

In a recent study we tested a wide range of T-cell-associated products for eosinophil chemotactic activity (ECA) and compared our findings with the documented granulocyte chemoattractants PAF, C5a, C5a des Arg, LTB4, and N-formyl-methionyl-leucyl-phenylalanine (fMLP) [15]. We have compared the relative potency of a wide range of mediators including

* Department of Allergy and Clinical Immunology, National Heart & Lung Institute, Dovehouse Street, London, SW3 6LY, United Kingdom.

PAF, C5a, C5a des Arg, LTB4, fMLP, recombinant interleukin (IL)-1, IL-2, tumour necrosis factor (TNF), interferon-γ, and granulocyte/macrophage-colony stimulating factor (GM-CSF), and a purified mononuclear-cell-derived chemotactic factor (M-CF) for their ability to promote eosinophil locomotion in vitro. To obtain M-CF, peripheral mononuclear cells were cultured for 48 hours, with 5 µg/ml phytohaemagglutinin (PHA), the supernatant concentrated 150-fold and the 10 kD activity isolated by gel filtration using FPLC (Superose 12 prep grade). M-CF had substantial neutrophil chemotactic activity, but eosinophils were relatively unresponsive. Maximal activity (cells/10 high power field) of the various chemotactic factors at their optimal concentrations (i.e., concentrations above these values giving high dose inhibition) were as follows: PAF (10^{-6} M) 725 ± 307; C5a (10^{-8} M) 352 ± 204; C5a des Arg (10^{-7} M) 243 ± 127; LTB4 (10^{-7} M) 37 ± 25; fMLP (10^{-7} M) 14 ± 14; M-CF (10^{-6} M) 28 ± 10; diluent 10 ± 7. IL-1-β (5–80 U/ml), IL-2 (1–1000 U/ml), interferon-γ (1–1000 U/ml), TNF (1–1000 U/ml), and GM-CSF (20–4000 pg/ml) gave eosinophil chemotactic counts of less than 11. Thus, among chemically characterized mediators PAF appears to be the most potent eosinophil chemotactic factor so far described.

Culture supernatants obtained from human peripheral blood mononuclear cells, stimulated with the T-cell mitogens PHA or concanavalin A (ConA) had substantial neutrophil chemotactic activity (NCA) but negligible ECA. Following gel filtration on Superose 12, the NCA of PHA supernatants eluted as a single peak together with proteins of a molecular size of 10 kD (M-NCF). This partially purified material also had trivial ECA. Similarly, supernatants from allergen-specific T-cells lines also lacked ECA but had considerable NCA. None of the recombinant cytokines studies (which included interleukin (IL)-1, IL-2, IL-5, interferon-γ, GM-CSF, and TNF) had appreciable ECA even when tested over a large dose range. The rank order of these substances in terms of neutrophil chemotaxis at optimal concentrations was PAF (10^{-6} M) > C5a (10^{-8} M) > C5a des Arg (10^{-7} M) = LTB4 (10^{-7} M) = M-NCF (11 µg protein/ml) = fMLP (10^{-7} M). PAF was a potent eosinophil chemotactic factor and was equally potent in eliciting eosinophil and neutrophil locomotion. The ECA of C5a and C5a des Arg were less than PAF. LTB4, M-CSF, and fMLP had negligible ECA. Thus, in our opinion, PAF remains the most potent eosinophilotactic agent so far characterized.

There are a number of selective PAF antagonists. Of particular interest is a family of terpenes isolated from the Chinese tree *Ginkgo biloba*, termed ginkgolides A, B, C, M, and J (BN 52020, BN 52021, BN 52022, BN 52023, and BN 52024, respectively) (reviewed in [16]). BN 52021 is the most efficient antagonist of PAF binding to washed rabbit and human platelets (IC50 approximately 10^{-7} M [17, 18] and is also effective in inhibiting PAF-induced aggregation of human and rabbit platelets [18, 19]. In a recent study, we studied the capacity of BN 52021 to inhibit PAF-induced chemotaxis of eosinophils and neutrophils [20]. We also compared BN 52021 with a number of anti-asthma agents including sodium cromoglycate, nedocromil sodium, salbutamol, and a corticosteroid (dexamethasone).

In response to an optimal concentration of PAF (10^{-6}) M) the drug was significantly more potent (p<0.001) in inhibiting eosinophil as compared to neutrophil locomotion. These inhibitory effects were observed in a dose-dependent manner, with an IC50 of 7.0 ($\pm$ 2.2) $\times 10^{-6}$ M and 2.3 ($\pm$ 0.2) $\times 10^{-5}$ M, for eosinophils and neutrophils, respectively. Sodium cromoglycate, nedocromil sodium, salbutamol and dexamethasone (preincubated with cells up to 6 hours) had no effect over a wide dose range (10^{-3} to 10^{-9} M). BN 52021 was significantly more effective in inhibiting chemotaxis when the cells were preincubated with the compound for up to 1 h before commencement of the locomotion assay, whereas washing the cells completely abolished this effect. Inhibition by BN 52021 was specific for PAF, in that it had no effect on chemotaxis induced by either LTB4, fMLP, or a purified human mononuclear cell-derived neutrophil chemotactic factor. BN 52021 also inhibited the specific binding of [^{3}H]-PAF (10^{-8} M) to eosinophils and neutrophils, in a concentration-dependent fashion, with an IC50 of 1.5 ($\pm$ 0.3) $\times 10^{-6}$ M and 9.1 ($\pm$ 2.5) $\times 10^{-7}$ M, respectively. These results suggest than BN 52021 has potential as an anti-inflammatory agent in conditions associated with PAF-induced accumulation of neutrophils and eosinophils.

Neutrophil Chemotactic Factors

There are a very large number of neutrophil chemotactic factors associated with allergy and asthma. In vivo IgE-dependent release of PAF and LTB4 can readily be demonstrable. Whether the source of these lipid mediators is predominantly from high-affinity IgE receptor bearing cells, i.e., basophils and mast cells, or those with $Fc_\varepsilon R_{II}$, i.e., macrophages, eosinophils, and possibly platelets, is still unclear. On the other hand, in vivo, i.e., clinical situations associated with allergy and asthma, the NCA most fully documented is the high molecular weight neutrophil chemotactic activity (HMW-NCA) observed in the serum during provoked models of asthma and in the acute severe form of the disease ("status asthmaticus"). We now have evidence that the apparent high molecular weight may be partly explained by the heating process, since samples require heating at 56°C for 30 minutes to distinguish them from heat-labile activity found in normal serum.

Furthermore, and most importantly, it seems likely that NCA observed in the serum in early- and late-phase and on-going asthma could be mononuclear cell-derived. However, most of the mononuclear cell-derived NCA is of low molecular weight, i.e., 10 kD. Our preliminary results are compatible with the hypothesis that HMW-NCA may be derived from the 10 kD material as an artefact of heating although this is not yet fully established.

The release of low molecular weight (10 kD) NCA from human PBMC stimulated with lipopolysaccharide [21] from human alveolar macrophages stimulated with aggregated human IgG or zymosan particles [22] and from adherent blood mononuclear cells in the absence of serum [23] has been reported. The cellular source of this activity has been controversial with both monocytes [21] and T lymphocytes [22] being suggested as the cell of origin. In a recent study using antigen specific T lymphocyte clones we confirmed that T-cells can release a neutrophil chemotactic factor of similar molecular weight (10 kD) [25]. Following direct stimulation of the T-cell antigen receptor by anti-CD3 antibody or specific antigen in association with MHC class II gene products NCA can be detected in serum-free culture supernatants. The ability of unfractionated PBMC to release NCA following stimulation with anti-CD3 suggests this is a general prop-

erty of T-cells and not unique to the clones analyzed here. Thus, our results conform the cellular nature of an apparently identical NCF of 10 kD form partially purified T-cells stimulated with mitogens which has been recently isolated and sequenced [23]. The smaller peaks of NCA derived from the T-cells and chromatographing in the fractions 51–54 from the Superose-12 column may be TNF, which shows, by gel filtration, an apparent MW of 45 kD [26].

Lymphokine generation has been reported following antigen stimulation of peripheral blood mononuclear cells (PBMC) form sensitized donors [27]. However, with the aeroallergens of D. farinae or grass pollen we observed only negligible production of NCA from PBMC of atopic individuals. This may reflect the paucity of sensitized T lymphocytes in the peripheral blood, since it has been reported that in individuals with house dust mite allergy only a small proportion (0.02%) of circulating lymphocytes are reactive with the specific mite allergen [28].

The generation of this NCF in vitro by antigen-specific T lymphocytes raises the possibility that it could be involved in the inflammatory events associated with allergic and infectious diseases, particularly allergen-induced asthma. The immediate events of atopic asthma may be attributable to acute mediator release via specific IgE mechanisms—in vitro house dust mite-specific cloned T lymphocytes can support specific antigen-dependent IgE synthesis from autologous B cells [29]. The sustained asthmatic response could in part be due to events triggered by the subsequent NCA release from the T-cells since an NCA was identified in the serum of asthmatic individuals during allergen-induced late-phase asthmatic reactions [30]. The asthma-associated serum NCA has recently been found to be heterogeneous in terms of size and molecular weight, and in some instances (e.g., acute severe asthma) a low MW (< 20 kD) peak of NCA was observed [31].

Very recently we studied peripheral blood mononuclear cells isolated from patients with acute severe asthma (ASA, "status asthmaticus"), for their ability to generate NCA spontaneously in culture [32]. PBMC were isolated from 14 patients on admission to hospital as an emergency with ASA, and in some cases 7 days later. PBMC were similarly isolated from control subjects (normals, mild asthma, chronic obstructive airways disease). PBMc from ASA patients elaborated significantly greater amounts of NCA into the culture supernatants after 24 h as compared with all control groups. In all ASA patients a reduction was observed in the amount of this PBMC-derived NCA after 1 week of therapy. Supernatants from ASA and normal controls were pooled, concentrated by freeze drying, and subjected to Superose-12 size fractionation and Mono P chromatofocusing using FPLC. A peak of NCA corresponding to a molecular size of 16–25 kD and pI of 6.8 was detectable in the concentrated ASA supernatants but completely absent from the control supernatants. Thus, the molecular size of NCA from cultured PBMC from asthma patients appears to be somewhat higher than the 10 kD material from antigen- or lectin-stimulated lymphocytes and monocytes. The relationship between all of these NCAs is at present unclear and must await the results of sequencing data currently in progress.

References

1. Clark, R. A. F., J. I. Gallin, and A. P. Kaplan. 1975. The selective eosinophil chemotactic activity of histamine. J. Exp. Med. 142: 1462.
2. Turnbull, L. W., and A. B. Kay. 1976. Eosinophils and mediators of anaphylaxis. Histamine and imidazole acetic acid as chemotactic agents for human eosinophil leucocytes. Immunology 31: 797.
3. Goetzl, E. J., and K. F. Austen. 1975. Purification and synthesis of eosinophilotactic tetrapeptides of human lung tissue: Identification as eosinophil chemotactic factor of anaphylaxis. Proc. Natl. Acad. Sci. USA 72: 4112.
4. Kay, A. B., and K. F. Austen. 1971. The IgE-mediated release of an eosinophil leukocyte chemotactic factor from human lung. J. Immunol. 107: 899.
5. Nagy, L., T. H. Lee, E. J. Goetzl, W. C. Pickett, and A. B. Kay. 1982. Complement receptor enhancement and chemotaxis of human neutrophils and eosinophils by leukotrienes and other lipoxygenase products. Clin. Exp. Immunol. 47: 541.
6. Salari, H., P. Borgeat, M. Fournier, J. Herbert, and G. Pelletier. 1985. Studies on the release of leukotrienes and histamine by human lung parenchymal and bronchial fragments upon immunologic and nonimmunologic stimulation. J. Exp. Med. 162: 1904.
7. Wardlaw, A. J., R. Moqbel, O. Cromwell, and A. B. Kay. 1986. Platelet-activating factor. A potent

chemotactic and chemokinetic factor for human eosinophils. J. Clin. Invest. 78: 1701.
8. Cohen, S., and P. A. Ward. 1971. In vitro and in vivo activity of a lymphocyte and immune complex-dependent chemotactic factor for eosinophils. J. Exp. Med. 133: 133.
9. Colley, G. 1973. Eosinophils and immune mechanisms: I. Eosinophil stimulation promotor (ESP): A lymphokine induced by specific antigen or phytohaemagglutinin. J. Immunol. 110: 1419.
10. Wadee, A. A., and R. Sher. 1980. The effect of a soluble factor released by sensitized mononuclear cells incubated with S. haematobium ova on eosinophil migration. Immunology 41: 989.
11. Tashiro, K., K. Sakata, M. Hirashima, and H. Hayashi. 1987. The regulation of tissue eosinophilia V. Induction of lymphocyte-derived eosinophil chemotactic inhibitory factor production by a macrophage product from complete adjuvant treated guinea pigs. Cell. Immunol. 104: 1.
12. Sanderson, C. J., D. J. Warren, and M. Strath. 1985. Identification of a lymphokine that stimulates eosinophil differentiation in vitro. Its relationship to interleukin-3 and functional properties of eosinophils produced in cultures. J. Exp. Med. 162: 60.
13. Lopez, A. F., C. J. Sanderson, J. R. Gamble, H. D. Campbell, I. G. Yough, and M. A. Vadas. 1988. Recombinant human interleukin 5 is a selective activator of human eosinophil function. J. Exp. Med. 167: 219.
14. Yamaguchi, Y., Y. Hayashi, Y. Sugama, Y. Miura, T. Kasahara, S. Kitamura, M. Torisu, S. Mita, A. Tominaga, K. Takatsu, and T. Suda. 1988. Highly purified murine interleukin 5 (IL-5) stimulates eosinophil function and prolongs in vitro survival. J. Exp. Med. 167: 1737.
15. Kurihara, K., A. J. Wardlaw, P. Maestrelli, J.-J. Tsai, and A. B. Kay. 1988. IL-1, IL-2, TNF, INF-γ, GM-CSF and PHA-stimulated leukocyte supernatants have negligible eosinophil chemotactic activity compared with platelet activating factor (PAF). FASEB J. 2: A1449.
16. Braquet, P. 1987. The ginkgolides: Potent platelet-activating factor angatonists isolated from Ginkgo biloba L.: Chemistry, pharmacology and clinical applications. Drugs of the Future 12: 643.
17. Korth, R., and J. Benveniste. 1987. BN 52021 displaces [^{3}H] PAF-acether from, and inhibits it binding to intact human platelets. Eur. J. Pharmacol. 142: 331.
18. Braquet, P., B. Spinnewyn, M. Braquet, R. H. Bourgain, A. Taylor Etienne, and K. Drieu. 1985. BN 52021 and related compounds: A new series of highly specific PAF-acether receptor antagonists isolated from Ginkgo biloba. Blood & Vessels 16: 558.

19. Nunez, D., M. Chignard, R. Korth, J. P. Le Couedic, X. Norel, B. Spinnewyn, P. Braquet, and J. Benveniste. 1986. Specific inhibition of PAF-acether-induced platelet activation by BN 52021 and comparison with the PAF-acether inhibitors Kadzurenone and CV3988. Eur. J. Pharmacol. 123: 197.

20. Kurihara, K., A. J. Wardlaw, R. Moqbel, and A. B. Kay. 1989. Inhibition of platelet activating factor (PAF)-induced chemotaxis, and PAF binding to human eosinophils and neutrophils by the specific gingkolide-derived PAF antagonist, BN 52021. J. Allergy Clin. Immunol., in press.

21. Yoshimura, T., K. Matsushima, J. J. Oppenheim, and E. J. Leonard. 1987. Neutrophil chemotactic factor produced by lipopolysaccharide (LPS)-stimulated human blood mononuclear leukocytes: Partial characterisation and separation from interleukin 1 (IL-1). J. Immunol. 139: 788.

22. Snyderman, R., L. Meadows, and D. M. Amos. 1977. Characterization of human chemotactic lymphokine production induced by mitogens and mixed leukocyte reactions using a new microassay. Cell. Immunol. 30: 225.

23. Kownatzki, A., A. Kapp, and S. Uhrich. 1986. Novel neutrophil chemotactic factor derived from human peripheral blood mononuclear leucocytes. Clin. Exp. Immunol. 64: 214.

24. Gregory, H., J. Young, J.-M. Schröder, U. Mrowietz, and E. Christophers. 1988. Structure determination of a human lymphocyte derived neutrophil activating peptide (LYNAP). Biochem. Biophys. Res. Comm. 151: 883.

25. Maestrelli, P., R. E. O'Hehir, J. R. Lamb, J.-J. Tsai, O. Cromwell, and A. B. Kay. 1988. Antigen-induced neutrophil chemotactic factor from cloned human T lymphocytes. Immunology, in press.

26. Aggarwal, B. B., W. J. Kohr, B. M. Hass, B. Moffat, C. A. Spencer, W. J. Henzel, T. S. Bringman, G. E. Nedwin, D. V. Goeddel, and R. N. Harkins. 1985. Human tumor necrosis factor. Production, purification, and characterization. J. Biol. Chem. 260: 2345.

27. Potter, J. W., and D. E. Van Epps. 1986. Human T-lymphocyte chemotactic activity: Nature and production in response to antigen. Cell. Immunol. 97: 59.

28. Halvorsen, R., and B. Bosnes. 1986. T cell responses to a *Dermatophagoides farinae* allergen preparation in allergics and healthy controls. Int. Arch. Allergy Appl. Immun. 80: 62.

29. O'Hehir, R. E., V. Bal, D. Quint, R. Moqbel, A. B. Kay, E. Zanders, and J. R. Lamb. 1988. IgE induction by human cloned T lymphocytes specific for house dust mite is IL-4 dependent. FASEB J. 2: A1442.

30. Nagy, L., T. H. Lee, and A. B. Kay. 1982. Neutrophil chemotactic activity in antigen-induced late asthmatic reactions. New Engl. J. Med. 306: 497.

31. Buchanan, D. R., O. Cromwell, and A. B. Kay. 1987. Neutrophil chemotactic activity in acute severe asthma ("status asthmaticus"). Am. Rev. Respir. Dis. 136: 1397.

32. Nagy, L., C. J. Corrigan, J.-J. Tsai, and A. B. Kay. 1989. Cultured peripheral blood mononuclear cells from patients with acute severe asthma elaborate a neutrophil chemotactic activity spontaneously. Clin. Exp. Allergy 19, in press.

Effects of Mediators on Leukocytes

*Marco Baggiolini**

Neutrophil leukocytes are chiefly involved in host defence against microorganisms. They are activated by chemotactic agonists which induce shape change and migration, enzyme release, and the respiratory burst. The mechanism of neutrophil activation by receptor agonists is described.

The main role of neutrophil leukocytes is the defence of the host organism against microbial invasion. To this end, these cells are capable of sensing chemotactic signals generated upon infection and of migrating out of microvessels into the infected tissues. Infectious microbes are usually phagocytosed and killed. Upon chemotactic and phagocatic activation, the neutrophils generate superoxide and H_2O_2 as well as a variety of bioactive lipids, and release enzymes and other storage proteins. Some of these products are required for the killing [1, 2], and some induce inflammation and tissue damage—typical consequences of neutrophil activation [3].

Like other white cells, the neutrophils circulate passively in the blood. They are called into play by chemotactic stimuli which promote their margination, adhesion and diapedesis. Five chemotactic agonists, acting via distinct receptors, have been characterized in recent years. They are the anaphylatoxin C5a formed upon complement activation via the classical or the alternative pathway [4], N-formyl-Met-Leu-Phe (fMLP) and other N-formylmethionyl peptides of bacterial origin [5], two bioactive lipids, platelet-activating factor (PAF) and leukotriene B4 (LTB4) [6, 7, 8], and a 72-amino acid peptide produced by human monocytes which was identified most recently [9]. Three major functional responses are characteristic for the response of neutrophils to all five chemotactic stimuli described, i.e., shape changes, the exocytosis of granule contents, and the respiratory burst. All three responses can be assessed in real time and can thus be used to evaluate the mechanism of signal transduction and response generation. Under physiological conditions, chemotactic stimulation leads in addition to a rapid, transient rise of the cytosolic-free calcium concentration ($[Ca^{2+}]_i$), which can also be monitored in real time. This situation makes the neutrophil a unique model for the study of white cell activation.

Neutrophil Activation

The mechanism of neutrophil activation by receptor-mediated signals is largely unknown. Two events are believed to be essential for eliciting a response: a transient enhancement of $[Ca^{2+}]_i$ and activation of protein kinase C. The role of $[Ca^{2+}]_i$ changes is suggested by the inability of calcium-depleted neutrophils—which cannot raise $[Ca^{2+}]_i$ unless extracellular calcium is supplied—to respond with exocytosis and a respiratory burst to stimulation with receptor agonists [10]. Protein kinase C appars to be involved since phorbol esters and permeant diacylglycerols elicit the respiratory burst [11]. Receptor-mediated neutrophil responses are prevented by pretreatment of the cells with *B. pertussis* toxin, showing that functional GTP-binding proteins are necessary [12]. Studies on the activation of the respiratory burst have shown in addition that continuous receptor occupancy by an agonist is a prerequisite to maintaining NADPH-oxidase activity [13].

From these observations, the minimum sequence of events leading to the activation of the respiratory burst is the following:

The process begins with the binding of the agonist to its receptor. This induces the interaction between the ligand-receptor complex and a GTP-binding protein with consequent activation of a phosphatidylinositol-specific phospholipase C [14]. The latter enzyme delivers inositoltrisphosphate (IP3) into the cytosol and diacylglycerol, which remains in the membrane. IP3 liberates calcium from intracellular stores raising $[Ca^{2+}]_i$. Together, diacylglycerol and Ca^{2+} induce the translocation of protein kinase C to the plasma membrane and its subsequent activation [15, 16].

---

*   Theodor-Kocher Institute, University of Bern, P. O. Box 99, CH-3000 Bern 9.

Our approach to the study of the mechanism of human neutrophil activation was based on real-time measurements of $[Ca^{2+}]_i$ changes and the release of respiratory burst H_2O_2.

$[Ca^{2+}]_i$ was measured in quin-2 or fura-2-loaded cells placed in the stirred cuvette of a specially constructed broad-band filter fluorimeter with a response time of 30 ms [17]. The cells were stimulated with the chemotactic agonist fMLP or the calcium ionophore ionomycin. Both stimuli led to a rise in $[Ca^{2+}]_i$, but the initial kinetics were different: The rise induced by ionomycin was immediate, while that induced by fMLP occurred after a distinct lag of at least 0.8 s, which increased markedly with decreasing agonist concentration. These results suggested that calcium release fro internal stores and calcium influx across the plasma membrane are regulated by a rate-limiting process [17]. Since calcium liberation is considered to depend on IP_3, the lag could reflect the time required for the generation of threshold levels of this second messenger.

The onset time of the respiratory burst (i.e., the time elapsing between stimulation and the beginning of product formation) can be used to assess the duration of the signal transduction process, provided assay method is sufficiently sensitive to detect very low amounts of product. For this purpose, we developed a highly sensitive chemiluminescence assay of the rate of H_2O_2 formation, which directly reflects NADPH-oxidase activity [18]. The respiratory burst responses to fMLP, C5a, PAF, and LTB_4 differed considerably in extent and duration. The onset time of the responses, however, was the same for all four agonists and averaged approximately 2.4 s. These observations suggested that signals from different receptors are transduced by similar or even identical processes [19]. The onset time of the respiratory burst induced by ionomycin or PMA was at least 3–5 times longer, indicating that receptor-dependent activation is much more rapid and, therefore, probably based on a different mechanism. Combination of PMA and ionomycin elicited a more rapid response, but the onset time was still markedly longer than that observed on stimulation with receptor agonists.

A significant shortening of the onset time of the respiratory burst response to receptor agonists was observed when the neutrophils were pretreated with threshold concentrations of PMA or other protein kinase C activator. The extent of the shortening depended on the interval between PMA and agonist addition. If the agonist was added with a respiratory burst had already been induced by PMA, the ensuing enhancement of H_2O_2 production was immediate, i.e., shorter than 0.2 s, the approximate time resolution of our instrument.

Under the latter experimental conditions, respiratory burst activation preceded the agonist-dependent rise in $[Ca^{2+}]_i$, indicating that once protein kinase C is active, receptor agonists can turn on the NADPH-oxidase without appreciable changes in $[Ca^{2+}]_i$. Thus, activation of protein kinase C could be the rate-limiting step in receptor-mediated induction of the respiratory burst.

The fact that agonists are much faster activators than PMA and ionophores and show synergism with PMA and other protein kinase C ligands suggests that receptor-dependent neutrophil activation involves a transduction process that does not rely on $[Ca^{2+}]_i$ changes and protein kinase C, in addition to the common Ca^{2+}- and protein kinase C-dependent transduciton sequence discussed above. A scheme of our present view of the induction of the respiratory burst along a branching signal transduction pathway is shown in Figure 1.

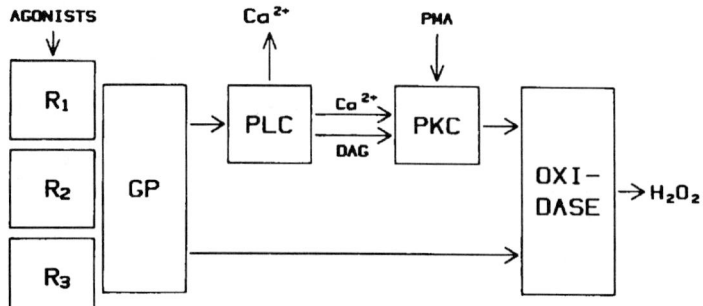

Figure 1. Signal transduction in the activation of the respiratory burst in human neutrophils. R_1, R_2 and R_3 designate different receptors. Upon agonist binding, they become coupled to a common type of GTP-binding protein. Downstream of the latter, the transduction pathway branches off into two sequences. See text for details.

Agonists acting on different receptors engage a common type of G-proteins. Downstream of this step, two separate processes can be distinguished, one leading to activation of phospholipase C delivers diacylglycerol and leads (via IP$_3$) to a rise in [Ca^{2+}]$_i$ and to the activation of protein kinase C. This process requires free Ca^{2+} and does not operate in calcium-depleted cells, but can be short-cutted with PMA or other protein kinase C ligands. The other process is still elusive in biochemical terms, but can be identified functionally as being fast and Ca^{2+} insensitive. The dependence of both processes on a similar class of G-proteins is indicated by their common sensitivity to *B. pertussis* toxin. It appears that both sequences must be functional and must operate in concert for transducing receptor-dependent signals since calcium depletion, which only affects the upper sequence of the scheme, blocks transduction. On the other hand, the shortening of the onset time of agonist-induced respiratory burst by PMA suggests a modulatory role for protein kinase C.

References

1. Babior, B. M. 1978. Oxygen-dependent microbial killing by phagocytes. New Engl. J. Med. 298: 659.
2. Baggiolini, M. 1984. Phagocytes use oxygen to kill bacteria. Experientia 40: 906.
3. Henson, P. M., and R. B. Johnston Jr. 1987. tissue injury in inflammation. J. Clin. Invest. 79: 669.
4. Fernandez, H. N., P. M. Henson, A. Otani, and T. E. Hugli. 1978. Chemotactic response to human C3$_a$ and C5$_a$ anaphylatoxins. I. Evaluation of C3$_a$ and C5$_a$ leukotaxis in vitro and under simulated in vivo conditions. J. Immunol. 120: 109.
5. Showell, H. J., R. J. Freer, S. H. Zigmond, E. Schiffmann, S. Aswanikumar, B. Corcoran, and E. L. Becker. 1976. The structure-activity relations of synthetic peptides as chemotactic factors and inducers of lysosomal enzyme secretion for neutrophils. J. Exp. Med. 143: 1154.
6. Ingraham, L. M., T. D. Coates, J. M. Allen, C. P. Higgins, R. L. Baehner, and L. A. Boxer. 1982. Metabolic, membrane and functional responses of human polymorphonuclear leukocytes to platelet-activating factor. Blood 59: 1259.
7. Ford-Hutchinson, A. W., M. A. Bray, M. V. Doig, M. E. Shipley, and M. J. H. Smith. 1978. Leukotriene B, a potent chemokinetic and aggregating substance released from polymorphonuclear leukocytes. Nature 286: 264.
8. Baggiolini, M., B. Dewald, and M. Thelen. 1988. Effects of PAF on neutrophils and mononuclear phagocytes. Progr. Biochem. Pharmacol. (Karger Series) 22: 90.
9. Lindley, I., H. Aschauer, J. M. Seifert, C. Lam, W. Brunowsky, E. Downatzki, M. Thelen, P. Peveri, B. Dewald, V. von Tscharner, A. Walz, and M. Baggiolini. 1988. Synthesis and expression in *E. coli* of the gene of NAF, a monocyte-derived neutrophil-activating factor. Biological equivalence between natural and recombinant NAF. Proc. Natl. Acad. Sci. USA, in press.
10. Grzeskowiak, M., V. Della Bianca, M. A. Cassatella, and F. Rossi. 1986. Complete dissociation between the activation of phosphoinositide turnover and of NADPH oxidase by formyl-methionyl-leucyl-phenylalanine in human neutrophils depleted of Ca^{2+} and primed by subthreshold doses of phorbol 12,myristate 13, acetate. Biochem. Biophys. Res. Commun. 135: 785.
11. Repine, J. E., J. G. White, C. C. Clawson, and B. M. Holmes. 1974. The influence of phorbol myristate acetate on oxygen consumption by polymorphonuclear leukocytes. J. Lab. Clin. Med. 83: 6761.
12. Okajima, F., T. Katada, and M. Ui. 1985. Coupling of the guanine nucleotide regulatory protein to chemotactic peptide receptors in neutrophil membranes and its uncoupling by islet-activating protein, pertussis toxin. A possible role for the toxin substrate in Ca^{2+}-mobilizing receptor-mediated signal transduction. J. Biol. Chem. 260: 6761.
13. Sklar, L. A., P. A. Hyslop, Z. G. Oades, G. M. Omann, A. J. Jesaitis, R. G. Painter, and C. G. Cochrane. 1985. Signal transduction and ligand-receptor dynamics in the human neutrophil. Transient responses and occupancy-response relations at the formyl peptide receptor. J. Biol. Chem. 260: 11461.
14. Smith, C. D., C. C. Cox, and R. Snydermann. 1986. Receptor-coupled activation of phosphoinositide-specific phospholipase C by an N protein. Science 232: 97.
15. Wolf, M., H. LeVine III, W. S. May Jr., P. Cuatrecasas, and N. Sahyoun. 1985. A model for intracellular translocation of protein kinase C involving synergism between Ca^{2+} and phorbol esters. Nature 317: 546.
16. Horn, W., and M. L. Karnovsky. 1986. Features of the translocation of protein kinase C in neutrophils stimulated with the chemotactic peptide f-Met-Leu-Phe. Biochem. Biophys. Res. Commun. 139: 1169.
17. von Tscharner, V., B. Prod'hom, M. Baggiolini, and H. Reuter. 1986. Ion channels in human neutrophils activated by a rise in free cytosolic calcium concentration. Nature 324: 369.
18. Wymann, M. P., V. von Tscharner, D. A. Deran-

leau, and M. Baggiolini. 1987. Chemiluminescence detection of H_2O_2 produced by human
neutrophils during the respiratory burst. Anal.
Biochem. 165: 371.

19. Wymann, M. P., V. von Tscharner, D. A. Deran-
leau, and M. Baggiolini. 1987. The onset of the
respiratory burst in human neutrophils. Real-
time studies of H_2O_2 formation reveal a rapid
agonist-induced transduction process. J. Biol.
Chem. 262: 12048.

Induction and Metabolism of Lipid Mediators in Inflammation

*Wolfgang König, Jochen Brom, Monika Raulf, and Manfred Köller**

Leukotrienes are potent mediators of inflammation and allergy and are generated by a variety of cells. Polymorphonuclear granulocytes can be activated by the classical stimuli C-ionophore A 23187, opsonized zymosan, fMLP, bacterial toxins, and by bacteria themselves to generate and metabolize leukotrienes. The profile of leukotriene generation and metabolization is dependent on the stimuli used. The LTB4 metabolization by granulocytes to 20-OH-LTB4 and 20-COOH-LTB4 is reduced by preactivation of the cells with phorbol myristate acetate; the decrease strictly correlates with the decreased expression of the LTB4 receptor. Tumor necrosis factors (TNFs) modulate the LTB4 receptor expression by transforming the high and low affinity subsets into receptors expressing a homologous subset of intermediate affinity. In contrast to granulocytes, the human lung macrophages transform LTB4 into the dihydro-LTB4 metabolite.

It appears that the extent of leukotriene formation and metabolization is controlled by the stimulus, the individual cells, as well as the cellular environment.

It is evident by now that leukotrienes are generated in the microenvironment for purposes of local action, rather than as for hormones, for an effect at a distal region. This involvement of chemical mediators in altering homeostasis of the microenvironment has implications for the diagnosis and management of various disease processes. An essential role of leukotrienes in allergic and inflammatory disease processes has been suggested from the fact that these mediators are generated by a variety of cells that have specific requirements of cell activation [1, 2]. In considering human disease processes, the term "inflammation" is the excessive formation or relatively inadequate inactivation of chemical mediators generated either by resident or inflitrating cell types. In this regard we directed our studies in order to further precisely analyze

Table 1. Leukotriene release induced by various stimuli (Ca-ionophore, opsonized zymosan, fMLP, alveolysin, streptolysin O).

| Stimulus | LTB4 | Leukotrienes (ng/10^7 PMN) | | | |
		20-OH-LTB4	20-COOH-LTB4	6-trans-LTB4	LTC4
Ca-ionophore A23187 (7.3µM)	108.2±4.3	164±8.5	38.4±5.2	28.4±2.5	37.2±3.6
opsonized zymosan (2 mg)	21.5±3.2	24.6±2.7	9.8±2.4	0	1.5±0.9
fMLP (18µM)	5.2±2.7	12.6±2.0	14.2±3.8	0	0
alveolysin (10 U)	3.8±0.6	n.d.	n.d.	1.9±0.9	25.1±5.4
streptolysin O (10 U)	2.2±1.9	n.d.	n.d.	1.8±1.1	16.8±1.5

PMNs ($1 \cdot 10^7$) were incubated for 15 min with the various stimuli in the presence of calcium and magnesium at 37°C. Analysis of cell-free supernatants was performed by reversed-phase HPLC. The results represent mean values calculated from five different experiments.
n.d. = not determined

*   Lehrstuhl für Medizinische Mikrobiologie and Immunologie, Arbeitsgruppe für Infektabwehrmechanismen, Ruhr-Universität Bochum, Universitätsstraße 150, D-4630 Bochum, Federal Republic of Germany.
    This work was supported by the Deutsche Forschungsgemeinschaft (DFG-Kö 7/4).

— the nature of stimuli that induce leukotriene formation

— the events that modulate or even impair the metabolism of leukotrienes.

Biochemistry of Leukotriene Formation

The profile of leukotriene generation and metabolization has been thoroughly analyzed in the neutrophil because of the feasibility of purification. The classical stimuli for leukotriene activation are the Ca-ionophore A 23187, opsonized zymosan, and the bacterial peptide fMLP. Stimulation of human neutrophils with either of the above stimuli induced a time- and dose-dependent generation of leukotrienes (20-COOH-LTB4, 20-OH-LTB4, LTB4, LTB4 isomers, and LTC4) (Table 1) [3]. The amount of leukotriene generation after stimulation with opsonized zymosan only comprised a small fraction (15%) of that obtained with the Ca-ionophore A 23187. The leukotriene release obtained after stimulation with opsonizes zymosan was completely dependent on the

presence of divalent cations. Only calcium concentrations above 1.25 mM induced LTB4 release that was detected by reversed-phase HPLC. In the presence of magnesium yet at a constant calcium concentration, leukotriene release was enhanced. In contrast, leukotriene release induced by the Ca-ionophore was not affected by magnesium [4].

Role of Lipid Mediators During Bacterial Inflammation

An important observation which supports the role of leukotrienes for the induction of inflammatory disease processes is the finding that these mediators are induced by bacterial toxins and bacteria themselves on cellular stimulation. In this regard it has been described that the sulfhydryl (SH)-activated cytolysins, among which the prototype is streptolysin O (SLO), leads to membrane damage as a result of cholesterol rearrangement within the cell membrane [5]. We provided evidence that the SLO induces leukotriene formation as well as PAF metabolism from human granulocytes. The predominant product from neutrophils was LTC4, which was unlike the activation in-

Table 2. Characterization of different P. aeruginosa strains (A) and the purified glycolipid (B).

(A) Bacteria Strain	Hemolysis (%)	PLC-act. (E404)	Histamine (%)	LTB4 (ng)	12-HETE (ng)
		Strains from cystic fibrosis patients			
P1	8±3	0.13±0.06	0	0	0
P3	11±5	0.19±0.10	0	0	0
P4	21±2	0.42±0.09	20±5	9.7±1.5	0
		Strains from burned patients			
B10	44±4	0.71±0.04	35±1	4.6±1.0	0
582 f	29±2	0.55±0.05	29±2	5.3±0.5	0

(B) Purified glycolipid (heat stable hemolysin) Glycolipid (μg)	Hemolysis (%)	Histamine (%)	LTB4 (ng)	12-HETE (ng)
50	97±2	95±3	0	190±70
25	78±5	97±5	0	28±3
10	3±2	95±4	0	20±6
2	3±2	8±3	0	1±1

(A) Characterization of different P. aeruginosa strains according to their bacterial bound hemolysin; PLC-activity, induction of histamine release from rat peritoneal mast cells (RPMC), leukotriene B4 (LTB4) release from PMNs and 12-HETE formation from human platelets.
(B) Effect of purified glycolipid (heat stable hemolysin) on the induction of histamine release from RPMC, on the generation of leukotrienes from PMNs and 12-HETE from human platelets.

itiated by the Ca-ionophore or opsonized zymosan [6]. The major product of granulocytes generated by the latter stimuli was LTB4 (Table 2).

A variety of bacteria which colonize the tissue subsequently invade the host and induce inflammatory reactions; these proceed via (a) specific attachment of the microorganisms to the tissue and (b) activation and damage of the appropriate target cells. We analyzed the role of genetically cloned strains as well as clinical isolates *E. coli, Pseudomonas aeruginosa* as well as *Listeria monocytogenes* [7]. These bacterial strains have in common that they produce exotoxins; because of the their property to lyse erythrocytes, the toxins have been named hemolysins. The membrane biochemical mechanism of the hemolysins for various cells are quite distinct. There was little information as to whether leukotrienes are involved in the pathogenesis of the above-mentioned bacteria-induced diseases as well as their toxin-mediated effects. Our studies with *E. coli* showed that distinct strains with defined adherence properties induce inflammatory mediator release, e.g., leukotrienes as well as histamine [8]. The coexpression of the strains for hemolysin even enhanced mediator release among which leukotriene B4 was the major component. With Pseudomonas aeruginosa strains (cystic fibrosis patients, patients from intensive-care units, heavily burned patients) it became evident that distinct hemolysins according to their heat stability induce differences as to the induction of leukotriene formation. Strains expressing heat-labile hemolysin (phospholipase C) initiated LTB4 release from human PMNs as well as histamine release from rat mast cells. Purified heat-stable hemolysin (glycolipid) was negative as to leukotriene generation, but induced histamine release and also 12-HETE formation from human platelets (Table 2). These results clearly suggested that phagocytes do respond toward bacterial toxins and the interacting bacteria; the granulocytes then provide according to the bacterial pathogenicity factors the mediators of inflammation.

Modulation of Leukotrienes by Enzymes

As has been suggested primarily the inflammatory response is also dependent on the

Figure 1. Time-dependent effect of PMA on the catabolism of exogenous LTB4. PMNs (1×10^7) were incubated for various times with PMA (0.23 μM) in the presence of calcium and magnesium at 37 °C. The cells were washed in PBS-buffer and LTB4 (300 pmol) was added. This incubation period was terminated after 15 min; the analysis was carried out using HPLC. The ordinate shows the percentage of the sum for LTB4 and the omega-oxidated products. The preincubation time of 0 min represents the control without prestimulation with PMA. All values were the mean ± SEM of four individual experiments.

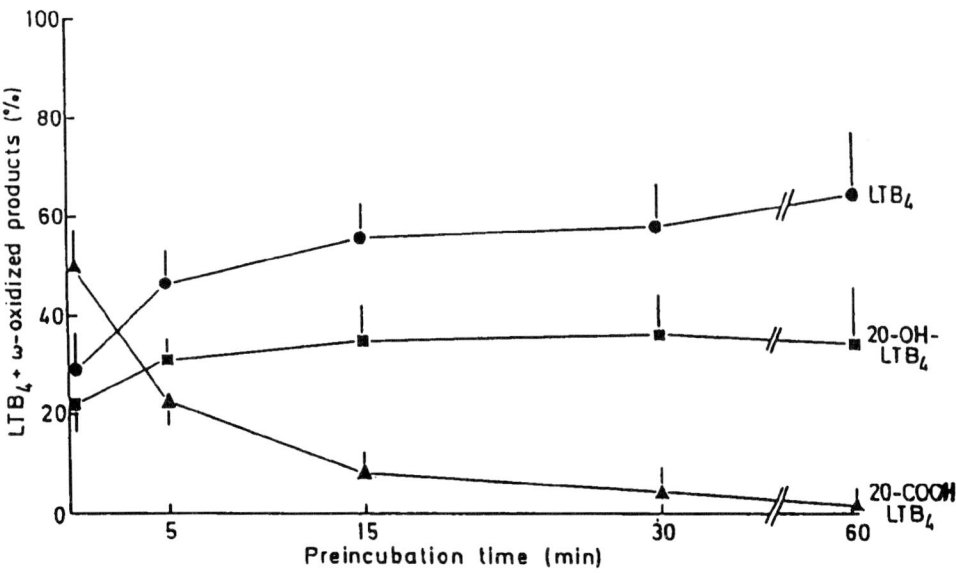

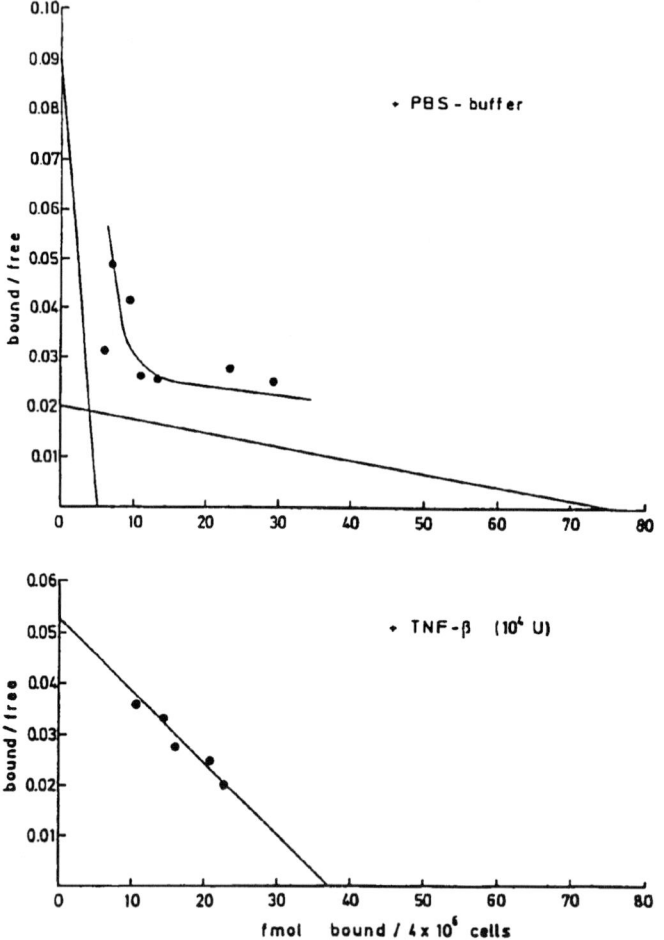

Figure 2. Scatchard plot analysis for the binding of (3H)LTB4. PMNs were incubated with TNF-β (104 U) or PBS-buffer for 30 min at 37°C, washed, and the specific binding of various concentrations of (3H)LTB4 was determined. Upper panel: neutrophils stimulated with PBS. Lower panel: neutrophils stimulated with TNF-β. The data represent a characteristic result of the individual experiments.

capacity to modulate or even inactivate the leukotrienes. Granulocytes inactivate LTB4 via a two-step reaction resulting in 20-OH-LTB4 and 20-COOH-LTB4, which express a reduced biological capacity compared to leukotriene B4 [9]. The initial reaction is carried out by the LTB4-omega-hydroxylase, which is localized within the microsomal fraction. The second step of the LTB4 inactivation pathway is catalyzed by the 20-OH-LTB4 dehydrogenase, an enzyme which is localized in the cytosol fraction. It has been suggested that the biological response of LBT4 is transmitted via a high- and a low-affinity receptor, the former transducing the chemotactic responses and the latter the degranulation response [20]. Preactivation of human PMNs with phorbol myristate acetate (Figure 1) or the Ca-ionophore showed a reduction of the LTB4 metabolization rate especially a decreased for-

mation of the omega-carboxy metabolite. The decreased LTB4 conversion strictly correlated with the decreased expression of the LTB4 receptor on the preactivated cells. These results suggested that the cellular preactivation induces the downregulation of the receptor, which subsequently leads to an impaired uptake of exogenous LTB4. The potency of the phorbol esters is suggestive for a central regulatory role of the proteinkinase C [11].

Interaction of Tumor Necrosis Factors (TNFs) with LTB4 Receptors

An important role during chronic inflammatory reactions has been recently attributed to cytokines. It is evident that various cyto-

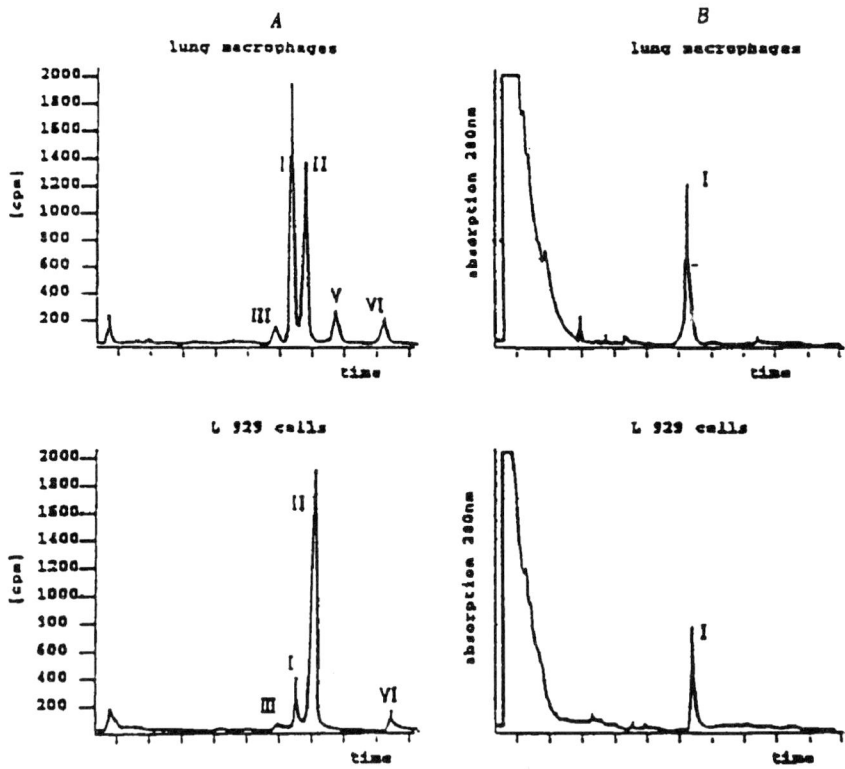

Figure 3. Comparison of the LTB4 metabolism in L929 cells and human lung macrophages; both cell types were incubated with (3H)LTB4 (1.8 kBq) for 60 min. A: radioactive HPLC; B: UV absorbance (280 nm) HPLC; Peak I: LTB4, Peak II: main metabolite (Dihydro-LTB4); Peak III: a metabolite which is more polar than LTB4; Peak IV: a further unpolar metabolite which is more polar than LTB4; Peak V: a further unpolar metabolite; Peak VI: a metabolite which is only found in the macrophage fraction.

kines interfere with the generation of lipid mediators. In this regard, tumor necrosis factors which are either derived from the monocyte-macrophage lineage (TNF-?-cachectin) or a product of the T lymphocytes and B lymphoblastoid cell lines (TNF-β-lymphotoxin) mediate multiple aspects of the host inflammatory response [12]. It has been reported that TNF augments the phagocytic activity, the degranulation, and the neutrophil adhesion to endothelial cells. Preincubation of human PMNs with the TNFs modulate the LTB4 receptor expression. The high- and low-affinity subsets are transformed into receptors expressing a homologous subset of intermediate affinity [13] (Figure 2). These data provided evidence that cytokines may control granulocyte influx and responses by their effect on receptors for leukotrienes. It is surprising that preactivation of granulocytes with toxins, e.g., streptolysin O, induces a reduced generation of leuko-trienes

after subsequent stimulation of the cells with the Ca-ionophore. An enhanced LTB4 conversion was obtained [14]. These results suggest that exogenous stimuli exert a regulatory control on the phagocyte's capacity to generate leukotrienes.

Release and Metabolism of LTB4 from Human Lung Macrophages

With human dispersed lung as well as tonsillar cells containing a purified macrophage preparation which are either activated by the Ca-ionophore or anti-IgE, a different pattern of LTB4 metabolism became apparent. Our studies showed that human lung macrophages transform LTB4 into the dihydro-LTB4 metabolite (5,12 dihydroxy-eicosatrienoic acid). This metabolite is also obtained when LTB4 is incubated with the fibroblast cell line L 929 [15]

(Figure 3). Similar results were also observed when tonsillar cells were studied [16]. In inflammatory processes of the lung it is obvious that granulocytes are also present within the bronchoalveolar space. Addition of LTB4 to the granulocytes containing alveolar cell population induced a rapid turnover of LTB4 into several products. The omega-oxidation products, the dihydro-LTB4 and still unknown metabolites were observed. It is presently unclear to which extent the metabolic pathway of LTB4 is modulated during various disease processes. Thus, our results provide evidence that the extent of leukotriene formation is controlled by the stimulus, the individual cells as well as the cellular environment. Soluble products that occur during inflammation may tune the inflammatory cascade initiated or perpetuated by leukotrienes. Future studies will be directed toward determining to which extent the pattern of leukotriene formation may characterize the actual disease processes.

References

1. Bray, M. A. 1986. Leukotrienes and inflammation. Agents Actions 19: 87.
2. Parker, C. W. 1987. Lipid mediators produced through the lipoxygenase pathway. Ann. Rev. Immunol. 5: 65.
3. Raulf, M., M. Stüning, and W. König. 1985. Metabolism of leukotrienes by L-γ-glutamyl-transpeptidase and dipeptidase from human polymorphonuclear granulocytes. Immunology 55: 135.
4. Raulf, M., M. Stüning, and W. König. 1986. Effect of cations on leukotriene release: Requirements for the metabolism of peptido-leukotrienes (leukotrienes C4, D4) by human polymorphonuclear granulocytes. Immunology 58: 479.
5. Alouf, J. E. 1986. Interaction of bacterial protein toxins with host defense mechanisms. In Bacterial Protein Toxins. P. Falmagne, J. E. Alouf, F. J. Fehrenbach, J. Jeljaszewicz, and M. Thelestam, eds. Gustav Fischer Verlag, Stuttgart, p. 121.
6. Bremm, K. D., W. König, P. Pfeiffer, I. Rauschen, K. Theobald, M. Thelestam, and J. E. Alouf. 1985. Effect of thiol-activated toxins (streptolysin O, alveolysin, and theta-toxin) on the generation of leukotrienes and leukotriene-inducing and -metabolizing enzymes from human polymorphonuclear granulocytes. Infect. Immun. 50: 844.
7. Scheffer, J., W. König, J. Hacker, and W. Goebel. 1985. Bacterial adherence and hemolysin freom Escherichia coli induces histamine and leukotriene release from various cells. Infect. Immun. 50: 271.
8. Scheffer, J., K. Vosbeck, and W. König 1986. Induction of inflammatory mediators from human polymorphonuclear granulocytes and rat mast cells by haemolysin-positive and -negative E. coli strains with different adhesion. Immunology 59: 541.
9. Hansson, G., J. A. Lindgren, S.-E. Dahlen, P. Hedqvist, and B. Samuelsson. 1981. Identification and biological activity of novel w-oxidized metabolites of leukotriene B4 from human leukocytes. FEBS Lett. 130: 107.
10. Goldman, D. W., and E. J. Goetzl. 1984. Heterogeneity of human polymorphonuclear leukocyte receptors for leukotriene B4. Identification of a subset of high affinity receptors that transduce the chemotactic response. J. Exp. Med. 159: 1027.
11. Brom, J., W. Schönfeld, and W. König. 1988. Metabolism of leukotriene B4 by activated human polymorphonuclear granulocytes. Immunology 64: 509.
12. Beutler, B., and A. Cerami. 1988. The common ediator of shock, cachexia, and tumor necrosis. Adv. Immunology 42: 213.
13. Brom, J., J. Knöller, M. Köller, and W. König. 1988. Tumour necrosis factors modulate the affinity state of the leukotriene B4 receptor on human neutrophils. Immunology, in press.
14. Bremm, K. D., W. König, M. Thelestam, and J. E. Alouf. 1987. Modulation of granulocyte functions by bacterial exotoxin and endotoxins. Immunology 62: 363.
15. Schlüter, B., W. Schönfeld, and W. König. 1988. Generation and metabolism of leukotrienes and release of histamine from human dispersed tonsillar cells. Scand. J. Immunol. 27: 451.
16. Schönfeld, W., B. Schlüter, and W. König. Leukotriene generation and metabolism in isolated human lung macrophages. Immunology, in press.

Role of Platelet-Activating Factor in Allergic Inflammation

*Jean-Michel Mencia-Huerta, David Hosford, Pierre Braquet**

Platelet-activating factor (PAF) is a phospholipid mediator of inflammatory processes whose role in allergic inflammation has been recently suggested. Indeed, PAF has been shown to induce long-lasting bronchial hyperreactivity in the guinea pig and in humans. In addition, PAF is capable of recruiting eosinophil in lung tissue and thus contributes to the local inflammation. Recently, long-term administration of PAF to the guinea pig via osmotic alzet minipumps has proved to be a valuable model for studying morphologic and cell infiltration induced by the mediator. Long-term administration of PAF results in the development of bronchial hyper-responsiveness to histamine associated with cell infiltration and morphologic alterations of the lung architecture including smooth muscle cell hyperplasia, metaplasia of the epithelium and presence of mucus obstruction. These alterations, probably resulting from the priming effect of PAF on the production of various cytokines implicated in the regulation of specific and nonspecific immune pro-cesses, may play a critical role in the development of bronchial hyperresponsiveness.

PAF and Allergy

The role of PAf in allergic reactions was initially suggested by the experiments of Pinckard et al. [1] and Vargaftig et al. [2], demonstrating platelet-activation during anaphylactic shock in the rabbit and the guinea pig. In both species, intravenous injection of synthetic or natural PAF evokes bronchopulmonary alterations resembling those observed during anaphylactic shock. In the guinea pig, the platelet dependency of the PAF-induced bronchoconstriction was demonstrated using a pharmacologic approach. Treatment of the animals with a cyclooxygenase blocker in combination with antihistamine and antiserotonin drugs abrogated PAF-induced bronchopulmonary alterations without affecting the hypotensive effect of the autacoid [3]. In addition, treatment of the animals with an antiplatelet antiserum or PGI_2 (which blocks platelet activation) also results in a marked decrease in the in vivo effect of the autacoid on lung tissue. Despite the fact that the mediator mimicks the symptoms occurring during antigen challenge of sensitized animals, the direct demonstration of its release at the time of in vivo antigen stimulation is still missing. However, the generation of PAF by lung tissue isolated from sensitized guinea pigs upon challenge with the specific antigen has been reported [4, 5]. Therefore, it is likely that besides alveolar macrophages [6], which also generates PAF, the lung tissue is also probably a source for this very potent autacoid.

PAF and Bronchial Hyperreactivity

Several lines of evidence indicate that PAF is a primary mediator involved in the development of bronchial hyperreactivity either in the animal model and in humans. Indeed, initial experiments by Mazzoni et al. [7] have shown that administration of PAF, either intravenous-ly or by aerosol, induced after 24 hours a bronchial hyperreactivity to further stimulation with histamine or methacholine. Cuss et al. [8] have also shown that in humans bolus administration of PAF by aerosol induces a bronchial hyperreactivity to methacholine lasting for at least several weeks. The pharmacologic modulation of the development of bronchial hyperreactivity has only been investigated in the animal model [9]. Since such a phenomenon is inhibited by various unrelated drugs, its development probably results from a very complex set of events. However, the role of platelet-derived growth factor (PDGF), of platelet factor 4 (PF4), and of the various monocyte-derived cytokines implicated in the specific and nonspecific immune processes are primary agents in the local initia-

---

*   Institut Henri Beaufour, 1 avenue des Tropiques, 91952 Les Ulis, France.

tion of inflammatory reactions leading to bronchial hyperreactivity.

The demonstration that PAF could play an important role in bronchial hyperreactivity in animal models has been provided by the use of PAF antagonists, including BN 52021. Indeed, antigen challenge of sensitized animals also leads to the development of bronchial hyperreactivity associated with cell infiltration in the lung tissue. In both the guinea pig and the rabbit, BN 52021 inhibits in a dose-dependent fashion the antigen-induced bronchial hyperresponsiveness to histamine, suggesting that PAF is generated during this process. In addition, cell infiltration in the lung tissue or in the bronchoalveolar lavages is markedly reduced upon treatment of the animals with BN 52021 (reviewed in [10]). Therefore, antigen provocation of sensitized animals leads to the local or systemic generation of PAF, which, in turn, is one of the primary agents involved in bronchial hyperreactivity.

Acute and Long-Term Effect of PAF

In most of the studies reported above, the mediator was administered by a bolus. This probably does not relate to what happens in atopic patients who are in constant stimulation with the antigen. Therefore, a new model for investigating the role of PAF in bronchial hyperreactivity has been established implicating the use of osmotic Alzet minipumps releasing the autacoid at a constant flow rate. Long-term administration of PAF leads to bronchial hyperresponsiveness, but not to hyperreactivity to histamine. Indeed, although the amplitude of the response is markedly higher in PAF-treated animals, the threshold dose inducing an increase in the pulmonary inflation pressure is similar in both PAF-treated and untreated animals. The bronchial hyperresponsiveness to histamine in the guinea pig is not observed when the animals are treated with the PAF antagonist, BN 52021 (15 mg/kg, twice a day) during the period of minipump implantation.

In addition to the alterations of the bronchopulmonary responsiveness noted in PAF-treated animals, changes in lung architecture and cell infiltrates are observed. Lungs from PAF-treated animals exhibit a congestive appearance associated with contraction of small bronchies, metaplasia of the epithelium, and hypersecretion of mucus. In addition, smooth muscle cell hyperplasia and hypertrophy are also noted. The number of eosinophils infiltrating lung tissue is markedly enhanced in PAF-treated animals as compared to those implanted with minipumps containing the solvent alone. Finally, the number of mast cells in peribronchial regions is markedly increased. Both the alterations in pulmonary architecture and in the number of eosinophils and mast cells in lung tissue are significantly lower in the group of animals receiving BN 52021 during the period of minipump implantation.

Recently, Touvay et al. [11] demonstrated that antigen administration via osmotic minipumps to sensitized guinea pigs also leads to bronchial hyperresponsiveness to histamine. As in the case of PAF, hyperresponsiveness rather than hyperreactivity to histamine is observed. In contrast, however, with histamine, the response to leukotriene D_4 and PAF itself are markedly and significantly increased in the antigen-treated animals. For these two lipid mediators, true hyperreactivity is noted since the threshold dose inducing a pulmonary response is markedly and significantly decreased.

Long-term administration of PAF to animals leads to various alterations that are probably unrelated to each other. Indeed, eosinophil infiltration in lung tissue is probably due to the direct chemotactic action of PAF on this cell type [12]. The hyperplasia of lung smooth muscle cells is probably related to various phenomena including the production of PDGF from PAF-activated platelets. In addition, the "priming" effect of PAF on various cell types including macrophages, polymorphonuclear neutrophils, and eosinophils could play a role in the smooth muscle cell hyperplasia. As well, PAF has been shown to enhance markedly the production of tumor necrosis factor by human monocytes stimulated with interferon-γ. Consistent with this effect, PAF at low doses also potentiates interleukin-1 production by lipopolysaccharide-stimulated monocytes. Both tumor necrosis factor and interleukin-1 are able to generate PAF from endothelial cells [13], which thus may be involved in a vicious cycle leading to an enhancement of vascular permeability and cell infiltration in various tissues, including lung.

Concluding Remarks

Via its numerous biological activities, PAF is a likely candidate in the development of bronchial hyperreactivity and inflammatory reactions in lung. Up to now, these activities have been solely demonstrated in in vitro experimental animals. However, with the use of potent and specific PAF antagonists, the precise role of this phospholipid in lung pathology will be probably determined and its relative importance compared to the other putative mediators of asthmatic reactions will be established.

References

1. Pinckard, R. N., M. Halonen, J. D. Palmer. L. M. McManus, J. O. Shaw, and P. M. Henson. 1987. Intravascular aggregation and pulmonary sequestration of platelets during IgE-induced systemic anaphylaxis in the rabbit: Abrogation of lethal anaphylactic shock by platelet depletion. J. Immunol. 119: 2185.
2. Vargaftig, B. B., J. Lefort, M. Chignard, and J. Benveniste. 1980. Platelet-activating factor induces a platelet-dependent bronchoconstriction unrelated to the formation of prostaglandin derivates. Eur. J. Pharmac. 65: 185.
3. Chignard, M., F. Wal, I. Lefort, and B. B. Vargaftig. 1982. Inhibition by sulphinpyrazone of the platelet-dependent broncho-constriction due to platelet-activating factor (PAF-acether) in the guinea pig. Eur. J. Pharmacol. 78: 71.
4. Fitzgerald, M. F., S. Moncada, and L. Parente. 1986. The anaphylactic release of platelet-activating factor from perfused guinea pig lungs. Br. J. Pharmacol. 88: 149.
5. Parente, L., M. F. Fitzgerald, and S. Moncada. 1987. Anaphylactic release of platelet-activating factor and eicosanoids from guinea-pigs sensitized to ovalbumine aerosol. In: Advances in prostaglandins, thromboxane and leukotrienes research. B. Samuelsson, R. Paoletti, P. Ramwell, eds. Raven Press, 17: 171.
6. Arnoux, B., D. Duval, and J. Benveniste. 1980. Release of platelet-activating factor (PAF-acether) from alveolar macrophages by the calcium ionophore A23187 and phagocytosis. Eur. J. Clin. Invest. 10: 437.
7. Mazzoni, L., J. Morley, C. P. Page, and S. Sanjar. 1985. Induction of hyperreactivity by platelet-activating factor in the guinea-pig. J. Physiol. 365: 107P.
8. Cuss, F. M., C. M. S. Dixon, and P. J. Barnes. 1986. Effects of inhaled platelet-activating factor on pulmonary function and bronchial responsiveness in man. Lancet ii: 189.
9. Morley, J., S. Sanjar, and C. P. Page. 1984. The platelet in asthma. Lancet ii: 1142.
10. Braquet, P., L. Touqui, T. Y. Shen, and B. B. Vargaftig. 1987. Perspectives in platelet-activating factor research. Pharmacol. Rev. 39: 97.
11. Touvay, C., B. Vilain, A. Pfister, C. Carré, V. Poisson, J. M. Hencia-Huerta, and P. Braquet. 1988. Effect of the platelet-activating factor (PAF) antagonist, BN 52021, on bronchial hyperresponsiveness induced by chronic infusion of antigen in sensitized guinea-pig (Abstract). 9th Eur. Immunology Meeting, Rome, September 14–17.
12. Wardlaw, A. J., and A. B. Kay. 1986. PAF-acether is a potent chemotactic factor for human eosinophils. J. Allergy Clin. Immunol. 77: 236.
13. Bussolino, F. Brevario, C. Tetta, M. Aglietta, A. Mantovani, and E. Dejana. 1986. Interleukin 1 stimulates platelet-activating factor production in cultured human endothelial cells. J. Clin. Invest. 77: 2027.

The Role of PAF in Allergic Inflammation

*Dom Spina, Anthony J. Coyle, Clive P. Page**

In 1966, Barbaro and Zweifler demonstrated the release of histamine in plasma following exposure of sensitised rabbits to allergen [1]. In 1972, Benveniste and coworkers demonstrated that histamine release was a consequence of IgE activation of rabbit basophils with the generation of a mediator capable of inducing platelet activation, which they termed platelet activating factor (PAF) [2]. In 1979, the structure of PAF was demonstrated to be 1-0-alkyl-2-acetyl-sn-glyceryl-3-phosphorylcholine by three independent group (reviewed in [3]).

With the availability of synthetic PAF, much attention has been focused on the possible involvement of this phospholipid in the pathogenesis of allergic inflammation. This article reviews the evidence that PAF may be an important mediator of the allergic response. It is anticipated that, with the recent availability of several classes of selective PAF antagonists, the role of PAF in allergic diseases will be more clearly defined in the near future.

Cellular Origins

PAF is formed de novo following both allergic and non-allergic stimuli in a number of inflammatory cells including alveolar macrophages, eosinophils, neutrophils and platelets (reviews in [3, 4]). The biosynthetic pathway involves activation of a calcium-dependent phospholipase A_2 which cleaves membrane-bound ether-linked phospholipids resulting in the formation of lyso-PAF, the precursor for PAF. Lyso-PAF has similar physiochemical properties to PAF, although it is devoid of any biological activity. Lyso-PAF may then be acted on by an acetyltransferase which acetylates lyso-PAF at the sn-2 position of the molecule [4].

PAF is very rapidly degraded in vivo because of the rapid metabolism by a cytosolic acetylhydrolase enzyme resulting in the formation of lyso-PAF. Thus, lyso-PAF is both the precursor and the major metabolite of PAF. Lyso-PAF may then be taken up by the membrane and re-incorporated into membrane lipids [4].

It is of interest that certain cells, most notably neutrophils, monocytes and lung mast cells, can synthesize PAF, but that much of the synthesized is retained within the cell and not released into the extracellular milieu. The precise role of intracellular PAF is at present unclear.

However, eosinophils from allergic individuals release PAF in greater amounts than eosinophils from normal subjects, which appears to involve a defect in the acetyltransferase enzyme, which no longer acts as the rate-limiting step in the biosynthetic pathway for PAF [4].

Since the eosinophil has been implicated as a central cell in the aetiology of allergy disease and PAF is very potent at activating eosinophils [5] (see below), these observations are of particular interest in our future understanding of the pathogenesis of allergic disease.

PAF Antagonists

A number of distinct chemical substances have now been described as PAF antagonists, which will be useful in furthering our understanding of the role of PAF in allergic diseases. The PAF antagonists currently available can be divided into three separate classes:

Synthetic Analogues of PAF

Following the discovery of the structure of PAF, many synthetic analogues have been produced which possess antagonist activity. The first compound described in this class was CV-3988 [6], which has now reached early clinical development [7]. Although this compound behaves as a PAF antagonist in humans, it will have limited usefulness clinically, because in common with other PAF analogues (e.g., SRI

* Department of Pharmacology, Chelsea Campus, Kings College, University of London, Manresa Rd, Chelsea, London SW3 4XL, England.

63-073, ONO-6240 and Ro193704), it has poor oral bioavailability (reviewed in [3]). Furthermore, CV-3988 has been reported to induce haemolysis [7].

Natural Products

One of the most interesting developments in the search for PAF antagonists has been the recognition that a number of Chinese medicinal herbs contain molecules that are active as selective PAF antagonists. Kadsurenone was the first molecule of this type to be discovered, isolated from the medicinal herb haifentang (*Piper futokadsura*) [8]. Kadsurenone is a natural tetrahydrofuran, and the discovery of this molecule has led to the synthesis of a number of more potent orally active analogues such as L-652,731 [9] and L-659,989 [10].

It has been recognised for centuries that the leaves of the Ginkgo biloba tree are useful in the treatment of various "chest complaints" [3]. Recently, it has been demonstrated that the leaves from this plant contain complex chemical structures belonging to the ginkgolide family of molecules [11]. The most potent and widely studied of the ginkgolides is BN 52021 or ginkgolide B [3]. This molecule is the most active constituent of a ginkgolide mixture (BN 52063), which is currently undergoing clinical investigation (see below) as it has recently been demonstrated to be a selective, orally active PAF antagonist in normal healthy volunteers [12].

Other naturally occurring PAF antagonists have been identified from fungi and certain microorganisms such as products derived from gliotoxin isolated from a wood fungus (FR-900452 and FR-49175) (reviewed in [11]).

Synthetic Structures

A wide range of chemical compounds have now been described that have selective PAF antagonistic activity, yet have structures distinct from PAF itself. One of the earliest compounds described in this class was 48740 RP [13] and some later derivatives (e.g., 52770 RP and 59227 RP) [14, 15]. These compounds have oral bioavailability, 48740 RP has recently been administered to normal volunteers [16]. Interestingly, other synthetic compounds that have

been described as PAF antagonists also possess other pharmacological properties. For instance, the triazolobenzodiazepines are widely prescribed as sedatives and anxiolytics, but it has recently been shown that some of these drugs (brotizolam, alprazolam, triazolam) are able to antagonize the biological actions of PAF. In contrast, classical benzodiazepines such as diazepam do not have this activity [17, 18]. A number of oral triazolobenzodiazepines have now been developed which retain the PAF antagonistic activity but without any sedative effect. An example of this type of PAF antagonist is WEB 2086 [19], which has recently initiated phase I trials in healthy volunteers [20].

Effect of PAF on Inflammatory Cells

PAF has a wide range of pharmacological activities. Many studies have shown that PAF is a potent activator of various inflammatory cells including platelets, neutrophils, eosinophils and macrophages [3]. Many PAF-induced effects can be inhibited by PAF antagonists, which suggests that PAF mediates its effects by recognition of a specific binding site on the target cell [3].

Although PAF has been described as being the most potent activator of human eosinophils [21] and initiating eosinophil infiltration into the skin of allergic subjects compared to that induced by antigen [22], recent evidence in experimental animals demonstrate that PAF-induced eosinophil accumulation in the lung is dependent upon platelet activation [23].

The effects of PAF on eosinophils can be inhibited by various PAF antagonists such as BN 52021 and WEB 2086 (reviewed in [3]), and it is noteworthy that PAF antagonists will also inhibit IgE-dependent activation and release of oxygen-free radicals from eosinophils highly suggestive of a central role for PAF in allergen-induced eosinophil activation [24].

Such a conclusion is reinforced by the numerous investigators who have reported that PAF will induce eosinophil infiltration into the lungs (reviewed in [3, 23]), and that the accumulation of eosinophils into the lung following exposure to PAF or antigen can be inhibited by the PAF antagonists WEB086, BN 52021 ad L-659,989 [23, 25–27].

57

The eosinophil contains many substances that are toxic to mammalian cells. In particular, eosinophil-derived major basic protein (MBP) has been shown to be toxic for respiratory epithelial cells [28], which may result in the loss of epithelial cell function (e.g., loss of epithelium-derived relaxant factor or loss of degradative enzymes for neuropeptides), loss of mucociliary function and exposure of sensory nerves [29]. Very recently, MBP has also been shown to induce hyperreactivity of airway smooth muscle in vitro, which suggests that loss of epithelial cell function may contribute to the non-specific bronchial hyperreactivity characterizing asthma [30].

It is therefore not surprising that PAF, administered by aerosol or intravenously, induces bronchial hyperreactivity to various spasmogens in a number of animal species (reviewed in [29]), including human beings [31]. Furthermore, treatment of the nasal cavity with PAF in individuals with allergic rhinitis results in an increase in nasal blockage to allergen compared with individuals not exposed to PAF [32], suggesting that PAF may also have a role in nasal hyperreactivity.

Clinical Studies with PAF Antagonists

Although a number of PAF antagonists have been demonstrated to inhibit allergic bronchoconstriction in experimental animals [3, 33–35], such studies have yet to be undertaken in humans. However, it is important to consider that most of the experimental systems have required the presence of H_1 antagonists and inhibitors of either cyclooxygenase and/or lipoxygenase metabolism of arachidonic acid before a beneficial effect of a PAF antagonist can be demonstrated, which suggests that PAF is unlikely to be a central determinant of allergen-induced bronchoconstriction.

PAF has considerable activity at inducing increased vascular permeability in a number of organs including the lung, which can be inhibited by PAF antagonists (reviewed in [3]). Recent preliminary clinical data have demonstrated that an oral dose of the ginkgolide mixture (BN 52063) inhibits the oedema induced by intradermal PAF in normal healthy [12] and atopic volunteers [36]. Perhaps of more interest is that in the latter study, an oral dose also

attenuates allergen-induced oedema 15 minutes after i.d. allergen in allergic subjects, which suggests that PAF may be one of the mediators contributing to the acute inflammatory response following allergen administration. No such investigations have been reported in the lung of allergic volunteers, although no inhibition of allergen-induced oedema formation in the bronchial circulation of sensitised guinea-pigs is observed in the presence of PAF antagonists [37, 38].

A preliminary clinical study has also revealed that the ginkgolide mixture BN 50263 is able to reduce the cutaneous late-onset response following local allergen challenge of atopic volunteers [36], an event known to be associated with both the infiltration of inflammatory cells and the release of PAF [39]. However, at this point in time, no direct clinical evidence has been reported demonstrating the effect of PAF antagonists on allergen-induced cellular infiltration in humans, although, as mentioned, various studies in experimental animals have reported an inhibitory effect of PAF antagonists on allergen-induced eosinophil infiltration.

Conclusions

Since the discovery of PAF in the early 1970s, a considerable body of evidence has accumulated on the putative role of this mediator in the allergic response. The ability of PAF to mimic just about all the features of allergic inflammation, particularly the ability of this phospholipid to induce eosinophil infiltration in a comparable manner to allergen, suggests that this mediator may be central to maintaining eosinophil infiltration characterizing allergic inflammatory lesions. The availability of a number of PAF antagonists should not only provide useful tools to test this hypothesis in the clinical arena, but will hopefully lead to the development of anti-allergic and anti-inflammatory drugs.

References

1. Barbaro, J. F., and N. J. Zweifler. 1966. Antigen-induced histamine release from platelets and rabbits producing homologous PCA antibody. Proc. Soc. Exp. Biol. Med. 122: 1245.

2. Benveniste, J., P. M. Henson, and C. G. Cochrane. 1972. Leucocyte histamine release from rabbit platelets: The role of IgE, basophils and a platelet activating factor. J. Exp. Med. 136: 1356.

3. Braquet, P., L. Touqui, T. Y. Shen, and B. B. Vargaftig. 1987. Perspectives in platelet-activating factor research. Pharmacol. Rev. 39: 97.

4. Synder, F. 1985. Chemical and biochemical aspects of platelet activating factor: A novel class of acetylated ether-linked choline phospholipids. Med. Res. Rev. 5: 107.

5. Lee, T., D. J. Lenihan, B. Malone, L. L. Roddy, and S. I. Wasserman. 1984. Increased biosynthesis of platelet-activating factor in activated human eosinophils. J. Biol. Chem. 259: 5526.

6. Terashita, Z., S. Tsushima, Y. Yoshioka, H. Nomura, Y. Inada, and K. Nishikawa. 1983. CV-3988, a specific antagonist of platelet activating factor (PAF). Life Sci. 32: 1975.

7. Arnout, J., A. Van Hecken, I. de Lepeleire, Y. Miyamato, I. Holmes, P. de Schepper, and J. Vermylen. 1988. Effectiveness and tolerability of CV-3988, a selective PAF antagonist, after intravenous administration to man. Br. J. Clin. Pharmacol. 25: 445.

8. Shen, T. Y., S.-B. Hwang, M. N. Chang, T. W. Doebber, M. H. T. Lam, M. S. Wu, X. Wang, G. G. Han, and R. Z. Li. 1985. Characterisation of a platelet activating factor receptor antagonist isolated from haifentent (*Piper futokadsura*): Specific inhibition of in vitro and in vivo platelet-activating factor-induced effects. Proc. Natl. Acad. Sci. U.S.A. 82: 672.

9. Hwang, S.-B., M.-H. Lam, T. Biftu, T. R. Beattie, and S. Y. Shen. 1985. Trans-2,5-bis(3,4,5-trimethoxyphenyl) tetrahydrofuran. An orally active specific and competitive receptor antagonist of platelet activating factor. J. Biol. Chem. 260: 15639.

10. Hwang, S.-B., M.-H. Lam, A. W. Alberts, R. L. Bugianesi, J. C. Chabala, and M. M. Ponpipom. 1988. Biochemical and pharmacological characterization of L-659,989: An extremely potent, selective and competitive receptor antagonist of platelet activating factor. J. Pharmacol. Exp. Ther. 246: 534.

11. Hosford, D., J. M. Mencia-Huerta, C. P. Page, and P. Braquet. 1988. Natural antagonists of platelet activating factor. Phytotherapy Res. 2: 1.

12. Chung, K. F., M. McCusker, C. P. Page, G. Dent, Ph. Guinot, and P. J. Barnes. 1987. Effect of a ginkgolide mixture (BN 52063) in antagonising skin and platelet responses to platelet activating factor in man. Lancet i: 248.

13. Lefort, J., P. Sedivy, S. Desquand, J. Randon, E. Coeffier, I. Maridonneau-Parini, A. Floch, J. Benveniste, and B. B. Vargaftig. 1988. Pharmacological profile of 48740 R.P., a PAF-acether antagonist. Eur. J. Pharmacol. 150: 257.

14. Robaut, C., G. Durand, C. James, D. Lave, P. Sedivy, A. Floch, S. Mondot, D. Pacot, I. Cavero, and G. Le Fur. 1987. PAF binding sites. Characterization by [^{3}H]52770 RP, a pyrrolo[1,2-c]thiazole derivative, in rabbit platelets. Biochem. Pharmacol. 36: 3221.

15. Robaut, C., S. Mondot, A. Floch, L. Tarhaoui, and I. Cavero. 1988. Pharmacological profile of a novel potent and specific PAF receptor antagonist, the 59227 RP. Prostaglandins 35: 838.

16. Sedivy, P., S. Weber, J. Gregoire, F. Gaisne, G. Strauch, D. de Lauture, and D. Floch. 48740 RP inhibits PAF-induced platelet aggregation and thromboxane B2 generation ex-vivo in volunteers. Clin. Exp. Physiol. Pharmacol., in press.

17. Kornecki, E., Y. H. Ehrlich, and R. H. Lenox. 1985. Platelet activating factor induced aggregation of human platelets specifically inhibited by triazolobenzodiazepines. Science 226: 1954.

18. Casals-Stenzel, J., and K.-H. Weber. 1987. Triazolobenzodiazepines: Dissociation of their PAF (platelet activating factor) antagonistic and CNS activity. Br. J. Pharmacol. 90: 139.

19. Casals-Stenzel, J., G. Muacevic, and K.-H. Weber. 1987. Pharmacological actions of WEB 2086, a new specific antagonist of platelet activating factor. J. Pharmacol. Exp. Ther. 241: 974.

20. Adamus, W. S., H. Heuer, C. J. Meade, V. Haselbarth, and H. M. Brecht. 1988. Tolerability, safety and efficacy of WEB 2086 in healthy human volunteers. Allergy (Suppl. 7) 43: 124.

21. Wardlaw, A. J., R. Moqbel, O. Cromwell, and A. B. Kay. 1986. Platelet activating factor: A potent chemotactic and chemokinetic factor for human eosinophils. J. Clin. Invest. 78: 1701.

22. Henocq, E., and B. B. Vargaftig. 1986. Accumulation of eosinophils in response to intracutaenous PAF-acether and allergens in man. Lancet ii: 1378.

23. Lellouch-Tubiana, A., J. Lefort, M.-T. Simon, A. Pfister, and P. B. Vargaftig. 1988. Eosinophil recruitment into guinea-pig lungs after PAF-acether and allergen administration. Am. Rev. Respir. Dis. 137: 948.

24. Capron, M., J. Benveniste, P. Braquet, and A. Capron. 1988. The role of Paf-acether in IgE-dependent activation of eosinophils. New Trends Lipid Mediator Res. 2: 10.

25. Coyle, A. J., S. C. Urwin, C. P. Page, C. Touvay, B. Villain, and P. Braquet. 1988. The effect of the selective PAF antagonist BN 52021 on PAF- and antigen-induced bronchial hyperreactivity and eosinophil accumulation. Eur. J. Pharmacol. 148: 51.

26. Hutson, P. A., S. T. Holgate, and M. K. Church. 1988. Effect of WEB 2086 on early and late airways responses to ovalbumin challenge in con-

59

scious guinea-pigs. Proc. Pharmacol. Soc., 7th–9th September, University of Nottingham, C76.

27. Smith, H. R., P. M. Henson, K. L. Clay, and G. L. Larsen. 1988. Effect of the PAF antagonist L-659,989 on the late asthmatic response and increased airway reactivity in the rabbit. Am. Rev. Respir. Dis. 137: 283.

28. Frigas, E., and G. J. Gleich. 1986. The eosinophil and the pathophysiology of asthma. J. Allergy Clin. Immunol. 77: 527.

29. Barnes, P. J., K. F. Chung, and C. P. Page. 1988. Inflammatory mediators and asthma. Pharmacol. Rev. 40: 49.

30. Flavahan, N. A., N. R. Slifman, G. J. Gleich, and P. M. Vanhoutte. 1988. Human eosinophil derived major basic protein causes hyperreactivity of respiratory smooth muscle. Am. Rev. Respir. Dis. 138: 685.

31. Cuss, F. M., C. M. S. Dixon, and P. J. Barnes. 1986. Effect of inhaled platelet activating factor on pulmonary function and bronchial responsiveness in man. Lancet ii: 189.

32. Andersson, M., and U. Pipkorn. 1988. Platelet activating factor: A mediator of nasal hyperreactivity. XIII International Congress of Allergology and Clinical Immunology. A778.

33. Darius, H., D. J. Lefer, B. Smith, and A. M. Lefer. 1986. Role of platelet activating factor in mediating guinea-pig anaphylaxis. Science 232: 58.

34. Casals-Stenzel, J. 1987. Effects of WEB 2086, a novel antagonist of platelet activating factor in active and passive anaphylaxis. Immunopharmacol. 3: 7.

35. Pretolani, M., J. Lefort, E. Malanchere, and B. B. Vargaftig. 1987. Interference by the novel PAF-acether antagonist WEB 2086 with the bronchopulmonary responses to PAF-acether and to active and passive anaphylactic shock in guinea-pigs. Eur. J. Pharmacol. 140: 311.

36. Roberts, N. M., C. P. Page, K. F. Chung, and P. J. Barnes. 1988. Effect of a PAF antagonist, BN 52063, on antigen-induced acute and late-onset cutaneous responses in atopic subjects. J. Allergy Clin. Immunol. 82: 236.

37. Evans, T. W., G. Dent, D. F. Rogers, B., Aursudkij, K. F. Chung, and P. J. Barnes. 1988. Effect of a Paf antagonist, WEB 2086, on airway microvascular leakage in the guinea-pig and platelet aggregation in man. Br. J. Pharmacol. 94: 164.

38. Evans, T. W., D. F. Rogers, B. Aursudkij, K. F. Chung, and P. J. Barnes. 1988. Inflammatory mediators involved in antigen-induced airway microvascular leakage in guinea-pigs. Am. Rev. Respir. Dis. 138: 395.

39. Michel, L., Y. Denizot, Y. Thomas, J. Benveniste, and L. Dubertret. 1988. Release of Paf-acether and precursors during allergic cutaneous reactions. Lancet ii: 404.

Activation of the Kinin-Forming Pathways in Allergic Diseases

*Allen P. Kaplan, Sesha Reddigari, Michael Silverberg**

Release of tissue kallikrein causes digestion of LMW-kininogen to release kalliden (lysyl bradykinin), which is converted to bradykinin by a plasma aminopeptidase. Bradykinin can be formed directly by contact activation of plasma. In this pathway, Hageman factor autoactivates upon contact with certain negatively charged molecules (e.g., connective tissue proteoglygrans or mast cell heparin), and converts prekallikrein to kallikrein. HMW-kininogen circulates bound to prekallikrein and acts as a co-factor to accelerate conversion to kallikrein. The HMW-kininogen is then digested by kallikrein to generate bradykinin. The enzymes, activated Hageman factor, and kallikrein are inactivated by plasma inhibitors while kininases such as carboxyreptidase N and angiotensin converting enzyme destroy bradykinin.

Assessment of this system in clinical disease can use newly developed assays, including quantitation of complexes which consist of activated Hageman factor-C1 INH, kallikrein-C1 IHN, and kallikrein-α_2 macroglobulin. Cleavage of HMW-kininogen is quantitated by immunoblotting using a monoclonal antibody directed to its light chain, and bradykinin is measured by radioimmunoassay. Tissue kallikrein is assessed by cleavage of synthetic substrates. There is evidence of formation of bradykinin and lysyl bradykinin upon antigen challenge of patients with allergic rhinitis during the acute response as well as the late phase reaction with evidence of tissue kallikrein release and plasma kallikrein formation. Late phase cutaneous reactions are associated with activation of the Hageman factor dependent pathway as assessed by the generation of activated HF-C1 INH and kallikrein-C1 INH complexes. Patients with hereditary angioedema lack C1-INH and have episodes of swelling that appear to be mediated by bradykinin. The plasma is readily activated such that HMW-kininogen is cleaved and bradykinin is generated under conditions in which normal plasma yields no demonstrable response. Kinin formation therefore appears to be among the vasoactive substances released in wide variety of allergic disorders as well as circumstances in which level of control proteins is diminished.

Introduction

Allergic reactions are associated with the release of a wide variety of vasoactive mediators, among which are histamine, leukotrienes C4 and D4, platelet-activating factor (PAF), and prostaglandin D2. As we have come to appreciate late phase reactions, it is clear that a more prolonged inflammatory response is possible because of the release of chemotactic factors and/or other substances that promote cell recruitment. These cells may become activated, and in some tissues, this is associated with a second wave of histamine release. Whenever there is an acute inflammatory response such as this with its attendant tissue injury, there may be release of tissue kallikrein to form bradykinin. As a result of the increase in vascular permeability, plasma dilution, and contact with either negatively charged surfaces or macromolecules, the plasma coagulation-kinin system may also be activated and thereby contribute to the inflammatory response. In this paper, I review the various mechanisms by which kinins can be generated, discuss the methods used to assess the system in human disease, and review recent data regarding bradykinin formation in IgE-mediated reactions and in C1 inactivator deficiency.

Formation and Degradation of Kinin

Bradykinin can be generated either by cleavage of low molecular weight (LMW) kininogen by tissue kallikrein or by activation of the plasma proteolytic cascade (Figure 1). This latter pro-

* Division of Allergy, Rheumatology, and Clinical Immunology, Department of Medicine, Health Sciences Center, SUNY—Stony Brook, Stony Brook, NY 11794.

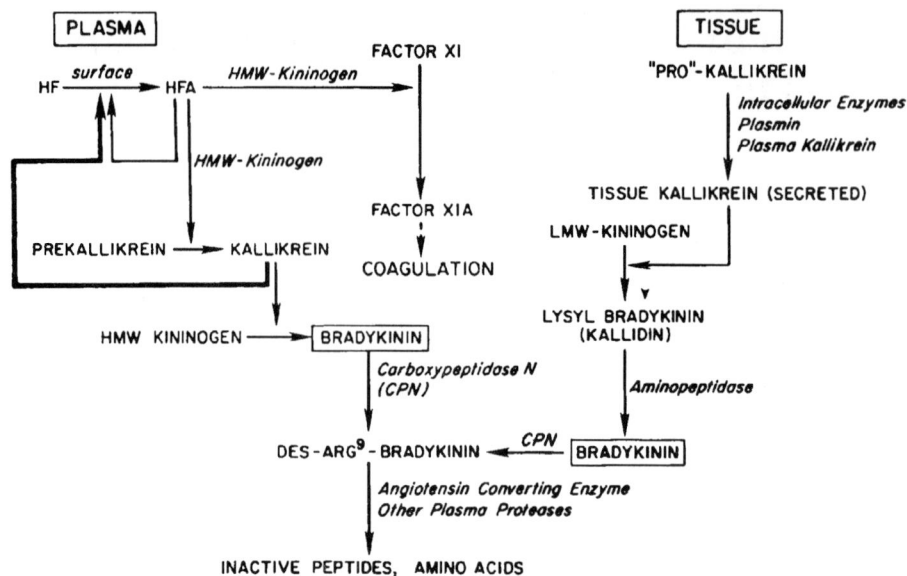

Figure 1. Schematic outline of the plasma and tissue pathways of kinin formation and degradation.

cess is known as "contact activation" as it is initiated by the interaction of plasma proteins with certain negatively charged surfaces and results in blood coagulation [1].

From the point of view of blood coagulation, the initiation step requires the interaction of three plasma proteins, namely, Hageman factor (Coagulation Factor XII), prekallikrein, and a high molecular weight form of kininogen (HMW-kininogen). These are the same three proteins that are requisite for the formation of bradykinin, and the interaction of all three is required for optimal activation of Hageman factor. The second step in blood coagulation is the conversion of Factor XI to Factor XIa by HFa; Factor XIa then activates Factor IX to continue the intrinsic coagulation pathway.

The initiating surface in an allergic reaction is likely to be connective tissue proteoglycans [2] or, perhaps, mast cell heparin [3]. Hageman factor (HF) binds directly to the surface [4], and circulating complexes of prekallikrein-HMW kininogen [5] and Factor XI-HMW kininogen [6] bind to adjacent sites. The Hageman factor can autoactivate once bound [7], and this may generate sufficient HFa for the reactions to proceed. As shown in Figure 1, prekallikrein is converted to kallikrein, and the attached HMW-kininogen (shown along the arrow) catalyzes the reaction, i.e., its presence accelerates the formation of kallikrein [9, 10]. Kallikrein,

once formed, then has a positive feedback reaction, in which it rapidly activates the remaining Hageman factor [11, 12]. The reaction is 50–100 times more rapid than the HF autoactivation, and it is therefore the major mechanism by which HFa is generated [12, 13]. By this feedback, HF activation is kallikrein-dependent and, indirectly, dependent upon HMW-kininogen. Kallikrein also cleaves the HMW-kininogen to form bradykinin while HFa then activates Factor XI. HMW-kininogen bound to the Factor XI substrate catalyzes this reaction in a fashion analogous to prekallikrein activation.

The tissue kallikrein cascade is dependent upon release of a kallikrein that is completely distinct from plasma kallikrein [14]. The same protein is found in various glandular tissues (salivary, pancreas, pituitary) as well as mucous/serous secreting glands; a kallikrein-like enzyme has also been described in basophils and mast cells [15], but it is not clear whether this is identical to tissue kallikrein. Tissue kallikrein is synthesized within the cell as a precursor, and cleavage of an amino-terminal peptide converts it to an active enzyme [16]. Once secreted, tissue kallikrein acts on low molecular weight kininogen (LMW-kininogen) to generate lysylbradykinin (kallidin). This kinin possesses most of the functions of bradykinin, but a plasma aminopeptidase rapidly removes the lysine to form bradykinin. The formation of lysyl bradykinin, therefore, implies release of a tissue kallikrein, while direct demonstration of bradykinin could occur by either pathway (or both). Bradykinin is rapidly inactivated by plasma proteases as well as tissue proteases (primarily pulmonary). In plasma, carboxypeptidase N rapidly removes the C-terminal arginine to form des-arg^9-bradykinin [17], and angiotensin converting enzyme (ACE) more slowly converts the eight amino acid peptide to a pentapeptide (arg-pro-pro-gly-phe) plus a tripeptide (ser-pro-phe) [18]; each of these is then further degraded such that arg-pro-pro and free amino acids are the final products [19]. In the pulmonary circulation, ACE predominates, and it removes the C-terminal phe-arg from bradykinin followed by ser-pro to form the above pentapeptide.

Assessment of the Kinin-Forming System in Human Disease

Since bradykinin is degraded rapidly, it is difficult to assess its generation in human disease. When experimental challenge can be done, meaningful results are more likely than when samples are taken during the course of an illness, since the course of bradykinin formation can be controlled and degradation can be prevented by adding kininase inhibitors to the samples. Regardless, sensitive and specific methods are needed so that the enzymes that generate kinin and the kininogen substrate can be assessed. Activated Hageman factor binds to C1-inactivator (C1-INH) to form a complex and kallikrein is inactivated by binding to C1-INH and to α_2 macroglobulin. We have developed assays for quantitation of each of these complexes in collaboration with Dr. Peter Harpel (Cornell Medical Center, New York). Tissue kallikrein can be quantified directly using synthetic substrates since its inactivation is relatively slow and no major plasma inhibitor has been identified. For each molecule of bradykinin that is generated, HMW-kininogen is cleaved to convert it from 140,000 in non-reduced SDS gels, to 103,000 and then 96,000 [20]. When reduced, the cleavage products fragment to a heavy chain of 60,000 and light chains of 56,000 and 49,000, respectively [20]. Using a monoclonal antibody to the light chain, we have recently developed an immunoblotting

assay for HMW-kininogen which can detect as little as 2% change in non-reduced gels. The sum of the 103,000 plus 96,000 bands divided by the 140,000 band gives the fraction cleaved [21]. A summary of these methods, as applied to human disease, is given in Table 1. An analogous assay for cleaved HMW-kininogen has not yet been developed, but would be an adjunct to assessment of the tissue kallikrein pathway. An assay for des-arg^9 bradykinin, the rate-limiting plasma degradation product, has been developed [22], but has not been applied to disease states; since tissue inactivation, in which ACE predominates, may be more rapid than plasma inactivation, the ultimate utility of this assay is uncertain.

Table 1. Assessment of kinin-forming pathways in human disease.

1. Assay for tissue kallikrein by cleavage of synthetic substrates [23].

2. Measure complex of activated Hageman factor and C1-INH by double antibody ELISA assay [24].

3. Measure complex of plasma kallikrein and C1-INH by double antibody ELISA assay [25].

4. Measure complex of plasma-kallikrein-α_2 by macroglobulin [26].

5. Quantitate cleaved HMW-kininogen by immunoblotting [21].

6. Measure bradykinin by radioimmunoassay [27].

The Role of Kinins in Allergic Disease

The Hageman factor-dependent pathway and the tissue kallikrein pathway have been shown to contribute to inflammation in a wide variety of diseases. Many of these are allergic in nature, i.e., either dependent initially upon IgE antibody or on inflammatory disorders commonly treated by allergist-immunologists. Antigen challenge of patients with allergic rhinitis has demonstrated that both bradykinin and lysylbradykinin are present in secretions [28] as is high and low molecular weight kininogen [29]. Since lysylbradykinin is present, a tissue kallikrein must be released, and further investigation has shown one or more enzymes with tissue kallikrein-like activity to be present [30].

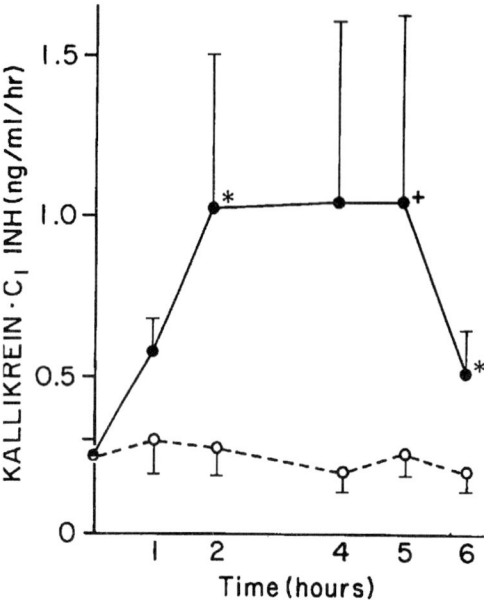

Figure 2. Kallikrein-C1 INH complexes (ordinate) detected in skin chamber fluid after antigen (●——●, mean and SEM) and buffer (O——O) incubation from 0 to 6 h (on abscissa) in the 10 subjects. *p < 0.056, Walsh test; +p < 0.025, Walsh test.

The source may be from mucosal glands which are stimulated to secrete, or from nasal mast cells. The bradykinin seen could result from aminopeptidase action on lysylbradykinin or from activation of the Hageman factor-dependent pathway. Plasma kallikrein was also then shown to be present in nasal secretions [31], suggesting that both kinin-forming pathways are involved. A similar assessment of bronchoalveolar lavage fluid of antigen-challenged asthmatics demonstrated the presence of tissue kallikrein and, to a variable degree, plasma kallikrein [32]. Such studies suggest that kinins may participate in the acute phase of virtually all allergic reactions; however, these studies have sought the presence of active enzymes in a challenge situation. The methods listed in Table 1 would allow a more global assessment of this cascade and are applicable to nonchallenged patients who are exposed to allergen by natural means. It is also of interest that a study of the antigen-induced late-phase reaction in the nose demonstrated release of the same group of vasoactive substances as did the acute reaction (except PGD_2) including the formation of kinin [33].

We have studied the late-phase cutaneous allergic reactions utilizing the skin blister chamber technique [34, 35] in collaboration with Drs. Paul Atkins and Burton Zweiman of the University of Pennsylvania. We have demonstrated the formation of complexes of kallikrein-C1-INH (Figure 2) and activated Hageman factor-C1-INH in the chambers between two and six hours, a time course that coincides with the development of late-phase reactions. The interstitial fluid of skin has been shown to possess the various proteins of the Hageman factor-dependent pathway, and the mast cell proteoglycan dilation by edema fluid and/or exposure to connective tissue elements serve to activate this cascade. Thus, although many cell types and vasoactive substances interact to cause the late-phase reaction, recruitment of the plasma kinin-forming pathway must also be considered contributory to the inflammatory reaction.

Hereditary angioedema is a disorder in which activation of the plasma kinin-forming system may be the key event that causes the swelling. Early studies by Talamo et al. [36] suggested elevated bradykinin levels in patients during attacks of swelling; however, the assay used was far less discriminatory than present methods. In recent years, induced skin

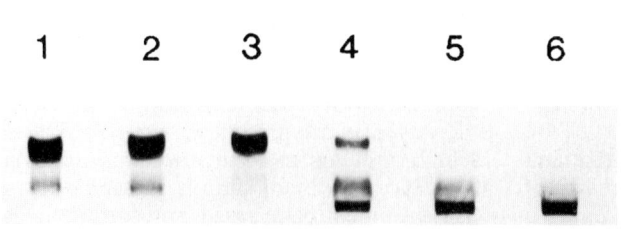

Figure 3. Cleavage of HMWK in HAE plasma upon activation by dextran sulfate. Effect of time of incubation with dextran sulfate. NHP (lanes 1 and 2) or HAE plasma (lanes 3–6) were incubated with 10 µg/ml dextran sulfate for 0 (lanes 1 & 3), 4 (lane 4), 8 (lane 5), and 16 (lanes 2 & 6) minutes at 37 °C.

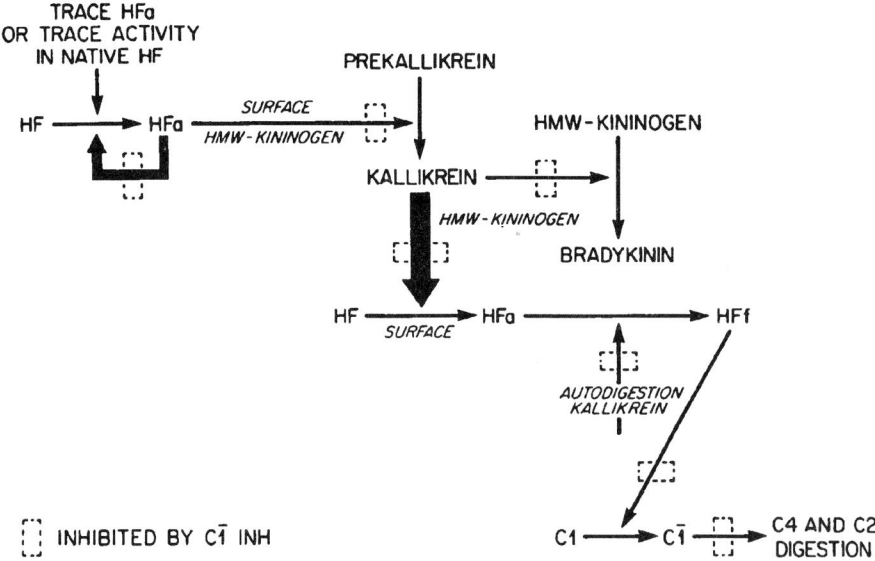

Figure 4. Diagrammatic representation of the plasma Hageman factor-dependent pathway to indicate all steps inhibitable by C1 INH. The HF autoactivation step is followed by the kallikrein feedback loop after which bradykinin is formed and HF is fragmented. Also shown is the ability of HFf to enzymatically cleave and activate the C1r subcomponent of C1 to thereby activate C1.

blisters of patients have been shown to contain plasma kallikrein when compared to control blisters [37], and the plasma of patients has been shown to be unstable and gradually evolve kinin upon incubation at 37°C [38, 39]. In Figure 3 is shown an immunoblotting assay for cleaved HMW-kininogen in hereditary angioedema plasma compared to normal plasma using a dose of dextran sulfate which is ineffective as a plasma activator when tested at 37°C. Whereas normal plasma showed no cleavage of HMW-kininogen after 16 min, progressive cleavage in hereditary angioedema plasma is evident. All such studies emphasize the ready activation of the Hageman factor-dependent cascades when C1-INH is absent on a familial basis (hereditary angioedema) or when it is depleted in acquired disorders such as lymphoma, connective tissue disorders, or production of autoantibody directed to C1-INH. While a Hageman factor-dependent kinin-like molecule has been reported to be a product of complement activation (either from C2 or C2b) [40, 41], the factor has never been identified.

In Figure 4 is shown a more detailed diagrammatic representation of the plasma kinin-forming system, indicating those steps that can be inhibited by C1-INH. The C1-INH is the sole effective inhibitor of activated Hageman factor in plasma and therefore inhibits HF autoactivation and the activation of prekallikrein by HFa. It is one of two plasma inhibitors of kallikrein and therefore inhibits the feedback activation of HF by kallikrein as well as the ability of kallikrein to cleave HMW-kininogen. Once HFa is formed, it can be cleaved further to active fragments (HFf) [42] that lack the binding site for the surface and are no longer effective activators of Factor XI, but do retain the ability to activate prekallikrein in the fluid phase [43]. HFf has also been shown to enzymatically activate the C1S subcomponent of complement [43]. Thus, although C1 is unstable and autoactivates in the absence of C1-INH [44], HFf can augment the process and all such steps are inhibited by C1-INH. It appears that C1-INH deficiency renders the kinin-forming pathway exceedingly labile, such that relatively minor trauma or other such insults can cause activation in hereditary angioedema. Since the hereditary disorder is inherited as a dominant trait, the remaining normal C1-INH gene is functional. But levels are far less than 50% of normal because of hypercatabolism

[45], and when the level is less than 25% of normal, attacks are much more likely to occur. Androgenic compounds not used to treat hereditary angioedema (Danazol, Stanazolol) appear to raise C1-INH levels and thereby dampen the process [46, 47].

References

1. Silverberg, M., and A. P. Kaplan. 1988. The coagulation-kinin pathway of human plasma. Blood 70: 1.
2. Silverberg, M., and S. Diehl. 1987. The autoactivation of Factor XII (Hageman factor) induced by low-mr heparin and dextran sulfate. Biochem. J. 248: 715.
3. Hojimay, C. G. Cochrane, R. C. Wiggins, K. F. Austen, and R. L. Stevens. 1984. In vitro activation of the contact (Hageman factor) system of plasma by heparin and chondoitin sulfate E. Blood 63: 1453.
4. Revak, S. D., and C. G. Cochrane. 1976. The relationship of structure and function in human Hageman factor, the association of enzymatic and binding activities with separate regions of the molecule. J. Clin. Invest. 57: 852.
5. Mandle, R. J., Jr., R. W. Colman, and A. P. Kaplan. 1976. Identification of prekallikrein and HMW-kininogen as a circulating complex in human plasma. Proc. Natl. Acad. Sci. 73: 4174.
6. Thompson, R. E., R. J. Mandle, Jr., and A. P. Kaplan. 1977. Association of factor XI and high molecular weight kininogen in human plasma. J. Clin. Invest. 60: 1376.
7. Silverberg, M., J. T. Dunn, L. Garen, and A. P. Kaplan. 1980. Autoactivation of human Hageman factor—Demonstration utilizing a synthetic substrate. J. Biol. Chem. 255: 7281.
8. Mandle, R. J., Jr., and A. P. Kaplan. 1977. Hageman factor substrates: Human plasma prekallikrein: Mechanism of activation by Hageman factor and participation in Hageman factor dependent fibrinolysis. J. Biol. Chem. 252: 6097.
9. Giffin, J. H., and C. G. Cochrane. 1976. Mechanisms for the involvement of high molecular weight kininogen in surface-dependent reactions of Hageman factor. Proc. Natl. Acad. Sci. 73: 2559.
10. Meier, H. L., J. V. Pierce, and A. P. Kaplan. 1977. Activation and function of human Hageman factor—The role of high molecular weight kininogen and prekallikrein. J. Clin. Invest. 60: 18.
11. Cochrane, C. G., and K. D. Wuepper. 1973. Activation of Hageman factor in solid and fluid phase. J. Exp. Med. 138: 1564.
12. Dunn, J. T., M. Silverberg, and A. P. Kaplan. 1982. The cleavage and formation of activated Hageman factor by autodigestion and by kallikrein. J. Biol. Chem. 257: 1779.
13. Tankersley, D. L., and J: S. Finlayson. 1984. Kinetics of activation and autoactivation of human factor XII. Biochem. 23: 273.
14. Fukushima, D., N. Kitamura, and S. Nakanishi. 1985. Nucleotide sequence of cloned c-DNA for human pancreatic kallikrein. Biochem. 24: 8037.
15. Proud, D., D. W. MacGlashan, Jr., H. H. Newball, E. S. Schulman, and L. M. Lichtenstein. 1985. Immunoglobulin E-mediated release of a kininogenase from purified human lung mast cells. Am. Rev. Resp. Dis. 132: 405.
16. Takada, Y., R. A. Skidgel, and E. G. Erdos. 1985. Purification of human urinary prekallikrein, identification of the site of activation by the metalloproteinase thermolysin. Biochem. J. 232: 851.
17. Sheikh, I., and A. P. Kaplan. 1986. Studies on the digestion of bradykinin, lysylbradykinin, and kinin degradation products by carboxypeptidases A, B., and N. Biochem. Pharmacol. 35: 1957.
18. Sheikh, I., and A. P. Kaplan. 1986. Studies of the digestion of bradykinin, lysylbradykinin, and des-arg^9-bradykinin by angiotensin converting enzyme. Biochem. Pharmacol. 36: 1951.
19. Sheikh, I., and A. P. Kaplan. 1988. The mechanism of digestion of bradykinin and lysylbradykinin (kallidin) in human serum: The role of carboxypeptidase, angiotensin converting enzyme, and determination of final degradation products. Biochem. Pharmacol., in press.
20. Reddigari, S., and A. P. Kaplan. 1988. Cleavage of human high-molecular weight kininogen by purified kallikreins and upon contact activation of plasma. Blood 71: 1334.
21. Reddigari, S., and A. P. Kaplan. A quantitative assay for cleaved human high molecular weight kininogen as assessed by immunoblotting with anti light chain monoclonal anti-ser. J. Immunol. Methods, in press.
22. Odya, C. E., P. Moreland, J. M. Stewart, J. Barabe, and D. C. Regoli. 1986. Development of a radioimmunoassay for des-arg^9 bradykinin. Biochem. Pharmacol. 35: 1951.
23. Geiger, R., and H. Fritz. 1981. In: Methods of enzymology, Vol. 80, Proteolytic enzymes, Part C. L. Lorand, ed. New York: Academic Press, pp. 466–492.
24. Kaplan, A. P., B. Gruber, and P. Harpel. 1985. Assessment of Hageman factor activation in human plasma: Quantification of activated Hageman factor-C1 inactivator complexes by an enzyme linked differential antibody immunosorbent assay. Blood 66: 636.
25. Lewin, M. F., A. P. Kaplan, and P. C. Harpel. 1983. Studies of C1 inactivator-plasma kallikrein complexes in purified systems and in plasma.

Quantification by an enzyme-linked differential antibody immunosorbent assay. J. Biol. Chem. 238: 6415.

26. Harpel, P. C., M. F. Lewin, and A. P. Kaplan. 1985. Distribution of plasma kallikrein between C1 inactivator and α_2 macroglobulin-kallikrein complexes. J. Biol. Chem. 260: 4257.

27. Shimamoto, K., I. Ando, I. Nakao, S. Tanaka, M. Sakuma, and M. Miyahora. 1978. A sensitive radioimmunoassay method for urinary kinins in man. J. Lab. Clin. Med. 91: 721.

28. Proud, D., A. Togias, R. M. Naclerio, S. B. Crush, P. S. Norman, and L. M. Lichtenstein. 1983. Kinins are generated in-vivo following nasal airway challenge of allergic individuals with allergen. J. Clin. Invest. 72: 1678.

29. Baumgarten, C. R., A. G. Togias, R. M. Naclerio, L. M. Lichtenstein, P. S. Norman, and D. Proud. 1983. Influx of kininogens into nasal secretions after antigen challenge of allergic individuals. J. Clin. Invest. 76: 191.

30. Baumgarten, C. R., R. C. Nichols, R. M. Naclerio, and D. Proud. 1986. Concentrations of glandular kallikrein in human nasal secretions increase during experimentally induced allergic rhinitis. J. Immunol. 137: 1323.

31. Baumgarten, C. R., R. C. Nichols, R. M. Naclerio, L. M. Lichtenstein, P. S. Norman, and D. Proud. 1986. Plasma kallikrein during experimental-induced allergic rhinitis: Role in kinin formation and contribution to TAME-esterase activity in nasal secretions. J. Immunol. 137: 977.

32. Christianson, S. C., D. Proud, and C. G. Cochrane. 1987. Detection of tissue kallikrein in the bronchoalveolar lavage fluids of asthmatic subjects. J. Clin. Invest. 79: 188.

33. Naclerio, R. M., D. Proud, A. G. Togias, N. F. Adkinson, Jr., P. A. Meyers, A. Kagey-Sabotka, M. Plaut, P. S. Norman, and L. M. Lichtenstein. 1985. Inflammatory mediators in late antigen-induced rhinitis. N. Engl. J. Med. 313: 65.

34. Talbot, S. F., P. C. Atkins, M. Valenzano, and B. Zweiman. 1980. Patterns of mast cell alterations and in-vivo mediator release in human allergic skin reactions. J. Allergy Clin. Immunol. 66: 417.

35. Atkins, P. C., G. Miragliotta, S. F. Talbot, B. Zweiman, and A. P. Kaplan. 1987. Activation of plasma Hageman factor and kallikrein in ongoing allergic reactions in the skin. J. Immunol. 139: 2744.

36. Talamo, R. C., E. Haber, and K. F. Austen. 1969. A radioimmunoassay for bradykinin in plasma and synovial fluid. J. Lab. Clin. Med. 74: 816.

37. Curd, S. G., L. D. Prograis, Jr., and C. G. Cochrane. 1980. Detection of active kallikrein in induced blister fluids of hereditary angioedema patients. J. Exp. Med. 152: 242.

38. Fields, T., B. Ghebrehiwet, and A. P. Kaplan. 1983. Kinin formation in hereditary angioedema plasma: Evidence against kinin derivation from C2 and in support of "spontaneous" formation of bradykinin. J. Allergy Clin. Immunol. 72: 54.

39. Curd, S. G., M. Yelvington, N. Burridge, N. P. Stimler, G. Gerard, L. J. Prograis, Jr., C. G. Cochrane, and H. J. Muller-Eberhard. 1983. Generation of bradykinin during incubation of hereditary angioedema plasma. Molec. Immunol. 19: 1365.

40. Donaldson, V. H. 1967. Mechanism of activation of C1 esterase in hereditary angioneurotic edema in vitro—The role of Hageman factor, a clot promoting agent. J. Exp. Med. 127: 411.

41. Donaldson, V. H., F. S. Rosen, and D. H. Bing. 1977. Role of the second component of complement (C2) and plasmin in kinin release in hereditary angioneurotic edema plasma. Trans. Assoc. Am. Physicians 40: 174.

42. Kaplan, A. P., and K. F. Austen. 1970. A prealbumin activator of prekallikrein. J. Immunol. 105: 802.

43. Ghebrehiwet, B., B. P. Randazzo, J. T. Dunn, M. Silverberg, and A. P. Kaplan. 1983. Mechanism of activation of the classical pathway of complement by Hageman factor fragment. J. Clin. Invest. 71: 1450.

44. Ziccardi, R. J. 1982. Spontaneous activation of the first component of human complement (C1) by an intramolecular autocatalytic mechanism. J. Immunol. 128: 2500.

45. Quastel, J., R. Harrison, M. Cicardi, C. A. Alper, and F. S. Rosen. 1983. Behavior in-vivo of normal and dysfunctional C1-inhibitor in normal subjects and patients with hereditary angioedema. J. Clin. Invest. 71: 1041.

46. Gelfand, J. A., R. J. Sherins, D. W. Alling, and M. M. Frank. 1976. Treatment of hereditary angioedema with danazol—Reversal of clinical and biochemical abnormalities. N. Engl. J. Med. 295: 1444.

47. Sheffer, A. L., D. T. Fearon, and K. F. Austen. 1987. Hereditary angioedema: A decade of management with stanazolol. J. Allergy Clin. Immunol. 80: 855.

Role of Nerves and Other Local Environmental Factors in Mast Cell Regulation

John Bienenstock, Michael G. Blennerhassett*, Yasunori Kakuta*,
Shinishi Kawabori*, Glenda MacQueen**, Jean S. Marshall*, Mary H. Perdue*,
Shepard Siegel**, Ron H. Stead*, Motoaki Tomioka**

Mast cells are often found in increased numbers in tissues in which inflammation is occurring. There is significant literature that suggests that mast cells and nerves are often found in close association. We present here some recent evidence suggesting a purposeful functional association between mast cells and nerves. Not only do mast cells communicate with nerves, but it appears that nerves can also communicate with mast cells. A hypothesis is suggested in which mast cells sensitized to environmental antigens through passive binding of IgE and IgG antibodies to their Fc receptors can communicate information to the peripheral, and thereby to the central nervous system, concerning the extent to which these local antigens are interacting with

them. Through this mechanism, axon reflexes can be initiated and influence the epithelium, smooth muscle, and other structures in their immediate vicinity. There is evidence—although it is controversial—that stimulation of nerves can cause mast cell degranulation. Furthermore, psychological conditioning of rats for mast cell degranulation upon exposure solely to the conditioning stimulus has recently been shown to occur. Thus, a bi-directional input between mast cells and the nervous system has been demonstrated. The extent to which this may be regulated and controlled, and the extent to which it occurs under normal physiological conditions, remains to be more completely evaluated.

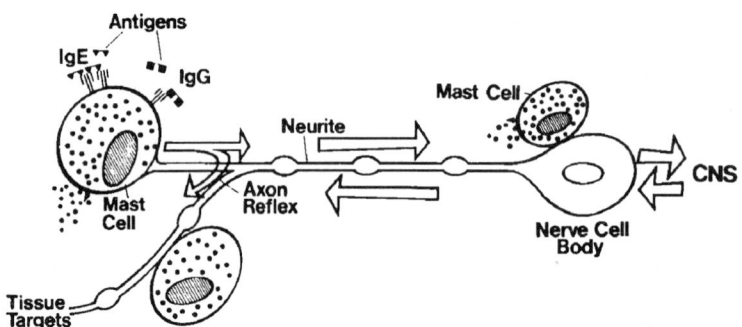

Figure 1. Mast cells become sensitized passively with IgE and IgG antibodies directed against predominantly environmental antigens. This schematic outline represents possible ways in which mast cells may act in this fashion as sensory receptors communicating information about the environment to the peripheral and central nervous system. Also shown in this figure is the possibility of two-way communication between the nervous system and mast cells. The psychological conditioning experiments referred to in the test indicate that the brain, in an as yet unknown manner, can communicate in an efferent fashion to peripheral mast cells. Reprinted from [3] by permission of Raven Press.

In this paper we indicate some of the evidence that mast cells and nerves communicate and interact in vivo so as to regulate their local environment. We review the data we have obtained in vivo, ex vivo, and in vitro to support this thesis. We believe that the evidence now clearly indicates a purposeful interaction between mast cells and nerves which serve both to control their local environment and communicate with the peripheral and central nervous system through mediator release [1–3]. This communication ap-

---

*   Molecular Virology and Immunology Program and Intestinal Disease Research Unit, Department of Pathology, McMaster University Medical Centre, Hamilton, Canada.
**   Department of Psychology, McMaster University, Hamilton, Canada.
      Acknowledgements: Medical Research Council of Canada, Fisons U.K. and the Council for Tobacco Research, USA Inc.

pears to be bi-directional, and under some circumstances it can be directly influenced by efferent or anti-dromic impulses, derived either from the central or the peripheral nervous system. Indeed, there is a significant body of literature suggesting that the mast cell may be involved in axon reflex production of vasodilatation and flare reaction in the skin. Antidromic stimulation of the saphenous nerve produces a wheal and flare reaction through substance P release in capsaicin-sensitive nerves, which is also sensitive to inhibition by anti-histaminics of the H1 type.

Our own interest in this area stems from a long-standing study of the mechanisms and expression of mucosal immunity both in the lung and gut. In the course of these studies, we became convinced that neuropeptides must be playing a role in the regulation of mucosal immunity [4, 5]. This conclusion was initially an emotional one based on the observation of Furness and Costa [6], who calculated that the total number of neurones within the spinal cord was about equivalent to those found in the gastrointestinal tract. This information, coupled with the known large amounts of certain neuropeptides within the GI and respiratory tracts, led us to investigate the effects of substance P (SP), vasointestinal polypeptide (VIP), and somatostatin (SOM). As a brief summary of an extensive body of work, we have shown that these neuropeptides, which can act as neurotransmitters, also appear in vivo and in vitro to influence the expression of mucosal immunity [7, 8]. The presence of specific receptors for these neuropeptides on lymphocytes supports this conclusion, although it is not clear at the present time whether these effects are exerted directly or indirectly, in whole or in part, on lymphocytes, antigen-presenting cells, or vascular endothelium.

Morphological Evidence

Our laboratory has for some years been interested in the characterization, both biochemically and functionally, of the mast cells found in mucosal tissues [9]. We carried out a series of experiments looking at the potential secretagogue role of SP, SOM, VIP, bombesin, endorphins, and other putative neurotransmitters. Of all the molecules tested, the only one that consistently caused significant histamine

release from rat intestinal mucosal mast cells was SP [10]. Accordingly, we carried out a careful morphometric study, looking for possible local mast cell/nerve interactions [11]. We found this both in the normal as well as in the nematode-infected rat intestine. Frequent interactions of this kind were seen with light microscopy, which appeared on ultrastructural examination to consist of membrane-membrane interactions between mast cells and nerves which often contained substance P or calcitonin gene-related peptide (CGRP) in dense core vesicles. This was statistically highly significantly.

Others have contributed to the literature and have proposed evidence for regular mast cell/nerve associations in a variety of tissue sites [12–15].

Experiments carried out by Perdue et al. [16] showed that anaphylactic degranulation of mast cells in vivo produces a local effect on function of the intestinal epithelium. These effects can be mimicked in vitro by antigen in Ussing chambers in which measurement of short-circuit current revealed changes that were dependent on the secretion of chloride ions. These could be blocked by drugs that were known to inhibit secretion by rat intestinal mucosal mast cells such as doxantrazole, whereas cromoglycate, which has no effect on these cells, also had no effect in the system being tested. Furthermore, these effects could be blocked by tetrodotoxin, a selective nerve poison. While there experiments were initially carried out in the rat intestine, we have more recently confirmed these effects in the rat trachea using a modified Ussing chamber [Sestine, Purdue, & Bienenstock, submitted]. In brief, these latter experiments show that luminal egg albumin to which rats have been sensitized by the use of alum and pertussis produces antigen-specific and -dependent short-circuit current changes similar to those found in the intestine. These were blocked by doxantrazole but not by sodium cromoglycate. Animals treated neonatally with capsaicin to deplete substance P in the sensory afferent nervous system failed, when examined as adults, to respond to antigen in Ussing chambers. No differences were seen in the levels of serum IgE antibody or the numbers and presence of mucosal tracheal mast cells between the capsaicin-treated and control groups. We have concluded that in the rat trachea an antigen-specific mast cell and nerve-dependent system exists in the sensitized rats which can regulate epithelial cell function.

In vivo Experiments

Similar experiments have been carried out in vivo using technetium-labelled DTPA as a measure of solute clearance and lung epithelial permeability [17]. In these experiments, we first established the normal clearance rate of technetium-labelled DTPA by the use of a computer-assisted gamma camera at 7.5 minutes after administration of the aerosol. We did this first of all in normal rats and subsequently in rats sensitized to egg albumin with alum and pertussis. Not surprisingly, a significant increase in clearance occurred following specific antigen administered by aerosol to sensitized animals relative to nonsensitized controls. We then looked at the question of solute clearance in animals that had been neonatally treated with capsaicin and found that they exhibited a very significant decrease of solute clearance relative to the sham-treated animals. We concluded from these studies that, as counterpart to the evidence quoted above in vitro for an antigen-specific, mast cell and nerve-dependent system operative in the lung of sensitized rats to regulate presumed epithelial cell function (as reflected by solute clearance).

McDonald [18] has shown that the stimulation of the rat vagus can cause neurogenic inflammation in rat trachea. Similarly, Leff et al. [19] showed that vagal stimulation could cause an enhancement of mast cell-derived histamine secretion after challenge with ascaris antigen in natively allergic dog lungs. Field stimulation of rat ileum caused a diminution in mast cell granularity and histamine release which was decreased by atropine or tetrodotoxin [20].

We have carried out experiments in Sprague-Dawley rats previously sensitized with egg albumin in alum and pertussis. Stimulation of the superior laryngeal nerve via a bi-polar electrode for 30 seconds caused significant increases of rat mast cell protease II (RMCP II) in the perfusate which were not seen in sham-stimulated animals [Kakuta, Perdue, Stead, Kawabori, & Bienenstock, submitted].

Capsaicin pretreatment or neonatal capsaicin inhibits the neurogenic inflammation re-sulting from anti-dromic nerve stimulation of the saphenous nerve, which otherwise causes mast cell degranulation in the skin [21–23]. However, more recent data by Kowalski and Kaliner [24] suggest that anti-dromic responses only promote mast cell degranulation if prolonged. Thus, the evidence concerning nerve stimulation causing mast cell degranulation is controversial, and further work must be done to clarify these differences.

Co-Culture Experiments

In addition, we have carried out a whole series of experiments in which primary culture of superior cervical ganglia from neonatal mice have been performed in association with mast cells of different types [Blennerhassett & Bienenstock, submitted]. These co-culture experiments have shown very striking nerve/mast cell interactions in which the sympathetic nerves have displayed specific and selective association with rat peritoneal mast cells and RBL 2H3 (the homologue of rat mucosal mast cells). Both cell types displayed neurotropic effects on the neurites growing out from the ganglia, whereas fibroblasts and a rat plasmacytoma cell line failed to show these characteristics.istics The mast cells became innervated in the sense that within a 16-hour period the majority of the 1000 mast cells in culture (60–80%) showed neuronal attachment. Once this had occurred, contact was preserved over a period of culture of up to 144 hours. The mast cells contacted by nerves stopped dividing, became more differentiated (more granules), and exhibited electrophysiological changes such as an increase in conductance when compared to mast cells in the same culture dish without such nerve contact. We again take this to indicate selective and functional nerve/mast cell interactions in vitro.

Effects of Psychological Conditioning

Lastly, we have examined the question of whether mast cells can be caused to secrete mediators by psychological cues to which the animals had been conditioned. In these experiments, rats were conditioned with an audiovisual conditioning stimulus which consisted of loud noise and flashing lights [25]. We paired this to antigen in the experimental groups. To maximize the readout of the experiment, which consisted of measurements of RMCP II mast cells in the circulation, we first gave all groups 3,000 larvae of the nematode *Nippostrongylus brasiliensis* to produce mucosal mast cell hyperplasia. The design of the experiment was such as to show that when the antigen stimulus was paired with the conditioning stimulus and the animals subsequently exposed to the conditioning stimulus alone, the serum level of RMCP II found within one hour was no different than the positive control consisting of antigen and the audiovisual cue. The negative control and an unpaired stimulus in which the audiovisual stimulus preceded the antigenic stimulus by 24 hours were significantly different at a P value of less than .001 in terms of RMCP II concentrations in the serum. Thus, we conditioned rats experimentally for mast cell degranulation and RMCP II release. We are not yet certain of the mechanism through which this release of a mucosal mast cell mediator was conditioned, although it is possible that this occurred by direct transmission of information from the central nervous system via the nerves to the mucosal mast cells in the respiratory and gastrointestinal tracts.

Conclusions

Mast cells are often found to be increased in a number of inflammatory situations [26]. Mast cells may be sensitized by both specific IgG and IgE antibodies via ligand binding to specific Fc receptors (Figure 1). Thus, they respond to a variety of antigens upon interaction with them. Mast cells can be found in association with nerves and may have a selective tendency to associate with them. Mast cells can cause activation of nerves locally through the release of mediators such as histamine or products of arachidonic acid metabolism and their action on those nerves [27]. It is less clear, though well documented, that nervous stimulation can, either through axon reflexes or other mechanisms, promote mast cell degranulation. We believe that our experiments with psychological conditioning of mast cell degranulation have some pertinence to our understanding of lung disease, especially asthma. We further believe that the mast cell can act as a sensory

receptor for antigens to which the organism is sensitized. This would be particularly related to environmental antigens at mucosal surfaces. In this way, and through mast cell degranulation, the brain would receive information about the presence of such antigens in the environment and the level of the exposure. It is well known that antigen-induced anaphylaxis produces EEG changes and direct effects on the central nervous system. In this way, the brain must be involved as well as the rest of the central nervous system in both afferent and efferent processing of information such as this. The mast cells would in this situation serve to focus informational transfer from the periphery. How these systems are further regulated and may be manipulated to promote therapeutic effects are now the subjects of intense study.

References

1. Bienenstock, J., M. Blennerhassett, M. Tomioka, J. Marshall, M. H. Perdue, and R. H. Stead. 1988. Evidence for mast cell/nerve interactions. In: Neuroimmune networks: Physiology and disease. E. Goetzl, ed. In press.
2. Bienenstock, J., M. Perdue, M. Blennerhassett, R. Stead, Y. Kakuta, P. Sestini, C. Vancheri, and J. Marshall. 1988. Inflammatory cells and the epithelium: Mast cell/nerve interactions in the lung in vitro and in vivo. Am. Rev. Resp. Dis., in press.
3. Bienenstock, J., M. Blennerhassett, Y. Kakuta, G. MacQueen, J. Marshall, M. Perdue, S. Siegel, T. Tsuda, J. Denburg, and R. Stead. 1988. Evidence for central and peripheral nervous system interaction with mast cells. In: Mast cell and basophil differentiation and function in health and disease. S. J. Galli and K. F. Austen, eds. New York: Raven Press, in press.
4. Stead, R., J. Bienenstock, and A. M. Stanisz. 1987. Neuropeptide regulation of mucosal immunity. Immunol. Rev. 100: 333.
5. Stanisz, A. M., D. Befus, and J. Bienenstock. 1986. Differential effects of vasoactive intestinal peptide, substance P, and somatostatin on immunoglobulin synthesis and proliferation by lymphocytes from Peyer's patch, mesenteric lymph node and spleen. J. Immunol. 136: 152.
6. Furness, J. B., and M. Costa. 1980. Commentary: Types of nerves in the enteric nervous system. Neuroscience 5: 1.
7. Stanisz, A. M., R. Scicchitano, P. Dazin, J. Bienenstock, and D. G. Payan. 1987. Distribution of substance P receptors on murine spleen and Peyer's patch T and B cells. J. Immunol. 139: 749.

8. Scicchitano, R., J. Bienenstock, and A. M. Stanisz. 1988. In vivo immunomodulation by the neuropeptide substance P. Immunology 63: 733.

9. Bienenstock, J. 1988. An update on mast cell heterogeneity including comments on mast cell/ nerve relationships. J. Allergy Clin. Immunol. 81: 763.

10. Shanahan, F., J. A. Denburg, J. Fox, J. Bienenstock, and A. D. Befus. 1985. Mast cell heterogeneity. Effects of neuroenteric peptides on histamine release. J. Immunol. 135: 1331.

11. Stead, R. H., M. Tomioka, G. Quinonez, G. T. Simon, S. Y. Felten, and J. Bienenstock. 1987. Intestinal mucosal mast cells in normal and nematode-infected rat intestines are in intimate contact with peptidergic nerves. Proc. Natl. Acad. Sci 84: 2975.

12. Skofitsch, G., J. M. Savitt, and D. M. Jacovowitz. 1985. Suggestive evidence for functional unit between mast cells and substance P fibres in the rat diaphragm and mesentery. Histochemistry 82: 5.

13. Newson, B., A. Dahlstrom, L. Enerback, and H. Ahlman. 1983. Suggestive evidence for a direct innervation of mucosal mast cells. An electron microscopic study. Neuroscience 10: 565.

14. Olsson, Y. 1988. Mast cells in the nervous system. Int. Rev. Cytol. 29: 27.

15. Heine, H., and F. J. Forster. 1975. Relationship between mast cells and preterminal nerve fibres. Z. Mikrosk.-Anat. Forsch. Leipzig 89: S934.

16. Perdue, M. H., M. Chung, and D. G. Gall. 1984. The effect of intestinal anaphylaxis on gut function in the rat. Gastroenterology 86: 391.

17. Sestini, P., M. Dolovich, C. Vancheri, R. H. Stead, J. S. Marshall, M. Perdue, J. Gauldie, and J. Bienenstock. 1988. Antigen-induced lung solute clearance in rats is dependent on capsaicin-sensitive nerves. Am. Rev. Resp. Dis., in press.

18. McDonald, D. M. 1987. Neurogenic inflammation in the respiratory tract: Actions of sensory nerve mediators on blood vessels and epithelium of the airway mucosa. Am. Rev. Resp. Dis. 136: 565.

19. Leff, A. R., N. P. Stimler, N. M. Munoz, T. Shioya, J. Tallet, and C. Dame. 1986. Augmentation of respiratory mast cell secretion of histamine caused by vagus nerve stimulation during antigen challenge. J. Immunol. 135: 1066.

20. Bani-Sacchi, T., M. Barattini, S. Bianchi, S. Blandina, P. Blandina, S. Brunelleschi, R. Fantozzi, P. F. Mannaioni, and E. Masini. 1986. The release of histamine by parasympathetic stimulation in guinea-pig auricle and rat ileum. J. Physiol. 371: 29.

21. Weisner-Menzel, L., B. Schulz, F. Vakilzadeh, and B. M. Czarnetzki. 1981. Electron microscopical evidence for a direct contact between nerve fibres and mast cells. Acta Dermatovener (Stockholm) 61: 465.

22. Kiernan, J. A. 1972. A pharmacological and histological investigation of the involvement of mast cells in cutaneous axon reflex vasodilatation. Q. J. Exp. Physiol. 57: 311.

23. Lembeck, F., and P. Holzer. 1979. Substance P as a neurogenic mediator of antidromic vasodilatation and neurogenic plasma extravasation. Naunyn-Schmiedelberg's Arch. Pharmacol. 310: 175.

24. Kowalski, M. L., and M. A. Kaliner. 1988. Neurogenic inflammation, vascular permeability, and mast cells. J. Immunol. 140: 3905.

25. MacQueen, G., J. S. Marshall, M. Perdue, S. Siegel, and J. Bienenstock. 1988. Pavlovian conditioning of rat mucosal mast cells to secrete rat mast cell protease II. Science, in press.

26. Bienenstock, J., M. Tomioka, R. Stead, P. Ernst, M. Jordana, J. Gauldie, J. Dolovich, and J. Denburg. 1987. Mast cell involvement in various inflammatory processes. Am. Rev. Resp. Dis. 135: S5.

27. Weinreich, D., and B. J. Undem. 1987. Immunological regulation of synaptic transmission in isolated guinea pig autonomous ganglia. J. Clin. Invest. 79: 1529.

Neuropeptides and Asthma

*Peter J. Barnes**

Many neuropeptides have now been identified in the respiratory tract [1]. Their precise physiological role in airways remains uncertain, but the potent effects of these neuropeptides on various aspects of airway function suggest that they may be involved in controlling airway tone, vasculature and secretions [2]. It is possible that defective function of peptidergic nerves might be involved in airway disease, and particular asthma [3].

Non-Adrenergic Non-Cholinergic (NANC) Nerves

Neural control of airways is more complex than previously recognised, and in addition to classical cholinergic and adrenergic pathways, neural mechanisms which are neither adrenergic nor cholinergic have been described [4]. There is increasing evidence that neuropeptides may be the neurotransmitters of these NANC nerves. Both excitatory and inhibitory NANC mechanisms have been described in airways, but the physiological significance of these pathways will remain uncertain until specific blockers become available. In human airways, inhibitory nerves are the only inhibitory nervous pathway, since direct adrenergic innervation of airway smooth muscle is lacking.

Vasoactive Intestinal Peptide

VIP, a 28 amino acid peptide originally discovered as a vasoactive substance in lung extracts, potently relaxes airway smooth muscle in vitro [5]. VIP has been localised to nerves in human and animal lungs; in human airways VIP-immunoreactive nerve fibres are associated with airway smooth muscle (particularly in large airways), submucosal glands, bronchial vessels, and cholinergic ganglia [6].

VIP relaxes human bronchi in vitro and is considerably more potent than isoprenaline, making it the most potent endogenous bronchodilator so far discovered [7]. In vivo, inhaled VIP is rather disappointing, since it has no bronchodilator effect and provides only weak protection against histamine-induced bronchoconstriction [8], probably because little of the nebulised peptide can reach receptors in the airway smooth muscle. VIP is a likely candidate for the neurotransmitter of NANC inhibitory nerves, since, in animal airways, it mimics the electrophysiological changes produced by NANC nerve stimulation and is released into the muscle bath when these nerves are stimulated electrically [5]. And when tolerance is induced by exposure to high concentrations of VIP, the NANC inhibitory nerve effects (but not the sympathetic inhibitory effects) are reduced. Histochemical studies show that VIP-immunoreactive nerves diminish in the smaller airways and are virtually absent from bronchioles. Interestingly, non-adrenergic relaxation is almost absent in small airways, and these airways fail to relax with VIP, although they do respond to isoprenaline [7]. All this evidence points toward VIP as a neurotransmitter of NANC inhibitory nerves, though certain proof must await the development of specific blockers.

In animals, VIP is also a potent stimulant of mucus secretion from airway glands [9] and ion transport in airway epithelium [10], suggesting that VIP-ergic nerves may also regulate airway secretions. VIP is a potent dilator of pulmonary vessels, and in the bronchial circulation, it might play an important role in regulation of airway perfusion. Mapping of VIP-receptors in human lung by autoradiography confirms the presence of receptors on airway glands, epithelium, and vascular smooth muscle, and also demonstrates the presence of receptors on smooth muscle of bronchi but not bronchioles [11].

* Professor and Chairman, Department of Thoracic Medicine, Cardiothoracic Institute, Dovehouse Street London SW3 6LY, and Honorary Consultant Physician, Brompton Hospital, London, United Kingdom.
Acknowledgements: Supported by the Medical Research Council and the Asthma Research Council, UK. I thank Madeleine Wray for typing the manuscript.

Ultrastructural studies suggest that VIP may be present in cholinergic nerves in the airways and may therefore function as a co-transmitter with acetylcholine [6]. VIP may modulate release of acetylcholine, or it may modify its effects. VIP reduces the contractile effect of exogenous acetylcholine on airway smooth muscle in vitro and may then act as a "braking" mechanism to cholinergic bronchoconstriction [3]. It is possible that VIP is co-released only under certain patterns of neural activation, such as high frequency firing, acting as a protective mechanism. Another possible physiological role for VIP could involve regulation of bronchial blood flow. If cholinergic nerve activity causes bronchoconstriction, release of VIP from activated cholinergic nerves may have an effect on adjacent bronchial vessels (which are very sensitive to VIP), so that bronchial blood flow increases as smooth muscle contracts, thus supplying oxygen to active smooth muscle cells.

Peptide Histidine Isoleucine (PHI) is a 27 amino acid with marked structural similarities to VIP and coded by the same gene. In humans, the sequence is slightly altered and peptide histidine methionine (PHM) has been identified. PHI/PHM is present in the same nerves as VIP and has rather similar effects. PHM is equipotent to VIP as a relaxant of airway smooth muscle [7], although it is less potent as a vasodilator than VIP, suggesting that it might act on separate receptors.

Whether any abnormality in NANC inhibitory nerves or VIP might contribute to bronchial hyperresponsiveness is uncertain. A defect in inhibiting control of airway smooth muscle would certainly account for some of the features of hyperresponsiveness. A primary defect in NANC innervation seems unlikely, since there is no abnormality in gastrointestinal sphincters or motility in asthmatic patients which would be expected in a generalised defect of this system. However, it is possible that a functional defect might develop as a result of airway inflammation, which appears to be related to the bronchial hyperresponsiveness which is so characteristic of asthma. Inflammatory cells identified in the asthmatic airway, such as neutrophils, eosinophils, and mast cells may release a variety of peptidases which would rapidly break down VIP and PHM. This would be like taking the brake off cholinergic nerves, resulting in exaggerated cholinergic bronchoconstrictor responses in the larger airways [3]. While this is unlikely to be the cause of asthma, it may be a contributory factor in the bronchial hyperresponsiveness associated with airway inflammation.

Sensory Neuropeptides

Substance P (SP) is localised to unmyelinated sensory nerves (C-fibres) in airways and has several actions which suggest that it may take part in the inflammatory response of asthma [12]. In addition to contraction of airway smooth muscle, SP also potently stimulates airway mucus secretion and increases airway microvascular permeability and exudation of plasma into the airway lumen. SP also degranulates mast cells of the skin, although this has not been demonstrated conclusively in lung, and it may have chemotactic effects on inflammatory cells. Non-cholinergic bronchoconstrictor nerves have been demonstrated in guinea-pigs. These nerves are antagonised by SP antagonists, suggesting that SP may be the excitatory neurotransmitter [12]. These studies raise the possibility that SP might be released from sensory nerve endings by retrograde activation, as in an axon reflex.

Capsaicin, the hot extract of pepper, releases SP from unmyelinated sensory nerve endings and, in rats and guinea-pigs, causes acute bronchoconstriction and airway microvascular leakiness [3, 12]. Chronic treatment with capsaicin leads to depletion of SP-immunoreactivity and is associated with a reduced bronchoconstrictor response to allergen in sensitised animals [13] and prevents irritants, such as cigarette smoke or mechanical stimulation of the airway from airway microvascular leakage [12]. While these effects of SP innervation are seen in rodents, the relevance of these findings to human airways is less certain. Reports of SP innervation of human airways are conflicting, but human lungs obtained at surgery are usually from older smokers in whom SP content may be reduced. Nevertheless, SP causes contraction of human airways in vitro, and capsaicin causes bronchoconstriction, albeit transiently, when inhaled [14].

Recently, two peptides related in structure to SP, neurokinin A and neurokinin B, have been localised to lung [12]. NKA is coded by the same gene as SP but has a different spectrum of effects, suggesting the existence of separate receptors. NKA is far more potent than SP in contracting airway smooth muscle, whereas SP is more potent than NKA in causing vasodilatation and microvascular leakage.

Another peptide that has recently been localised to sensory nerves is calcitonin gene-related peptide (CGRP), which may also be co-stored with SP. CGRP is a potent vasodilator and contracts human airways in vitro [15].

Because sensory neuropeptides, such as SP, neurokinins and CGRP produce many of the features of asthma, it is tempting to speculate that they may be involved in its pathogenesis, and the idea of neurogenic inflammatory mechanisms in asthma is attractive [16]. Damage to airway epithelium (possibly as a result of toxic eosinophil products) may occur even in relatively mild asthmatics, exposing afferent nerve endings. These nerve endings may then be stimulated by inflammatory mediators. Bradykinin, an inflammatory peptide formed by enzymatic cleavage from a plasma precursor, is likely to be formed in the asthmatic airway by the action of enzymes released from inflammatory cells on exudated plasma. Bradykinin selectively stimulated C-fibre endings and may release sensory neuropeptides. Bradykinin is a potent bronchoconstrictor in asthmatics and acts indirectly, possibly by stimulating sensory nerve endings [17]. This may result in the retrograde release of sensory neuropeptides such as SP, neurokinins, and CGRP from collaterals, via an axon reflex. This could result in bronchoconstriction, mucus hypersecretion, and microvascular leakage leading to oedema of the airway wall and extravasation of plasma in the lumen.

Other Neuropeptides

Several other neuropeptides have been identified in human airway nerves [1], but their physiological role is far from certain [2].

Neuropeptide Y is co-localised with noradrenaline in adrenergic nerves of the lung. It may play a role in regulating bronchial blood flow and cholinergic neurotransmission, rather than airway smooth muscle directly, since sympathetic nerves do not directly supply airway smooth muscle in humans. *Galanin* appears to be co-localised with VIP in airway nerves, but has little known effect on airway smooth muscle. It may have a neuromodulatory role.

Cholecystokinin has also been found in airways and is a potent bronchoconstrictor of large airways.

The presence of so many neuropeptides in airways raises questions about their physiological role. It seems most likely that they may act as subtle regulators under physiological conditions, but in inflammatory diseases of the airways, such as asthma, they may have a pathogenetic role. Specific antagonists are needed to elucidate the contribution of these potent neuropeptides in human diseases such as asthma.

Therapeutic Prospects

It is certainly possible that pharmacological agents which interact with neuropeptides may be developed for the treatment of such diseases in the future. VIP is a potent bronchodilator in vitro, yet has little effect in vivo, probably because of rapid degradation. Stable analogues might therefore be useful, although it is likely that they would be less effective than beta-agonists, since they do not act on small airways. Drugs that permit degradation of VIP may suffer from a similar disadvantage.

Drugs that block sensory neuropeptide receptors are not very effective at present. In the future, it may be possible to develop non-peptide antagonists, but since many peptides are released from sensory nerves (some of which have not yet been identified), it may be more useful to develop drugs that inhibit the release of sensory neuropeptides. Recent studies show that morphine via u-opioid receptors may inhibit sensory neuropeptide release in airways.

References

1. Polak, J. M., and S. R. Bloom. 1986. Regulatory peptides of the gastrointestinal and respiratory tracts. Arch. int. Pharmacodyn. 280: 16–49.
2. Barnes, P. J. 1987. Neuropeptides in the lung, localization, function and pathophysiological implications. J. Allergy Clin. Immunol. 79: 285–295.
3. Barnes, P. J. 1987. Airway neuropeptides and asthma. Trends Pharm. Sci. 8: 24–27.
4. Barnes, P. J. 1986. Neural control of human airways in health and disease. Am. Rev. Respir. Dis. 134: 1289–1314.

5. Said, S. I. 1982. Vasoactive peptides in the lung, with special reference to vasoactive intestinal peptide. Exp. Lung Res. 3: 343–348.

6. Laitinen, A., M. Partanen, A. Hervonen, M. Peto-Huikko, and L. A. Laitinen. 1985. VIP-like immunoreactive nerves in human respiratory tract. Light and electron microscopic study. Histochemistry 82: 313–319.

7. Palmer, J. B., F. M. C. Cuss, and P. J. Barnes. 1986. VIP and PHM and their role in non-adrenergic inhibitory responses in isolated human airways. J. Appl. Physiol. 61: 1322–1328.

8. Barnes, P. J., and C. M. S. Dixon. 1984. The effect of inhaled vasoactive intestinal peptide on bronchial hyperreactivity in man. Am. Rev. Respir. Dis. 130: 162–166.

9. Peatfield, A. C., P. J. Barnes, C. Bratcher, J. A. Nadel, and B. Davis. 1983. Vasoactive intestinal peptide stimulates tracheal submucosal gland secretion in ferret. Am. Rev. Respir. Dis. 128: 89–93.

10. Nathanson, I., J. H. Widdicombe, and P. J. Barnes. 1983. Effect of vasoactive intestinal peptide on ion transport across dog traceal epithelium. J. Appl. Physiol. 55: 1844–1848.

11. Carstairs, J. R., and P. J. Barnes. 1986. Visualization of vasoactive intestinal peptide receptors in human and guinea pig lung. J. Pharmacol. Exp. Ther. 239: 249–255.

12. Lundberg, J. M., and A. Saria. 1987. Polypeptide-containing neurons in airway smooth muscle. Ann. Rev. Physiol. 49: 557–572.

13. Andersson, R. G. G., and N. Grundstrom. 1983. The excitatory non-cholinergic, non-adrenergic nervous system of the guinea-pig airways. Eur. J. Respir. Dis. 64: 141–157.

14. Fuller, R. W., C. M. S. Dixon, and P. J. Barnes. 1985. The bronchoconstrictor response to inhaled capsaicin in humans. J. Appl. Physiol. 85: 1080–1084.

15. Palmer, J. B. D., F. M. C. Cuss, P. K. Mulderry, M. A. Ghatei, D. R. Springall, A. Cadieux, A., S. R. Bloom, J. M. Polak, and P. J. Barnes. 1987. Calcitonin gene-related peptide is localised to human airway nerves and potently constricts human airways smooth muscle. Br. J. Pharmacol. 91: 95–101.

16. Barnes, P. J. 1986. Asthma as an axon reflex. Lancet i: 242–245.

17. Fuller, R. W., C. M. S. Dixon, F. M. C. Cuss, and P. J. Barnes. 1987. Bradykinin-induced bronchoconstriction in man: Mode of action. Am. Rev. Respir. Dis. 135: 176–180.

18. Belvisi, M. G., K. F. Chung, D. M. Jackson, and P. J. Barnes. 1988. Opioid modulation of non-cholinergic neural bronchoconstriction in guinea-pig in vivo. Br. J. Pharmacol., in press.

Effect of Neuropeptides on Human Skin Mast Cells

Martin K. Church, Mark A. Lowman, Paul H. Rees, C. Robinson,
*R. Christopher Benyon**

The release of preformed mediators, such as histamine and neutral proteases, and the generation of eicosanoids including prostaglandin D_2 (PGD_2) and leukotriene C_4 (LTC_4) from activated mast cells provides the initiating stimulus for the immediate hypersensitivity response. Research into activation-secretion coupling in human mast cells has concentrated on the cross-linkage of membrane-bound IgE by allergen as the stimulator for mediator release. However, in many allergic reactions or pseudoallergic responses, there is no obvious link with an extrinsic allergen. In the skin such diseases include chronic idiopathic urticaria, heat-induced urticaria, cold-induced urticaria, and cholinergic urticaria, all of which may be reduced in severity by therapy with histamine H_1-antagonists, suggesting that mast cell-derived histamine is involved in their etiology.

The reduction of the severity of heat- and cold-induced urticaria by capsaicin [1], the irritant substance from chilli peppers, which depletes the skin of neuropeptides [2], and the observations that neuropeptides such as substance P may induce a weal and flare response when injected intradermally [3] have suggested a neurogenic basis for these diseases. The ability of histamine H_1-antagonists to reduce partially the weal and inhibit the flare induced by substance P [4] indicates that the neurogenic effects may, at least in part, be mediated through mast cell mediators. In order to increase our understanding of the relationships between neuropeptides and mast cells, we have studied mediator release from human dispersed skin mast cells. This review concentrates on three aspects of these studies: the heterogeneity of mast cell responsiveness to neuropeptides, the nature of the mast cell activation site, and the characteristics of the secretory response to neuropeptides.

Heterogeneity of Mast Cell Responsiveness to Neuropeptides

The concept of mast cell heterogeneity, although documented initially more than 80 years ago by Maximow [5], has become widely accepted since the classical papers of Enerback in 1966 describing differences in fixation, staining, amine composition, and responsiveness to compound 48/80 between mast cells of rat connective tissues and intestinal mucosa [6–9]. Numerous workers have extended these studies, and today it is recognized that rat mast cells may be largely divided into those associated with connective tissues such as the peritoneal cavity and those associated with mucosal surfaces. In addition to the differences described above, these cells may be distinguished by size, differences in proteoglycan and neutral protease contents, and responsiveness to secretagogues and modulatory drugs [10–12]. Furthermore, unlike mast cells derived from mucosal surfaces, those obtained from connective tissues are responsive to a wide range of basic secretagogues including neuropeptides [13, 14]. Heterogeneity within human mast cells, however, appears to be more complex. The recent availability of specific antibodies against the mast cell neutral endoproteases, tryptase and chymase [15–17] has allowed a sub-division of human mast cells according to their immunocytochemical characteristics. In the lung and intestinal mucosa, the majority of the mast cells contain only tryptase and are signified MC$_T$. Like mast cells of the rodent intestinal mucosa [18,19], human intestinal mast cells appear to be dependent on T-lymphocyte-derived products for their maturation [20]. In contrast, mast cells of the skin

* Immunopharmacology Group, Clinical Pharmacology, Centre Block, Southampton General Hospital, Southampton SO9 4XY, U.K.
These studies have been supported in part by a Medical Research Council Project Grant. M.A.L. is a SERC-CASE award student in collaboration with Roussel Laboratories, and P.H.R. is supported by a University of Southampton studentship.

Table 1. Sensitivity of human mast cells to immunological and nonimmunological stimulation.

| Mast cell source | Secretory response to | | Mast cell sub-type |
	Anti-IgE	Substance P	
Lung	+	−	$MC_{TC} \ll MC_T$
Skin	+	+	$MC_{TC} \gg MC_T$
Colon mucosa*	+	−	$MC_{TC} \cong MC_T$
Colon muscle	+	−	$MC_{TC} > MC_T$

*mast cells dispersed from mucosal and sub-mucosal layers of human colon

Table 2. Responsiveness of human skin mast cells to neuropeptide tachykinins and analogues.

Neuropeptide	Response	SP analogue	Response
Substance P	++++	$SP_{2\text{-}11}$	+++
Somatostatin	++++	$SP_{3\text{-}11}$	++
VIP	++++	$SP_{4\text{-}11}$	±
Neurotensin	−	$SP_{1\text{-}4}$ −	
Neurokinin A	+	$[D\text{-}Pro^2, DTrp^{7,9}]SP$	++++
Neurokinin B	−	$[D\text{-}Pro^4, DTrp^{7,9,10}]SP_{4\text{-}11}$	−
Eledoisin	−		
Physalaemin	±		
CGRP	−		
Bradykinin	−		

and intestinal sub-mucosa contain both tryptase and chymase and are signified MC_{TC}. The persistence of MC_{TC} in the intestinal walls in lymphocyte deficiency diseases [20] would suggest that, like the connective tissue associated mast cells of the rodent, their maturation is independent from T-lymphocyte-derived lymphokines.

To examine the relationship between protease content and responsiveness of human mast cells to neuropeptides, we have compared cells dispersed from human skin, lung, colonic mucosa, and immediate submucosal layers (henceforth referred to colon mucosa) and colonic muscle layers. To avoid differences in dispersion techniques from influencing mast cell responsiveness, all tissues were dispersed with collagenase and hyaluronidase using similar protocols [21]. Whereas the predominancy of MC_{TC} and MC_T in skin and lung dispersates is well established [17, 22], the proportions of MC_T and MC_{TC} in mast cells preparations obtained by dispersal of intestinal tissue is less predictable. Therefore, in collaboration with Drs. Irani and Schwartz, we determined the protease content of our dispersed colonic mast cells. The results demonstrated the presence of chymase in 63% of the mast cells from the colonic mucosa and 74% of cells from the muscle layers, indicating the predominance of MC_{TC} in both layers.

Mast cells from the skin, lung, and colon all released histamine in response to stimulation with anti-IgE or calcium ionophore A23187 [21, 23, 24]. However, when stimulated with substance P, there was a marked heterogeneity of response that did not correlate with chymase content [25], the mast cells of the skin releasing histamine, while those of the lung and both layers of the colon did not (Table 1). A similar spectrum of sensitivity was observed with morphine and the polybasic secretagogues, compound 48/80, and poly-L-lysine [21, 23].

The Nature of the Neuropeptide Activation Site

Three tachykinin neuropeptide receptors, NK1, NK2 and NK3 [26] have been identified in smooth muscle. These may be distinguished by the relative concentrations of substance P, eledoisin, physalaemin, neurokinin A, and neurokinin B required to stimulate them. The observation [27] that, of these ligands, substance P was the only one to induce the release of significant amounts of histamine (Table 2) indicates that the activation site on skin mast cells is dissimilar to those found on smooth muscle.

Studies in rat peritoneal mast cells have demonstrated that both the positively charged N-terminal tetrapeptide and the lipophilic amide substituted C-terminal heptapeptide are required for histamine release, but the absolute configuration of these elements is not critical [14, 28, 29]. We have confirmed this observation in human skin mast cells [27]. The stepwise removal of N-terminal amino acids led to a progressive reduction in mast cell stimulant activity, the relative potencies of substance P (SP): $SP_{2-11} : SP_{3-11}$ being 1:0.46:0.16, with SP_{4-11} having negligible activity (Table 2). The requirement for a lipophilic moiety was indicated by the observation that the N-terminal tetrapeptide SP_{4-11} did not release histamine. The lack of a precise structural requirement for this lipophylic portion was illustrated by the ability of the substance P analogue [D-Pro^2,D-Trp^{7,9}]SP to release histamine.

The ability of skin mast cells may be stimulated by a range of tachykinins, including substance P, somatostatin, and vasoactive intestinal peptide (VIP), and polybasic secretagogues suggest the nonspecific association of these basic substances with structural components of the cell membrane. However, evidence that they may in fact act through a true receptor stems from the observations that the effect of these secretagogues, but not that of anti-IgE, is blocked by the substance P antagonist [D-Pro^4,D-Trp^{7,9,10}]SP$_{4-11}$. However, further definition of this receptor site must await the development of more potent and specific agonists and antagonists.

Histamine release initiated by substance P and other neuropeptides is rapid, reaching completion within 20 seconds [23]. Furthermore, release may progress in the absence of extracellular calcium indicating a basic difference from activation-secretion initiated by anti-IgE. That neuropeptide-induced histamine release is prevented by incubation of the cells with 2-deoxy-D-glucose and antimycin A demonstrates an obligatory requirement for intact pathways of glycolysis and oxidative phosphorylation, strongly suggesting that it is not a cytotoxic process. This is supported by observations that neuropeptide-induced release may be suppressed by the receptor antagonist [D-Pro^4,D-Trp^{7,9,10}]SP$_{4-11}$ [23, 27] and by the β-adrenoceptor stimulant salbutamol [30].

IgE-dependent and neuropeptide stimuli also differ in their ability to generate eicosanoids from skin mast cells [31]. Studies with mast cells radiolabelled with [^{3}H$_8$]-arachidonic acid and enriched up to 80% homogeneity by differential centrifugation through discontinuous gradients of Percoll (1.051—1.100 g/ml) have shown prostaglandin D$_2$ (PGD$_2$) and leukotriene C$_4$ (LTC$_4$) to be the major cyclooxygenase and lipoxygenase products to be released into the supernatant following stimulation with either calcium ionophore A23187 or ε-chain specific anti-human IgE [32, 33].

Table 3. Production of PGD$_2$ and LTC$_4$, from human skin mast cells following stimulation with 25 µg/ml anti-IgE or 10 µM substance P.

	Mediator generation (pmol/10^6 mast cells)		
Stimulus	Histamine	PGD$_2$	LTC$_4$
Anti-IgE	3188 ± 291	112 ± 41	8.7 ± 0.7
Substance P	4279 ± 665	6 ± 2	0.5 ± 0.1

Characteristics of the Secretory Response to Neuropeptides

IgE-dependent activation of human skin mast cells induces a relatively slow secretion of the preformed mediator histamine, requiring six minutes to reach completion. This secretory mechanism has an obligatory requirement for extracellular calcium and intact pathways of glycolysis and oxidative phosphorylation [23].

In further experiments using unlabelled cells [31], the release of these eicosanoids has been quantified by radioimmunoassay (Table 3). Following activation with 25 µg/ml ε-specific anti-IgE, human skin mast cells generated histamine, PGD$_2$ and LTC$_4$ in a molar ratio of 1000:35:3. However when the cells were stimulated with substance P at a concentration of 10 µM, negligible amounts of PGD$_2$ and LTC$_4$ were released into the supernatant during the

30 minute incubation period. These differences in eicosanoid generation with anti-IgE and substance P stimulation suggest fundamental differences in the biochemical mechanisms coupling cell stimulation to mediator secretion.

Conclusions

Our studies have shown that skin mast cells, but not those from lung or intestine, respond to neuropeptide stimulation with the secretion of histamine in the virtual absence of eicosanoid generation. This suggests that the phenotypical development of human skin mast cells is influenced by their local environment, mainly blood vessels, nerves and connective tissues [34, 35], to produce a cell with a homeostatic role such as control of blood flow or angiogenesis [36, 37]. This contrasts with the defensive role usually associated with mast cells at mucosal surfaces. Further knowledge about the functional heterogeneity of human mast cells and their relationships with neuropeptides and blood vessels in the skin will advance our understanding of mast cell mediated diseases and enable us to develop more appropriate therapy.

References

1. Toth-Kasa, I., G. Jancso, F. Obal, S. Husz, and N. Simon. 1983. Involvement of sensory nerve endings in the cold and heat urticaria. J. Invest. Dermatol. 80: 34.
2. Theriault, E., M. Otsuka, and T. Jessel. 1979. Capsaicin-evoked release of substance P from primary sensory neurones. Brain Res. 170: 209.
3. Hagermark, O., T. Hokfelt, and B. Pernow. 1978. Flare and itch induced by substance P in human skin. J. Invest. Dermatol. 71: 233.
4. Foreman, J. C., and W. Piotrowski. 1984. Peptides and histamine release. J. Allergy Clin. Immunol. 74: 127.
5. Maximow, A. 1906. Über die Zellformen des lockeren Bindegewebes. Arch. F. Mikr. Anat. (Bonn) 67: 680.
6. Enerback, L. 1966. Mast cells in the gastrointestinal mucosa. I. Effects of fixation. Acta Path. Microbiol. Scand. 66: 289.
7. Enerback, L. 1966. Mast cells in the gastrointestinal mucosa. II. Dye binding and metachromatic properties. Acta Path. Microbiol. Scand. 66: 303.
8. Enerback, L. 1966. Mast cells in the gastrointestinal mucosa. III. Reactivity towards compound 48/80. Acta Path. Microbiol. Scand. 66: 313.
9. Enerback, L. 1966. Mast cells in the gastrointestinal mucosa. IV. Monoamine storing capacity. Acta Path. Microbiol. Scand. 67: 365.
10. Lee, T. D. G., M. Swieter, J. Bienenstock, and A. D. Befus. 1985. Heterogeneity in mast cell populations. Clin. Immunol. Rev. 4: 143.
11. Enerback, L. 1986. Mast cell heterogeneity: The evolution of the concept of a specific mucosal mast cell. In: Mast Cell Differentiation and Heterogeneity. A.D. Befus, J. Bienenstock, and J. A. Denburg, eds. New York: Raven Press, p. 1.
12. Gibson, S., and H. R. P. Miller. 1986. Mast cell subsets in the rat distinguished immunohistochemically by their content of serine proteinases. Immunology 58: 101.
13. Shanahan, F., J. A. Denburg, J. Fox, J. Bienenstock, and A. D. Befus. 1985. Mast cell heterogeneity: Effects of neuroenteric peptides on histamine release. J. Immunol. 135: 1331.
14. Foreman, J. C., and W. Piotrowski. 1985. Some effects of substance P antagonists on mast cells. In: Tachykinin Antagonists. R. Hakanson and F. Sundler, eds. Amsterdam: Elsevier, p. 405.
15. Schwartz, L. B. 1985. Monoclonal antibodies against human mast cell tryptase demonstrate shared antigenic sites on subunits of tryptase and selective localization of the enzyme to mast cells. J. Immunol. 134: 526.
16. Schechter, N. M., J. K. Choi, D. A. Slavin, D. T. Deresienski, S. Sayama, G. Dong, R. M. Lavaker, D. Proud, and G. S. Lazarus. 1986. Identification of a chymotrypsin-like proteinase from human mast cells. J. Immunol. 137: 962.
17. Irani, A. A., N. M. Schechter, S. Craig, G. DeBlois, and L. B. Schwartz. 1986. Two types of human mast cells that have distinct neutral protease compositions. Proc. Natl. Acad. Sci. USA. 83: 4464.
18. Haig, D. M., T. A. McKee, E. E. E. Jarrett, R. Woodbury, and H. R. P. Miller. 1982. Generation of mucosal mast cells is stimulated in in vitro by factors derived from T cells of helminth infected rats. Nature 300: 188.
19. Ihle, J. N., J. Keller, S. Oroszlan, L. E. Henderson, T. D. Copeland, F. Fitch, M. B. Prytsowsky, E. Goldwasser, J. W. Schrader, E. Palaszynski, M. Dy, and B. Lebel. 1983. Biological properties of homogeneous interleukin 3: Demonstration of WEHI-3 growth factor activity, mast cell growth factor activity, P-cell stimulating factor activity, colony-stimulating activity and histamine producing cell stimulating factor activity. J. Immunol. 131: 282.
20. Irani, A. A., S. S. Craig, G. DeBlois, C. O. Elson, N. M. Schechter, and L. B. Schwartz, 1987. Deficiency of the tryptase-positive chymase-negative mast cell type in gastrointestinal mucosa of patients with defective T-lymphocyte function. J. Immunol. 138: 4381.

21. Lowman, M. A., P. H. Rees, R. C. Benyon, and M. K. Church. 1988. Human mast cell heterogeneity: Histamine release from mast cells dispersed from skin, lung, adenoids, tonsils and intestinal mucosa in response to IgE-dependent and non-immunological stimuli. J. Allergy Clin. Immunol. 81: 590.

22. Schwartz, L. B., A. A. Irani, K. Roller, M. Castells, and N. M. Schechter. 1987. Quantitation of histamine, tryptase, and chymase in dispersed human T and CT mast cells. J. Immunol. 138: 2611.

23. Benyon, R. C., M. A. Lowman, and M. K. Church. 1987. Human skin mast cells: their dispersion, purification and secretory characterization. J. Immunol. 138: 861.

24. Rees, P. H., K. Hillier, and M. K. Church. 1988. The secretory characteristics of mast cells isolated from human large intestinal mucosa and muscle. Immunology, in press.

25. Church, M. K., R. C. Benyon, P. H. Rees, M. A. Lowman, A. M. Campbell, C. Robinson, and S. T. Holgate. 1989. Functional heterogeneity of human mast cells. In: Mast cell and basophil differentiation and function in health and disease. S. J. Galli and K. F. Austen, eds. New York: Raven Press, in press.

26. Lee, C. M., L. L. Iverson, M. B. Hanley, and B. E. B. Sandberg. 1982. The possible existence of multiple receptors for substance P. Naunyn Schmiedebergs Arch. Pharmacol. 318: 281.

27. Lowman, M. A., R. C. Benyon, and M. K. Church. 1988. Characterization of neuropeptide-induced histamine released from human dispersed skin mast cells. Br. J. Pharmacol. 95: 121.

28. Foreman, J. C., C. C. Jordan, P. Oehme, and H. Renner. 1983. Structure-activity relationships for some substance P-related peptides that cause wheal and flare reactions in human skin. J. Physiol. (Lond.) 335: 449.

29. Repke, H., W. Piotrowski, M. Bienert, and J. C. Foreman. 1987. Histamine release induced by Arg-Pro-Lys-Pro(CH$_2$)$_{11}$CH$_3$ from rat peritoneal mast cells. J. Pharmacol. Exp. Ther. 243: 317.

30. Lowman, M. A., R. C. Benyon, and M. K. Church. 1988. Human skin mast cells: Effects of salbutamol and sodium cromoglycate on histamine release induced by anti-IgE and substance P. J. Skin Pharmacol. 1: 63.

31. Benyon, C. R., C. Robinson, and M. K. Church. 1988. Mediator release from human skin mast cells: differences between IgE-dependent and non-immunological stimuli. Br. J. Pharmacol., in press.

32. Robinson, C., R. C. Benyon, S. T. Holgate, and M. K. Church. 1987. The calcium- and IgE-dependent release of eicosanoids from human cutaneous mast cells. Br. J. Pharmacol. 92 (Proceedings Suppl.): 516P.

33. Benyon, R. C., C. Robinson, S. T. Holgate, and M. K. Church. 1987. Prostaglandin D$_2$ release from human skin mast cells in response to ionophore A23187. Br. J. Pharmacol. 92: 635.

34. Eady, R. A. J., T. Cowen, T. F. Marshall, V. Plummer, and M. W. Greaves. 1979. Mast cell population density, blood vessel density and histamine content of normal human skin. Br. J. Dermatol. 100: 623.

35. Wiesner-Menzel, L., B. Schulz, F. Vakilzadeh, and B. M. Czarnetzki. 1981. Electron microscopical evidence for a direct contact between nerve fibres and mast cells. Acta Derm. Venereol. (Stockh.) 61: 465.

36. Schayer, R. W. 1962. Evidence that induced histamine is an intrinsic regulator of the microcirculatory system. Am. J. Physiol. 202: 66.

37. Marks, R. M., Roche, W. R., Czerniecki, M., Penny, R. and Nelson, D. S. 1986. Mast cell granules cause proliferation of human microvascular endothelial cells. Lab Invest 55: 289.

Interaction Between Neuropeptides and Classical Mediators of Allergy

*John C. Foreman**

In human skin, certain types of inflammation involve a neurogenic component. The nerves involved appear to be neuropeptide-containing C fibres which receive inputs from polymodal nociceptors responding to firm mechanical pressure, to heat intense enough to cause pain, and to some chemicals. Neurogenic inflammation to some types of stimulus can be blocked by antagonists of histamine at H_1 receptors, and this has suggested a role for mast cells in neurogenic inflammation. In this paper it is shown that carbachol-induced flare in human skin is blocked by antihistamine, which is consistent with the hypothesis that peptides liberated in an axon reflex can release histamine which contributes to the inflammatory response. It has also been shown that PGE_2 potentiates the wheal induced by substance P in human skin, indicating the possibility of interactions between various mediators in neurogenic inflammation.

There is evidence that neuropeptide-containing primary afferent neurones are capable of fulfilling an *effector* function, and one example of a physiological response in which such neurones are recruited and exert an effector function is in the axon reflex-mediated vasodilatation response to injury in the skin.

It has been shown that application of mustard oil to skin induces an inflammatory response consisting of vasodilatation, plasma extravasation, and the phagocytosis of particles released from the circulation into the tissue. The inflammatory response was suppressed by local anaesthesia and, more specifically, by transection of sensory nerves distal to the dorsal root ganglion [1]. Sensory neurones appear, therefore, to be involved in the inflammatory response to mustard oil. Nociceptor information is carried largely in C fibres, and direct recording from C fibres has shown that polymodal nociceptors respond to firm pressure, heat intense enough to cause pain, and to chemical stimulation by a variety of agents such as histamine [2]. As much as 80% of all C fibres receive inputs from polymodal nociceptors, which themselves can have receptive fields with a diameter of 1 mm to 1 cm. Primary afferent neurones have been shown to contain the peptides somatostatin, substance P, neurokinin A, and calcitonin gene-related peptide, and it is likely that the latter three neuropeptides coexist in a single class of neurones [3]. Substance P is present in the peripheral ends of these neurones and can be released by stimulation [4, 5].

The drug capsaicin is able to cause the release of neuropeptides from primary afferent neurones, and it also causes depletion of the peptides from the neurones. It has been shown that capsaicin pretreatment of human skin abolishes the axon reflex-induced vasodilatation, which is consistent with the view that neuropeptides released from primary afferent neurones are mediators of this vasodilatation [6, 7]. In rat skin, capsaicin has also been shown to prevent heat-induced plasma extravasation [8]. Thus, inflammatory responses can, in some circumstances, have a neurogenic component involving neuropeptide release from primary afferent neurones.

Of course, there are many inflammatory mediators, and what is generally accepted about inflammation suggests that in a variety of inflammatory responses, several interacting mediators are involved to produce the overall response.

Lewis [9] originally suggested an involvement of histamine as a mediator of axon reflexes. Histamine is mainly contained within mast cells, and there is evidence for mast cell-neurone interaction in neurogenic inflammation in skin, although the exact nature of such an interaction is controversial. One hypothesis is that injury to the skin causes mast cell damage and the release of histamine. The histamine activates primary afferent neurones through H_1 receptors, and neuropeptides are released by axon reflex to cause an inflam-

*   Department of Pharmacology, University College London, Gower Street, London WC1E 6BT, United Kingdom

matory response [10]. An alternative view is that stimulation of a primary afferent neurone by whatever means initiates an axon reflex and the release of neuropeptides, which then act upon mast cells to release histamine. In this case, the final response is caused by histamine, though the neuropeptide may also contribute [11]. The two hypotheses are not mutually exclusive. Evidence for a role for mast cells and histamine at the distal end of the axon reflex, as in the second hypothesis given above, can be summarized as follows:

1. Substance P-containing neurones form close associations with mast cells [12].

2. Substance P releases histamine from mast cells, though not in all tissues and species [13].

3. H_1 histamine antagonists or compound 48/80 pretreatment blocks inflammation induced by stimulating primary afferent nerves [15, 16].

Against this hypothesis and favouring the first hypothesis given above are the data showing that inflammation induced by capsaicin, i.e., chemically induced neuropeptide release, is not blocked by H_1 antagonists [10].

In this paper, data are presented on experiments designed to answer the following questions:

1. What is the effect of an H_1 antagonist on vasodilatation induced by initiating an axon reflex through cholinoceptor stimulation?

2. Does substance P interact with PGE2, a classical mediator of inflammation?

Methods

The protocol used in these experiments was approved by the Ethics Committee of University College London. The subjects were healthy adult volunteers of both sexes in the age range 20 to 40 years. Subjects were receiving no medication at the time of or immediately prior to the experiments, and none of them had a history of atopic disease.

Substance P was prepared from a frozen stock solution of about 1 mM in 0.1% acetic acid which was thawed, neutralized with 1 M sodium hydroxide, and diluted in sterile, buffered saline (pH 7.5). PGE2 was dissolved in ethanol to give a stock solution of about 1 mM and diluted in sterile, buffered saline. Carbachol was dissolved in sterile, buffered saline, and was made up freshly before the experiments.

Solutions were drawn up into 1 ml plastic syringes fitted with a 21-gauge needle. A volume of 25 µl was placed intradermally into the skin of the volar surface of the forearm. No more than 4 injections were made into one forearm, and injections were randomly located. The identify of the injection was not known to the individual making the measurements of responses.

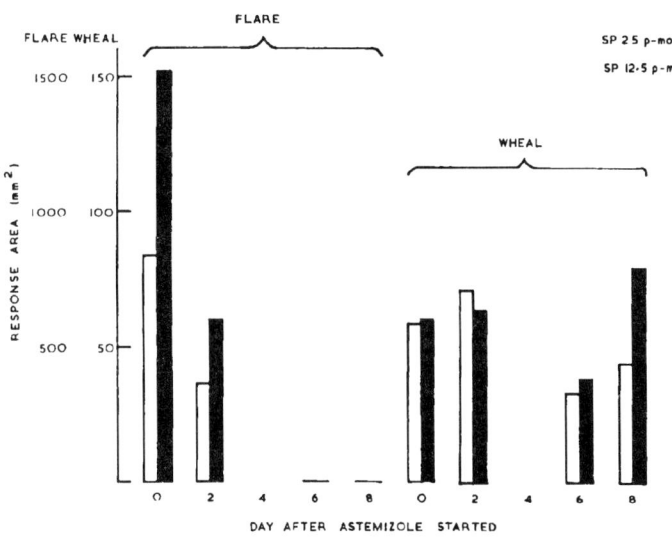

Figure 1. The effect of astemizole on wheal and flare reactions in human skin induced with substance P. Astemizole 30 mg was given orally on day 0.

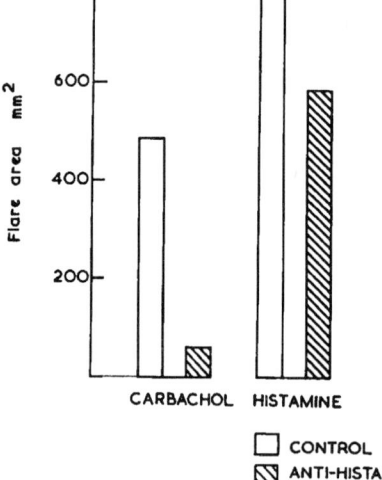

Figure 2. The effect of pretreatment of subjects with astemizole (30 mg orally) before intradermal injection of carbachol (750 p-mol) or histamine (750 p-mol). The area of the flares induced at 3 min after the injection is shown before and after antihistamine treatment in the same group of three subjects.

Wheal and flare responses, measured at the times indicated in the results, were quantified by measuring their diameter in two directions at right angles. The average diameter was used to calculate the area of the response in mm^2. Data from several subjects were pooled. The areas of wheals and flares have been corrected by subtraction of the areas of the vehicle controls.

In experiments involving astemizole, the commercial formulation "Hismanal" (Janssen) was given orally at least two hours after food. Substance P was obtained from Peninsula, St Helens; PGE_2 from Sigma, Poole; carbachol and histamine acid phosphate from B.D.H., Poole.

Results

Figure 1 shows the time course of the effect of orally administered astemizole on the wheal and flare responses to two doses of substance P injected intradermally. Two days after astemizole, the flare response to substance P is reduced, but the wheal response is unchanged. Six and eight days after the astemizole, the flare response is abolished, but the wheal response is little changed.

Figure 2 shows the flare response to both histamine and carbachol before and after pretreatment of the subjects with astemizole. The histamine antagonist inhibited the flare response to carbachol and to histamine.

Figure 3 shows the interaction between prostaglandin E_2 and substance P in the generation of wheal. The dose of PGE_2 was chosen, on the basis of preliminary experiments, to produce a degree of vasodilatation at the lower end of the dose-response curve. Similarly, the substance P doses were chosen from the lower end of the dose-response curve. It can be seen that PGE_2 produced virtually no wheal by itself, but when mixed together and injected with substance P, the prostaglandin potentiates the wheal responses to substance P.

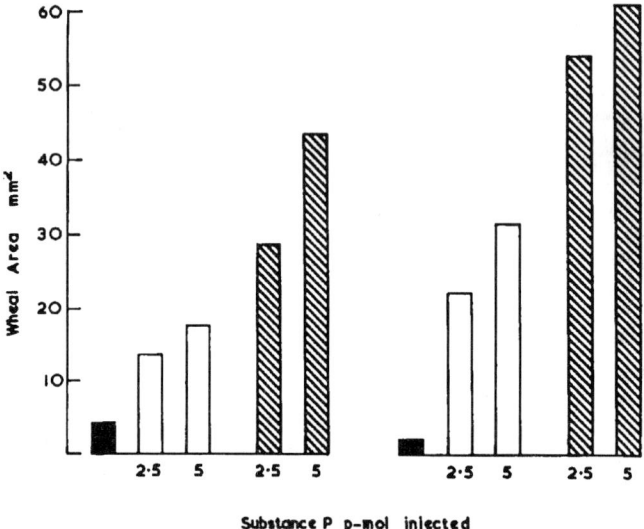

Figure 3. The interaction between substance P (SP) and prostaglandin E_2 (PGE_2) in the generation of wheal in human skin. The data grouped on the left of the figure was obtained from measurements 15 min after injection, and that grouped on the right of the figure from measurements at 45 min after injection. ■ PGE_2 6.25 p-mol; □ SP 2.5 or 5 p-mol; ▢ PGE_2 6.25 p-mol plus SP 2.5 or 5 p-mol. Each value is the mean of data from three subjects.

Discussion

The data presented show that initiation of an axon reflex in human skin by nicotinic cholinoceptor stimulation is inhibited by the H_1 antagonist astemizole which is itself devoid of anticholinergic activity. Assuming carbachol does not release histamine—and there is no evidence that it does—it follows that the axon reflex induces histamine release. According to the hypothesis presented above, it is suggested that the data are consistent with a model of the axon reflex in which substance P released from the neurone by cholinoceptor stimulation causes mast cells to release histamine and induce vasodilatation. This conflicts with other data [10] in which it was shown that capsaicin-induced axon reflex vasodilatation is not inhibited by antihistamine. The resolution of the conflict may be explained by an involvement of mast cells in the distal arm of the axon reflex which is dependent on the nature of the stimulus activating the axon reflex. Clearly, the nature of mast cell involvement in axon reflex vasodilatation has yet fully to be determined.

The second part of the data presented indicates the importance of considering mediator interactions in neurogenic inflammation. Calcitonin gene-related peptide (CGRP), which may be co-released with substance P, is unlikely to be a mediator of flare in human skin because of its slow time course of action [17], but it does potentiate the effects of several inflammatory mediators which produce increased vascular permeability [18]. It is clear that PGE_2, a vasodilator that is more rapidly acting than CGRP, can potentiate oedema induced by substance P. Whether such interactions are of physiological significance remains to be established.

References

1. Jancsó, N., A. Jancsó-Gábor, and J. Szolcsanyi. 1967. Direct evidence for neurogenic inflammation and its prevention by denervation and by pretreatment with capsaicin. Br. J. Pharmacol. 31: 138.
2. Torebjörk, H. E., and R. G. Hallin. 1974. Idenfication of afferent C units in intact human skin. Brain Res. 67: 387.
3. Nawa, H., T. Hirose, H. Takashima, S. Inayama, and S. Nakanishi. 1983. Nucleotide sequences of cloned cDNAs for two types of bovine brain substance P precursor. Nature 306: 32.
4. Hökfelt, T., J. O. Kellerth, G. Nilsson, and B. Pernow. 1976. Experimental immunohisto-chemical studies on the localization and distribution of substance P in cat primary sensory neurones. Brain Res. 100: 235.
5. Thériault, E., M. Otsuka, and T. Jessel. 1979. Capsaicin-evoked release of substance P from primary sensory neurones. Brain Res. 170: 209.
6. Bernstein, J. E., R. M. Swift, K. Soltani, and A. L. Lorincz. 1981. Inhibition of axon reflex vasodilation by topically applied capsaicin. J. Invest. Dermatol. 76: 394.
7. Foreman, J. C., C. C. Jordan, P. Oehme, and H. Renner. 1983. Structure-activity relationships for some substance P-related peptides that cause wheal and flare reactions in human skin. J. Physiol. 335: 449.
8. Saria, A., and J. M. Lundberg. 1983. Capsaicin pretreatment inhibits heat-induced oedema in the rat skin. Naunyn Schmiedeberg's Arch. Pharmacol. 323: 341.
9. Lewis, T. 1927. The blood vessels of the human skin and their responses. Shaw & Sons, London.
10. Barnes, P. J., M. J. Brown, C. T. Dollery, R. W. Fuller, D. J. Heavey, and P. W. Ind. 1986. Histamine is released from skin by substance P but does not act as the final vasodilator in the axon reflex. Br. J. Pharmacol. 88: 741.
11. Fewtrell, C. M. S., J. C. Foreman, C. C. Jordan, P. Oehme, H. Renner, and J. M. Stewart. 1982. The effect of substance P on histamine and 5-hydroxytryptamine release in rat. J. Phys. 330: 393.
12. Skofitsch, G., J. M. Savitt, and D. M. Jacobowitz. 1985. Suggestive evidence for a functional unit between mast cells and substance P fibres in the rat diaphragm and mesentery. Histochemistry 2: 5.
13. Johnson, A. R., and E. G. Erdös. 1973. Release of histamine from mast cells by vasoactive peptides. Proc. Soc. Exp. Biol. Med. 142: 1253.
14. Kiernan, J. A. 1972. The involvement of mast cells in vasodilatation due to axon reflexes in injured skin. Q. Jl. Exp. Physiol. 57: 311.
15. Graham, B. H., and F. Lioy. 1973. Histaminergic vasodilatation in the hindlimb of the dog. Pflügers Arch. Physiol. 342: 307.
16. Lembeck, F., and P. Holzer. 1979. Substance P as neurogenic mediator of antidromic vasodilation and neurogenic plasma extravasation. Naunyn Schmiedeberg's Arch. Pharmacol. 310: 175.
17. Piotrowski, W., and J. C. Foreman. 1986. Some effects of calcitonin gene-related peptide in human skin and on histamine release. Br. J. Dermatol. 114: 37.
18. Brain, S. D., and T. J. Williams. 1985. Inflammatory oedema induced by synergism between calcitonin gene-related peptide (CGRP) and mediators of increased vascular permeability. Br. J. Pharmacol. 86: 855.

Neuroendocrine Peptide Mediators of Hypersensitivity and Inflammation

*Edward J. Goetzl, Setu P. Rangi, Maria H. Serwonska, Sunil P. Sreedharan**

Mast cells, macrophages, lymphocytes, and other elements of the immune system generate peptide mediators similar or structurally identical to neuroendocrine peptides encoded by the same genes. Such peptides from neuroendocrine and immune sources exert effects in both systems through receptors specific for the mediator and the target cell. Further elucidation of the roles of these families of neuropeptide mediators in immunity and hypersensitivity may provide new diagnostic techniques and avenues for therapy.

Neuropeptides, neuropeptide-like factors, and other neuromediators have been implicated in the pathogenesis of immediate hypersensitivity, other immunological reactions, and inflammation [1, 2]. Substance P (SP) has been identified by direct assays in inflamed tissues of rats with experimental arthritis [1] and in pulmonary airways of guinea pigs induced to exhibit hyperreactivity analogous to asthma [3]. In these models, elevations of the concentrations of SP paralleled the development of disease temporally and regionally, surgical and pharmacological reductions of the level or local effects of SP diminished the severity of disease, and administration of SP at sites of mild disease enhanced the tissue reactions [1, 3]. In human diseases, studies have been limited to observations of increases in the lesional fluid concentrations of SP in cutaneous bullous diseases [4], SP and calcitonin gene-related peptide (CGRP) in ascites evoked by interleukin 2 and lymphokine-activated killer cells during intraperitoneal treatment of carcinoma [5], and CGRP and somatostatin (SOM) in nasal secretions elicited by ryegrass antigen challenge of allergic patients [6]. SP and some other neuropeptides are capable of evoking classical wheal and flare reactions in human skin, partly as a result of recruiting cutaneous mast cells [7].

Some mechanisms of neuromediation of immunity, hypersensitivity, and inflammation have been elucidated recently by the definition of critical cellular and molecular constituents. The roles of SP and other tachykinins in inflammation, the structures of the neuropeptides and neuropeptide-like factors from immune cells, and the characteristics of receptors on immune cells that recognize neural signals specifically are better understood.

Tachykinins as Mediators of Allergy, Inflammation, and Tissue Repair

SP, substance K (SK), and neuromedin K are usually present together in primary afferent and other neurons selectively, and upon release into tissues evoke various responses typical of neurogenic inflammation [8]. SP contracts gastrointestinal and pulmonary airway smooth muscle from many species with nanomolar potency [8, 9], dilates systemic arteries and arterioles [8], and enhances airway secretions in guinea pigs, rats, dogs, and ferrets, with far less effect in humans [10]. SP also recruits and activates leukocytes, with a distinctly high potency for monocytes [11]. SP stimulates the proliferation and some synthetic activities of lymphocytes [1], and SP and SK have similar effects on many fixed tissue constituents, such as smooth muscle cells, fibroblasts, endothelial cells, and synoviocytes [12]. Mast cells, but not basophils, are stimulated by SP to release histamine and, in some instances, other mediators by IgE-independent mechanisms [7]. The cellular activities of SP are attributable to distinct subsets of receptors in every system examined, although their specificity varies with the type of cell [3]. Interactions between tachykinins and neuropeptides of other classes are common, and may be inhibitory or facilitory. The

* Howard Hughes Medical Institute and the Department of Medicine and Microbiology-Immunology University of California Medical Center, San Francisco, California.

86

vasodilator CGRP, for example, lacks perceptible vasopermeability activity, but augments this function of SP. SP conversely shortens the duration of the vasodilatory action of CGRP [13].

Neuropeptide Mediators from Immunological Cells

Adrenocorticotrophic hormone, corticotropin-releasing hormone, human chorionic gonadotropin, and β-endorphin from lymphocytes are identical to the corresponding neural forms [2]. In contrast, variants of many different neuroendocrine peptides have been identified in immunological cells, but not detected by similar techniques in the nervous system.

Enkephalins from different subsets of lymphocytes are quite heterogeneous and include forms that are extended amino- and carboxy-terminally, presumably as a result of peptidolysis of a different precursor generated by alternative transcription. The SP from eosinophils and monocytes is identical to the nonapeptide from neural sources, whereas that from mast cells and some basophils is a mixture of the parent forms, as well as SP_{1-7} and SP_{8-11} from the action of chymase on SP_{1-11} [14, 15].

Efferent autonomic neurons in many tissues and some other neuroendocrine cells produce vasoactive intestinal peptide (VIP_{1-28}), which serves as a potent mediator of smooth muscle relaxation, vasodilatation, secretion, cellular division and differentiation [16]. The recent appreciation of the immunological effects of VIP_{1-28} led to the demonstration of native and variant forms of VIP_{1-28} in extracts of unstimulated cultured rat basophilic leukemia (RBL) cells, rat serosal mast cells, and supernatant fluids from RBL stimulated by ionophore [17]. Identical extracts of eosinophils and PMN leukocytes contained an immunoreactive VIP peptide that proved to be the same as the VIP_{1-28} derived from neuroendocrine sources [14]. In contrast, the immunoreactive VIP peptides from mast cells consisted principally of VIP_{10-28} free acid and, to a lesser extent, of two amino-terminally extended forms of VIP_{1-28} [17]. Only a minor amount of VIP_{1-28} was detected in rat mast cells and none was found in the RBL cells. The VIP_{10-28} and other variant forms of VIP were not generated by peptidolysis of VIP_{1-28} or prepro-VIP. Mast cell tryptase

and chymase cleave VIP_{1-28} into VIP_{1-14}, VIP_{15-20}, VIP_{15-28}, VIP_{21-28}, and VIP_{23-28}, but not VIP_{10-28} [15]. The results of preliminary studies suggest that the variants of VIP from mast cells may be attributable to alternative splicing of messenger RNA resulting in a pre-pro-VIP susceptible to a unique cleavage. The possible functional significance of a structurally diverse representation of some neuropeptides in the immune system will only be known when the differences between the recognition mechanisms for these neuropeptides are elucidated in the two systems.

Lymphocyte Receptors for VIP_{1-28} and SOM

SOM and VIP_{1-28} are potent and selective inhibitors of a range of lymphocyte functions, including proliferation and generation of immunoglobulins other than IgG [18], by receptor-dependent mechanisms. Flow cytometric analyses of the binding of fluorescent conjugates of neuropeptides by Jurkat human T-lymphocytes and U266 human myeloma cells indicated that the majority of these lymphocytes recognized SOM and VIP_{1-28}. The presence of an excess of unlabeled SOM or VIP_{1-28} prevented more than 50% of the respective fluorescent labeling of the cells. Computer-based analyses of the specific binding of $[^{125}I\text{-}Tyr^{11}]SOM$ or $[^{125}I\text{-}Tyr^{10}]VIP_{1-28}$ to Jurkat and U266 cells revealed 10^2 and 10^3 high affinity sites for SOM with Kd values of 3 pM and 5 pM, respectively, and a large number of low affinity sites with Kd values of 66 nM and 100 nM, respectively. VIP_{1-28} bound to 10^4 high affinity sites per Jurkat and U266 cell with Kd values of 5.2 nM and 7.6 nM, respectively.

Analogs of SOM, including the naturally occurring twenty-eight amino acid variant SOM 28, mono-iodinated $[Tyr^{11}]SOM$ and $[D\text{-}Trp^8, D\text{-}Cys^{14}]SOM$ also inhibited the binding of $[^{125}I\text{-}Tyr^{11}]SOM$ to both cell lines. Similarly, the principal mast cell-derived variant VIP_{1-28}, L-8-K and $[Ac\ Tyr^1, D\text{-}Phe^2]GRF_{1-29}$ amide peptide analogs of VIP_{1-28} displaced $[^{125}I\text{-}Tyr^{10}]VIP_{1-28}$ from Jurkat and U266 cells, respectively. VIP_{10-28} exhibited an affinity 1/10 that of VIP_{1-28} for lymphocyte receptors, whereas it had only 1/10,000 the affinity of VIP_{1-28} for neural receptors. SP, CGRP, and VIP_{1-28} failed to competitively inhibit the binding of [^{125}I-Tyr^{11}]SOM to Jurkat and U266 cells, respectively, while SP and SOM had no effect on the binding of [^{125}I-Tyr^{10}]VIP$_{1-28}$ to either cell line.

Mast Cell Mediators of Lymphocyte Proliferation, Differentiation and Function

The evidence currently available does not permit assignment of the relative importance of any one mediator from mast cells in the regulation of lymphocytic function in host defense or any specific disease state. The overall effect of the array of mediators released from activated mast cells, however, appears to be suppression of the functions of T-cells and antibody-producing cells. Histamine activates a subset of suppressor T-cells (Ts) by an H$_2$-dependent mechanism. Prostaglandin (PG) D$_2$ is generated by the cyclo-oxygenation of arachidonic acid and, like PGE$_2$, suppresses helper T-cell (TH) activity, enhances Ts activity, facilitates the conversion of pre-Ts to Ts, and inhibits the production of immunoglobulin by cells of B-lineage. Leukotriene (LT) B$_4$ is synthesized from arachidonic acid by the 5-lipoxygenase pathway and exhibits the same activities as PGD$_2$/E$_2$, except for a lack of effect on the immunoglobulin-synthesizing activities of plasma cells. Both PGD$_2$/E$_2$ and LTB$_4$ not only shift the regulatory functions of T-cells toward a suppressor role, but also inhibit proliferative and some synthetic capacities of T-cells. As for PGD$_2$/E$_2$ and histamine, neuroendocrine-derived VIP$_{1-28}$ also appears to inhibit T-cell and B-cell activities, in part through cyclic AMP-dependent mechanisms, but VIP$_{1-28}$ exhibits an immunoglobulin isotypic preference for non-IgG classes. The functional roles of mast cell-derived VIP$_{10-28}$ remain to be elucidated, but may either encompass the same primary reactions as VIP$_{1-28}$ or instead be devoid of such actions and exhibit solely an effect antagonistic to VIP$_{1-28}$.

References

1. Levine, J. D., E. J. Goetzl, and A. I. Basbaum. 1987. Contribution of the nervous system to the pathophysiology of rheumatoid arthritis and other polyarthritides. Rheum. Dis. Clin. N.A. 13: 369.

2. Goetzl E. J., S. P. Sreedharan, and W. S. Harkonen. 1988. Pathogenetic roles of neuroimmunologic mediators. Immunol. & Allergy Clin. N.A. 8: 183.

3. Lundberg, J. M., A. Saria, E. Brodin, S. Rosell, and K. Folkers. 1983. A substance P antagonist inhibits vagally induced increase in vascular permeability and bronchial smooth muscle contraction in the guinea pig. Proc. Natl. Acad. Sci. U.S.A. 80: 1120.

4. Wallengren, D., R. Ekman, and H. Moller. 1986. Substance P and vasoactive intestinal peptide in bullous and inflammatory skin disease. Acta Derm. Venereol. (Stockh.) 66: 23.

5. Schiogolev, S. A., E. J. Goetzl, W. J. Urba, and D. L. Longo. 1988. Appearance of neuropeptides in ascitic fluid after peritoneal therapy with interleukin 2 and lymphokine-activated killer cells for intraabdominal malignancy. J. Clin. Immunol., in press.

6. Walker, K. B., M. H. Serwonksa, F. H. Valone, W. S. Harkonen, O. L. Frick, K. H. Scriven, W. D. Ratnoff, J. G. Browning, D. G. Payan, and E. J. Goetzl. 1988. Distinctive patterns of release of neuroendocrine peptides after nasal challenge of allergic subjects with ryegrass antigen. J. Clin. Immunol. 8: 108.

7. Foreman, J. C., C. C. Jordan, and W. Piotrowski. 1982. Interaction of neurotensin with the substance P receptor mediating histamine release from rat mast cells and the flare in human skin. Br. J. Pharmacol. 77: 531.

8. Pernow, B. 1983. Substance P. Pharmacol. Rev. 35: 85.

9. Lundberg, J. M., C.-R. Martling, and A. Saria. 1982. Substance P and capsaicin-induced contraction of human bronchi. Acta Physiol. Scand. 119: 49.

10. Borson, D. B., R. Corrales, S. Varsano, W. Gold, N. Viro, G. Caughey, J. Ramachandran, and J. A. Nadel. 1987. Enkephalinase inhibitors potentiate substance P-induced secretion of 35S04-macromolecules from ferret trachea. Exp. Lung. Res. 12: 21.

11. Ruff, M. R, S. M. Wahl, and C. B. Pert. 1985. Substance P receptor-mediated chemotaxis of human monocytes. Peptides 6: 107.

12. Nilsson, J., A. M. Von Euler, and C. J. Dalsgaad. 1985. Stimulation of connective tissue cell growth by substance P and substance K. Nature 315: 61.

13. Brain, S. D., and T. J. Williams. 1988. Substance P regulates the vasodilation activity of calcitonin gene-related peptide. Nature 335: 73.

14. Aliakbari, J., S. P. Sreedharan, C. W. Turck, and E. J. Goetzl 1987. Selective localization of vasoactive intestinal peptide and substance P in

human eosinophils. Biochem. Biophys. Res. Commun. 148: 1440.

15. Caughey, G. H., F. Leidig, N. F. Viro, and J. A. Nadel. 1988. Substance P and vasoactive intestinal peptide degradation by mast cell tryptase and chymase. J. Pharmacol. Exp. Ther. 244: 133.

16. Said, S. I. 1984. Vasoactive intestinal polypeptide (VIP): Current status. Peptides 5: 143.

17. Goetzl, E. J., S. P. Sreedharan, and C. W. Turck 1988. Structurally distinctive vasoactive intesti-

nal peptides from rat basophilic leukemia cells. J. Biol. Chem. 263: 9083.

18. Stanisz, A. M., D. Befus, and J. Bienenstock. 1986. Differential effects of vasoactive intestinal peptide, substance P, and somatostatin on immunoglobulin synthesis and proliferations by lymphocytes from Peyer's patches, mesenteric lymph nodes, and spleen. J. Immunol. 136: 152.

The Mast Cell Receptor for Immunoglobulin E: Prospects for Therapy 1988

*Henry Metzger, Jean-Pierre Kinet, Uli Blank, Larry Miller, Chisei Ra, Juan Rivera, Kenneth White**

The receptor with high affinity for immunoglobulin E (IgE) is a potentially useful target at which to direct drugs in order to prevent and/or halt allergic attacks. Recently, cDNAs corresponding to the α, β, and γ subunits that comprise the receptor have been cloned and expressed in transfected cells. These results provide the tools with which to analyze the structural basis of IgE binding, and to screen for inhibitors of IgE binding efficiently. Similarly, these results provide new ways to explore the mechanism by which the receptor initiates degranulation and should therefore assist in the development of inhibitors of receptor-mediated degranulation.

Three years ago, at the 12th Congress in Washington, D.C., one of the authors presented a paper entitled "The Mast Cell Receptor for Immunoglobulin E: Prospects for Therapy" [1]. That paper assessed how increasing knowledge about the high-affinity receptors for IgE on mast cells and basophils could lead to the development of new treatments for allergic diseases. Two principal categories of intervention were considered: (1) interfering with the binding of IgE to the high-affinity receptor and (2) interfering with the early biochemical signals that result from activation of these receptors. In this paper, we summarize new results that have brought us closer to developing such new therapeutic strategies. We focus on four principal aspects of the receptor: the tissue distribution of the receptor, its binding properties, its peptide structure, and its topology in the membrane. Each of these four is directly relevant to the prospects of using information about the receptor to develop new therapies.

Distribution of Receptor

The localization of the high-affinity receptor was initially determined by IgE binding and other studies. These suggested its presence on mast cells and basophils exclusively [2–4]. The availability of molecular genetic probes as well as monoclonal antibodies permits us to extend these analyses, particularly with respect to those subunits of the receptor that cannot be assessed by simple binding studies using IgE [5–7]. We currently have rather convincing evidence that the γ subunits (below) may be found in cells other than basophils and mast cells [Ra et al., unpublished results]. Therefore, if eventually one wished to use drugs to interfere with the function of those subunits, one must be prepared for the possibility that one will also interfere with the function of proteins other than the high-affinity receptor for IgE.

Binding Properties

The binding properties of the high-affinity receptor have been substantially characterized [8, 9]. We wish to reemphasize the importance of the rate constants. The slow dissociation of IgE from its receptor means that it will take many hours for an inhibitor to displace IgE from cells—not matter how effective it may be as an inhibitor of binding. This subject has been dealt with at greater length in Dr. Hans Spiegelberg's contribution [10]. The subject of ligand specificity has also been dealt with elsewhere in this volume [11]. Here, we simply note that the possibility of defining the sites on the Fc region of IgE with which the receptor interacts [11] will likely enhance the ability to discover suitable inhibitors for that interaction. The results we summarize here will, we believe, demonstrate that such investigations can now be made much more practical than before.

* Section on Chemical Immunology, Arthritis and Rheumatism Branch, National Institute of Arthritis and Musculoskeletal and Skin Diseases, National Institutes of Health, Bethesda, Maryland 20892, USA.
U. B. was supported by a grant from the Deutsche Forschungsgemeinschaft (FRG).

Peptide Structure

The peptide structure of the receptor on rat basophilic leukemia cells was initially explored by protein chemical analysis. Those studies demonstrated that the receptor consisted of three types of polypeptide chains—an α subunit, which by itself is sufficient to bind IgE, an associated single β chain, and two disulfide-linked γ chains [12].

More recently, we have identified the nucleic acid sequences that code for each of the subunits. In each case the same strategy was used: The subunit was purified, selected tryptic peptides were sequenced, oligonucleotide probes were synthesized based on such sequences, and the probes used to screen a gt11 cDNA library prepared from mRNAs of rat basophilic leukemia cells. Positive colonies were cloned and the open reading frame of the selected cDNA determined. For each cDNA presumptively coding for a particular subunit, a variety of structural and immunological criteria were used to verify that the correct gene had been isolated. Characterization of the cDNA coding for the α chain was first published in mid-1987 [13; see also 14, 15], that for the β chain has just been published [5], and a manuscript describing our isolation of the cDNA coding for the γ chains will appear shortly [7]. In each case the sequence predicted by the cDNA was found to be fully consistent with the chemical and immunologic data.

Topology

Analysis of the amino acid sequence by so-called hydropathicity plots [16] as well as by other statistical analyses [17] allows one to make predictions about the topology of a membrane protein. These predictions can be further tested by assessing the exposure of the protein on intact and permeabilized cells by labeling reagents, by the use of proteolytic enzymes, and by the use of antibodies directed to specific regions of the protein. We have employed all of these techniques to develop a working model of the receptor [7], which is shown in Figure 1. In this model, each of the 589 amino acid residues of which the expressed receptor is composed is shown as a circle with the cysteines highlighted. In the diagram, the exterior of the cell would be at the top, the plasma membrane

in which the receptor is embedded would be in the middle, and the interior of the cell toward the bottom. Each of the polypeptide chains—the α on the left, the β chain in the middle, and the two γ chains on the right—contains one or more transmembrane segments. We shall comment briefly about some of the details of the model.

The α chain is thought to contain two intrachain disulfide loops, and the sequences of these loops show considerable homology with immunoglobulins [13–15]. Thus, the α subunit is another member of the immunoglobulin superfamily [18]. The extracellular and transmembrane segments of the α chain show considerable homology with the immunoglobulin binding chain of Fc receptors that bind IgG [19], but the intracellular cytoplasmic tail is quite different. We have not indicated the carbohydrate residues that are covalently attached to the extracellular portion of the α chain. There are seven potential sites for N-linked carbohydrates [13, 14], but which of these are actually used by the cell remains to be determined. We, and others, have data that indicate that the carbohydrate is not essential for the binding of IgE by this chain [20; Rivera & Metzger, unpublished data].

The β chain contains four transmembrane segments [5], and our studies with monoclonal antibodies [5, 6] show that the amino- and carboxy-terminii, which are respectively 59 and 43 residues long, protrude from the cytoplasmic face of the plasma membrane. Similarly, the γ chains have an extensive intracellular extension, but only very limited exposure to the exterior [7]. The arrangement of the chains in this diagram is not entirely arbitrary: We have a variety of direct and indirect data to support specific aspects of this model [7], though much further work will be required to test our proposal.

Expression of the Transfected Genes

When we first isolated the cDNA for the IgE binding α subunit, we naturally tried to express it by transfecting nonreceptor-containing cells with a plasmid containing the cDNA sequence for the α subunit. We [13], and subsequently others [14], were unsuccessful. Similarly, when we isolated the cDNA for the β

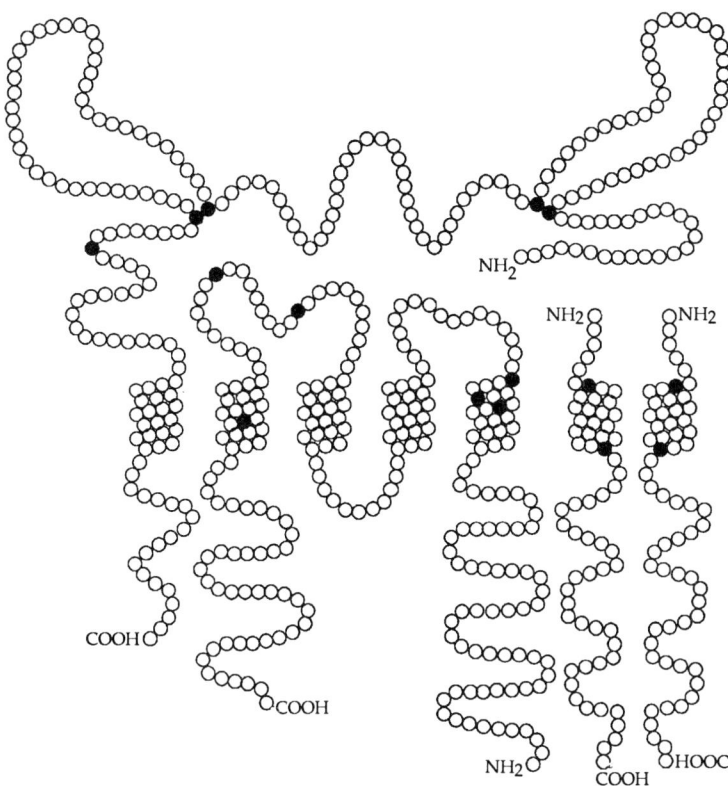

Figure 1. Model of tetrameric receptor. The α chain is shown on the left, the β in the middle, and the two disulfide-linked γ chains on the right. The cysteines are highlighted. This is a simplified version of that given in [7].

subunit, cotransfection of α and β failed to allow the α chain to be expressed [5]. Recently, having isolated the cDNA for the γ chain, we attempted a triple transfection with the cDNAs for the α, β, and γ chains [7]. We analyzed the cells both for specific messenger RNA production as well as for their ability to bind a hapten-specific IgE. In turn, the presence of bound IgE was detected by exposing the cells to haptenated sheep red blood cells in a rosetting technique. The results were clearcut: In each case the transfection worked insofar as the appropriate messenger RNA was synthesized, but only those populations that were transfected with the cDNAs for all three subunits simultaneously contained cells capable of binding [7]. When excess nonspecific IgE was present, complete inhibition was observed as expected.

Our ultimate goal is, of course, to analyze not only the rat receptor for IgE, but also—and more importantly—the human receptor. We and others have identified and sequenced cDNAs for the α subunit of the human IgE receptor [14, 15]. There is an overall homology of about 47%, but an almost 70% homology in the presumed transmembrane domains. In fact, in the central portion of the transmembrane domains, there is a stretch of ten consecutive residues that are completely identical.

Since the transmembrane segment is the region of the α chain that is most likely to interact with the β and γ chains, it was reasonable to hope that the human α chain would be expressible, if transfected, along with the rat β and γ chains. We have recently been successful in this regard [L. Miller et al., submitted]. That is, we were able to express human IgE binding by Cos cells transfected simultaneously with the human α and the rat β and γ subunits. It will be advantageous, of course, to have permanently transfected cells lines, and for such lines, one will want to utilize the human β and γ subunits. We are well along in identifying the coding sequences for these subunits, so that preparing such transfectants should be straightforward. Thus, with the materials available now, it is already practical to search for peptide inhibitors of human IgE binding in vitro. To make the assay suitable for truly mass screening of drugs will require apparently minor extensions of our current work.

The genetic work, of course, provides much more than an assay, as important as the latter may be. Through directed mutation, it will, in addition, allow one to develop further information about the critical binding regions. Potentially, therefore, rational drug design will become possible.

Functional Analysis

We wish to comment briefly about the function of the receptor in signal transduction, and what one can reasonable expect in the short-term future. The importance of this area is such that it could be a therapeutic target for *aborting* allergic attacks—not just *preventing* them. To the extent to which the mechanism of signal transduction is at all receptor-specific, one can anticipate that interrupting it will not induce extensive side effects.

In our introductory remarks we referred to the discussion of this subject presented at the Congress in Washington [1]. Regrettably, we must conclude that the field has not progressed in any fundamental way over the last three years. Some of the previously described phenomena have been discarded as unlikely to represent significant steps in the pathway to degranulation; others have not really been further extended or extended substantially [21–23]. Despite considerable efforts by our own group, adequate membrane preparations capable of exhibiting receptor-mediated reactions still elude us. We continue to feel that such preparations are likely to be required to make major new advances.

Nevertheless, the progress in the molecular genetics of the receptor may allow one to develop new approaches to the problem. For example, by directed mutagenesis one may be able to influence selectively one or more of the many perturbations induced by the receptor. In turn, by relating these to subsequent degranulation of the cells, one may be able to assess the significance of the biochemical changes. For such studies it will be important to transfect receptors into cells that will respond to the activation of the receptor in a manner similar to that used by mast cells and basophils. We have set this as a major priority for our laboratory in the coming years.

References

1. Metzger, H. 1986. The mast cell receptor for immunoglobulin E: Prospects for therapy. In Proc. XII Int. Cong. Allerg. Clin. Immunol. C. E. Reed, ed. St. Louis, MO: C.V. Mosby, p. 308.
2. Graham, H. T., O. H. Bowry, F. Wheelwright, M. A. Lenz, and H. H. Parrish. 1955. Distribution of histamine among leukocytes and platelets. Blood J. Hematol. 29: 467.
3. Ishizaka, K., H. Tomioka, and T. Ishizaka. 1970. Mechanisms of passive sensitization. I. Presence of IgE and IgG molecules on human leukocytes. J. Immunol. 105: 1459.
4. Sullivan, A. L., P. M. Grimley, and H. Metzger. 1971. Electron microscopic localization of immunoglobulin E on the surface membrane of human basophils. J. Exp. Med. 134: 1403.
5. Kinet, J.-P., U. Blank, C. Ra, K. White, H. Metzger, and J. Kochan. 1988. Isolation and characterization of cDNAs coding for the β subunit of the high-affinity receptor for immunoglobulin E. Natl. Acad. Sci. 85: 6483.
6. Rivera, J., J.-P. Kinet, J. Kim, C. Pucillo, and H. Metzger. 1988. Studies with a monoclonal antibody to the β subunit of the receptor with high affinity for immunoglobulins E. Mol. Immunol. 25: 647.
7. Blank, J., C. Ra, L. Miller, K. White, H. Metzger, and J.-P. Kinet. 1989. The complete structure of the Fc receptor with high affinity for immunoglobulin E and its surface expression in transfected cells. Nature, in press.
8. Kulczycki, A. Jr., and H. Metzger. 1974. The interaction of IgE with rat basophilic leukemia cells. II. Quantitative aspects of the binding reaction. J. Exp. Med. 140: 1676.
9. Conrad, D., J. R. Wingard, and T. Ishizaka. 1983. The interaction of human and rodent IgE with the human basophil IgE receptor. J. Immunol. 130: 327.
10. Spiegelberg, H. D. 1989. Does IgE receptor blockade have a chance for treatment of allergy? In this volume.
11. Helm, B. 1989. The mast cell binding site on human IgE. In this volume.
12. Metzger, H., G. Alcaraz, R. Hohman, J.-P. Kinet, V. Pribluda, and R. Quarto. 1986. The receptor with high affinity for immunoglobulin E. Ann. Rev. Immunol. 4: 419.
13. Kinet, J.-P., H. Metzger, J. Hakimi, and J. Kochan. 1987. A cDNA presumptively coding for the α subunit of the receptor with high affinity for immunoglobulin E. Biochemistry 26: 4605.
14. Shimizu, A., I. Tepler, P. N. Benfey, E. H. Berenstain, R. P. Siraganian, and P. Leder. 1988. Human and rat mast cell high- affinity immunoglobulin E receptors: Characterization of putative α-chain gene products. Proc. Natl. Acad.

Sci. USA 85: 1907.

15. Kochan, J., L. F. Pettine, J. Hakimi, K. Kishi, and J.-P. Kinet. 1988. Isolation of the gene coding for the α subunit of the human high affinity IgE receptor. Nucleic Acids Res. 16: 3584.

16. Engelman, D. M., T. A. Steitz, and A. Goldman. 1986. Identifying nonpolar transbilayer helices in amino acid sequences of membrane proteins. Ann. Rev. Biophys. Chem. 15: 321.

17. von Heijne, G. 1988. Transcending the impenetrable: How proteins come to terms with membranes. Biochim. Biophys. Acta 947: 307.

18. Williams, A. F., and A. N. Barclay. 1988. The immunoglobulin superfamily—Domains for cell surface recognition. Ann. Rev. Immunol. 6: 381.

19. Ravetch, J. V., A. D. Luster, R. L. Weinshank, J. Kochan, A. Pavlovec, D. A. Portnoy, J. Hulmes, Y. E. Pan, and J. C. Unkeless. 1986. Structural heterogeneity and functional domains of murine immunoglobulin G Fc receptors. Science 234: 718.

20. Hempstead, B. L., C. W. Parker, and A. Kulczycki, A. Jr. 1981. The cell surface receptor for immunoglobulin E—Effect of tunicamycin on molecular properties of receptor from rat basophilic leukemia cells. J. Biol. Chem. 256: 10717.

21. Beaven, M. A., and J. R. Cunha-Melo. 1988. Membrane phosphoinositide-activated signals in mast cells and basophils. Prog. Allergy 42: 123.

22. Oliver, J. M., R. F. Seagrave, R. F. Stump, J. R. Pfeiffer, and G. G. Deanin. 1988. Signal transduction and cellular responses in RBL-2H3 mast cells. Prog. Allergy 42: 185.

23. Metzger, H. 1988. Molecular aspects of receptors and binding factors for IgE. Adv. Immunol. 43: 277.

The Mast Cell Binding Site on Human IgE: A Single ε-Chain Can Engage the High-Affinity (FcεR1) Receptor

Birgit A. Helm*, Nicolas J. Short*, Raif S. Geha**

We reinvestigated the proposal that one of the interchain disulphide bonds in CH2 of human IgE was necessary for binding to the high-affinity receptor (FcεR1) on mast cells and basophils. Since deletion of sequences upstream of Gln 301, which include Cys 241, do not affect target cell interaction [1, 2, 3], we replaced, by site-directed mutagenesis, Cys 328 by a Ser and a Met residue. Ser substitution does not inhibit the binding of IgE to FcεR1, and rE2-4 Ser 328, unlike wild-type rE2-4, does not lose biological activity following reductive alkylation. In contrast, replacement of Cys 328 by Met mimics the loss of biological activity observed with reduced-alkylated IgE. This demonstrates that none of the Cys residues in IgE are required for mast-cell interaction, and that a monomer can form the binding site. It also shows that the structural integrity of the site occupied by Cys 328 is critical for receptor binding, since alkylation of this residue or its replacement by Met is associated with loss of biological activity.

A series of overlapping recombinant human epsilon (ε) chain fragments was employed to map the site(s) on human IgE that interact with the class-specific high-affinity (FcεR1) present on mast cells and basophils. The outcome of these studies showed that the receptor binding site on IgE is located within a 67 amino-acid (a.a.) fragment spanning the carboxy(C)-terminal Cε2 and the amino(N)-terminal Cε3 domain [1]. The interaction requires sequences C and N terminal to a.a. 336, since ε-chain fragments containing the separate sequences (a.a. 218–336 and a.a. 340–547) are inactive. These sequences may contain either a.a. involved in the interaction with the receptor, or provide structural scaffolding. Structural analysis of biologically active recombinant human ε-chain fragments showed that both covalently linked dimers and apparently monomeric fragments can bind FcεR1, sensitize and inhibit the passive sensitization of mast cells and basophils [1, 2, 3].

The acceptance of monomeric ε-chain fragments by FcεR1 was difficult to reconcile with a number of earlier observations, which had demonstrated the sensitivity of reaginic antibodies to the action of thiols [4, 5, 6]. The most detailed study on the effects of reduction followed by alkylation on the biological activity of myeloma IgE (PS) was published in 1975 by Takatsu et al. [7]. Since the a.a. sequence of the ε-chain had been determined in 1974 [8], and the high-affinity binding site was known to reside in the Fc fragment, the authors attempted to correlate progressive reduction followed by alkylation with the loss of biological activity. Their data showed the following:

1) Reductive alkylation of the Cys residues involved in the formation of light-epsilon chain bonds does not adversely affect biological activity.

2) Alkylation of one of the Cys residues forming the intrachain bonds in Cε1 results in a conformational change that modifies the idiotypic antigenic determinants and leads to a reduction in cytotropic activity. However, when the Fc portion was prepared from this fragment, a recovery in biological activity occurred, suggesting that the cleavage of disulphide bonds in the Fab portion induced

---

* Department of Biophysics, King's College, University of London; Present address: Department of Biochemistry, Division of Biomolecular Sciences, University of Sheffield.
** Division of Immunology, The Children's Hospital and Dept. of Pediatrics, Harvard Medical School, Boston, MA. We wish to thank Drs. K. and T. Ishizaka for the generous gift of IgE(PS) and their helpful discussions, I. Chrétien for the gift of anti-epsilon monoclonal antibodies, N. Sarner for helpful technical assistance, and Prof. H. J. Gould for provision of laboratory facilities. The work at King's College was supported by grants from the MRC and CRC, that at Harvard Medical School by the USPHS, the National Foundation, and the March of Dimes.

conformational changes which reduced the affinity of the Fc portion for target cells.

3) Reduction of IgE with 10 mM dithiothreitol (DDT) followed by alkylation led to the cleavage of five disulphide bonds. This is accompanied by the loss of both sensitizing and blocking activities. These observations led to the proposal that one of the inter-epsilon chain disulphide bonds, and thus a dimeric structure, was crucial to the maintenance of an active conformation. Furthermore, since the second Cys residue involved in interchain disulphide bond formation at the N-terminal end of the Ce2 domain appears to remain intact, they suggested that this disulphide bond is most resistant to reduction and may preserve a dimeric, though inactive structure. An alternative proposal was that the cleavage of the C-terminal inter-epsilon chain disulphide bond might change the conformation of the Fc portion involved in receptor binding [7].

Directly connected with the question whether a monomeric or dimeric conformation of IgE-Fc is required for FcεR1 interaction is the nature of the inter-epsilon chain disulphide bond arrangement in Cε2. Current models [9, 10] for human IgE-Fc envisage a crossed disulphide bond pairing, i.e., Cys 241 on one epsilon chain binds to Cys 328 on the opposite chain. The demand for a dimeric conformation is incompatible with a crossed disulphide bond arrangement since sequences N-terminal to a.a. 301 and thus Cys 241 do not contribute to receptor binding [1, 2, 3].

The postulated requirement for a covalent dimer originated from investigations in which the activity of reduced-alkylated IgE had been compared with that of native IgE. Our own observations had consistently shown that reductive alkylation does indeed destroy the biological activity of recombinant dimeric (rE2-4) and monomeric (rE2'-3') fragments. Since studies on the role of disulphide bonds on the conformation of, for example, Cλ, indicate that no significant conformational change occurs upon reduction of disulphide unless SH groups are alkylated [11], we speculated that a conformational

change effected by alkylation, rather than the cleavage of a disulphide bond and the destruction of a dimeric structure, might account for the loss of cytotropic activity.

In order to test this hypothesis, it was decided to replace, by site-directed mutagenesis [12], Cys 328 by a Ser and a Met residue. The former is thought to mimic the effect of reduction on this Cys residue, but eliminates the potential for re-oxidation and thus the reformation of a covalent interchain disulphide bond, while the latter should produce an effect on structure closely resembling that which the introduction of an alkyl group might have.

The observations reported here demonstrate that the sensitizing and blocking activity of rE2-4 and rE2'-3', which is lost upon alkylation, is not affected by the replacement of Cys 328 by Ser. Furthermore, rE2-4 Ser 328, when alkylated, retains full biological activity. In contrast, replacement of Cys 328 by Met is associated with a loss of biological activity characteristic of reductive alkylation.

Materials and Methods

Recombinant ε-chain fragments rE2-4 and rE2'-3' were isolated from lysates of *E. coli* and affinity purified as previously described [2, 13].

Oligonucleotide-directed site-specific mutagenesis was performed by the method of Inouye [12], and the mutations were confirmed by DNA sequencing [14].

Table 1. The effect of reduction-alkylation on the capacity of wild-type and mutant rFcε to inhibit the Prausnitz-Kustner reaction. Skin sites in the forearm of a normal donor were injected one hour before sensitization with recombinant ε-chain peptides. Here, rE2-4, rE2-4 Ser 328, and reduced-alkylated rE2-4 Ser 328 are compared with rE2-4 Met 328 and reduced alkylated rE2'-3' for their capacity to inhibit passive cutaneous anaphylasis. A 1:100 dilution of reaginic serum E.C. was used to sensitize skin sites which were challenged 48 h later with ragweed antigen (experimental details are given in [2, 16]).

	Control native protein	Test alkylated protein
IgE(PS)	active	inactive
rE2-4	active	inactive
rE2'-3'	active	inactive
rE2-4 Ser 328	active	active
rE2-4 Met 328	inactive	not tested

97

Reduction and alkylation of recombinant wild type and mutant rFcε fragments was carried out by a method of Crestfield et al. [15], and the concentration of monomers, dimers, and oligomers was monitored by polyacrylamide gel electrophoresis [16].

The inhibition of the Prausnitz-Kustner (P-K) reaction by recombinant ε-chain fragments used in the present study was carried out as previously described [17].

Results

The biological activity of recombinant wild-type and mutant ε-chain peptides to inhibit passive sensitization in vivo are summarized in Table 1. The data presented here clearly show that the biological activity of human myeloma or recombinant IgE-derived peptides is lost upon reduction followed by alkylation, although we have shown in previous studies [2] that apparently monomeric recombinant ε-chain fragments possess similar binding ability and are almost as potent in inhibiting IgE effector functions as native IgE. The outcome of the present study shows that this paradox can be resolved by substituting Cys 328 by a Ser and a Met residue. Though the mutant epsilon

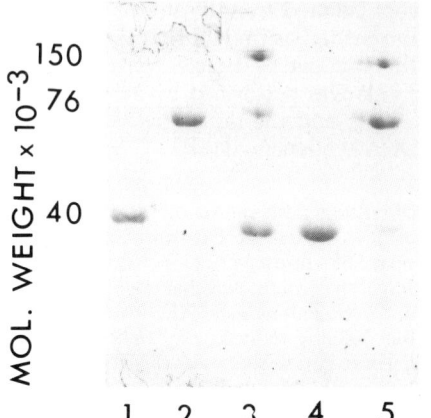

Figure 1. Polyacrylamide gel electrophoresis of recombinant ε-chain peptides used in the present study. The samples were run in SDS under nonreducing conditions. Order of sample application: 1. rE2-4 (monomer), 2. rE2-4 (dimer), 3. rE2-4 Ser 328 (32% tetramer, 23% dimer, 45% monomer), 4. reduced alkylated rE2-4 Ser 328 (monomer), 5. rE2-4 Met 328 (28% tetramer, 612% dimer, 11% monomer). The peptides were isolated from *E. coli* and affinity purified as described previously [2, 16].

chain fragments did not dimerize as efficiently as rE2-4 and give rise to tetramers (Figure 1), in vitro experiments (see Table 2) showed that a preparation of rE2-4 Ser 328 can spontaneously trigger and sensitize peripheral blood basophils for antibody-induced mediator release. After reductive alkylation, however, monomer-ic rE2-4 Ser 328 displays similar activity as rE2-4 in inhibiting the P-K reaction or in the passive sensitization of peripheral blood basophils while rE2-4 Met 328 is completely inactive.

Table 2. Spontaneous triggering and passive sensitization of peripheral blood basophils by rFcε peptides in vitro. Leucocytes isolated from the plasma of a non-atopic individual (BH) were concentrated to $1–2 \times 10^7$ cells ($1–2 \times 10^5$ basophils) per ml by dextran sedimentation according to instructions accompanying the Photometric Allergy Degranulation Test Kit (Boehringer-Mannheim). To measure the spontaneous triggering of basophils, cells were incubated at 37°C with 2 µg/ml IgE(PS), 0.8 µg/ml rE2-4 and mutant r2-4, and 0.4 µg/ml rE2'-3'. After 90 min, 200 µl of ice cold phosphate-buffered EDTA was added and the cells were centrifuged for 5 min at 900g. The spectrophotometric change in absorbance at 405 nm of the supernatant caused by the release of a basophil specific protease, liberating p-NO2-analide from chromozym TH, was measured. For passive sensitization, peptides were incubated with the white blood cell fraction as described above for 90 min at 4°C. Subsequently, the cells were washed with RPM1 1940 medium and suspended in 10 mM Hepes-buffered Tyrode solution, and incubated for 30 min with 0.5 µg/ml mAB IC27 [18]. The reaction was stopped, and the protease activity was measured as described above. Total protease activity present in aliquots of lysed cells resulted in an increase in A_{405nm} of 8.3 units (100%) in 30 min. (Data shown represent the mean of two determinations carried out in duplicate.)

	% of total protease released	
	A	B
	spontaneous triggering	passive sensitization
IgE(PS)	4.85	29.8
rE2-4	8.9	27.9
rE2-4 Ser 328	18.3	23.4
reduced alkylated rE2-4 Ser 328	2.1	28.2
rE2'-3'	9.4	22.3
reduced alkylated rE2'-3'	1.1	3.4
rE2-4 Met 328	0.9	3.8
control	1.1	3.2

Discussion

The data presented here clearly show that the biological activity of human IgE or recombinant IgE-derived peptides is lost upon reduction followed by alkylation, although monomeric recombinant ε-chain fragments possess similar bindability and are almost as potent in inhibiting IgE effector functions as native IgE [1, 2, 3].

Earlier studies [4, 5, 6, 7], in which the effect of progressive reduction followed by alkylation on the biological activity of human IgE was measured, led to the proposal that one of the interchain disulphide bonds in CH2, and thus a dimeric structure, was important for biological activity. Since Cys 241 is not required for FcεR1 interaction, we investigated the effect of two point mutations at a.a. 2328 on the biological activity of IgE.

The present study demonstrates the following: Replacement of Cys 328 by Ser does not adversely affect biological activity. Reduction of this mutant, followed by alkylation, produces a monomeric Fcε fragment with no potential for covalent dimerization, and yet this material is as active as rE2-4. This clearly indicates that none of the Cys residues on IgE are required for the interaction of this molecule with its high-affinity receptor. In contrast, the replacement of Cys 328 by Met is associated with a complete loss of biological activity.

The following interpretation of these data offers an entirely self-consistent explanation for these findings:

1) Binding of IgE to FcεR1 does not require the assembly of ε-chains into disulphide-linked dimers, i.e., a monomeric fragment suffices to form the binding site.

2) The structural integrity of the site occupied by Cys 328, but not Cys 241 is critical for receptor binding since alkylation of Cys 328, but not Cys 241 is associated with loss of receptor binding.

3) Although a monomeric FcεR1 binding site on IgE is compatible with a crossed interchain disulphide bond arrangement proposed by current model structures for human IgE-Fc, the biological activity of alkylated rE2-4 Ser 328 is difficult to reconcile with these models, since only alkylation of Cys 328 destroys the FcεR1 binding site on IgE. The alkylation of all other Cys residues, including Cys 241, which forms a covalent bond with Cys 328 according to the model structures, has no effect on mast cell interaction.

Furthermore, the relative resistance of Cys 241 to reduction observed by both Bahr-Lindstrom and Bennich [8] as well as by Takatsu et al. [7] argues against an asymmetric disulphide bond pairing. This puts into perspective the usefulness of current IgE-Fc models [9, 10], which in the absence of a crystal structure determination should provide a 3-D framework for discussing the properties of the molecule, including the effect of mutations on structure [9]. Clearly the arrangement of the interchain disulphide bonds in human IgE requires clarification and should be determined by 2-disulphide bond mapping.

References

1. Marsh, P., B. Helm, and H. Gould. 1988. IgE in allergic inflammation. Allergy, in press.
2. Helm, B., P. Marsh, D. Vercelli, E. Padlan, H. Gould, and R. Geha. 1988. The mast cell binding site on human IgE. Nature 331: 180.
3. Lui, F.-T., K. A. Albrandt, C. G. Bry, and T. Ishizaka. 1984. Expression of a biologically active fragment of human IgE epsilon chain in E. coli. Proc. Natl. Acad. Sci. USA. 81: 5369.
4. Rockey, J. H., and H. G. Kunkel. 1962. Unusual sedimentation and sulphydryl sensitivity of certain isohemaglutinins and skin-sensitizing antibody. Proc. Soc. Exp. Biol. Med. 110: 101.
5. Ishizaka, K., and T. Ishizaka. 1968. Physico-chemical properties of human reaginic antibodies. VIII. Effect of reduction and alkylation on ε antibodies. J. Immunol. 102: 69.
6. Stanworth, D. R., J. Housely, H. Bennich, and S. G. O. Johansson. 1970. Effect of reduction upon the tissue-binding activity of immunoglobulin E. Immunochemistry 7: 321.
7. Takatsu, K., T. Ishizaka, and K. Ishizaka. 1975. Biologic significance of disulphide bonds in human IgE molecules. J. Immunol. 114: 1838.
8. Bennich, H., and H. von Bahr-Lindstrom. 1974. Structure of Immunoglobulin E (IgE). Prog. Immunol. 11, Vol. 1: 49.
9. Padlan, E. A., and D. R. Davies. 1986. A model of the Fc of immunoglobulin E. Mol. Immunol. 23: 1063.
10. Pumphrey, R. 1986. Computer models of human immunoglobulins. Immunol. Today 7: 174.
11. Ashihari, Y., Y. Arata, and K. Hamaguchi. 1985. pH-induced unfolding of the constant fragment

of the immunoglobulin light chain: effect of reduction on the intrachain disulfide bond. J. Biochem. Tokyo 97: 517.

12. Morinaga, Y., T. Franceshini, S. Inouye, and M. Inouye. 1984. Improvement of oligonucleotide-directed site-specific mutagenesis using double-stranded plasmid DNA. Biotechnology, July 1984: 636.

13. Kenten, J., B. Helm, T. Ishizaka, P. Cattini, and H. J. Gould. 1984. Properties of a human immunoglobulin ε-chain fragment synthesized in *Escherischia coli*. Proc. Natl. Acad. Sci. 81: 2955.

14. Messing, J. 1983. New M13 vectors for cloning. In: Methods in enzymology, Vol. 101, 20. W. R. Grossman, and K. Moldave, eds. New York: Academic Press.

15. Crestfield, A. M., S. Moore, and W. H. Stein. 1963. The preparation and enzymatic hydrolysis of reduced and S-carboxymethylated protein. J. Biol. Chem. 238: 622.

16. Laemmli, U. K. 1971. Cleavage of structural proteins during the assembly of the head of bacteriophage T4. Nature 227: 680.

17. Geha, S. R., B. Helm, and H. Gould. 1985. Inhibition of the Prausnitz-Kustner reaction by an immunoglobulin ε-chain fragment synthesized in *E. coli*. Nature 315: 577.

18. Chrétien, B. Helm, P. Marsh, E. Padlan, J. Wijdenes, and J. Banchereaux. 1988. A monoclonal anti-IgE antibody against an epitope in the CH3 domain inhibits IgE binding to the low-affinity IgE receptor (CD23). J. Immunol., in press.

The IgE Binding Site for Low-Affinity Fcε Receptors

Donata Vercelli, Birgit Helm**, Philip Marsh**, Eduardo Padlan***,
Hannah Gould**, Raif S. Geha**

Using a series of recombinant ε-chain fragments, expressed in *E. coli*, we mapped the binding site for the B cell Fcε receptor on human IgE to the Leu 340-Lys 547 region. The site is likely to be located in the N-terminal part of Cε3. The B cell IgE receptor does not require glycosylation of its ligand. The requirements for IgE binding to the mast cell and the B cell Fcε receptors are distinct.

Two types of receptors for the Fc portion of human IgE (FcεR) have been identified on the surface of human cells. These two types of receptors differ in their affinity for IgE as well as in their cellular distribution and function [1]. High-affinity FcεR (FcεR1, K_a: 10^9 M^{-1}) are detectable on mast cells and basophils. The reaction between allergens and IgE found to FcεR1 induces degranulation of basophils and mast cells, with release of chemical mediators responsible for their clinical manifestations of allergy [2]. By contrast, low-affinity FcεR (FcεR2, K_a: 10^7–10^8 M^{-1}) are present on monocytes/macrophages, B lymphocytes, platelets, and eosinophils. The binding of IgE to FcεR2 on monocytes, eosinophils, and platelets activates a variety of effector functions in these cells [3–5]. FcεR2 on B lymphocytes has been implicated in the transduction of growth signals and in B cell activation [6].

Using a series of recombinant human ε-chain fragments expressed in *E. coli*, we recently mapped the FcεR1 binding site on human IgE to within a 76 amino acid sequence (Gln 301–Arg 376), spanning the junction of the Cε2 and Cε3 domains [7]. We have now used a similar approach to locate the IgE binding site for the B cell FcεR2.

Table 1. Comparison between the FcεR1 and FcεR2 binding ability of the recombinant ε-chain fragments.

Ligand	FcεR1	FcεR2
IgE	+	+
rE2-4	+	+
rE2'-4	+	+
rE3-4	–	+
rE2-3	+	–
rE2'-3'	+	–
rE2	–	–
rE4	–	–

The reactivity of the rE peptides with the mast cell FcεR1 has been previously characterized [7].

Materials and Methods

The recombinant ε-chain (rE) peptides used in this study have been previously described in detail [7]. The rE peptides are named according to the domains they contain, with primed numbers indicating a truncated domain. For indirect immunofluorescence, 0.5×10^6 RPMI 8866 cells (>99% FcεR2-positive) in RPMI 1640–2.5% fetal bovine serum–0.01% azide were incubated with various concentrations of purified rE fragments or native IgE (PS) (a kind gift of K. Ishizaka, Baltimore, MD) for 40 min at 4 °C. After washing, the cells were incubated for 30 min at 4 °C with the appropriate fluorescein isothiocyanate (FITC)-conjugated anti-Fcε mAb or with an affinity-purified goat anti-human IgE antibody (10 µg/ml). After extensive washing, the percentage of cells binding IgE or the rE fragments was evaluated by a FACScan (Becton Dickinson, Mountain View, CA).

* Division of Immunology, The Children's Hospital and Department of Pediatrics, Harvard Medical School, Boston, MA, USA.
** Department of Biophysics, King's College, London, U.K.
*** Laboratory of Molecular Biology, National Institute of Diabetes and Digestive and Kidney Diseases, National Institutes of Health, Bethesda, MD, USA.

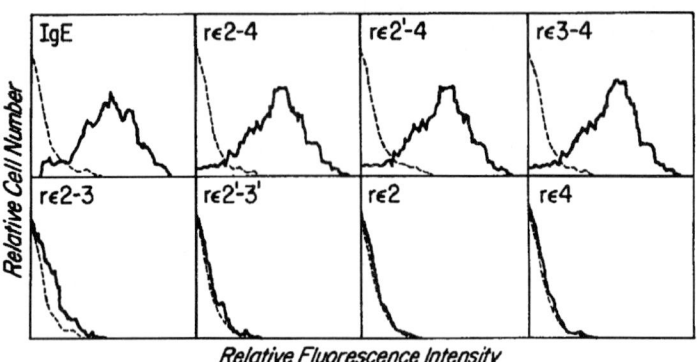

Figure 1. Binding ability of recombinant ε-chain peptides, as assessed by indirect immunofluorescence.

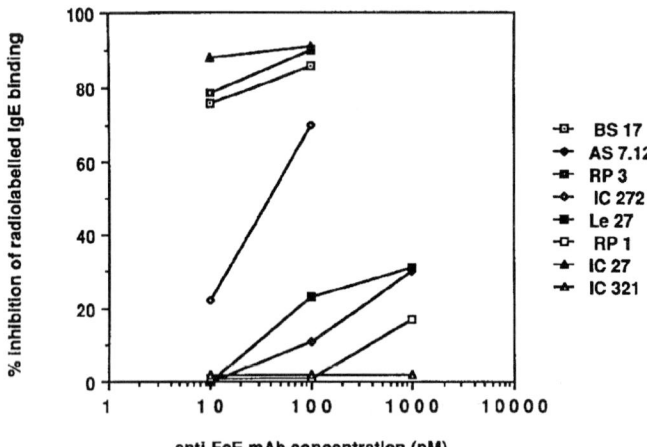

Figure 2. Inhibition of ^{125}I-IgE binding to B cells by anti-Fcε mAbs.

Results

For the mapping of the FcεR2 site on IgE, mAb BS17 and Le27 were kindly provided by B. Stadler, Bern; mAb 7.12 was a kind gift of A. Saxon, Los Angeles, CA; mAb RP1 and RP3 were kindly provided by R. Pumphrey, Manchester; mAb IC 272, IC 27, and IC 321 were a gift of J. Banchereau, Dardilly.

The specificity of the anti-Fcε mAbs has been previously characterized [8, 9]. To test the ability of the anti-Fcε mAbs to inhibit the binding of IgE to FcεR2, ^{125}I-IgE labelled by the chloramine-T method (15 ng in 50 µl, specific activity: 8000 cpm/ng) in PBS-0.5% BSA was mixed with a 10, 100, 1000 M excess of anti-Fcε mAb for 1 h at 37°C and then added to 1×10^6 RPMI 8866 cells in 0.1 ml. After incubation for 2 h at 4°C, the cells were spun through serum and the cell-bound radioactivity was counted. Maximal binding was determined by incubating the cells with ^{125}I-IgE in the presence of medium alone.

Like the myeloma protein IgE (PS), r2-r (ASp 218–Lys 547) rE2'-4 (Gln 301–Lys 547), and rE3-4 (Leu 340–Lys 547) bound to ≥90% of FcεR2-positive RPMI 8866 B cells, as assessed by indirect immunofluorescence (Figure 1). By contrast, there was no detectable binding of rE2-3 (Asp 218–Pro 439), rE2'-3' (Gln 310–Arg 376), rE4 (Arg 440–Lys 547), and rE2 (Asp 218–Val 336). The binding of the rE peptides was specific, since it could be completely inhibited by preincubation of the cells with two anti-FcεR2 monoclonal antibodies (mAb 135 and anti-BLAST-2), but not by control IgG1 of unrelated specificity. Moreover, there was no binding to the FcεR2-negative cell lines Jurkat and Raji (data not shown).

We then compared the relative activities of different ε-chain fragments. To this purpose, we measured the peptide concentration required for 50% binding to B cells. rE2-4 was highly active (7.2×10^{-10} M), indeed perceptibly more so than myeloma IgE (9.0×10^{-10} M). This elevated affinity is presumably the result of the absence of carbohydrate, since deglycosylation of IgE (PS) with N-glycosydase F increased its activity (4.8×10^{-10} M). rE3-4, which lacks Cϵ2 and nine amino acids from Cϵ3, displayed a much lower activity than rE2-4 (5.8×10^{-7} M). A truncated peptide, rE2'-4', retaining the C-terminal 30 amino acids of Cϵ2, by contrast, was almost as active as the full Fcϵ sequence (2.6×10^{-9} M).

Thus, the FcϵR2 binding site is contained in the rE3-4 peptide (Leu 340–Lys 547) and does not require the Cϵ2 domain. Both Cϵ3 and Cϵ4 are required for B cell binding, although all three Fcϵ domains appear to contribute to optimal activity. For a further definition of the FcϵR2 binding site, we need to establish whether the site is formed by sequences contributed by both Cϵ3 and Cϵ4, or is located in Cϵ3, the isolated Cϵ4 being unable to bind to B cells. In the latter case, Cϵ4 may be required to generate an appropriate structure. In this respect, it should be stressed that (a) the rE fragments able to bind to B cells are all dimeric; (b) only the rE peptides containing Cϵ4 can form dimers [7]. This suggests that the non-covalent association in Cϵ4 is required to place the thiols in register in Cϵ2, so that disulphide bond formation can occur. Dimerization of the ϵ-chains may in turn be required to generate an active FcϵR2 binding site. This hypothesis is presently being tested.

To map the FcϵR2 binding site more precisely, we have used monoclonal antibodies (mAbs) against epitopes in the Fcϵ region and measured their efficacy in inhibiting the binding of ^{125}I-labelled IgE to B cells. The various epitopes recognized by the antibodies were mapped to the rE peptides by Western blotting, and the locations of the peptides in the sequence were related to their positions in our model model of Fcϵ [7, 10]. The results are summarized in Figure 2. Three of the eight monoclonal antibodies strongly inhibited the binding of ^{125}I-IgE to B cells. The epitopes for mAb BS 17 and RP 3 lie in the C-terminal region of Cϵ2 (between Gln 301 and Thr 315), and that for the third, IC 27, is at the N-terminal end of Cϵ3 (comprising Lys 367–Val 370). The three sites are located within or near the cleft between the Cϵ2 and Cϵ3 domains in the

model of Fcϵ. A fourth Mab, IC 272, which binds to an intervening sequence (Thr 315–Val 336) in the loop separating the two β-strands that line the cleft between the Cϵ2 and Cϵ3 domains was only weakly inhibitory. Two other mAbs, RP 1 and Le 27, which bind within a second intervening sequence (Leu 340–Val 361), had no inhibitory effect. The whole of this peptide segment points away from the cleft. Two other mAbs, AS 7.12 and IC 321, which bind to epitopes outside the Cϵ2–Cϵ3 junction region, in Cϵ2 and Cϵ4, did not inhibit receptor binding. Taken together with the results of the fragment binding assay, these data suggest that FcϵR2 may bind to the Cϵ3, in the vicinity of ASP 362–Val 370. Since Cϵ2 does not contribute sequences to the binding site, inhibition by anti-Cϵ2 mAbs can result only from steric hindrance.

Discussion

We have shown that the FcϵR2 binding site on human IgE is contained in the sequence Leu 340–Lys 547 and is likely to be in the N-terminal region of Cϵ3, close to Cϵ2 in our three-dimensional model of Ccϵ [7]. The requirements for the binding of IgE to FcϵR1 and FcϵR2 are distinct [7]: FcϵR1, but not FcϵR2, binds to rE2-3 and rE2'-3', whereas FcϵR2, but not FcϵR1, binds to rE3-4 (Table 1). This indicates that some part of the sequence between Gln 301 and Leu 340 is required for Fcϵr1, but not for FcϵR2 binding. The sites may overlap in Cϵ3, in the region between Val 362 and Lys 367, which forms the C-terminal boundary of the FcϵR1 site [Marsh et al., in preparation], but the FcϵR2 site may extend further toward the C-terminal side, or indeed the sites may be totally separate. Higher-resolution mapping is required to establish the N-terminal boundary of the FcϵR2 binding site and thus determine the extent, if any, of common sequence. The finding that the requirements for FcϵR1 and FcϵR2 binding are different is not surprising, since FcϵR1 and FcϵR2 are unrelated proteins; FcϵR1 belongs to the immunoglobulin superfamily, like all other immunoglobulin receptors so far described [11]. FcϵR2 is unique, in that it is homologous to the asialoglycoprotein receptor [12, 13, 14], although it recognizes unglycosylated sequences.

103

References

1. Capron, A., J. P. Dessaint, M. Capron, M. Joseph, J. C. Ameisen, and A. B. Tonnel. 1986. From parasites to allergy: A second receptor for IgE. Immunol. Today 7: 15.
2. Ishizaka, T., and K. Ishizaka. 1975. Biology of immunoglobulin E. Prog. Allergy 19: 60.
3. Rankin, J. A., M. Hitchcock, W. Merrill, M. K. Bach, J. R. Brashler, and P. W. Askenase. 1982. IgE-dependent release of leukotriene C4 from alveolar macrophages. Nature 297: 329.
4. Capron, M., H. L. Spiegelberg, L. Prin, H. H. Bennich, A. E. Butterworth, R. J. Pierre, M. A. Ouaissi, and A. Capron. 1984. Role of IgE receptors in effector function of human eosinophils. J. Immunol. 132: 462.
5. Cines, D. B., H. v.d. Keyl, and A. I. Levinson. 1986. In vitro binding of an IgE protein to human platelets. J. Immunol. 136: 3433.
6. Wang, F., C. D. Gregory, M. Rowe, A. B. Rickinson, D. Wang, M. Birkenbach, H. Kikutani, T. Kishimoto, and E. Kieff. 1987. Epstein-Barr virus nuclear antigen 2 specifically induces expression of the B-cell activation antigen CD23. Proc. Natl. Acad. Sci. USA 84: 3452.
7. Helm, B., P. Marsh, D. Vercelli, E. Padlan, H. Gould, and R. S. Geha. 1988. The mast cell binding site on human immunoglobulin E. Nature 331: 180.
8. Chretien, I., B. A. Helm, P. J. Marsh, E. A. Padlan, J. Wijdenes, and J. Banchereau. A monoclonal anti-IgE antibody against an epitope (A.A. 367-376) in the CH3 domain inhibits IgE binding to the low affinity IgE receptor (CD23). J. Immunol.
9. Vercelli, D., B. Helm, P. Marsh, E. Padlan, R. S. Geha, and H. Gould. The B cell binding site on human immunoglobulin E. Submitted for publication.
10. Padlan, E., and D. R. Davies. 1986. A model of the Fc of immunoglobulin E. Molec. Immun. 23: 1063.
11. Williams, A. R., and A. N. Barclay. 1988. The immunoglobulin superfamily—Domains for cell surface recognition. Ann. Rev. Immunol. 6: 381.
12. Kikutani, H., S. Inui, R. Sato, E. L. Barsumian, H. Owaki, K. Yamasaki, T. Kaisho, N. Uchibayashi, R. R. Hardy, T. Hirano, S. Tsunasawa, F. Sakiyama, M. Suemura, and T. Kishimoto. 1986. Molecular structure of human lymphocyte receptor for immunoglobulin E. Cell 47: 657.
13. Ikuta, K., M. Takam, C. W. Kim, T. Honjo, T. Miyoshi, Y. Tagaya, T. Kawabe, and J. Yodoi. 1987. Human lymphocyte Fc receptor for IgE: Sequence homology of its cloned cDNA with animal lectins. Proc. Natl. Acad. Sci. USA 84: 819.
14. Suter, U., R. Bastos, and H. Hofstetter. 1987. Molecular structure of the gene and the 5'-flanking region of the human lymphocyte immunoglobulin E receptor. Nucl. Acid Res. 15: 7295.

Exploitation Of Synthetic Epsilon Chain Peptides in the Elucidation of the Role of IgE Antibodies in Allergic Reactions

*Denis R. Stanworth**

For almost the whole of my researching life I have been interested in the characterization of anaphylactic antibodies responsible for the mediation of immediate-type hypersensitivity responses. This endeavour has, of course, been greatly facilitated in the last 20 years or so by the availability of myeloma forms of human IgE and IgG4, which has permitted, for instance, what I have referred to as the "fragmentation approach" to the location of mast cell (and basophil) binding sites. But it is the advent of a strategy based on the synthesis of peptides with ε-chain sequences representative of putative Fc effector sites which has enabled us to really start to "get to grips" with the molecular pathology of these fascinating cytophilic antibodies.

I am going to outline briefly the manner in which we have been exploiting such peptides in the delineation of the role of IgE antibody molecules in mast cell triggering. And let me say right away: I shall not be considering "water imprinting" nor any other paranormal phenomenon! I will, however, be providing evidence in support of the contention that the IgE antibody does indeed play an instructional role in the triggering of mast cells. In other words, it is not a "silent" participant in those signalling events which culminate in the exocytosis of the mast cell granules and the release of their mediators.

But it is our use of synthetic ε-chain peptides and anti-peptide antibodies as structural probes into the location and nature of the mast cell binding site(s) within the human and rat IgE molecule which are of particular relevance to the themes of the other papers being presented in this symposium. Moreover, we, too, have been employing synthetic ε-chain peptides in parallel studies on the site of binding of human IgE to the low affinity receptor on B lymphocytes. This I mention briefly at the end.

Identification Of the IgE Mast Cell Binding Site

Our first incursion into the synthesis of human ε-chain peptides was prompted by my receipt from Bob Hamburger of a pre-print of his 1975 *Science* paper, in which he reported the inhibition of the Prausnitz-Küstner reaction by a synthetic pentapeptide analogue of a human Cε2 domain sequence. We synthesised—at that time by the classical technique—right away a similar peptide and confirmed (unlike some other laboratories) that it was partially inhibitory, in the PK system; and, also, in a human IgE-mediated PCA reaction in baboons. I have never been convinced, however, that the partial inhibition effects which we observed were attributable to the blocking of binding of IgE to its high affinity receptor on skin mast cells.

With the availability of our own solid-phase peptide synthesis facility, first using t-Boc amino acid derivatives and later based on Fmoc active ester chemistry on polyamide resins (in a fully automated Biolynx synthesiser), we decided to adopt a systematic approach to the identification of the mast cell binding site on rat IgE. Short linear peptides, comprising 7 different sequences within the Fc domain of rat IgE were synthesised initially. These were selected on the predictability of their location within accessible regions of the immunoglobulin Fc dimer, on the assumption of a three dimensional structural homology between the rat Cε3 and Cε4 domains and the human Cγ2 and Cγ3 domains (as defined by the X-ray studies of Diesenhofer, 1981); and on the basis of their content of a high number of polar residues.

Peptides representative of equivalent sequences within the Fc region of human IgE have been likewise synthesised and purified. And both the series of rat and human ε-chain

*   Rheumatology and Allergy Research Unit, University of Birmingham, Birmingham B15 2TJ, England.

peptides have been conjugated to a carrier protein (KLH) and used in the immunization of rabbits; the resultant polyclonal antisera being characterized by ELISA. Whilst, in addition, monoclonal murine antibodies are now being produced against the same peptides. Thus, we have built up a very useful repertoire of structural probes, which are providing an insight into the nature of the high-affinity Fc receptor binding sites on both the human and rat IgE molecules (Burt & Stanworth, 1987; Burt et al., 1987).

In vitro testing of the capacity of the synthetic peptides to inhibit the binding of ^{125}I-labelled rat immunocytoma IgE to purified rat peritoneal mast cells revealed that four of the seven peptides (comprising one C_H3 and three C_H4 domain sequence) possessed substantial blocking activity; whereas the three other ε-chain peptides tested (representative of one C_H3 and two C_H4 domain sequences) proved to possess no inhibitory activity, as did non-IgE control peptides. Significantly, the heating of rat immunocytoma IgE at 56°C for 1 hour (treatment which is known to abrogate the immunoglobulin's cytophilicity for mast cells) was found (by ELISA) to enhance its reactivity with rabbit antibodies against those four rat ε-chain peptides which inhibited IgE binding to mast cells in vitro; but it had no effect on the reactivity of the IgE with antisera directed against the three non-inhibitory rat ε-chain peptides. These findings are consistent with the previous findings of Dorrington and Bennich (1978), based mainly on physico-chemical studies of thermally induced structural changes of human IgE, which suggested that such treatment results in irreversible conformation changes within regions in both the C_H3 and C_H4 domains. So it is tempting to speculate that one or more of the peptides in question (comprising rat ε-chain residues 414–428, 459–472, 491–503, and 542–557) which are representative of surface accessible regions of the Cε3 and Cε4 domains, may form part of the heat-sensitive cytophilic site.

How then does one envisage the precise manner in which the IgE molecule binds to the high-affinity receptor on mast cells, on the basis of these findings? It is tempting to speculate that sites within the Cε3 and Cε4 domains combine with the complementary sites within the two immunoglobulin domain-like structures, which receptor cloning studies (referred to by Henry Metzger) have shown to occur within the mast cell α-chain. In an attempt to throw more light on this question, we have also adopted another approach to the employment of anti-ε-chain peptide antibodies as IgE structural probes. This has involved comparing the pattern of binding of the various anti-rat ε-chain antibodies to affinity purified rat IgE in solution and to rat mast cell bound IgE, as revealed by the subsequent measurement of histamine release. Somewhat surprisingly, we found that antibodies directed against most of the C_H3 and C_H4 domain surface epitopes represented by the synthesised peptides, including that constituting the rat Cε4 domain terminal sequence, are still capable of binding to receptor-occupied IgE. These findings argue against the commonly held notion of a "pocket" receptor for IgE on mast cells, in which both the C_H3–C_H4 domains are masked, and the docked IgE molecule lies perpendicularly to the mast cell membrane surface. Rather, on the basis of the data which I am now discussing (and of that of other groups), we suggest that only one of the identical pairs of ε-chain sequences which we postulate comprise the high-affinity receptor binding site actively interact with the receptor, thereby leaving the symmetry related set accessible and available for subsequent combination with their specific anti-peptide antibodies. Interestingly, computer graphic studies (undertaken with the help of Dr Brian Sutton, at that time in Oxford) indicate that sites of which the four mast cell binding peptides are representative form a contiguous three-dimensional array comprising three (one C_H3 and two C_H4 domain) sites within one of the pairs of Fc ε-chains and one (C_H4 domain) site in the other.

Nature Of IgE Mast Cell Triggering Site

As I have pointed out on many occasions such as this, it is important to recognise that the binding of IgE antibody molecules to high-affinity receptors on mast cells is a "null event", and that it is not until two antibody molecules are cross-linked, by antigen or artificially (by anti-IgE, lectins, etc.), that the mobilisation of intracellular calcium occurs (most probably as the result of the G protein regulated activation of phospholipase C, and the break-down of phosphatidyl inositol 4,5 bi-phosphate into inositol triphosphate and diacyl glycerol). So, unlike the situation as far as many polypeptide hormone receptor interactions are concerned, it is not enough for the IgE antibody to merely "address" the target mast cell in the manner which I have discussed already.

Contrary to the view—put forward initially by Ishizaka and Ishizaka, 1978—that the IgE antibody molecules merely act as surrogate receptors, facilitating the association of the Fc(ε)RI receptors as a result of their cross-linking by antigen, we have growing evidence to suggest that the antibody provides triggering information to the sensitized mast cell. Most of our experimental evidence in support of this idea has already been published (see, for instance, Stanworth, 1984), so I will only summarize it here.

The main points I want to bring out are as follows:

1. We predicted the likely chemical features of such a mast cell triggering site, on the basis of comprehensive structure activity studies on model histamine releasing peptides (synthetic ACTH analogues and melittin cleavage products).

2. A sequence within (the C_H4 domain) of only the IgE of the five major human immunoglobulin isotypes was found to possess such structural characteristics and peptides (octa, nona, and deca) representative of this sequence were synthesized, and shown to elicit the non-cytolytic release of histamine from non-sensitized rat mast cells in a manner that closely resembled the natural immunological stimulatory process.

3. Subsequent detailed structure activity studies on a wide range of synthetic peptide analogues of this sequence (Stanworth et al., 1984) have provided precise information about the structural characteristics of this direct mast cell triggering site. This turns out to be composed of a positively charged N-terminal "head" separated by three amino acid residues from a hydrophobic C-terminal "tail" (viz: Lys-Thr-Lys-Gly-Ser-Gly-Phe-Phe-Val-Phe). Furthermore, its overall length seems to be relatively critical, as does the relative disposition of the cationic and hydrophobic regions. In other words, it seems that a certain degree of specificity (which I have termed "second grade") is necessary

for direct mast cell triggering, although, unlike the situation with respect to peptide hormone ligands, primary structural specificity is not essential.

4. Significantly, substance P, a neuropeptide released from primary afferent neurones (in response to antidromic stimuli), where it appears to act on neighbouring mast cells to induce histamine release, has remarkably similar primary structural characteristics to the human ε-chain decapeptide, namely, a hydrophilic N-terminal region separated by three residues from a C-terminal hydrophobic region. It seems possible (on the basis of the results of model membrane studies) that both peptides exert their direct triggering action on mast cells by inserting into the lipid bilayer of the plasma membrane via the C-terminal hydrophobic region, leaving the N-terminal cationic end available for reacting with oppositely charged groups on membrane proteins, thereby perhaps contributing to the conveyance of the "second message".

This is where speculation takes over, with regard to the manner in which the antigen-cross-linked IgE antibody molecules provide a triggering signal. But it is, nevertheless, tempting to suggest that the region comprising the ε-chain decapeptide—which computer graphics shows is partially accessible in active monomeric IgE—becomes exposed as a result of a conformational change, which possibly leads to its cleavage by a plasma membrane protease. We have preliminary evidence, from the analysis of atopics' nasal fluids, that such a selective cleavage process does indeed occur in vivo.

Concluding Comments

In this contribution, an insight has been provided into how we are employing both synthetic peptides and anti-peptide antibodies to probe into the molecular pathology of the IgE molecule. Obviously, the picture is by no means complete yet. Nevertheless, I hope that I have provided enough evidence of the advantages of the approach.

We are now adopting a similar strategy in an investigation of the manner in which human IgE binds to the low affinity receptor on human B lymphocytes. Here, too, we are finding that certain peptides representative of both C_H3 and C_H4 domain sequences are capable of inhibiting the binding of human IgE to B cells (in rosette and radioimmunoassays). But there is not complete concordance with the equivalent rat ε-chain peptides which inhibit the binding of rat IgE to rat mast cells. The histamine-releasing human ε-chain decapeptide, shows, however, interesting direct stimulatory effects on human B-lymphocytes, proving capable of enhancing the expression of Fc(ε)RII with a potency comparable to that of IL-4 (Ghadieri and Stanworth: to be published).

It is hoped that another outcome of our work will prove to be the development of novel, and more effective, ways of abrogating IgE-mediated clinical hypersensitivity responses. Already, we have obtained some promising pointers toward the realisation of such a goal. Moreover, our findings of striking structural similarities between substance P and the synthetic human ε-chain decapeptide, suggest intriguing possibilities for functional interchanges between these two peptides, in immunomodulation as well as in the mediation of hypersensitivity responses.

References

1. Dorrington, K. J., and H. H. Bennich. 1978. Structure-function relationships in human immunoglobulin. E. Immun. Rev. 4: 3–25.

2. Burt, D. S., G. Z. Hastings, J. Healy, and D. R. Stanworth. 1987. Analysis of the interaction between rat immunoglobulin E and rat mast cells using anti-peptide antibodies. Molec. Immunol. 24: 379–389.

3. Burt, D. S., and Stanworth, D. R. 1987. Inhibition of binding of rat IgE to rat mast cells by synthetic IgE peptides. Eur. J. Immunol. 17: 437–440.

4. Ishizaka, T., and K. Ishizaka. 1978. Triggering of histamine release from rat mast cells by divalent antibodies against IgE receptors. J. Immunol. 120: 800–805.

5. Stanworth, D. R. 1984. The role of non-antigen receptors in mast cell signalling processes. Molec. Immunol. 21: 1183–1190.

6. Stanworth, D. R., J. W. Coleman, and Z. Khan. 1984. Essential structural requirements for triggering of mast cells by a synthetic peptide comprising a sequence in the Cε4 domain of human IgE. Molec. Immunol. 21: 243–247.

Results of Clinical Trials of the IgE Pentapeptide

*Robert N. Hamburger, Gary S. Hahn, Anne E. Daigle, Kathryn F. Rangus, Thomas O. Thayer**

IgE pentapeptide is a five amino-acid peptide, L-Asp-Ser-Asp-Pro-Arg, derived from the Fc region of human IgE. This compound was recently assigned the generic name "pentigetide" by the United States Adopted Names Council which will be used in this manuscript.

Pentigetide has been studied extensively in both preclinical animal safety studies and in human clinical trials since 1981. Three routes of administration have been studied in humans, subcutaneous injection, a nasal solution and an ophthalmic solution, and a fourth, bronchial inhalation, will soon begin safety studies in mild asthmatics. Safety results from all controlled clinical trials and efficacy results from recently completed pivotal trials will be presented in this manuscript.

The pharmacologic activity of pentigetide in vitro shows inhibition of A23187 mast cell degranulation, no inhibition of 48/80 induced degranulation and no effect on T or B cell function. In vivo, pentigetide inhibits PCA in humans, rats, rabbits, baboons, and dogs; inhibits antigen-induced conjunctivitis in a guinea pig model, inhibits antigen-induced asthma in guinea pig and dog; and inhibits Substance-P, carrageenan and DTH-induced inflammation in a mouse footpad model.

As expected for a peptide derived from a naturally occurring molecule, pentigetide has not shown toxicity in animal safety studies different from placebo. Studies have been conducted in mice, rats, rabbits, and primates for up to two years. Results from animals treated with up to 250 times the effective clinical dose of pentigetide are no different from placebo-treated animals. General fertility and reproduction, and teratology studies have demonstrated no pentigetide induced effects. In acute studies, pentigetide administered subcutaneously to mice, rats, and dogs resulted in no mortality at 5 g/kg. Results from human trials have shown no evidence of toxicity measured by changes or shifts in vital signs, complete blood count with differential, clinical chemistries, urinalyses, or physical examinations.

In clinical trials of all dosage forms, no differences in adverse effects between pentigetide and placebo groups were found. In six clinical trials of the injectable dosage form, 8% (49/625) patients receiving pentigetide and 8% (21/273) patients receiving placebo reported adverse effects. Most adverse effects reported were related to the route of administration and not qualitatively or quantitatively different between treatment groups.

In six trials studying the nasal solution, 15% (58/376) of the patients receiving pentigetide and 18% (56/311) of the patients receiving the vehicle control (preserved, phosphate-buffered saline) reported adverse effects. In eleven trials studying the ophthalmic solution, 20% (87/446) of the patients receiving pentigetide and 23% (63/274) of the patients receiving the vehicle control reported adverse effects. Again most effects were related to the route of administration and there were no differences between the two groups.

Efficacy results from recent pivotal trials for each dosage form studied will be presented. All trials used a randomized, double-blind, placebo or active-controlled design. More patients were randomized to the pentigetide groups to increase safety data. Patients in all trials were symptomatic for allergic rhinitis or conjunctivitis with positive skin tests or RAST. All patients were between the ages of 12 and 65.

* Immunetech Pharmaceuticals, San Diego, California.
Acknowledgements: We thank Robert N. Hamburger, M.D., for presenting these results at the XIII ICACI. We also thank the following principal investigators who participated in these clinical trials: M. B. Abelson, S. R. K. Dennis, S. R. Findlay, Z. H. Haddad, F. C. Hampel, D. P Huston, J. G. Kalpaxis, W. T. Kniker, H. C. Mansmann, E. O. Meltzer, B. M. Prenner, P. H. Ratner, J. P. Rosen, R. R. Rosenthal, D. G. Tinkelman, R. T. Wold, and R. W. Ziering.

Table 1. Pentigetide for injection: Patient disposition.

	Pentigetide (n=138)		Placebo (n=59)	
	n	%	n	%
Enrolled	143	(100)	62	(100)
Completed	138	(97)	59	(95)
Discontinued	5	(3)	3	(5)

Table 2. Pentigetide for injection: Physician-assessed symptom frequency.

	Percent reduction (intake-outtake)		
	Pentigetide n=138	Placebo n=59	ANOVA p
Sneezing	44	26	0.01
Nasal congestion	33	9	0.001
Rhinorrhea	52	27	0.003

Table 3. Pentigetide for injection: Patient daily diary symptoms.

	Percent reduction (intake-outtake)		
	Pentigetide n=138	Placebo n=59	ANOVA p
Sneezing	50	25	0.01
Nasal congestion	54	31	0.001
Rhinorrhea	57	35	0.03

Table 4. Pentigetide for nasal solution: Patient disposition.

	Pentigetide		Placebo	
	n	%	n	%
Enrolled	214	(100)	217	(100)
Completed	203	(95)	203	(94)
Discontinued	11	(5)	14	(6)

Table 5. Pentigetide for nasal solution: Physician-assessed symptom frequency.

	Percent reduction (intake-outtake)		
	Pentigetide n=203	Placebo n=303	ANOVA p
Sneezing	25	10	0.006
Nasal congestion	22	10	0.01

Pentigetide for Injection

Results are presented for a six-center trial of 7 weeks duration. One week of baseline was followed by 6 weeks of pentigetide 20 mg or placebo subcutaneously administered twice weekly. Table 1 gives the patient disposition including the number of patients enrolled, completed, and discontinued.

Treatment groups were comparable for age, gender ratio, family history of allergy, other allergic conditions, severity of allergic disease at intake, and immunotherapy.

Pentigetide significantly reduced symptom scores when rated by the physician or by the patient in a daily diary. Table 2 presents the percent improvement over baseline for the nasal symptoms of sneezing, nasal congestion, and rhinorrhea assessed by the physician. Table 3 presents the percent improvement over one week untreated baseline for the same nasal symptoms as rated by the patient in a daily diary. All comparisons favor pentigetide treatment, are statistically significant, and demonstrate the clinical efficacy of pentigetide in reducing allergic symptoms. The physician assessment of symptoms and the patient diary ratings are remarkably consistent.

Both physicians and patients independently rated the therapeutic response of patients. Significantly more patients in the pentigetide group (68%) were rated improved by the physician compared to the placebo group (47%), (Mann-Whitney Test, p=0.001). Significantly (p=0.05) more patients rated themselves improved in the pentigetide group (71%) compared to the placebo group (56%).

Pentigetide reduced the use of antihistamines when compared to placebo. Figure 1 demonstrates a steady decline in antihistamine usage in the pentigetide group during the six weeks of treatment while usage in the placebo group remains at the same level. Few patients used decongestants in either group and no trends were observed.

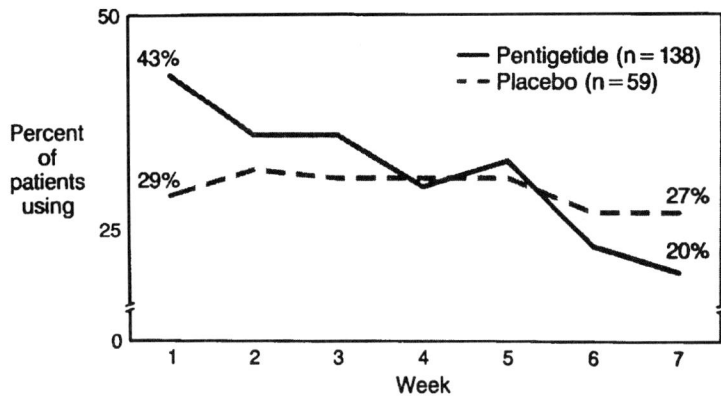

Figure 1. Pentigetide for injection. Concomitant medication—antihistamines.

Decongestants: <15% patients used; no consistent trends

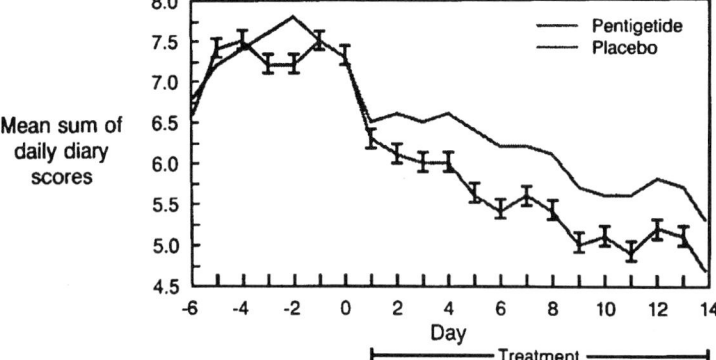

Figure 2. Pentigetide for nasal solution. Patient daily diary symptom means ten-center trial.

Daily Means - Pentigetide & Placebo with Standard Error for Pentigetide

Pentigetide for Nasal Solution

Results from a three-week trial at ten centers are presented. After a one week baseline, patients administered 2 sprays per nostril, 4 times per day of either Pentigetide Nasal Solution 0.5% or the vehicle control for two weeks. Table 4 gives the patient disposition including the number of patients enrolled, completed, and discontinued.

Patients were comparable for age, gender ratio, family history of allergy, other allergic conditions, severity of allergic disease at intake, and immunotherapy.

Table 5 demonstrates that for the nasal symptoms of sneezing, nasal congestion, and rhinorrhea, the pentigetide group experienced substantially more reduction in symptoms. Pentigetide Nasal Solution significantly reduced physician-rated sneezing and nasal congestion.

Figure 2 demonstrates that daily symptoms rated by the patient were immediately reduced in the pentigetide group compared to the placebo group. Comparisons did not achieve statistical significance. Standard error bars are presented for the pentigetide daily means.

The physicians assessed significantly more patients improved in the pentigetide group (62%) compared to the placebo group (47%), (p=0.003). Patient assessments did not demonstrate significant differences between the groups.

Pentigetide for Ophthalmic Solution

In an ocular antigen model, 26 patients were randomly assigned to receive Pentigetide Ophthalmic Solution (either 2.5, 5.0, 10.0, 20.0, or 30.0 mg/ml) in one eye and the vehicle control

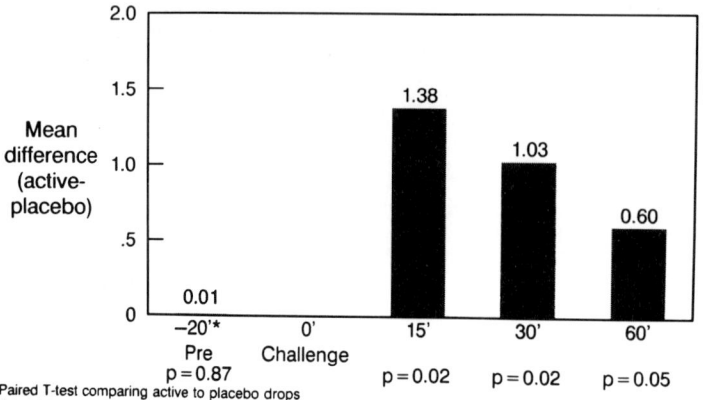

Figure 3. Pentigetide for ophthalmic solution. Antigen challenge results (n = 26).

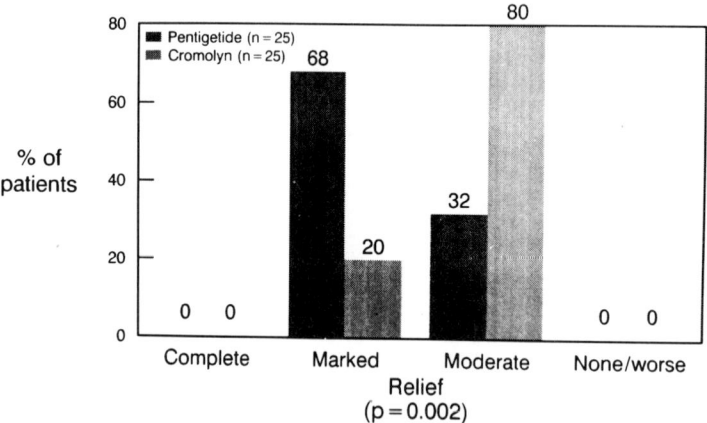

Figure 4. Pentigetide for ophthalmic solution. Ocular assessment at outtake by physician.

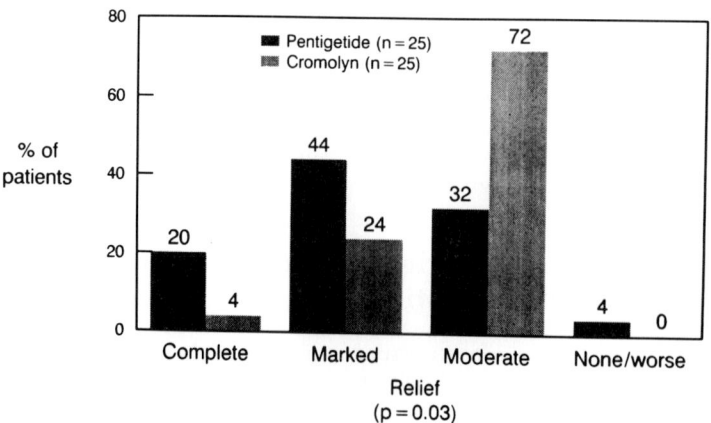

Figure 5. Pentigetide for ophthalmic solution. Ocular assessment at outtake by patient.

in the contralateral eye. A baseline titration challenge to elicit 2+ itching and redness to cat dander was performed. Two weeks after the baseline challenge, eyes were dosed as above and rechallenged with the baseline concentration of cat dander. The 26 eyes dosed with any concentration of pentigetide and the 26 placebo eyes were compared to ascertain efficacy. Figure 3 demonstrates that total symptom scores after antigen challenge were significantly reduced after 15, 30, and 60 minutes by Pentigetide Ophthalmic Solution.

In a single-center, active-controlled, two-week trial in patients presenting with the signs and symptoms of allergic conjunctivitis, the physician assessed 68% of the pentigetide-treated and 20% of the cromolyn-treated patients as demonstrating marked ocular relief. Figure 4 demonstrates that no patients were assessed as achieving complete relief or no re-lief by the physician, and that the differences between the groups significantly favored pentigetide (p = 0.002). Patient assessments of their ocular condition demonstrated more pentigetide patients as experiencing complete or marked relief. Figure 5 demonstrates that more patients in the pentigetide group assessed their ocular condition as complete or marked relief (64%) compared to those in the cromolyn group (28%) (p=0.03).

The therapeutic efficacy of pentigetide in the treatment of allergic rhinitis and conjunctivitis has been demonstrated in numerous clinical trials. Safety has been well established in both animal and human studies. The physician will have a unique new clinical entity to treat allergic patients without the side effects associated with antihistamines and decongestants. Pentigetide holds promise for the treatment of asthma and other allergic diseases.

Does IgE Receptor Blockade Have a Chance for Treatment of Allergy?

*Hans L. Spiegelberg**

The ability of injections of the rat IgE myeloma protein IR162 to inhibit passive cutaneous anaphylaxis (PCA) was compared with its effect on active cutaneous anaphylaxis in ovalbumin (OVA) sensitized rats. It was shown that the PCA reaction is relatively easily inhibited if IgE IR162 is injected i.p. before skin sensitization or i.c. as a mixture of IgE IR162 and IgE anti-OVA antibodies. In contrast, the cutaneous hypersensitivity reaction elicited in the skin of OVA immunized rats was not prevented despite injection of IgE IR162 leading to one to three thousand-fold excess of the IgE IR162 serum levels over the IgE anti-OVA antibody level. The data indicate that it is relatively easy to inhibit the PCA reaction but difficult if not impossible to block IgE Fc receptors on mast cells with myeloma IgE in actively immunized rats. Therefore, it appears unlikely that administration of human IgE Fc fragment-derived synthetic or recombinant DNA-produced peptides will prevent allergic reactions even if they have an affinity for the mast cell IgE Fc receptor identical to native IgE.

IgE antibodies are mainly responsible for allergic diseases in humans [1]. These antibodies bind to Fc receptors (FcεR) on mast cells [2] and persist on these cells for long periods of time [3] because the mast cell Fcε has a very high affinity for IgE antibodies [4]. When the allergen reaches the IgE bound to mast cells, it causes cross-linking of the FcεR, which induces the release of vasoactive substances such as histamine and leukotrienes that are responsible for the allergic reaction [1, 2]. In theory, IgE-mediated allergic reactions could be prevented if a compound were found that binds to the FcεR and blocks the IgE antibodies from attaching to the mast cells. In 1975, Hamburger reported that he had synthesized a peptide having an amino acid sequence derived from the human IgE Fc fragment that blocked the passive cutaneous human skin (Prausnitz-Kust-ner) reaction in man [5]. This observation has stimulated a great interest in the possibility of preventing allergic disorders with either synthetic peptides or recombinant DNA-produced IgE Fc fragment pieces [6] that could be administered to allergic patients. However, to date, 15 years after the initial report, the question whether FcεR blockade is a suitable approach for finding a new therapy for allergic disorders has not been definitely answered. Also, the inhibition of binding of IgE to Fcε by the pentapeptide [5] is still controversial [7, 8]. To determine the feasibility of preventing allergic reactions by Fcε blockade, it is important to study the effect of a potential Fcε blocker on anaphylactic reactions in actively immunized animals, since they mimic allergic disease more closely than the PCA reaction. However, relatively few such studies have been performed in the past. Jarrett et al. [9] reported that "nonspecific" IgE induced in rats infected with the helminth *Nippostrongylus brasiliensis* (Nbr) inhibits neither skin nor general anaphylaxis in rats immunized with ovalbumin. However, this model may not have proven whether IgE without known antibody activity fails to block hypersensitivity reactions. First, the Nbr infection does not allow an accurate control of the parasitically induced IgE serum level. Second, and more importantly, the Nbr infection may have induced IgE anti-parasite antibodies that cross-react with OVA or may have induced an anamnestic IgE response to OVA resulting from dietary immunization. For these reasons, we investigated the effect of rat IgE IR162 on the passive and active cutaneous reaction to OVA in rats [10]. This allowed us to quantitate the amount of IR162 IgE in the serum of the treated animals and to estimate the ratio of non-antibody to anti-OVA antibody specific IgE which would be necessary to block FcεR.

* Department of Immunology, Research Institute of Scripps Clinic, La Jolla, California.
Supported by U.S. Public Health Service grant AI 10734, Biomedical Research Support Program grant RRO-5514, and by a grant from the Eli Lilly Co. (publication no. 5598-IMM from the Research Institute of Scripps Clinic).

In a first set of experiments, the effect of injections of IgE IR162 on the PCA reaction was tested. As little as 2.5 mg IgE/100 g body weight (bwt) injected i.p. 24 h before skin sensitization completely inhibited a PCA reaction. The IgE serum level in these rats reached a peak of >100 µg IgE/ml which is 5–10-fold more than the in vitro FcεR saturation level [4]. Similarly, when the myeloma IgE was mixed with IgE anti-OVA antibodies and injected into the skin, the PCA reaction was completely inhibited at a ratio of myeloma:antibody IfE of 100:1. These experiments showed that the PCA reaction can be inhibited relatively easily when the myeloma IgE is injected before or with the specific IgE antibodies (Table 1) presumably by occupying most of the mast cells FcεR. In contrast, when the IgE anti-OVA was injected into the skin before the i.p. injection of the myeloma IgE, it had no effect on the PCA reaction. Apparently the IgE anti-OVA, once bound to mast cells in the skin, could not be displaced by the large excess of nonspecific IgE given at 10 mg/100 g bwt for almost a week (Table 1).

Next, we investigated the effect of IgE IR162 injections on the skin reaction of actively OVA sensitized rats. The Lewis rats were immunized i.p. with 100 µg OVA in B. pertussis adjuvant and treated for 13 days with daily injections of 2.5 mg IgE IR162/100 g bwt. The animals were then skin tested with 0.1, 1 and 10 µg OVA in 0.1 ml saline followed by an i.v. injection of Evans blue. As shown in Table 2, all control and IgE IR162-treated rats showed positive skin reactions. Although the diameters of the blueing reaction of the treated rats was smaller than those of the control rats, the differences were statistically not significant. To determine the approximate ratio of IgE IR162 to IgE anti-OVA in these rats, the IgE antibodies were quantitated in the control rats. These data showed that the rats formed approximately 20 ng IgE anti-OVA. The rats injected with 2.5 mg IgE/100 g bwt had peak levels of 180–215 µg IgE/ml decreasing with a half-life of 11 h to 30–70 µg IgE/ml over a 24 h period. However, even at the lowest levels, the rats had >1000-fold more IgE IR162 than IgE anti-OVA in the serum. The fact that this large excess of myeloma IgE was unable to block the skin reactions shows how effective small quantities of IgE antibodies are in sensitizing mast cells.

Our experiments confirm those of Jarrett et al. [9] and show that myeloma IgE having no known antibody activity, like parasitically induced IgE, cannot prevent mast cell sensitization for an anaphylactic reaction in actively sensitized rats. Apparently, even a small amount of IgE antibodies present in the serum and extravascular body fluids still has a chance to bind to vacant FcεR despite a >1000-fold excess of competing non-antibody IgE. Furthermore, once bound to the FcεR, the specific IgE antibodies cannot easily be displaced even with a large excess of myeloma IgE as shown by the failure to prevent the PCA reaction by myeloma IgE treatment after skin sensitization.

In summary, our experiments show that it is not possible to inhibit an immediate type hypersensitivity reaction by inducing serum levels of nonspecific IgE exceeding the 10–20 µg IgE/ml in vitro mast cell FcεR saturation level [4]. Because IgE is the natural ligand for the FcεR, it is unlikely that a compound or peptide will be found that will compete more efficiently than IgE itself for

Table 1. Effect of myeloma IgE injections on PCA reactions given before or after i.p. skin sensitization.

Treatment	Positive PCA/total rats tested IgE anti-OVA serum dilution		
	1:20	1:40	1:80
Controls			
mg IgE/100 g bwt before skin sensitization			
2.5 mg, day -1	0/5	0/5	0/5
0.3 mg, day -1	1/3	1/3	0/3
mg IgE/100 g bwt after skin sensitization			
2.5 mg days 1 through 6	4/4	4/4	4/4
10 mg days 1 and 2	4/4	4/4	4/4

Table 2. Effect of myeloma IgE injections on anaphylactic skin reaction in OVA immunized rats.

Treatment	Positive skin test/total rats tested µg OVA injected		
	0.1	1	10
Controls	12/13	12/13	13/13
2.5 mg IgE, days 3 through 13	7/7	7/7	7/7
2.5 mg IgE, days 0 through 13	5/5	5/5	5/5

115

binding to FcεR on mast cells. In contrast to the lack of inhibition of the skin reaction in actively immunized mice, the PCA reaction was relatively easily inhibited both by injecting IgE IR162 before skin sensitization and by mixing the myeloma protein with the IgE anti-OVA antibodies. The reason for this good inhibition may be a relatively poor efficiency of mast cell sensitization by intracutaneous injection of IgE antibodies. It is likely that most of the injected IgE antibodies diffuse from the injection site into the circulation before they have a chance to bind to mast cells because of the presence of an excess of myeloma IgE. Therefore, a successful inhibition of the Prausnitz-Kustner reaction in humans with an IgE peptide or fragment does not allow the conclusion that this peptide will be useful for the treatment of allergic patients.

References

1. Ishizaka, K., and T. Ishizaka. 1978. Mechanisms of reaginic hypersensitivity and IgE antibody response. Immunol. Rev. 41: 109.
2. Dreskin, S. C., and H. Metzger. 1988. The high-affinity receptor for immunoglobulin E. JAMA 260: 1265.
3. Cass, R. M., and B. R. Anderson. 1968. The disappearance rate of skin-sensitizing antibody activity after intradermal administration. J. Allergy Clin. Immunol. 42: 29.
4. Kulczycki, A., and H. Metzger. 1974. The interaction of IgE with rat basophilic leukemia cell receptor for IgE. II. Quantitative aspects of binding reaction. J. Exp. Med. 140: 1676.
5. Hamburger, R. N. 1975. Peptide inhibition of the Prausnitz-Kustner reaction. Science 189: 389.
6. Geha, R. S., B. Helm, and N. Wood. 1987. IgE sites relevant for binding to type 1 Fc epsilon (FcεR) receptors on mast cells. J. Allergy Clin. Immunol. 79: 129.
7. Bennich, H., U. Ragnarsson, S. G. O. Johansson, K. Ishizaka, T. Ishizaka, D. A. Levy, and L. M. Lichtenstein. 1977. Failure of the putative IgE pentapeptide to compete with IgE for receptors on basophils and mast cells. Int. Arch. Allergy Appl. Immunol. 53: 459.
8. Burt, D. S., and D. R. Stanworth. 1987. Inhibition of binding of rat IgE to rat mast cells by synthetic IgE peptides. Eur. J. Immunol. 17:437.
9. Jarrett, E., S. Mackenzie, and H. Bennich. 1980. Parasite-induced "nonspecific" IgE does not protect against allergic reactions. Nature 283: 302.
10. Spiegelberg, H. L., K. M. Canning, M. Scheetz, G. Koppel, and J. M. Chiller. 1986. Effect of myeloma IgE injections on passive and active cutaneous anaphylaxis in rats. J. Immunol. 136: 131.

Genetic and Immunochemical Studies of Human Immune Responsiveness: The Allergy Model

*David G. Marsh, Patty Zwollo, Aftab A. Ansari**

We studied the genetics of human immune responsiveness using two model systems, the *Amb* V allergens in which responsiveness is associated with DR2/Dw2, and the *Lol p* I, II, and III allergens in which responsiveness is associated with DR3. We used amino acid sequencing of the allergens and computer analysis for amphipathic sequences to identify putative major Ia/T-cell epitopes on both sets of molecules. DNA typing and sequencing of HLA-D-region gene segments was used to identify which polymorphic DNA sequences may encode the binding sites for specific Ia/T-cell epitopes on the allergen molecules. The isolation of relevant polymorphic HLA-D-region gene segments has been greatly facilitated by the use of a revolutionary new gene-amplification technology, the polymerase chain reaction (PCR). Either HLA-DR or DQ molecules associated with Dw2 could be implicated in the binding of major Ia/T-cell epitopes of the *Amb* V allergens; a DR3-associated Ia molecule is implicated in the binding of a major epitope on the *Lol p* allergens. Further experiments to test these hypotheses will include the use of allergen-specific T-cell clones.

An issue that is central to our understanding of the genetics of immune responsiveness is the study of the trimolecular complex, which bridges the antigen-presenting cell (APC) and the helper T cell and leads to the initiation of the immune response. In the case of humoral immune responses, this complex usually involves a major histocompatibility complex (MHC) class II (Ia) molecule, a fragment of the antigen involved in the response and the T-cell receptor (TcR) on helper cells of the CD4 phenotype [1, 2] (Figure 1). The Ia molecule is comprised of α and β polypeptide chains, each of which have two extracellular domains, the first, non-immunoglobulin-like domains of each chain being involved in the IaAgTcR complex. From mouse studies, several different types of APCs have been implicated in antigen

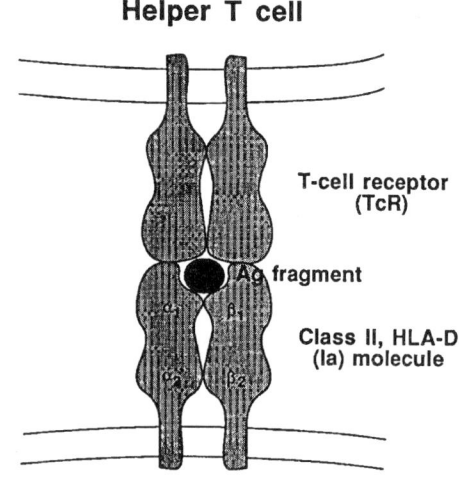

Helper T cell

T-cell receptor (TcR)

Ag fragment

Class II, HLA-D (Ia) molecule

Antigen-Presenting Cell (APC)

Figure 1. The Ia-Ag-TcR complex—a simplified model. The α and β polypeptide chains of the Ia molecule both contain non-immunoglobulin-like domains, α_1 and β_1, which are involved in binding to the Ag fragment, and essentially non-polymorphic, immunoglobulin-like domains, α_2 and β_2. The α and β polypeptide chains of the TcR both contain two immunoglobulin-like domains; the α_1 and β_1 domains are polymorphic, and the α_2 and β_2 domains are essentially non-polymorphic. Reprinted by permission from Marsh [3].

presentation, including macrophages, monocytes, dendritic cells and B cells [1, 4]. For our human studies, we have selected atopic allergy as a model for reasons discussed in detail elsewhere (5–7) and summarized in Figure 2. Because of the low antigen dosages involved in inhalant allergy (typically <1 ng/h) [5], B cells are probably the APCs primarily involved, since they carry immunoglobulin-like B-cell receptors (BcRs) on their cell surfaces. Thus, certain B cells have the potential to interact (via their specific BcRs) with surface B-cell epitopes

---

* Johns Hopkins University School of Medicine, Good Samaritan Hospital, Baltimore, Maryland 21239, USA.
Supported by NIH grants Nos. AI 19727, AI 20059, and AI 25372

1. Common disease — afflicts 20–30% of Caucasoids.

2. Familial aggregation established.

3. Many highly purified allergens available for study.

4. Possibility of "fingerprinting" human immune responsiveness to the different allergens.

5. Natural exposure is to highly limiting Ag doses, typically <1µg/yr.

6. Can study all classes of humoral as well as cellular immune responses.

7. Study of gene interactions (eg, IgE-regulating and HLA-linked *Ir* genes).

Figure 2. Features of the allergy model for studies of human immune responsiveness.

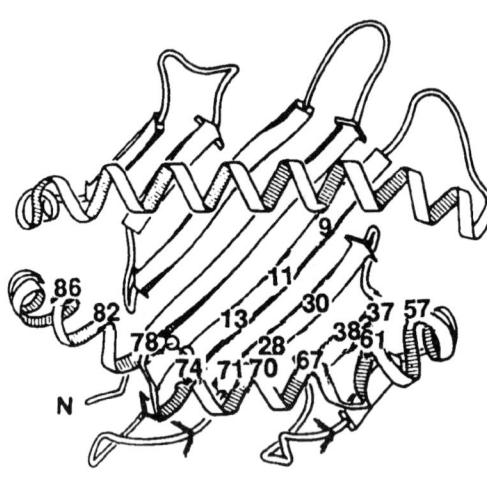

Figure 3. Ribbon diagram of the Ag-binding "groove" of the HLA-A2 class I molecule, as the TcR would "see" it during presentation of the Ag fragment. The groove is comprised of the α_1 and α_2 domains of the molecule, which together form a β-pleated sheet at the bottom of the groove and α-helices at either side of the groove. The α_1 and α_2 domains of class I molecules show sequence homology with the α_1 and β_1 domains of class II molecules, respectively. The residue numbers of the (usually highly polymorphic) residues of the DRβ1 polypeptide which, according to computer modeling, point into the groove, and which are implicated in binding to the Ag fragment, are superimposed on the model. Residues 9, 11, 13, 28, 30, 37, and 38 form part of the β-pleated sheet structure; the remaining marked residues lie on the α-helix forming one wall of the groove. (Residues 60 and 85 on the α-helix may also point into the groove.) The DRα1 domain forms the other part of the class-II groove (i.e., left-hand half of the β-pleated sheet structure and the upper α-helix). Reprinted by permission from [12, 13].

on the antigen/allergen (Ag) molecule and, thereby, function as efficient APCs [3].

The following discussion provides a simplified summary of the events that are then believed to take place within, and on the surface of, the APC [1, 4, 8–10]. The AgBcR complex formed on a B cell with affinity for the native Ag is internalized and the Ag is "processed," which involves proteolytic breakdown and probably, in some cases, breakage of disulfide bonds. A specific peptide fragment (an Ia/T-cell epitope) of the Ag, which has sufficient affinity toward one of the individual's specific Ia molecules (encoded by HLA-D-region genes), may then form a stable IaAg fragment complex which is transported to the surface of the APC. This complex then interacts with a specific TcR on a helper T cell, causing T-cell activation. The resultant release of lymphokines from the T cell, in turn, activates the neighboring B cell, which differentiates into a plasma cell capable of secreting antibody (Ab) of the same specificity as the BcR originally involved in Ag binding. By analogy with mouse studies [11], it seems probable that a TH2-like T cell is involved in facilitating IgE biosynthesis, and that IL-4 is an important T-cell lymphokine involved in the stimulation of B cells which become committed to IgE Ab biosynthesis.

A major recent advance has been the elucidation of the three-dimensional X-ray crystallographic structure of a class I MHC molecule [12], which has allowed computer modeling of approximate structures for the Ag-binding "grooves" of the homologous class II (Ia) molecules involved in Ag fragment/TcR binding [13] (Figure 3). Figure 4 presents a diagram of the HLA-D region, a typical gene, DRB1 from this region, and the first domain of the encoded DRβI polypeptide. The polymorphic regions of this domain of DRβI that fold to form part of

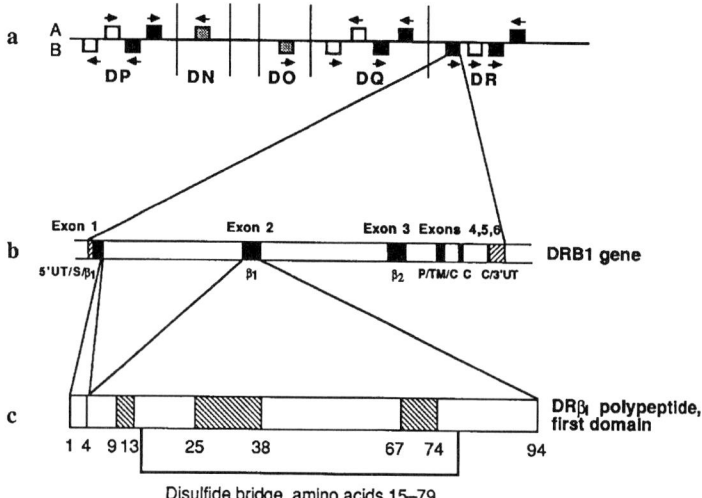

Figure 4.

(a) The human HLA-D region and its sub-regions. The genes shown by solid boxes are expressed as protein products; those shown by open boxes are not expressed. The genes shown by stippled boxes are weakly expressed and/or produce inactive products. Arrows indicate the direction of gene transcription from the 5′ to the 3′ end of one or the other anti-parallel DNA strands. The class II *Ir* genes include both A (formerly called α) genes, upper boxes, and B (formerly β) genes, lower boxes. The number of unexpressed B "pseudogenes" within the DR sub-region varies somewhat among the different DR subtypes, but most have two expressed B genes, DRB1 and DRB3.

(b) The arrangement of exons (which produce RNA transcripts) and introns (non-expressed regions) of the DRB1 gene. Untranslated regions and encoded peptides of the DRβI chain are indicated as follows: 5′ UT, the untranslated region located at the 5′ end of the gene; S, signal (or leader) peptide (which is removed upon formation of the mature DRβI polypeptide); β1 and β2, the two extracellular domains of the DRβI polypeptide; P, the connecting peptide between the extracellular β2 domain and the trans-membrane (TM) peptide; C, the cytoplasmic peptide; 3′ UT, the untranslated region located at the 3′ end of the gene. The other HLA-D-region genes have exon arrangements quite similar to DRB1.

(c) A schematic representation of the first domain of the DRβI polypeptide, emphasizing the hypervariable regions (shaded), which are involved in binding to the Ag fragment and the TcR (cf. Figure 1). Other expressed HLA-D genes have similar hypervariable regions, except DRA which is essentially invariant. Data from [14–17]; diagram reprinted by permission from Marsh [3].

the Ag-binding groove are shown in Figure 4c; the specific residues predicted, from computer modeling [13], to point into the groove (and which are implicated in Ag-binding) are indicated by residue numbers in Figure 3.

Ia/T-Cell Epitopes of Allergen Molecules

For our molecular studies of human immune responsiveness, we focused on two model allergen systems, the *Amb* V (Ra5) homologues from three species of *Ambrosia* (ragweed) pollen and the *Lol p* I, II, and III allergens from *Lolium perenne* (rye grass) pollen. Within each set, there are two non-cross-reacting pairs and

one cross-reacting pair of allergens (*Amb t* V is virtually non-cross-reactive with the cross-reactive pair *Amb a* V/*Amb p* V [18, 19], and *Lol p* I is non-cross-reactive with the cross-reactive pair *Lol p* II/III [20]). We compared the amino acid sequences of the Ags within the two sets. Similar peptide segments containing *amphipathic* segments (which contain separated hydrophilic and hydrophobic regions) were identified (Figure 5). Berzofsky and his collaborators [25] have previously shown that 78% (18/23) of the Ia/T-cell antigenic epitopes recognized by mouse T cells are amphipathic, usually helical peptides. From these analyses, we predict that the related epitopes within each set of Ags would bind to the same HLA-D-associated Ia molecule(s). We will see that this

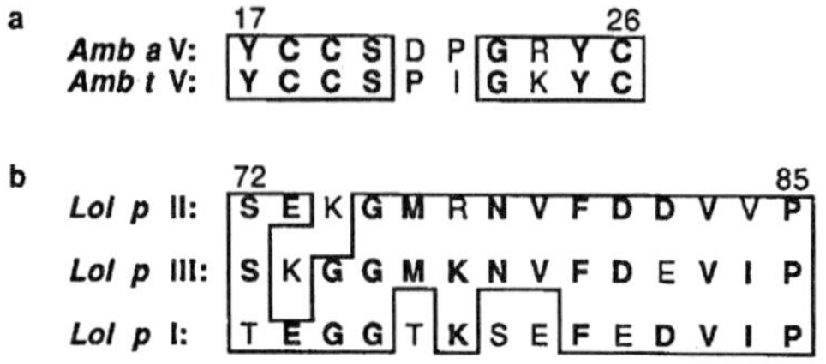

a
```
              17                    26
Amb a V:  | Y C C S | D  P | G R Y C |
Amb t V:  | Y C C S | P  I | G K Y C |
```

b
```
              72                              85
Lol p II:   | S E | K | G M R N V F D D V V P |
Lol p III:  | S K | G | G M K N V F D E V I P |
Lol p I:    | T E  G G | T | K | S E | F E D V I P |
```

Figure 5. Comparison of homologous regions having amphipathic segments for the *Amb* V homologues and the *Lol p* allergens using the Berzofsky-DeLisi algorithm [25]. Residues that are either identical or closely homologous are boxed; identical residues are shown in bold type.

(a) Amb a V and *Amb t* V comparison. Segments 21–24 (*Amb a* V) and 19–24 (*Amb t* V) are amphipathic (using blocks of 7 amino acids); Segments 24–26 (*Amb a* V) and 9–23 (*Amb t* V) are amphipathic (using blocks of 11 amino acids). The corresponding sequence of *Amb p* V is presently unknown, but from the similarity of amino acid composition and the strong cross-reactivity between *Amb a* V and *Amb p* V, it is believed to be similar to that of *Amb a* V. See [7, 22, 23].

(b) Lol p II, III and I comparison. Using *Lol p* II numbering throughout, segments 74–83 (*Lol p* II) and 72–83 (*Lol p* III) are amphipathic (using blocks of 7 amino acids); segments 73–81 (*Lol p* II) and 70–83 (*Lol p* III) are amphipathic (using blocks of 11 amino acids). Only a 28-residue segment was available for *Lol p* I [24], which was insufficient to confirm amphipathicity for the segment shown for this Ag. The *Lol p* I sequence has a variant with valine (V) at position 80. Data from [Ansari, Shenbagamurthi and Marsh, submitted, and 24].

postulate is completely consistent with the observed HLA-immune response association data discussed below. It should be emphasized that an identical HLA association for immune responsiveness to the non-cross-reactive Ags within a set can not be attributed to antigenic cross-reactivity.

Antigen-Binding Sites in Ia Grooves

Recombinant DNA technology has provided the most economical approach toward deriving amino acid sequence information of the polymorphic regions of Ia molecules (shaded in Figure 4c). We used a revolutionary new methodology, the polymerase chain reaction (PCR) [26, 27] (Figure 6), for rapid amplification of the second exons of the DRB1, DRB3, DQB1, and DQA genes from a large number of allergic subjects. The DRA gene was not studied because it is essentially non-polymorphic [14]. The PCR-amplified gene segments were dot-blotted onto nylon membranes and radiolabeled sequence-specific oligonucleo-tides (SSOs) having sequences corresponding to the polymorphic regions of different HLA-DR and DQ alleles were used for specific typing [27]. Since this method can discriminate between sequences differing by a single nucleotide (after highly stringent washing of the filters), it has allowed us to deduce the precise amino acid

1. To ~1μg genomic DNA add large excess of:
   a. Primer oligonucleotides corresponding to the sequences of ~18 – 22 bases at each 5' end of the opposite DNA strands flanking the region of interest.
   b. All 4 deoxynucleoside triphosphates.

2. Denature/inactivate sample (95° for 10 min)

3. Cool and add *Taq* DNA polymerase (from the thermophilic bacterium *Thermus aquaticus*).

4. Heat sample at 95° for 2 min to ensure that DNA is single-stranded.

5. Anneal the primers (2 min at 37°– 55°).

6. Extend DNA strands (1–3 min at 72°).

7. Repeat steps #4 – 6 approx 24 times.

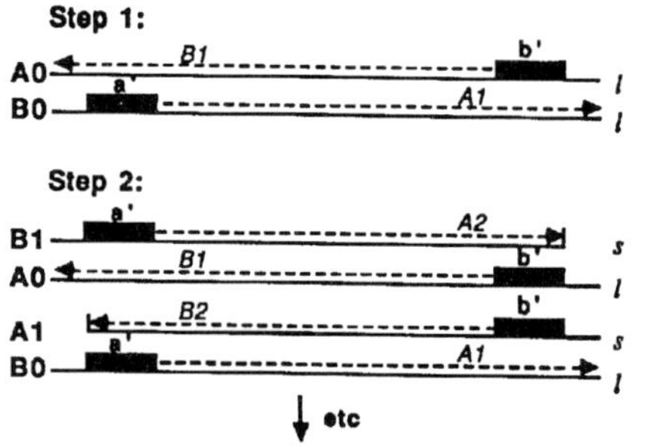

Step 1:
```
A0 ◄------ B1 -------------------- b'
   a                                    l
B0 ■■■ -------------------------- A1 ►
                                        l
```

Step 2:
```
      a'                    A2
B1 ■■■ ------------------------- ►◄
A0 ◄------ B1 ------------------- b'     s
                                          l
A1 ◄-- B2 ----------------- b'
B0 ■■■ ----------------------- A1 ►     s
                                          l
```
↓ •tc

Theoretical number of short ('s') strands produced at step 'n' = $2^n - 2$.
25 steps should produce ~3 x 10^7 short strands. (Yield ~ 10^6 strands.)

Figure 6. The polymerase chain reaction (PCR). The tem-perature selected for the annealing Step 5 is optimized for the particular primers being used. This figure is reprinted by permission from [29].

120

sequences of the polymorphic regions of the respective Ia molecules. Where further information was needed, the PCR-amplified fragments were cloned into the M13 vector and sequenced by the dideoxy procedure. These approaches are allowing us to deduce the possible structures of the grooves of the Ia molecules possessed by *Amb* V or by *Lol p* I, II, and III responders [28, 30, Zwollo et al., unpublished; Ansari et al., unpublished]. Such Ia molecules may be implicated in the binding of particular Ia/T-cell epitopes of these Ags, perhaps those illustrated in Figure 5. This approach allows us to formulate hypotheses which can be directly tested in future cellular immunological experiments. We have focused on the investigation of HLA-D-region sequences which may be implicated in the binding of common Ia/T-cell epitopes on the *Amb* V Ags and on the *Lol p* Ags.

HLA-D and Responsiveness to *Amb* V Homologues

We previously studied the DR and Dw typings of people who make IgE and IgG Abs from ultra-low-dose natural exposure to *Amb a* V (from *Ambrosia artemisiifolia,* short ragweed) resulting from the inhalation of the pollen. We found that 36 of 38 white subjects [31] and two black subjects [unpublished] who made IgE Ab to *Amb a* V typed DR2/Dw2. These data were generally consistent with subsequent DNA restriction fragment length polymorphism (RFLP) mapping studies, except that one of the DR2/Dw2 responders (who had an equivocal Dw2 typing, "Dw2$^{\pm}$") exhibited an RFLP pattern for a DQB probe that is characteristic of Dw2$^-$ subjects [32]. We also investigated IgG Ab responses to higher doses of *Amb a* V used in ragweed immunotherapy (Rx) of our allergic patients [33]. All DR2/Dw2 made good IgG Ab responses to *Amb a* V; some non-DR2/Dw2 made moderate or weak responses. In further studies, we found three atypical DR2/Dw2 subjects who do not respond after Rx.

In recent SSO and sequencing studies of 69 selected Caucasoid subjects who had received Rx [28, Zwollo et al., unpublished], we found that all who typed DR2/Dw2 (including the one Dw2$^{\pm}$), had DRB1 and DRB3 second-exon sequences characteristic of the Dw2-associated subspecificity, DR2.2. These subjects include

both *Amb a* V$^+$ and *Amb a* V$^-$ subjects after Rx. All except the aforementioned Dw2$^{\pm}$, *Amb a* V$^+$ subject and one of the Dw2$^+$, *Amb a* V$^-$ individuals had typical Dw2-associated DQB1 sequences; the exceptional subjects (including the Dw2$^{\pm}$ subject) had different DQB1 sequences (one characteristic of Dw21 and one not yet fully defined). Thus, we could not discriminate between the Dw2$^+$,*Amb a* V$^+$ and the Dw2$^+$, *Amb a* V$^-$ subjects by RFLP and SSO typing, or by sequencing. These results suggest that a Dw2-associated Ia molecule recognizes the major Ia/T-cell epitope on the *Amb a* V molecule; this Ia molecule is usually a necessary, but not sufficient, requirement for Ab responsiveness to *Amb a* V. The non-responsiveness to natural exposure with *Amb a* V of many Dw2$^+$ subjects, and the three cases of non-responsiveness following Rx, can be explained both by environmental causes and by the requirement for other genes determining responsiveness.

Weaker IgG Ab responses after prolongued Rx were associated with DR2.21 (a DR2 variant found in low frequency in the Caucasoid population) and with certain subtypes of DR4 and DQw3 [Zwollo et al., unpublished]. Interestingly, the sequences of the two exceptional non-DR2/Dw2, *Amb a* V$^+$ subjects, who responded following natural *Amb a* V exposure, had typical DR8, 9/ DQw4, 3.3 and DR3, 4.14/ DQw2, 3.2 sequences. These data suggest that Ia molecules associated with Dw21 and DR4/DQw3 also serve Ag receptors; either they recognize a minor Ia/T-cell determinant, or they bind less avidly to the major determinant. Presently, it is not possible to discriminate between whether DR and/or DQ molecules are *Ir* gene products for different or the same Ia/T-cell determinants. Our current hypotheses are summarized in Table 1.

We have also found that IgG Ab responses to immunotherapy with *Amb t* V (from *Ambrosia trifida,* giant ragweed) and *Amb p* V (from *Ambrosia psilostachya,* western ragweed) are both primarily associated with Dw2 [18, 19, Marsh et al., unpublished], suggesting that the postulated major Ia/T-cell epitopes on these molecules (cf. Figure 5 a) are involved in the binding to the same Dw2-associated Ia molecule as the respective epitope of *Amb a* V. We are developing Ag-specific T-cell clones to test this hypothesis, along with those presented in Table 1.

Table 1. Where do the *Amb a* V-*Ir* genes map? Conflicting hypotheses in favor of DR vs. DQ from studies of 69 allergic caucasoids.

DR hypotheses[1]	
DRB1*2.2 (Dw2-associated sequence):	Present in all 22 Dw2$^+$ high responders (before and/or after Rx[2]) and 1 Dw2$^\pm$ high responder studied[3]; two of these subjects (including one Dw2$^\pm$) do not have DQB1 sequences typically associated with Dw2. **May encode an Ia segment that binds to the major *Amb* V Ia/T-cell epitope.**
DRB1*2.21 (Dw21-associated sequence):	Found in four low-to-high responders after extensive Rx[3]. DRB1*2.21 contains sequences identical or similar to DRB1*2.2 in 1st and 2nd polymorphic regions. **May encode an Ia segment that binds to the major *Amb* V Ia/T-cell epitope, but more weakly than DRB1*2.2.**
DRB1*4 (all DR4 sub-type sequences):	Present in a DR2$^-$ responder before Rx (1 of 2 atypical people), and a majority of moderate responders after extensive Rx (at least 6 of 8 people).[4] Sequences of all DR4 subtypes are identical in 1st and 2nd polymorphic regions. **May encode Ia segment that binds a minor *Amb* V Ia/T-cell epitope.**
DQ hypotheses	
DQA1*1.2/DQB1*1.2 (Dw2-associated):	Present in 21 of 22 Dw2$^+$ high responders studied.[5] **May encode the binding site for the major Ia/T-cell *Amb* V epitope.**
DQA1*1.2/DQB1*1.21 (Dw21-associated):	Present in the Dw2$^\pm$ high responder and all four DR2$^+$Dw2$^-$ low-to-high responders after Rx.
DQA1*1.2 is	common to this group and the preceding group. **DQA1*1.2 may encode an important part of a major DQ binding site for the major *Amb* V epitope, modulated by the influence of the different DQβ chains, 1.2 vs. 1.21.**
DQA1*3(DQB1*3 (DQw3), *non*-DR5:	Present in all 10 DR2$^-$ responders, including two atypical responders before Rx and 8 moderate responders after prolonged Rx.[6] **May encode the binding site for a minor Ia/T-cell *Amb* V epitope.**

[1]DRA is non-polymorphic for residues forming the binding groove; therefore, it has no influence on the DR hypotheses [14].
[2]Immunotherapy with short ragweed Ags, including *Amb a* V.
[3]Among DR2$^+$ *non*-responders after Rx, three possess DRB1*2.2 and two have DRB1*2.21.
[4]Data not yet complete.
[5]The exceptional subject has a DQw1 subtype (not yet sequenced) that is not usually associated with Dw2.
[6]Thirteen non-responders (after Rx) also possess DQw3*non*-DR5 subspecificities.
The remaining subjects studied possess none of the above sequences and were all non-responders after extensive ragweed Rx.

HLA and *Lol* p I, II, and III Associations

An interesting analogy can be drawn between the *Amb* V immune response associations discussed above and the findings of significant HLA-DR3 associations with responsiveness to the *Lol p* I, II, and III Ags. As noted earlier, one molecule, *Lol p* I crossreacts neither with *Lol p* II nor *Lol p* III. Nevertheless, immune responsiveness to all three molecules is significantly associated with HLA-DR3 [29, 34]. This result suggests that the postulated homologous

major Ia/T-cell epitopes on these molecules may be involved in binding to the same, DR3-associated Ia molecule.

Additionally, in the case of responsiveness to the *Lol p* III allergen, we found a secondary, significant association with HLA-DR5 [30]. This finding led to the hypothesis that the sequence, EYSTS, which is present in the first polymorphic region (positions 9–13) of both DR3 and DR5 might be important in antigen presentation [30]. Analyses of HLA-D DNA sequences and PCR dot-blots are currently in progress to examine this question further. Also, the relationship between these results and data concerning the other two *Lol p* allergens will be tested at the cellular level using T-cell clones specific for the individual *Lol p* allergens.

Discussion and Conclusions

The foregoing examples illustrate how the allergy model can be used for molecular studies of the genetic basis of human immune responsiveness. From these studies, we have generated hypotheses that can be tested directly by cellular immunological studies employing Ag-specific T-cell clones, defined peptides corresponding to the postulated Ia/T-cell epitopes, and specified Ia molecules on defined B-cell lines. L cells transfected with specified HLA-D genes will also be used to investigate the influence of individual Ia molecules more selectively. Also, we will test the binding of the specified antigenic peptides to relevant Ia molecules, which will either be the isolated Ia molecules themselves [4, 9], or Ia molecules on B cells (EBV-transformed lines), as recently employed by Rothbard, Lamb and their collaborators [unpublished].

In the future, we will need to study the sequences of the hypervariable regions of the α and β chains of the TcRs involved in binding to particular Ia-Ag complexes. The PCR will provide a rapid method of amplifying the relevant gene segments. As further automation of DNA sequencing becomes available, molecular studies of all of the molecules involved in the Ia-Ag-TcR complex will be greatly facilitated. Furthermore, the techniques of X-ray crystallography, nuclear magnetic resonance spectroscopy, and computerized structure modeling will provide invaluable tools for exploring the molecular nature of the Ia-Ag-TcR complex more fully. Indeed, it is likely that the three-dimensional structure of an IaAg complex will soon be determined and, eventually, the structure of an entire Ia-Ag-TcR complex will be deduced. Using these technologies, together with relevant experiments using T-cell clones, we believe that it will be possible to define more clearly the molecular basis of immune responsiveness to defined allergen molecules. Since there are so many different allergen molecules available for study, many of which have already been defined by physical, chemical, and immunologic criteria, allergy offers the unique model for studying the molecular basis of human immune responsiveness toward a wide variety of different macromolecules. This approach will not only help in the understanding and treatment of allergy, but also of many other immunologic diseases which afflict humans.

References

1. Schwartz, R. H. 1985. T-lymphocyte recognition of antigen in association with gene products of the major histocompatibility complex. Ann. Rev. Immunol. 3: 237.
2. Marrack, P., and J. Kappler. 1987. The T-cell receptor. Science 238: 1073.
3. Marsh, D. G. 1989. Immunogenetic and immunochemical factors determining immune responsiveness to allergens: studies in unrelated subjects. In: Genetic and environmental factors in clinical allergy. D. G. Marsh and M. N. Blumenthal, eds. University of Minnesota Press, in press.
4. Unanue, E. R., and P. M. Allen. 1987. The basis for the immunoregulatory role of macrophages and other accessory cells. Science 236: 551.
5. Marsh, D. G. 1975. Allergens and the genetics of allergy. In: The antigens, Vol. III. M. Sela, ed. New York: Academic Press, p. 271.
6. Marsh, D. G. 1976. Allergy: A model for studying the genetics of human immune response. In: Molecular and Biological Aspects of the Acute Allergic Reaction. S. G. O. Johansson, K. Strandberg, K. and B. Uvnas, eds. Nobel Symposium No. 33. New York: Plenum Publishing Co., p. 23.
7. Marsh, D. G. 1986. Defining human immune response fingerprints toward ultra-pure allergens: Immunochemical and genetic aspects of responsiveness toward the *Amb* V (Ra5) homologues. In: Proc. XII Internatl. Congress Allergol. Clin. Immunol., Washington, D.C. C.E. Reed, ed. St. Louis: C.V. Mosby. J. Allergy Clin. Immunol. 78 (Suppl.): 242.
8. Babbitt, B. P., P. M. Allen, G. Matsueda, E. Haber, and E. R. Unanue. 1985. Binding of immunogenic peptides to Ia histocompatibility molecules. Nature 317: 359.
9. Buus, S., A. Sette, S. M. Colon, et al. 1987. The relation between major histocompatibility complex (MHC) restriction and the capacity of Ia to bind immunogenic peptides. Science 235: 1353.
10. Guillet, J. G., M. Z. Lai, T. J. Briner et al. 1987. Immunological self, nonself discrimination. Science 235: 865.
11. Snapper, C. M., and W. E. Paul. 1987. Interferon-γ and B cell stimulatory factor-1 reciprocally regulate Ig isotype production. Science 236: 944.

123

12. Bjorkman, P. J., M. A. Saper, B. Samraoui, W. S. Bennett, J. L. Strominger, and D. C. Wiley. 1987. Structure of the human class I histocompatibility antigen, HLA-A2. Nature 329: 506.

13. Brown, J. H., T. Jardetsky, M. A. Saper, B. Samraoui, P. J. Bjorkman, and D. C. Wiley. 1988. A hypothetical model of the foreign antigen binding site of Class II histocompatibility molecules. Nature 332: 845.

14. Trowsdale, J., J. A. T. Young, A. P. Kelly, et al. 1985. Structure, sequence and polymorphism in the HLA-D region. Immunol. Rev. 85: 5.

15. Hardy, D. A., J. I. Bell, E. O. Long, T. Lindsten, and H. O. McDevitt. 1986. Mapping of the class II region of the human major histocompatibility complex by pulsed-field gel electrophoresis. Nature 323: 453.

16. Andersson, G., D. Larhammar, E. Widmark, B. Servenius, and P. A. Petersen. 1987. Class II genes of the human major histocompatibility complex: organization and evolutionary relationship of the DRβ genes. J. Biol. Chem. 262: 8748.

17. Jonsson, A. K., J. Hyldig, J. J. Nielsen, B. Servenius et al. 1987. Class II genes of the human major histocompatibility complex: Comparisons of the DQ and DX α and β genes. J. Biol. Chem. 262: 8767.

18. Roebber, M., D. G. Klapper, L. Goodfriend, W. B. Bias, S. H. Hsu, and D. G. Marsh. 1985. Immunochemical and genetic studies of Amb.t.V (Ra5G), an Ra5 homologue from giant ragweed pollen. J. Immunol. 134: 3062.

19. Marsh, D. G., L. R. Freidhoff, D. B. K. Golden et al. 1987. Genetic studies of immune response to the Amb V homologues. Fed. Proc. 46: 1047 (Abstract).

20. Ansari, A. A., T. K. Kihara, and D. G. Marsh. 1987. Immunochemical studies of Lolium perenne (rye grass) allergens Lol p I, II and III. J. Immunol. 139: 4034.

21. Ansari, A. A., P. Shenbagamurthi, and D. G. Marsh. 1988. Comparison of amino acid sequences of Lolium perenne allergens Lol p II and III. J. Allergy Clin. Immunol. 81: 307.

22. Mole, L. E., L. Goodfriend, C. B. Lapkoff et al. 1975. The amino acid sequence of allergen Ra5. Biochem. 14: 1216.

23. Goodfriend, L., A. M. Choudhury, D. G. Klapper et al. 1985. Ra5G, a homologue of Ra5 in giant ragweed pollen: Isolation, HLA-DR-associated activity and amino acid sequence. Mol. Immunol. 22: 899.

24. Esch, R. E., and D. G. Klapper. 1989. Isolation and characterization of a major cross-reactive grass Group I allergenic determinant. Mol. Im-

munol., in press.

25. Margalit, H., J. L. Spouge, J. L. Cornette, K. B. Cease, C. DeLisi, and J. A. Berzofsky. 1987. Prediction of immunodominant helper T-cell antigenic sites from the primary sequence. J. Immunol. 138: 2213.

26. Saiki, R. K., S. Scharf, F. Faloona et al. 1985. Enzymatic amplification of β-globin genomic sequences and restriction site analysis for diagnosis of sickle cell anemia. Science 230: 1350.

27. Erlich, H. A., E. L. Sheldon, and G. Horn. 1986. HLA typing using DNA probes. Biotechnology 4: 975.

28. Zwollo, P., T. Kihara, A. A. Ansari, H. A. Erlich, and D. G. Marsh. 1988. sequence differences in HLA-DRβ genes between Amb a V responders and non-responders. J. Allergy Clin. Immunol. 81: 307 (Abstract).

29. Marsh, D. G., P. Zwollo, and A. A. Ansari. 1989. Toward a total human immune response fingerprint: The allergy model. In: First DPC Symposium on Allergy and Molecular Biology. S. El Shami and T. Merrett, eds. Oxford: Pergamon Press, in press.

30. Ansari, A. A., L. R. Freidhoff, D. A. Meyers, W. B. Bias, and D. G. Marsh. 1989. Human immune responsiveness to Lolium perenne (rye) grass pollen allergen Lol p III (Rye III) is associated with HLA-DR3 and DR5. Hum. Immunol., in press.

31. Marsh, D. G., S. H. Hsu, M. Roebber, E. E. Kautzky, L. R. Freidhoff, D. A. Meyers, M. K. Pollard, and W. B. Bias. 1982. HLA-Dw2: a genetic marker for human immune response to short ragweed pollen allergen Ra5. I. Response resulting primarily from natural antigenic exposure. J. Exp. Med. 155: 1439.

32. Zwollo, P., A. A. Ansari, and D. G. Marsh. 1989. Association of class II DNA restriction fragments with responsiveness to Ambrosia artemisiifolia (short ragweed) pollen allergen Amb a V in ragweed-allergic patients. J. Allergy Clin. Immunol., in press.

33. Marsh, D. G., D. A. Meyers, L. R. Freidhoff, E. E. Kautzky, M. Roebber, P. S. Norman, S. H. Hsu, and W. B. Bias. (1982). HLA-Dw2: A genetic marker for human immune response to short ragweed pollen allergen Ra5. II. Response after ragweed immunotherapy. J. Exp. Med. 155: 1452.

34. Freidhoff, L. R., E. E. Kautzky, D. A. Meyers, S. H. Hsu, W. B. Bias, and D. G. Marsh. 1988. Association of HLA–DR3 and total serum immunoglobulin E level with human immune response to Lol p I and Lol p II allergens in allergic subjects. Tissue Antigens 31: 211.

Mast Cell and Basophil Activation by Human Anti-IgE Autoantibodies

Gianni Marone*, Vincenzo Casolaro*, Isabella Quinti**, Roberto Paganelli**, Giuseppe Spadaro*, Cristiana Stellato*

The "reverse-type" of anaphylaxis in vitro is based on the challenge of human basophils or mast cells with rabbit or goat anti-human IgE (R-aIgE). R-aIgE bridges the high-affinity IgE receptor of human basophils/mast cells by interacting with the Fc portion of IgE. This leads to cell activation and mediator release. In patients with allergic rhinitis and asthma, there is an excellent correlation between the maximum percent histamine release caused by anti-IgE and the release of histamine caused by antigen challenge of basophils. Furthermore, an increased IgE-mediated releasability can be found in patients with atopic dermatitis, allergic rhinitis, and extrinsic asthma. One out of 6 IgG obtained from patients with atopic dermatitis associated with elevated anti-IgE activity (H-aIgE) induced histamine and peptide leukotriene C4 (LTC4) release from human basophils and mast cells. The release reaction caused by H-aIgE was Ca^{2+}- and temperature-dependent. There was an excellent correlation between the maximum percent histamine release caused by R-aIgE and H-aIgE from human basophils. Lactic acid removal of IgE from basophils blocked the releasing activity of both R-aIgE and H-aIgE. H-aIgE specifically desensitizes basophils to a subsequent challenge with both R-aIgE and H-aIgE and vice versa. Purified IgE myeloma isolated from three different patients dose-dependently blocked the histamine-releasing activity of both R-aIgE and H-aIgE. These results indicate that naturally occurring autoantibodies IgG anti-IgE from a patient with atopic dermatitis induce mediator release from human basophils/mast cells through a "reverse-type" of anaphylaxis.

The discovery of the IgE and its physicochemical characterization [1, 2] boostered the study of allergic reactions in vitro and in vivo. In the 1960s it was widely held that most of the pathophysiological manifestations of allergic diseases could be attributed directly or indirectly to the IgE antibodies present in serum and capable of sensitizing high-affinity receptors on human basophils and mast cells. This concept was supported by the finding that serum concentrations of IgE were increased in patients with atopic dermatitis, allergic rhinitis, and bronchial asthma [3, 4].

Evidence that IgE antibodies are involved in the pathogenesis of allergic reactions was also obtained at a cellular level. Lichtenstein and Osler observed histamine release from isolated leukocytes of atopic patients under allergen challenge [5], and Levy and Osler showed passive sensitization of normal leukocytes with reaginic serum for antigen-induced histamine release [6]. Also, studies conducted with the "reverse-type" anaphylactic reaction model indicated that IgE antibodies were associated with histamine release. In fact, incubation of leukocytes from atopic patients and some normal individuals with IgG isolated from serum of rabbits immunized with purified IgE myeloma (rabbit anti-human IgE) resulted in the release of histamine [7]. It was also demonstrated that the injection of appropriate doses of allergens in patients undergoing hyposensitization led to an increase of IgG ("blocking") antibodies against the allergens [8].

It was then noted that patients with the same degree of skin mast cell reactivity to allergens or serum concentration of specific IgE and IgG had different degrees of clinical manifestations. This is typically observed in patients with insect allergy. In fact, patients with identical levels of IgE anti-venom antibodies, and similar skin tests can be stung with opposite results [9]. It was also demonstrated in vitro that baso-

---

*   Division of Clinical Immunology, Department of Medicine, University of Naples, Second School of Medicine, Naples, Italy.
** Division of Clinical Immunology, Department of Medicine, University of Rome "La Sapienza," School of Medicine, Rome, Italy.
Supported by grants from the C.N.R. (86.00088.04 and 88.00559.04), the M.P.I., and the Italian Ministry of Health (Rome).

phils with 5,000 IgE molecules on the surface released the same percentage of histamine as those with 500,000 molecules [10]. Furthermore, different patients with the same number of IgE molecules/cell released a different percentage of histamine (from 10% to 95%). An explanation for this enigma is that the sensitivity of basophils and mast cells to release chemical mediators (i.e., histamine, leukotrienes, etc.) is influenced by something other than the serum concentrations of specific IgE and IgG antibodies. This is the concept of basophil and mast cell "releasability": a kind of "black box" that controls—independently of the number of the IgE molecules on the membrane surface— the response of these cells to allergens or anti-IgE [11].

The pathogenesis of allergic disease is characterized by three hallmarks: increased IgE synthesis, increased releasability of chemical mediators from basophils and mast cells, and hyperresponsiveness of end organs such as bronchial smooth muscle and skin vessels [12]. Increased basophil and mast cell releasability has been mainly documented with IgE-mediated stimuli. In most studies rabbit or goat antibodies against human monoclonal IgE have been used to challenge basophils and mast cells. These antibodies cross-link the Fc portions of IgE molecules on the surface of these cells and trigger the release of preformed (histamine) and de novo synthesized (peptide leukotriene C_4) mediators from human basophils and mast cells [13]. Anti-IgE has been of great importance in documenting an increased IgE-mediated releasability of basophils from young patients with atopic dermatitis [14], allergic rhinitis [12] and bronchial asthma [15]. Increased IgE-mediated releasability of mast cells obtained from bronchoalveolar lavage (BAL) has also been demonstrated in patients with bronchial asthma compared to controls [15]. The rationale of using rabbit or goat anti-IgE is the assumption that releasability of these cells in response to anti-IgE is correlated to the response to the relevant allergen. Recently, we have documented an excellent linear correlation between the maximum percent histamine release induced by anti-IgE and that induced by the purified P1 antigen in patients with allergic rhinitis or bronchial asthma and skin test positive to *Dermatophagoides pteronyssinus* [12]. In addition, anti-IgE autoantibodies have been found in a variety of allergic disorders [16–21].

Autoantibodies against IgE were first described by Williams et al. [16]. These naturally occurring antibodies belonged exclusively to the IgM class and were found in various groups of patients, the highest incidence being among patients with allergic and parasitic diseases. IgM anti-IgE did not induce histamine release from basophils, nor did they block antigen-induced histamine release. After this initial report, several groups have described the presence of autoantibodies directed against IgE in several conditions, mostly related to atopy [17–21]. The interest in such autoantibodies derives from their potential triggering of mediator release from mast cells and basophils and therefore their participation in the pathogenesis of allergic disorders. Several studies have tried, without success, to obtain histamine release from basophils challenged in vitro with affinity-purified IgG anti-IgE [22, 23]. More recently, however, the group of Allen Kaplan has confirmed the presence of autoantibodies of IgG and IgM classes directed against myeloma IgE in approximately 50% of patients with urticarial syndromes [24]. In addition, they reported that several sera containing these autoantibodies induced histamine release from human basophils.

We extended the latter observation in an attempt to clarify the apparently discordant results as to the role of anti-IgE antibodies in human sera. Quinti et al. [21] have previously shown that patients with atopic dermatitis contain significant amounts of IgG directed toward the Fc portion of IgE. Therefore, we tested the effect of IgG antibodies isolated from patients with atopic dermatitis and from normal donors on histamine release from human basophils and mast cells isolated from skin and lung tissues. Purified IgG from normals did not induce release from these cells. In contrast, affinity-purified IgG anti-IgE (H-aIgE) (10^{-4} to 2 µg/ml) from 1 out of 6 atopic dermatitis patients with high levels of IgG anti-IgE antibodies induced the release of histamine from basophils of 4 different donors (Figure 1 A). The histamine release reaction caused by H-aIgE was Ca^{2+}- and temperature-dependent: little or no release occurred at 22 °C or 4 °C, respectively, and maximal release occurred at 37 °C. Moreover, IgG from this patient induced histamine release from human basophils in the presence of 1 to 5 mM Ca^{2+} in the extracellular medium. We also found an excellent correlation between

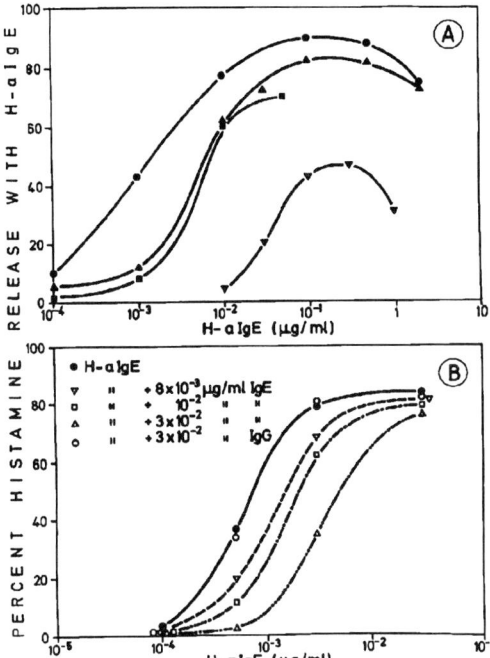

Figure 1. (A) Effect of increasing concentrations of IgG purified from patient D. A. with atopic dermatitis with a high level of anti-IgE activity (H-aIgE) on histamine release from human basophils isolated from four different donors. Each line represents the release obtained with the cells of a single donor. (B) The effect of H-aIgE, alone or in combination with purified IgE myeloma (∇, 8×10^{-3} μg/ml; $\square$, 10^{-2} μ/ml; $\triangle$, 3×10^{-2} μg/ml) or purified polyclonal IgE (O, 3×10^{-2} μg/ml) on the percentage histamine release from human basophils. The cells were preincubated 5 min with monoclonal IgE or polyclonal IgG. H-aIgE was then added and the cells were incubated for an additional 45 min at 37°C. Each point represents the mean of duplicate determinations.

the maximum percent histamine release caused by rabbit anti-IgE and IgG from this patient, suggesting that the IgG containing anti-IgE activity might interact with the IgEs present on the basophil membrane. Desensitization of basophils with rabbit anti-IgE abolishes the subsequent response with both rabbit anti-IgE and human IgG containing anti-IgE activity. Similarly, preincubation with human IgG anti-igE abolishes the release on challenge with both rabbit anti-IgE and the human IgG anti-IgE.

Further evidence that IgG from the atopic dermatitis patient induces histamine release by binding IgE was based on the inability to in-

duce histamine release from basophils from which IgE had been dissociated by treatment with lactic acid. Finally, we found that IgE purified from three different patients with myeloma blocked in a competitive fashion the histamine releasing activity of both rabbit anti-IgE and human IgG with anti-IgE activity. Figure 1 B shows a typical experiment in which increasing concentrations of purified monoclonal IgE shifted in parallel to the right of the dose-response curve caused by graded concentrations of human IgG with anti-IgE activity. Human polyclonal IgG, used as control, did not affect the releasing activity of human IgG anti-IgE.

The IgG autoantibodies to IgE present in this patient with atopic dermatitis also caused the de novo synthesis of peptide leukotriene C_4 from human basophils. There was an excellent correlation between the maximum percent histamine release and the synthesis of LTC_4 caused by human IgG anti-IgE from basophils. We also found that human IgG anti-IgE induces the release of histamine from mast cells isolated from lung parenchyma and skin tissue.

The foregoing observations suggest a number of implications for anti-IgE autoantibodies naturally occurring in patients with atopic dermatitis, asthma, and urticarial syndromes. However, the real prevalence of functional anti-IgE autoantibodies in these allergic syndromes should be evaluated in larger groups of patients. In fact, we found functional IgG anti-IgE only in 1 out of 6 patients with atopic dermatitis with high levels of IgG anti-IgE. It is possible that, in most patients, IgG or IgM anti-IgE are complexed with high affinity with IgE and that they are practically unable to activate basophil/mast cell-bound IgEs. Alternatively, the affinity of IgG or IgM for IgE might be very low in most patients. A third possibility is a very low prevalence of functionally active anti-IgE autoantibodies in allergic syndromes. These three hypotheses are compatible with the findings obtained in patients with urticarial syndromes [24] and in our group of atopic dermatitis patients. In both studies the prevalence of anti-IgE autoantibodies that activated basophils was very low. Whatever the prevalence and the biological significance of anti-IgE autoantibodies in patients with allergic syndromes, our results demonstrate that at least in a small percentage of patients with atopic dermatitis, IgG anti-IgE induces the release of chemical mediators from human basophils and tissue mast cells by interacting with cell-bound IgE.

References

1. Ishizaka, K., T. Ishizaka, and M. M. Hornbrook. 1966. Physicochemical properties of reaginic antibody. V. Correlation of reaginic activity with E globulin antibody. J. Immunol. 97: 840.
2. Johansson, S. G. O., and H. Bennich. 1967. Immunological studies of an atypical (myeloma) immunoglobulin. Immunology 13: 381.
3. Juhlin, L., S. G. O. Johansson, H. Bennich, C. Hogman, and N. Thyresson. 1969. Immunoglobulin E in dermatoses: levels in atopic dermatitis and urticaria. Arch. Dermatol. 100: 12.
4. Johansson, S. G. O. 1967. Raised levels of a new immunoglobulin class (IgND) in asthma. Lancet 2: 951.
5. Lichtenstein, L. M., and A. G. Osler. 1964. Studies on the mechanisms of hypersensitivity phenomena. IX. Histamine release from human leukocytes by ragweed pollen antigen. J. Exp. Med. 120: 507.
6. Levy, D. A., and A. G. Osler. 1966. Studies on the mechanisms of hypersensitivity phenomena. XIV. Passive sensitization in vitro of human leukocytes to ragweed pollen antigen. J. Immunol. 97: 203.
7. Ishizaka, T., K. Ishizaka, S. G. O. Johansson, and H. Bennich. 1969. Histamine release from human leukocytes by anti-γE antibodies. J. Immunol. 102: 884.
8. Platts-Mills, T. A. E., R. K. von Maur, K. Ishizaka, P. S. Norman, and L. M. Lichtenstein. 1976. IgA and IgG anti-ragweed antibodies in nasal secretions. Quantitative measurements of antibodies and correlation with inhibition of histamine release. J. Clin. Invest. 57: 1041.
9. Hunt, K. J., M. D. Valentine, A. K. Sobotka, A. W. Benton, F. J. Amodio, and L. M. Lichtenstein. 1978. A controlled trial of immunotherapy in insect hypersensitivity. N. Engl. J. Med. 299: 157.
10. Conroy, M. C., N. F. Adkinson Jr., and L. M. Lichtenstein 1977. Measurement of IgE on human basophils: Relation to serum IgE and anti-IgE-induced histamine release. J. Immunol. 118: 1317.
11. Marone, G. 1986. Modulation of basophil/mast cell functions in vivo: the releasability concept. In: Proceedings of the XII Congress of Allergology and Clinical Immunology. C. E. Reed, J. Bellanti, R. J. Davies, S. Friedlaender, A. Oehling, and R. G. Slavin, eds. St. Louis: C. V. Mosby, p. 175.
12. Marone, G., V. Casolaro, F. Ayala, G. Melillo, and M. Condorelli. 1989. The concept of releasability in allergic disorders. In: Clinical Immunology, Vol. 2. G. Melillo, P. S. Norman, and G. Marone, eds. Toronto: B. C. Decker, in press.
13. Marone, G., M. Columbo, M. Triggiani, R. Cirillo, A. Genovese, and S. Formisano. 1987. Inhibition of IgE-mediated histamine and peptide leukotriene release from human basophils and mast cells by forskolin. Biochem. Pharm. 36: 13.
14. Marone, G., R. Giugliano, G. Lembo, and F. Ayala. 1986. Human basophil releasability. II. Changes in basophil releasability in patients with atopic dermatitis. J. Invest. Dermatol. 87: 19.
15. Casolaro, V., D. Galeone, A. Giacummo, A. Sanduzzi, G. Melillo, and G. Marone. 1989. Human basophil/mast cell releasability. V. Functional comparisons of cells obtained from peripheral blood, lung parenchyma and by bronchoalveolar lavage in asthmatics. Am. Rev. Respir. Dis., in press.
16. Williams, R. C. Jr., R. W. Griffiths, J. D. Emmons, and R. C. Field. 1972. Naturally occurring human antiglobulins with specificity for γE. J. Clin. Invest. 51: 955.
17. Carini, E., and J. Brostoff. 1983. An antiglobulin: IgG anti-IgE. Occurrence and specificity. Ann. Allergy 51: 251.
18. Inganäs, M., S. G. O. Johansson, and H. Bennich. 1981. Anti-IgE antibodies in human sera: occurrence and specificity. Int. Archs. Allergy appl. Immunol. 65: 51.
19. Nawata, Y., T. Koike, T. Yanagisawa, I. Iwamoto, T. Itaya, S. Yoshida, and H. Tomioka. 1984. Anti-IgE autoantibody in patients with bronchial asthma. Clin. exp. Immunol. 58: 348.
20. Nawata, Y., T. Koike, H. Hosokawa, H. Tomioka, and S. Yoshida. 1985. Anti-IgE autoantibody in patients with atopic dermatitis. J. Immunol. 135: 478.
21. Quinti, I., C. Brozek, N. Wood, R. S. Geha, and D. Y. M. Leung. 1986. Circulating IgG autoantibodies to IgE in atopic syndromes. J. Allergy Clin. Immunol. 77: 586.
22. Johansson, S. G. O. 1986. Anti-IgE antibodies in human serum. J. Allergy Clin. Immunol. 77: 555.
23. Johansson, S. G. O., C. G. M. Magnusson, and P. H. Larsson. 1986. Occurrence, specificity, and putative roles of anti-IgE antibodies in human serum. In: Proceedings of the XII International Congress of Allergology and Clinical Immunology. C. E. Reed, J. Bellanti, R. J. Davies, S. Friedlaender, A. Oehling, and R. G. Slavin, eds. St. Louis: C. V. Mosby, p. 193.
24. Gruber, B. L., M. L. Baeza, M. J. Marchese, V. Agnello, and A. P. Kaplan. 1988. Prevalence and functional role of anti-IgE autoantibodies in urticarial syndromes. J. Invest. Dermatol. 90: 213.

A New Approach to Suppressing the IgE Antibody Response to Allergen

Kimishige Ishizaka, Makoto Iwata, Claudio Carini, Toru Takeuchi*

The glycosylation inhibiting factor (GIF), a T-cell-derived lymphokine with phospholipase-inhibitory activity, facilitates the generation of antigen-specific suppressor T cells from antigen-primed T cell population. Activation of spleen cells of antigen-primed mice by the antigen, followed by propagation of the activated T cells by IL-2 in the presence of GIF, resulted in the selective development of antigen-specific suppressor T cells. T cell hybridomas constructed from the T cell population produce antigen-specific GIF upon antigenic stimulation, and the factors could suppress the antibody response of the donor of spleen cells in a carrier-specific manner. The same principle applies to human lymphocytes of patients allergic to bee venom. Antigenic stimulation of peripheral blood lymphocytes of such patients, followed by propagation of T cells by IL-2 in the presence of recombinant lipocortin resulted in the development of suppressor T cells that form allergen-specific GIF. T cell hybridomas from such T cells would produce lymphokines effective for the suppression of antibody response in the donor of peripheral blood.

Before the last International Congress of Allergology, we presented evidence that the biologic activities of IgE-binding factors are controlled by two T cell factors, i.e., glycosylation enhancing factor (GEF) and glycosylation inhibiting factor (GIF), which regulate the post-translational glycosylation process of IgE-binding peptide [1]. Subsequent experiments revealed that GIF has immunosuppressive effects. Repeated injections of affinity-purified GIF from rodent T cell hybridoma into BDF1 mice suppressed both the primary and on-going IgE and IgG antibody responses of mice to alum-absorbed ovalbumin (OVA) [2]. In the past 10 years, several different approaches have been made to control the IgE antibody formation. Modified allergen, such as polyethylene glycol conjugates of allergen and urea-denatured antigen, successfully suppressed the primary IgE

antibody response to the native antigen in experimental animals [3]. However, the on-going IgE antibody formation was difficult to control by such modified antigens. As the suppression of on-going IgE antibody formation by GIF was unique, we analyzed the mechanisms involved in the immunosuppression by GIF. Thus, two groups of BDF1 mice were immunized with alum-absorbed OVA, and one group was treated by intravenous injections of GIF given every 2 days. Two weeks after the priming, when IgE antibody titer of untreated mice reached maximum, they were sacrificed and their spleen cells were stimulated by antigen. As expected, spleen cells of untreated mice produced IgE-potentiating factor and GEF, while those of GIF-treated mice formed IgE-suppressive factor and GIF. Thus, GIF treatment switches the spleen cells from the formation of IgE-potentiating factor to the formation of IgE-suppressive factor. Furthermore, we realized that GIF released from the spleen cells of the OVA-primed GIF-treated mice had affinity for ovalbumin [2]. Our previous experiments have shown that the major cell source of antigen-specific GIF is antigen-specific suppressor T cells [4]. Indeed, ovalbumin-specific suppressor T cells were detected in the spleen of the OVA-primed GIF-treated mice. Thus, it appears that GIF treatment of antigen-primed mice facilitated the generation of antigen-specific suppressor T cells, and these cells were responsible for the immunosuppression.

We anticipated that GIF may facilitate the generation of antigen-specific suppressor T cells in vitro and determined whether the principles obtained with mouse T cells apply to human lymphocytes. Here, we would like to summarize the results of the experiments to prove the hypothesis and suggest a new approach to the control of IgE antibody response of allergic patients.

First of all, we tried to reproduce the effect

*   Johns Hopkins University School of Medicine, Baltimore, MD 21239, USA.
    This work was supported by research grants AI-11202 and AI-14784 from the United States Human and Health Service.

129

Figure 1.

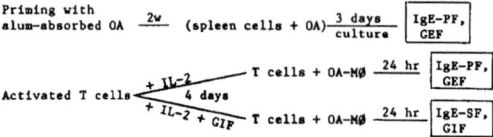

Figure 2.

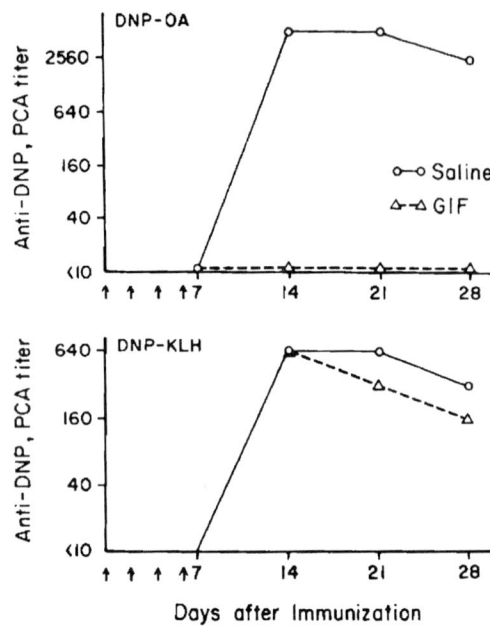

Days after Immunization

of GIF in vitro, using mouse lymphocytes. As shown in Figure 1, BDF1 mice were immunized with alum-absorbed ovalbumin for the IgE antibody response, and their spleen cells were obtained 2 weeks after the immunization, when the IgE antibody titer reached maximum. The spleen cells were cultured with ovalbumin to activate T cells, and the activated T cells were propagated by Il-2 in the presence or absence of GIF for 4 days. Since antigen-specific T cells should have selectively proliferated during the culture, the cells recovered from the cultures were stimulated with ovalbumin-pulsed syngeneic macrophages. Upon antigenic stimulation, the original spleen cells as well as T cells propagated in the absence of GIF produced IgE-potentiating factor and GEF. In contrast, the same T cells propagated in the presence of GIF produced IgE-suppressive factor and GIF (Figure 1). The GIF was detected in the culture supernatant bound to OVA-coupled sepharose and was recovered by elution at acid pH. Since GIF added to T cells together with IL-2 during their propagation did not have affinity for OVA, GIF detected in the antigen-stimulated T cell cultures does not appear to be a carryover of the GIF added in previous cultures. The results indicated that the addition of nonspecific GIF during the propagation of antigen-specific T cells facilitated the generation of antigen-specific T cells that produce their own GIF [5].

Separate experiments in our laboratory indicated that antigen-specific GIF is similar to antigen-specific suppressor T cell factors in their molecular characteristics and biologic activities [6]. If this is the case, one may expect that the antigen-specific GIF obtained in the culture may suppress the antibody response of the donor of spleen cells. To test this possibility, OVA-primed T cells were propagated in the presence of GIF, and such T cells were fused with BW 5147 cells to construct hybridomas. Among 32 hybridomas obtained, 14 hybrid clones constitutively formed GIF, and 7 out of the 14 hybridomas responded to ovalbumin-

pulsed syngeneic macrophages to form OVA-specific GIF. Thus, we selected one representative hybridoma and cultured the cells with OVA-pulsed macrophages. OVA-specific GIF in culture supernatants were purified by using OVA-sepharose and tested for immunosuppressive activity. In the experiment shown in Figure 2, groups of BDF1 mice were immunized with either alum-absorbed DNP-OVA or DNP-KLH, and they were treated by 4 i.v. injections of OVA-specific GIF from the hybridoma. It is evident that OVA-specific GIF suppressed the anti-hapten IgE antibody response to DNP-OVA without affecting the antibody response to DNP-KLH [7]. It appears that OVA-specific GIF suppressed the antibody response in a carrier-specific manner.

The series of the experiments provides a maneuver to obtain antigen-specific suppressor factor from antigen-primed T cell population. We wondered whether this protocol can be used to generate antigen-specific suppressor T cells from lymphocytes of allergic patients. As an experimental model, we chose patients allergic to honey bee venom. As the major allergen in honey bee venom is phospholipase A_2, we took peripheral blood mononuclear cells from allergic patients and cultured the

Figure 3.

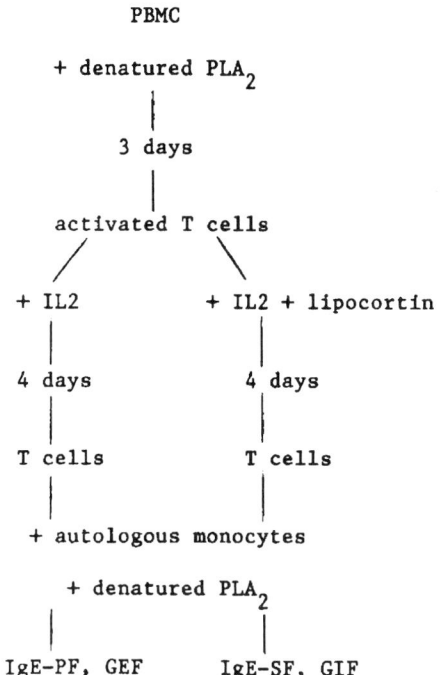

PBMC

+ denatured PLA$_2$

|

3 days

|

activated T cells

/ \

+ IL2   + IL2 + lipocortin

| |

4 days   4 days

| |

T cells   T cells

| |

+ autologous monocytes

+ denatured PLA$_2$

| |

IgE-PF, GEF   IgE-SF, GIF

cells with bee venom phospholipase A$_2$ that had been denatured by treatment with guanidine hydrochloride in the presence of reducing reagent (Figure 3). This treatment completely inactivated the enzymatic activity of the allergen [8], but the denatured antigen should maintain the sequence of peptide that would associate with MHC produces and stimulate antigen-specific T cells. T cells activated by the antigen were divided into two portions and propagated by IL-2, in the presence or absence of recombinant human lipocortin [9]. Since we did not have human GIF, we employed lipocortin that has GIF activity. T cells propagated under the conditions were recovered and incubated with autologous monocytes in the presence of denatured phospholipase A$_2$. Culture supernatants were then assessed for the presence of IgE-binding factors and GEF or GIF. As expected, T cells propagated by IL-2 alone produced IgE-potentiating factor and GEF, while those propagated in the presence of lipocortin produced IgE-suppressive factor and GIF. Similar results were obtained with peripheral blood mononuclear cells of 4 out of 5 patients.

We tested whether the GIF has affinity for bee venom phospholipase A$_2$. Peripheral blood mononuclear cells of bee venom-sensitive patients were stimulated by denatured PLA$_2$, and antigen-activated T cells were propagated in the presence of lipocortin. The cells were then cultured with autologous monocytes and denatured antigen, or with monocytes alone. IgE-BF was detected only when the cells were stimulated by antigen-pulsed monocytes. The culture supernatants were absorbed with IgE-sepharose, and filtrates were fractionated on phospholipase-coupled sepharose, to determine the distribution of GIF between the effluent and eluate fractions. It is apparent that the T cells constitutively release nonspecific GIF lacking affinity for PLA$_2$, but antigen stimulation of the same cells results in the formation of GIF, which has affinity for PLA$_2$. GIF present in culture supernatant of antigen-stimulated cells bound to phospholipase-sepharose and was recovered by elution at acid pH. As the stimulation of the T cells by antigen should go through T cell receptors, we anticipated that stimulation of the same T cells with OKT 3 may induce the formation of antigen-specific GIF. Indeed, the T cells cultured in OKT 3-coated wells formed IgE-binding factors and GIF, which had affinity for bee venom phospholipase A$_2$. Thus, we succeeded in generating antigen-specific suppressor T cells, which form antigen-specific GIF from peripheral blood T cells of bee venom-sensitive patients.

Finally, attempts were made to construct human T cell hybridomas that produce GIF. Peripheral blood mononuclear cells of a bee venom-sensitive patient were stimulated with denatured PLA$_2$, and the cells were propagated by IL-2 in the presence of human lipocortin. The cells were then fused with BUC cells. Only four T cell hybridomas were obtained in the experiments; however, two of them constitutively produced GIF. One of the hybridomas was expanded and cultured for PLA$_2$-sepharose. As we do not have an appropriate system for the measurement of antibody response of human peripheral blood lymphocytes to bee venom PLA$_2$, we cannot evaluate immunosuppressive activity of antigen-specific GIF. Considering that antigen-specific GIF from mouse T cells suppress the in vivo antibody response of syngeneic mice in a carrier-specific manner, we suspect that allergen-specific GIF from human T cell hybridomas will suppress the antibody response of the donor of parent T cells to specific allergen.

References

1. Ishizaka, K. 1988. IgE-binding factors and regulation of the IgE antibody response. Ann. Rev. Immunol. 6: 513.
2. Akasaki, M., P. Jardieu, and K. Ishizaka. 1986. Immunosuppressive effects of glycosylation inhibiting factor on the IgE and IgG antibody response. J. Immunol. 136: 3172.
3. Sehon, A. H. 1982. Suppression of IgE antibody responses with tolerogenic conjugates of allergens and haptens. Prog. Allergy 32: 161.
4. Jardieu, P., T. Uede, and K. Ishizaka. 1984. IgE-binding factors from mouse T lymphocytes. III. Role of antigen-specific T cells in the formation of IgE suppressive factor. J. Immunol. 133: 3266.
5. Iwata, M., and K. Ishizaka. In vitro modulation of antigen-primed T cells by a glycosylation inhibiting factor that regulates the formation of antigen-specific suppressor factor. Proc. Natl. Acad. Sci. USA 84: 2444.
6. Jardieu, P., M. Akasaki, and K. Ishizaka. 1987. Carrier-specific suppression of antibody responses by antigen-specific glycosylation inhibition factors. J. Immunol. 138: 1494.
7. Iwata, M., and K. Ishizaka. 1988. Construction of antigen-specific suppressor T cell hybridomas from spleen cells of mice primed for the persistent IgE antibody formation. J. Immunol., in press.
8. King, T. P., A. K. Sobotka, L. Kochonmain, and L. M. Lichtenstein. 1976. Allergens of honey bee venom. Arch. Biochem. and Biophys. 172: 661.
9. Wallner, B. P., R. J. Mallalicano, C. Hession, R. L. Cate et al. 1986. Cloning and expression of human lipocortin, a phospholipase A_2 inhibitor with potential anti-inflammatory activity. Nature 320: 77.

Human IgE-Binding Factors

G. Delespesse*, M. Sarfati*, H. Hofstetter**, M. Letellier**, R. Peleman*

In addition to a brief review of the literature, the authors report their most recent findings regarding FcεRII and IgE-binding factors. Hence, it was clearly shown that, by contrast to the mouse system, human CD5[+] B cells may express FcεRII. Definitive evidence that this receptor may also be expressed on some normal T cells was provided by the observation that FACS-sorted T cells contained FcεRII mRNA and reacted with monoclonal antibodies to FcεRII. We next reported that IgE-BFs, known to be the soluble fragments of FcεRII, are generated by an autoproteolytic mechanism. Finally, highly purified native and recombinant IgE-BFs were shown to potentiate the spontaneous and the IL4-induced synthesis of human IgE in an isotype-specific manner.

The possible role of B cell-derived IgE-binding factors (IgE- BFs) in the regulation of human IgE synthesis was suggested several years ago [1, 2]. It was observed that the culture supernatant (CSN) of several B cell lines expressing FcεRII was capable of both potentiating the spontaneous synthesis of IgE by B cells from atopic patients and of inhibiting the binding of IgE to FcεRII-bearing cells. Since these two activities could be specifically adsorbed on IgE-immunoadsorbent columns from which they could be recovered, it was suggested that they were mediated by IgE- BFs. Moreover, such IgE-BFs were detected only in the CSN of FcεRII bearing cells and not in the CSN of FcεRII negative cells, suggesting that IgE-BFs were derived from FcεRII. This prompted us to produce monoclonal antibodies to FcεRII (MabER) with a view of obtaining antibodies cross-reacting with IgE-BFs. The availability of these MabER has permitted a significant progress in our understanding of the structure and the biology of FcεRII and of IgE-BFs [3]. It was found that MabER and anti-CD23 antibodies react with the same molecules, demonstrating the identity between FcεRII and CD23, which was known as a B cell-specific differentiation antigen [4].

Cellular Expression of FcεRII

It is now accepted that FcεRII is expressed on B lymphocytes, monocytes/macrophages, eosinophils, and platelets [5, 6]. On B lymphocytes, this receptor is selectively expressed on sIgM/sIgD double bearing cells and it is lost after isotype switching [7]. The majority of circulating B cells from normal individuals are FcεRII positive, and in allergic patients the cellular density of FcεRII is increased [8, 9]. By opposition to a recent study in the mouse system we found that CD5[+] B cells are capable of expressing FcεRII [10]. The expression of FcεRII on T cells is still controversial [11–15]. In a most recent study, T cells obtained by cell-sorting from the blood of normal donors were shown to express FcεRII both at the phenotypic and at the mRNA level [Nutman et al., manuscript in preparation]. Accumulating evidence suggests that FcεRII may also be expressed on epidermal Langerhans cells [16]. Upon incubation at 37 °C, in the absence of stimulant, FcεRII rapidly disappears from the surface of normal B cells. This phenomenon is specifically blocked by IgE, even in the presence of protein synthesis inhibitors [11]. The disappearance of FcεRII from the cell surface is accounted for by two mechanisms: (i) its cleavage into soluble fragments that may be detected in the CSN [17], and (ii) the disappearance of FcεRII mRNA [18]. Hence, the expression of FcεRII by normal B cells is not constitutive, and additional observations have shown that it requires the presence of IL4.

Structure of FcεRII

This receptor is made of a single chain consisting of a 45 KD sialoglycoprotein containing one N-linked carbohydrate chain of the complex type [19–21]. When this molecule is isolated in the absence of protease inhibitors, it is rapidly cleaved into IgE-binding fragments

---

*   University of Montreal, Notre-Dame Hospital, Research Center.
** CIBA-GEIGY, Biotechnology, Basel, Switzerland.

with mol. wt. of 37 KD, 33 KD, 25 KD, and 16 KD. FcεRII is spatially associated with HLA DR [22]. The cDNA coding for FcεRII has been cloned and functionally expressed [23–25]; it predicts for a protein of 321 amino acids. This transmembrane protein has an inverted orientation, with the N- terminus being intracellular. The predicted amino acid sequence displays a striking homology with several animal lectins.

Interestingly, the homology region was recently shown to contain the IgE-binding site of FcεRII [H. Hofstetter, unpublished observations]. On the other hand, some of these animal lectins were shown to bind carbohydrates via the same homology region. These two observations, suggesting that FcεRII binds to IgE through its carbohydrates, are in contrast with the finding that recombinant and nonglycosylated IgE binds to FcεRII (26). It is of note that FcεRII cDNA has no homology with the cDNA encoding rodent IgE-BFs [27], indicating that FcεRII and its soluble fragments, i.e., IgE-BF/soluble CD23, are unrelated to the T cell-derived IgE-BFs described in the animal model. Since human T cell-derived IgE-BFs with similar biochemical characteristics to rodent IgE-BFs have also been described [9, 28], it is possible that there is more than one family of IgE-binding proteins. The data reviewed hereafter refer exclusively to the B cell-derived IgE-BFs or soluble CD23.

Mechanisms of Formation of IgE-BFs

IgE-BFs were purified to homogeneity by a combination of affinity-chromatography and ion exchange or reverse phase chromatography [29]. These molecules display some micro heterogeneity with mol. wt. ranging from 25 to 27 KD and pI comprised between 4.5 to 5.2. IgE-BFs are O- but not N-linked glycosylated. The sequence of the first 20 N-terminal amino acids of IgE-BFs perfectly matches with a stretch of the FcεRII sequence, demonstrating that IgE-BFs are cleavage fragments of FcεRII. It was subsequently shown that the cleavage of FcεRII into IgE-BFs occurs at the cell surface, and that it is not an intracellular post-transcriptional process [17, 20]. Our most recent observations further indicate that IgE-BFs are formed by the autoproteolysis of FcεRII [Delespesse et al., unpublished observations].

Moreover, IgE-BFs appear to be more heterogeneous than previously thought. They are comprised not only of molecules with mol. wt. of 25–27 KD but also of 37 KD, 33 KD, and 16 KD. The 25 KD IgE-BFs are derived from soluble 37 KD and 33 KD precursor molecules, and the enzyme involved in their cleavage is the 45 KD FcεRII itself. The mechanisms leading to the formation of 16 KD IgE-BFs are currently being analyzed. The above fragments of FcεRII are capable of binding to IgE as shown by the following three observations: (i) They inhibit the binding of IgE to FcεRII-bearing cells; (ii) they are retained on IgE-immunoadsorbent; and (iii) they react in a sandwich RIA employing MabER, IgE and monoclonal anti-IgE antibodies [30]. In this assay, a solid-phase is first coated with some MabER reacting with an epitope located outside the IgE-binding site of FcεRII. Purified preparations of IgE-BFs are then incubated with the MabER-coated solid phase; after washing out the unbound molecules, the solid-phase is successively reacted with IgE and radiolabeled anti-IgE. Hence, by opposition to the mouse system, some soluble fragments of FcεRII are indeed capable of binding to IgE.

Regulation of FcεRII Expression and of IgE-BFs Production

The expression of FcεRII and the production of IgE- BFs by B cells and monocytes have been analyzed in some detail. As already mentioned, normal lymphocytes rapidly lose FcεRII when incubated at 37 °C in the absence of stimulant, and this is accompanied by the disappearance of FcεRII mRNA. The only cytokine capable of re-inducing FcεRII expression and IgE- BF production by these cultured B cells is IL4. IL4 exerts this effect on both B cells and monocytes [24, 31, 32, 33]. When B cells are co- stimulated with IL4 and anti-IgM (or phorbol esthers), there is a super-induction of IgE-BFs production (and of FcεRII expression). However, co-stimulation of the same B cells with a-IgM and either low mol. wt. BCGF, IL2 or IFN-γ does not induce production by these cells. This clearly indicates that FcεRII is not a general marker of B cell activation. The expression of FcεRII and the release of IgE-BFs by IL4- stimulated highly purified B cells is inhibited by IFN-γ, IFN-α and PGE2 [31, 34] as well as by hydrocortisone.

134

IFN- γ increases the production of IgE-BFs by adherent cells and by the monocytic cell line U937 [31, 35]. When added to IL4- stimulated peripheral blood mononuclear cells, IFN-γ does not suppress IgE-BFs production; indicating that its inhibiting effect on B cells is masked by its enhancing effect on monocytes. IFN- α suppresses both the IL4-and the IFN-γ- induced production of IgE-BFs by PBMC, indicating that it is active both on B cells and on monocytes. Because IgE-BFs are breakdown products of FcεRII, one would expect that the production of IgE-BFs is directly correlated with the expression of surface FcεRII. However, in view of the following two observations such a direct relationship does not always exist. First, upon incubation with tunicamycin, FcεRII-bearing cells express much less FcεRII but release more IgE-BFs [20]. This observation is taken to indicate that N-linked carbohydrates have an inhibiting effect on the autoproteolytic cleavage of FcεRII into IgE-BFs. Secondly, IgE stabilizes FcεRII, resulting in an apparent increase of the cellular density of this receptor and a concomitant decrease of the release of IgE-BFs [36]. A similar dissociation between FcεRII expression and IgE-BFs production was recently reported by Kawabe et al. [35]. These authors observed that IFN-γ downregulates the IL4-induced expression of FcεRII on the JIJOYE B cell line, whereas it increases the release of IgE-BFs by these cells. The mechanisms regulating FcεRII expression on eosinophils have not been analyzed to date, although it is known that this receptor is preferentially expressed on activated and hypodense eosinophils [5]. Finally, the expression of FcεRII on platelets is increased by IFN-γ[37].

Function of FcεRII and of IgE-BF

The function of FcεRII depends upon the cells on which it is expressed. On eosinophils, platelets and monocytes, it is mediating the IgE-dependent cytotoxicity against parasites [5]. It may also be involved in the allergen-induced release of inflammatory mediators by the same cells [38]. The function of FcεRII on B cells is unknown, and the hypothesis that it may serve as the receptor for the low mol. wt. BCGF has now been abandoned [39]. Our own hypothesis is that FcεRII is a membrane-bound precursor of soluble biologically active molecules. Hence,

soluble fragments of FcεRII (containing a mixture of 25 KD and 12 KD molecules) displayed both an autocrine activity on EBV- transformed B cells and a BCGF-activity on anti-IgM stimulated B cells [40]. We were able to repeat these observations by using affinity- purified fragments of FcεRII; however, such preparations contained several families of molecules differing by their mol. wt. as shown by SDS-PAGE analysis. At this stage it is not yet possible to relate this BCGF activity to a well-defined and highly purified fragment of FcεRII. The role of FcεRII or its soluble fragments in B cell proliferation is also suggested by the following observations. Hence, the proliferation of B cells co- stimulated with anti-IgM and IL4 is specifically blocked by MabER or its F(ab')2 fragments, but not by unrelated monoclonal antibodies of the same IgG subclass. Moreover,the same MabER have no effect on the proliferative response of anti-IgM activated B cells to either IL2, IFN-, or the low mol. wt. of BCGF. Finally, soluble IgE induces a moderate but significant inhibition of both the proliferation of B cells co-stimulated by anti-IgM and IL4 and of the release of IgE-BFs by the same cells.

Our earlier observations indicating that B cell-derived IgE-BF are capable of potentiating the synthesis of human IgE have been recently confirmed by others [41]. Since semi-purified preparations of IgE-BFs were used in those experiments, it was most important to shown that both highly purified native and recombinant IgE-BFs do indeed display the same activity. These observations were made independently by three laboratories including our own [35; Delespesse et al., unpublished data; deVries et al., in preparation]. Hence, such preparations of IgE-BFs were shown to potentiate both the spontaneous production of IgE by B lymphocytes from allergic donors and the IL4-induced IgE synthesis by normal PBMC. The potentiating activity was observed at very low concentrations of IgE-BFs (less than 1 nM/l); at higher concentrations there was either no effect or a suppression of IgE production. The activity of IgE-BFs was isotype-specific, and, as expected, it could be blocked by MabER but not by unrelated monoclonal antibodies of the same IgG subclass. The role of FcεRII/IgE-BFs in the regulation of human IgE was further shown by the observation of an inhibiting effect of MabER on the spontaneous and the IL4-induced IgE synthesis [30]. Also in this case, the action of

135

MabER was isotype-specific. Current studies aim to relate the BCGF activity of FcεRII fragments to their IgE-potentiating effects.

References

1. Sarfati, M., E. Rector, K. Wong, M. Rubio-Trujillo, A. H. Sehon and, and G. Delespesse. 1984. In vitro synthesis of IgE by human lymphocytes. II. Enhancement of the spontaneous IgE synthesis by IgE- binding factors secreted by RPMI 8866 lymphoblastoid B cell line. Immunology. 53:197.

2. Sarfati, M., E. Rector, M. Rubio-Trujillo, K. Wong, A. H. Sehon, and G. Delespesse. 1984. In vitro synthesis of human IgE. III. IgE potentiating activity of culture supernatants from Epstein-Barr virus (EBV) transformed B cells. Immunology. 53:207.

3. Rector, E., T. Nakajima, C. Rocha, A. H. Sehon, and G. Delespesse. 1985. Detection and characterization of monoclonal antibodies specific to IgE receptors on human lymphocytes by flow cytometry. Immunology. 55: 481.

4. Bonnefoy, J. Y., J. P. Aubry, C. Peronne, J. Wijdenes, and J. Banchereau. 1987. Production and characterization of a monoclonal antibody specific for the human lymphocyte low affinity receptor for IgE: CD23 is a low affinity receptor for IgE. J. Immunol. 138: 2970.

5. Capron, A., J. P. Dessaint, M. Capron, M. Joseph, J. C. Ameisen, and A. B. Tonnel. 1986. From parasites to allergy: A second receptor for IgE. Immunol. Today 7: 15.

6. Spiegelberg, H. L. 1981. Lymphocytes bearing Fc receptors for IgE. Immunol. Rev. 56: 199.

7. Kikutani, H., M. Suemura, H. Owaki, H. Nakamura, R. Sato, K. Yamasaki, E. L. Barsumian, R. R. Hardy, and T. Kishimoto. 1986. Fcε receptor, a specific differentiation marker transiently expressed on mature B cells before isotype switching. J. Exp. Med. 164: 815.

8. Spiegelberg, H. L. 1987. The expression of IgE Fc receptors on lymphocytes of allergic patients. Int. Rev. Immunol. 2: 63.

9. Suemura, M., and J. Kishimoto. 1987. IgE class-specific regulatory factors and Fcε receptors on lymphocytes. Int. Rev. Immunol. 2:27.

10. Lebrun, P., C. L. Sidman, and H. L. Spiegelberg. 1988. IgE formation and Fc Receptor-Positive lymphocytes in normal, immunol-deficient, and auto-immune mice infected with nippostrongylus brasiliensis. J. of Immunol. 141: 249.

11. Delespesse, G., M. Sarfati, M. Rubio-Trujillo, and T. Wolowiec. 1986. IgE receptors on human lymphocytes. II. Detection of cells bearing IgE receptors in unstimulated mononuclear cells by means of a monoclonal antibody. Eur. J. Immunol. 16:1043.

12. Nutman, T. B., G. Delespesse, M. Sarfati, and D. J. Volkman. 1987. IgE binding factors of T cell origin. I. Cloned and transformed T cells producing IgE-binding factors. J. Immunol. 139: 4049.

13. Huff, T. F., and K. Ishizaka. 1981. Formation of IgE- binding factors by human T cell hybridomas. Proc. Natl. Acad. Sci. 81: 1692.

14. Prinz, J. C., N. Endres, G. Rank, J. Ring, and E. P. Rieber. 1987. Expression of Fcε receptors on activated human T lymphocytes. Eur. J. Immunol. 17: 757.

15. Suemura, M., H. Kikutani, H. Owaki, H. Makamura, R. Sato, E.L. Yamasaki, E. L. Barsumian, R. R. Hardy, and T. Kishimoto. 1986. Monoclonal anti-Fcε receptor antibodies with different specificities and studies on the expression of FcεR on human B and T cells. J. Immunol. 137: 1214.

16. Barker, J. N. W. N., V. A. Alegre, and D. M. MacDonald. 1988. Surface bound immunoglobulin E on antigen-presenting cells in cutaneous tissue of atopic dermatitis. J. Inv. Dermatol. 90: 117.

17. Nakajima, T., M. Sarfati, and G. Delespesse. 1987. Relationship between human IgE-binding factors and lymphocyte receptors for IgE. J. Immunol. 139: 848.

18. Delespesse, G., H. Hofstetter, M. Sarfati, U. Suter, T. Nakajima, H. Frost, M. Letellier, R. Peleman, and E. Kilchherr. 1988. Human FcεRII. Molecular, biological and clinical aspects. Progress in Allergy, in press.

19. Nakajima, T., and G. Delespesse. 1986. IgE receptors on human lymphocytes. I. Identification of the molecules binding to monoclonal anti-Fcε receptor antibodies. Eur. J. Immunol. 16: 809.

20. Letellier, M., T. Nakajima, and G. Delespesse. 1988. IgE receptor on human lymphocytes (FcεRII). IV. Further analysis of its structure and the role of N-linked carbohydrates. J. Immunology 141: 2374.

21. Peterson, L. H., and D. H. Conrad. 1985. Fine specificity, structure and proteolytic susceptibility of the human lymphocyte receptor for IgE. J. Immunol. 135: 2654.

22. Bonnefoy, J. Y., O. Guillot, H. Spits, D. Blanchard, K. Ishizaka, and J. Banchereau. 1988. The low-affinity receptor for IgE (CD23) on B lymphocytes is spatially associated with HLA-DR antigens. J. Exp. Med. 167:57.

23. Ludin, C., H. Hofstetter, M. Sarfati, C. Levy, U. Suter, D. Alaimo, E. Kilchherr, E. Frost, and G. Delespesse. 1987. Cloning and expression of the cDNA coding for a human lymphocyte IgE receptor. EMBO Journal. 6: 109.

24. Kikutani, H., S. Inui, R. Sato, E. L. Barsumian, H. Owaki, K. Yamasaki, T. Kaisho, N. Uchibayasi,

R. R. Hardy, T. Hirano, S. Tsunasawa, F. Sakiyama, M. Suemura, and T. Kishimoto. 1986. Molecular structure of human lymphocyte receptor for immunoglobulin E. Cell. 47: 657.

25. Koichi, I., M. Takami, C. Won Kim, T. Honjo, T. Miyoshi, U. Tagaya, T. Kawabe, and J. Yodoi. 1987. Human lymphocyte Fc receptor for IgE: Sequence homology of its cloned cDNA with animal lectins. Proc. Natl. Acad. Sci. USA 84: 819.

26. Vercelli, D., M. D. Gould, H. Silk, D. Y. Leung, and R. S. Geha. 1987. IgE sites relevant for binding to type 2 Fc epsilon receptors (FcεR) on B cells. J. All. Clin. Immunol. 79: Abst. No. 21.

27. Martens, C., T. F. Huff, P. Jardieu, M. L. Trounstine, R. L. Coffman, K. Ishizaka, and K. V. Moore. 1985. cDNA clones encoding IgE-binding factors from a rat-mouse T cell hybridoma. Proc. Natl. Acad. Sci. USA 82: 2460.

28. Young, M. C., D. Y. Leung, and R. S. Geha. 1984. Production of IgE-potentiating factor in man by T cell lines bearing Fc receptors for IgE. Eur. J. Immunol. 14: 871.

29. Sarfati, M., T. Nakajima, H. Frost, E. Kilchherr, and G. Delespesse. 1987. Purification and partial biochemical characterization of IgE-binding factors secreted by lymphoblastoid B cell line. Immunology. 60: 539.

30. Sarfati, M., and G. Delespesse. 1988. Possible role of FcεRII (CD23) or its soluble fragments in the in vitro synthesis of human IgE. J. Immunology. 141: 2195.

31. Delespesse, G., M. Sarfati, and R. Peleman. 1989. Influence of recombinant interleukin 4, interferon α and interferon γ on the production of human IgE-binding factors. J. Immunology, in press.

32. Defrance, T., J.P. Aubry, F. Rousset, B. Vanbervliet, J. Y. Bonnefoy, N. Arai, Y. Takebe, T. Yokota, F. Lee, K. Arai, J. E. deVries, and J. Banchereau. 1987. Human recombinant interleukin 4 induces Fcε receptors (CD23) on normal B lymphocytes. J. Exp. Med. 165: 1459.

33. Vercelli, D., H. H. Jabara, B. W. Lee, N. Woodland, R. Geha, and D. Y. M. Leung. 1988. Human recombinant interleukin 4 induces FcεRII/CD23 on normal human monocytes. J. Exp. Med. 167: 1406.

34. Pène, J., F. Rousset, F. Brière, I. Chrétien, J. Y. Bonnefoy, H. Spits, T. Yokota, N. Arai, K. Arai, Banchereau, J., and J. E. deVries. IgE production by normal human lymphocytes is induced by IL-4 and suppressed by interferons α, and prostaglandin E 2. Proc. Natl. Acad. Sci. USA, in press.

35. Kawabe, T., M. Takami, M. Hosoda, Y. Maeda, S. Sato, M. Mayumi, H. Mikawa, K.-I. Arai, and J. Yodoi. 1988. Regulation of FcεRII/CD23 gene expression by cytokines and specific ligands. J. of Immunol. 141: 1376.

36. Delespesse, G., M. Sarfati, and M. Rubio-Trujillo. 1987. In vitro production of IgE-binding factors by human mononuclear cells. Immunology. 60: 103.

37. Pancré, V., M. Joseph, A. Capron, J. Wietzerbin, and J. P. Kusnierz. 1988. Recombinant human interferon-γ induces increased IgE receptor expression on human platelets. Eur. J. Immunol. 18: 829.

38. Rankin, J.A. 1986. IgE immune complexes induce leukotriene B4 release from rat alveolar macrophages. Ann. Inst. Pasteur 137C: 364.

39. Gordon, J., A. J. Webb, L. Walker, G. R. Guy, and M. Rowe. 1986. Evidence for an association between CD23 and the receptor for a low molecular weight B cell growth factors. Eur. J. Immunol. 16: 1627.

40. Swendeman, S., and D. A. Thorley-Lawson. 1987. The activation antigen Blast 2, when shed, is an autocrine BCGF for normal and transformed B cells. EMBO J. 6:1637.

41. Pène, J., F. Rousset, F. Brière, I. Chrétien, J. Wideman, J.-Y. Bonnefoy, and J. E. De Vries. 1988. Interleukin 5 enhances interleukin 4-induced IgE production by normal human B cells. The role of soluble CD23 antigen. Eur. J. Immunol. 18:929.

T Cells and T Cell Factors Active in Human IgE Synthesis

*Sergio Romagnani, Enrico Maggi, Gianfranco Del Prete, Antonio Tiri, Donatella Macchia, Paola Parronchi, Priscilla Biswas, Mario Ricci**

The understanding of mechanisms regulating the IgE antibody response is of primary importance to evaluation of the possible alterations responsible for IgE-mediated allergic disorders in humans and to obtaining more successful therapeutical strategies of atopic diseases. Previous studies in rodents suggested that IgE production might be regulated not only by antigen-specific helper and suppressor T cells, but also through isotype-specific factors showing affinity for IgE (IgE binding factors) [1]. More recently, however, a different pathway of IgE regulation essentially based on the reciprocal role of interferon-gamma (IFN-γ) and IL-4 has been described in mice [2].Little is known about the mechanisms involved in the control of human IgE production, since in vivo studies analogous to those performed in rodents are not feasible. In this paper we summarized different models for the study of human IgE synthesis in vitro, as well as our findings in their application to the understanding of mechanisms regulating IgE synthesis in physiological and pathological conditions.

T Cell Clone-Induced IgE Synthesis

The first unambiguous demonstration of in vitro induced IgE synthesis in normal B cells was provided by the use of alloreactive human T cell clones (TCC) [3]. The alloreactive TCC we used was able to induce proliferation of B cells derived from the original donor of the stimulating cells, with the production of considerable amounts of all immunoglobulin classes, including IgE. In addition, this clone induced IgE synthesis even in B cell cultures from other normal or atopic individuals, provided they shared the appropriate alloantigen [3]. Successful induction of IgE synthesis in

vitro by the use of selected autoreactive T cell clones has also been reported [4]. Unfortunately, such in vitro models, although very elegant, can be applied only to a limited number of B cell donors.

To overcome these difficulties, we recently assessed the ability to induce IgE synthesis in vitro of TCC obtained by stimulation of single T cells with phytohemagglutinin (PHA), followed by repeated addition of interleukin 2 (IL-2). To date, the activity of a total number of 643 TCC so obtained from the peripheral blood (PB) or tonsil of 12 nonatopic donors has been evaluated. Following activation with PHA, 117 (18%) TCC were found to provide helper function for IgE, as well as for IgG and IgM, synthesis in B cells from all donors tested [5, 6]. Furthermore, stimulation of clonal T cells with anti-CD3 (OKT3) MoAb developed a helper activity for IgE synthesis comparable to that displayed by the same TCC following activation with PHA [6]. From these data, we concluded that the helper function of these clones on IgE synthesis was mediated by a direct activation of the CD3 molecular complex. Thus, by developing an in vitro system of IgE production which bypasses both antigen-specificity and MHC-antigen restriction, we achieved a model suitable for extensive investigations on IgE regulatory mechanisms in humans.

Soluble Factors Produced by TCC Induce IgE Synthesis in vitro and IL-4 Is the Essential Mediator for this Phenomenon

After we were successful in establishing TCC providing helper function for IgE synthesis, attempts were made to generate clonal soluble

* Allergology and Clinical Immunology Department, University of Florence, Florence, Italy.
  This work was supported by funds of the Italian Ministry of Education (12.02.00944), by Consiglio Nazionale delle Ricerche (87.01508.04), and by A.I.R.C. Donatell Macchia and Antonio Tiri were supported by a fellowship from the Italian Association for Cancer Research (A.I.R.C.).

factor(s) able to induce or enhance IgE production. Upon stimulation with PHA for 24 h, supernatants (SUPs) of TCC, derived from normal individuals and selected for their helper function on IgE (TCC SUPs), were found to induce IgE synthesis in both normal and atopic B cells showing low or undetectable spontaneous IgE production in vitro. In contrast, TCC SUPs derived from PHA-stimulated TCC unable to provide helper function for IgE synthesis consistently failed to elicit or enhance production of IgE [7]. Partial physicochemical characterization izationof the factor(s) in TCC SUPs providing helper function for IgE showed that it apparently had a m.w. between 10 and 50 Kd and did not bind to immobilized IgE. Interestingly, the IgE helper activity of TCC SUPs was strongly inhibited by the addition to B cell cultures of human recombinant IFN-γ [7].

It has recently been shown that IL-4, a pleiothropic lymphokine previously described as B cell stimulatory factor 1 (BSF-1), is a strong stimulant of IgG1 and IgE secretion by mouse B cells treated with lypopolysaccharide (LPS) [2]. In this system IFN-γ induces LPS-stimulated B cells to develop into IgG2a-secreting cells, and is able to inhibit the switching to IgG1 and IgE induced by IL-4. The recent availability of human recombinant IL-4 and the use of an appropriate immunoenzymatic assay to measure it in biological fluids allowed us to test the possibility that such a lymphokine was indeed, at least in part, responsible for the IgE helper activity of our TCC SUPs. To do this, the property to induce IgE synthesis in vitro in human B cells of 109 CD4 TCC was compared with their ability to produce IL-2, IL-4 and IFN-γ in their SUPs following 24 h-stimulation with PHA. A significant positive correlation (r = 0.725) was found between the property of TCC to induce IgE synthesis and their ability to release IL-4. In contrast, there was an inverse relationship (r = –0.348) between the IgE helper activity of TCC and their ability to release IFN-γ. In contrast, no statistical correlation between the property to induce IgE synthesis and to produce IL-2 was observed [8].

The ability to induce IgE synthesis in B cells of SUPs from 71 of these CD4 TCC was also investigated. Twenty-nine SUPs (all derived from TCC active on IgE synthesis) induced production of substantial amounts of IgE in target B cells. There was a correlation between the amount of IgE synthesized by B cells in response to these SUPs and their IL-4 content. An even higher correlation (r = 0.94) was found between the IgE synthesis induced by these SUPs and the ratio between the amount of IL-4 and IFN-γ present in the same SUPs [8].

Like IL-4-containing SUPs, recombinant IL-4 (rIL-4) was also found to be able to induce IgE production in B cells from both atopic and nonatopic donors [8]. More importantly, the addition to B cell cultures of anti-IL-4 antibody virtually abolished not only the IgE synthesis induced by rIL-4, but also that stimulated by active TCC and their SUPs [8]. In contrast, the IgG synthesis induced by TCC SUPs was not or only slightly inhibited by the presence in culture of anti-IL-4 antibody [8]. Taken together, these data indicate that in humans as in mice, IL-4 and IFN-γ play an important and reciprocal role in the regulation of IgE synthesis.

Other Signals Are Required for the IL-4-Induced IgE Synthesis

The main message coming from our work in the human system is consistent with that derived from the murine model. However, at least two substantial differences seem to exist between humans and mice. The first important difference arose when we asked whether besides B cells other cell types were required in culture for the IL-4-mediated IgE synthesis. Evidence was obtained that rIL-4, which was active on unfractionated tonsillar mononuclear cells, was consistently unable to induce IgE synthesis in highly purified B cells from the same tonsils [8]. On the other hand, readdition of appropriate concentrations of both untreated and mitomycin C-treated autologous T cells enabled tonsillar B cells to synthesize IgE in response to rIL-4 (Figure 1). Taken together, our results suggest that the presence in culture of T cells is necessary for the IL-4-mediated IgE synthesis in human B cells.

At least two possible explanations may be provided for these findings. The first is that T-cell-derived lymphokines other than IL-4 are also involved in the induction of IgE synthesis. To explore this possibility we tested the effect on the IgE synthesis stimulated by TCC SUPs of the addition to B cell cultures of specific antibodies to different interleukins, such as IL-

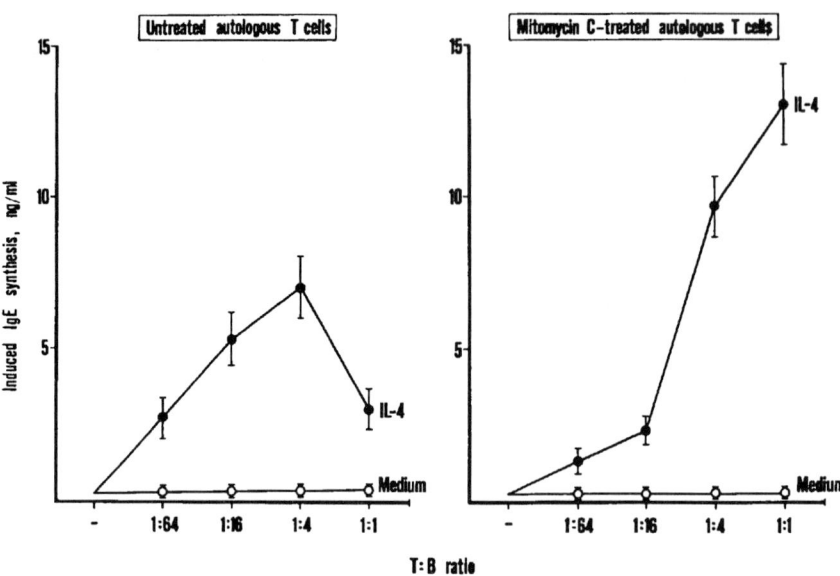

Figure 1. Readdition of untreated or mitomycin C-treated autologous T cells enables purified tonsillar B cells to synthesize IgE in response to recombinant IL-4. Untreated (left panel) or mit.C-treated (right panel) tonsillar T cells were cultured for 10 days with purified autologous B cells (2×10^5) in medium alone or in the presence of IL-4 (2 ng/ml). Supernatant from these cultures assayed for their IgE content. The results represent the mean values of triplicate determinations of duplicated culture supernatants.

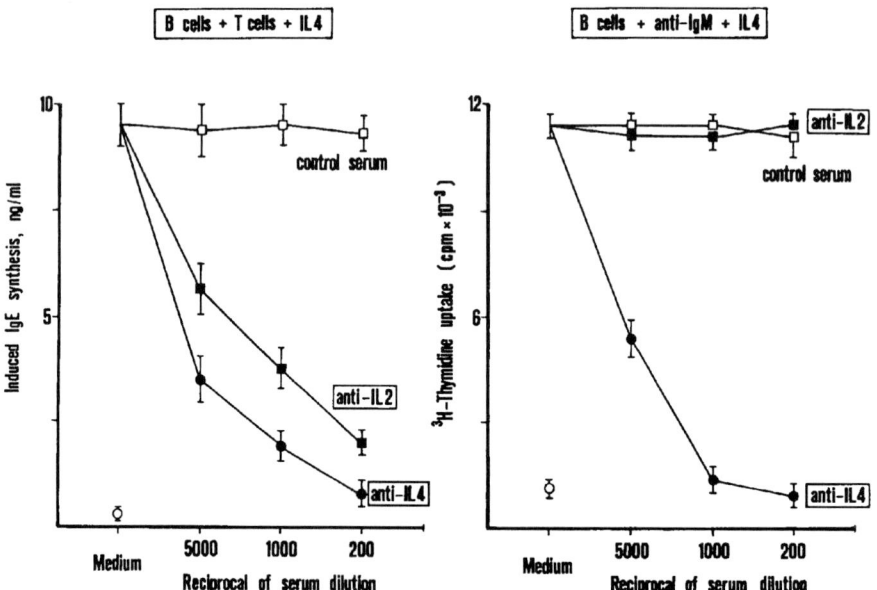

Figure 2. Addition in culture of anti-IL-2 antibody inhibits the IL-4-induced IgE synthesis (left panel), but has no effect on the B cell proliferation induced by IL-4 in the costimulatory assay with anti-IgM (right panel). Culture conditions for IgE synthesis in vitro were the same as described in the legend of Figure 1. The assay for IL-4-induced proliferation was performed with purified tonsillar B cells (10^5 / well) cultured in the presence of suboptimal concentrations of F(ab')2 fragments of rabbit IgG anti-μ chain. After pulsing with 3H-Thymidine, cultures were harvested and the radionuclide uptake measured by scintillation counting.

140

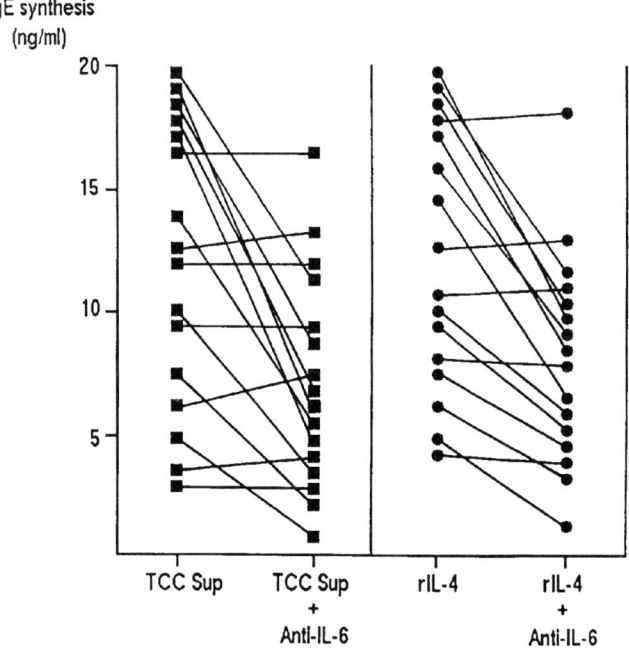

IgE synthesis
(ng/ml)

Figure 3. Inhibitory effect of anti-IL-6 antibodies on the IgE synthesis induced by T cell clone supernatants (TCC Sup) or by recombinant IL-4 (rIL-4). The culture conditions for IgE synthesis were the same as described in Figure 1. Polyclonal rabbit IgG anti-recombinant IL-6 was used at 5 128mg/ml (final dilution).

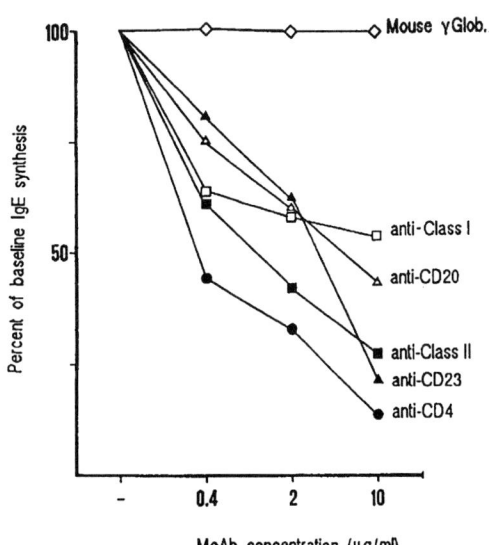

Figure 4. Inhibitory effect of monoclonal antibodies against B and/or T cell surface molecules on the IL-4-induced IgE synthesis. Tonsillar T and B cells were cultured (at a ratio of 1:4) in the presence of IL-4 (2 ng/ml) and MoAbs at three different concentrations. Purified mouse gamma-globulins were used as control.

2 and IL-6. We found that the addition in culture of anti-IL-2 antibody consistently exerted a strong inhibitory effect on the IL-4-induced IgE synthesis, whereas it had no effect on the B cell proliferation induced by IL-4 in the co-stimulatory assay with anti-IgM antibody (Figure 2). Even though less consistently, anti-IL-6 antibody was also inhibitory (Figure 3). These data suggest that IL-2 and possibly IL-6 play a role in the IL-4-mediated IgE synthesis. Interestingly, purified human IL-6 was able to potentiate the spontaneous IgE synthesis by B cells from a number of atopic subjects (data not shown). These latter observations suggest that at least some B cells in advanced stage of differentiation, which have probably already switched to IgE synthesis in vivo, may be directly induced by either IL-6 to secrete detectable amounts of IgE in vitro.

Another possibility, which is now being investigated in our laboratory, is that a T-B cell to cell contact is necessary for the IL-4-induced IgE synthesis. Moabs specific for several surface antigens of T and B cells (Anti-CD4, Anti-CD20, Anti-ClassII, Anti-CD23, etc.) were able to inhibit IgE synthesis induced by IL-4 in a dose related fashion (Figure 4). In addition, when cultures were performed with T and B cells separated by a membrane filter, no pro-

141

Table 1. T-B cell contact is required for IgE synthesis in vitro.

Culture conditions*		IgE synthesis in vitro (ng/ml)**		
Upper chamber	Lower chamber	Exp. 1	Exp. 2	Exp. 3
B cells	T cells	0.3	0.7	0.4
B + T cells	Medium	0.4	0.7	0.5
B cells + IL4	T cells + IL4	0.2	0.6	0.5
B + T cells + IL 4	Medium + IL4	6.5	10.5	3.4

*T and B cells were cultured in distinct chambers separated by a millipore filter (0.45 μ).
**B cells (10^6/ml) were cultured for 10 days in the presence of T cells (3×10^5/ml) and of recombinant IL4 (4 ng/ml).

Table 2. Effect on the IgE synthesis of the sequential addition of T cells and IL-4 to autologous B cells.

Time of addition		IgE synthesis in vitro (ng/ml)*		
Day 0	Day 4	Exp. 1	Exp. 2	Exp. 3
Medium	Medium	0.6	0.3	0.4
T cells	Medium	0.5	0.3	0.3
IL-4	Medium	0.8	0.4	0.5
T cells + IL-4	Medium	3.7	4.3	1.8
IL-4	T cells	0.7	0.5	0.4
T cells	IL-4	11.0	8.9	6.0

*Culture conditions were the same as described in Table 1.

duction IgE antibody was seen (Table 1), either IL-4 was added in the chamber containing T cells or B cells. This data suggests that T-B cell contact plays a crucial role in the induction of IgE synthesis in vitro. Lastly, sequential addition of T cells and IL-4 in culture had shown that T cells are needed in the first hours of the culture, whereas the maximum activity on IgE synthesis was obtained when IL-4 was added on day four (Table 2), confirming that this molecule is active after T-B cell contact. Obviously such two possibilities (T-B cells contact and additional signals mediated by lymphokines such as IL-2 and IL-6) are not mutually exclusive.

The second main difference between the mouse and the human IgE system is that we could not find in humans a so well defined dichotomy between type 1 (Th1) and type 2 (Th2) helper T cells as reported in mice [2]. Mouse Th1 cells are able to produce IL-2, IFN-γ lymphotoxin (LT), but not IL-4, whereas Th2 synthesize IL-4 and IL-5 but not IL-2, IFN-γ and LT. Only Th2 cells were found to be able to induce IgE production by LPS-stimulated murine B cells [3]. A detailed analysis of the pattern of lymphokine activity performed by us in a series of more than 500 CD4-positive clones derived from 14 different donors and from 4 different sources, such as Pb, tonsils, lymph nodes, and spleens, clearly indicated that human T lymphocyte populations not only consist of Th1- and TH2-like clones, but also of T helper clones able to produce at the same time IL-4 and IFN-γ, IL-4 and IL-2 or all the three lymphokines [9].

Mechanisms Possibly Involved in the Disregulation Of IgE Synthesis in Pathological Conditions Characterized by Hyperproduction of IgE.

Having provided new and meaningful information on the basic mechanisms that probably regulate the human IgE synthesis, we asked whether alterations of such mechanisms were at least in part responsible for the altered regulation of IgE antibody production in patients with atopic diseases or other disorders characterized by hyperproduction of IgE. To answer this question, we attempted a preliminary ap-

Table 3. Functional profile of CD4+ T cell clones derived from nonatopic subjects and from patients with common atopy or hyper-IgE syndrome.

Diagnosis	No. of CD4+ clones tested	No. of clones showing:		
		Production of IL-4*	Production of IFN-γ*	Helper function for IgE
Nonatopic subjects	336	146 (43%)[a]	185 /55%)[d]	56 (17%)[g]
Patients with				
Common atopy	357	216 (61%)[b]	145 (41)[e]	104 (29%)[h]
Hyper-IgE syndrome	142	67 (47%)[c]	17 (12%)[f]	79 (55%)[i]

*IL-4 was evaluated in the supernatant of PHA-induced T cell clones by an ELISA. IFN-γ production was evaluated by a calibrated RIA.
chi^2 analysis: b vs. a = $p < 0.0005$; e vs. d = $p < 0.0005$; h vs. g = $p < 0.0005$; f vs. d = $p < 0.0005$; i vs. g = $p < 0.0005$.

proach based on the analysis of the functional activity of a high number of T cell clones derived from normal donors, patients with common atopy or patients with the hyper-IgE syndrome.

When we looked at patients with common atopy or with the hyper-IgE syndrome, we found that they possessed in their peripheral blood a significantly higher number of T cells able to provide helper function for IgE synthesis in comparison with nonatopic donors. There was also a significant decrease in the proportion of IFN-γ producing clones in patients with common atopy in comparison with that of nonatopic donors (Table 3). In addition, interestingly, we found that four children with the hyper-IgE syndrome had in their peripheral blood a very low number of T cells able to produce IFN-γ (Table 3). When we looked at the ability of T cell clones of patients with common atopy to produce IL-4, we found that they possessed in their blood a significantly higher proportion of both CD4-positive and CD8-positive T cells potentially inducible to IL-4 production [10], whereas there was no significant difference in the proportion of IL-4-producing clones between nonatopic donors and patients with hyper-IgE syndrome. These data provide a reasonable explanation of why patients with common atopy possess in their blood a significantly higher proportion of T cells able to provide helper function for IgE than nonatopics, as well as of why this type of helper T cells is even more common in the peripheral blood of patients with the hyper-IgE syndrome. Taken together, these data suggest that an enhanced aptitude to produce IL-4 may represent one of the defects allowing the ele-

vated and prolonged IgE production seen in patients with common atopy, whereas the normal capacity to produce IL-4 combined with a severe deficiency in T cells able to produce IFN-γ, which negatively regulates the production of IgE, might be the prominent feature of patients with the hyper-IgE syndrome.

Summary and Conclusions

The studies on human IgE synthesis summarized here provide further insight into the cellular and molecular mechanisms involved in the IgE regulation as well as in the alterations responsible for IgE disregulation in some pathological conditions. They have clearly demonstrated that IL-4 is the essential factor for the induction of human IgE synthesis, since no substantial IgE production in vitro could be obtained in the absence of this lymphokine. Another T-cell-derived lymphokine, IFN-γ, negatively regulates the IgE synthesis induced by IL-4. These two lymphokines can be produced by different T helper cells, as shown in mice, but they can also be the product of the same T cell clones. In such a case, the possibility that a given clone provides helper function for IgE seems to be dependent on the balance between the amounts of the two lymphokines produced. Additional cellular and/or molecular signals, such as T-B cell to cell contact and activity of IL-2 and IL-6, seem to be involved in the IL-4-induced IgE synthesis, but their precise role in this process still needs to be determined. Finally, alterations of one or more of these regulatory mechanisms begin to be detected in patients with pathological conditions characterized by hyperproduction of IgE. In particular, the increased prevalence of T cell clones able to produce IL-4 appears to be a distinctive feature of patients with common atopy, whereas a reduction in the proportion of IFN-γ-producing T cells seems to be peculiar of patients with hyper-IgE syndrome.

References

1. Ishizaka, K., J. Yodoi, M. Suemura, and M. Hirashima. 1983. Isotype-specific regulation of the IgE response by IgE-binding factors. Immunol. Today 4: 192.
2. Coffman, R. L., B. W. Seymour, D. A. Lebman, D. D. Hiraki, J. A. Christiansen, B. Shader, H. M. Cherwinski, H. F. J. Savelkoul, F. D. Filkelman, M. W. Bond, and T. R. Mosmann. 1988. The role of helper T cell products in mouse B cell differentiation and isotype regulation. Immunl. Rev. 102: 5.
3. Ricci, M., G. F. Del Prete, E. Maggi, A. Lanzavecchia, P. G. Sala, and S. Romagnani. 1985. In vitro synthesis of human IgE: reappraisal of a 5-year study. Int. Archs. Allergy Appl. Immun. 77: 32.
4. Umetsu, D. T., D. Y. M. Leung, R. Siraganian, H. H. Jabara, and R. S. Geha. 1985. Different requirements of B cells from normal and allergic subjects for the induction of IgE synthesis by an alloreactive T cell clone. J. Exp. Med. 162: 202.
5. Del Prete, G. F., E. Maggi, D. Macchia, A. Tiri, P. Parronchi, M. Ricci, and S. Romagnani. 1986. Human T cell clones can induce in vitro IgE synthesis in normal B cells regardless of alloantigen recognition or specificity for peculiar antigens. Eur. J. Immunol. 16: 1509.
6. Romagnani, S., G. F. Del Prete, E. Maggi, and M. Ricci. 1987. Activation through CD3 molecule leads a number of human T cell clones to induce IgE synthesis in vitro by B cells from allergic and nonallergic individuals. J. Immunol. 138: 1744.
7. Maggi, E., G. F. Del Prete, A. Tiri, D. Macchia, P. Parronchi, M. Ricci, and S. Romagnani. 1988. T cell clones providing helper function for IgE synthesis release soluble factor(s) that induce IgE production in human B cells: possible role for interleukin 4 (IL-4). Clin. Exp. Immunol. 73: 57.
8. Del Prete, G. F., E. Maggi, P. Parronchi, I. Chretien, A. Tiri, D. Macchia, M. Ricci, J. Banchereau, J. De Vries, and S. Romagnani. 1988. IL-4 is an essential factor for the IgE synthesis induced in vitro by human T cell clones and their supernatants. J. Immunol. 140: 4193.
9. Maggi, E., G. F. Del Prete, D. Macchia, P. Parronchi, A. Tiri, I. Chretien, M. Ricci, and S. Romagnani. 1988. Profiles of lymphokine activities and helper function for IgE in human T cell clones. Eur. J. Immunol. 18: 1045.
10. Romagnani, S., G. F. Del Prete, E. Maggi, P. Parronchi, A. Tiri, D. Macchia, M. G. Giudizi, F. Almerigogna, and M. Ricci. 1988. Role of interleukins in induction and regulation of human IgE synthesis. Clin. Immunol. Immunopath., in press.

Regulation of Human IgE Synthesis

*Donata Vercelli, Haifa H. Jabara, Raif S. Geha**

The requirements for the induction of IgE synthesis by human B cells differ from those for the induction of other Ig isotypes. Powerful polyclonal B cell activators—such as pokeweed mitogen (PWM), Epstein-Barr virus (EBV), and Staphylococcus aureus Cowan I (SAC)—have consistently failed to induce IgE production by B cells from both normal and allergic donors, even after removal of CD8+ cells. This suggested two possibilities:

1) IgE precursor cells are absent from the circulation of normal donors, or

2) the activation of IgE producing B cells requires signals not generated by normal T cells under experimental conditions known to stimulate the differentiation of IgG-producing B cells.

Experiments from several laboratories, including our own, over the last 3 years clearly demonstrated that B cells from both normal and allergic donors could be induced to synthesize Ig of all isotypes, including IgE, under conditions of cognate stimulation by selected alloreactive [1, 2] or autoreactive T cell clones [3]. In addition, IgE synthesis has been induced in bystander B cells by PHA- or anti-CD3-activated clones derived from blood or tonsil T cells cultured by limiting dilution [4]. These results conclusively show that circulating B cells from normal donors can be induced to differentiate into IgE-producing cells.

More recently, it has become clear that the T-cell-derived lymphokine interleukin-4 (IL-4) plays a key role in the regulation of IgE synthesis. IL-4 is a multifunctional lymphokine, the receptors of which are present on many different cell types [5–7]. In mice, IL-4 induces IgE and IgG1 production in vitro by lipopolysaccharide-stimulated blasts [8, 9], and the in vivo administration of an anti-IL-4 antibody inhibits the IgE response [10, 11].

In humans, we and others have recently reported that IL-4 induces IgE synthesis by normal peripheral blood mononuclear cells

Table 1. Induction of IgE synthesis by clone A1 supernatants and rIL-4.

Stimulus	Net IgE synthesis (pg/ml)		
	Exp. 1	Exp. 2	Exp. 3
Medium	200	<150	200
A1 Sup	1100	1400	1100
A1 Sup + anti-IL-4 Ab	<150	600	ND
rIL-4	4400	2200	2800

PBMC (1.5×10^6 cells/ml) were incubated with complete medium, clone A1 supernatants (25%) or human rIL-4 (100 U/ml). A rabbit anti-IL-4 antibody was added at a 1:500 dilution. Control cultures were set up in the presence of cycloheximide (100 µg/ml). After 10 days, the culture supernatants were collected and assayed by RIA for their IgE content.

(PBMC), both when present in T cell clone supernatants and in a recombinant form [12–16].

In particular, we have studied the IgE-inducing ability of the supernatants of a human alloreactive T cell clone, A1, which secretes IL-4 and IL-5, but not IL-2 or interferon-γ (IFN-γ). This clone may thus represent the human equivalent of a murine Th2 clone [17]. Supernatants of clone A1 readily induced IgE synthesis by human PBMC (Table 1). This was blocked by an anti-IL-4 antibody. rIL-4 also induced IgE synthesis by normal PBMC [13]. Thus, the presence of IL-4 in clone A1 supernatants was necessary and sufficient for IgE induction. By contrast, A1 supernatants—but not rIL-4—vigorously induced IgG synthesis by normal PBMC. This indicates that B cell growth and/or differentiation factors other than IL-4 are involved in IgG induction by clone A1 supernatants.

Moreover, supernatants from clone A1 induced eosinophil differentiation from progenitors in normal human cord blood, supporting the complete maturation of the eosinophil lineage, as determined by electron microscopy.

* Division of Immunology, The Children's Hospital, and the Department of Pediatrics, Harvard Medical School, Boston, MA, USA.

The lymphokine in A1 supernatant responsible for this effect is likely to be IL-5, because rIL-5, but not the other lymphokines known to be secreted by clone A1 (i.e., IL-4, GM-CSF), induced substantial differentiation of eosinophilic myelocytes by 2 and 3 weeks of culture.

The coordinate synthesis and secretion by a single alloreactive T cell clone of IL-4 and IL-5 has important implications. IL-4 induces not only IgE synthesis, but also the expression of low-affinity Fcε receptors (FcεR2/CD23) on B cells [18] and monocytes [19]. The interaction between IgE and FcεR2/CD23 induces the release of monocyte mediators, and has been postulated to modulate signal transduction by B cell growth factors [20]. IL-5 induces eosinophil maturation [21, 22]. Upon activation, eosinophils express FcεR2. Cross-linking of FcεR2 by antigen-bound IgE results in the release from eosinophils of biologically active mediators [23, 24]. Thus, the synthesis of both IL-4 and IL-5 by a single T cell clone may be important in the activation of multiple components of the immune response. Moreover, it is consistent with the clinical observation that increased production of IgE is often associated with blood eosinophilia in a number of diseases, including allergic and parasitic disease, acute graft-versus-host disease and some immunodeficiency diseases.

Clone A1 supernatants also induced FcεR2/CD23 on normal human monocytes, as detected by both immunofluorescence and immunoprecipitation [25]. CD23 induction by A1 supernatants was IL-4 dependent, since it was blocked by preabsorption with anti-IL-4 antibody coupled to Protein A-Sepharose 4B. These results are consistent with our previous observation that human rIL-4 is the only lymphokine that induces CD23 expression on normal human monocytes. None of the other interleukins tested (IL-1, IL-2, IL-3, IL-5, IL-6, GM-CSF, IFN-γ) was able to increase CD23 expression [19]. These results may provide the basis for the clinical observation that increased numbers of circulating CD23+ monocytes are frequently observed in atopic patients [26].

We have subsequently studied the mechanisms and requirements for the IL-4-dependent induction of human IgE synthesis [27]. Purified B cell populations stimulated with rIL-4 could not be induced to produce IgE. The addition of T cells fully restored IL-4 responsiveness. Thus, IL-4-induced IgE synthesis is T cell dependent.

Furthermore, monocytes are required for an optimal IgE induction by IL-4, since depletion of monocytes from PBMC resulted in a strong decrease in IL-4-dependent IgE production.

These results indicated that rIL-4 cannot induce IgE synthesis by acting exclusively on the B cells, although resting B cells are known to bear receptors for IL-4 [5, 7]. Additional signals, derived from both T cells and monocytes, are required for IL-4-induced IgE synthesis to proceed. In an attempt to characterize these signals, we assessed the role played in IL-4-dependent IgE induction by several T cell- and monocyte-derived lymphokines (i.e., IL-5, IL-6, IL-2, IL-1, and TNFα) known to regulate B cell maturation. Our results showed that IL-5 and IL-6 upregulate the IgE response induced by IL-4 in PBMC. IgE upregulation by rIL-5 (5%) was more evident when suboptimal concentrations of rIL-4 (25 U/ml) were used, while rIL-6 (100 U/ml) could upregulate IgE synthesis even in the presence of high concentrations of rIL-4 (100 U/ml). The effects of the combination of rIL-4, rIL-5, and rIL-6 were additive in some experiments and clearly synergistic in others. By contrast, IL-2, IL-1, and TNFα had no amplifying effect.

Most interestingly, we found that endogenous IL-6 is crucially involved in IL-4-dependent IgE induction, since an anti-IL-6 antibody completely inhibited the production of IgE induced by IL-4 (Table 2). Thus, our data indicate that a cytokine cascade may play an important role in the regulation of human IgE synthesis. Isotype specificity may be provided by IL-4, which seems to act as an early IgE-specific switching signal [28], possibly by in-

Table 2. A polyclonal anti-IL-6 antibody inhibits rIL-4-dependent IgE synthesis by PBMC.

| Stimulus | Net IgE synthesis (pg/ml) | |
	Exp. 1	Exp. 2
Nil	<150	150
rIL-4	11200	2200
rIL-4 + anti-IL-6 Ab	300	700
rIL-4 + control rabbit serum	10900	2000

Unfractionated PBMC (1.5×10^6 cells/ml) were cultured with rIL-4 (100 U/ml), in the presence or absence of a rabbit polyclonal anti-IL-6 antibody or a control rabbit serum (100 µg/ml). After 9 days the culture supernatants were harvested and assessed by RIA for their IgE content.

creasing the accessibility of the ε switch region to a common recombinase [29]. In addition, IL-4 may contribute to the activation of B cells, which is known to be required for the induction of IL-6 responsiveness and the expression of IL-6 receptors [30]. It is not yet known whether IL-4 is also directly responsible for IL-6 secretion. IL-6 may provide a late signal for IgE synthesis. It has recently been shown that an anti-IL-6 antibody inhibits PWM-induced IgE synthesis [31]. IL-6 may therefore represent a non-isotype-specific, late-acting amplification signal for Ig synthesis by B cells. IL-5 has been recently implicated in IgE production [32] and in IgA synthesis as a late-acting signal for post-switch IgA B cells [33]. The role of endogenous IL-5 in human IgE synthesis will have to be further defined.

This hypothesis is consistent with a recent model [34] according to which the maturation of human B cell is sequentially regulated by T cell- and monocyte-derived cytokines: IL-4 activates resting B cells, IL-5 promotes the growth and the differentiation of activated B cells, and IL-6 amplifies and enhances the terminal differentiation into high-rate Ig secreting cells, with no effect on cell proliferation.

However, none of the cytokines tested, alone or in combination, induced purified normal B cells to synthesize IgE. Furthermore, IL-4 responsiveness of monocyte-depleted PBMC could not be restored by a combination of IL-6 and IL-1. It is unlikely that other IL-4 induced cytokine(s) so far unidentified are needed, since supernatants from T or T+B cell populations stimulated with IL-4 could not induce IgE synthesis by purified B cells [35]. Thus, the requirement for the presence of T cells and monocytes could not be bypassed by soluble signals. This strongly suggests that cytokine-mediated signals, although essential, are not sufficient for the IL-4-dependent induction of IgE synthesis. Experiments currently in progress in our laboratory indicate that cell-cell interactions are also required for the IL-4-dependent induction of IgE synthesis [35].

References

1. Lanzavecchia, A., and B. Parodi. 1984. In vitro stimulation of IgE production at a single precursor level by human alloreactive T-helper clones. Clin. Exp. Immunol. 55: 197.

2. Umetsu, D. T., D. Y. M. Leung, R. Siraganian, H. H. Jabara, and R. S. Geha. 1985. Differential requirements of B cells from normal and allergic subjects for the induction of IgE synthesis by an alloreactive T cell clone. J. Exp. Med. 162: 202.

3. Leung, D. Y. M., M. C. Young, and R. S. Geha. 1986. Induction of IgG and IgE synthesis in normal B cells by autoreactive T cell clones. J. Immunol. 136: 2851.

4. Romagnani, S., G. F. D. Prete, E. Maggi, and M. Ricci. 1987. Activation through CD3 molecule leads a number of human T cell clones to induce IgE synthesis in vitro by B cells from allergic and nonallergic individuals. J. Immunol. 138: 1744.

5. Ohara, J., and W. E. Paul. 1987. Receptors for B-cell stimulatory factor-1 expressed on cells of haematopoietic lineage. Nature 325: 537.

6. Nakajima, K., T. Hirano, K. Koyama, and T. Kishimoto. 1987. Detection of receptors for murine B cell stimulatory factor 1 (BSF-1): presence of functional receptors on CBA/N splenic B cells. J. Immunol. 139: 774.

7. Park., L. S., D. Friend, H. M. Sassenfeld, and D. L. Urdal. 1987. Characterization of the human B cell stimulatory factor 1 receptor. J. Exp. Med. 166: 476.

8. Coffman, R. L., and J. Carty. 1986. A T cell activity that enhances polyclonal IgE production and its inhibition by Interferon-γ. J. Immunol. 136: 949.

9. Coffman, R. L., J. Ohara, M. W. Bond, J. Carty, A. Zlotnik, and W. E. Paul. 1986. B cell stimulatory factor-1 enhances the IgE response of lipolysaccharide-activated B cells. J. Immunol. 136: 4538.

10. Finkelman, F. D., I. M. Katona, J. F. Urban, C. M. Snapper, J. Ohara, and W. E. Paul. 1986. Suppression of in vivo polyclonal IgE responses by monoclonal antibody to the lymphokine B-cell stimulatory factor 1. Proc. Natl. Acad. Sci. USA 83: 9675.

11. Finkelman, F. D., I. M. Katona, J. F. Urban, J. Holmes, J. Ohara, A. S. Tung, J. v. Sample, and W. E. Paul. 1988. IL-4 is required to generate and sustain in vivo IgE responses. J. Immunol. 141: 2335.

12. Jabara, H. H., R. S. Geha, and D. Vercelli. 1988. Induction of IgE synthesis by human recombinant IL-4. FASEB J. 2: 6652.

13. Jabara, H. H., S. J. Ackerman, D. Vercelli, T. Yokota, K. Arai, J. Abrams, A. M. Dvorak, M. C. Lavigne, J. Banchereau, J. deVries, D. Y. M. Leung, and R. S. Geha. 1988. Induction of IL-4 dependent IgE synthesis and IL-5 dependent eosinophil differentiation by supernatants of a human helper T cell clone. J. Clin. Immunol., in press.

14. Del Prete, G. F., E. Maggi, P. Parronchi, I. Chretien, A. Tiri, D. Macchia, M. Ricci, J. Banchereau, J. deVries, and S. Romagnani. 1988.

IL-4 is an essential factor for the IgE synthesis induced in vitro by human T cell clones and their supernatants. J. Immunol. 140: 4193.

15. Pene, J., F. Rousset, F. Briere, I. Chretien, J. Y. Bonnefoy, H. Spits, T. Yokota, N. Arai, K. Arai, J. Banchereau, and J. deVries. 1988. IgE production by normal human lymphocytes is induced by interleukin 4 and suppressed by interferons γ and α and prostaglandin E2. Proc. Natl. Acad. Sci. USA 85: 6880.

16. Sarfati, M., and G. Delespesse. 1988. Possible role of human lymphocyte receptor for IgE (CD23) or its soluble fragments in the in vitro synthesis of human IgE. J. Immunol. 141: 2195.

17. Mosmann, T. R., H. Cherwinski, M. W. Bond, M. Giedlin, and R. L. Coffman. 1986. Two types of murine helper T cell clone. I. Definition according to profiles of lymphokine activities and secreted proteins. J. Immunol. 136: 2348.

18. Defrance, T., J. Aubry, F. Rousset, B. Vanbervliet, J. Bonnefoy, N. Arai, Y. Takebe, T. Yokota, F. Lee, K. Arai, J. deVries, and J. Banchereau. 1987. Human recombinant interleukin 4 induces Fcε Receptors (CD23) on normal B lymphocytes. J. Exp. Med. 165: 1459.

19. Vercelli, D., H. H. Jabara, B. Lee, N. Woodland, R. S. Geha, and D. Y. M. Leung. 1988. Human recombinant interleukin 4 induces FcεR2/CD23 on normal human monocytes. J. Exp. Med. 167: 1406.

20. Wang, F., C. D. Gregory, M. Rowe, A. B. Rickinson, D. Wang, H. Birkenbach, H. Kikutani, T. Kishimoto, and E. Kieff. 1987. Epstein-Barr virus nuclear antigen 2 specifically induces expression of the B cell activation antigen CD23. Proc. Natl. Acad. Sci. USA 84: 3542.

21. Campbell, H. D., W. Q. Tucker, Y. Hort, M. E. Martinson, G. Mayo, E. J. Clutterbuck, C. J. Sanderson, and I. G. Young. 1987. Molecular cloning, nucleotide sequence and expression of the gene encoding human eosinophil differentiation factor (interleukin 5). Proc. Natl. Acad. Sci. USA 84: 6629.

22. Saito, H., K. Hatake, A. Dvorak, K. Leiferman, A. Donnenberg, N. Arai, K. Ishizaka, and T. Ishizaka. 1988. Selective differentiation and proliferation of hematopoietic cells induced by recombinant human interleukins. Proc. Natl. Acad. Sci. USA 85: 2288.

23. Capron, M., A. Capron, J. Dessaint, A. Torpier, S. Johansson, and L. Prin. 1981. Fc receptors for IgE on human and rat eosinophils. J. Immunol. 126: 2087.

24. Khalife, J., M. Capron, J. Cesbron, P. Tai., H. Taelman, L. Prin, and A. Capron. 1986. Role of specific IgE antibodies in peroxidase (EPO) release from human eosinophils. J. Immunol. 137: 1659.

25. Vercelli, D., D. Y. M. Leung, H. H. Jabara, and R. S. Geha. 1988. Interleukin 4 dependent induction of IgE synthesis and CD23 expression by the supernatants of a human helper T cell clone. Int. Arch. Allergy Appl. Immunol., in press.

26. Spiegelberg, H. L. 1984. Structure and function of Fc receptors for IgE on lymphocytes, monocytes and macrophages. Adv. Immunol. 35: 61.

27. Vercelli, D., H. H. Jabara, K. Arai., T. Yokota, and R. S. Geha. Endogenous IL-6 plays an obligatory role in IL-4 induced human IgE synthesis. Submitted for publication.

28. Lebman, D. A., and R. L. Coffman. 1988. Interleukin 4 causes isotype switching to IgE in T cell-stimulated clonal B cell cultures. J. Exp. Med. 168: 853.

29. Lutzker, S., P. Rothman, R. Pollock, R. Coffman, and F. W. Alt. 1988. Mitogen- and IL-4-regulated expression of germ-line Ig g2b transcripts: Evidence for directed heavy chain class switching. Cell 53: 177.

30. Taga, T., Y. Kawanishi, R. R. Hardy, T. Hirano, and T. Kishimoto. 1987. Receptors for B cell stimulatory factor 2. Quantitation, specificity, distribution and regulation of their expression. J. Exp. Med. 166: 967.

31. Muraguchi, A., T. Hirano, B. Tang, T. Matsuda, Y. Horii, K. Nakajima, and T. Kishimoto. 1988. The essential role of B cell stimulatory factor 2 (BSF-2/IL-6) for the terminal differentiation of B cells. J. Exp. Med. 167: 332.

32. Pene, J., F. Rousset, F. Briere, I. Chretien, J. Wideman, J. Y. Bonnefoy, and J. E. deVries. 1988. Interleukin 5 enhances interleukin-4-induced IgE production by normal human B cells. The role of soluble CD23 antigen. Eur. J. Immunol. 18: 929.

33. Harriman, G., D. Y. Kunimoto, J. F. Elliott, V. Paetkau, and W. Strober. 1988. The role of IL-5 in B cell differentiation. J. Immunol. 140: 3033.

34. Kishimoto, T., and T. Hirano. 1988. Molecular regulation of B lymphocyte response. Ann. Rev. Immunol. 6: 485.

35. Vercelli, D., H. H. Jabara, K. Arai, and R. S. Geha. Induction of human IgE synthesis requires interleukin 4 and T/B cell interactions involving the T cell receptor/CD3 complex and MHC class II antigens. Submitted for publication.

The Role of Lymphokines in IgE and IgG Subclass Formation

Hubert G. Nüsslein and Hans L. Spiegelberg*

Peripheral blood mononuclear cells (PBMC) from healthy nonallergic donors were incubated with recombinant human interleukin-4 (rIL-4) and the level of all isotypes secreted into the cell supernatant was determined. Concentration of 10 to 1000 U rIL-4/ml induced significant IgG4 and IgE secretion. In contrast, rIL-4 had no effect on IgG1, IgG2, IgG3, IgM, IgA1, and IgA2 secretion. As shown by Percoll density centrifugation, rIL-4 induced high density B cells to secrete IgG4 and IgE, suggesting that rIL-4 most likely induced the switch from IgM to IgG4 and IgE secretion rather than expand IgG4 and IgE in vivo precommitted cells. Addition of pokeweed mitogen, lipopolysaccharide or *Staphylococcus aureus* Cowan II to the PBMC abolished the rIL-4 induced IgE secretion presumably by inducing secretion of inhibitors of IL-4 such as interferon-γ from non-B cells. The data demonstrate that human IL-4, like murine IL-4, induces B cells to secrete IgE and IgG4, the IgG subclass that is most likely the subclass corresponding to mouse IgG1 since both are increased together with IgE in chronic helminthic infections. The concomitant induction of IgE and IgG4 suggests that the regulation of these two isotypes may be linked.

It has recently been demonstrated that interleukins secreted by T helper cells play an important role in the switch mechanism from IgM to other isotypes. Murine interleukin-4 (IL-4) induces lipopolysaccharide (LPS)-activated B cells to secrete IgG1 and IgE [1, 2]. Similarly, interferon-γ (IFN-γ) induces LPS-activated mouse B cells to secrete IgG2a [3]. In contrast to mice, relatively little is known about the role of human interleukins on the isotype secreted by B cells. The reason for this may be because isolated human B cells incubated with polyclonal B cell activators and IL-4 do not secrete an IgG subclass and IgE, as is the case in the mouse [4, 5]. However, when IL-4 is added to peripheral blood mononuclear cells (PBMC) containing B cells, T cells, and monocytes, human natural or recombinant IL-4 (rIL-4) induces IgE secretion without affecting IgM, IgG, and IgA formation [6–9]. Whether human rIL-4 induces the secretion of an IgG subclass analogous to murine IgG1 has not been investigated. Therefore, we cultured unfractionated PBMC with rIL-4 (kindly provided by Drs. M. Schreier and H. P. Kocher, Sandoz Co., Basel, Switzerland) and measured the secretion of the different human Ig isotypes [10].

The IgE and IgG subclass secretion by PBMC (2×10^6 cells/ml) from five nonallergic healthy normal donors (IgE serum levels < 150 ng/ml) that were incubated with 100 U rIL-4/ml (10 ng/ml) is shown in Figure 1. In the absence of rIL-4, the cells secreted < 0.4 ng IgE/ml. However, the addition of rIL-4 induced the PBMC from all donors tested to secrete IgE in quantities ranging from 10 to 120 ng IgE/ml in different donors and cultures. Without rIL-4, PBMC secreted a mean of 5 ng IgG4/ml, whereas in about 60 ng IgG4/ml. In contrast, rIL-4 had no significant effect on IgG1, IgG2, and IgG3 or IgM, IgA1, and IgA2 secretion (data not shown).

Dose-response analysis showed little or no IgE/IgG4 secretion at 1 U rIL-4/ml, whereas concentrations of 10 to 1000 U rIL-4/ml induced IgE/IgG4 formation similar to the 100 U rIL-4/ml shown in Figure 1. The rIL-4-induced IgE and IgG4 secretion was completely inhibited by addition of the protein-synthesis inhibitor cycloheximide and the RNA and DNA inhibitors actinomycin D and mitomycin C. Kinetic studies showed no IgE/IgG4 secretion on day 5, whereas about 50% of the IgE/IgG4 found in day 15 cell supernatants was secreted by day 7. Fractionation of the PBMC by Percoll density gradient centrifugation showed that rIL-4-stimulated high-density B cells to secrete IgE/IgG4, whereas it had a slight suppressive

---

*   Department of Immunology, Research Institute of Scripps Clinic, La Jolla, California.
    Supported by U.S. Public Health Service grant AI 10734, Biomedical Research Support Program grant RRO-5514, and a grant from Eli Lilly Co. (publication no. 5596-IMM from the Research Institute of Scripps Clinic).

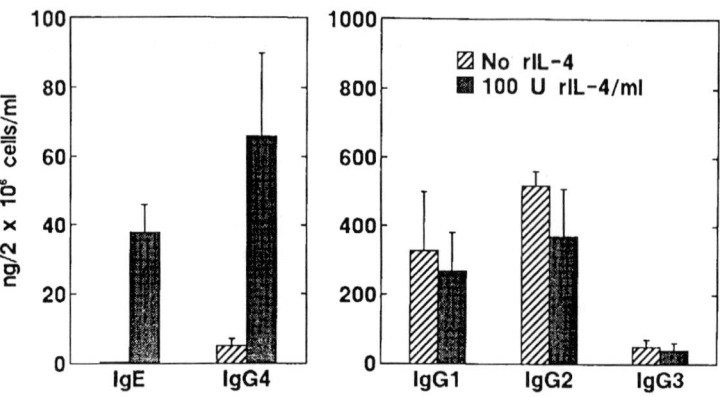

Figure 1. Effect of human rIL-4 on IgE and IgG subclass secretion (day 10) by B cells in peripheral blood mononuclear cells from 5 normal donors (mean ± SEM).

Table 1. Effect of polyclonal B cell activators on rIL-4-induced IgE secretion by PBMC from normal humans.

Activator	rIL-4 (U/ml)	IgE (ng/ml) Exp. 1	Exp. 2
None	–	<1	<1
None	100	27	89
5 µg PWM	100	<0.4	<0.4
10 µg LPS	100	<0.4	<0.4
SAC (1:100,000)	100	<0.4	<0.4

Table 2. Effect of myeloma IgE injections on anaphylactic skin reaction in OVA immunized rats.

Treatment	Positive skin test/total rats tested µg OVA injected		
	0.1	1	10
Controls	12/13	12/13	13/13
2.5 mg IgE, days 3–13	7/7	7/7	7/7
2.5 mg IgE, days 0–13	5/5	5/5	5/5

effect on IgG4 secretion by low-density B cells. To determine whether the rIL-4-induced IgE secretion could be enhanced with polyclonal B cell activators, we added PWM, LPS, and SAC to the PBMC cultures. As can be seen in Table 1, all three activators completely inhibited the IgE secretion. The mechanism of this inhibition is presently not understood. It is conceivable that the activators induced non-B cells to secrete inhibitors of IL-4 such as IFN-γ and PGE2 [8]. The nature of non-B cells that are required for rIL-4 induced IgE/IgG4 secretion has not

been fully explored. In preliminary studies, depletion of monocytes (< 1%) abolished IgE/IgG4 secretion, whereas removal of 98% of the T cells had no significant effect.

The in vitro induction of IgG4 and IgE by rIL-4 strikingly parallels the murine IL-4-induced IgG1 and IgE secretion and suggests that the induction of IgG4/IgG1 formation is linked both in man and mice to that of IgE, presumably by interaction with T helper cells secreting IL-4 [11]. Evidence for such a linkage has also been obtained in vivo. In mice, infections with helminth parasites induce a large increase of both the IgG1 and IgE serum levels [13, 14]. Similarly, it has been reported that humans with chronic filariasis [14] or schistosomiasis [15] show specific and concomitant increases in the IgG4 and IgE serum levels.

The IgG subclass of antibodies to pollen or insect venom allergens is restricted to IgG1 and IgG4 with IgG1 formation being more common to nonallergic humans and preceding IgG4 formation [reviewed in 16]. Patients occasionally stung by a bee and novice beekeepers form IgG1 antibodies to phospholipase A2 (PLA2) of honey bee venom (HBV), whereas patients on HBV immunotherapy and beekeepers have almost exclusively IgG4 anti-PLA2 antibodies [17]. To our knowledge, accurate quantitative kinetic studies of IgE, IgG1, and IgG4 antibody formation are not available, as it is difficult to quantitate the small amount of specific IgE without first removing the IgG antibodies. Therefore, it is unknown whether IgE antibody formation parallels IgG1 or IgG4 antibody formation in normal or atopic humans. However, it was reported that a patient's predominant IgG4 response after immunotherapy resulted in a poor amelioration of clinical symptoms [18], which implies that they probably formed both IgE and IgG4 antibodies to the allergen injections. At present the role of IgG4 anti-allergen antibodies is not fully understood, and it is unknown whether IgG4 antibody production is always accompanied by some IgE antibody formation. Since our in vitro studies suggest that IgG4 and IgE formation may be linked, it will be important to study and compare quantitatively the IgG4 and IgE responses to antigens such as grass pollen allergen in nonallergic and allergic individuals. It is conceivable that atopic patients show a lower ratio of IgG4:IgE antibodies than nonatopic humans, because IL-4 may be more effective in inducing the IgM to IgE switch in allergic than in nonallergic humans.

References

1. Isakson, P. C., E. Pare, E. S. Vitetta, and P. H. Krammer. 1982. T cell derived B cell differentiation factor(s): Effect on the isotype switch of murine B cells. J. Exp. Med. 155: 734.

2. Coffman, R. L., J. Ohara, M. W. Bond, J. Carty, A. Zlotnik, and W. E. Paul. 1986. B cell stimulatory factor-1 enhances the IgE response of lipopolysaccharide-activated B cells. J. Immunol. 136: 4638.

3. Snapper, C. M., and W. E. Paul. 1987. Interferon-γ and B cell stimulatory factor-1 reciprocally regulate Ig isotype production. Science 236: 944.

4. Jelinek, D. F., and P. E. Lipsky. 1988. Inhibitory influence of IL-4 on human B cell responsiveness. J. Immunol. 141: 164.

5. Nüsslein, H. G., and H. L. Spiegelberg. 1988. Secretion of Ig of different classes and subclasses by human B cells stimulated with different polyclonal activators and lymphokines. Fed. Proc. 47: A1250.

6. Jabara, H. H., R. S. Geha, and D. Vercelli. 1988. Induction of IgE synthesis by human recombinant IL-4. FASEB J. 2: 6652.

7. Del Prete, G., E. Maggi, P. Parraonchi, I. Chretien, A. Tiri, D. Macchia, M. Ricci, J. Banchereau, J. De Vries, and S. Romagnani. 1988. IL-4 is an essential factor for the IgE synthesis induced in vitro by human T cell clones and their supernatants. J. Immunol. 140: 4193.

8. Pène, J., F. Rousset, F. Briere, I. Chretien, J.-Y. Bonnefoy, H. Spits, T. Yokota, N. Arai, K.-I. Arai, J. Banchereau, and J. E. De Vries. 1988. IgE production by normal human lymphocytes is induced by interleukin 4 and suppressed by interferons γ and α and prostaglandin E2. Proc. Natl. Acad. Sci. USA 85: 6880.

9. Pène, J., F. Rousset, F. Briere, I. Chretien, J. Widemann, J. Y. Bonnefoy, and J. E. De Vries. 1988. Interleukin-5 enhances interleukin-4 induced IgE production by normal human B cells. The role of soluble CD23 antigen. Eur. J. Immunol. 18: 929.

10. Nüsslein, H. G., and H. L. Spiegelberg. 1989. Human recombinant interleukin-4 induces both IgG4 and IgE secretion. J. Exp. Med., in press.

11. Mosmann, R. R., H. Cherwinski, M. W. Bond, M. A. Giedlin, and R. L. Coffman. 1986. Two types of murine helper T cell clones. I. Definition according to profiles of lymphokine activities and secreted proteins. J. Immunol. 136: 2348.

12. Lebrun, P., and H. L. Spiegelberg. 1987. Concomitant immunoglobulin E and immunoglobulin G1 formation in Nippostrongylus brasiliensis-infected mice. J. Immunol. 139: 1459.

13. Zakroff, S. G. H., L. Beck, E. G. Platzner, and H. L. Spiegelberg. 1989. The polyclonal and antigen specific IgE, IgG1, and IgG2a response of mice infected with four different helminth parasites. Cell. Immunol., in press.

14. Otteson, E. A., F. Skvaril, S. P. Tripathy, R. W. Poindexter, and R. Hussain. 1985. Prominence of IgG4 in the IgG antibody response to human filariasis. J. Immunol. 134: 2707.

15. Iskander, R., P. K. Das, and R. C. Aalberse. 1981. IgG4 antibodies in Egyptian patients with schistosomiasis. Int. Arch. Allergy Appl. Immunol. 66: 200.

16. Djurup, R. 1985. The subclass nature and clinical significance of the IgG antibody response in patients undergoing allergen-specific immunotherapy. Allergy 40: 469.

17. Aalberse, R. C., R. van der Gaag, and J. van der Leeuwen. 1983. Serologic aspects of IgG4 antibodies. I. Prolonged immunization results in an IgG4-restricted response. J. Immunol. 130: 722.

18. Djurup, R., H.-J. Malling, I. Sondergaard, and B. Weeke. 1985. The IgE and IgG subclass antibody response in yellow jacket sting-allergic patients undergoing different regimens of venom immunotherapy. J. Allergy Clin. Immunol. 76: 46.

The Inflammatory Basis of Bronchial Asthma

Stephen T. Holgate, William Roche, Richard C. Beasley*

The relationship between intermittent airways obstruction, bronchial hyperresponsiveness and the symptoms of asthma may be unified by inflammatory processes. Bronchoalveolar lavage (BAL) before and at time intervals after allergen provocation indicates important contributions by mast cells, eosinophils, neutrophils, T-lymphocytes and macrophages. Pharmacological studies support the view that mast-cell mediators account for much of the early allergen response, whereas activated eosinophils are responsible for late-phase airway events. Endobronchial biopsies in patients with mild asthma confirm that existence of ongoing inflammation involving all the cell types found in BAL and in addition show evidence for increased subepithelial collagen synthesis. These findings extend those studies on the pathology of the airways in patients who have died from asthma, also confirming the existence of acute and chronic inflammatory events in mild asthma.

Asthma is defined clinically in terms of reversible airways obstruction. Two other important factors contribute to the symptoms of asthma: bronchial hyperresponsiveness and a specific form of airways inflammation focused on mucosa and submucosa. Provocation testing in patients with all forms of asthma with agents such as histamine and methacholine reveal an increased response when compared to non-asthmatic airways. Hyperresponsiveness, frequently defined as the provocative concentration or dose of agonist reducing FEV_1 by 20% (PC_{20}, PD_{20}) is not a fixed abnormality. Indeed, within a 24-hour period and between days, large variations in PC_{20} may be observed in patients with asthma, and it is considered responsible for much of the symptomatology of nocturnal, exercise, and cold-air-induced asthma and bronchial irritability in general.

Pathologists have long known that patients who have died from asthma exhibit an extensive inflammatory response in the airways. The inflammatory reaction stops abruptly at the respiratory bronchioles and within involved airways is mostly centred on the airway epithelium and submucosa. At post mortem, the characteristic features include mucus plugging, plasma exudation, epithelial disruption, eosinophil and mononuclear cell infiltration, mucosa gland hypertrophy, apparent thickening of the basement membrane and hypertrophy of airways smooth muscle. What is somewhat surprising is that these changes are only just being related to asthma on a day-to-day basis.

Pathological Changes in Mild Asthma

Bronchoalveolar Lavage

The advent of the fibre-optic bronchoscope has brought a new approach to studying asthma. The use of bronchoalveolar lavage (BAL) has focused attention on abnormalities occurring at the surface of the airways in asthma. Several studies have shown that metachromatic cells—now identified as mucosal-type mast cell—are increased in BAL from patients with atopic and non-atopic asthma [1]. Although these cells comprise only a minor proportion of the total nucleated cell content of BAL (0.01–1%), their ultrastructural appearance indicates that they are in an activated state. The presence of increased concentrations of histamine [2] and tryptase [3] (a neutral protease unique to human mast cells) in the cell-free BAL fluid supports the view that mast cell mediator secretion is an ongoing event in clinical asthma. Mast cell numbers and basal secretion have been correlated with the degree of their basal airways observation and non-specific bronchial responsiveness [1].

In addition to mast cells, eosinophil leukocytes are present in BAL from patients with asthma in increased numbers [4, 5]. In some respects this is hardly surprising, since it has long been known that sputum eosinophilia is a

_____

*   Immunopharmacology Group, Level D, Centre Block, Southamptom General Hospital, Southampton SO9 4XY, England.

hallmark of asthma and not infrequently is typified by the additional presence of Charcot-Leyden crystals, composed of lysolecithinase from degenerate eosinophils. Eosinophils recovered by BAL are mostly of the hypodense type when subjected to density flotation through Percoll. Their presence suggests active recruitment of these cells from the systemic circulation which provides a rich vascular network to the airways submucosa. Peripheral blood eosinophilia is another clinical feature of asthma and has been correlated with asthma severity and increased bronchial responsiveness [6]. At one time it was thought that eosinophils served a protective function in allergic tissue responses. While these cells may contribute toward the degradation of mast-cell-derived mediators such as histamine, leukotrienes and heparin, their major function appears to be as proinflammatory aggressors. Eosinophils, when suitably activated, release a wide array of preformed and newly generated mediators of inflammation relevant to asthma pathogenesis. Among these are included major basic protein, cationic protein and eosinophil-derived neutoroxin and peroxidase, which are cytotoxic to epithelial and other formed elements of the airways, platelet-activating factor (PAF), which has a myriad of vaso- and broncho-active functions, and the sulphidopeptide leukotriene (LT) C_4, which in its own right of after conversion to LTD_4 is among the most potent contractile agonists for human airways smooth muscle known.

Bronchoalveolar lavage (BAL) in asthma has also revealed the fragility of the ciliated pseudostratified bronchial epithelium by demonstrating increased numbers of epithelial cells in the lavagate in proportion to the extent of nonspecific hyperresponsiveness [5, 7]. Many of these cells retain their motile cilia indicating their viability. Their presence in BAL probably reflects weak attachment to the basement membrane although whether this defect in adherence is a primary abnormality in asthma or occurs secondarily to inflammatory events is not known. The recent discovery of an epithelial-derived relaxant factor (Ep-DRF) for airways smooth muscle [8] and the presence of large numbers of β_2-adrenoceptors, purinoreceptor and receptors for sulphidopeptide leukotrienes and tachykinins on epithelial cells emphasises their importance as regulators of normal airway function. It follows that any disturbance of this epithelial integrity as occurs in asthma might have profound effects on airway function.

Other features of BAL in asthma that draw attention to inflammatory mechanisms are the presence of activated macrophages [9], increased numbers of T-helper lymphocytes [10] and neutrophil granulocytes [11]. The presence of serum proteins in BAL of asthmatics including albumin, kininogen, transferin, α_1-antitrypsin, fibrinogen, complement proteins indicate increased leakage of the submucosal microvasculature, an abnormality that is prominent in all forms of tissue inflammation.

Endobronchial Biopsies

Direct biopsy of the bronchial mucosa provided further valuable information concerning inflammatory mechanisms in asthma. Biopsies obtained via the rigid bronchoscope led Laitinen and coworkers to the conclusion that disruption of the pseudostratified ciliated columnar epithelium is a characteristic feature of clinical asthma [12]. With increasing experience of fibre-optic bronchoscopy in asthma, a number of laboratories have undertaken studies on endobronchial biopsies. Our own study [7] was conducted on 8 atopic, mildly asthmatic subjects whose asthma was controlled with β_2 agonist along (n = 6) or did not require any therapy (n = 2). When compared to 4 nonasthmatic subjects, subcarinal biopsies showed widespread infiltration of the submucosa with mononuclear cells and eosinophils. Many of the eosinophils had the appearance of hypodense cells, with loss of the granule crystalloid core of major basic protein (Figure 1). In the nonasthmatic subjects, mast cells were observed predominantly beneath the basement membrane and exhibited the characteristic granule scroll structure identifying them as "tryptase-only" (mucosal) mast cells in contrast to tryptase- and chymase-containing mast cells characteristic of connective tissue sites [13]. Almost invariably when mast cells were observed in the asthma biopsies they showed evidence of partial degranulation (Figure 2), confirming the view that mediator release from these cells contributes to disordered airway function.

Another striking feature of bronchial biopsies in asthma was the amount of collagen deposited beneath the basement membrane

154

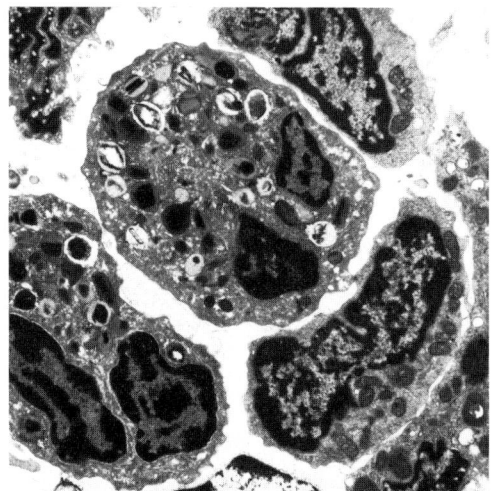

Figure 1. Transmission electron micrograph of leucocytes infiltrating the bronchial submucosa of a patient with mild asthma. Note the heterogeneity of secretory granule structure of the eosinophils and the selective loss of the dense crystalloid containing major basic protein. Magnification ×10,000.

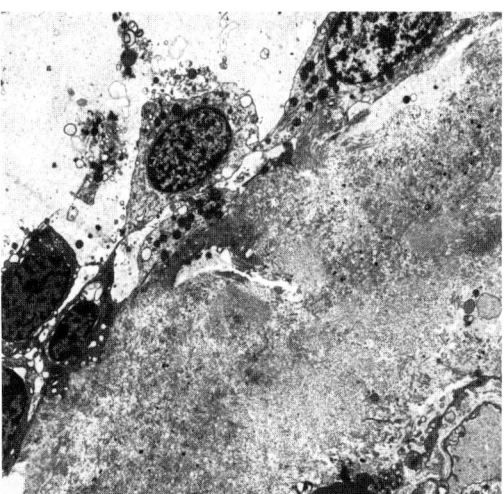

Figure 3. Transmission electron micrograph of the epithelium of an endobronchial biopsy for a patient with mild atopic asthma. Note the normal subepithelial basement membrane beneath which is deposited an extensive amount of type III and type V collagen. Magnification ×5,000.

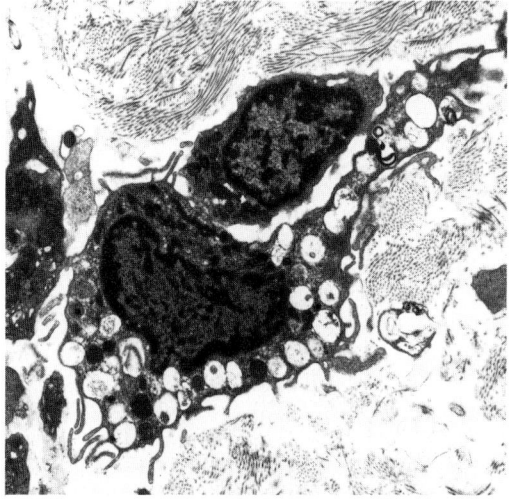

Figure 2. Typical appearance of a mast cell in the bronchial submucosa of a patient with mild asthma showing evidence of partial degranulation and preformed mediator release. Magnification ×10,000.

(Figure 3). Immunohistochemically, this band of collagen, which is frequently and incorrectly referred to as "thickened basement membrane," stains positively for Types 3 and 5 collagens and fibronectin, but not for Type 4 collagen and laminin, indicating its likely origin from submucosal fibroblasts rather than epithelial cells. Increased deposition of collagen was also noted throughout the submucosa, indicating that the inflammatory processes in asthma may not be as reversible and benign as originally thought. The possibility exists that part of the pathology of chronic persistent asthma includes submucosal fibrosis which might contribute to irreversible airways obstruction [14].

The rich blood supply to the bronchial submucosa provides ready access to plasma proteins and circulating leukocytes. Even in the mild asthmatic subjects biopsied, there was ample evidence of leukocyte adherence to postcapillary venule endothelial cells. In this situation eosinophils, neutrophils, monocytes and platelets were observed in close association with endothelial cells, suggesting that all these cell types contribute toward the complex pattern of inflammation in asthma. It is likely that their recruitment and activation for mediator release occurs following the release of chemoattractants from activated cells within the bronchial epithelium.

Attention has recently focused on the potentially important role of the lymphocyte whose numbers in the submucosa are markedly increased in asthma [15]. Immunohistochemical staining of endobronchial biopsies has shown that the majority of these cells are of the helper-T4 type. The capacity of this lymphocyte population to release cytokines that modify the growth and function of inflammatory cells located at the same site is a possibility and provides a cellular basis for the efficacy of immune-modulating drugs such as corticosteroids and methotrexate in asthma. Clearly further studies are required to define in more detail processes involved in the induction of the asthma process and in particular the role of antigen processing and presenting cells which includes dendritic cells, macrophages and T-lymphocytes.

Bronchial Provocation Testing

The majority of asthma in children and young adults occur in association with atopy. Inhalation provocation of sensitised airways causes both early- and late-phase bronchial obstruction. Direct measurement of chemical mediators, BAL and the use of selective pharmacological agents has permitted the dissection of those processes thought to be important in the pathogenesis of these events.

Early Asthmatic Reaction

From both in vitro and in vivo animal studies, and confirmed in certain human tissues such as skin, mast cells have been considered of prime importance in the pathogenesis of the immediate Type I response. Immediate bronchoconstriction provoked by allergen is no exception. Following challenge, histamine or its N-methyl-metabolite have been isolated in increased amounts from BAL fluid, blood and urine. The newly formed oxidative metabolites of arachidonic acid prostaglandin (PG) D_2 and leukotriene (LTC_4) are also released from airway mast cells in pharmacologically relevant concentration and may be recovered as the parent mediators or their metabolites from BAL fluid following challenge [16, 17]. Histamine, PGD_2 and the sulphidopeptide LTs (LTC_4, LTD_4 and LTE_4) are all bronchoconstrictor agents with asthmatic airways being hyperresponsive to them.

Selective histamine H_1-receptor antagonists such as terfenadine and astemizole attenuate the allergen-provoked early reaction by up to 50%, implicating a major role for histamine [18]. Potent cyclooxygenase inhibitors such as flurbiprofen and the thromboxane receptor antagonist GR32191 (which is also active as PGD_2 receptor) attenuate the early response by 30% [18, 19]. Finally, receptor antagonists of LTD_4, which include LY171883 and L-649,923, attenuate bronchoconstriction during the later time points of the early response, suggesting some role for the sulphidopeptide LTs. Other mediators that also contribute to this response include bradykinin, secondary prostaglandins, e.g., $PGF_{2\alpha}$, TxA_2, platelet-activating factor (PAF) and the tachykinin class of sensory neuropeptides (reviewed in [20]).

Mast-cell mediators also play an important role in acute bronchoconstriction provoked by exercise, hypertonic saline and adenosine, and indicate that these cells are primed to respond to a wide variety of secretory stimuli. However, in contrast to the immediate allergen response, and with the possible exception of exercise, these other forms of acute bronchoconstriction are not followed by a second, later phase of airways narrowing and an accompanying increase in non-specific bronchial responsivness.

Late Asthmatic Response

Studies in a variety of animals and indirect observations in human asthma indicate that late phase bronchoconstriction occurs following the recruitment into the airways of effector leukocytes especially eosinophils. In being difficult to reverse with a β_2-receptor agonist, late-phase bronchoconstriction is likely to comprise oedema of the airway wall, exudation of plasma proteins and hypersecretion of mucus into the airway lumen. Bronchoalveolar lavage during the late reaction has revealed an influx of neutrophils and to a greater extent eosinophils which appear to be of the "hypodense" type. The capacity of these leukocytes to secrete a wide array of pharmacologically active mediators places them as prime candidates for effecting the late-phase bronchial obstruction, although final proof of this is still wanting.

Interest in the cellular events of the late-phase reaction increased when it was realised that prior to and throughout its onset, the airways acquire an increased responsiveness to a wide variety of non-specific stimulants. Since hyperresponsiveness is such an important feature of asthma, its association with late-phase bronchial obstruction has focused attention on its inflammatory basis. A number of mediators are thought to contribute toward the functional abnormality, but at the time of writing, platelet-activating factor (PAF) [21] and LTE_4 [22] are prime candidates, both having been shown to increase airways responsiveness to challenge after inhalation. Only with the development of potent and selective inhibitors and antagonists will it be possible to know for certain whether an individual mediator or mediator class contribute as causative factors of hyperresponsiveness. The observation that a component of bronchial hyperresponsiveness can be passively transferred, and that a component of hyperresponsiveness is asthma may be inherited even in subjects without symptomatic asthma indicates the complexity of this measurement.

Current opinion points to an important role for sensory nerves in the pathogenesis of hyperresponsiveness [23]. Damage to the respiratory epithelium as occurs in asthma would render the submucosa vulnerable to exogenous stimuli. The rich sensory nerve supply to the epithelium and submucosa and the known potent pro-inflammatory actions of their neurotransmitters such as substance P, neurokinin-A and calcitonin gene-related peptide provides a mechanism whereby an inflammatory stimulus applied to the surface of the airways could be magnified.

Concluding Remarks

An inflammatory basis for bronchial asthma provides a rational explanation of how drugs such as corticosteroids or sodium cromoglycate modify the disease. Although space does not permit a detailed analysis of the proposed mechanisms of these drugs, inhibitory actions of both drugs have been shown on a large number of the inflammatory cells mentioned in this brief review. An important corollary of this is that if inflammatory events are of such importance in asthma mechanisms, both patients and physicians should consider treatment aimed at modifying inflammation rather than relying on symptomatic bronchodilator remedies. If the data on the long-term damaging consequences of mucosal inflammation in asthma are confirmed, then the use of disease-modifying drugs such as topical corticosteroids and sodium cromoglycate earlier in the course of the disease also becomes important.

References

1. Flint, K. C., K. B. P. Leung, B. N. Hudspith, J. Brostoff, F. L. Pearce, and N. M. I. Johnson. 1985. Bronchoalveolar mast cells in intrinsic asthma: A mechanism for the initiation of antigen specific bronchoconstriction. Br. Med. J. 291: 923–926.
2. Tomioka, M., S. Ida, S. Yariko, T. Ishihara, And T. Takashima. 1984. Mast cells in bronchoalveolar lumen of patients with bronchial asthma. Am. Rev. Respir. Dis. 129: 1000–1005.
3. Dworski, R., G. A. Fitzgerald, C. J. Roberts II, L. B. Schwartz, and J. R. Sheller. 1988. Eicosanoid formation in atopic lung. Effect of indomethacin. Am. Rev. Respir. Dis. 173: 375 (Abstract).
4. Metzger, W. J., H. B. Richerson, K. Warden, M. Monick, and G. W. Hunninghake. 1986. Bronchoalveolar lavage of allergic asthmatic patients following allergen provocation. Chest 89: 477–483.
5. Wardlaw, A. J., S. Dunette, G. Gleich, J. V. Collins, and A. B. Kay. 1988. Eosinophils and mast cells in bronchoalveolar lavage in mild asthma: Relationship to bronchial hyperreactivity. Am. Rev. Respir. Dis. 137: 61–69.
6. Horn, B. R., E. D. Robin, J. Theodore, and A. Van Kessell. 1975. Total eosinophil counts in the management of bronchial asthma. N. Engl. J. Med. 292: 1152–1155.
7. Beasley, R., W. R. Roche, J. A. Roberts, and S. T. Holgate. 1988. Cellular events in the bronchi in mild asthma and after bronchial provocation. Am. Rev. Respir. Dis., in press.
8. Goldie, R. G., L. B. Fernandes, P. J. Rigby, and J. W. Paterson. 1988. Epithelial dysfunction and airway hyperreactivity in asthma. Progr. Clin. Biol. Res. 263: 317–329.
9. Metzger, W. J., D. Zavala, H. B. Richerson, P. Moseley, P. Iwamota, M. Monick, K. Sjoerdsma, and G. W. Hunninghake. 1987. Local allergen challenge and bronchoalveolar lavage of allergic asthmatic lungs. Description of the model and local airway inflammation. Am. Rev. Respir. Dis. 135: 433–440.
10. Gonzalez, C., P. Diaz, F. Galleguillos, P. Ancic, and O. Cromwell. 1987. Allergen-induced recruitment of bronchoalveolar T-helper (OKT4) and T suppressor (OKT8) cells in asthma: Relative increase in OKT8 cells in single early as compared to late-phase responders. Am. Rev. Respir. Dis.

11. Kelly, C., C. Ward, C. S. Stenton, G. Bird, D. J. Hendrick, and E. H. Walters. 1988. Number and activity of inflammatory cells in bronchoalveolar lavage fluid in asthma and their relation to airway responsiveness. Thorax 43: 684–692.

12. Laitinen, L. A., M. Heino, A. Laitinen, T. Kava, and T. Haahtela. 1985. Damage of the airway epithelium and bronchial reactivity in patients with asthma. Am. Rev. Respir. Dis. 131: 599–606.

13. Craig, S. S., N. M. Schechter, and L. B. Schwartz. 1988. Ultrastructural analysis of human T and TC mast cells identified by immunoelectron microscopy. Lab. Invest. 58: 582–591.

14. Connolly, C. K., N. S. Chan, and R. J. Prescott. 1988. The relationship between age and duration of asthma and the presence of persistent obstruction in asthma. Postgrad. Med. J. 64: 422–425.

15. Poulter, L. W., C. Burke, E. Gallagher, and J. Kidney. 1988. Does a cell mediated immune reaction contribute to asthma? Thorax (Abstract).

16. Murray, J. J., A. B. Tonnel, and A. R. Brash. 1986. Release of prostaglandin D_2 into human airways during antigen challenge. N. Engl. J. Med. 315: 800–804.

17. Lum, S., H. Chan, J. C. Le Riche, M. Chan-Yeung, and H. Salari. 1988. Release of leukotrienes in patients with bronchial asthma. J. Allergy Clin. Immunol. 81: 711–717.

18. Curzen, N., P. Rafferty, and S. T. Holgate. 1987. Cyclooxygenase inhibition and H_1-histamine receptor antagonism alone and in combination on allergen-induced bronchoconstriction in man. Thorax 42: 946–952.

19. Beasley, C. R. W., R. L. Featherstone, M. K. Church, P. Rafferty, J. G. Varley, A. Harris, C. Robinson, and S. T. Holgate. The effect of thromboxane receptor antagonist GR32191 on PGD_2- and allergen-induced bronchoconstriction. J. Appl. Physiol., submitted.

20. Holgate, S. T., and J. P. Finnerty. 1988. Recent advances in understanding the pathogenesis of asthma and its clinical implications. Quart. J. Med. 66: 5–19.

21. Cuss, F. M., C. M. Dixon, and P. J. Barnes. 1986. Effect of platelet activating factor on pulmonary function and bronchial responsiveness in man. Lancet ii: 189–192.

22. Arm, J. P., B. W. Sur, and T. H. Lee. 1987. Leukotriene E_4 (LTE_4) enhances airway histamine responsiveness in asthmatic subjects. Thorax 42: 220 (Abstract).

23. Barnes, P. J. 1986. Asthma as an axon reflex. Lancet i: 242–244.

The Mechanisms of Airflow Obstruction in Asthma

*Michael A. Kaliner**

Airflow obstruction in asthma is due to at least four components: airway edema and inflammation, mucus secretion and muscle contraction. It is likely that physicians have placed undue attention on muscle contraction as the cause of asthma to the detriment of patient care. As we enter a new decade, our approach to asthma is also changing. Pharmacologic agents capable of stabilizing mast cells, reversing or preventing airway inflammation, reversing edema, and relaxing smooth muscles will play equal roles in therapy. Such a balanced approach is certain to benefit patient care and may reduce asthma mortality.

Asthma may be defined as reversible airway obstruction clinically manifested as wheezing and caused by verious combinations of smooth muscle spasm, mucosal edema, cellular infiltration, and excessive mucus secretion. The clinical course, as every physician knows, varies [1].

After death from *status asthmaticus*, the lungs remain inflated—in fact, they may spill out of the chest when the thorax is opened. Muscles, like all contractile tissue, relax at the time of death. The lung has considerable elastic recoil and should relax back to its resting state. Thus, airflow obstruction in fatal asthma is not due to muscle spasm alone. In fatal *status asthmaticus*, the airflow obstruction is fixed, due to mucus inspissation and blockage of the airways by thickened airway walls which are edematous and inflamed.

Mucus Secretion

Mucus secretion may be attributed to the actions of histamine, prostaglandins, HETEs, leukotrienes, and prostaglandin-generating factor (PGF-A) [2]. With regard to the relative level of activity of these agonists, histamine is by far the least active molecule at causing mucus se-

cretion, followed by prostaglandins. The HETEs are about 1,000 to 10,000 times more active than histamine on a molecular basis, while leukotrienes are about 10 times more active than HETEs. The airway produces 5- and 15-HETE spontaneously at all times; during inflammation, this production increases dramatically. Because leukotrienes do not appear to be produced spontaneously by the airways, we must assume that the HETEs are much more important in the normal regulation of mucus secretion than are leukotrienes, while the latter may be more important when allergic mechanisms are involved. Platelet-activating factor (PAF) is also capable of causing mucus secretion. PAF may act by causing the formation of lipoxygenase products including leukotrienes.

The autonomic nervous system is capable of inducing mucus secretion in two ways: through parasympathetic stimulation involving muscarinic receptors, which results in both serous and mucus secretion, and through alpha-adrenergic stimulation, which tends to be responsible only for serous secretion. Of the neuropeptides, substance P, which may be released along with acetylcholine in response to sensory stimuli, is a potent stimulus for mucus secretion.

Vascular Permeability

The role of vascular permeability in acute asthma has unfortunately been largely overlooked. We know that vascular permeability is the hallmark of mast cell degranulation in all tissues. Mast cells, which are located near vessel walls, cause the vascular beds to leak, the primary site of action being the endothelial cells of postcapillary venules. Histamine released from tissue mast cells stimulates these cells to contract upon themselves, creating pores to develop between adjacent cells through which proteins extravasate from the plasma. Water

*   Head, Allergic Diseases Section, Laboratory of Clinical Investigation, National Institute of Allergy and Infectious Diseases, National Institutes of Health, Bethesda, MD 20892, USA.

159

then passively follows the protein as a result of oncotic pressure, leading to edema [3].

In the airway, edema forms first in the lamina propria but then begins to spread to areas of least resistance. As it reaches the basal layer of epithelium, the overlying cells are lifted off, forming Creola bodies.

Edema occurs because of the release of histamine, leukotrienes, prostaglandins, PAF, and other mediators. Each of these molecules, in addition to causing edema, can also induce smooth muscle contraction. Substance P, which can be released in response to mast cell mediators, can cause vascular permeability directly—independent of activation of the mast cell [4].

The question remains, therefore: What are the respective roles of vascular permeability and smooth muscle contraction in asthma? Certainly there is considerable evidence to support the contribution of smooth muscle contraction:

1. It occurs rapidly;

2. it is reversible with many of the drugs known to be effective in treating asthma; and

3. it has been demonstrated in vitro.

However, there is no direct evidence for muscle contraction in humans in vivo. Since the layer of bronchial smooth muscle is hundreds of microns beneath the airway surface, it is hard to anticipate direct contact with antigen or mast cell mediators. Bronchoscopy of an obstructed airway after an antigen challenge reveals no muscles crisscrossing the epithelium to account for this effect. Instead, one sees edema, indicating vascular permeability.

Some of the drugs used to treat asthma, such as beta agonists, theophylline, and corticosteroids, prevent vascular permeability as well as possibly affecting smooth muscle. There is no direct evidence that theophylline relaxes smooth muscle at the concentrations achieved in humans in vivo. Corticosteroids have no direct effect on smooth muscle contraction, although they do exert a number of indirect effects, such as promoting the formation of new beta-adrenergic receptors and potentiating beta-adrenergic stimulation. However, corticosteroids are effective in preventing vascular permeability.

Like smooth muscle contraction, vascular permeability occurs rapidly in response to a challenge. Vascular permeability is prevented by all the classic antiasthmatic drugs. More importantly, bronchoscopy reveals vascular permeability as reflected in mucosal edema after an antigen challenge in patients with allergy. Although it would be impossible at this point to determine the relative contributions of vascular permeability versus smooth muscle contraction in asthma, both these effects must be considered important factors in causing airflow obstruction.

Late-Phase Allergic Reactions

After an antigen challenge, the lung responds with an immediate decrease in airflow, spontaneous resolution, and then a second period of airflow obstruction. Mast-cell mediators cause the classic allergic reaction—the immediate hypersensitivity response. This response is characterized by smooth muscle contraction, increased vascular permeability, flushing, hypotension, mucus secretion, and pruritus. In addition, mediators derived from the mast cell granule matrix remain at the site of mast cell degranulation and produce the late-phase reaction, which becomes apparent within 2 to 8 hours and is characterized histologically by infiltration with neutrophils and eosinophils. As this first stage of the delayed reaction matures, a more persistent mononuclear infiltration takes place that in many cases can last 72 hours or more [5] (Figure 1).

The mechanism believed to underlie these late-phase reactions is understood to follow these steps: When a mast cell releases its mediators, the rapidly eluted, but short-lived mediators, such as histamine and leukotrienes, increase vascular permeability and initiate neutrophil chemotaxis, among other responses. The mast cell granule matrix consists of heparin and other proteoglycans (depending on the type of mast cell), proteolytic enzymes, and molecules termed "inflammatory factors of anaphylaxis." These granule-related mediators remain at the site of mast cell degranulation and provide a continuing source of chemoattraction, bringing neutrophils to the site of mast cell degranulation. By some still undefined process, the neutrophil then attracts mononuclear cells, presumably through the release of additional chemotactic factors. Eosinophils are also attracted, especially in patients with eosinophilia, as occurs in atopic individuals.

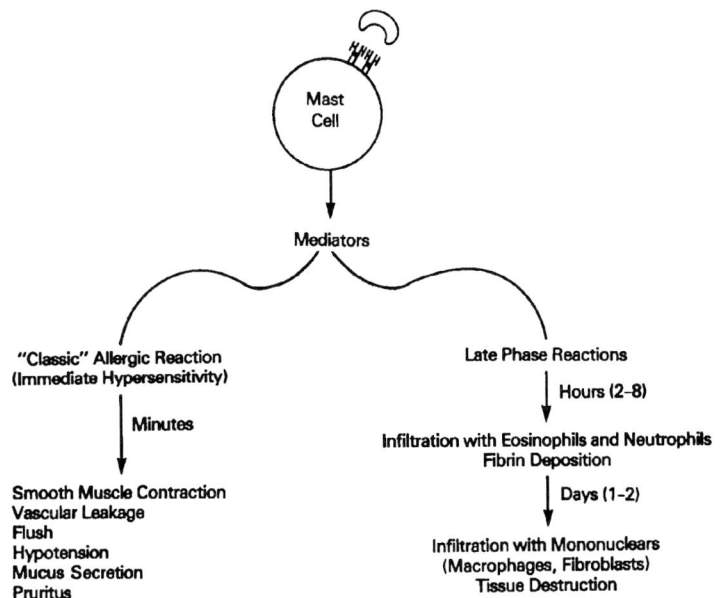

Figure 1. Consequences of mast cell-mediator release can be divided temporally into immediate and late-phase reactions. Late-phase reactions develop over a period of hours and are characterized histologically by an early influx of polymorphonuclear leukocytes and fibrin deposition followed later by infiltration of mononuclear cells. (Reprinted with permission from [5].)

The late-phase reaction is associated with renewed histamine release which may contribute to the recrudescence of airflow obstruction. We have conjectured that neutrophils, which are the first type of cell to arrive at the site of mast cell degranulation, might release a factor termed "histamine-releasing factor from neutrophils" (or HRA- N) that might reactivate mast cell degranulation [6].

Indeed, it has now been found that not only neutrophils, but also eosinophils, monocytes, lymphocytes, platelets, and endothelial cells produce histamine-releasing factors. Thus, the projected model for the late-phase reaction is as follows: Mast cells degranulate, causing the immediate and late-phase reactions, and attracting eosinophils and neutrophils. Each of these cells then generates its own histamine-releasing activity. These histamine-releasing factors induce renewed mast cell degranulation and airflow obstruction due to edema and vascular permeability occurs. As lymphocytes and macrophages infiltrate the area around the mast cell, they too contribute histamine-releasing activity, so that the response persists.

References

1. Kaliner, M. A., P. A. Eggleston, and K. P. Mathews. 1987. Rhinitis and asthma. JAMA 258: 2851.

2. Shelhamer, J. H., B. Borson, C. Patow, Z. Marom, J. Nadel, and M.A. Kaliner. 1987. Respiratory mucus: Chemistry, physiology and pharmacology. In: The airways: Neural control in health and disease. M.A. Kaliner and P.J.Barnes, eds. New York: MarcelDekker, p.575.

3. Persson, C. G. A. 1986. Role of plasma exudation in asthmatic airways. Lancet: 1126.

4. Kowalski, M. L., and M. A. Kaliner. 1988. Neurogenic inflammation, vascular permeability and mast cells. J.Immunol. 140: 3905.

5. Oertel, H., and M. A. Kaliner. 1981. The biologic activity of mast cell granules: Purification of inflammatory factor of anaphylaxis (IF-A) responsible for causing late phase reactions. J. Immunol. 127: 1398.

6. White, M. V., and M. A. Kaliner. 1987. Neutrophils and mast cells. I. Human neutrophil-derived histamine-releasing activity. J. Immunol. 139: 1624.

Cellular Activation and Bronchial Asthma

*P. Godard, M. Damon, J. L. Pujol, P. Chanez, M. Rabier, J. Bousquet, F. B. Michel**

Bronchial asthma is characterized by the patho-physiological triad of airway smooth muscle contraction, inflammation, and hypersecretion, which are thought to contribute to the clinical manifestations of airflow obstruction with dyspnea and cough. These cardinal features of asthma, that is to say reversible airway obstruction, nonspecific bronchial hyperreactivity, and bronchial inflammation, are promoted by the action of chemical mediators on airways. They exert their effects directly by stimulation of receptors on target cells, or indirectly by stimulation of receptors on afferent nerve endings [15]. In the human lung, mast cells, which are known to be activated at the early stage of the lung inflammation process, exist freely in the bronchoalveolar lumen, though always in a low proportion. The activation of these cells is considered as the first cellular event. On the other hand, alveolar macrophages (AM) are the principal resident phagocytes; they play a major role in the local defense against environmental agents and are involved in the development and expression of humoral and cell-mediated immune response.

In a very nice and important piece of work, R. Patterson [14] demonstrated that bronchoalveolar cells obtained by bronchoalveolar lavage (BAL) in sensitized monkeys and injected into the trachea of unsensitized syngenic monkeys were able to promote bronchial asthma after specific inhalation challenge. Since AM accounted for about 90% to 95% of the cells recovered by BAL, a potential role for AM could be suggested. We would like to overview the evidences which outline that AM play an important role in the pathophysiology of human bronchial asthma [10], and by this example emphasize the role of cellular activation.

1. AM are able to synthesize and release chemical mediators which are involved in the pathophysiology of bronchial asthma; they can be activated by IgE, phagocytosed particules (zymosan and opsonized zymosan) or small peptides (such as fMLP which can be released by bacteria) dependent mechanisms relevant to bronchial asthma.

2. AM are activated in vivo in asthmatic patients and the activation correlates with the severity of the disease (bronchial obstruction and nonspecific airway reactivity); this concept of releasability seems to be very important; AM could be primed in vivo by the action of inflammatory mediators which are released by cells or nerve endings.

Alveolar Macrophages Activation

AM can be obtained safely and easily by BAL in asthmatic patients and cultured in vitro under various conditions in the presence or absence of different concentrations of agonists or antagonists. It has been shown that they are able to synthesize and release great quantities of chemical mediators, mainly from membrane phospholipids.

Activation by Various Relevant Stimuli

Activation of AM involves a variety of stimuli (Figure 1). Some years ago, M. Joseph, A.B. Tonnel, and A. Capron et al. [11] were able to show, in vitro and then in vivo, that AM from allergic asthmatics have surface-bound IgE molecules and can be specifically triggered by contact with the sensitizing allergens. J. MacDermot showed that IgE-anti-IgE complexes mediate a selective activation of AM with release of arachidonic acid-derived mediators and lysosomal hydrolases, but not accompanying oxygen burst [13].

AM can be activated also by other stimuli which are relevant for pathological conditions such as bronchial asthma, namely, phagocytosis of Zymosan and opsonized Zymosan, but also fMLP or complement components.

The role of substance P (SP) in the pathogenesis of asthma is unclear. As assessed by TXB_2 release, we studied in vitro the activation of AM after addition of four concentrations of SP (10^{-7}, 10^{-6}, 10^{-5}, 10^{-4} M) in 6 normal subjects

* Clinique des maladies respiratoires, Avenue Major Flandre, 34059 Montpellier cedex, France.

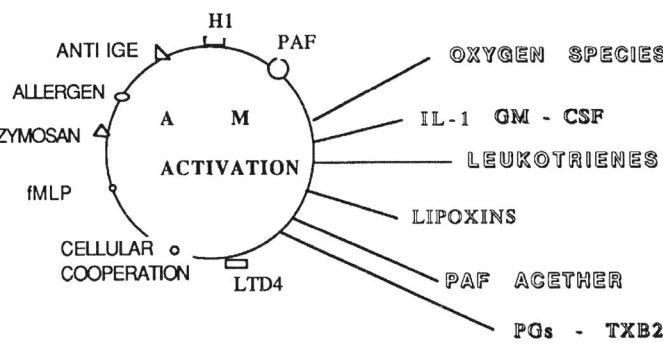

Figure 1. Alveolar macrophages activation and mediator release.

and 7 asthmatics; SP stimulated AM only from 1/7 asthmatics.

Arachidonic Acid Metabolites

Via the cyclooxygenase pathway, AM from healthy subjects and asthmatic patients released mainly TXB_2 as compared to PGE_2 and PF_{2a}. By the lipoxygenase pathway, AM were able to release 5 HETE, LTB_4 and sulfidopeptide leukotrienes, and lipoxins.

In comparison to the peripheral blood monocytes, the human AM from both normal and allergic asthmatic donors were on average capable of generating 3- to 5-fold as much LTB_4 in response to A23187 and developed the capacity to respond preferentially to an opsonized particule, opsonized zymosan, relative to a non opsonized particule, Zymosan, with biosynthesis of LTB_4.

As assessed by HPLC in the supernatants and in the cells after a 90 min culture in the presence of opsonized zymosan, AM were able to generate 5HETE (Table 1). 5HETE remained mainly in the cells in healthy subjects and in asthmatics and was significantly higher in allergic asthmatics than in healthy subjects.

Table 1. 5HETE synthesis and release by opsonized zymosan-stimulated alveolar macrophages ($ng/10^6$ AM).

	Supernatants	Cells	Total
Healthy subjects	13± 7	30±8	43± 14
Allergic asthmatics	6±3	72±15	78±14
p	NS	<0.05	0.03

Platelet Activating Factor

PAF acether is a unique class of lipid which derives from membrane phospholipids. It aggregates platelets and induces the release of their vaso-active amines, induces an important bronchoconstriction, and has pro-inflammatory properties because of the eosinophils it is able to attract into the bronchoalveolar lumen. It is able to induce a nonspecific bronchial hyperreactivity in normal healthy volunteers. It seems that a lot of its action is mediated by other mediators such as leukotrienes and histamine.

Calcium ionophore-stimulated AM released quantities of paf-acether and lyso paf-acether, making these cells and mediator candidates to recrute and activate eosinophils in the lung, specially in asthmatic patients. AM obtained from asthmatic patients release paf-acether, its derivative and precursor nonacetylated lyso paf-acether when stimulated by various allergens [1].

Alveolar Macrophages Releasability

The Concept of Releasability in Asthmology

This concept has been known for a long time and has been demonstrated with peripheral blood cells, such as basophils and neutrophils [6]. In 1981, we observed that mast cells were present in the bronchoalveolar lavage fluid, and that they were able to be activated to release histamine after incubation with specific allergens. Calcium ionophore-stimulated bronchoalveolar cells released histamine and PGD_2;

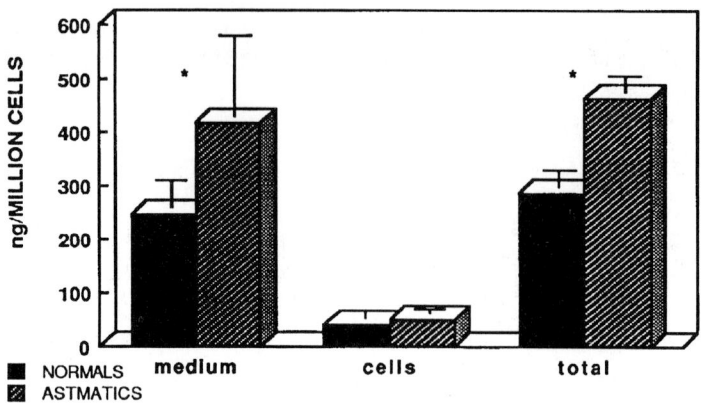

Figure 2. A23187 induced LTB₄ release by AM.

the release of these two mediators was correlated; net maximal histamine release averaged $28 \pm 17\%$ in asthmatics and was significantly higher (p < 0.02) than in healthy subjects ($10 \pm 9\%$) [12]. Flint et al. [7, 8] were able to show that the BAL fluid histamine content was increased and was correlated to bronchial hyperreactivity as assessed by PC$_{20}$ histamine. But it seems that cooperation with other cells, namely AM, is an important step to induce histamine release. AM could prime mast cells.

Tryptase is an enzyme that characterizes T mast cells; it has been shown that tryptase content in BAL fluid was higher in allergic asthmatics as compared to healthy subjects; activation of these cells at baseline was increased by instillation of the specific allergen into the bronchi [17].

AM Releasibility

In a series of experiments with AM we observed

1. that AM from asthmatics released higher quantities of LTB$_4$, 5 HETE, LTD$_4$ and oxygen species than AM from healthy subjects and

2. that the release of oxygen species was correlated to the severity of asthma.

LTB$_4$ was assessed by HPLC in the supernatants and in the cells after a 30-min culture in the presence of 2.5 mM A23187 [9]. The generation of LTB4 was significantly higher in asthmatics than in healthy subjects; calcium ionophore A23187 induced a synthesis and

mainly a release of LTB$_4$; LTB$_4$ averaged $247 + 51$ ng/10^6 AM in healthy subjects in medium (versus $41 + 12$ ng/10^6 AM in the cells) and was significantly higher in asthmatics: $415 + 153$ ng/10^6 AM (p < 0.05).

On the other hand, equivalent quantities of 5HETE were assessed in the cells (64 ± 16 ng/10^6 AM) and in the supernatants (81 ± 30 ng/10^6 AM), in healthy subjects; in asthmatics 5HETE was assessed mainly in the cells (137 ± 28 versus 47 ± 27 ng/10^6 AM in the cells and in the supernatants, respectively) and in significantly higher quantities as compared to normals (p < 0.02).

LTD$_4$ generation was studied [4] in preparations of purified human alveolar macrophages from healthy subjects (n = 5), symptomatic and untreated allergic asthmatics (n = 9) and chronic bronchitis patients (n = 7). AM were incubated for 6 to 24 hours in the presence of labeled arachidonic acid and for an additional 5 hours without labeled AA; the study of the metabolites showed that the most abundant sulfidopeptide leukotriene was LTD4 as ana-

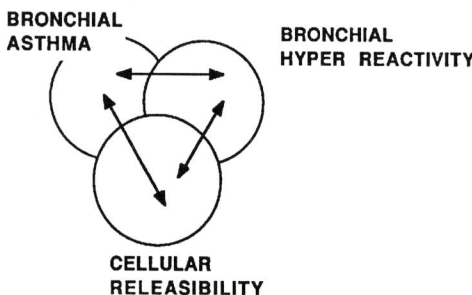

Figure 3. Cellular activation and bronchial asthma.

lyzed by thin layer chromatography and identified by reversed phase HPLC. The release was time dependent and was significantly higher (p < 0.01) in AM from asthmatics (from 180% to 200%) and from patients with chronic bronchitis (from 110% to 150%) than in those from healthy subjects.

The release of superoxide anion (O_2.-) by fMLP-stimulated AM was studied in 8 mild asthmatics and 9 normal subjects. After purification by adherence on plastic dishes during a 2-h culture, AM were stimulated with fMLP (10^{-7} M) in the presence of ferricytochrome C (80 μM) with or without superoxide dismutase (SOD: 30 mg/ml) for 60 min. O_2.- release was assessed 0, 5, 15, 30 and 60 min after the addition of fMLP and averaged 7.3 ± 1.3 nM/10^6 AM in asthmatics versus 1.7 ± 0.4 nM/10^6 AM in healthy subjects (p < 0.05) at the 5th min [3].

M. Cluzel et al. studied the capacity of AM to release oxygen species during zymosan phagocytosis; it was correlated to the severity of asthma: Both in asthmatics and healthy subjects, the maximal value of luminol-enhanced chemiluminescence was obtained after 10–13 min of stimulation by opsonized zymosan. Baseline values and maximal chemiluminescence of AM values were significantly increased (p < 0.03 and p < 0.01) in asthmatic subjects. There was a significant (p < 0.01) correlation between maximal chemiluminescence of AM and the severity of asthma, as assessed by a clinical score defined by Aas (r = 0.87; p < 0.01). The BAL eosinophils percentage was significantly correlated (p < 0.01) for all subjects with the peak of chemiluminescence of AM.

Phospholipids Metabolism in AM

Arachidonic acid (AA) metabolism was studied in preparation of purified AM from healthy subjects and asthmatics. AM were incubated for 6 to 24 hours in the presence of labelled AA. TLC analysis of radioactivity distributed between different lipid classes at 24 hours revealed more labelling in AM phospholipids from asthmatics than those from healthy subjects and was reflected in phosphatidylethanolamine and phosphatidylinositol species [4].

In an other study [5], we compared the phosphatidylinositol turnover and the production of O_2.- in quiescent (healthy subjects) and activated AM (asthmatics) stimulated in vitro by the N-formyl-leucyl-phenylalanine (fMLP). AM from asthmatics showed a Li+-sensitive continuous higher production of IP1, indicating that these cells were activated in a continuous manner. Furthermore, whereas IP1, IP2, and IP3 increased rapidly (within 1 min) up to 125–175% in fMLP stimulated AM from healthy subjects, the stimulation of cells from asthmatics promoted only a low increase in these inositol phosphates. This moderate production could be due to a permanent state of activation leading to depleted pool of phosphoinositides, corroborating the higher capacity of these cells to generate superoxide anion after stimulation by chemoattractant. This activation state could be explained by the action of priming inflammatory mediators that are known to be released into inflammatory sites. The primary action of fMLP was to stimulate the hydrolysis of IP2 to yield diacylglycerol (DAG) and IP3.

We studied the gamma GT activity of AM by analyzing the transformation of LTC4 into LTD4; the enzymatic activity was determined on sonicated cell suspension by a colorimetric method; the LTD4 production was evaluated by reversed phase HPLC after AM incubation with LTC4. The data showed that AM developped an enzymatic activity to transform LTC4 into LTD4 and LTE4. This activity could be correlated with the severity of local bronchial inflammation as assessed by an endoscopic score.

Cooperation of Cells and Mediators

In the bronchoalveolar lumen, AM act in cooperation with other cells, mainly lymphocytes but also mast cells and eosinophils. During pathological conditions, other cells can be recruited, and the cellular sociology is one of the main routes to understanding the inflammatory processes.

AM and Mast Cells

It has been shown that human lung macrophages could elicit mast cell degranulation via the release of one or several histamine releasing factors (Il-1, GM-CSF).

165

In the bronchoalveolar lumen, these cells exist and could act in cooperation; one could prime the other one, in a kind of vicious circle, to increase inflammatory mediator releasability and generation after specific or nonspecific activation.

Histamine could activate alveolar macrophages via H_1 receptor, to increase cGMP concentrations [18].

AM and Lymphocytes

In healthy subjects, the AM/lymphocytes ratio is about 10/1, and it has been extensively proved that AM suppress the ConA and PHA lymphoproliferative response. In allergic asthma, we showed that this suppressive activity was decreased [2].

In another set of experiments we have studied the in vitro secretion of interleukine 1 (Il-1) from AM; 7 nonsmoker healthy volunteers and 12 asthmatic patients were studied. After purification by adherence, AM were cultured for 20 h in the presence or absence of LPS (5 and 10 μg/ml). Supernatants were tested for Il-1 activity (units) by the thymocyte co-mitogenic assay; they were also controlled for the absence of Il-2 activity. AM from nonsmoker volunteers did not spontaneously produce Il-1; on the other hand, in asthmatics AM released high quantities of Il-1: 48 $\mu/10^6$ AM (versus 5 units/10^6 AM in normals; $p < 0.05$). But by western blotting, we were unable to evidence Il-1alpha or Il-1a protein.

AM and Eosinophils

Eosinophils play an important role in the pathophysiology of bronchial asthma. They are recruited by activated cells and mediators into the bronchoalveolar lumen and release their own mediators, which are able to amplify the inflammation [16].

AM recruit and activate eosinophils mainly by PAF, but also by LTB$_4$ and probably IL1; it is not impossible that AM cooperate with eosinophils by the way of an other mediator, namely GM-CSF (T. Lee & Ph. Godard, personal data, not published).

Conclusion

Between the various and numerous clinical stimuli able to induce an asthma attack and the target tissue and organ, that is to say the bronchi and moreover the bronchoalveolar tree, cells such as mast cells and alveolar macrophages are stimulated to release mediators and induce the inflammatory cascade which lead to the airway obstruction. To the concept of bronchial hyper reactivity we would like to propose this one of cellular hyperreactivity which induces a continuous release of inflammatory mediators and, in the absence of adequate regulation, an asthma attack.

Membrane phospholipids abnormalities could explain a number of mechanisms involved in the pathophysiology of bronchial asthma and justify much attention and therapeutic consideration.

References

1. Arnoux, B., M. Joseph, M. H. Simoes et al. 1987. Antigenic release of paf-acether and beta glucuronidase from alveolar macrophages of asthmatics. Bull. Eur. Physiopathol. Respir. 23: 119–124.
2. Aubas, P., B. Cosso, Ph. Godard et al. 1984. Decreased suppressor cell activity of alveolar macrophages in bronchial asthma. Am. Rev. Resp. Dis. 130: 875–878.
3. Cluzel, M., M. Damon, P. Chanez et al. 1987. Enhanced alveolar cell luminol dependent chemiluminescence in asthma. J. Allergy Clin. Immunol. 80: 195–201.
4. Damon, M., C. Chavis, A. Crastes de Paulet et al. 1987. Arachidonic acid metabolism in alveolar macrophages. A comparison of cells from healthy subjects, allergic asthmatics, and chronic bronchitis patients. Prostaglandins 34: 293–308.
5. Damon, M., H. Vial, A. Crastes de Paulet et al. 1988. Phosphoinositide breakdown and superoxide anion release in formyl- peptide-stimulated human alveolar macrophages: Comparison between quiescent and activated cells. FEBS Letter, in press.
6. Findlay, S. R., and L. M. Lichtenstein. 1980. Basophil "releasabilityF in patients with asthma. Am. Rev. REsp. Dis. 122: 53–59.
7. Flint, K. C., K. B. P. Leung, B. N. Hudspith et al. 1985. Broncho alveolar mast cells in extrinsic asthma: A mechanism for the initiation of antigen specific bronchoconstriction. Br. Med. J. 291: 923–926.

8. Flint, K. C., K. B. P. Leung, F. L. Pearce et al. 1985. Human mast cells recovered by bronchoalveolar lavage: Their morphology, histamine release and the effect of sodium cromoglycate. Clin. Science 68: 427–432.

9. Godard, Ph., M. Damon, F. B. Michel et al. 1983. Leukotriene B4 production from human alveolar macrophages. Clin. Res. 31: 548A.

10. Godard, Ph., M. Damon, and Ph. Vago. 1987. Alveolar macrophages. In: Highlights in asthmology. F. B. Michel, Ph. Godard, J. Bousquet, eds. Berlin: Springer, pp. 186194.

11. Joseph, M., A. B. Tonnel, G. Torpier et al. 1983. The involvement of IgE in the secretory processes of alveolar macrophages from asthmatic patients. J. Clin. Invest. 71: 221–230.

12. Lebel, B., J. Bousquet, P. Chanez et al. 1988. Spontaneous and non-specific releasability of histamine and PGD2 by bronchoalveolar lavage cells from asthmatic and normal subjects: Effect of nedocromil sodium. Clin. Allergy, in press.

13. MacDermot, J., and R. W. Fuller. 1988. Macrophages. In: Asthma: Basic mechanisms and clinical management. P. J. Barnes, I. W. Rodger, and N. C. Thomson, eds. London: Academic Press, pp. 97–114.

14. Patterson, R., I. M. Susko, and K. E. Harris. 1978. The in vivo transfer of antigen induced airway reactions by bronchial lumen cells. J. Clin. Invest. 61: 519–524.

15. Pujol, J. L., Ph. Godard, J. Bousquet et al. 1987. Les mécanismes inflammatoires de l'asthme bronchique. Rev. Fr. Mal. Respir. 4: 111–120.

16. Tonnel, A. B., L. Prin, M. Capron et al. 1985. Infiltrats pulmonaires éosinophiles. Etude comparée des éosinophiles sanguins et alvéolaires. In: Traitement de l'asthme. Ph. Godard, J. Bousquet, and F. B. Michel, eds. Paris: Masson, pp. 21–30.

17. Wenzel, S. E., A. A. Fowler, and L. B. Schwartz. 1988. Activation of pulmonary mast cells by bronchoalveolar allergen challenge: In vivo release of histamine and tryptase in atopic subjects with and without asthma. Am. Rev. Resp. Dis. 137: 1002–1008.

18. White, W. V., and M. A. Kaliner. 1988. Histamine. In: Asthma: Basic mechanisms and clinical management. P. J. Barnes, I. W. Rodger, and N. C. Thomson, eds. London: Academic Press, pp. 231–258.

167

Regulation of IgE Responses to Allergen Deposited on the Respiratory Epithelium

Patrick G. Holt, Christine McMenamin, Michael A. Schon-Hegrad, Geoffrey A. Stewart*

Exposure of healthy animals to aerosols containing non-pathogenic environmental antigens leads to the activation of specific suppressor T-cells which confer long-lived protection against subsequent allergic sensitisation to the same antigens. This "inhalation tolerance" process appears to be the respiratory tract equivalent of oral tolerance in the GIT. The efficiency of inhalation tolerance is genetically determined, but is subject to modulation by a variety of host and environmental factors, including hormonal status, age, respiratory virus infections, and inhaled irritants. The precise mechanism of suppressor cell activation, which occurs initially in the regional lymph nodes draining the upper respiratory mucosa, remains to be defined. Recent studies on the nature of respiratory mucosal presenting/transporting cells suggest an important role for epithelial dendritic cells in the process.

It is now generally accepted that overall IgE-responsiveness is genetically determined, and that it is controlled via the activity of specialised populations of T-lymphocytes [1, 2]. However, it is also recognised that the ultimate expression of the IgE-responder phenotype is subject to modulation by a variety of environmental factors, including those that exert their effects either in specific target tissues or at sites of initial allergen challenge.

Consequently, in the case of the respiratory tract, it is logical to propose that cellular processes occurring at the level of the respiratory mucosa play potentially important roles in allergic sensitisation to aeroallergens. The recent identification of highly specialised populations of T-cells [3, 4] and antigen presenting cells [5, 6] associated with mucosal sites, further argues for the need for more detailed analysis of local immunological processes in the respiratory tract, in relation to allergy.

Our laboratory is focussing upon local tissue-related factors involved in down-regulation of IgE responses to environmental allergens in the respiratory tract in the steady-state. For this purpose, we have developed two experimental models, one concentrating upon regulation of antigen presenting cell func-

Table 1. Influence of genetic background on the development of inhalation tolerance to aeroallergens.

| | IgE responder phenotype | |
	High responders	Low responders
Ease of tolerance induction	+	+++
Allergen threshold for tolerance	µg	ng
Transient IgE response seen during tolerance induction	+	–
Tolerance transfer with serum	–	–[a]
Tolerance transfer with T-cells	+	+
Suppressor T-cell phenotype	CD4⁻CD8⁺	n.d.
Overall immune status post tolerance:		
(1) IgE response	persistent	tolerised
(2) Secretory IgA response	+	biphasic (eventual tolerance)
(3) DTH reactivity	not affected	tolerised

[a]may transfer tolerance for DTH

* Clinical Immunology Research Unit, Princess Margaret Hospital, Subiaco 6008, Western Australia. Supported by grants from the W. A. Asthma Foundation and the Princess Margaret Children's Medical Research Foundation.

tion(s) at the level of the respiratory mucosa, the other upon control of T-helper cell activation in the regional lymph nodes of the respiratory tract in response to inhaled allergens.

In the latter system, we are exposing experimental animals acutely and chronically to aeroallergens, under conditions approximating natural environmental exposure, viz. low levels of allergens (nanogram zone) delivered via aerosols.

The current status of this work is summarised in Table 1 as per our recent review [7]. It is now evident that the natural response of the respiratory mucosal immune system to exposure to an aeroallergen not previously encountered is the activation of a population of allergen-specific suppressor T-cells, which render the host anergic to restimulation with the same allergen [8–11]. This state of immunological tolerance is inducible with classical aeroallergens such as ragweed [12] and Der p I from house dust mite [13], and confers specific protection against subsequent allergic sensitisation to the initial eliciting allergen. In this respect it closely parallels oral tolerance in the GIT, which provides protection against sensitisation to food antigens [14], and has accordingly been termed Inhalation Tolerance [15].

The overall sensitivity of this process is primarily determined by genetic factors, as under identical conditions of exposure up to 10^4 fold differences have been demonstrated in aeroallergen thresholds required for tolerogenesis of high-IgE-responder (microgram doses) versus low-IgE-responder (nanograms) strains of rats and mice [16, 17]. Corresponding qualitative differences have also been described in the tolerance process. These include the presence of transient IgE responses during early aeroallergen exposure of high but not low-responders [8, 9, 18], and comparable variations in effects upon IgG [8–10, 16], DTH (118) and secretory IgA (137).

Despite the importance of background genetics in the inhalation tolerance process, a variety of environmental and pharmacological agents have been demonstrated to be capable of circumventing the tolerance induction process, and can be thus ascribed potential "risk factor" status in relation to primary sensitisation to aeroallergens. These include disturbances in hormone levels [17], respiratory virus infections [20], chemical (e.g., NO_2) and pharmacological agents (e.g., histamine) that affect

the integrity of the respiratory epithelium and/or adjacent vascular endothelium [17], and immunological immaturity (viz. infancy [21])—it is noteworthy that many of these factors have previously been suggested to be associated with increased risk of respiratory allergy in man [15]. The precise relationship of the T-cells which mediate inhalation tolerance to those producing IgE-T-suppressor factor (TSF) in the Ishizaka system [1] remains to be formally established, but it seems likely that the present process may represent a major route for activation of the IgE-TSF producers that are relevant to protection against respiratory allergy.

Can this system be exploited, in the context of immunotherapy? That is, can this "natural" route of IgE-suppressor T-cell activation be employed to superimpose tolerance upon ongoing IgE responses?

Without further dissection of the precise mechanisms underlying the induction of inhalation tolerance, the answer is clearly no, as aerosol exposure of pre-primed animals simply boosts IgE production [8]. Accordingly, we are proceeding with a more detailed analysis of how inhaled allergen deposited on the respiratory epithelium is normally translated into a tolerogenic signal by the systemic T-cell system.

This phase of the work is guided by earlier results obtained on the kinetics of IgE-T-suppressor cell induction in aerosol-exposed rats, which demonstrated that initial "recognition" of inhaled allergen, and initial suppressor cell activation, occurred in the regional lymph nodes draining the oropharyngeal mucosa [11, 18]. Thus, tolerogenesis must involve initial trapping of inhaled allergen at the intact respiratory epithelium, followed by lymphatic transport to regional nodes and presentation to T-cells, by mechanisms that have yet to be defined.

We have based our approach to this aspect of the problem on the results of earlier experiments on cell-mediated transport of antigen from the GIT in rats [5], in which we demonstrated the passage of large numbers of antigen-bearing dendritic cells (DC) from the gut wall to regional (mesenteric) lymph nodes. These antigen-bearing DC were also shown to be highly efficient in transmitting antigen-specific activation signals to T-cells, much more so than macrophages in this species [5]. The many

169

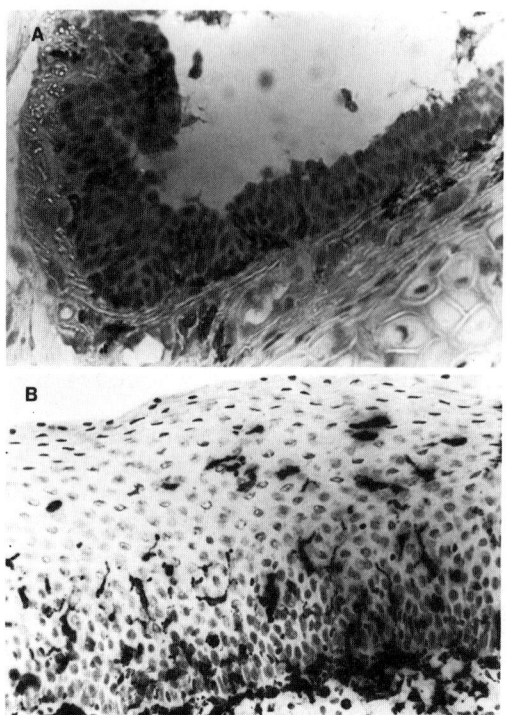

Figure 1. Frozen sections of (A) rat tracheal mucosa and (B) human oropharyngeal mucosa stained via immunoperoxidase employing monoclonal antibodies against rat and human Ia antigens. Note darkly stained dendritic cells within epithelia.

known similarities between the mucosal immune system in the gastrointestinal and respiratory tracts prompted us to seek a similar DC population within the respiratory mucosa. Employing immunoperoxidase staining of frozen sections of rat airway mucosa (Figure 1A) with a bank of monoclonal antibodies against macrophage and DC markers, we have identified a large population of MHC class II antigen (Ia)-bearing DC within (and below) the airway epithelium, closely associated with the basement membrane [6, 22]. These DC appear to form a network comparable to the Langerhans cell system in the skin. Similar cells are apparent in tissue sections of the human oropharyngeal mucosa (Figure 1B) and the bronchial mucosa (not shown).

Functional studies on these DC in rat are currently in progress. Preliminary experiments [6] involving harvest and subsequent dissociation of tracheal epithelial sheets from aerosol-exposed rats indicate that these cells are capable of trapping inhaled allergen in immunogenic form and subsequently presenting it to immune T-cells. If these epithelial DC can be shown to transport allergen to the regional lymph nodes draining upper respiratory tract mucosa in an analogous fashion to their counterparts in the gut wall, then it could be logically assumed that they play a pivotal role in T-cell regulation in response to inhaled antigens, and our experiments are proceeding with this possibility in mind. We are currently seeking information on the origin and dynamics of these DC, in particular the nature of the factor(s) which regulate their egress from the epithelium.

References

1. Ishizaka, K. 1984. Regulation of IgE synthesis. Ann. Rev. Immunol. 2: 159.
2. Katz, D. H. 1980. Recent studies on the regulation of IgE antibody synthesis in experimental animals and man. Immunology 41: 1.
3. Janeway, C. A. 1988. Frontiers of the immune system. Nature 333: 804.
4. Goodman, T., and L. Lefrancois. 1988. Expression of the $\gamma\delta$ T-cell receptor on intestinal $CD8^+$ intraepithelial lymphocytes. Nature 333: 855.
5. Mayrhofer, G., P. G. Holt, and J. M. Papadimitriou. 1986. Functional characteristics of the veiled cells in afferent lymph from the rat intestine. Immunology 58: 379.
6. Holt, P. G., M. A. Schon-Hegrad, and J. A. Oliver. 1988. MHC class II antigen-bearing dendritic cells in pulmonary tissues of the rat: Regulation of antigen presentation activity by endogenous macrophage populations. J. Exp. Med. 167: 262.
7. Holt, P. G., and J. D. Sedgwick. 1987. Suppression of IgE responses following antigen inhalation: A natural homeostatic mechanism which limits sensitisation to aeroallergens. Immunology Today 8: 14.
8. Holt, P. G., J. E. Batty, and K. J. Turner. 1981. Inhibition of specific IgE responses in mice by pre-exposure to inhaled antigen. Immunology 42: 409.
9. Sedgwick, J. D., and P. G. Holt. 1983. Induction of IgE-isotype specific tolerance by passive antigenic stimulation of the respiratory mucosa. Immunology 50: 625.
10. Holt, P. G., and S. Leivers. 1982. Tolerance induction via antigen inhalation: Isotype specificity, stability and involvement of suppressor T-cells. Int. Arch. Allergy appl. Immun. 67: 155.
11. Sedgwick, J. D., and P. G. Holt. 1985. Induction of IgE-secreting cells and IgE-isotype-specific

suppressor T-cells in respiratory tract lymph nodes of rats exposed to an antigen aerosol. Immunol. 94: 182.

12. Fox, P. C., and R. P. Siraganian. 1981. IgE antibody suppression following aerosol exposure to antigens. Immunology 43: 227.

13. Stewart, G. A., and P. G. Holt. 1987. The immunogenicity and tolerogenicity of a major house dust mite allergen, Der p I in mice and rats. Int. Arch. Allergy appl. Immun. 83: 44.

14. Tomasi, T. B. Jr. 1980. Oral tolerance. Transplantation 29: 353.

15. Holt, P. G., and C. McMenamin. 1988. Defence against allergic sensitisation in the healthy lung: the role of Inhalation Tolerance. Clin. Exp. Immunol., in press.

16. Sedgwick, J. D., and P. G. Holt. 1984. Suppression of IgE responses in inbred rats by repeated respiratory tract exposure to antigen: Responder phenotype influences isotype specificity in induced tolerance. 14: 893.

17. Holt, P. G., D. Britten, and J. D. Sedgwick. 1987. Suppression of IgE responses by antigen inhalation: Studies on the role of genetic and environmental factors. Immunology 60: 97.

18. Sedgwick, J. D., and P. G. Holt. 1986. Induction of IgE secreting cells in the lymphatic drainage of the lungs of rats following passive antigen inhalation. Int. Arch. allergy appl. Immunol. 79: 329.

19. Holt, P. G., M. F. Reid, D. Britten, J. D. Sedgwick, and H. Bazin. 1987. Suppression of IgE responses by passive antigen inhalation: Dissociation of local (mucosal) and systemic immunity. Cell Immunol. 104: 434.

20. Holt, P. G., J. Vines, and N. Bilyk. 1988. Effect of influenza virus infection on allergic sensitisation to inhaled antigen. Int. Archs. Allergy appl. Immun. 86: 121.

21. Holt, P. G., J. Vines, and D. Britten. 1988. Suppression of IgE responses by antigen inhalation: failure of tolerance mechanisms in newborn rats. Immunology 63: 591.

22. Holt, P. G., and M. A. Schon-Hegrad. 1988. Localisation of T cells, macrophages and dendritic cells in respiratory tract tissue: Implications for immune function studies. Immunol. 62: 349.

Participation of Fc-εRII Positive Cells in Asthma

*A. B. Tonnel, P. Gosset, M. Capron, M. Tomassini, M. Joseph, A. Capron**

The identification of a second class of receptors for IgE (FcεRII) on inflammatory cells present in airways supports the hypothesis that FcεRII positive cells can be directly activated by an IgE-dependent stimulation. Concerning alveolar macrophages (AMs), the % of cells expressing the Fcε receptor is higher in allergic asthmatics, they are able to produce after IgE triggering a large variety of mediators (PGE2, PGF2α, LTB4, PAF-acether) as well as monokines susceptible to regulate the local immune response to inhaled allergens. The proportion of eosinophils bearing the FcεRII is also elevated in patients with increased serum IgE levels or after previous incubation in the presence of chemotactic factors.

Triggering through the Fcε receptor also induces a specific release of mediators: MBP, eosinophil peroxidase, or other lipid derived mediators. On the other hand, the level of mediator release is clearly enhanced in hypodense eosinophils, although the relationship between density and the presence of FcεRII remains to be defined clearly. As for platelets, if the concept of platelet activation by an IgE-stimulus cannot be denied, its relevance in allergic asthma remains controversial and based more on experimental data than on clinical arguments.

Many of the characteristics of bronchial asthma may be explained on the basis of inflammatory processes induced by mediators released after antigen-IgE interaction. The rapid release of mast cell-associated mediators probably plays a major role in the early clinical manifestations of asthma, and immediate reactions are largely the result of bronchoconstriction by consecutive to the released histamine, PGD2, or leukotrienes. But other cells are also involved in the pathogenesis of allergic asthma, namely, in the development of the local inflammatory response that occurs after repeated exposure to allergens or during the late phase reaction, leading progressively to bronchial hyperresponsiveness; besides mast cells that have a high affinity receptor for IgE, other cell types like alveolar macrophages, eosinophils, and even platelets can be directly activated by an IgE-dependent stimulation.

Parallel to studies on the control of IgE response which clearly showed that T and B cells bore receptors for IgE, various experiments, including rosette formation with IgE-coated erythrocytes, labeled IgE binding, use of monoclonal anti Fcε receptor antibodies have allowed the demonstration of a specific receptor for IgE expressed on inflammatory cells. This second receptor named FcεRII [1] differs from the classical mast cell receptor by a lower affinity ($Ka\ 10^7$ versus $10^9 M^{-1}$), a distinct antigenicity as shown by the absence of cross-reactivity with mast cell receptors, and its modulation by IgE itself, the number of FcεRII positive cells increasing in all experimental or pathological situations associated with high IgE levels.

Alveolar Macrophages and Asthma

Mast cells probably initiate type I hypersensitivity reactions, though bronchial asthma cannot be fully explained by this only cell type. Less than 0.25% of the cells recovered from the airway lumen by bronchoalveolar lavage (BAL) are mast cells, and paradoxically the highest levels of mast cells and histamine are recovered from patients with interstitial pulmonary diseases [2]. In fact, the most abundant cell type present in the lumen of the respiratory tract is the alveolar macrophage (AM). Indeed, AM is present not only at the level of alveoli, but also throughout the bronchial tree at the surface of bronchiolar and bronchial mucosa: Using a new technique to isolate a human large airway in vivo, Rankin detected, in bronchial wash, cellular components largely different from BAL but with two prominent cell types, macrophages and neutrophils that, together, represent almost 60% of the total cell count [3].

* Centre d'Immunologie et Biologie Parasitaire, Institut Pasteur de Lille, F-Lille 59019, France.
Supported in part by Réseau de Recherche Clinique INSERM No. 850027.

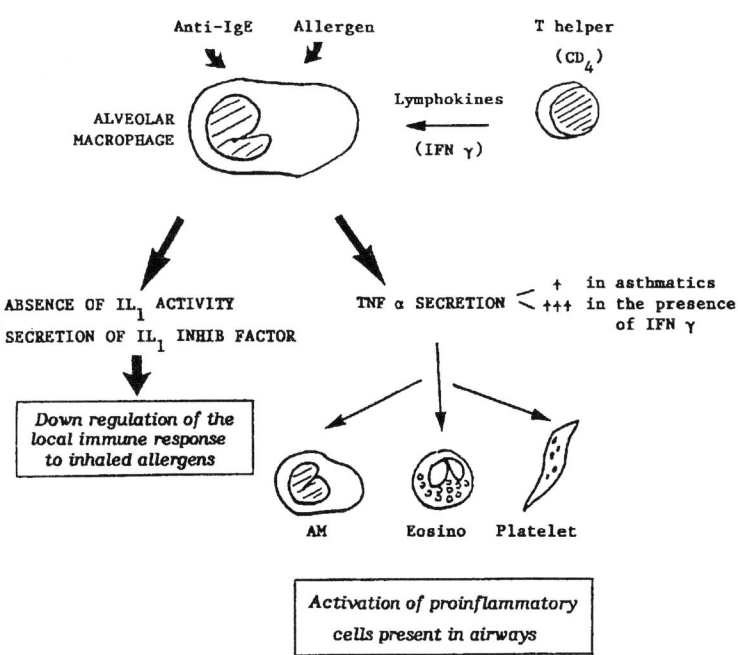

Figure 1. Hypothesis on cytokine network in asthma.

Involvement of Alveolar Macrophages in Allergic Asthma: Mediator Release

Several studies have identified the presence of receptors for IgE on the mononuclear phagocyte surface and their increased number in atopic disorders. Concerning alveolar macrophages, the percentage of human AMs expressing the Fcε receptor was found to be approximately 18–20% in allergic asthmatics, versus 6–8% in controls [4]. Additional evidence for the presence of surface IgE on AMs was provided by electron microscopy with colloidal gold conjugated anti-IgE [5].

Moreover, AMs, known as potent secretory cells, can be directly implicated in hypersensitivity mechanisms by releasing mediators after anti-IgE or allergen triggering. In experimental models [6, 7], IgE immune complexes stimulated rodent peritoneal macrophages to generate LTC_4 and other arachidonic acid metabolites. In man, Fuller [5] showed after AM stimulation with anti-IgE the secretion of TxB_2, $PGF2\alpha$ and LTB_4 that appeared within the first 15 minutes. The data suggest that the in vivo release might effectively occur within the timespan necessary to initiate bronchospasm after challenge in sensitive patients. AMs retrieved from asthmatic patients were also shown to be potent producers of PAF-acether [8], a lipid-derived mediator known to act as a chemotactic factor for human eosinophils and also as an inducer of severe and prolonged bronchial hyperreactivity when given by inhalation in man. After incubation with anti-IgE or specific allergens, AMs were also able to secrete a low molecular weight chemotactic factor for neutrophils and eosinophils, probably related to LTB_4 [9]. Lastly, a recent study demonstrated that human lung macrophages secreted a factor susceptible to induce calcium-dependent histamine release from human basophils and lung mast cells [10]. Therefore, all these findings point to the human alveolar macrophage as a potential source of mediators implicated in the local inflammatory response, more especially as some of them can be released after local bronchial challenge test [11].

Alveolar Macrophages and Monokine Production after IgE-Dependent Stimulation

The role of AMs in allergic asthma is not restricted to the secretion of lipid-derived mediators: AMs can also act as regulatory cells. In order to study the possible role of AMs in the development of the local immune response, our interest was recently focused on *monokine* production, Interleukin 1 (IL1) and Tumor necrosis factor α (TNFα) after IgE-dependent stimulation.

Mononuclear phagocytes are known to produce *Interleukin 1*, a molecule considered as playing a crucial role in inflammatory processes and in lymphocyte proliferation. To appreciate the possible role of AMs in the local response to inhaled allergens, we compared IL1 production by peripheral blood monocytes and AMs from allergic asthmatics and controls [12]. When stimulated by lipopolysaccharide, AMs and blood monocytes released IL1 in similar amounts (148 ± 47 and 160 ± 78

IL1 units/ml) but in response to anti-IgE or allergens, at variance of monocytes that generated significant amounts of IL1, AM supernatants contained *no detectable IL1 activity*. On the contrary, in the same experimental conditions, AMs secreted preferentially an IL1 inhibitory factor independent from prostaglandin E2, with a molecular weight of 40–50 kD. Thus, these results demonstrate that, on the contrary to some stimuli like endotoxins, which are able to induce IL1 production, AMs after IgE-dependent stimulation deliver a negative signal for lymphocyte proliferation, suggesting an potential *in situ* limitation of the immune response to common inhaled allergens.

In parallel with Interleukin 1, another monokine, (TNFα) has been recently investigated. Spontaneously, AMs directly retrieved from the lung of asthmatics released significantly more TNFα (0.96 ± 0.50 ng/ml) than AMs from controls. After IgE-dependent stimulation, performed in vitro by addition of allergen or anti-IgE, the levels of TNFα present in supernatants raised up to 2.8 ± 0.9 ng/ml. It is also interesting to note a significant amplification ($\times 3$) of monokine production in the case of costimulation with Interferon γ. These results concerning the measurements of TNFα production were clearly corroborated by the evaluation of TNFα mRNA expression. These high levels of TNFα secretion seen in asthma as well as its potentiation by IFNγ suggest a possible interaction with lymphocytes present in airways. The recruitment of T lymphocytes after inhalation challenge [13], the presence of a high proportion of activated T lymphocytes, with a predominant CD4 "helper-inducer" subset, shown in blood of patients suffering from acute severe attack of

asthma [14] raise the possibility of interactions between AMs and T lymphocytes present in airways, interactions susceptible to contribute to a subsequent activation of other cells recruited in the respiratory tract (Figure 1).

Eosinophils and Asthma

Although peripheral blood eosinophilia is currently associated with allergic disorders, contribution of eosinophils has yet to be fully appreciated. Early studies centered on its ability to down-regulate immediate hypersensitivity reactions, but convincing data have more recently focused interest on the role of eosinophils as effector cells for killing parasites but also for causing bronchial and/or lung damage [15, 16].

The Eosinophil Fcε Receptor and Its Relationship to Cell Density

Eosinophils are known to express on their surface receptors for IgE, the demonstration of which was obtained after binding with labeled myeloma IgE, by rosette formation and by flow-microfluorometry, with a significant correlation between all methods [17, 18]. Inhibition experiments using aggregated IgE or IgG confirmed the specificity of the binding, without any cross-reactivity of the binding sites between IgE and IgG. Thus was it possible to evaluate the proportion of eosinophils bearing the Fcε receptor: in humans 20% to 55% of blood eosinophils express the IgE receptor; the percentage of FcεRII positive cells is more elevated in patients with increased serum IgE levels. Rise in FcεRII bearing eosinophils seems also linked to the presence of chemotactic factors such as PAF-acether susceptible to enhance the receptor expression on normal eosinophils.

The relationship between expression of the Fcε receptor and eosinophil density is not definitely established. However, hypodense eosinophils, recovered from tissues, for example, from the lung by bronchoalveolar lavage, have a greater proportion of receptors occupied in vivo by IgE than corresponding circulating eosinophils [19]. Whether the proportion of FcεRII positive cells, evaluated by rosette assay, was not significantly different in normo- and hypodense cells, the number of receptor sites per cell and their affinity were increased in low-density eosinophils. This demonstration of a large proportion of hypodense eosinophils with surface bound IgE suggests that an increased expression of Fcε receptor might represent one of the markers of eosinophil activation.

Eosinophil Fcε and Mediator Release

The eosinophil is known to release a large variety of substances able to cause cellular and tissular damage in bronchial asthma. Among cationic proteins, Major Basic Protein (MBP) mediates damages that mimick the pathology of asthma. MBP concentrations as low as 10 µg/ml produced ciliostasis with disruption of the epithelium and damage to the cells present in the lumen. With higher MBP concentrations (50–100 µg/ml) ciliated cells were progressively exfoliated to the level of the basal membrane. In parallel, measurements of MBP showed that patients with acute asthma had high levels of MBP in sputum, compatible with cell alterations observed in vitro [20]. Other eosinophil derived products are potentially active in asthma, such as eosinophil peroxidase (E.P.O.) localized in the granule matrix, that can, in the presence of H_2O_2 and halide, induce mast cell degranulation. Among lipid-derived mediators, leukotriene C_4 [21], and PAF-acether [22] are preferentially produced by activated eosinophils: Hypodense eosinophils produce more PAF-acether in response to calcium ionophore than cells with normal density; lung eosinophils obtained by BAL produced 1000-fold more PAF after incubation with anti-IgE than the corresponding blood eosinophils from the same patients. A selective release of eosinophil peroxidase (EPO) was also observed after incubation of hypodense eosinophils with anti-IgE antibodies, while no effect could be obtained after incubation with anti-IgG, which seems to demonstrate a preferential release of EPO through the Fcε receptor. These data primarily seen in filariasis [23] were confirmed recently in the case of patients sensitized to common inhaled allergens.

Participation of Eosinophils in Asthmatic Patients

A series of recent clinical studies, focused either on peripheral blood eosinophils or on resident eosinophils recovered by bronchoalveolar lavage, have brought interesting data on the eosinophil involvement in asthma.

Based on density and metabolic activity, peripheral blood eosinophils appeared as a heterogeneous population in allergic disorders [24, 25, 26]. A significant higher proportion of blood eosinophils (defined as density < 1.081 gm/ml) was observed in patients with allergic asthma ($40.8 \pm 5.8\%$ hypodense eosinophils) or allergic rhinitis (30.0 ± 5.0), versus $9.0 \pm 1.9\%$ in controls. In addition, increased percentage of hypodense eosinophils were detected more often in patients with severe symptoms, suggesting a possible connection between hypodense cells and the development of symptoms. This eosinophil heterogeneity in atopy was also reflected in differences in leukotriene production [27]. Hypodense eosinophils demonstrated different profiles in leukotriene C_4 (LTC_4) production according to the stimulus used: Reduced LTC_4 release after triggering with calcium ionophore, increased LTC_4 production with opsonized zymosan particles, which is compatible with a modified expression of C_3b receptors in low density eosinophils. But no information was brought in this work concerning the role of IgE molecules.

By studying blood eosinophils highly purified on density gradient, we have shown in asthmatics the release of EPO (manuscript in preparation) after triggering by the specific related allergen: grass pollen and/or *Dermatophagoides pteronyssinus*. The specificity of EPO release was clearly demonstrated by a parallel mediator release in the presence of anti-IgE and allergen, while anti-IgG antibodies were ineffective. Interestingly, in a control group of nonatopic patients with high eosinophilia (mean blood eosinophil count: 42%—range 8–85% compared to 12.5%—range 5–20% in asthmatics) no EPO could be detected after allergen stimulation, which renders highly probable the mediator release through the Fcε receptor.

Another way to evaluate the role of eosinophils in asthma is represented by the bronchoalveolar lavage (B.A.L.) which gives access to resident cells present in the airways. In patients with mild asthma, the differential cell count showed, besides an increased proportion of mast cells, a significant elevation in eosinophils as well as a higher concentration of MBP in BAL fluid only detected in symptomatic patients. In addition, it must be stressed that a significant inverse correlation did exist between bronchial hyperresponsiveness (PC 20) and the percentage of eosinophils (p < 0.01) but also of desquamated epithelial cells [28].

In conjunction with allergen challenge, B.A.L. gave accurate information on the influx of eosinophils during the late phase reaction. In patients exhibiting early and late asthmatic reactions, de Monchy [29] found in BAL performed 5–7 h after allergen inhalation a mean value of 30.0 ± 9% eosinophils. The presence of eosinophils was also corroborated with elevated levels of eosinophil cationic protein in the lavage fluid. In a similar study Metzger [30] detected an increased number of eosinophils within 4 h after bronchoprovocation, but with a concomitant recruitment of neutrophils; moreover, electron microscopy of BAL-cells fluid revealed degranulated eosinophils with loss of the dense cores of granules. So eosinophils considered for a long time as secondary cells are capable not only to be mobilized at the sites of the allergen conflict but also directly triggered through their specific IgE receptors in the release of various mediators.

Platelets and Allergic Asthma

While the participation of inflammatory cells expressing the low affinity Fcε receptor like eosinophils or mononuclear phagocytes is largely accepted, the exact role of platelets in allergic diseases, and more precisely in asthma, remains controversial.

In the context of allergic asthma, platelets isolated from patients with mite or grass pollen sensitivity exhibited after incubation with anti-IgE or the related allergen an activation evaluated both by the release of cytocidal mediators and the generation of oxygen metabolites. Similar results were obtained with platelets from healthy donors previously sensitized with IgE-rich sera of allergic patients. Furthermore, the involvement of IgE could be demonstrated by the total inhibition of both activation parameters after IgE removal or after platelet preincubation with anti FcεRII monoclonal or polyclonal antibodies. Similar criteria of plate-

let activation could also be demonstrated in non allergic situations like aspirin-sensitive asthma in the presence of aspirin or other cyclooxygenase inhibitory drugs [31].

Nevertheless, if the concept of platelet activation cannot be denied, its relevance in vivo has to be confirmed. In animal studies, platelet activation was considered as an important parameter during bronchospastic responses produced by PAF-acether or allergen [32]. In guinea pigs, changes in airway resistance and platelet accumulation in pulmonary vasculature have been reported either after PAF-acether or allergen inhalation [33]. In baboons, PAF-acether induced a transient bronchoconstriction, which was associated with an accumulation of platelets within the pulmonary vessels [34]. In humans, several investigators [35, 36] have reported the release into plasma of platelet specific proteins such as platelet factor 4 (PF4) or β-thromboglobulin after allergen challenge or exercise—data not confirmed by other investigators [37]. In asthmatics, the turnover of circulating platelets was shown to be accelerated, falling to nearly 50% of its value in normal donors, suggesting a continuous in vivo activation [38]. Platelets were also found in the bronchoalveolar lavage fluid immediately after local antigen challenge and during the late phase response [39]. Likewise, patients who had died from status asthmaticus had megakaryocytes present in abundance in the lungs. Another indirect argument for platelet involvement in allergy is the inhibitory effect of antiallergic drugs on platelet reactivity. Drugs like disodium cromoglycate or nedocromil sodium, known for their clinical efficacy in allergic asthma, strongly inhibited in vitro parameters of platelet activity but were also able to reproduce the same effect in ex vivo experiments when given by aerosols. Nevertheless, it must be pointed out that these drugs were acting not only on platelets but on all cells expressing the Fcε receptor. In fact, at the present time, additional investigations are necessary to definitively include platelets among the cells implicated in pathophysiology of asthma.

Conclusion

Taken together, these series of observations clearly indicate that mast cells and basophils can no longer be considered the only target cell in IgE-dependent processes. Inflammatory cells through the expression of FcεRII and the presence of cytophilic IgE on their surface can directly participate as effector cells in the pathophysiology of asthma and particularly in its inflammatory components.

References

1. Capron, A., J. P. Dessaint, M. Capron, M. Joseph, J. C. Ameisen, and A. B. Tonnel. 1986. From parasites to allergy. The second receptor for IgE (FcεRII). Immunology Today 7: 15–18.
2. Rankin, J. A., M. Kaliner, and H. Y. Reynolds. 1987. Histamine levels in bronchoalveolar lavage from patients with asthma, sarcoidosis and idiopathic pulmonary fibrosis. J. Allergy Clin. Immunol. 79: 371–377.
3. Rankin, J. A., T. Marcy, S. Smith, J. Olchowski, J. Sussman, and W. W. Merrill. 1988. Human airway lining fluid (ALF): cellular and protein constituents. Am. Rev. Respir. Dis. 137: suppl. p. 5 (Abstract).
4. Joseph, M., A. B. Tonnel, G. Torpier, A. Capron, B. Arnoux, and J. Benveniste. 1983. Involvement of IgE in the secretory processes of alveolar macrophages from asthmatic patients. J. Clin. Invest. 71: 221–230.
5. Fuller, R. W., P. K. Morris, R. Richmond, D. Sykes, I. M. Varndell, D. M. Kemeny. P. J. Cole, C. T. Doller, and J. Macdermot. 1986. Immunoglobulin E-dependent stimulation of human alveolar macrophages: significance in type 1 hypersensitivity. Clin. Exp. Immunol. 65: 416–426.
6. Rouzer, C. A., W. A. Scott, A. L. Hamill, F. T. Liu, D. H. Katz, and Z. A. Cohn. 1982. Secretion of leukotriene C4 and other arachidonic acid metabolites by macrophages challenged with IgE immune complexes. J. Exp. Med. 156: 1077–1082.
7. Rankin, J. A., M. Hitcock, W. W. Merrill, S. S. Huand, J. R. Braschler, M. K. Bach, and P. W. Askenase. 1984. IgE immune complexes induced immediate and prolonged release of leukotriene C4 (LTC4) from rat alveolar macrophages. J. Immunol. 132: 1993–1997.
8. Arnoux, B., D. Duval, and J. Benveniste. 1980. Release of platelet activating factor (PAF-acether) from alveolar macrophages by the calcium ionophore A 23187 and phagocytosis. Eur. J. Clin. Invest. 10: 437–441.
9. Gosset, P., A. B. Tonnel, M. Joseph, L. Prin, A. Mallart, J. Charon, and A. Capron. 1984. Secretion of a chemotactic factor for neutrophils and eosinophils by alveolar macrophages patients. J. Allergy Clin. Immunol. 74: 827–834.
10. Schulman, E. S., M. C. Liu, D. Proud, D. W. MacGlashan, L. H. Lichtenstein, and M. Plaut.

11. Tonnel, A. B., P. Gosset, M. Joseph, E. Fournier, and A. Capron. 1983. Stimulation of alveolar macrophages in asthmatic patients after local provocation test. Lancet i: 1406–1408.
12. Gosset, P., P. Lassalle, A. B. Tonnel, J. P. Dessaint, B. Wallaert, L. Prin, J. Pestel, and A. Capron. 1988 Production of an interleukin 1 inhibitory factor by human alveolar macrophages from normal and allergic patients. Am. Rev. Respir. Dis. 138: 40–46.
13. Gonzales, C., P. Diaz, F. Galleguillos, P. Ancic, O. Cromwell, and A. B. Kay. 1987. Allergen induces recruitment of bronchoalveolar helper (OKT4) and suppressor (OKT8) cells in asthma. Relative increases in OKT8 cells in single early responders compared with those in late phrase responders. Am. Rev. Respir. Dis. 136: 600–604.
14. Corrigan, C. J., A. Hartnell, and A. B. Kay. T lymphocyte activation in acute severe asthma. Lancet i: 1129–1132.
15. Frigas, E., and G. Gleich. 1986. The eosinophil and the pathophysiology of asthma (Postgrad course). J. Allergy Clin. Immunol. 77: 527–537.
16. Davis, B. W., A. G. Fells, S. Wiu-Hong, E. J. Gadek, A. Venet, and R. G. Crystal. 1984. Eosinophil-mediated injury to lung parenchymal cells and interstitial matrix. J. Clin. Invest. 74: 269–278.
17. Capron, M., H. C. Spiegelberg, L. Prin, H. Bennich, A. E. Gutterworth, R. J. Pierce, A. Ouassi, and A. Capron. 1984. Role of IgE-receptor in effector function of human eosinophils. J. Immunol. 132: 462–468.
18. Capron, M., J. P. Kusnierz, L. Prin, H. L. Spiegelberg, G. Ovlaque, P. Gosset, A. B. Tonnel, and A. Capron. 1985. Cytophilic IgE on human blood and tissue eosinophils: Detection by flow microfluorometry. J. Immunol. 134: 3013–3018.
19. Prin, L., M. Capron, P. Gosset, B. Wallaert, P. Kusnierz, O. Bletry, A. B. Tonnel, and A. Capron. 1986. Eosinophil lung disease: Immunological studies of blood and alveolar eosinophils. Clin. Exp. Immunol. 63: 249–257.
20. Frigas, E., D. A. Loegering, G. O. Solley, G. M. Farrow, and G. J. Gleich. 1981. Elevated levels of the eosinophil granule major basic protein in the sputum of patients with bronchial asthma. Mayo Clinics Proceedings 63: 249–257.
21. Shaw, R. J., O. Cromwell, G. M. Walski, and A. B Kay. 1985. Activated human eosinophils generate SRS-leukotrienes after physiological (IgG-dependent) stimulation. Fed. Proc. 44: 1185.
22. Jouvin-Marche, E., J. M. Grzych, C. Boullet, M. Capron, and J. Benveniste. 1984. Formation of PAF-acether by human eosinophils. Fed. Proc. 43: 1924.

23. Khalife, J., M. Capron, J. Y. Cesbron, Po Chun Tai, H. Taelman, L. Prin, and A. Capron. 1986. Role of specific IgE antibodies in peroxidase (EPO) release from human eosinophils. J. Immunol. 137: 1659–1664.

24. Fukuda, T., S. L. Dunnette, C. E. Reed, S. J. Ackerman, M. S. Peters, and G. J. Gleich. 1985. Increased number of hypodense eosinophils in the blood of patients with bronchial asthma. Am. Rev. Respir. Dis. 132: 981–985.

25. Shult, P. A., M. Lega, S. Jadidi, R. Vrtis, T. Warner, F. M. Graziano, and W. W. Busse. 1988. The presence of hypodense eosinophils and diminished chemiluminescence response in asthma. J. Allergy Clin. Immunol. 82: 119–125.

26. Frick, W. E., J. B. Sedgwick, and W. W. Busse. 1988. Hypodense eosinophils in allergic rhinitis. J. Allergy Clin. Immunol. 82: 119–125.

27. Kauffman, H. F., B. van der Belt, J. G. R. de Monchy, H. Boelens, G. H. Koeter, and K. de Vries. 1987. Leukotriene C4 production by normal-density and low-density eosinophils of atopic individuals and other patients with eosinophilia. J. Allergy Clin. Immunol. 79: 611–619.

28. Wardlaw, A. J., S. Dunnette, G. J. Gleich, J. V. Collins, and A. B. Kay. 1988. Eosinophils and mast cells in bronchoalveolar lavage in subjects with mild asthma. Relationship to bronchial hyperreactivity. Am. Rev. Respir. Dis. 137: 62–69.

29. De Monchy, J. G. R., H. F. Kauffman, P. Venge, G. H. Koeter, H. M. Jansen, H. J. Sluiter, and K. de Vries. 1985. Bronchoalveolar eosinophilia during allergen-induced late asthmatic reactions. Am. Rev. Respir. Dis. 131: 373–379.

30. Metzger, W. J., H. B. Richerson, B. S. Worden, M. Monick, and G. W. Hunninghake. 1986. Bronchoalveolar lavage of allergic asthmatic patients following allergen bronchoprovocation. Chest 89: 477–483.

31. Capron, A., J. C. Ameisen, M. Joseph, C. Auriault, A. B. Tonnel, and J. Caen. New functions for platelets and their pathological implications. Int. Archs. Allergy Appl. Immunol. 77: 107–114.

32. Vargaftig, B. B., J. Lefort, M. Chignard, and J. Benveniste. 1980. Platelet activating factor induces a platelet-dependent bronchoconstriction unrelated to the formation of prostaglandin derivates. Eur. J. Pharmacol. 65: 185–192.

33. Page, C. P. 1988. The involvement of platelets in non thrombotic processes. T. I. P. S. 9: 66–71.

34. Arnoux, B., A. Denjean, C. P. Page, D. Nolibe, J. Morley, and A. Benveniste. 1988. Accumulation of platelets and eosinophils in baboon lung after PAF-acether challenge. Inhibition by Ketotifen. Am. Rev. Respir. Dis. 137: 855–860.

35. Knauer, K. A., L. M. Lichtenstein, N. F. Adkinson, and J. E. Fish. 1981. Platelet activation during antigen induced airway reaction in asthmatic subjects. New Engl. J. Med. 304: 1404–1407.

36. Johnson, C. E., P. W. Belfield, S. Davis, N. J. Cooke, A. Spencer, and J. A. Davies. 1986. Platelet activation during exercise induced asthma: Effect of prophylaxis with cromoglycate and salbutamol. Thorax 41: 290–294.

37. Durham, S. R., J. Dawes, and A. B. Kay. 1985. Platelet in asthma. Lancet ii: 36.

38. Taytard, A., H. Guenard, L. Vuillemin, J. L. Bouror, J. Vergeret, D. Ducassou, Y. Piquet, and P. Freour. 1986. Platelet kinetics in stable atopic asthmatic patients. Am. Rev. Respir. Dis. 134: 983–985.

39. Metzger, W. J., G. W. Hunninghake, and H. B. Richerson. 1985. Late asthmatic responses: inquiry into mechanisms and significance. Clin. Rev. Allergy 3: 145–165.

Evaluation of Asthma and Airway Hyperresponsiveness by Cytology of Bronchoalveolar Lavage or Sputum

Frederick E. Hargreave, Peter G. Gibson, E. Helen Ramsdale, Jerry Dolovich, Judah Denburg*

In asthma, the physiological abnormalities of variable airflow limitation and airway hyperresponsiveness appear to be secondary to airway inflammation; however, they can also occur in cigarette smokers with chronic airflow limitation who are considered to have a different pathogenesis. Examination for the inflammation by cytology of bronchoalveolar lavage in mild stable asthmatics demonstrates small increases in eosinophils and/or metachromatic cells (mast cells or basophils). These cells occur in greater numbers in the sputum during exacerbations of asthma; in comparison, there are few or none in the sputum of smokers with simple chronic bronchitis. Further studies relating airway cytological (or histopathological) characteristics to the various clinical and physiological features are required to improve our understanding of asthma and other airway conditions.

The Ciba Foundation Study Group on the Identification of Asthma in 1971 could not reach agreement on the definition of asthma [1]. In ignorance of the pathogenesis, an arbitrary definition was adopted: Asthma was defined as a disease characterized by wide variations over short periods of time in resistance to flow in intrapulmonary airways [2]. In other words, it was defined by a disorder of airway function—referred to here as variable airflow limitation. The variability can be observed spontaneously as in diurnal variation, by improvement after anti-asthma treatment, or by deterioration after various bronchoconstrictive stimuli. An increase in the bronchoconstrictive response to various nonallergic or nonsensitizing stimuli is called airway hyperresponsiveness.

Measurements of airway responsiveness to histamine or methacholine have improved our understanding of asthma in a number of ways [3]. They have contributed to the current hypothesis that asthma and airway hyperresponsiveness can be secondary to airway inflammation [3]. However, they have demonstrated discrepancies between responsiveness and symptoms [4–6]. Moreover, methacholine hyperresponsiveness does not seem to be specific for asthma when there is chronic airflow limitation [7].

Here, we present recent observations of the cytology of bronchoalveolar lavage (BAL) and sputum in asthma and other airway diseases. We suggest that continuing comparison of such methods with various clinical features including airway responsiveness will be useful to improve our understanding of asthma.

Cytology of BAL in Mild Stable Asthma

Inflammatory cells such as eosinophils and/or metachromatic cells (mast cells or basophils) are increased in the BAL from mild asthmatics (with methacholine airway hyperresponsiveness), when compared to that from atopic or nonatopic nonasthmatic subjects with normal methacholine responsiveness [8,9]. An increase in metachromatic cells appears to be an early abnormality. The magnitude of increase in metachromatic cells, eosinophils, and epithelial cells correlates with the magnitude of hyperresponsiveness to methacholine. Hence, there is evidence of airway inflammation even when asthma is mild and stable.

*   Departments of Medicine and Pediatrics, McMaster University, Hamilton, Ontario, Canada.
    Supported by Medical Research Council of Canada and Boehringer Ingelheim Inc.
    Acknowledgements: We thank Mrs. Laurie Whitely for typing the manuscript.

Cytology of Sputum in Exacerbations of Asthma and in Simple Chronic Bronchitis

Recently, we reconsidered the use of sputum to study the pathogenesis of asthma and other airway diseases [Gibson et al, submitted for publication], based on analogous models demonstrating similar findings in mucosae and secretions in allergic rhinitis [10]. The accumulation of effector cells such as mast cells, basophils, and eosinophils in rhinitis and in nasal polyposis appears to involve kinetic changes in blood progenitors and the elaboration of growth and differentiation factors by nasal epithelium [11, 12].

We initially established methods to determine total cell and differential cell counts in sputum. There was a high level of reproducibility within selected plugs from the same sputum specimen and between plugs from specimens on two consecutive days. Then, sputum cell counts in patients with an exacerbation of asthma were compared with counts in cigarette smokers with cough and sputum consistent with chronic bronchitis. The asthmatics had methacholine airway hyperresponsiveness or airflow limitation. The sputum and any airflow limitation were reversed by treatment with corticosteroid. The bronchitics had normal spirometry, normal methacholine responsiveness and no improvement in sputum after treatment with corticosteroid. There was no overlap in the cell counts. The sputum of all of the asthmatics was characterized by a marked eosinophilia and an increase in metachromatic cells; the bronchitics had few or no eosinophils or metachromatic cells.

These studies show that the cytology of sputum can be reproducible when methods of examination are standardized, and that the cytology of the sputum of asthma is quite different to the sputum in smokers with simple chronic bronchitis. The results, in conjunction with the BAL studies, suggest that an increase in eosinophils and metachromatic cells are characteristic of the mucosal inflammation of asthma.

Cytology of Sputum of Chronic Cough Reversed by Corticosteroids

The sputum sampling methods developed were then applied to the examination of the sputum of a group of nonsmokers who presented with chronic cough and sputum, and with normal spirometry and normal methacholine responsiveness, yet in whom there was subsequently a reversal of the symptoms by treatment with corticosteroid [Gibson et al., manuscript in preparation]. The sputum was examined before the onset of corticosteroid treatment, and the findings were similar to those seen in asthmatics during an exacerbation. The results of these studies, which help to characterize the airway inflammation in chronic cough patients, suggest a pathogenesis similar or identical with asthma; the one exception is that the patients failed to acquire methacholine hyperresponsiveness. The results raise the possibility that the asthmatic process need not be accompanied by variable airflow limitation or airway hyperresponsiveness to methacholine.

Airway Responsiveness in Asthma and Chronic Airflow Limitation

Measurement of airway responsiveness to histamine or methacholine in cigarette smokers with or without chronic airflow limitation demonstrates a linear relationship between FEV_1 and the provocation concentration of methacholine to cause a fall in FEV_1 of 20% (PC_{20}); the lower the FEV_1, the lower the PC_{20} [7]. Similar observations have been made by others [13–17]. In the study by Ramsdale and coworkers [14], an FEV_1 of less than about 70% of the vital capacity was always associated with a PC_{20} in the asthmatic range indicating airway hyperresponsiveness to methacholine. By contrast, only three of these subjects bronchoconstricted after hyperventilation of cold dry air. These results differ from those observed in a group of asthmatics who were selected because their FEV_1 was similar to the smokers but was completely normal after bronchodilator [7]. The PC_{20} was decreased in the asthmatics who had a normal FEV_1, and the severity of hyperresponsiveness in those with a reduced FEV_1 was greater than in the smokers with a comparable reduction of FEV_1. Furthermore, hyperventilation of cold dry air caused bronchoconstriction in all but one of the asthmatic group. The results raise the possibility that

1. hyperresponsiveness to methacholine, which is considered to act chiefly by a direct effect on receptors on airway smooth muscle, can be a result of reduced airway caliber;

2. hyperresponsiveness to hyperventilation, which is considered to act indirectly via release of chemical mediators [12], is more specific for the presence of asthma.

Both of these suggestions are supported by other recent observations. Lim and co-workers [17] have shown in a longitudinal study of smokers that the FEV_1 and PC_{20} fell together, and Woolcock and co-workers [19] have found that smokers with chronic airflow limitation, unlike asthmatics do not bronchoconstrict after inhalation of propranolol. Also, in common with other nonasthmatics [20], they demonstrated a maximal response plateau on the methacholine dose-response curve [21]. The interpretation of these discrepancies may be clarified by an examination of the cytology of the sputum or of BAL in relation to these clinical characteristics.

References

1. Fletcher, C. M., J. B. L. Howell, J. Pepys, and J. G. Scadding. 1971. Addendum. Report of the working group on the definition of asthma. In Identification of asthma. Ciba Foundation. Study Group No. 38. R. Porter, and J. Birch, eds. Edinburgh and London: Churchill Livingstone, p. 172.

2. Scadding, J. G. 1983. Definition and clinical categories of asthma. In: Asthma (2nd ed.) T. J. H. Clark and S. Godfrey, eds. Cambridge: Chapman and Hall Ltd., p. 1.

3. Hargreave, F. E., E. H. Ramsdale, J. G. Kirby, and P. M. O'Byrne. 1986. Asthma and the role of inflammation. Eur. J. Respir. Dis. 69 (Suppl 147): 16.

4. Ramsdale, E. H., M. M. Morris, R. S. Roberts, and F. E. Hargreave. 1985. Asymptomatic bronchial hyperresponsiveness in rhinitis. J. Allergy. Clin. Immunol. 75: 573.

5. Adelroth, E., F. E. Hargreave, and E. H. Ramsdale. 1986. Do physicians need objective measurements to diagnose asthma? Am. Rev. Respir. Dis. 134: 704.

6. Woolcock, A. J., J. K. Peat, C. M. Salome, K. Yan, S. D. Anderson, R. E. Schoeffel, G. McCowage, and T. Killalea. 1987. Prevalence of bronchial hyperresponsiveness and asthma in a rural adult population. Thorax 42: 361.

7. Ramsdale, E. H., R. S. Roberts, M. M. Morris, and F. E. Hargreave. 1985. Differences in responsiveness to hyperventilation and methacholine in asthma and chronic bronchitis. Thorax 40: 422.

8. Kirby, J. G., F. E. Hargreave, G. J. Gleich, and P. M. O'Byrne. 1987. Bronchoalveolar lavage cell profiles of asthmatic and nonasthmatic subjects. Am. Rev. Respir. Dis. 136: 379.

9. Wardlaw, A. J., S. Dunnett, G. J. Gleich, J. V. Collins, and A. B. Kay. 1988. Eosinophils and mast cells in bronchoalveolar lavage in subjects with mild asthma. Relationship to bronchial hyperreactivity. Am. Rev. Respir. Dis. 137: 62.

10. Otsuka, H., J. A. Denburg, J. Dolovich, D. Hitch, P. Lapp, R. S. Rajan, J. Bienenstock, and D. Befus. 1985. Heterogeneity of metachromatic cells in human nose: significance of mucosal mast cells. J. Allergy Clin. Immunol. 76: 695.

11. Otsuka, H., J. Dolovich, D. Befus, S. Telizyn, J. Bienenstock, and J. A. Denburg. 1986. Basophilic cell progenitors, nasal metachromatic cells, and peripheral blood basophils in ragweed-allergic patients. J. Allergy Clin. Immunol. 78: 365.

12. Otsuka, H., J. Dolovich, M. Richardson, J. Bienenstock, and J. A. Denburg. 1987. Metachromatic cell progenitors and specific growth and differentiation factors in human nasal mucosa and polyps. 136: 710.

13. Bahous, J., A. Cartier, G. Ouimet, L. Pineau, and J.-L. Malo. 1984. Nonallergic bronchial hyperexcitability in chronic bronchitis. Am. Rev. Respir. Dis. 129: 216.

14. Ramsdale, E. H., M. M. Morris, R. S. Roberts, and F. E. Hargreave. 1984. Bronchial responsiveness to methacholine in chronic bronchitis: relationship to airflow obstruction and cold air responsiveness. Thorax 39: 912.

15. Yan, K., C. M. Salome, and A. J. Woolcock. 1985. Prevalence and nature of bronchial hyperresponsiveness in subjects with chronic obstructive pulmonary disease. Am. Rev. Respir. Dis. 132: 25.

16. Mullen, J. B. M., B. R. Wiggs, J. L. Wright, J. C. Hogg, and P. D. Pare. 1986. Nonspecific airway reactivity in cigarette smokers. Relationship to airway pathology and baseline lung function. Am. Rev. Respir. Dis 133: 120.

17. Lim, T. K., R. G. Taylor, A. Watson, H. Joyce, and N. B. Pride. 1988. Changes in bronchial responsiveness to inhaled histamine over four years in

middle aged male smokers and ex-smokers. Thorax 43: 599.

18. Pauwels, R., G. Joos, and M. van der Straeten. 1988. Bronchial hyperresponsiveness is not bronchial hyperresponsiveness is not bronchial asthma. Clin. Allergy 18: 317.

19. Woolcock, A. J., W. Cheung, and C. Salome. 1986. Relationship between bronchial responsiveness to propranolol and histamine. Am. Rev. Respir. Dis. 132: A177.

20. Sterk, P. J., E. E. Daniel, N. Zamel, and F. E. Hargreave. 1985. Limited bronchoconstriction to methacholine using partial flow-volume curves in nonasthmatic subjects. Am. Rev. Respir. Dis. 132: 272.

21. Du Toit, J. I., A. J. Woolcock, C. M. Salome, R. Sundrum, and J. L. Black. 1986. Characteristics of bronchial hyperresponsiveness in smokers with chronic air-flow limitation. Am. Rev. Respir. Dis. 134: 498.

Bronchial Hyperresponsiveness in Clinical Asthma

*Romain A. Pauwels**

Patients with asthma have an increased responsiveness to many different stimuli. The mechanisms involved in the acute bronchoconstrictor response can be divided into direct smooth muscle activation and the triggering of intermediary cells such as neurons and inflammatory cells. Methacholine and histamine may act directly on bronchial smooth muscle when given by inhalation. Other stimuli such as exercise, distilled water, propranolol, adenosine, neurokinin A, etc., act partially via indirect mechanisms. A distinction between direct and indirect bronchial responsiveness may be useful in the study of the relationship between bronchial responsiveness and clinical asthma. Histamine and/or methacholine responsiveness are related to the diurnal variation in peak flow and the need for anti-asthmatic medication in asthmatics. Epidemiological studies suggest however that the correlation between histamine hyperresponsiveness and the presence of clinical asthma is rather poor. Studies on the effect of drugs on bronchial hyperresponsiveness must take into account the two types of bronchial hyperresponsiveness. Further investigations are necessary to judge the clinical value of different agents for the assessment of bronchial responsiveness.

Bronchial hyperresponsiveness to several non-allergic stimuli is a major physiopathological characteristic of bronchial asthma [1]. There is a good correlation between the responsiveness to histamine and the diurnal variation in Peak Expiratory Flow Rate, and between the methacholine or histamine responsiveness and the severity of the asthmatic disease in asthmatic patients [2, 3]. A reduction of the nonspecific bronchial hyperresponsiveness is therefore generally accepted to be a rational goal in the treatment of bronchial asthma. The present paper discusses the relationship between bronchial hyperresponsiveness and clinical asthma on the one hand, and reviews the possibilities of therapeutic modulation of the nonspecific bronchial hyperresponsiveness on the other.

The first question that can be raised is the following: Can we equate clinical asthma with airway hyperresponsiveness? The answer is evidently no. Several studies have observed that there is an overlap in histamine or methacholine responsiveness between asthmatic and nonasthmatic subjects. Studies in a small number of individuals had already demonstrated the presence of asthma in the absence of an increased airway responsiveness to histamine or acetylcholine [5].

Epidemiological studies have now demonstrated that there is indeed a rather poor correlation between the epidemiology of bronchial hyperresponsiveness to methacholine or histamine and the epidemiology of asthma. In a study on 815 9-year-old children in New Zealand, Sears et al. [6] observed that 8% of the children had no respiratory symptoms despite an increased airway responsiveness to methacholine. 35% of the children with current or previous wheezing did not respond to any dose of methacholine. When the children with bronchial hyperresponsiveness but without symptoms were reinvestigated two years later, 50% were no longer hyperresponsive, 25 had a decreased level of responsiveness, and less than 20% had developed symptoms of asthma.

Salome et al. [7] explored the relationship between bronchial hyperresponsiveness to histamine, respiratory symptoms, and diagnosed bronchial asthma in a group of 2363 school children aged 8 to 11 years; 17.9% of all children had bronchial hyperresponsiveness. However, 37% of the hyperresponsive children had no symptoms or a previous diagnosis of asthma, and 5.6% of all children had a diagnosis of asthma but had no bronchial hyperresponsiveness.

Josephs et al. [8] did not find any significant relationship between bronchial responsiveness to methacholine and baseline airway caliber, diurnal variation in peak expiratory flow rate, or symptom score in 19 asthmatics who were followed up over a period of 2 to 18 months.

The second question that we may ask is then: Can we find a method to assess bronchial responsiveness that correlates better with clinical

---

*   Department of Respiratory Diseases, University Hospital, De Pintelaan 185, B-9000 Ghent, Belgium.

asthma? There is no answer at the moment to this question, though ongoing studies may soon yield relevant data. What are the options? In asthmatics acute bronchoconstriction can be provoked by several stimuli including allergens, exercise, cold air, fog, air pollutants, cigarette smoke, the intake of drugs such as aspirin, etc. The mechanisms involved in the acute bronchial response to these triggers are partially understood. The bronchoconstrictor response to different stimuli is mediated via interaction with receptors situated on the bronchial smooth muscle cells, or with receptors on inflammatory cells such as mast cells and macrophages leading to the liberation of mediators that act on the smooth muscle cells or nerve receptors, or by stimulation of the sensory nerve receptors leading to local axon reflexes or vagally mediated central nervous reflexes. In vitro investigations in humans have shown that there are interindividual differences in the responsiveness of isolated bronchial smooth muscle, but that these differences cannot explain the hyperresponsiveness in asthmatics. There is in most studies a very poor correlation between in vivo and in vitro responsiveness of the airways [9–12].

It is easily conceivable that most of the stimuli causing symptoms in asthmatics do not act directly on the bronchial smooth muscle cell. The mucosa and the submucosa act as a barrier between the inspired air and the bronchial smooth muscle layer. Damage to the epithelium may cause a better penetration of stimuli in the airway wall [13]. Many bronchoconstrictor stimuli act indirectly, either by activation of mast cells and other inflammatory cells or by stimulating irritant receptors and causing nervous reflexes. There are at least two types of reflexes involved: the local axon reflex and the central vagally mediated reflex. The local axon reflex arises by stimulation of a sensory nerve ending and the antidromical release of one or more transmitters from axon collaterals [14]. The transmitters of these axon reflexes are not known, but there are reasons to believe that both neuropeptides and adenosine may be involved. The presence of neuropeptides, such as substance P and neurokinin A, and of nucleosides, more specifically ATP that is rapidly degraded to adenosine upon release, has been demonstrated in neurons of the airways [15, 16]. Neuropeptides, including neurokinin A, cause bronchoconstriction both in experimental animals and in humans [17, 18]. Adenosine has been shown to cause bronchoconstriction in rats and in asthmatic patients [19, 20]. There is now evidence that both the neuropeptides and adenosine cause bronchoconstriction by an interaction with specific receptors on vagal nerve endings and mast cells. The simultaneous release of acetylcholine from nerve endings and smooth muscle constricting agents from mast cells causes a synergistic bronchoconstriction. The influence of various pharmacological agents on the bronchoconstriction induced by different nonspecific stimuli supports the hypothesis of a role for inflammatory cells and the vagal nerve as opposed to a direct effect on smooth muscle cells [21]. There is in general a good correlation between bronchial responsiveness to histamine and to methacholine [22]. The bronchial responsiveness to methacholine is less well or rather poorly correlated to the bronchial responsiveness to exercise [23, 24, 25], distilled water [26], propranolol [27], adenosine [28], bradykinin [29], or neurokinin A [30]. We therefore suggest that in studies on the relationship between asthmatic symptoms and bronchial responsiveness and in studies on the effect of anti-asthmatic drugs, a distinction should be made between the so-called direct and indirect bronchial responsiveness. We define direct responsiveness as the bronchial reaction to agents that act directly on bronchial smooth muscle cells, e.g., methacholine; indirect bronchial responsiveness involves besides the smooth muscle cell other cell types such as mast cells and neurons. Adenosine-monophosphate, bradykinin, neurokinin A, propranolol, distilled water, hyperventilation of cold air and exercise are challenges that probably involve indirect mechanisms. The acute symptoms in asthma are seldom related to a direct activation of the bronchial smooth muscle cell. Although further studies are clearly needed, we would predict that the day-to-day symptoms in asthma will probably be more related to indirect bronchial responsiveness than to direct responsiveness [8].

We also suggest that measurements of indirect bronchial responsiveness should be included in studies on the short- and long-term effects of drugs on bronchial hyperresponsiveness. Published data illustrate the usefulness of this concept. Single-dose treatment with sodium cromoglycate inhibits exercise-induced bronchoconstriction, but has nearly no effect on histamine or methacholine responsiveness [31, 32]. One month of treatment with inhaled steroids significantly attenuates the exercise-induced bronchoconstriction, though a prolonged treatment with high doses of steroids is necessary to obtain a moderate decrease of the bronchial responsiveness to histamine [33, 34]. After 4 weeks of treatment with 1 mg of inhaled budesonide per day, there is no correlation between the inhibitory activity of this treatment on the exercise-induced bronchoconstriction and the modification of the histamine responsiveness [R. Dahl: personal communication].

The third question relevant to the topic of this paper is: How might treatment affect bronchial responsiveness? Clinical, epidemiological, and experimental data suggest that the bronchial responsiveness is determined both by genetic and exogenous factors. The degree of bronchial responsiveness is not fixed and is modulated by various exogenous factors. Airway inflammation has been hypothesized to play an important role in the modulation of nonspecific bronchial responsiveness, and in particular neutrophils, eosinophils, and platelets have been put forward as cells involved in this process [35, 36, 37]. The role of inflammation in the pathogenesis of bronchial hyperresponsiveness is suggested by the following observations: Factors known to increase bronchial responsiveness such as viral infections, exposure to air pollutants, allergens or occupational agents are inducing airway inflammation; steroids, potent antiinflammatory agents, reduce the bronchial responsiveness in asthmatics; airway inflammation is a common pathological feature in asthmatics [38].

Drugs may modify the airway responsiveness either by inhibiting the acute airway response to bronchoconstrictory stimuli or by preventing and decreasing the airway inflammation and the associated increase in airway responsiveness. Many investigators have studied the effect of anti-asthmatic drugs on the acute bronchoconstrictor reaction to different stimuli, including the indirect stimuli (Table 1). The effect of anti-asthmatic drugs on airway inflammation and nonspecific bronchial responsiveness is presently the subject of intensive research in various centers. The late asthmatic reaction is a valuable model for the investigation of the effect of drugs on the inflammatory response in the airways. The late asthmatic reaction is characterized by the development of airway inflammation and an increased responsiveness to histamine and methacholine [39–42]. Steroids inhibit the late reaction following allergen challenge [43]. Both sodium cromoglycate and nedocromil sodium have been shown to inhibit the late asthmatic reaction [44–45]. Adachi et al. [46] demonstrated that ketotifen in rather high doses also inhibits the late asthmatic reaction following allergen challenge. We have demonstrated that theophylline at therapeutic serum concentrations has only a marginal effect on the immediate bronchoconstriction following allergen challenge, but completely inhibits the late reaction [47]. All these clinical data suggest that several anti-asthmatic drugs may have an effect on airway inflammation. Cockcroft [48] recently demonstrated that sodium cromoglycate and inhaled steroids—but not sympathomimetics—prevent the increase in bronchial responsiveness following the late asthmatic reaction.

It has been repeatedly shown that steroids, either inhaled or taken orally, reduce bronchial hyperresponsiveness in asthmatics [49–50]. This effect is not very impressive but certainly significant. Sodium cromoglycate and nedocromil sodium have been shown to pre-

Table 1. Inhibitory effect of drugs on the bronchoconstrictor activity of different stimuli.

Drug	Exercise	Osmotic	SO_2	Cold air	Adenosine	NKA	Propranolol
Sympathomimetics	++++	+++	+++	+++			
Theophylline	++	++		++	+++		
Anticholinergics	+	++	+++	++	±	±	+
Steroids	-/+++						
SCG	+++	+++	+++	+++	+++		+++
Nedocromil	+++	+++	+++	+++	+++	+++	
Ketotifen	++	++		++			
H_1-antagonists	++				++		

vent the seasonal increase in bronchial responsiveness observed in pollen asthmatics [51–52]. Ketotifen has been shown to decrease the responsiveness to acetylcholine in asthmatic patients allergic to house dust mite [53].

No study has yet looked in asthmatics at the relationship between the therapeutic effect on airway inflammation, on nonspecific bronchial responsiveness, and on clinical symptoms and outcome. The tools for performing such a study are becoming available. We may, therefore, expect that in the coming years the answer to the fourth question—Is there a link between airway inflammation, bronchial hyperresponsiveness, and clinical asthma?—will be given.

References

1. Nadel, J., R. Pauwels, and P. D. Snashall. 1987. Bronchial hyperresponsiveness. Osford: Blackwell Sci. Publ.

2. Hargreave, F. E., G. Ryan, N. C. Thomson, P. M. O'Byrne, K. Laitinen, E. F. Juniper, and J. Dolovich. 1981. Bronchial responsiveness to histamine or methacholine in asthma: Measurement and clinical significance. J. Allergy Clin. Immunol. 68: 347.

3. Woolcock, A. 1988. Asthma. In: Textbook of respiratory medicine. J. F. Murray and J. A. Nadel, eds. Philadelphia: W. B. Saunders Co., p. 1030.

4. Townley, R. G., and R. J. Hopp. 1988. Measurement and interpretation of nonspecific bronchial reactivity. Chest 94: 452.

5. Stanescu, D. C., and A. Frans. 1982. Bronchial asthma without increased airway reactivity. Eur. J. Respir. Dis. 63: 5.

6. Sears, M. 1986. Epidemiology of asthma. In: Recent advances in respiratory medicine. D. Flenley, D. and T. Petty, eds. 4: 1.

7. Salome, C. M., J. K. Peat, W. J. Britton, and A. J. Woolcock. 1987. Bronchial responsiveness in two populations of Australian school children. I. Relation to respiratory symptoms and diagnosed asthma. Clin. Allergy 17: 271.

8. Josephs, I. K., I. Gregg, D. J. G. Bain, and S. T. Holgate. 1987. A longitudinal study of non-specific bronchial responsiveness in asthma. Thorax 42: 711.

9. Vincenc, K. S., J. L. Black, K. Yan, C. L. Armour, P. D. Donnelly, an dA. J. Woolcock. 1983. Comparison of in vivo and in vitro responses to histamine in human airways. Am. Rev. Respir. Dis. 128: 875.

10. Roberts, J. A., D. Raeburn, I. W. Rodger, and N. C. Thomson. 1984. Comparison of in vivo airway responsiveness and in vitro smooth muscle

11. Goldie, R. G., D. Spina, P. J. Henry, K. M. Lulich, and J. W. Paterson. 1986. In vitro responsiveness of human asthmatic bronchus to carbachol, histamine, beta-adrenergic agonists and theophylline. Br. J. Clin. Pharmac. 22: 669.

12. Cerrina, J., M. Le Roy Ladurie, C. Labat, B. Raffestin, A. Bayol, and C. Brink. 1986. Comparison of human bronchial muscle responses to histamine in vivo with histamine and isoproterenol agonists in vitro. Am. Rev. Respir. Dis. 134: 57.

13. Laitinen, L. A., M. Heino, A. Laitinen, T. Kava, and T. Haahtela. 1985. Damage of the airway epithelium and bronchial reactivity in patients with asthma. Am. Rev. Respir. Dis. 131: 599.

14. Barnes, P. J. 1986. Asthma as an axon reflex. Lancet i: 242.

15. Martling, C. R., E. Theodorsson-Norheim, and J. M. Lundberg. 1987. Occurrence and effects of multiple tachykinins: SP, NKA and NPK in human lower airways. Life Sci. 40: 1633.

16. Burnstock, G. 1986. Purines as cotransmitters in adrenergic and cholinergic neurones. In: Progress in Brain Research, Vol. 68. T. Hökfelt et al., eds. Amsterdam: Elsevier, p. 193.

17. Joos, K., J. Kips, R. Pauwels, and M. Van Der Straeten. 1986. The effect of tachykinins on the conducting airways of the rat. Arch. Int. Pharmacodyn. Suppl 280: 176.

18. Joos, G., R. Pauwels, and M. Van Der Straeten. 1987. Effect of inhaled substance P and neurokinin A on the airways of normal and asthmatic subjects. Thorax 42: 779.

19. Pauwels, R., and M. Van Der Straeten. 1987. An animal model for the adenosine induced bronchoconstriction. Am. Rev. Respir. Dis. 136: 374.

20. Cushley, M. J., A. E. Tattersfield, and S. T. Holgate. 1984. Adenosine-induced bronchoconstriction in asthma. Am. Rev. Respir. Dis. 129: 380.

21. Pauwels, R., Joos, G., and Van Der Straeten, M. 1988. Bronchial hyperresponsiveness is not bronchial hyperresponsiveness is not bronchial asthma. Clin. Allergy 18: 317.

22. Juniper, E. F., P. A. Frith, C. Dunnett, D. W. Cockcroft, and F. E. Hargreave. 1978. Reproducibility and comparison of responses to inhaled histamine and methacholine. Thorax 33: 705.

23. Anderton, R. C., M. T. Cuff, P. A. Frith, D. W. Cockcroft, J. C. L. Morse, N. L. Jones, and F. E. Hargreave. 1979. Bronchial responsiveness to inhaled histamine and exercise. J. Allergy Clin. Immunol. 63: 315.

24. Eggleston, P. A. 1979. A comparison of the asthmatic response to methacholine and exercise. J. Allergy Clin. Immunol. 63: 104.

25. Neijens, H. J., T. Wesselius, and K. F. Kerrebijn. 1981. Exercise-induced bronchoconstriction as an expression of bronchial hyperreactivity: A

study of its mechanisms in children. Thorax 36: 517.

26. Anderson, S. A., and R. E. Scoeffel. 1985. The inhalation of ultrasonically nebulized aerosols as a provocation test for asthma. In: Airway responsiveness. F. E. Hargreave and A. J. Woolcock, eds. Mississauga: Astra Pharmaceuticals Canada Ltd., p. 39.

27. Foresi, A., A. Chetta, G. M. Corbo, A. Cuomo, and D. Olivieri. 1987. Provocative dose and dose-response curve to inhaled propranolol in asthmatic subjects with bronchial hyperresponsiveness to methacholine. Chest 92: 455.

28. Mann, J. S., S. T. Holgate, A. G. Renwick, and M. J. Cushley. 1986. Airway effects of purine nucleosides and nucleotides and release with bronchial provocation in asthma. J. Appl. Physiol. 62: 1667.

29. Fuller, R. W., C. M. S. Dixon, F. M. C. Cuss, and P. J. Barnes. 1987. Bradykinin-induced bronchoconstriction in humans. Am. Rev. Respir. Dis. 135: 176.

30. Joos, G. 1988. The role of neuropeptides in the pathogenesis of asthma. Ph.D. Thesis, University of Ghent.

31. Davies, S. E. 1968. Effect of disodium cromoglycate on exercise-induced asthma. Brit. Med. J. 3: 593.

32. Lemire, I., A. Cartier, J. Malo, L. Pineau, H. Ghezzo, and R. R. Martin. 1984. Effect of sodium cromoglycate on histamine inhalation tests. J. Allergy Clin. Immunol. 73: 234.

33. Henriksen, J. M., and R. Dahl. 1983. Effects of inhaled budesonide alone and in combination with low-dose terbutaline in children with exercise-induced asthma. Am. Rev. Respir. Dis. 128: 993.

34. Kerrebijn, K. F., E. E. M. van Essen-Zandvliet, and H. Neijens. 1987. Effect of long-term treatment with inhaled corticosteroids and beta-agonists on the bronchial responsiveness in children with asthma. J. Allergy Clin. Immunol. 79: 653.

35. Nadel, J. A. 1984. Inflammation and asthma. J. Allergy Clin. Immunol. 73: 651.

36. Wardlaw, A. J., and A. B. Kay. 1987. The role of the eosinophil in the pathogenesis of asthma. Allergy 42: 321.

37. Morley, J., S. Sanjar, and C. P. Page. 1984. The platelet in asthma. Lancet ii: 1142.

38. Hogg, J. C. 1985. The pathology of asthma. In: Glucocorticosteroids, inflammation and bronchial hyperreactivity. J. C. Hogg, R. Ellul-Micalef, and R. Brattsand, eds. Amsterdam: Excerpta Medica, pp. 3"10.

39. De Monchy, J. G. R., H. F. Kaufmann, P. Venge, G. H. Koëter, H. M. Jansen, J. H. Sluiter, and K. de Vries. 1985. Bronchoalveolar eosinophilia during allergen induced late asthmatic reactions. Am. Rev. Respir. Dis. 131: 373.

40. Metzger, W. J., H. B. Richerson, K. Worden, M. Monick, and G. W. Hunninghake. 1986. Bronchoalveolar lavage of allergic asthmatic patients following allergen bronchoprovocation. Chest 89: 477.

41. Cockcroft, D. W., R. E. Ruffin, J. Dolovich, and F. E. Hargreave. 1977. Allergen induced increase in non-allergic bronchial reactivity. Clin. Allergy 7: 503.

42. Cartier, A., M. C. Thomson, P. A. Frith, R. Roberts, and F. E. Hargreave. 1982. Allergen-induced increase in bronchial responsiveness to histamine: Relationship to the late asthmatic response and change in airway caliber. J. Allergy Clin. Immunol. 70: 170.

43. Booij-Noord, H., N. G. M. Orie, and K. de Vries. 1971. Immediate and late bronchial obstructive reactions to inhalation of house dust and protective effects of disodium cromoglycate and prednisolone. J. Allergy Clin. Immunol. 48: 344.

44. Pepys, J., F. E. Hargreave, M. Chan, and D. S. McCarthy. 1968. Inhibitory effects of disodium cromoglycate on allergen- inhalation tests. Lancet ii: 134.

45. Dahl, R., and B. Pedersen. 1986. Influence of nedocromil sodium on the dual asthmatic reaction after allergen challenge: A double-blind, placebo-controlled study. Eur. J. Respir. Dis. 69 (Suppl. 147): 263.

46. Adachi, M., H. Kobayashi, N. Aoki, M. Iijima, F. Kokubu, A. Furuya, and T. Takahashi. 1984. A comparison of the inhibitory effects of ketotifen and disodium cromoglycate on bronchial response to house dust, with special reference to the late asthmatic reaction. Pharmatherapeutica 4: 36.

47. Pauwels, R., D. Van Renterghem, M. Van Der Straeten, N. Johannesson, and C. G. A. Persson. 1985. The effect of theophylline and enprofylline on allergen-induced bronchoconstriction. J. Allergy Clin. Immunol. 76: 583.

48. Cockcroft, D. W., and K. Y. Murdock. 1987. Comparative effects of inhaled salbutamol, sodium cromoglycate and beclomethasone dipropionate on allergen-induced early asthmatic responses, late asthmatic responses, and increased bronchial responsiveness to histamine. J. Allergy Clin. Immunol. 79: 734.

49. Sotomayor, H., M. Badier, D. Vervloet, and J. Orehek. 1984. Seasonal increase of carbachol airway responsiveness in patients allergic to grass pollen. Am. Rev. Respir. Dis. 130: 56.

50. Kraan, J., G. H. Koëter, T. W. van de Mark, H. J. Sluiter, and K. de Vries. 1985. Changes in bronchial hyperreactivity induced by 4 weeks of treatment with antiasthmatic drugs in patients with allergic asthma: A comparison between budesonide and terbutaline. J. Allergy Clin. Immunol. 765: 628.

187

51. Löwhagen, O., and S. Rak. 1985. Modification of bronchial hyperreactivity after treatment with sodium cromoglycate during pollen season. J. Allergy Clin. Immunol. 75: 460.

51. Altounyan, R. E. C., M. Cole, and T. B. Lee. 1986. Effect of nedocromil sodium on changes in bronchial hyperreactivity in non- asthmatic, atopic rhinitic patients during the grass pollen season. Eur. J. Respir. Dis. 69 (Suppl. 147): 271.

52. Dorward, A. J., J. A. Roberts, and N. C. Thomson. 1986. A preliminary report on the effect of nedocromil sodium on histamine airway responsiveness in patients allergic to grass pollen. Eur. J. Respir. Dis. 69 (Suppl. 147): 299.

52. Girard, J. P. 1981. Ketotifen and bronchial hyperreactivity in asthmatic patients. Clin. Allergy 11: 449.

Relationship Between Bronchial Hyperreactivity to Cold Air and Blood IgE Levels and Eosinophils in an Asthmatic Population

Leonardo Greiding, Guachalla Castro, Emilio J. A. Roldán*

Bronchial hyperreactivity (BHR) is considered as "a severe alteration of bronchomotor tone, measured as changes produced in certain functions related to resistance of the airway" [1]. Asthma is the pathology most closely related to BHR. Several drugs, such as metacholine, histamine, leukotriene, PAF, etc., as well as physical factors, such as distilled water, physical exercise, hyperventilation, cold air ventilation, etc., have proved to cause BHR. In our environment (Buenos Aires City), temperature changes are very frequent, so asthmatic patients undergo deterioration of their disease during lower temperature periods.Under experimental conditions, BHR was studies in 47 atopic asthmatic patients with a cold-air generator ($-15\,°C$ to $-20\,°C$). Decreases with respect to values of FEV 1 or FEF 25–75 above 10% from baseline were considered positive, and patients responding with decreases below 10% were considered non-responders, by means of an isocapnic maximum inspiratory ventilation test, with 8 breaths per minute. IgE (IU/ml) and eosinophils (cells/mm^3) blood values were related to BHR indexes. For this purpose, patients were classified in accordance with their BHR to cold air as follows:

1. non-responders,
2. responders with decreases ranging from 10– 20%,
3. responders with decreases from 21% to 30%,
4. responders with decreases of more than 31%.

The following results were obtained:

1. non-responders (n=18): eosinophils 399 ± 86; IgE 310.2 ± 85;
2. responders 10–20% (n=13): eosinophils 334 ± 131, IgE 388 ± 172;
3. responders 21–30% (n=9): eosinophils 431 ± 194, IgE 448 ± 105;
4. responders above 31% (n=7): eosinophils 684 ± 181, IgE 567 ± 276.

Correlation coefficient of the mean values, according to Kendall's partial tests, gave the following statistical results: 1.0 between BHR and IgE and 0.67 between BHR and eosinophils. Therefore, in our atopic asthmatic population, exacerbation of BHR because of cold temperature is parallel to higher IgE and eosinophilia. Thus, it is supposed that maximum control of allergic inflammation will reduce spontaneous BHR from cold temperature.

In asthmatic patients, bronchoobstructive response can be obtained by means of specific agents when it is challenged with the related antigen; by unspecific elements when chemical agents are used, such as histamine, metacholine (the most frequent); by physical activities, such as physical exercise; by distilled water or by cold air inhalation.

This bronchoobstructive response can be quantified by means of several functional procedures, measurement of FEV 1 and FEF 25–75 decreases being the most frequent.

In this study, we evaluated the relationship between intensity in FEV 1 and FEF 25–75 decreases and IgE and eosinophilia blood levels after exposure to cold air, in samples taken at provocation time from atopic asthmatic patients.

The study of this relationship was undertaken because of the frequent clinical observation that, in a climate like that in Buenos Aires, sudden temperature drops often provoke asthma attacks in patients, some of them being atopic of extrinsic asthmatic one. We also wanted to study the role of eosinophils as an inflammatory-cytotoxic factor.

Methods

Selection of Patients

A total of 47 atopic asthmatic patients who agreed to take part in this trial were selected, taking into consideration their family and per-

---

*   Argentine Institute of Allergy and Immunology, Medrano 291, 1178 Buenos Aires, Argentina.

189

sonal history; they presented with at least two intense reactions to 20 of the most common allergens in a prick test and had an IgE value of more than 2 SD from mean of a normal population, according to age.

Patients were told not to use bronchodilators 24 h before commencement of the study; corticoids and teophylline intake as well as topic corticoids or CGDS application were to be suspended 48 h before the study. Patients were free from respiratory infections for at least 21 days.

Cold Air Generator

This consisted of an iron-clad motor compressor of 1/5 power, an air-refrigerated condensation battery, an evaporator with a serpentine immersed into 6 l of ethylenglycol, liquid acting as cold transmission to the 20 l deposit, which had a natural air entrance, with a filter and a with 4 cm^2 exit tube. In the cold air expulsion tube, there was a thermometer measuring the air temperature at a distance of 7 cm from the patient's mouth. This temperature ranged from –15 °C to –20 °C (Figure 1).

Spirography

Basal spirographic values, which were never less than 65% of the expected ones, were estimated by means of a computerized spirograph, Vitalograf brand, Compact model.

VC, FEV 1, and FEF 25–75 were recorded before cold air exposure and 10 min thereafter, with controls from the first minute to 10 min, performed every 2 min.

Provocation Method

In a previous study, hyperventilation had been used. The correlation between hyperventilation and cold air to induce bronchospasm has been demonstrated [2]. Therefore, each patient was told to inhale cold air deeply with a maximum frequency of inhalatory ventilations (VMI) per minute, for 3 min. Once maximum inhalation of cold was finished, the patients withdrew their mouth from the mouthpiece and exhaled air. This technique enabled us to determine different FEV 1 and FEF 25–75 reduction levels. Thus, in normal subjects, maximum PD reduction was 10% from the first min-

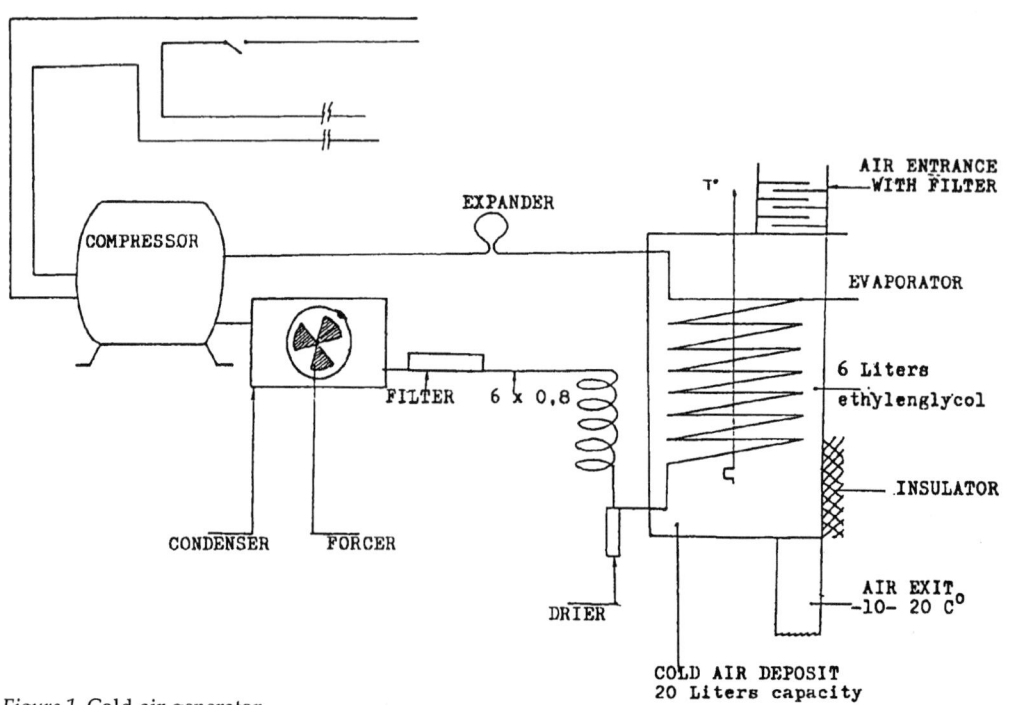

Figure 1. Cold-air generator.

Groups	% decrease of FEV 1 or FEF 25–75			
	Non-responders	Responders		
	<10	10–20	21–30	>31
Patients (n)	18	13	9	7
Eosinophils (cells/mm^3)	399	334	431	684
IgE (IU/l)	310	388	448	567
Age (yrs)	33.5	29	22	23

Table 1. Patients exposed to a cold-air generator. Response is considered as a decrease in FEV 1 or FEF 25–75 above 10% of previous values. Values of eosinophils, IgE, and age are given as means (see text for SEM).

ute of provocation up to 10 min, considering PD as that showing the maximum FEV 1 or FEF 25–75 decrease of the different controls performed, with PD as decrease percentage.

Patients were classified into four groups according to their decrease percentages or PD as follows:

— Group 1: Non-responders, with PD lower than 10

— Group 2: Responders, with PD from 10 to 20

— Group 3: Responders, with PD from 21 to 30

— Group 4: Responders, with PD higher than 31.

Blood Determination

Total IgE was calculated by means of Prist (Phadebas) Test, and eosinophilia in samples taken before the respiratory study.

Statistics

Values are given as mean ± SEM. Kendall's partial test was employed to correlate mean values of BHR response, age, IgE, and eosinophils.

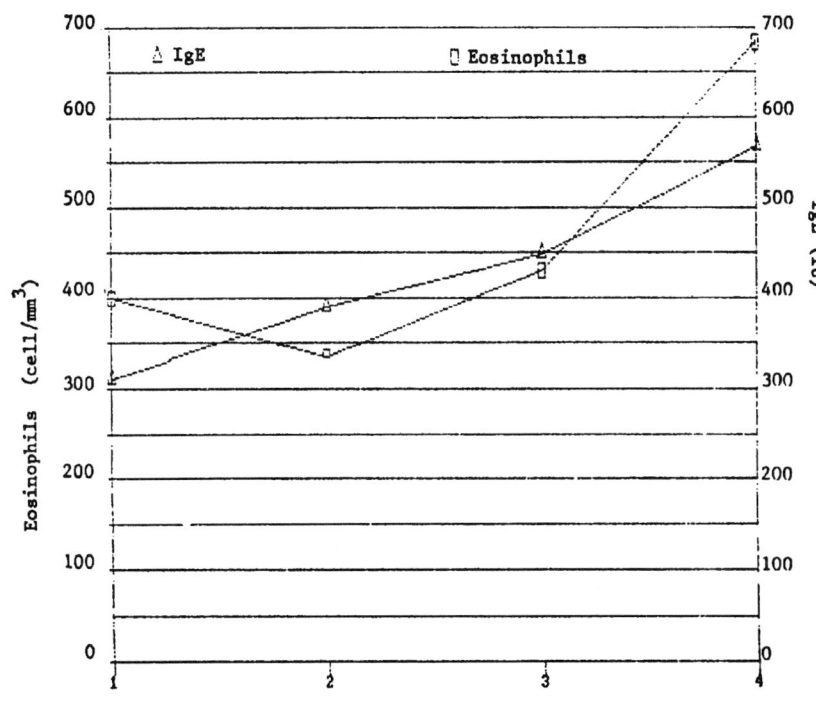

Groups of responders

Figure 2. Correlation among group of responders (see text), eosinophils and IgE values in asthmatic patients exposed to cold air.

191

Results

In group 1 (non-responders), there were 18 patients who had an eosinophils average of 399 ± 86, IgE 310 ± 85, age 33.5 ± 3.9 years.

Group 2 (responders with PD from 10 to 20) consisted of 13 patients with eosinophilia of 334 ± 131, IgE of 388 ± 172, and age of 29 ± 6.8 years.

In group 3 (responders with PD from 21 to 30), there were 9 patients, eosinophilia being 431 ± 194, IgE 448 ± 105, age 22 ± 4.4 years.

Group 4 (responders with PD higher than 31) was formed by 7 patients with eosinophilia 684 ± 181, IgE 567 ± 276, age 23 ± 4.5 years.

The statistical study determined a significant correlation between non-responders and maximum responders, with IgE 1.0 and eosinophils 0.67, and IgE/eosinophils 0.67 ($p < 0.05$ for all variables).

Discussion

BHR investigation can be carried out by means of several techniques, nebulizing pharmacological mediators such as histamine and metacholine, or others such leukotrienes, PAF, prostaglandins, etc. [1], which determined FEV 1 decrease in asthmatic patients. Nebulizations with distilled water and physical exercise are also used, but to lesser extent, in other groups, i.e., allergic rhinitic or chronic bronchial patients. Physical exercise is associated with asthma through cold air in its physiopathogenic mechanism; this technique postulates a degranulation of respiratory mucosa mast cells, determined by the hyperosmolarity produced by heat loss, which leads to evaporation of secretory liquid [1]. Several studies have established a good correlation between BHR investigation by means of cold air and that performed with metacholine or histamine, obtaining a dose-response curve with an obstruction plateau for the former [3–7].

The question is whether BHR is merely "a severe alteration of the bronchomotor tone, measured as changes produced in some functions related to resistance of the airway," or whether it evidences a related IgE reaction, which should add the immunologic aspect to the functional definition.

Fink et al. [8] have experimentally demonstrated the possibility of passive transfer from humans to monkey of the ability to respond with BHR to metacholine by injection of IgE from BHR positive patients. In addition, Souhrada [9] showed the correlation between BHR in guinea pigs and IgE response to egg albumin.

Woolcock et al. [10] demonstrated an evident correlation between atopy, familiar history of asthma, allergen exposure, and BHR degree in Australian children. Cockcroft [11] expressed the importance of allergic inflammation as a factor aggravating BHR.

Other authors mention the presence of high IgE and eosinophilia in BHR studies performed in asthmatic patients with metacholine and histamine [5, 12, 13].

We have tried to develop a simple technique, reproducing natural conditions of exposure to cold air in our patients. Since in this case we did not intend to use it for asthma diagnosis, hyperventilation was avoided because it may limit a bronchoobstructive response in asthmatic patients [2]. A maximum inhalation was sought to take the maximum cold air volume, with a slow exhalation reaching the forced vital capacity volume, in a slow frequency of 8 breaths per minute. This procedure determines wider threshold responses, so the number of non-responder patients is higher, amounting to 18 out of a total of 47 (38%), considering that the $80 \pm 10\%$ of the asthmatic population is reached with hyperventilation is used [1].

In addition, this technique usually demonstrates in non-asthmatic, non-allergic persons a PD of up to 10% during the first minutes after provocation with cold air, meaning that cold normally produces a bronchoconstriction response, soon neutralized by bronchodilator reflexes, which is not the case in asthmatic persons, who have a greater and more permanent degree of obstruction.

We divided up the population of patients into different groups of responders and non-responders, according to the PD obtained. As the relationship between FEV 1 or FEF 25–75 decrease degree was evaluated, taking the maximum PD obtained, a statistically significant correlation between provoked IgE mean level, patients' mean eosinophilia, and degree of obstruction could be observed. It should be noted that, except for age variables, eosinophils and IgE show great variability among patients, and the average values analyzed in this study may represent responses corresponding to those found in many patients but not in all. This individual variability should be studied using broader samples.

Therefore, we conclude that allergic inflammation mediated by IgE and where eosinophils become important through release of basic protein, peroxidase and neurotoxins, all conducting larger inflammation and epithelial injury, it is directly associated with the obstructive response obtained in the sample of atopic asthmatic patients.

Even though causes are multiple, we think that the presence of an atopic component, or at least of a given IgE reaction, contributes to enhance or accompany the process of spontaneous obstruction or of BHR in bronchoobstructive asthma responses and probably in those of other pathologies.

References

1. Boushey, H. 1985. Bronchial challenge by physical agents. Clin. Rev. Allergy 3: 411–426.
2. Castro, G., and L. Greiding. 1987. In: Actas XIII Congreso Nacional de Alergia e Inmunología. Greiding, Grinstein, Cortigiani, eds. pp. 270–274.
3. Heaton, R. W., A. Henderson, and J. Costello. 1986. Cold air as a bronchial provocation technique. Reproducibility and comparison with histamine and metacholine inhalation. Chest 6: 810–814.
4. O'Byrne, P., G. Ryan, M. Morris, D. McCormack, N. Jones, J. Morse, and F. Hargreave. 1982. Asthma induced by cold air and its relation to nonspecific bronchial responsiveness to metacholine. Am. Rev. Respir. Dis. 125: 281–285.
5. Witt, C., M. S. Stuckey, A. J. Woolcock, and A. L. Dawkins. 1986. Positive allergy prick tests associated with bronchial histamine responsiveness in an unselected population. J. Allergy Clin. Immunol. 77: 698–702.
6. Zach, M., and G. Polgar. 1987. Cold air challenge of airway hyperreactivity in children: Dose-response interrelation with a reaction plateau. J. Allergy Clin. Immunol. 80: 9–17.
7. Tessier, P., H. L. Ghezzo, J. Archeveque, A. Cartier, and J. Malo. 1987. Shape of the dose-response curve to cold air inhalation in normal and asthmatic subjects. Am. Rev. Respir. Dis. 136: 1416–1423.
8. Fink, J. N., D. P. Schlueter, and J. J. Barboriak. 1987. Passive transfer of metacholine sensitivity from man to monkey. J. Allergy Clin. Immunol. 79: 427–432.
9. Souhrada, M., and J. F. Souhrada. 1984. Immunologically induced alterations of airway smooth muscle cell membrane. Science 225: 723.
10. Salome, C. M., J. K. Peat, J. Britton, and A. Woolcock. 1987. Bronchial hyperresponsiveness in two populations of Australian school children. Clinical Allergy 17: 271–281.
11. Cockcroft, D. W. 1987. Airway hyperresponsiveness: Therapeutic implications. Annals of Allergy, 291–300.
12. Blecker, E. 1985. Airways reactivity and asthma. J. Allergy Clin. Immunol. 75: 21–23.
13. Burrows, B., M. D. Lebowit, and R. Barbee. 1976. Respiratory disorders and allergy skin test reactions. Ann. Intern. Med. 84: 134–139.

Childhood Asthma in the Third World

*Eugene G. Weinberg**

Varying reports of the prevalence of asthma in Third World children have appeared. In these countries the proportion of children under 15 years of age constitutes almost half of the population. The tendency toward urbanization is increasing rapidly. Childhood asthma also appears to be increasing in urban communities in underdeveloped countries.Unique problems face health professionals in the diagnosis, treatment, and prevention of asthma in the Third World. These problems, while often difficult to overcome, present a unique opportunity for research into asthma in populations previously unaffected by this disorder.

In contrast to the developed countries of the world, in which children under 15 years constitute approximately 22% of the population, in Third World countries children form 45–50% of the population. By 1990 there will be 1.5 billion Third World children under 15 years, compared to 300 million in the developed countries [1]. Urbanization is also increasing at a very rapid rate in underdeveloped countries. The health problems of these children remain overwhelmingly those of poor education, poor housing, and poor nutrition, with malnutrition and the ravages of the common infectious diseases still being rife. Increasingly, however, these children will also manifest the illnesses more prevalent in the developed countries, such as the atopic disorders and asthma. Health professionals are faced with unique problems in the diagnosis and management of asthma, but also great opportunities for studying the emergence of asthma in populations previously unaffected by this illness.

Prevalence of Asthma

The epidemiology of asthma has suffered from the absence of a widely accepted definition of the condition. Much confusion has also resulted from the many revisions to the International Classification of Diseases (ICD).

A wide variation has been reported in the prevalence of asthma in developed countries, but the average prevalence rate is thought to be approximately 5% of the childhood population [2]. Similarly widely varying rates have been reported from underdeveloped countries, though many studies are inaccurate, being based on inadequate population samples. In rural Africa the reported incidence has usually been low in young children. Asthma was virtually absent from rural communities in Gambia [3]. A similar finding was the virtual absence of childhood asthma in rural Transkei [4]. Various reasons have been sought for this low prevalence. Among factors mentioned are those of a lack of Western influence, the role of parasitic infection, lack of wind- borne pollination, a high death rate in young children, and the protective effect of breast-feeding. Areas of higher incidence occur possibly as a result of local allergies such as the green nimitti midges [5] or high housedust mite counts [6]. It is known that asthma is not uncommon among adults in the rural areas and is certainly an increasing problem among both adults and children in Third World cities. In Zaria, Nigeria, childhood asthma is hardly ever seen, but in Ibadan, the capital, there is a greater prevalence of asthma among adults and children [7]. A common feature of studies in Africa has been the reversal of the normal male to female ratio of childhood asthma [4]. This may result from exposure to allergens within the home or from chores such as grinding wheat or maize usually performed by females. Differences in asthma prevalence have also been described in New Guinea. As in Africa, the incidence in adults is often higher, and again an adult onset of disease is apparent [8].

The effect of urbanization appears to be very important to the prevalence of asthma. Comparison of asthma using exercise challenge testing in Xhosa children living in rural Transkei, South Africa, revealed only one asthmatic among 671 children. Their urbanized counter-

*   Allergy Service, Red Cross Children's Hospital and Institute of Child Health, University of Cape Town, Rondebosch 7700, South Africa.

parts in Guguletu, a township near Cape Town, had a prevalence of asthma of 3.1% [4]. In 1966, a hurricane devastated Tokelau, a group of islands in the Pacific Ocean. Half of the population went to New Zealand, where in 1975 children examined there were found to have a prevalence of asthma similar to New Zealand children. Their counterparts who had remained in Tokelau had a much lower prevalence [9]. In Birmingham, immigrants from the West Indies and Africa had a low prevalence of asthma, while their children had a similar prevalence to that of English children [10].

High asthma prevalences have been reported in several isolated island communities among adults and children. These include Tristan da Cunha [11] and the Maldives [12]. Inbreeding of the population, weather conditions and high mite exposure are thought to be responsible for the increased prevalence of asthma. The number of children presenting to the Children's Hospital in Cape Town with acute severe asthma has shown a three-fold increase over the past 10 years.

Asthma Diagnosis

The diagnosis of asthma in children from underdeveloped populations in southern Africa is not a simple process. This is especially so in recently urbanized children where social, language, and cultural barriers create many problems. The maxim becomes "All that wheezes is not asthma—especially in the African child." The diagnosis has to be made only after careful exclusion of other causes of wheezing, specifically excluding tuberculosis, pneumonia, bronchiolitis, and round worm infestation.

The usual approach to asthma diagnosis in developed countries would include a careful history, physical examination, pulmonary function tests, skin testing for common allergens, possible IgE estimation and eosinophil counts, and bronchial challenge tests. Each of these investigations presents its own problem in the populations seen at the Children's Hospital in Cape Town.

The History

This normally valuable approach to diagnosis may present unique problems. Language barriers may be considerable as in the majority of African dialects no word exists for "Asthma" or for "wheezing." Parents are not impressed by a doctor who spends a long time asking them all about their child's condition. They want to know what is wrong with their child and not to tell the doctor. They may turn to traditional healers for their child's illness.

In Third World communities, and among the urban poor in developed countries, a matriarchal society commonly occurs [13]. For various reasons, men often abandon their families. The children are reared by their mothers and grandmothers. Mothers often have to go out to work in order to survive, and the grandmother may bring the child to the hospital. Even the best of grandmothers is seldom able to give a good review of the child's illness. In addition, that valuable pointer to diagnosis, a positive family history, is frequently absent. Thus, in many cases the history is an unrewarding and often frustrating exercise.

Examination

As so often occurs, when the child is seen no wheezing may be detectable on auscultation, and testing response to bronchodilators is not possible. Valuable pointers to the fact that one is dealing with an atopic condition such as associated allergic rhinitis or atopic eczema are excessively rare in African children. Poor growth and any degree of chest deformity often bear no relation to asthma or to therapy, but are the result of poor nutrition and infections.

Specific attention must be paid to excluding other possible causes of wheezing, and tuberculosis is specifically sought and excluded. Chest radiographs are an essential component of the examination. Stool samples are examined for parasites in all cases to exclude the possibility of round worm infestation.

Pulmonary Function Tests

The apparatus used is the Wright peak flow meter and the Vitalograph spirometer. It is not difficult to teach recently urbanized or rural children from as young as 5 years to use the apparatus correctly. Some problems may arise with the interpretation of results. Reports have indicated that there is a difference in the normal values accepted for Black and White children [14]. Our practice has been to use normal tables developed in Britain and the United States, and no problems have been experienced in the interpretation of normal and abnormal pulmonary function tests.

Skin Testing

Skin tests in children with dark skin requires a great deal of experience. The procedure is often regarded as a therapeutic and not a diagnostic process by the parents and explanations have to be carefully given. There is difficulty in observing flare reactions in dark skins, and positive results depend on wheal size alone. Comparing wheal size with the histamine positive control may be difficult, since many children—for unknown reasons—do not react to the histamine control. A useful technique is to wet the skin with a damp cloth. This indicates positive sites clearly by showing up the wheals more sharply.

IgE Estimates and Eosinophil Counts

In Cape Town townships many children are infested with ascaris lumbricoides or other intestinal parasites. This makes interpretation of IgE levels and eosinophil counts extremely difficult and of dubious value. An additional problem is that normal IgE levels for African children are not available. Normal values used in Europe and derived from Scandinavian children are of little help. Ethiopian children have IgE levels many times that of Swedish children [15]. Orren and Dowdle [16], using blood donor samples, found normal IgE concentrations to be three times higher in Black compared to White adults. As total eosinophil counts are also influenced by parasitic infestation, their value as a diagnostic test in children in underdeveloped communities is also in doubt.

Tests of Bronchial Hyperreactivity

While of undoubted value in establishing or identifying the asthmatic child, metacholine, histamine, or cold-air challenge tests are too time-consuming or expensive for use in busy outpatient clinics and community health centers. Far more useful, although not as accurate, is the exercise challenge test. The child runs as fast as possible on the level for 6 minutes. A positive diagnosis is made if the post-exercise peak flow falls by 15% or more when compared to the pre-exercise value. This test is often the only way to make the diagnosis if any doubt exists. It is simple, costs nothing, and is ideal for the Third World situation.

Treatment

The usual treatment of asthmatic children includes advice about environmental control and a decision regarding the use of medication.

Environmental Control

Third World children often live in the most rudimentary housing in overcrowded poor conditions. There are often 2 or 3 children to a bed. Cooking over open fires or kerosene stoves may be done in the same room. Smoking among adults is common. The homes seldom have the benefit of electricity. Mothers of children from such environments find lectures on environmental control or instructions drawn up in developed countries on housedust control of little use. Expensive methods of avoiding housedust cannot be advised, and vacuum cleaning is simply not possible. The best method of reducing housedust mite exposure is to hang the bedding out in the sunlight as often as possible. Pillows and bedding may be stuffed with cheap foam chips instead of feathers or kapok. Changes in cooking practices such as constructing a simple outside shelter for this purpose and advising against smoking in the child's presence are also of value.

Medication

If the disadvantaged asthmatic child requires regular medication, due regard must be paid to cultural, socio-economic, and educational factors. Simply following the recommendations of First World asthma experts is not advisable. Many Third World countries have a limited budget for medicines and restrict these accordingly. It is often completely impossible to recommend a home nebulizer for patients or to use any complex inhaler systems including aerosols. Parents may be illiterate, so that graphically illustrated labeling of medicines is often of great benefit. Storage of medication is a problem, and it should be known if the medication prescribed is susceptible to change by damp conditions, heat, or sunlight. The color of medicines is important, and the opposite preferences of parents is found to that of First World countries. Thus, a great favorite would be a red or other brightly colored solution. Compliance in medication usage is also a problem. Once the child stops wheezing, there is immense difficulty in persuading the parents that ongoing medication may be essential. The simplest of medicines must be prescribed, oral medication being preferred by many. It is always best to use treatment twice a day if possible. Once frequency of medication has to be increased, compliance in administration falls off greatly.

Special nurses are employed in all clinics to aid in the training of asthmatic children in medication usage. They follow these children at home and monitor their correct usage of medications. Children are taught to use their medicines independently of parental supervision. Much effort goes into the education of both parents and children as to the nature and treatment of asthma through illustrated booklets.

Asthma Deaths

As in other parts of the world, and especially New Zealand [17], an increase in the number of young people dying of asthma has also been experienced in Cape Town [18]. Unfortunately, several of these patients came from the less affluent section of the population. Reduced access to medical services and the expense of services are important factors. A problem here, as elsewhere, is that many asthmatics go undiagnosed or undertreated [19].

Patients with severe asthma, those on regular steroid therapy, and those with a history of frequent presentation with acute severe asthma to the Children's Hospital are given the right to "patient self-admission." They are monitored at home using diary cards and daily recording of their peak-flow readings. Very helpful has been the establishment of small clinics and Day Hospitals situated close to the homes of the children where access to nebulized bronchodilators and other therapy is available on a round-the-clock basis.

Prediction and Prevention of Asthma

The use of cord blood IgE levels as a predictor of atopy is of no value in Black South African infants [20]. The lack of early warning signs in these infants, such as atopic eczema, is an additional problem. More is to be learnt from these children when comparing urban and rural counterparts. How is it possible that the rural Xhosa child, who lives in a mud hut with a thatched roof and dung floor with animals roaming in and out and a fire burning day and night, does not develop asthma? One important difference is that these children are not exposed to housedust mites. They sleep on mats that are aired in the sun daily in which no mites are to be found. In Cape Town children sleep on mattresses, and mites are found on every mattress.

The role of breast-feeding in the prevention of allergy and asthma may be important. Rural Xhosa mothers all breast-feed their infants, compared to only 70% of their urban counterparts [4]. There is also a tendency for urban mothers to breast-feed for a much shorter period than do rural mothers. Another important initiating factor may be routine pertussis immunization [21].

The diagnosis and management of childhood asthma in an underdeveloped country presents its own unique problems but also great opportunities. Pliny said "Ex Africa semper aliquid novi." The children of Africa can teach us much about the development of asthma in communities previously free of this illness. These factors, once identified, could possibly be avoided in both developed and underdeveloped communities to the ultimate benefit of all.

References

1. Morley, D., and H. Lovel. 1986. My name is today. London: Macmillan.

2. Cookson, J. B. 1987. Prevalence rates of asthma in developing countries and their comparison with those in Europe and North America. Chest. 91: 97.
3. Godfrey, R. C. 1975. Asthma and IgE levels in rural and urban communities in Gambia. Clin Allergy 5: 201.
4. Van Niekerk, C. H., E. G. Weinberg, S. C. Shore, H. de V. Heese, and D. J. Van Scalkwyk. 1979. Prevalence of asthma: A comparative study of urban and rural Xhosa children. Clin Allergy. 9: 319.
5. Kay, A. B., C. M. U. Maclean, A. H. Wilkinson, and M. O. Gad el Rab. 1983. The prevalence of asthma and rhinitis in a Sudanese community seasonally exposed to a potent airborne allergen (the "green nimitti" midge: *cladotanytarsus lewisi*). J. Allergy Clin. Immunol. 71: 345.
6. Cookson, J. B., and G. Makoni. 1975. Seasonal asthma and the housedust mite in tropical Africa. Clin Allergy. 5: 375.
7. Abdurrahman, M. B., and A. M. Taqi. 1982. Childhood bronchial asthma in Northern Nigeria. Clin Allergy. 12: 379.
8. Woolcock, A. J., G. K. Dowse, K. Temple, H. Stanley, M. P. Alpers, and K. J. Turner. 1983. The prevalence of asthma in the South Fore people of Papua, New Guinea. A method for field studies of bronchial hyperreactivity. Eur. J. Respir. Dis. 64: 571.
9. Waite, D. A., E. F. Eyles, S. L. Tonkin, and T. V. O'Donnel. 1980. Asthma prevalence in Tokelauan children in two environments. Clin. Allergy. 10: 71.
10. Smith, J. M., L. K. Harding, and G. Cumming. 1971. The changing prevalence of asthma in school children. Clin. Allergy. 1: 57.
11. Citron, K. M., and J. Pepys. 1964. An investigation of asthma among the Tristan da Cunha is-landers. Br. J. Dis. Chest. 58: 119.
12. Wolstenholme, R. J. 1979. Bronchial asthma in the Southern Maldives. Clin. Allergy. 9: 325.
13. Lewis, O. 1966. The culture of poverty. Scientific American. 215: 19.
14. Hsu, K. H. K., D. E. Jenkins, B. P. Hsi, E. Bour-hofer, V. Thompson, N. Tanakawa, and G. S. J. Hsieh. 1979. Ventilatory functions of normal children and young adults—Mexican-American, white and black. I. Spirometry. J. Pediatrics. 95: 14.
15. Johansson, S. G. O., T. Mellbin, and B. Vahlquist. 1968. Immunoglobulin levels in Ethiopian pre-school children with special reference to high concentration of immunoglobulin E. Lancet. i: 1118.
16. Orren, A., and E. B. Dowdle. 1975. The effects of sex and age on Serum IgE concentrations in three ethnic groups. Int. Archs. Allergy appl. Immun. 48: 824.
17. Jackson, R. T., R. Beaglehole, H. H. Rea, and D. C. Sutherland. 1982. Mortality from asthma: a new epidemic in New Zealand. Br. Med. J. 285: 771.
18. Benatar, S. R., and G. M. Ainslie. 1986. Deaths from asthma in Cape Town, 1980–1982. S. Afr. Med. J. 69: 669.
19. Speight, A. N. P., D. A. Lee, and E. N. Hey. 1983. Underdiagnosis and undertreatment of asthma in childhood. Br. Med. J. 286: 1253.
20. Haus, M., H. de V. Heese, E. G. Weinberg, P. C. Potter, J. M. Hall, and D. Malberbe. 1988. The influence of ethnicity, an atopic family history and maternal ascariasis on cord blood serum IgE concentrations. J. Allergy Clin. Immunol. 82: 179.
21. Haus, M., and E. G. Weinberg. 1988. Specific IgE antibodies to bordetella pertussis after immuni-zation in infancy. Lancet. i: 1393.

Chronic Steroid Therapy in Severe Childhood Asthma

Simon Godfrey*, Natan Noviski*, Ariel Rosler**

Chronic perennial childhood asthma affects about 25% of all children with asthma, and of these about one-third require chronic steroid therapy at some stage in order to achieve adequate control of their disease. At present, the decision to use steroids is based on inadequate control with nonsteroid medication, but this requirement may be relaxed as the safety of steroid therapy becomes more generally recognized. The type of steroid used depends upon the ability of the child to cooperate with treatment, but the inhaled route is to be preferred. Recent developments have made available a topically active steroid that can be administered through a nebulizer and is effective in very young children. With inhaled steroids there is some biochemical evidence of adrenal suppression, but this has not been associated with clinical problems.

Asthma is a common problem throughout childhood, and various studies suggest that it affects at least 10% of all school age children at some time. About 20% of asthmatic children already have symptoms in the first year of life, 40% by the end of the second year, and 80% by the end of the fourth year [1–2]. From large community-based surveys [3] it seems that about 25% of children with asthma will have chronic perennial symptoms at some stage of their disease which require continuous prophylactic medication. About two-thirds of these children can be managed with nonsteroidal prophylaxis, but some 8% of asthmatic children and almost 1% of all children require continuous prophylaxis with corticosteroids at some time during childhood [4].

Indications for Steroid Therapy

At the present time, it is generally accepted that chronic steroid therapy should be reserved for those asthmatic children whose disease cannot be otherwise controlled. In adults, the criteria for the use of steroids are generally less stringent. To be considered for steroid therapy, the child should have symptoms on most days and/or nights for prolonged periods which interfere significantly with everyday life. The symptoms are likely to cause children to miss school, to keep them awake at night, and prevent them from keeping up with their peers at play. In addition, it must be established that these symptoms cannot be adequately controlled by conventional nonsteroidal therapy. This would normally consist of the regular administration of sodium cromoglycate or slow release theophylline with supplementary inhaled β agonist. It is important to be sure that the child is truly receiving the prescribed medication in the correct manner for an adequate period of observation—a month is usually long enough. Inhalation techniques should be checked and blood theophylline levels measured.

Available Steroid Regimens

Once it has been determined that the child has chronic perennial asthma that cannot be controlled by adequate nonsteroidal medication, the decision must be made as to which of the alternative forms of steroid therapy is to be used. Because of the adverse effect on growth and adrenal function, regular daily oral steroid medication is unsuitable for chronic therapy and can only be safely used for short, 5–7-day courses up to 3–5 times a year. Injections of corticotropin were popular at one time, but children dislike injections; pituitary suppression is also produced, and the steroidal side effects are probably just as severe as with daily oral steroids.

By giving oral steroids every other morning (single dose alternate morning, SDAM, therapy), it has proved possible to control asthma in children with minimal side effects [5]. The advantages of this form of treatment include its

*   Department of Pediatrics and **Deparment of Endocrinology, Hadassah University Hospital, Jerusalem, Israel.

relative efficacy, cheapness, and suitability for children of all ages. The disadvantages include poor control of the asthma on the nontreatment day, the (rare) complication of cataracts [6], and some biochemical evidence of adrenal suppression [7].

For almost 20 years topically active inhaled steroids have been available for the treatment of asthma. They have been shown to be especially useful for children [8] because they can be given twice daily without clinical side effects and with generally excellent control of the asthma. The disadvantages of this type of treatment are the need for a near perfect inhalation technique, relatively high cost and some biochemical evidence of adrenal suppression [7]. The problem of the inhalation technique has been overcome to a large extent by the advent of powder inhaler devices and valved spacers for use with regular metered dose inhalers. Recently, suspensions have been produced that can be delivered through regular nebulizers and given even to very young children [9–10].

Do Inhaled Steroids Produce Side Effects in Children?

Given that the inhaled route is generally preferred for children because of the excellent control it usually gives with twice or three times daily medication, it remains to be determined whether this type of therapy is associated with significant side effects. The chief concerns are the possibility of decreased rate of growth in height and adrenal suppression. Evaluation of growth is far from simple in children with asthma because there is some evidence that the disease itself is associated with slower than normal growth before puberty, with a tendency to delayed puberty and with eventual catch-up growth after puberty [11]. Thus, if children are studied over relatively short periods, especially before puberty, then any drug they are receiving may be suspected as causing growth retardation, and only long-term studies extending past puberty will reveal the true situation [12]. In our own studies of long-term treatment with beclomethasone dipropionate, BDP, we found no evidence of significant growth suppression [8].

In the past, adrenal function in children taking inhaled steroids has usually been measured simply in terms of the early morning cortisol level and the response to tetracosactrin. Using these tests, we found no evidence of adrenal suppression after one year of treatment with BDP in children [13]. Others using the excretion of free cortisol in urine or the pituitary/adrenal response to insulin or metyrapone found some evidence of adrenal suppression in children taking inhaled steroids [7, 14] and we confirmed this more recently for treatment both with BDP and a newer inhaled steroid, budesonide, BUD [15]. In fact, many believe that the best index of adrenal function is the 24-hour integrated plasma cortisol level (24ICO) or the area under the cortisol/time curve, which is very similar [16]. Using a partial overnight area under the curve approach, a dose-related reduction in adrenal function in children taking BDP has been reported [17]. We have now studied a group of infants between 1 and 5 years of age taking either single dose alternate morning prednisone, inhaled nebulized BUD, or no steroid medication by means of 24ICO tests. We found no evidence of adrenal suppression on either prednisone or BUD. We found low levels of 24-hour integrated growth hormone (24IGH) compared to the levels in older normal children, but these levels were similar whether or not the children were receiving steroids. These values for 24IGH may be normal for children <5 years, or they may reflect lower than normal values due to the asthma and not to its treatment.

Conclusion

Steroid therapy is available for all children with asthma that cannot be adequately controlled by other means. Correctly administered, steroids are not associated with significant clinical side effects in asthmatic children, though they may be associated with minor biochemical evidence of adrenal suppression. The safety and efficacy of long-term steroid therapy is such that it is necessary to consider whether this type of treatment should not be offered earlier to children with chronic perennial asthma.

References

1. Cserhati, E., G. Mezei, and J. Kelemen. 1984. Late prognosis of bronchial asthma in children. Respir. 46: 160.

2. Dawson, B., G. Horrobin, R. Illesley, and R. Mitchell. 1969. A survey of childhood asthma in Aberdeen. Lancet 1: 827.
3. McNicol, K. N., and H. E. Williams. 1973. Spectrum of asthma in children: Clinical and physiological components. Br. Med. J. 4: 7.
4. Godfrey, S. 1983. Childhood asthma. In: Asthma. T. J. H. Clark and S. Godfrey, eds. London: Chapman and Hall Ltd.
5. Falliers, C. J., H. Chai, L. Molk, H. Bane, and R. R. de A. Cardoso. 1972. Pulmonary and adrenal effects of alternate day corticosteroid therapy. J. Allergy Clin. Immunol. 49: 156.
6. Bhagat, R. G., and H. Chai. 1984. Development of posterior subcapsular cataracts in asthmatic children. Pediatrics 73: 626.
7. Wyatt, R. J. Waschek, M. Weinberger, and B. Sherman. 1978. Effects of inhaled beclomethasone dipropionate and alternate-day prednisone on pituitary-adrenal function in children with chronic asthma. N. Engl. J. Med. 299: 1387.
8. Godfrey, S., L. Balfour-Lynn, and M. Tooley. 1978. A three-to-five year follow-up of the use of the aerosol steroid beclomethasone dipropionate in childhood asthma. J. Allergy Clin. Immunol. 62: 335.
9. Storr, J., C. A. Leeney, and W. Leeney. 1986. Nebulized beclomethasone dipropionate in preschool asthma. Arch. Dis. Child 61: 270.
10. Godfrey, S., A. Avital, A. Rosler, A. Mandelberg, and K. Uwyyed. 1988. Nebulized budesonide in severe infantile asthma. (letter) Lancet 2: 851.
11. Hauspie, R. C. Susanne, and F. Alexander. 1977. Maturational delay and temporal growth retardation in asthmatic boys. J. Allergy Clin. Immunol. 59: 200.
12. Balfour-Lynn, L. 1985. Childhood asthma and puberty. Arch. Dis. Child 60: 231.
13. Godfrey, S., and P. Konig. 1974. Treatment of childhood asthma for 13 months and longer with beclomethasone dipropionate aerosol. Arch. Dis. Child 49: 591.
14. Vaz, R., B. Senior, M. Morris, and A. Binkiewicz. 1982. Adrenal effects of beclomethasone inhalation therapy in asthmatic children. J. Pediatr. 100: 660.
15. Springer, Ch., A. Avital, Ch. Maayan, A. Rosler, and Godfrey, S. 1987. Comparison of budesonide and beclomethasone dipropionate for treatment of asthma. Arch. Dis. Child 62: 815.
16. Zadik, Z., L. De Lacerda, A. H. De Carmargo, B. P. Hamilton, C. J. Migeon, and A. A. Kowarski. 1980. A comparative study of urinary 17-hydroxycorticosteroids, urinary free cortisol, and the integrated concentration of plasma cortisol. J. Clin. Endocrinol. Metab. 51: 1099.
17. Law, C. M., J. L. Marchant, J. W. Honour, M. A. Preece, and J. O. Warner. 1986. Nocturnal adrenal suppression in asthmatic children taking inhaled beclomethasone dipropionate. Lancet 1: 942.

Perspectives for Therapy of Reactions Dependent on Neuropeptide Release

Martin K. Church, Mark A. Lowman, Paul H. Rees, R. Christopher Benyon*

Following the identification of IgE in 1967 [1], research into the mechanisms of allergic diseases has concentrated on IgE-dependent stimulation of mast cell mediator release as the primary initiating stimulus. Release of histamine, prostaglandins, and leukotrienes in particular have been implicated as effectors of the immediate response, whilst the ability of chemotactic and chemokinetic factors to attract and activate inflammatory cells has been used to explain late-phase responses. It is now becoming clear, however, that the interaction of inflammatory cells with sensory neurones may also play a major role in the progression of the inflammatory response. Although the study of neurogenic inflammation is still in its infancy, there is some evidence that angioneurotic oedema, chronic idiopathic urticaria, heat-induced urticaria, cold-induced urticaria, and cholinergic urticaria involve both mast cell mediator release and a neurogenic component. This article explores the interrelationships between mast cells and neurones in human skin.

Evidence for Neuropeptide Involvement in Cutaneous Inflammation

The association with nerves and inflammation is not new. In 1874, Golz [2] suggested the capability of peripheral nerves to cause vasodilatation in the skin. This activity was localized further at the turn of the century by Langley [3], who proposed the existence of the axon reflex, and by Bayliss [4], who provided evidence that antidromic stimulation of peripheral nerves could induce vasodilatation. These studies provided the basis for the classical paper by Lewis in 1927 [5], who described the triple response to an intradermal injection of histamine and proposed that, whilst the wheal response was likely to be a direct effect of histamine in causing oedema, the flare response had a neurogenic mechanism probably involving axon reflexes in primary afferent neurones. More recently, these have been shown to be unmyelinated C fibers [6], which have polymodal nociceptors capable of responding to diverse stimuli including pressure, heat and histamine [7–9].

Neuropeptides are synthesized in the cell body of sensory neurones and migrate preferentially toward the sensory endings from which they are released during axon reflexes [10]. Although the undecapeptide substance P was the first neuropeptide tachykinin demonstrated to be released following antidromic stimulation [11, 12], it is not the only one—others, including somatostatin, neurokinin A (NKA), and calcitonin gene-related peptide (CGRP), have also been demonstrated in mammalian skin [13, 14]. Furthermore, there is some evidence that substance P, neurokinin A, and CGRP may co-exist in the same sensory neurones [15], whereas somatostatin is probably contained in separate nerves [16].

A link between neuropeptides, mast cells and inflammatory diseases of the skin is suggested by two observations. First, provocation challenge of patients with either cold- or heat-induced urticaria or cholinergic urticaria leads to an elevation of histamine levels in the venous effluent from challenged but not unchallenged arms [17–19]. Second, depletion of neuropeptides from cutaneous sensory neurones by capsaicin [20] reduces the severity of both heat- and cold-induced urticaria in man [20] and heat-induced oedema in rats [21].

* Immunopharmacology Group, Clinical Pharmacology, Centre Block, Southampton General Hospital, Southampton SO9 4XY, U.K.

These studies have been supported in part by a Medical Research Council Project Grant. MAL is a SERC-CASE award student in collaboration with Roussel Laboratories and PHR is supported by a University of Southampton studentship.

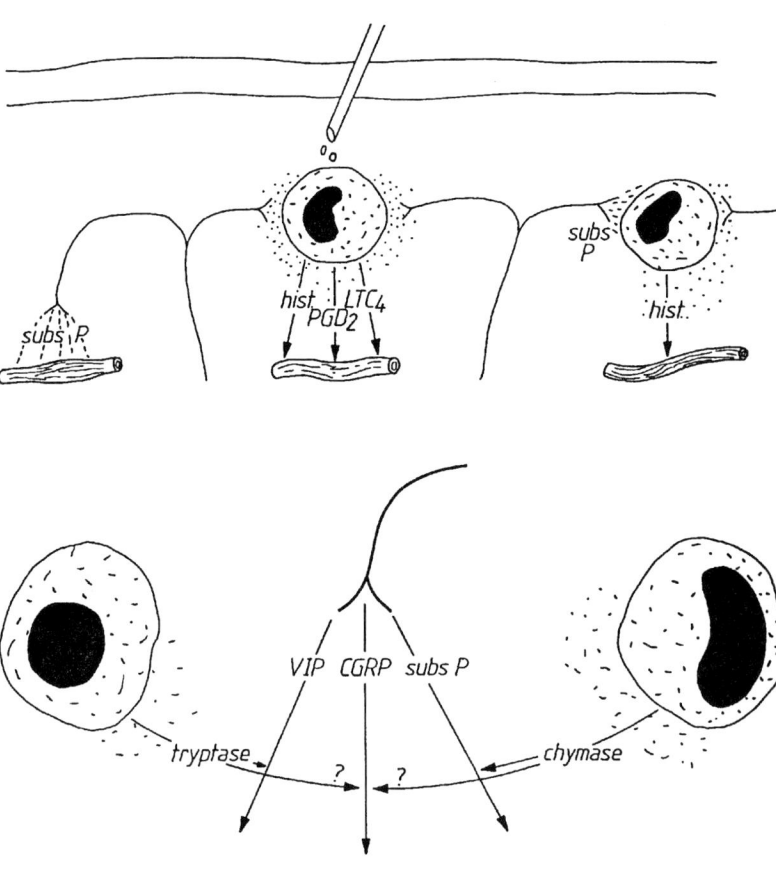

Figure 1. Interrelationships between mast cells, neurones, and blood vessels.

Figure 2. Selective metabolism of neuropeptides by mast cell proteases.

Interactions Between Neuropeptides, Mast Cells, and Blood Vessels in the Skin

In order to discuss the complex relationship between mast cells, cutaneous nerves, and inflammatory processes in the skin, it is first necessary to consider the possible mechanisms of the wheal and flare response (Figure 1). Intradermal injection of histamine induces a rapid oedematous response, indicative of increased blood flow and leakage of intravascular proteins, at the site of injection. That this response is also stimulated by the injection of allergen in sensitive recipients strongly suggests the involvement in the response of mediators derived from cutaneous mast cells.

The mechanism of development of the flare, or area of vasodilatation surrounding the wheal, is less well understood. The ability of

local anaesthetics [22] and depletion of neuropeptides from the skin with capsaicin [23] to inhibit the response clearly implicates axon reflexes in sensory cutaneous nerves in its propagation. Three questions regarding this response remain largely unanswered. First, how are the axon reflexes stimulated? The ability of histamine H_1-antagonists to effectively reduce flare suggests the direct stimulation of neurones by histamine, though definitive evidence for the existence of such receptors is lacking. The second question that arises relates to the mechanism by which axon reflexes cause vasodilatation. Two mechanisms have been proposed: vasodilatation induced by mast cell mediators following their release by neuropeptides [23] and a direct effect of neuropeptides on the cutaneous vasculature [24]. The former is supported by the effectiveness of H_1-antagonists in preventing the flare [23], histological evidence of mast cell degranulation in biopsies

203

taken from the flare area surrounding mechanical injury in experimental animals [25], and the ability of neuropeptides to stimulate histamine release from dermal mast cells [26]. However, a direct effect of neuropeptides on the vasculature is suggested by the failure of a histamine H_1-antagonist to abrogate the flare response because of the direct release of neuropeptides by capsaicin [24]. The third question, to which no satisfactory answer has been proposed, relates to the control of spread of the flare response. Although it is well established that the diameter of the flare response is related to the concentration of histamine or allergen initiating the wheal response, little is known about either the quantitative aspects of its propagation or its control.

A further mechanism of interaction between neuropeptides and mast cells has been suggested from the recent observations that mast cell proteases may degrade neuropeptides (Figure 2). Brain and Williams [27] have reported that intradermal injection of substance P with CGRP shortens the duration of the CGRP-induced erythema from about 4 h to less than 1 h. Co-incubation of CGRP with supernatants from stimulated rat mast cells suggested that mast cell proteases were responsible for the degradative inactivation. In a separate study, Caughey and colleagues [28] have investigated the differential degradation of substance P and vasoactive intestinal peptide (VIP) by dog mastocytoma proteases. They reported that tryptase degraded VIP whilst chymase catabolized substance P. This has particular relevance to pulmonary diseases, as the bronchodilator VIP would be preferentially metabolized by the tryptase-containing mast cells in that tissue [29], leaving the bronchoconstrictor actions of substance P unopposed.

Interactions of Neuropeptides with Mast Cells

The ability of intradermal injections of neuropeptide tachykinins to induce a wheal and flare response suggests that they are capable of inducing mediator release from cutaneous mast cells. To demonstrate this directly, we dispersed mast cells from human foreskin and breast skin by enzymatic digestion of the tissues with collagenase and hyaluronidase to obtain isolated cells in free suspension [26]. Mast

cells may then be purified to more than 80% homogeneity by density sedimentation through discontinuous gradients of Percoll [26].

In initial experiments [26, 30], substance P was found to induce a concentration-related release of histamine between 3 and 100 μM, net releases at 30 μM being 12.9±1.4% and 24.8±2.3% from mast cells from juvenile foreskin and adult breast skin, respectively. Subsequent experiments [31] have shown that somatostatin and vasoactive intestinal peptide (VIP) also stimulate skin mast cells whereas calcitonin gene-related peptide (CGRP), neurokinins A and B, and bradykinin cause little or no mediator release. Interestingly, somatostatin and VIP, like substance P, may initiate a wheal and flare response when injected intradermally, whereas CGRP causes a local erythema of prolonged duration and neurokinin A and bradykinin localized vasodilator responses [32].

The characteristics of IgE-dependent activation and that stimulated by neuropeptides show major differences [31]. Anti-IgE-induced histamine release is slow, taking some six minutes to reach completion, and dependent on extracellular calcium and intact pathways for glycolysis and oxidative phosphorylation. In contrast, substance P-induced release is rapid, being complete within 20 sec and largely independent of extracellular calcium. However, like IgE-dependent stimulus-secretion coupling, it is dependent on intact pathways for glycolysis and oxidative phosphorylation. Furthermore, whereas IgE-dependent activation induces the release of the eicosanoids prostaglandin D_2 and leukotriene C_4 in addition to histamine, mast cell activation by neuropeptides stimulates the preferential release of histamine [33].

Modulation of Histamine Release from Human Skin Mast Cells

The studies of Ting and colleagues [34] have shown that β-adrenoceptor stimulants reduce the wheal and flare response and histological evidence of mast cell degranulation following the intradermal injection of antigen. These results have been confirmed using isolated skin mast cells [35], salbutamol (0.01–100 μM) causing a concentration-related inhibition of histamine release following activation with both anti-IgE and substance P. Against anti-IgE, inhibition was significant (p<0.02) at 0.01 µM salbutamol and was maximum at 1 µM when 31.0±4.0% inhibition was observed. Against substance P, inhibition was significant (p<0.02) at 0.01 µM and reached a maximum of 27.7±4.9% at 10 µM. The methylxanthine phosphodiesterase inhibitor isobutylmethylxanthine (IBMX), in the concentration range 0.01–1 mM, also inhibited secretion induced by anti-IgE and substance P, suggesting that both secretory mechanisms are sensitive to agents which elevate intracellular levels of cyclic AMP.

In contrast to human lung [36] and intestinal [37] mast cells, human skin mast cells are refractory to the inhibitory effects of the anti-allergic drug sodium cromoglycate. In isolated mast cells, sodium cromoglycate in concentrations of 0.1–1000 µM had no significant effect on histamine release stimulated by either anti-IgE or substance P [35]. This would explain the failure of sodium cromoglycate to reduce the wheal and flare response and mast cell degranulation following challenge by intradermal injection of antigen [38].

Effects of Neurotropin

Whilst clinical studies have demonstrated that neurotropin inhibits the flare response following the intradermal injection of allergen [39], such studies give little indication of its mode of action. Several possibilities may be considered, including suppression of mediator release from human skin mast cells, prevents of cutaneous nerve stimulation by mast cell mediators, interference with signal transmission in the nonmyelinated peptidergic neurones which conduct the axon reflex, or prevention of neuro peptide release from these neurones. We have examined one of these mechanisms by investigating the effects of neurotropin on mast cells dispersed from human skin by tissue digestion with collagenase and hyaluronidase [26]. Histamine release was stimulated by incubations of cell aliquots for 15 min at 37°C with either 2.5 µg/ml ε-chain-specific anti-human IgE or 10 µM substance P. Histamine was assayed by automated spectrofluorimetry, and net release expressed as a percentage of total cell histamine corrected for spontaneous release. The results showed that neurotropin, freshly fil-

tered through a 0.44 µm filter and diluted with physiological buffer solution to final concentrations of 0.01–1 mg/ml, did not inhibit either IgE-dependent or substance P-induced histamine release when preincubated with skin mast cells for 5 min before challenge. In the same experiments, 1 µM salbutamol used as a positive control, inhibited release induced by anti-IgE and substance P by 23±7% and 27±6%, respectively. In further experiments, prolongation of the preincubation time of cells with neurotropin to 30 min before challenge also failed to induce an inhibitory effect.

These results, together with the observations of the analgesic effects of neurotropin [39], suggest an action on cutaneous C-fibers which at high rates of stimulation are associated with nociception and at low rats of stimulation may induce vasodilatation characteristic of the flare response.

References

1. Ishizaka, K., and T. Ishizaka. 1967. Identification of gamma-E antibodies as a carrier of reaginic activity. J. Immunol. 99: 1187.
2. Golz, F. 1874. Über gefäßerweiternde Nerven. Pflugers Arch. 9: 174.
3. Langley, J. N. 1900. On axon reflexes in the preganglionic fibres of the sympathetic system. J. Physiol. (Lond.) 25: 364.
4. Bayliss, W. M. 1901. On the origin from the spinal cord of the vasodilator fibres of the hind limb, and on the nature of these fibres. J. Physiol. (Lond.) 26: 173.
5. Lewis, T. 1927. The blood vessels of the human skin and their responses. London: Shaw.
6. Celander, O., and B. Folkow. 1953. The nature and distribution of afferent fibres provided with the axon reflex arrangement. Acta Physiol. Scand. 29: 359.
7. Van Hees, J., and J. M. Gybels. 1972. Pain related to single afferent C fibres from human skin. Brain Res. 48: 397.
8. Torebjork, H. E., and R. G. Hallin. 1974. Identification of afferent C units in intact human skin. Brain Res. 67: 387.
9. Kenins, P. 1981. Identification of the unmyelinated sensory nerves which evoke plasma extravasation in response to antidromic stimulation. Neurosci. Lett. 25: 137.
10. Hokfelt, T., J. O. Kellerth, G. Nillson, and B. Pernow. 1975. Experimental immunohistochemical studies on the localization and distribution of substance P in cat primary sensory neurones. Brain Res. 100: 235.

205

11. Keen, P., A. J. Harmar, F. Spears, and E. Winter. 1982. Biosynthesis, axonal transport and turnover of neuronal substance P. In: Substance P in the nervous system. Ciba Foundation Symposium, Vol. 91. R. Porter and M. O'Connor, eds. London: Pitman, p. 145.

12. Brodin, E., B. Gazelius, J. M. Lundberg, and L. Olgart, L. 1983. Substance P in trigeminal nerve endings: Occurrence and release. Acta Physiol. Scand. 111: 501.

13. Hartschuh, W., E. Weihe, and M. Reinecke. 1983. Peptidergic (neurotensin, VIP, substance P) nerve fibres in the skin. Immunohistochemical evidence of an involvement of neuropeptides in nociception, pruritis and inflammation. Br. J. Dermatol. 109 (Suppl. 25): 14.

14. Brain, S. D., J. R. Tippins, H. R. Morris, I. MacIntyre, and T. J. Williams. 1986. Potent vasodilator activity of calcitonin gene-related peptide in human skin. J. Invest. Dermatol. 87: 533.

15. Fisher, J., W. G. Forssman, T. Hokfelt, J. M. Lundberg, M. Rienecke, F. A. Tschopp, and Z. Wiesenfeld-Hakin. 1985. Immunoreactive calcitonin gene-related peptide and substance P: coexistence in sensory neurones and behavioural interaction after intrathecal administration in the rat. J. Physiol. (Lond.) 362: 29P.

16. Hokfelt, T., Elde, R., Johansson, O., Luft, R., Nillson, G. and Arimura, A. 1976. Immunohistochemical evidence for separate populations of somatostatin-containing and substance P-containing primary afferent neurones in the rat. Neuroscience 1: 131.

17. Heavey, D. J., A. Kobza-Black, S. E. Barrow, C. G. Chappell, M. W. Greaves, and C. T. Dollery. 1986. Prostaglandin D2 and histamine release in cold urticaria. J. Allergy Clin. Immunol. 78: 458.

18. Koro, O., J. S. Dover, D. M. Francis, A. Kobza-Black, R. W. Kelly, R. M. Barr, and M. W. Greaves. 1986. Release of prostaglandin D2 and histamine in a case of localized heat urticaria and effects of treatments. Br. J. Dermatol. 115: 721.

19. Kaplan, A. P., L. Gray, R. E. Shaff, Z. Horakova, and M. A. Beaven. 1975. In vivo studies of mediator release in cold urticaria and cholinergic urticaria. J. Allergy Clin. Immunol. 55: 394.

20. Toth-Kasa, I., G. Jancso, F. Obal, S. Husz, and N. Simon. 1983. Involvement of sensory nerve endings in the cold and heat urticaria. J. Invest. Dermatol. 80: 34.

21. Saria, A., and J. M. Lundberg. 1983. Capsaicin pretreatment inhibits heat-induced oedema in rat skin. Naunyn Schmiedebergs Arch. Pharmacol. 323: 341.

22. Foreman, J. C., and C. C. Jordan. 1983. Histamine release and vascular changes induced by neuropeptides. Agents Actions 13: 105.

23. Foreman, J. C. 1987. Neuropeptides and the pathogenesis of allergy. Allergy 42: 1.

24. Barnes, P. J., M. J. Brown, C. T. Dollery, R. W. Fuller, D. J. Heavey, and P. W. Ind. 1986. Histamine is released from skin by substance P but does not act as the final vasodilator in the axon reflex. Br. J. Pharmacol. 88: 741.

25. Kiernan, J. A. 1972. The involvement of mast cells in vasodilatation due to axon reflexes in injured skin. Q. J. Exp. Physiol. 57: 311.

26. Benyon, R. C., M. A. Lowman, and M. K. Church. 1987. Human skin mast cells: Their dispersion, purification and secretory characterization. J. Immunol. 138: 861.

27. Brain, S. D., and T. J. Williams. 1988. Substance P regulates the vasodilator activity of calcitonin gene-related peptide. Nature 335: 73.

28. Caughey, G. H., F. Leidig, N. F. Viro, and J. A. Nadel. 1988. Substance P and vasoactive intestinal peptide degradation by mast cell tryptase and chymase. J. Pharmac. Exp. Ther. 244: 133.

29. Irani, A. A., N. M. Schechter, S. Craig, G. DeBlois, and L. B. Schwartz. 1986. Two types of human mast cells that have distinct neutral protease compositions. Proc. Natl. Acad. Sci. USA 83: 4464.

30. Lowman, M. A., P. H. Rees, R. C. Benyon, and M. K. Church. 1988. Human mast cell heterogeneity: Histamine release from mast cells dispersed from skin, lung, adenoids, tonsils and intestinal mucosa in response to IgE-dependent and non-immunological stimuli. J. Allergy Clin. Immunol. 81: 590.

31. Lowman, M. A., R. C. Benyon, and M. K. Church. 1988. Characterization of neuropeptide-induced histamine released from human dispersed skin mast cells. Br. J. Pharmacol. 95: 121.

32. Fuller, R. W., T. B. Conradson, C. M. S. Dixon, D. C. Crossman, and P. J. Barnes. 1987. Sensory neuropeptide effects in human skin. Br. J. Pharmacol. 92: 781.

33. Benyon, C. R., C. Robinson, and M. K. Church. 1988. Mediator release from human skin mast cells: Differences between IgE-dependent and non-immunological stimuli. Br. J. Pharmacol., in press.

34. Ting, S., B. Zweiman, and R. M. Lavker. 1983. Terbutaline modulation of human allergic skin reactions. J. Allergy Clin. Immunol. 71: 437.

35. Lowman, M. A., R. C. Benyon, and M. K. Church. 1988. Human skin mast cells: Effects of salbutamol and sodium cromoglycate on histamine release induced by anti-IgE and substance P. J. Skin Pharmacol. 1: 63.

36. Church, M. K. and J. Hiroi. 1987. Inhibition of IgE-dependent histamine release from human dispersed lung mast cells by anti-allergic drugs and salbutamol. Br. J. Pharmacol. 90: 421.

37. Church, M. K., R. C. Benyon, P. H. Rees, M. A. Lowman, A. M. Campbell, C. Robinson, and S.

T. Holgate. 1989. Functional heterogeneity of human mast cells. In: Mast cell and basophil differentiation and function in health and disease. S. J. Galli and K. F. Austen, eds. New York: Raven Press, in press.

38. Ting, S., B. Zweiman, and R. M. Lavker. 1983. Cromolyn does not modulate human allergic skin reactions in vivo. J. Allergy Clin. Immunol. 71: 12.

39. De Weck, A. L. 1988. Effect of neurotropin on immediate type allergic reactions. NER Allergy Proc., in press.

Histamine and Other Mediators in Asthma

Wolfgang Schmutzler, Stefan Glück, Klaus P. Riesener, Frings Mariola*

The role of histamine in experimental and clinical asthma has been discussed since its discovery at the beginning of this century. Histamine fulfills also all of Henry Dale's criteria for a mediator, even though the study of inhibitors gave evidence that in addition to histamine, there are one or more other mediators in asthma: 5-hydroxytryptamine, bradykinin, acetylcholine, prostaglandins, thromboxane, leukotrienes (SRS-A), PAF-acether, neuropeptides, oxygen radicals, etc. have been discovered, brought into context with asthma, and, after some time, assigned a certain role.

Histamine remains the only substance that has been continually regarded as being an important mediator in asthma. From in vitro experiments H_1-blockers were expected to inhibit the release of histamine and other mediators. This turned out to be true for human basophils but not for human mast cells. On the other hand, comparative studies revealed striking differences between several H_1-blockers with respect to their affinity for H_1-receptors and their duration of action.

Asthma is a widespread disease characterized by bronchial hyperreactivity and signs of partial or total bronchial obstruction [1]. Attacks of asthma can be provoked by allergens or nonallergens, e.g., infections of the airways or drugs. It was acknowledged a long time ago that those mechanisms involve the release of endogenous substances with pharmacological actions in different effector cells. The expression of the disease is, however, modified by a multitude of modulating factors [2].

Asthma research has always been hindered by the lack of animal models covering all relevant aspects of the disease. Some of the problems concerning the involvement of mediators have been worked out using the model of local or systemic anaphylaxis: In 1910 Dale and Laidlaw [3] described the similarity of histamine and anaphylactic shock in the guinea pig. Twenty-four years later, Dale [4] referred to histamine when he postulated the prereq-

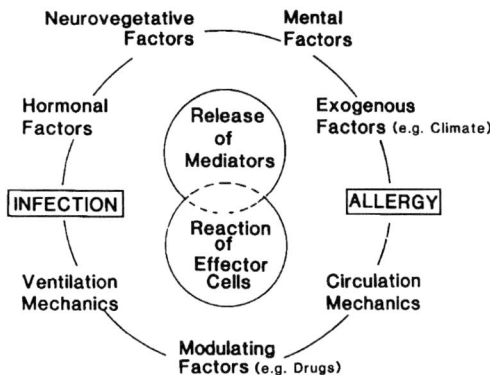

Figure 1. Factors influencing asthma (from [2]).

uisites for the acknowledgment of a mediator substance in a given reaction or disease: first, presence and release of the substance in pharmacogically active form; second, mimesis of the given reaction by the effects of the suspected substance; third, suppression of the reaction by a specific inhibitor of the suspected mediator.

The use of H_1-blockers (as they are called today) brought definite proof that the bronchial obstruction in both the anaphylatoxin and the anaphylactic reaction was caused by histamine [5]. The fact that higher doses of the antihistamine were required in anaphylaxis was explained by Dale as resulting from the different sources of the histamine, "intrinsic" in the case of anaphylaxis, "extrinsic" in the case of the anaphylatoxin reaction. The H_1-blockers did not prevent protracted death in a considerable proportion of the anaphylactic guinea pigs. This protracted death was not due to a late asthmatic reaction, but to anaphylactic heart failure. Nevertheless, this observation has always been taken as strong evidence that histamine was not the only mediator in anaphylaxis [7].

There was another point that caused a formidable problem. Code [8] described an in-

* Institute of Pharmacolgy, Medical Faculty, Rheinisch-Westfälische Technische Hochschule, D-5100 Aachen, Federal Republic of Germany.

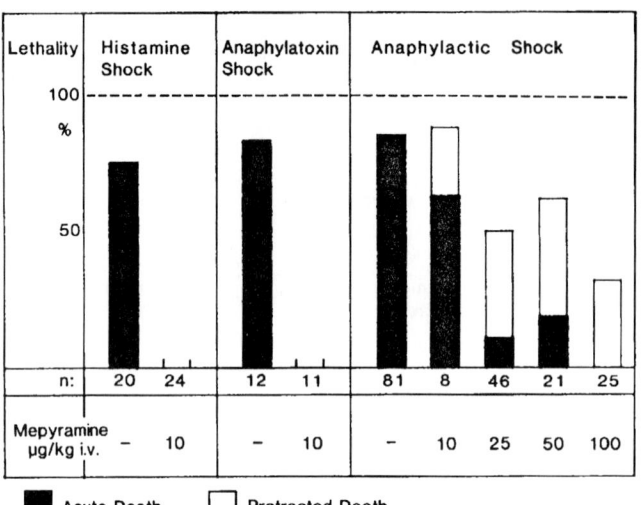

Figure 2. Effects of the H_1-anti-histamine on the histamine, anaphylatoxin, and anaphylactic reaction in the guinea pig. *Acute death:* death caused by bronchoconstriction within 15 min after challenge. *Protracted death:* death within 120 min without signs of bronchoconstriction.

Table 1. Histaminase activity (mU/ml) in human plasma before and after intravenous injection of heparin (500 IU/kg b.z.). Single values, mean ± S.E.M. (from [2]).

Probands	Before heparin	After heparin i.v.		
		30 min	60 min	120 min
W.Sch.	0.000	0.436	0.987	0.526
J.Kn.	0.013	0.411	0.798	0.252
P.Kr.	0.047	0.195	1.219	1.018
H.La.	0.000	0.000	0.107	0.169
Mean ± S.E.M.	0.012 ±0.009	0.247 ±0.080	0.736 ±0.162	0.523 ±0.152

crease of histamine content in whole blood of anaphylactic guinea pigs and dogs: The demonstration of increased plasma histamine was possible only after the discovery that the heparin released from the mast cells together with the histamine increased the histaminase content of the plasma [9]. This meant that without inhibition of the histamine metabolism in blood, the determination of correct histamine levels was impossible.

This point is very relevant for the reevaluation of histamine in asthma. In humans, the increase in the histaminase content in plasma is, in contrast to the guinea pig, slow in onset [10, 11], but it is strong enough to destroy at least a proportion of the released histamine.

It is, therefore, not surprising that some of the recent workers could not detect an appro-priate correlation between the plasma histamine levels and the severity of the clinical symptoms [12, 13]. This is important since plasma histamine levels in humans are very small and could be detected only using sophisticated methods that have been developed during the last 20 years [14, 15].

Previously, no histamine release during asthma could be found, and since the older H_1-blockers did not attenuate the symptoms of asthma, many clinical investigators came to the conclusion that histamine was entirely irrelevant in human asthma, and that H_1- blockers thus had no place in asthma therapy [16, 17]. Instead, a number of other putative mediators have been discovered and discussed [18]: 5-hydroxytrypamine, bradykinin, acetylcholine, neuropeptides, prostaglandins, thromboxane, leukotrienes PAF-acether, oxygen radials, and so forth—all of which may play a certain role in asthma. None of them, however, fulfills Dale's criteria equally well as histamine does.

From the results in rat models, some of the modern H_1-blockers have been expected to inhibit mast-cell degranulation and, thereby, mediator release [19, 20]. This was confirmed for ketotifen and oxatomide in human basophils [21, 22]. In human tissue mast cells, azelastine

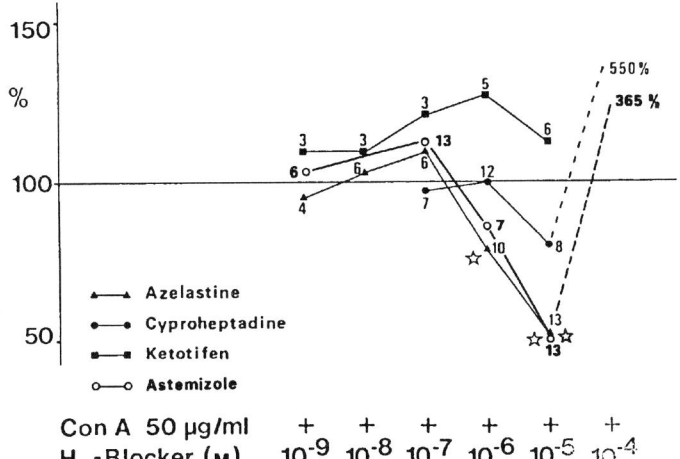

Figure 3. Influence of the H_1-antihistamines azelastine, cyproheptadine, ketotifen, and astemizole on the Concanavalin A-induced histamine release from human mast cells in vitro. Values stated as percent deviation of the respective (100%) control release in the absence of inhibitor. Mean values from the number of experiments stated. *$\alpha = 5\%$.

and astemizole at relatively high concentrations were found to possess histamine release inhibiting properties. A slight further increase in the antihistamine concentration reversed their action from inhibition to promotion of the histamine release presumably by a cytotoxic effect.

H_1-antihistamines at relatively high concentrations cannot be used therapeutically for an entirely different reason: Most of them block the main histamine metabolizing enzyme in humans, the histamine-N-methyltransferase. This phenomenon has been observed with all H_1-blockers so far studied [23, 24, 25]. It certainly limits the doses applicable in man.

The H_1-blockers available today differ from the older ones not just by their non-sedative properties, but also by their longer plasma half-time and their longer duration of action [27, 28]. In our own recent studies we found that mepyramine, pyrrobutamine, clemastine, mebhydroline and dimetindene could be washed out from the guinea pig ileum within 1 1/2–2 hrs. The more recent H_1- blockers, e.g., oxatomide, tefenadine, azelastine, and astemizole, had a much longer action period, and some showed rather irreversible effects.

From these results one should expect that H_1-blockers act in humans by their histamine antagonistic effects in the end organs which might be sustained best by rather low doses of long acting varieties. The results of recent clinical studies seem to substantiate this view.

References

1. McFadden Jr., E. R., and K. F. Austen. 1983. Asthma. In: Harrison's principles of internal medicine. McGraw-Hill Book Company Japan Ltd., p. 1512.
2. Aas, K. 1972. The biochemical and immunological bases of bronchial asthma. Springfield: IL: C.C. Thomas.
3. Dale, H. H., and P. P. Laidlaw. 1910. The physiological action of β-iminazol ethylamine. J. Physiol. (Lond.) 41: 318–344.
4. Dale, H. H. 1933. Progress in autopharmacology. Bull. Johns Hopkins Hosp. 53: 297–347.
5. Giertz, H., F. Hahn, I. Jurna, and W. Schmutzler. 1961. Vergleichende Untersuchungen über den anaphylaktischen Schock und den Anaphylatoxinschock am intakten Meerschweinchen. Naunyn-Schmiedeberg's Arch. exp. Path. Pharmak. 242: 65–75.
6. Dale, H. H. 1948. Antihistamine substances. Brit. med. J. 2: 281–283.
7. Hahn, F. 1977. Antianaphylactic and antiallergic effects. In: Handbook of experimental pharmacology 13/2. G. V. R. Born, O. Eichler, A. Farah, H. Herken, and A. D. Welch, eds, pp. 439–504.
8. Code, C. F. 1939. The histamine content of the blood of guinea pigs and dogs during anaphylactic shock. Amer. J. Physiol. 127: 78–93.
9. Schmutzler, W., O. Goldschmidt, K. P. Bethge, and J. Knop. 1969. The release of guinea pig liver histaminase and some of its properties. Int. Archs. Allergy 36: 45–55.
10. Hansson, R., C. G. Hohnberg, G. Tibbling, N. Tryding, H. Westling, and H. Wetterquist. 1966. Heparin-induced diamine oxidase increase in human blood plasma. Acta med. scand. 180: 533–536.

211

11. Schmutzler, W. 1968. Das Verhalten der Histaminase, Diaminoxydase und Benzylaminoxydase im Blutplasma von Meerschweinchen und Mensch nach intravenöser Injektion von Heparin. Klin. Wschr. 46: 953–956.

12a. Durham, S. R., T. H. Lee, O. Cromwell, R. J. Shaw, T. G. Merrett, J. Merrett, P. Cooper, and A. B. Kay. 1984. Immunologic studies in allergen-induced late-phase asthmatic reactions. J. Allergy Clin. Immunol. 74: 49–60.

12b. Howath, P.H., S. R. Durham, A. B. Kay, and S. T. Holgate. 1987. The relationsship between mast cell-mediator release and bronchial reactivity in allergic asthma. J. Allergy Clin. Immunol. 80: 703–711.

13. Iikura, Y., T. Nagakura, G. M. Walsh, K. Akimoto, M. Kisida, T. Kondon, Y. Odajima, M. Okuma, A. Akazawa, and T. Yukishita. 1988. Role of chemical mediators after antigen and exercise challenge in children with asthma. J. Allergy Clin. Immunol. 81: 1050–1055.

14. Lorenz, W. 1975. Histamine release in man. Agents & Actions 5: 402–415.

15. Fischer, B., and W. Schmutzler. 1980. Quantitative Methoden der Allergologie. I. Bestimmung von Mediatorsubstanzen der Allergie: Histamin.

16. Feinberg, S. M., S. Malkiel, and E. R. Feinberg. 1950. The antihistamines. Chicago: The Yearbook Publishers Inc.

17. Douglas, W. W. 1975. Histamine and antihistamines; 5- hydroxytryptamine and antagonists. In: The pharmacological basis of therapeutics (5th ed.). L. S. Goodman and A. Gilman, eds. New York / Toronto / London: Macmillan Publishing Co. Inc., pp. 590–629.

18. McFadden, E. R. 1984. Pathogenesis of asthma. J. Allergy Clin. Immunol. 73: 413.

19. Martin, U., and D. Römer. 1978. The pharmacological properties of a new, orally active antianaphylactic compound: Ketotifen, a benzocy-clohepta thiophene. Arzneim.-Forschg. 28: 770–782.

20. Borges, M., M. De Brabandes, J. van Reempts, F. Awouters, and P. A. J. Janssen. 1978. Morphological evaluation of oxatomide—A new antiallergic drug in guinea pig anaphylaxis. Int. Archs. Allergy appl. Immun. 56: 507–516.

21a. Bierman, C. W., E. S. K. Assem, and J. L. Mongar. 1979. Inhibition and stimulation of histamine release by oxatomide. Int. J. Immunopharmac. 1: 227–231.

21b. Church, M. K., and C. F. Gradidge. 1980. Oxatomide: Inhibition and stimulation of histamine release from human lung and leukocytes in vitro. Agents & Actions 10: 4–7.

22. Radermecker, M. 1981. Inhibition of allergen mediated histamine release from human cells by ketotifen and oxatomide. Respiration 41: 45–55.

23. Netter, K.J., and K. Bodenschatz. 1967. Inhibition of histamine-N-methylation by some antihistamines. Biochem. Pharmacol. 16: 1627–1631.

24. Barth, H., I. Niemeyer, and W. Lorenz. 1973. Studies on the mode of action of histamine H_1- and H_2-receptor antagonists on gastric histamine methyltransferase. Agents & Actions 3: 138–147.

25. Beaven, M. A., and R. E. Shaff. 1979. New inhibitors of histamine-N-methyltransferase. Biochem. Pharmacol. 28: 183–188.

26. Reinhardt, D., and U. Borchard. 1982. H_1-receptor antagonists: Comparative pharmacology and clinical use. Klin. Wschr. 60: 983–990.

27. Schmutzler, W. 1988. Grundlagen der Arzneimittel-Therapie. In: Manuale Allergologicum. E. Fuchs and K.H. Schulz, eds. Deisenhofen: Dustri-Verlag Dr. K. Feistle.

28. Bürger, I., and W. Schmutzler. Vergleichende Untersuchung in vitro alter und neuer H_1-Antihistaminika. Allergologie, in press.

Characterization of Pulmonary Histamine Receptors

*Pier Francesco Mannaioni and Emanuela Masini**

The taxonomy of the pulmonary H_1, H_2, and "atypical" histamine receptors is outlined, describing the receptor moiety present in pulmonary vascular and airway smooth muscle. Special focus is put on receptors distributed on membranes of lung mast cells which modulate further release of inflammatory mediators, and the cholinergic reflex action of histamine, aiming to identify asthma as a receptor disease.

A rehearsal of the role of histamine in the pathophysiology of asthma is warranted by the natural history of the release of histamine by lung tissues. That exogenous administration of histamine to guinea pigs evokes signs and symptoms of respiratory distress very much alike those appearing after challenge with the specific antigen has become common knowledge since the pioneering work of Dale and Laidlaw [1]. In 1932, Bartosch and colleagues first convincingly demonstrated that histamine was released during anaphylaxis from guinea pig lung [2], and isolated human asthmatic lung and bronchial tissues have been shown to release histamine since the paper by Schild and coworkers in 1951 [3]. Subsequently, the liberation of mast cell histamine in experimental pulmonary hypersensitivity and in clinical allergic states (e.g., asthma) has been firmly established and thoroughly reviewed [5].

According to Scadding [6] and the Ciba Foundation Guest Symposium [7], asthma is defined as "a disease characterized by a wide variation over short periods of time in resistance to flow in the airways of the lungs" [6].

In this context, the main concept in the taxonomy of the disease is the suddenness of the asthmatic attack resulting in explosive pathophysiological changes. One explosive event that differentiates asthmatics from nonasthmatics is the increased "releasability" of histamine from storage cells. In vitro studies have shown that isolated basophils from approxi-

mately 70% of asthmatics released histamine in response to the microtubule aggregating agent D_2O, while this occurred in fewer than 5% of normal individuals [8]. The histamine "releasability" from leukocytes challenged in vitro with unspecific histamine release (e.g., Ca^{2+} ionophore A 23187) was significantly higher in a group of asthmatics than in the healthy population [9].

The other event that is also typical of asthmatics is the increased bronchial reactivity. Inhalation tests with histamine have been used for many years to measure nonspecific bronchial reactivity: Virtually all asthmatics demonstrate increased bronchial response during such provocation tests [10]. Therefore, the abrupt "variation . . . in resistance to flow in the airway" (see the definition of the disease) might be accounted for by an increase of both histamine (and other mediators) "releasability" from lung mast cells, and the bronchial hyperreactivity to the released histamine. There are reasons to believe that both these conditions, which are characteristics of the disease, may rely upon an imbalance among histaminergic, adrenergic, and cholinergic receptors localized within the pulmonary tissue. Hence, we take this opportunity to review the taxonomy of pulmonary histamine receptors, with the aim of defining asthma as a receptor disease.

Pulmonary Histamine Receptors in Integrated Structures

Lungs are made up of integrated structures such as the pulmonary vasculature and airways, and by connective tissue containing different moieties of free cells (mast cell and other "inflammatory" cells). When mapped with the usual pharmacological tools (pharmacodynamic analysis: PA_2 and PD_2; "binding" analysis: B_{max} and K_m) [11], histaminergic receptors

* Department of Preclinical and Clinical Pharmacology, University of Florence, Viale G.B. Morgagni 65, 50134 Florence, Italy.

in pulmonary integrated structures appear to belong to the H_1 and H_2 subtypes. To our knowledge, no clearcut evidence of pulmonary H_3 receptors has been provided, although "atypical" histamine receptors have been inferred.

The actions of histamine on pulmonary blood vessels are biphasic—or "amphibaric" using the terminology of Page and McCubbin to describe the vascular effects of 5-hydroxytryptamine. Histamine may exert both vasoconstriction and vasodilatation in pulmonary blood vessels. In most animal species, vasoconstriction, with accompanying pulmonary hypertension, is the predominant effect, related to H_1 histamine receptor subtype since it is mimicked by H_1 receptor agonists and competitively blocked by traditional (anti-H_1) antihistamines [13, for a review]. Histamine reportedly also dilates the pulmonary vascular bed in situ. The vasodilator response to histamine is made more apparent after the blockade of H_1 receptors.

The pulmonary vasodilator action of histamine in the presence of mepyramine can be blocked by H_2-antagonists, thus establishing the vasodilator mechanism as being mediated by H_2 receptors [13]. The sheep is the only animal species in which "atypical" H_2 (or H_3?) receptors have been demonstrated, since the pulmonary vasodilator response to histamine cannot be blocked by currently available antihistamines [14]. Although histamine has long been suspected as a possible mediator of increased pulmonary microvascular permeability, it did not affect lung capillary membrane permeability in the dog [15]. However, Pietra et al. [16] found that histamine caused bronchial vessels, although not pulmonary vessels, to leak colloidal carbon in the dog.

A dual action of histamine is also apparent from its effects on airway smooth muscle. Histamine contracts tracheobronchial smooth muscle in vitro and in vivo by stimulation of H_1 receptors [17]. However, histamine stimulates H_2 receptors mediating relaxation of tracheobronchial smooth muscle from a variety of different species, including human beings [18]. Also, antagonists acting at H_2 receptors enhance the response of guinea pig bronchial smooth muscle to histamine [19]. In keeping with the observations relevant to the pulmonary vascular system, the bronchorelaxant effects of histamine in the trachea of some animal species were completely resistant to the action of all the H_2 receptor antagonists presently available, thus suggesting the presence of isoreceptors of H_2, or H_3 receptors mediating the "atypical" effect [13]. A final pathological change characterizing the status asthmaticus is the diffuse secretion of mucus. By employing human airways cultured in the presence of amino sugars, labeled glycoproteins synthesized in vitro have been quantitated and accounted for by an H_2 response, at least in this model of mucous secretion [20].

In conclusion, the application of selective histamine H_1 and H_2 receptor agonists and antagonists has established that H_1 receptors mediate actions such as bronchoconstriction, vasoconstriction, and edema formation (effects that may be deleterious in nature). Stimulation of pulmonary H_2 receptors, on the other hand, seems to play an important modulating role by causing bronchodilatation and increasing mucous secretion (Figure 1). The inhibition of the further release of mediators by H_2 receptor agonists calls for a thorough evaluation of histamine receptors on membranes of "inflammatory" cells.

Figure 1. Cholinergic reflex actions of histamine.

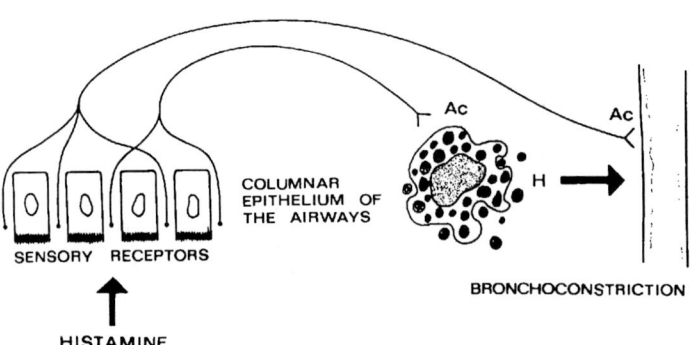

Histamine Receptors on Mast Cell: A Prospective Role in Asthma

In the human lung, mast cells are present in concentrations from 1 to $7 \cdot 10^6$ cells per gram of lung tissue [21], comprise up to 2% of alveolar cells, and are located in the connective tissue beneath the airway basement membrane surrounding glands and blood vessels, throughout the muscle bundles, and in the interalveolar septum as well as the bronchial lumen. Mast cells represent a physiological system of secretory cells, the homeostatic link with the environment being accomplished through receptors present on mast cell membranes. Among them, histaminergic and cholinergic receptors may be central to pathophysiological events leading to the asthmatic attack. H_1 receptors are present on rat serosal mast cells, which bind ^{3}H-pyrilamine specifically, rapidly, and reversibly in a saturable fashion to a receptor of the H_1 type, as shown by the specific displacement of the ligands [22]. Neither the chemical structure nor the physiological significance of the H_1 mast cell receptors has been clarified at the moment. H_2 receptors have been reported to be present on the mast cells of the guinea pig, but are apparently absent or nonfunctional in rat mast cells. However, specific binding sites for ^{3}H-cimetidine have been demonstrated in rat mast cell membrane preparations with Lineweaver-Burk analysis revealing a homogeneous population of specific binding sites [23]. Moreover, H_2 receptor agonists diminish the release of histamine by 48/80, dextran, and acetylcholine, in a fashion surmounted by H_2 receptor antagonists, thus showing a functional presence of H_2 receptors in isolated rat serosal mast cells [24]. As far as the pathophysiological function of mast cell H_2 receptors is concerned, mast cells isolated from sensitized guinea pigs release histamine when challenged in vitro with the specific antigen. The anaphylactic histamine release is dose-dependently inhibited by H_2 receptor agonists, the inhibiting effect being fully counteracted by H2 receptor antagonists [25].

Mast cell heterogeneity does not allow for the extrapolation of data obtained in different organs from different animal species; therefore, the inhibition of immunological mast cell histamine release by H_2 receptor activation, observed in serosal guinea-pig mast cells, is not straightforwardly relevant to human lung mast cells. However, the anaphylactic reaction in the guinea pig is reminiscent of human anaphylaxis, making possible the tentative hypothesis that the activation of mast cell H_2 receptors would also inhibit the further release of mediators in human lung mast cells.

Bronchial Asthma as a Model Receptor Disease

Besides the H_1/H_2 receptor moiety located on cell membranes of pulmonary vascular and airway smooth muscle and of mast cells, the activation of which is responsible for direct effects (such as the modulation of vessels and airway caliber and mediator release), a further histaminergic receptor, which mediates the cholinergic reflex actions of histamine, is relevant to the pathophysiology of asthma (Figure 2). A network of nerve fibers ramifying between the cells of the columnar epithelium of the airway has been repeatedly described [26]. These fibers are now thought to be the terminals of sensory receptors which respond to histamine

AIRWAY HISTAMINE RECEPTORS

Figure 2.

 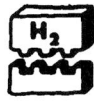 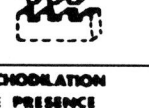

| CONSTRICTION OF SMOOTH MUSCLE IN TRACHEA, PRIMARY BRONCHUS AND LUNG STRIPS | RELAXATION OF CARBACHOL PRECONTRACTED TRACHEOBRONCHIAL SMOOTH MUSCLES | BRONCHODILATION IN THE PRESENCE OF MEPYRAMINE, EVOKED BY H2 AGONISTS BUT INSENSITIVE TO H2 ANTAGONISTS |

INCREASED FORMATION OF CYCLIC GMP

DEFICIENCY IN ASTHMA

with cholinergic bronchoconstriction reflex. Evidence for this reflex pathway is based on the fact that atropine or vagotomy reduced histamine-induced bronchoconstriction [26], and that H_1 receptor antagonists inhibit the histamine-induced stimulation of the afferent vagal sensory receptors [27]. Therefore the afferent part of the reflex mechanism may be classified as an H_1 receptor excitatory response consistent with the H_1 receptor-mediated direct bronchoconstrictor action of histamine. As far as the efferent part of the reflex is concerned, acetylcholine may directly evoke bronchoconstriction. In addition, it is worth remembering that there also exist cholinergic mechanisms that may facilitate the release of mediators themselves. In isolated rat serosal mast cells, acetylcholine possesses the ability to stimulate the secretion of histamine at concentrations as low as 10^{-12} M. The secretion of mast cell histamine by acetylcholine has the characteristic features of sequential exocytosis, is blocked by atropine, adrenaline and H_2 receptor agonists, and is enhanced by the presence of IgE on mast cell membrane [28, 29, 23]. It is therefore conceivable that acetylcholine released at the parasympathetic nerve endings would in turn evoke the secretion of histamine from mast cells, leading to bronchoconstriction. The concepts of mast cells as "paraneurons" [23] and of the innervation of mast cells are becoming better understood [23, 30, 31], in view of the explanation of terms such as "neuronal inflammation", "exercise-induced asthma," "learned histamine release" [32, 33, 34]. Moreover, the presence of the described diastaltic reflex could produce an "endless circle" (histamine, activation of the cholinergic reflex, cholinergic histamine release) perpetuating the pathophysiological features of the asthmatic attack.

It has already been hypothesized that asthma may be viewed as a disease characterized by a deficiency of adrenergic beta receptors. Increased bronchial sensitivity to histamine in mice vaccinated with *Bordetella pertussis* organism was found to be associated with a decrease in the beta adrenergic response; hence the proposal that increased airway sensitivity found in asthma was the result of a generalized beta receptor unresponsiveness [35]. The hypothesis is strengthened by the well-known pro-asthmatic side effects of beta-blockers. Accordingly, a decrease of the H_2 receptors would possibly enhance the H_1 response, leading to

increased airway constriction: Asthma subjects have a 100-fold decrease of H_2 response in granulocytes, in keeping with a 100-fold increase in sensitivity to histamine [36].

In conclusion, it is seductive to envisage the sudden asthmatic attack as the result of acquired and/or genetic down-regulation of H_2 and $beta_2$ receptors (leading to impaired bronchodilatation, potentiation of bronchoconstriction, progressive loss of the feedback mechanism inhibiting the further release of mediators), tentatively coupled to up regulation of H_1 and cholinergic muscarinic receptors (leading to bronchoconstriction and supporting the cholinergic histamine release). Within this framework, the drugs of choice would entail muscarinic anticholinergic compounds, H_2 receptor agonists, and H_1 receptor antagonists, suitable for reaching useful concentrations within the lung because of the paucity of the traditional side effects related to the lack of penetration in the central nervous system (astemizole, terfenadine).

References

1. Dale, H. H., and P. P. Laidlaw. 1910. The physiological action of beta-imidazolyl-ethyl amine. J. Physiol. 41: 318.
2. Bartosch, R., W. Feldberg, and E. Nagel. 1932. Das Freiwerden eines histaminähnlichen Stoffes bei der Anaphylaxie des Meerschweinchens. Pfluegers Arch. Gesamte Physiol. 230: 120.
3. Schild, O. H., D. R. Hawkins, J. L. Mongar, and H. Herxheimer. 1951. Reactions of isolated human asthmatic lung and bronchial tissue to a specific antigen. Histamine release and muscular contraction. Lancet 261: 376.
4. Kaliner, M. 1985. Mast cell mediators and asthma. Chest. 875: 25.
5. Friedman, M. M., and M. A. Kaliner. 1987. Human mast cells and asthma. Am. Rev. Respir. Dis. 135: 1157.
6. Scadding, J. C. 1976. Definition and clinical categorization. In: Bronchial Asthma. Mechanisms and Therapeutics. E. B. Weiss, M. S. Segal, eds. Boston: Little Brown & Company, p.19.
7. Ciba Foundation Guest Symposium. 1959. Terminology, definitions and classification of chronic pulmonary emphysema and related conditions. Thorax 14: 286.
8. Tung, R., and L. M. Lichtenstein. 1982. In vitro histamine release from basophils of asthmatic and atopic individuals in D_2O. J. Immunol. 128: 2067.

9. Neijens, H. J., H. C. Raatgeep, H. J. Degenhert, and K. F. Kerrebijn. 1982. Release of histamine from leukocytes and its determinants in vitro in relation to bronchial responsiveness to inhaled histamine and exercise in vivo. Clin. Allergy, 12: 577.

10. Cockroft, D. W. 1980. Clinical assessment of non-specific bronchial reactivity using a standardized histamine inhalation test: Relevance in early diagnosis. In: Occupational pulmonary disease. Focus on grain dust and health. Academic Press, Inc., p. 161.

11. Goldestein, A., L. Aronow, and S. M. Kalman. 1969. Principles of drug action. New York/London/Sidney/Toronto: John Wiley & Sons.

12. Page, H. I., and J. W. McCubbin. 1953. The variable arterial pressure response to serotonin in laboratory animals and man. Circ. Res. 1: 354.

13. Eyre, P., and N. Chand. 1982. Histamine receptor mechanisms of the lung. In: Pharmacology of histamine receptors, C.R. Ganellin and M.E. Parsons, eds. Wright PSG, p. 298.

14. Ahmed, T., and M. King. 1986. Suppression of pulmonary and systemic vascular histamine H_2 receptors in allergic sheep. J. Appl. Physiol. 60: 791.

15. Drake, R. E., and J. C. Gabel. 1980. Effect of histamine and alloxan on canine pulmonary vascular permeability. Am. J. Physiol. 238: 96.

16. Pietra, G. G., G. P. Szidon, M. M. Leventhal, and A. P. Fishman, 1971. Histamine and interstitial pulmonary edema in the dog. Circ. Res. 29: 323.

17. Chand, N., and P. Eyre. 1975. Classification and biological distribution of histamine receptor subtypes. Agents Actions 5: 277.

18. Foreman, J. C., T. J. Rising, and S. E. Webber, 1985. A study of the histamine H_2-receptor mediating relaxation of the parenchymal lung strip preparation of the guinea pig. Br. J. Pharmac. 86: 465.

19. Drazen, J. M., C. S. Venugopalan, and N. W. Schneider. 1980. Alteration of histamine response by H_2 receptor antagonism in the guinea-pig. J. Appl. Physiol. Resp. Environ. Exercise Physiol. 48: 613.

20. Shelhamer, J. H., Z. Marom, and M. Kaliner. 1980. Immunological and neuropharmacological stimulation of mucous glycoprotein release from human airways in vitro. J. Clin. Invest. 66: 1400.

21. Wasserman, S. I. 1980. The lung mast cells: Its physiology and potential relevance to defense of the lung. Envir. Health Perspect. 35: 153.

22. Wescott, S. L., W. A. Hunt, and M. Kaliner. 1982. Histamine H_1-receptors on rat peritoneal mast cells. Life Sci. 31: 1911.

23. Masini, E., R. Fantozzi, P. Blandina, S. Brunelleschi, and P.F. Mannaioni. 1985. The riddle of cholinergic histamine release from mast cells. Progr. Med. Chem. 22: 268.

24. Masini, E., P. Blandina, and P. F. Mannaioni. 1982. Mast cell receptors controlling histamine release: Influence on the mode of action of drugs used in the treatment of adverse drug reactions. Klin. Wochenschr. 60: 1031.

25. Mannaioni, P. F., R. Fantozzi, E. Giannella, and E. Masini. 1988. Pathophysiological significance of the distribution of histamine receptor subtypes in inflammation and in type I hypersensitivity reactions. Agents Actions 24: 26.

26. Widdicombe, J. G. 1975. Reflex control of airway smooth muscle. Postgrad. Med. J. 36: 36.

27. Vidruk, E. H., and S. R. Samson. 1978. H_1 histamine receptors on rapidly adapting vagal afferents in canine lungs. Fed. Proc. 37: 689.

28. Fantozzi, R., E. Masini, P. Blandina, P. F. Mannaioni, and T. Bani Sacchi. 1978. Release of histamine from rat mast cells by acetylcholine. Nature 273: 473.

29. Blandina, P., R. Fantozzi, P. F. Mannaioni, and E. Masini. 1980. Characteristics of histamine release evoked by acetylcholine in isolated rat mast cells. J. Physiol. 301: 281.

30. Skofitsch, G., J. M. Savitt, and D. M. Jacobowits. 1985. Suggestive evidence for a functional unit between mast cells and substance P fibers in the rat diaphragm and mesentery. Histochemistry 82: 5.

31. Dimitriadov, V., P. Aubineau, J. Taci, and J. Seylaz. 1987. Ultrastructural evidence for a functional unit between nerve fibers and type II cerebral vascular wall. Neuroscience 82: 5.

32. Edmunds, A. T., M. Tooley, and S. Godfrey. 1978. The refractory period after exercise induced asthma: its duration and relation to the severity of the exercise. Am. Rev. Respir. Dis. 177: 247.

33. Russell, M., K. A. Dark, R. W. Cummings, G. Ellman, E. Callaway, and H. V. S. Peeke. 1984. Learned histamine release. Science 225: 733.

34. Casale, T. B., T. M. Keahey, and M. Kaliner. 1986. Exercise induced anaphylactic syndromes. Insights into diagnostic and pathophysiological features. J. Amer. Med. Ass. 255: 2049.

35. Szentivany, A. 1968. The beta-adrenergic theory of the atopic abnormality in asthma. J. Allergy 42: 203.

36. Busse, W. W., and J. Sosman. 1977. Decreased H_2 histamine response of granulocytes of asthmatic patients. J. Clin. Invest. 59: 1080.

Therapeutic Effects of H_1 Receptor Antagonists in Asthma

*Paul Rafferty**

Early trials of antihistamines in the treatment of asthma were largely unsuccessful, and this may have been because of the unpleasant anticholinergic and sedative side effects of the older preparations which limited the doses that could be used. The emergence of the non-sedating antihistamines has permitted much more effective histamine blockade to be achieved. In a double-blind, placebo-controlled, parallel-group crossover study in grass pollen-sensitive asthmatics, terfenadine was found to reduce significantly symptoms of cough and wheeze, to reduce bronchodilator inhaler use, and to increase peak expiratory flow rates.

Histamine was first recognised as an important effector agent in allergic disease when Dale and Laidlaw [1] found that intravenous histamine could reproduce many of the features of anaphylaxis. High concentrations of histamine were subsequently found in lung tissue [2], and the association with asthma was made when Weiss [3] demonstrated that intravenous histamine could produce bronchoconstriction in asthmatics.

By the 1940s suitable histamine antagonists had been developed for use in man. They proved to be of value in the treatment of urticaria, allergic rhinitis and conjunctivitis, but were largely unhelpful in the treatment of asthma. However, a number of open studies using diphenhydramine and pyribenzamine reported subjective improvement in 12 to 50% of patients [4, 5].

In a early objective study utilizing antihistamnies, Curry [6] found that the fall in vital capacity produced in an asthmatic by the intravenous injection of histamine could be significantly attenuated by diphenhydramine. Subsequently, both parenteral and inhaled antihistamines have been shown to inhibit the bronchoconstriction following inhaled histamine, allergen, or after exercise [7, 8, 9]. Several authors have also been able to demonstrate a bronchodilator effect using pyribenzamine, thiazinium, chlorpheniramine, and clemastine [10–13]. Popa [12] noted that the greatest bronchodilator effect was seen in those subjects who had the largest initial reduction in baseline FEV_1 levels.

Since oral antihistamines were poorly tolerated, inhaled preparations were assessed. A single 200 µg dose of clemastine was shown to improve the peak expiratory flow rate by 6.5% in a group of schoolchildren, but the addition of regular inhaled clemastine to their current therapy resulted in no significant objective or symptomatic improvement [14].

The poor results of clinical studies using the older antihistamines may be the result of the relatively weak antihistaminic effect of these

Table 1. The relative potency of antihistamine assessed by their displacement of the histamine-concentration response (HCR) curve.

Preparation	Dosage	Route	Displacement of histamine CR curve	Reference
Diphenhydramine	20 mg	Neb	3.5	7
Chlorpheniramine	10 mg	IV	4.0–8.0	17
Clemastine	0.5 mg	Neb	4	8
Clemastine	1 mg	Neb	10	13
Astemizole	10 mg	Oral	17	16
Terfenadine	60 mg	Oral	14.8	18
Terfenadine	120 mg	Oral	22.9	18
Terfenadine	180 mg	Oral	34.3	18

* Deparment of Respiratory Medicine, Western Infirmary, Glasgow, Scotland, U.K.

Table 2. The effect of terfenadine on symptom scores, inhaler use, and PEFR.

Variable	Placebo	Terfenadine	%Improvement	P-value
Cough	0.3019	0.0697	76.9	0.005
Wheeze	0.5131	0.2723	46.9	0.026
Breathlessness	0.3057	0.2543	16.8	0.539
Chest tightness	0.4823	0.3361	30.3	0.121
Inhaler use (puff/day)	1.974	1.1795	40.3	0.203
PEFR am (l/min)	378.9	399.6	5.5	0.001
PEFR pm (l/min)	405.3	430.4	6.2	0.003

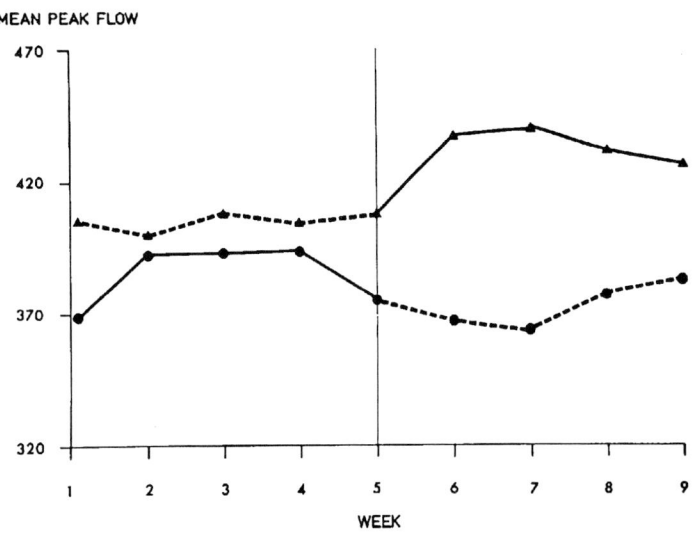

Figure 1. The effect of terfenadine and placebo on mean peak expiratory flow rates during the study. Solid lines = terfenadine treatment. Broken lines = placebo treatment.

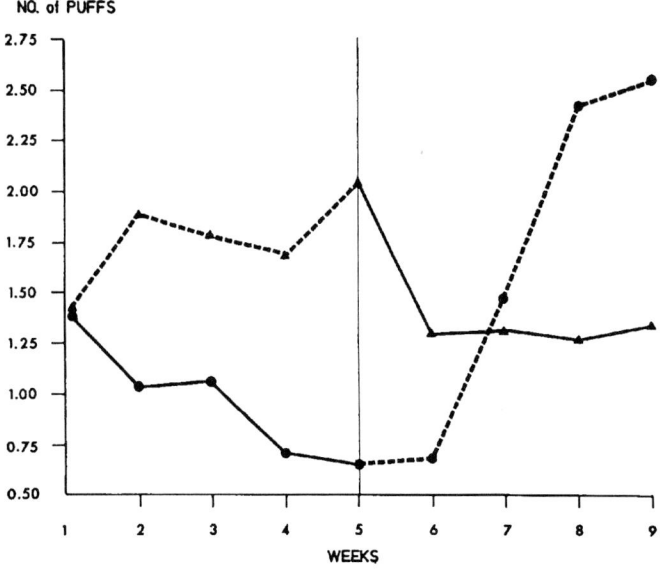

Figure 2. The effect of terfenadine and placebo on bronchodilator inhaler use during the study. Solid lines = terfenadine treatment. Broken lines = placebo treatment.

preparations and their associated unpleasant anticholinergic and sedative effects that limited the doses that could be tolerated. In recent years, the arrival of the non-sedating antihistamines, terfenadine and astemizole, has allowed more effective H_1 receptor antagonism to be achieved (Table 1). In view of their potency relative to the older preparations, a reassessment of their role in asthma is taking place.

Both terfenadine and astemizole have been found to reduce the early bronchoconstrictor reaction to inhaled allergen by 50% [15, 16]. In a clinical study in asthmatics with allergic rhinitis and conjunctivitis, astemizole was found to reduce significantly symptoms of wheezing experienced by the patients [16].

In Southampton, we recently carried out a double-blind, parallel-group crossover study to assess the efficacy of terfenadine 180 µg three times daily in the treatment of grass pollen-sensitive asthmatics during the pollen season. Eighteen mild, atopic asthmatics participated in the study. Their only medication was inhaled B_2 adrenoreceptor agonists. The first week of the study consisted of a run-in phase during which both groups of patients received placebo medication. This was followed by 4 weeks of terenadine or placebo. During the last 4 weeks of the study, patients received the alternate medication. Asthma symptoms were assessed each day by scoring the symptoms of cough, wheeze, breathlessness, and chest tightness on a scale from 0–3 (no symptoms to severe symptoms). In addition, twice daily peak expiratory flow rates were recorded. Throughout the study patients attended the laboratory each week where methacholine inhalation challenge tests were performed to assess any changes in airway reactivity.

All symptoms were reduced when patients were receiving terfenadine. Cough was reduced by 76.9% ($p<0.01$) and wheeze by 46.9% ($p<0.05$). Breathlessness and chest tightness were also reduced, though they did not reach statistical significance (Table 2). Bronchodilator inhaler use also fell by 40%, while at the same time morning and evening peak flow rates increased by 5.5% and 6.2% respectively ($p<0.01$) (Figures 1 and 2). Throughout the study there was a small increase in airway reactivity to methacholine; this was not significantly affected by treatment with terfenadine.

These results cannot be automatically extrapolated to more severe asthmatics. This group of mild asthmatics had a mean FEV_1 of 98% of the predicted value, and patients with more severe airway limitation could have a greater potential for further bronchodilation. The encouraging results of this preliminary study in mild asthmatics now warrant further investigation of the role of these potent antihistamines in the treatment of more severe asthma.

References

1. Dale, H. H., and P. P. Laidlaw. 1919. Histamine shock. J. Physiol. 52: 355.
2. Best. C. H., H. H. Dale, H. W. Dudley, and W. V. Thorpe. 1927. The nature of vasodilator constituents of certain tissue extracts. J. Physiol. 62: 397–417.
3. Weiss, S., G. P. Robb, and L. B. Ellis. 1932. The systemic effects of histamine in man with special reference to the response of the cardiovacular system. Arch. Int. Med. 49: 360–396.
4. Eyerman, C. H. 1946. Clinical experience with a new antihistamine drug. J. Allergy. 17: 210.
5. Bernstein, T. B., J. M. Rose, and S. M. Feinberg. 1947. New antihistamine drugs in hay fever and other allergic conditions. Ill. Med. J. 92: 90.
6. Curry, J. J. The effect of antihistamine substances and other drugs on histamine bronchoconstriction in asthmatic subjects. J. Clin. Invest. 25: 792–799.
7. Casterline, C. L., and R. Evans. Further studies on the mechanisms of histamine-induced asthma. 1977. J. Allergy Clin. Immunol. 59: 420–424.
8. Phillips, M., S. Ollier, C. A. L. Gould, and R. J. Davies. 1984. Effect of antihistamines and antiallergic drugs on responses to allergen and histamine provocation tests in asthma. Thorax. 39: 345–351.
9. Harley, J. P. R., and S. G. Norgrady. 1980. Effect of inhaled antihistamine on exercise induced asthma. Thorax. 35: 657–679.
10. Herxheimer, H. Antihistamines in bronchial asthma. 1949. Brit. Med. J. 901–905.
11. Booij-Noord, H., N. M. G. Orie, W. C. Berg, and K. de Vries. 1970. Protection tests on bronchial allergen challenge with disodium cromoglycate and thiazinium. J. Allergy. 46: 1–11.
12. Popa, V. T. 1977. Bronchodilating activity of an H_1 blocker, chlorpheniramine. 1977. J. Allergy Clin. Immunol. 59: 54–63.
13. Norgrady, S. G., and C. Bevan. 1978. Inhaled antihistamines: bronchodilation and effects on histamine and methacholine induced bronchoconstriction. Thorax. 33: 700–704.
14. Henry, R. L., I. G. C. Hodges, A. D. Milner, and G. M. Stokes. 1983. Bronchodilating effects of

the H_1 receptor antagonist clemastine. Arch. Dis. Childhood. 58: 304–305.

15. Rafferty, P., C. R. Beasley, and S. T. Holgate. 1987. The contribution of histamine to bronchoconstriction produced by inhaled allergen and adenosine 5′ monophosphate in asthma. Am. Rev. Resp. Dis. 136: 369–373.

16. Howarth, P. H., and S. T. Holgate. 1985. Astemizole, an H_1 antagonist, in allergic asthma. J. Allergy Clin. Immunol. 75 1: 166 (A).

17. Popy, V. T. 1980. Effect of an H_1 blocker, chlorpheniramine, on inhalation tests with histamine and allergen in allergic asthma. Chest. 78 3: 442–451.

18. Rafferty, P., and S. T. Holgate. 1987. Terfenadine (Seldane) is a potent and selective H_1 histamine receptor antagonist in asthmatic airways. Am. Rev. Resp. Dis. 135: 181–184.

Bronchodilator Activity of H_1 Receptor Antagonists

K. R. Patel and S. K. Ghosh*

The mechanism of histamine hyperresponsiveness in patients with asthma remains unclear. Histamine acts on the bronchial smooth muscle by interaction with at least two distinct receptors: H_1- and H_2-receptors, and probably through stimulation of the rapidly adapting irritant receptors.

In single-dose studies we have observed that the H_1-receptor antagonists clemastine, cetirizine, ketotifen, and azelastine produce small but significant bronchodilator effects in patients with extrinsic asthma suggesting "histamin tone" due to locally released histamine in the lung. In order to examine the dose-response relationship of H_1-antagonists on the bronchomotor tone in asthma, we compared the effect of terfenadine at doses of 60 mg, 120 mg, and 180 mg with placebo in 19 patients (aged 16 to 58 years) with mild extrinsic asthma (mean ± SEM of predicted FEV_1 88.0 ± 2.8%) and 7 patients (aged 26 to 62 years) with moderately severe asthma (mean predicted FEV_1 60.2 ± 4.3%) for up to 8 hours in double-blind, randomized studies.

Terfenadine produced a small but significant bronchodilatation in the patients studied, and the effect was present for up to 8 hours. Although the bronchodilator response was more marked in patients with moderately severe asthma, no dose-response relationship was observed. These results suggest the presence of histamine tone which is dependent on local endogenous histamine release.

Patients with asthma are hyperresponsive to histamine, and the capacity of histamine to induce bronchoconstriction has been known since 1929 [1–5]. The involvement of histamine in asthma is also supported by the finding of increased plasma histamine levels in acute asthma [6–8] and following exercise [9] and allergen inhalation challenges [10] in patients with asthma. Histamine acts directly on H_1 and H_2 histamine receptors on the bronchial smooth muscle and probably through stimulation of the vagal receptor to cause subsequent bronchoconstriction. Histamine-induced bronchoconstriction can be blocked by H_1 histamine antagonists, whereas atropine has no effect [11–14]. H_1 histamine receptor antagonists, chlorpheneramine [14, 15], clemastine [16, 17], terfenadine [18], and cetirizine have been reported to have a bronchodilator activity, and this is also true of ketotifen [19] and azelastine [20], antiallergic compounds with potent antihistaminic properties. The dose response effect of H_1 antagonists have not been studied previously because of CNS side effects observed with classical antihistamines. Terfenadine is a potent H_1-receptor antagonist, and as it does not cross the blood-brain barrier, it is devoid of major CNS side effects observed with classical antihistamines.

In order to examine the dose-response effect of terfenadine on the resting bronchomotor tone, we examined the effect of placebo and terfenadine 60 mg, 120 mg, and 180 mg on the FEV_1 in double-blind, crossover, randomized studies in 19 patients with mild extrinsic bronchial asthma over 4-hour periods, and in further 7 patients with moderately severe asthma over 8-hour periods.

Patients and Methods

Study 1

Nineteen patients (aged 16–58 years, mean 33.8 years, 6 females) with mild extrinsic asthma (mean (SEM) FEV_1 88 (2.8)%) of predicted normal values and reversible airflow obstruction were studied. Cromolyn sodium was stopped for 48 hours, and inhaled bronchodilator drugs were stopped for at least 12 hours prior to each test. Patients receiving oral corticosteroids, oral

---

* Department of Respiratory Medicine, Western Infirmary, Glasgow G11 6NT, Scotland, United Kingdom.
   Acknowledgements: We thank Dr. Malcolm Boyce of Merrill-Dow Pharmaceuticals Ltd. for statistical analysis, Miss Aileen Vetters for technical assistance, and Mrs. J. Peter for typing the manuscript.

Table 1. Percent change in FEV$_1$ from baseline in 19 patients with mild asthma.

| | Baseline | % change in FEV$_1$ in mild asthma (liters) | | | | |
		30 min	1 h	2h	3h	4h
Placebo	3.11 ± 0.19	−1.0	−0.3	−1.8	−1.8	−1.8
60 mg terfenadine	3.17 ± 0.19	0.2	3.3	7.2**	7.5*	6.9*
120 mg terfenadine	3.11 ± 0.21	2.2	7.9	10.6*	12.6**	11.1*
180 mg terfenadine	3.10 ± 0.20	1.0	6.0	9.2*	7.6**	8.0**

*p<0.05, **p<0.01

Table 2. Percent change in FEV$_1$ from baseline in seven patients with moderately severe asthma.

| | Baseline | % change in FEV$_1$ in mild asthma (liters) | | | | | | |
		30 min	1 h	2 h	3 h	4 h	6 h	8 h
Placebo	2.10 ± 0.24	−5.0	−3.0	−3.9	−6.5	−9.2	−13.9	−17.4
60 mg terfenadine	1.88 ± 0.22	7.7	9.6	15.3	20.5*	21.7*	17.7	12.1
120 mg terfenadine	1.91 ± 0.29	8.8	10.0*	20.6*	26.7*	23.0*	21.1*	18.3**
180 terfenadine	1.91 ± 0.21	5.4	14.6*	20.2*	22.7**	29.1**	24.8**	24.8**

*p<0.05, **p<0.01

bronchodilators, antihistamines, and anticholinergic drugs were excluded. The study was approved by the hospital ethics committee, and an informed consent was obtained in each case.

This was a double-blind, randomized, crossover study with placebo and terfenadine 60 mg, 120 mg, and 180 mg administered in single doses after a light breakfast. At least 48 hours were allowed to elapse between treatments. FEV$_1$ was measured on a dry wedge spirometer (Vitalograph, Buckingham, U.K.). Spirometry was repeated at 15, 30, 60, 120, 180, and 240 minutes after treatment. The best of three attempts was recorded for analysis. Ten of these patients underwent exercise challenge, and the remaining 9 patients methacholine inhalations. Results of the exercise and methacholine challenges have been reported previously [18, 23].

Study 2

Using an identical protocol, the effect of placebo and terfenadine was studied in 7 patients (aged 26–62 years, mean 45.7 years, all male) with moderately severe asthma (mean predicted FEV$_1$ 54 (8.7)%) and reversible airflow obstruction. FEV$_1$ was measured on a dry wedge spirometer before treatment and then at 15, 30, 60, 120, 180, 240, 360, and 480 minutes.

Statistical Analysis

The changes in FEV$_1$ at each time point were compared between different treatments and placebo with analysis of variance. Period effect, carry-over effect, and treatment × period interaction were also examined with analysis of variance.

Results

Study 1

The mean baseline FEV$_1$ values before treatment on 4 days of testing were comparable, and no statistical difference was noted (Table 1). The changes in the mean (SEM) percentage FEV$_1$ were −0.31 (1.0)%, 3.3 (1.3)%, 7.9 (2.6)%, and 6 (1.5)% with placebo, terfenadine 60 mg, 120 mg, and 180 mg, respectively, at 60 minutes, and by 250 minutes the changes were −1.8 (1.3)%, 6.9 (2)%, 11.1 (3.8)%, and 8.0 (2.9)%, respectively (Figure 1). The bronchodilator effect of terfenadine compared to placebo was highly significantly (p < 0.0001).

223

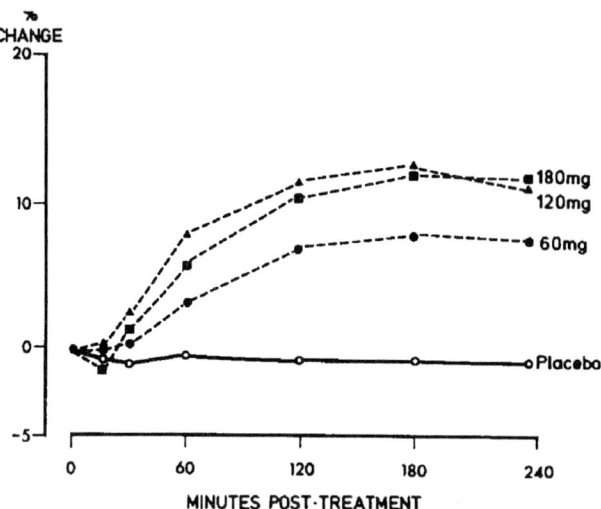

Figure 1. Terfenadine produced small but significant bronchodilatation in patients with mild asthma. No dose-response relationship was observed.

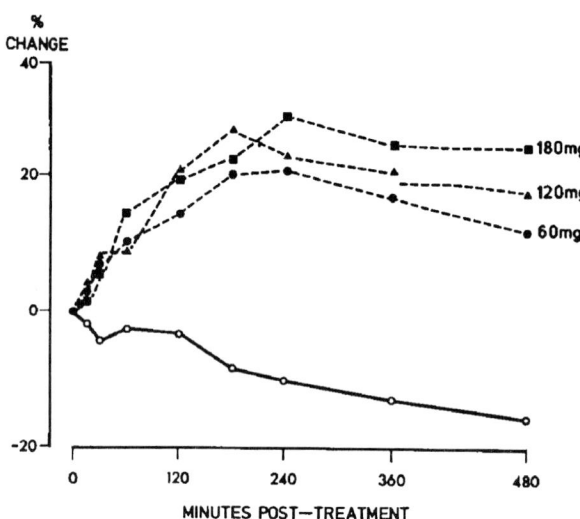

Figure 2. Terfenadine produced greater bronchodilatation in patients with moderately severe asthma compared to patients with mild asthma.

Study 2

In the second study in patients with moderately severe asthma, the mean baseline values before treatment on 4 days of testing were comparable and no statistical difference was noted (Table 2). The mean percentage changes in FEV_1 were –3.0 (4.4)%, 9.6 (6)%, 10 (1.8)%, and 14.6 (5.2)% with placebo and terfenadine 60 mg, 120 mg, and 180 mg, respectively, at 60 minutes, and by 240 minutes the changes were –9.2 (5.2)%, 21.7 (12.6)%, 23.0 (6.4)%, and 29.1 (6.8)%, respectively (Figure 2). The bronchodilator effect of terfenadine was still present at 8 hours, and changes with placebo and terfenadine 60 mg, 120 mg, and 180 mg were –17.4 (5.2)%, 12.1 (15.0)%, 18.3 (8.9)%, and 24.8 (11.1)%, respectively. The bronchodilator effect of terfenadine was significant compared to placebo ($p < 0.001$ at 240 minutes, $p < 0.01$ at 480 minutes).

Single dose of terfenadine 60 mg, 120 mg, and 180 mg caused bronchodilatation of at least 8 hours in duration. The profile of response was similar regardless of dose. The patients with more severe asthma tended to respond more than those with mild asthma. No significant adverse events were reported apart from two patients who complained of dryness of mouth.

Discussion

Dall and Laidlaw [21] first reported the physiological effects of histamine in 1911 and the ability of histamine to contract smooth muscle. Asthmatic patients are hyperresponsive to inhaled and injected histamine, an observation reported frequently since 1929 [1–5]. Raised plasma levels of histamine in acute asthma [7] and following exercise [8, 9] and allergen challenges [10] in asthmatic patients has been frequently cited as one possible mechanism of acute bronchoconstriction in asthma. H_1 antagonists have been reported to inhibit histamine [13–15], exercise [22, 23], and also allergen- induced bronchoconstriction [24].

The use of H_1-receptor antagonists in the treatment of asthma has been avoided in the past because a small proportion of asthmatic children [25] develop airflow obstruction with H_1-receptor antagonists, and also because of a theoretical risk that anticholinergic effects of antihistamine would cause airway drying and inspissation of mucus in the airways. These concerns, however, have not proved to be of clinical significance. Indeed, numerous studies [13–18] have shown that H_1-receptor antagonists to produce a bronchodilator response with improvement in lung function. Norgady and colleagues [16] found that inhaled clemastine, an H_1 histamine antagonist, was as effective as β_2 agonist, salbutamol in producing bronchodilatation in asthmatic subjects.

The questions addressed by the present studies were: (a) Does terfenadine produce bronchodilatation over 4- and 8-hour periods? (b) Is the response to terfenadine dose-related? (c) Does asthma severity affect the response to terfenadine? Compared with placebo, terfenadine produced bronchodilatation with highly significant increases in FEV_1. In fact, placebo treatment was associated with a fall in FEV_1 as the result of withholding patients' usual bronchodilator therapy. This deterioration in lung function was more marked in moderately severe asthmatics. The bronchodilator effect of terfenadine was present at least 8 hours post-dosing. No dose-response relationship was observed. Although patients with severe asthma achieved greater bronchodilatation compared to patients with mild asthma, the difference did not reach statistical significance because of the small numbers of subjects studied.

The bronchodilator effect of terfenadine together with its ability to modify exercise and allergen-induced asthma suggest that this drug merits further clinical investigation in the management of some patients with asthma. Furthermore, terfenadine and other non-sedating H_1 histamine antagonists can be administered in larger doses to achieve adequate H_1-receptor blockade in the airways without causing untoward CNS side effects seen with classical antihistamines.

References

1. Weiss, S., G. P. Robb, and H. L. Blumgart. 1929. The velocity of blood flow in health and disease as measured by the effect of histamine on the minute vessels. Am. Heart J. 4: 664–691.
2. Weiss, S., G. P. Robb, and L. B. Ellis. 1932. The systemic effects of histamine in man with special reference to the responses of the cardiovascular system. Arch. Intern. Med. 49: 360–379.
3. Curry, J. J. 1946. The action of histamine on the respiratory tract in normal and asthmatic subjects. J. Clin. Invest. 25: 785–791.
4. Curry, J. J. 1947. Comparative action of acetyl-betamethyl choline and histamine on the respiratory tract in normals, patients with hay fever, and subjects with bronchial asthma. J. Clin. Invest. 26: 430–438.
5. Itkin, I. H. 1967. Bronchial hypersensitivity to mecholyl and histamine in asthma subjects. J. Allergy 40: 245–256.
6. Simon, R. A., D. D. Stevenson, C. M., Arroyave, and E. M. Tan. 1977. The relationship of plasma histamine to the activity of bronchial asthma. J. Allergy Clin. Immunol. 60: 312316.
7. Bruce, C., R. Weatherstone, and W. H. Taylor. 1976. Histamine levels in plasma, blood and urine in severe asthma and the effect of corticosteroids. Thorax 31: 724–729.
8. Barnes, P. J., P. W. Ind, and M. J. Brown. 1982. Plasma histamine and catecholamines in stable asthmatic subjects. Clin. Sci. 62: 661665.
9. Lee, T. H., T. Nagakura, N. Papgeorgiou, Y. Likura, and A. B. Kay. 1983. Exercise induced late asthmatic reactions with neutrophil chemotactic activity. N. Engl. J. Med. 308: 1502–1505.
10. Durham, S. R., T. H. Lee, O. Cromwell et al. 1984. Immunologic studies in allergen-induced late-phase asthmatic reactions. J. Allergy Clin. Immunol. 74: 49–60.
11. Casterline, C. L., R. Evans, and G. W. Ward. 1976. The effect of atropine and albuterol on the human bronchial response to histamine. J. Allergy Clin. Immunol. 58: 607–613.

12. Casterline, C. L., R. Evans, and G. W. Ward. 1976. Further studies on the mechanism of human histamine-induced asthma. J. Allergy Clin. Immunol. 59: 420–424.

13. Eiser, N. M., J. Mills, P. D. Snashall, and A. Guz. 1981. The role of histamine receptors in asthma. Clin. Sci. 60: 363–370.

14. Thomson, N. C., and J. W. Kerr. 1980. Effect of inhaled H_1 and H_2 receptor antagonists in normal and asthmatic subjects. Thorax 35: 428–434.

15. Nathan, R. A., N. Segali, and A. L. Schocket. 1981. A comparison of the actions of H_1 and H_2 antihistamines on histamine induced bronchoconstriction and cutaneous wheal response in asthmatic patients. J. Allergy Clin. Immunol. 67: 171–177.

16. Nogrady, S. G., J. P. R. Hartley, P. D. J. Handslip, and N. P. Hursh. 1978. Bronchodilatation after inhalation of the antihistamine clemastine. Thorax 33: 479–482.

17. Dorward, A. J., and K. R. Patel. 1982. Comparison of ketotifen with clemastine, ipratropium bromide and sodium cromoglycate in exercise-induced asthma. Clin. Allergy 12: 355–361.

18. Patel, K. R. 1987. Effect of terfenadine on methacholine induced bronchoconstriction. J. Allergy Clin. Immunol. 79: 355–358.

19. Dorward, A. J., and K. R. Patel. 1985. Effect of inhaled ketotifen in exercise-induced asthma—a negative report. Eur. J. Resp. Dis. 67: 378–380.

20. Albazzaz, M. K., and K. R. Patel. 1988. Effect of azelastine on LTC_4 and histamine induced bronchoconstriction in patients with extrinsic asthma. Thorax 43: 306–311.

21. Dall, H. H., and P. P. Laidlaw. 1911. The physiologic action of beta imidazolylethylamine. J. Physiol. (London) 41: 318–344.

22. Hartley, J. P. R., and B. H. Davies. 1980. Effect of an inhaled antihistamine on exercise-induced asthma. Thorax 35: 675–679.

23. Patel, K. R. 1984. Terfenadine in exercise-induced asthma. Br. Med. J. 288: 1496–1497.

24. Phillips, M. J., S. Ollier, C. Gould, and R. J. Davies. 1984. Effect of antihistamines and antiallergic drugs on the responses to allergen and histamine provocation tests in asthma. Thorax 39: 345–351.

25. Schuller, D. R. 1983. Adverse effects of brompheniramine on pulmonary function in onset of asthmatic children. J: Allergy Clin. Immunol. 72: 175–179.

Understanding the Pathogenesis of Allergic Rhinitis

Robert M. Naclerio*/**, Alkis G. Togias*, David Proud*, Anne Kagey-Sobotka*, Lawrence M. Lichtenstein*

Nasal challenge with antigen and cold, dry air (CDA) was used to study the mechanism of allergic inflammation. Mast cell activation is suggested by an increase in the levels of histamine and prostaglandin D_2 and could also partly account for elevations in leukotrienes, TAME-esterase activity, and kinins in recovered nasal lavages following the early response (ER) to both stimuli. Topical azatadine, an H_1 antihistamine, inhibits the ER to antigen but not to CDA, indicating different roles for histamine and different mechanisms of mast cell activation. Both ERs, however, are followed in some individuals by a second increase in symptoms and mediators in 3 to 11 hours, suggesting that late-phase reactions (LPR) are the consequence of mast cell activation. The implications of these observations are discussed.

To understand the pathogenesis of an illness, it is necessary to observe the events occurring between exposure to the initiating stimulus and the development of pathologic changes with their associated symptomatology. After observing a change from baseline, the relevance of that change must be determined. Pharmacologic interventions assist in this endeavor as well as in the study of related diseases.

Here, we explore the pathophysiology of allergic rhinitis. The importance of pollen antigen and the prior development of specific IgE antibodies is assumed. Nasal lavage is used to observe the events between antigen exposure and the development of symptoms. Antihistamines are used to intervene pharmacologically, and the rhinitis secondary to the inhalation of CDA is used for parallel studies.

Methods

Subjects

Adult volunteers with a history of allergic rhinitis who previously responded positively to nasal antigen challenge, and individuals reporting nasal symptoms upon exposure to cold and windy environments who also demonstrated a positive response to 15-minute nasal challenge with CDA, were included in the studies. A positive response was defined as the occurrence of symptoms in association with a threefold increase in the levels of histamine and TAME-esterase activity in nasal secretions. All participants were asymptomatic and off all medication for at least two weeks prior to nasal challenge. The studies were approved by the Joint Committee on Clinical Investigation of the Johns Hopkins Medical Institutions and all subjects gave informed consent before participating.

Challenges

The technique of stimulating the nasal mucosa with CDA has been described in detail [1]. Briefly, subjects inhaled compressed air through a pediatric face mask placed over the nose for 15 minutes at a flow rate of 22.5 l/min. Prior to inhalation, the air was conditioned to a temperature ranging between -7 to $-10\,°C$ and a relative humidity of 0–10% for the CDA challenge or to 30–32 °C and 99% relative humidity for the warm, moist air (WMA) challenge.

---

*   Department of Medicine, Division of Clinical Immunology, Johns Hopkins University School of Medicine, Baltimore, Maryland.
** Department of Otolaryngology—Head & Neck Surgery, Johns Hopkins University School of Medicine, Baltimore, Maryland.
     From the O'Neill Laboratories at The Good Samaritan Hospital, 5601 Loch Raven Boulevard, Baltimore, Maryland 21239.
     Supported by grants NS 22488, HL 37119, HL 32272, AI 08270, AI 20136 from the National Institutes of Health, Bethesda, Maryland.

The protocol for antigen challenge is described in detail elsewhere [2]. In brief, after four baseline lavages the subjects received intranasal oxymetazoline spray (Afrin®, 0.1 ml of a 0.05% solution). They were then challenged twice with diluent (phosphate-buffered saline), followed by three doses of the antigen (10, 100 and 1000 PNU) to which they were allergic. Nasal lavages followed each dose of drug, diluent or antigen. After the third antigen challenge (t = 0), nasal lavages were performed at 10 and 20 minutes. To study LPRs, the lavages were continued hourly for the next 10 hours. All individuals remained in the laboratory throughout the experiments to limit their exposure to antigens.

To avoid any influence of one challenge on another, an interval of at least 7 days was allowed between sequential challenges. Nasal symptoms were rated by the volunteers before every nasal lavage. Rhinorrhea, congestion, and other symptoms—pruritus of the nose and eyes, headache, and postnasal drip—were rated on a scale from 0 (no symptoms) to 3 (severe symptoms). Episodes of sneezing were counted.

Mediator Measurements

Nasal lavages were performed by instilling 2.5 or 5.0 ml of saline, prewarmed to 37 °C, into each nostril. Lactated Ringer's solution was substituted for saline when cells were evaluated to preserve morphology. Ten seconds after instillation, the fluid was expelled into a plastic tray and transferred to a 15-ml polypropylene tube, which was stored on ice until the end of the experiment. The lavages were centrifuged to separate the sol from the gel phase, and the supernatants were divided into aliquots. Samples for histamine were mixed with 8% perchloric acid at a ratio of 4:1 respectively to precipitate proteins. The mixture was kept at 4 °C for 24 hours, centrifuged for 10 min at 1000 G, and the histamine levels in the supernatant were measured by an automated fluorometric assay [3] sensitive to 1 ng/ml. TAME-esterase activity was measured by a radiochemical assay which provides linear measurements to 20,000 CPM [4]. The appearance of TAME-esterase activity in nasal lavages has been shown to highly correlate with the symptomatology of the ER to nasal challenge

with CDA [1]. During the ER to antigen, the TAME-esterase activity represents approximately 75% plasma kallikrein complexed to alpha 2 macroglobulin, 25% mast cell tryptase, and a small amount of glandular kallikrein [5, 6]. The samples (0.5 ml) for prostaglandin (PGD$_2$) and leukotriene (LTC$_4$) were mixed with 95% ethanol at a ratio of 1 part sample to 4 parts ethanol. The samples for kinin determination were made 40 mM with respect to EDTA. All samples for the determination of kinins, PGD$_2$ and LTC$_4$ were stored at –80 °C until assayed. The leukotrienes detected in the ER of asymptomatic subjects challenged out of season are predominately LTC$_4$ with some LTD$_4$, whereas in the LPR, LTE$_4$ predominates [7, 8]. The kinins are a mixture of lysylbradykinin and bradykinin [9]. For challenges with histamine, albumin levels in the lavage fluids were measured using a radioimmunoassay [10] sensitive to 1 ng/ml.

The cell pellets were resuspended in Hanks buffer and then incubated with 10% N-acetyl cysteine for 45 minutes at 37 °C to dissolve the mucus, leading to single cell suspensions. The cells were washed three times in Hank's balanced salt solution, divided into aliquots, and counted in a hemocytometer before cytocentrifugation. At least one slide was stained with Diff Quick (a modified Wright's stain) and one with alcian blue pH 1 [11, 12].

Data Analysis and Statistics

The Wilcoxon Matched-Pairs Signed-Ranks test was used for comparison of the response during either the ER or LPR after challenge with CDA or antigen.

Results

Antigen Challenge

Early Reaction

In vitro studies of human mast cells and basophils have established their capacity to release potent mediators of inflammation. In vivo studies of allergic rhinitis have repeatedly shown that the intranasal presentation of antigen to susceptible individuals produces a

Table 1. Comparison between the early nasal reaction to antigen and to cold, dry air.

	Antigen	Cold, dry air
Sneezing	+	+/–
Rhinorrhea	+	+
Congestion	+	+
Histamine	+	+
TAME esterase	+	+
Kinins	+	+
PGD2	+	+
Leukotrienes	+	+

physiologic response manifested by sneezing, rhinorrhea, and nasal obstruction. Therefore, we rationalized that, if mast cell/basophil degranulation were central to the pathophysiology of allergic rhinitis, then these in vitro mediators should be present during the physiologic response. Therefore, we developed an in vivo model in which increasing concentrations of histamine, TAME-esterase activity, PGD2, LT C4/D4/E4, bradykinin and lysylbradykinin could be measured in nasal secretions during the immediate response to antigen. There is, however, no reason to believe that other mediators not presently measured in nasal secretions are not important.

Over 90% of individuals had an ER to nasal antigen challenge with respect to symptoms and mediators [13]. There was a significant association between both the amount of mediators and the total number of sneezes generated during the ER, and the response to skin test, ragweed-specific IgE levels and the amount of ragweed needed to induce half maximal basophil histamine release (BHR-50%); each parameter, however, only partially predicted the response in individual subjects.

Late Reaction

To study whether a LPR followed the immediate response, we initially selected allergic individuals who, after acute challenge, developed nasal symptoms hours after the initial response to antigen challenge. Following an ER, the characteristics of which are described above, all mediators declined toward baseline over a couple of hours. Beginning hours later, and peaking at different times postchallenge, the concentration of histamine, kinins, leukotrienes and TAME-esterase activity increased,

but PGD2 remained at baseline levels [14]. Nonallergic subjects challenged with antigen as well as individuals with late phase reactions who were challenged with placebo served as controls in these studies.

During the LPR, we evaluated the cellular content of the recovered lavages. Eosinophils showed a significant increase within 1–2 hours after antigen challenge and peaked 7–10 hours later. Neutrophils entered nasal secretions somewhat later, but they represented the greatest number of infiltrating cells during the LPR. Mononuclear cells were increased hours after the challenge, while epithelial cells showed little change [12]. We also evaluated the influx of alcian blue positive cells [11]. Although they represent approximately 1% of the incoming cells, the total number and the percentage of these cells increased significantly during the LPR. Dr. Stephen Galli reviewed the slides in a blinded manner and found, using previously established criteria, that approximately 70% of the alcian blue positive cells were basophils, less than 10% were mast cells, the remainder being indeterminate. The small percentage and total number of these cells precluded the use of electron microscopic evaluation.

Dr. Gerald Gleich measured the level of major basic protein (MBP), a cytotoxic constituent of eosinophils, in the nasal lavages. During the late phase reaction, the levels of MBP increased dramatically and were much greater than those found during the ER. Most importantly, the increase in the levels of MBP correlated with the total number of eosinophils found in the

Table 2. Comparison between the late nasal reaction to antigen and to cold, dry air.

	Antigen	Cold, dry air
Histamine	+	+
TAME esterase	+	+
Kinins	+	N.D.
PGD2	–	N.D.
Leukotrienes	+	N.D.
Major basic protein	+	N.D.
Eosinophil influx	+	+[1]
Neutrophil influx	+	+[1]
Basophil influx	+	N.D.
Reactivity to histamine	⇑	⇔[1]

[1]preliminary observations

lavage fluid during the same time period (r = .89, p < .01) [15]. The number of alcian blue positive cells also correlated significantly with the level of histamine in the LPR (r = .72; p < .01) [11]. Thus we can conclude that eosinophils and basophils not only enter nasal secretions during LPRs but also degranulate.

Subjects without symptoms of a late reaction did not show an increase in the levels of any of the evaluated mediators. Some of these subjects had a late increase in the number of cells, but, compared to individuals with both an early and a late reaction (dual responders), this increase was smaller, particularly with respect to eosinophils.

Our initial studies, like those published by others, used individuals known to have a dual response to test a hypothesis or therapeutic regimen. This approach fostered the idea that allergic individuals can be divided easily by their response to nasal challenge into those with only an ER and those with both an ER and a LPR. To test the validity of this concept as well as to establish the prevalence of late reactions, we studied the response to nasal challenge in 55 previously unchallenged patients with a history of ragweed hay fever and a positive intradermal skin test to ragweed allergens [13]. Some individuals clearly showed a dual response, whereas others clearly had only an ER. However, a spectrum of responses between these extremes was noted. To avoid an arbitrary separation into groups, we compared the total amount of mediators and symptoms present during the ER and LPR. There was a significant correlation between the intensity of each parameter in both the ER and LPR, suggesting an association between the two responses. Skin-test sensitivity, ragweed-specific IgE antibody levels, and basophil histamine release to ragweed did not correlate with the occurrence of a LPR.

In an attempt to define further the relationship between the ER and LPR, we defined a LPR as a twofold increase above baseline in two of three mediators (histamine, TAME-esterase activity or kinins). With this definition, we found a 43% prevalence of LPRs in the whole group, or a 48% prevalence in those having an ER. Interestingly, the antigen dose that first induced a positive response during the ER was not related to the presence or absence of a LPR. None of the four subjects who failed to demonstrate an ER showed evidence of LPR.

Cold, Dry Air

Early Reaction

We posed the question whether nasal challenge with cold, dry air (CDA) could provoke the release of mediators commonly associated with allergic reactions. Twelve subjects with a history of nasal symptoms upon cold or dry environmental exposure were challenged by nasal breathing of CDA and WMA. Two trials were performed on each subject, with the order of the challenge reversed. CDA caused a significant increase in symptom scores (p < .01) as compared to baseline and to WMA, regardless of the challenge sequence. Levels of histamine, TAME-esterase activity, kinins, leukotrienes and PGD_2 were also higher after CDA, compared to baseline or to WMA (p < .01 for each). WMA did not cause an increase in symptom scores or mediator levels except for a marginal increase in kinins. Changes in mediators correlated with one another, and histamine and PGD_2 levels correlated with symptom scores. Five subjects without nasal symptoms had no significant change in mediators after CDA or WMA [1, 16].

Late Reaction

Since the ER to CDA produces the same pattern of mediator release as the ER to antigen, we asked whether a LPR followed the early response to CDA. We selected individuals who described recurrence of symptoms after a previous challenge and exposed them to WMA on one occasion and to CDA on another. Significantly more symptoms and more histamine and TAME-esterase activity were recovered during the first 10 hours after CDA as compared to WMA [17].

Pharmacologic Studies with Antihistamines

Antigen

Azatadine, a tricyclic antihistamine, inhibits IgE-mediated release of histamine and leukotrienes from human lung mast cells in vivo [18]. To assess the clinical relevance of these findings and to compare in vitro mast cell data with results obtained in vivo, nasally instilled

Table 3. The effect of a topical tricyclic anti-histamine* on the early nasal reaction to antigen and cold, dry air.

	Antigen	Cold, dry air
Histamine	⇓	⇔
TAME esterase	⇓	⇔
Kinins	⇓	N.D.
Symptoms	⇓	⇔

*Azatadine base

azatadine was tested in a double-blind, placebo-controlled clinical trial in which nasal challenge with antigen was performed in eight allergic individuals. Pretreatment with azatadine significantly suppressed the number of sneezes following antigen stimulation and inhibited the associated elevations of histamine, TAME-esterase activity and kinins, whereas placebo was inactive [18]. These experiments suggested that topically applied azatadine, at high concentrations, inhibited the allergic response by suppressing antigen-induced mast cell activation.

Cold, dry air

We also studied the effect of topically administered azatadine on nasal challenge with CDA [19]. Ten subjects were premedicated with either azatadine or placebo, and sequentially challenged with CDA and histamine. The response to CDA was evaluated by symptom scores and the levels of histamine and TAME-esterase activity, whereas the response to challenge with histamine was monitored by symptom scores and by the level of albumin, an indicator of vascular permeability. Azatadine effectively inhibited the response to histamine challenge, but was ineffective against CDA. These data, coupled with the antigen challenge findings, suggest that the mechanisms of nasal mast cell activation by the two stimuli differ, and that pharmacologic control is stimulus dependent.

Discussion

Although allergic rhinitis constitutes a significant health problem affecting approximately 17% of the U.S. population and is the subject of considerable research, new developments for treating this condition have been limited. Non-sedating antihistamines and modifications of the antigens used in immunotherapy have led to modest therapeutic advances. With the long-term goal of developing new therapies, we developed a novel model to investigate the pathophysiology of allergic rhinitis by studying the response to nasal challenge with antigen.

Because the unknown dilutional effect of lavage makes the exact quantification of mediators in surface secretions difficult, we have viewed our measurements as a semiquantitative parameter and have chosen to focus on the pattern of mediators in lavages as a predictor of the underlying pathophysiology. By observing these different patterns in the early LPR, we predicted that basophils enter nasal secretions during the LPR. We have since shown this to be the case [11].

We were also able to correlate the influx of eosinophils and basophils with the levels of major basic protein and histamine, respectively. These cells not only enter the nose but are also activated. In addition, treatment with corticosteroids [8, 12] and immunotherapy [20], both effective modalities in allergic rhinitis, decreased the clinical LPR and its accompanying cellular influx. These observations strengthen the potential role of eosinophils and basophils in the inflammatory reaction and question the role of mast cells during the LPR.

However, mast cell degranulation seems to be very important in the initiation of events leading to LPR. Our evidence of mast cell degranulation, i.e., the release of histamine and PGD_2 during the ER to nasal challenge, combined with the response to pharmacologic manipulation, is in agreement with the biopsy studies of Kawabori and associates [21] and Gomez et al. [22]. The pattern of mediator release after CDA stimulation also suggests mast cell activation. Furthermore, the demonstration of a LPR following CDA stimulation supports our hypothesis that LPR is initiated by mast cell degranulation.

The possibility does exist, however, that antigen or the stimulus leading to CDA induced rhinitis may interact with receptor systems on other cell types to cause the subsequent inflammation. If this scenario were correct, blocking mast cell activation would mask the immediate symptoms of antigen exposure but would permit the consequences of the LPR.

Although the contents of nasal lavages have been predictive of underlying changes, we realize that differences may exist between cells in secretions and cells in the mucosa. In humans, some studies have revealed similarities between the cellular content of bronchoalveolar lavage and transbronchial biopsies of the lung parenchyma [23, 24]. Similar findings have been reported in animal models, with an interesting exception: Blythe et al. showed increases in neutrophils in alveolar lavage before the detection of changes in the lung parenchyma of rats [25]. Since biopsies sample small areas, whereas lavage covers the entire mucosa, the latter may be a more sensitive technique. In addition, histology only describes the presence of cellular types, whereas lavage can offer information about their functional status as well.

In preliminary studies, we have observed some additional similarities as well as some differences between the inflammation induced by CDA and antigen. The appearance of a LPR following CDA challenge, as shown by mediators and symptoms, is accompanied by a cellular influx which includes eosinophils, a similarity to antigen-induced LPRs. However, the increased sensitivity to nasal challenge with histamine, which occurs following antigen provocation, does not occur following CDA provocation. These results parallel those in the lung: antigen-induced LPRs are associated with increased reactivity to histamine, whereas bronchoprovocation with CDA is not. These studies point to the heterogeneity of inflammation and underline our inability to generalize. Furthermore, it is possible that the development of increased reactivity secondary to antigen challenge, in contrast to the LPR, is not a consequence of mast cell activation.

The difference between the effect of a topically applied antihistamine on the ER to antigen and CDA further distinguishes the two stimuli. Sneezing characterizes the ER to antigen whereas it rarely occurs following CDA. This may be explained by a qualitative difference in the stimuli or by interaction of the stimuli with different elements of the nasal mucosa. Although mast cells are activated, as suggested by the pattern of mediator release and the development of a LPR, other cells may also be stimulated. The ineffectiveness of azatadine in inhibiting the ER to CDA points to the limited role of H_1 activity in that reaction.

In summary, we believe that the ER to nasal challenge with antigen does not adequately represent the clinical disease of allergic rhinitis and that one must understand the subsequent inflammation and its consequences. We hypothesize that the LPR may result, in part, from mast cell degranulation; however, hyperreactivity to histamine may not. Parallel experiments with CDA uncovered similarities and differences which have helped us to better understand allergic inflammation.

References

1. Togias, A. G., R. M. Naclerio, D. Proud, J. E. Fish, N. F. Adkinson Jr., A. Kagey-Sobotka, P. S. Norman, and L. M. Lichtenstein. 1985. Nasal challenge with cold, dry air results in release of inflammatory mediators: Possible mast cell involvement. J. Clin. Invest. 76: 1375.

2. Naclerio, R. M., H. L. Meier, A. Kagey-Sobotka, N. F. Adkinson Jr., D. A. Meyers, P. S. Norman, and L. M. Lichtenstein. 1983. Mediator release after nasal airway challenge with allergen. Am. Rev. Respir. Dis. 128: 597.

3. Siraganian, R. 1974. An automated continuous flow system for the extraction and fluorometric analysis of histamine. Anal. Biochem. 57: 283.

4. Beaven, V. H., J. V. Pierce, J. J. Pisano. 1971. A sensitive isotopic procedure for the assay of esterase activity: measurement of human airway kallikrein. Clin. Chim. Acta. 32: 67.

5. Baumgarten, C. R., R. C. Nichols, R. M. Naclerio, L. M. Lichtenstein, P. S. Norman, and D. Proud. 1986. Plasma kallikrein during experimentally-induced allergic rhinitis: Role in kinin formation and contribution to TAME-esterase activity in nasal secretions. J. Immunol. 137: 977.

6. Baumgarten, C. R., R. C. Nichols, R. M. Naclerio, and D. Proud. 1986. Concentrations of glandular kallikrein in human nasal secretions during experimentally-induced allergic rhinitis. J. Immunol. 137: 1323.

7. Creticos, P. S., S. P. Peters, N. F. Adkinson Jr., R. M. Naclerio, E. C. Hayes, P. S. Norman, and L. M. Lichtenstein. 1984. Peptide leukotriene release after antigen challenge in patients sensitive to ragweed. N. Engl. J. Med. 310: 1626.

8. Pipkorn, U., D. Proud, L. M. Lichtenstein, R. P. Schleimer, S.P. Peters, N. F. Adkinson Jr., A. Kagey-Sobotka, P. S. Norman, and R. M. Naclerio. 1987. Effect of short-term systemic glucocorticoid treatment on human nasal mediator release after antigen challenge. J. Clin. Invest. 80: 957.

9. Proud, D., A. Togias, R. M. Naclerio, S. A. Crush, P. S. Norman, and L. M. Lichtenstein. 1983. Kinins are generated in vivo following na-

sal airway challenge of allergic individuals with allergen. J. Clin. Invest. 72: 1678.

10. Baumgarten C. R., A. G. Togias, R. M. Naclerio, L. M. Lichtenstein, P. S. Norman, and D. Proud. 1985. Influx of kininogens into nasal secretions following antigen challenge of allergic individuals. J. Clin. Invest. 76: 191.

11. Bascom, R., M. Wachs, R. M. Naclerio, U. Pipkorn, S. J. Galli, and L. M. Lichtenstein. 1988. Basophil influx occurs after nasal antigen challenge: Effects of topical corticosteroid pretreatment. J. Allergy Clin. Immunol. 80: 580.

12. Bascom, R., U. Pipkorn, L. M. Lichtenstein, and R. M. Naclerio. 1988. The influx of inflammatory cells into nasal washings during the late response to antigen challenge: Effect of systemic steroid pretreatment. Am. Rev. Respir. Dis.138: 406.

13. Iliopoulos, O., D. Proud, L. M. Lichtenstein, A. Kagey-Sobotka, P. S. Creticos, N. F. Adkinson Jr., S. M. MacDonald, P. S. Norman, and R. M. Naclerio. 1987. Relationships between early (ER), late (LPR) and rechallenge (RCR) responses to nasal challenge. J. Allergy Clin. Immunol.79: 253.

14. Nalerio, R. M., D. Proud, A. G. Togias, N. F. Adkinson Jr., D. A. Meyers, A. Kagey-Sobotka, M. Plaut, P. S. Norman, and L. M. Lichtenstein. 1985. Inflammatory mediators in late antigen-induced rhinitis. N. Engl. J. Med. 313(2): 65.

15. Bascom, R., U. Pipkorn, G. Gleich, L. M. Lichtenstein, and R. M. Naclerio. 1986. Effect of systemic steroids on eosinophils (EOS) and major basic protein (MBP) during nasal antigen challenge. J. Allergy Clin. Immunol. 77S: 246.

16. Togias, A. G., R. M. Naclerio, S. P. Peters, I. Nimmagadda, D. Proud, A. Kagey-Sobotka, N. F. Adkinson Jr., P. S. Norman, and L. M. Lichtenstein. 1986. Local generation of sulfidopeptide leukotrienes upon nasal provocation with cold, dry air. Am. Rev. Respir. Dis. 133: 1133.

17. Iliopoulos, O., D. Proud, P.S. Norman, L. M. Lichtenstein, A. Kagey-Sobotka, and R. M. Naclerio. 1988. Nasal challenge with cold, dry air induces a late phase reaction. Am. Rev. Respir. Dis. 138: 400.

18. Togias, A. G., R. M. Naclerio, J. Warner, D. Proud, A. Kagey-Sobotka, I. Nimmagadda, P. S. Norman, and L. M. Lichtenstein. 1986. Demonstration of inhibition of mediator release from mast cells by azatadine base: In vivo and in vitro evaluation. JAMA 255: 225.

19. Togias, A. G., D. Proud, A. Kagey-Sobotka, P. Norman, L. M. Lichtenstein, and R. M. Naclerio. 1987. The effect of a topical tricyclic antihistamine on the response of the nasal mucosa to challenge with cold, dry air and histamine. J. Allergy Clin. Immunol.79: 599.

20. Iliopoulos, O., D. Proud, A. Kagey-Sobotka, P. S. Creticos, P. S. Norman, L. M. Lichtenstein, and R. M. Naclerio. 1988. Effects of immunotherapy on early and late reactions to nasal challenge. J. Allergy Clin. Immunol. 81: 291.

21. Kawabori, S., M. Okuda, and T. Unno. 1983. Mast cells in allergic nasal epithelium and lamina propria before and after provocation: An electron microscopic study. Clin. Allergy 13: 181.

22. Gomez, E., O. J. Corrado, D. L. Baldwin, A. R. Swanston, and R. J. Davies. 1986. Direct in vivo evidence for mast cell degranulation during allergen-induced reactions in man. J. Allergy Clin. Immunol. 78:637.

23. Hunninghake, G. W., O. Kawanami, V. J. Ferrans, R. C. Young Jr., W. C. Roberts, and R. G. Crystal. 1981. Characterization of the inflammatory and immune effector cells in the lung parenchyma of patients with interstitial lung disease. Am. Rev. Respir. Dis. 123: 407.

24. Campbell, D. A., L. W. Poulter, and R. M. DuBois. 1985. Immunocompetent cells in bronchoalveolar lavage reflect the cell populations in transbronchial biopsies in pulmonary sarcoidosis. Am. Rev. Respir. Dis. 132: 1300.

25. Blythe, S., B. England, B. Esser, P. Junk, and R. F. Lemanski Jr. 1986. IgE antibody mediated inflammation of rat lung: Histologic and bronchoalveolar lavage assessment. Am. Rev. Respir. Dis. 134: 1246.

Overview: Role of Histamine in Rhinitis

Niels Mygind, Hans Bisgaard, Henrik Grønborg*

When histamine is sprayed into the nasal cavity, it causes immediate itching, sneezing, rhinorrhea, and blockage. The change in nasal airway patency is mainly caused by a direct effect on vascular H_1 and H_2 receptors, while the other effects are the result of indirect reflex activity, probably mediated by nervous H_1 receptors. A high dose of histamine is necessary to mimic the allergic response, which, in addition, is characterized by a late influx of eosinophils and an increase in mucosal reactivity.

The new potent, nonsedating H_1 antihistamines are almost as effective in relieving itching, sneezing, and watery rhinorrhea in allergic rhinitis as the steroid sprays, indicating that histamine is by far the most important mediator of these symptoms. As antihistamines have little or no effect on nasal blockage, other mediators probably contribute to this symptom. Interestingly, antihistamines are often effective in nonallergic rhinitis, provided the patient is a "sneezer" and not a "blocker."

This chapter summarizes what we know about the role of histamine in allergic rhinitis and its mode of action in the human nose. We can get knowledge about the role of histamine in three ways: (1) by nasal histamine provocation testing, (2) by measuring the concentration of histamine in nasal secretions, following allergen provocation, and (3) by analyzing the effect of specific histamine receptor antagonists.

Histamine Compared with Allergen Provocation

When histamine is sprayed into the human nose, it will, within a few seconds, give rise to itching, followed by a few sneezes and by watery rhinorrhea [1]. However, the symptoms are usually less severe than following allergen provocation, where up to 20 sneezes can be heard (maximum number in our laboratory is 32).

The histamine challenge is, like the allergen test, followed by increased nasal airway resis-

tance, which lasts for hours. In contrast to allergen, however, histamine does not appear to cause local eosinophilia, and, importantly, the provocation is not followed by an increase in nonspecific reactivity [2]. Thus, there are striking similarities, but also some differences, between the nasal response to histamine and to allergen challenge (Table 1).

Table 1. Results of histamine and allergen provocation tests.

	Histamine	Allergen
Itching and sneezing	+	+
Rhinorrhea	+	+
Blockage	+	+
Eosinophilia	−	+
Hyperreactivity	−	+

Okuda [3] has elegantly demonstrated that histamine induces itching, sneezing, and hypersecretion by an effect on the mucosal surface, as these symptoms were produced when he placed a droplet of histamine on the mucosa and not when it was injected into the mucous membrane.

The action on the sensory nerve endings can be inhibited by pretreatment with an H_1 but not with an H_2 histamine receptor antagonist [4], indicating that nervous H_1 histamine receptors are stimulated by histamine. Their existence in the nose, however, has not been directly demonstrated by ligand-binding studies. It is of interest that histamine provocations with 5-min intervals result in the development of tachyphylaxis [4], which resembles the rapidly adapting response of irritant receptors.

M. Okuda and N. Mygind [5] found that unilateral histamine provocation in the nose of 13 patients with perennial rhinitis resulted in 0.94 ml of secretion on the provoked side, and 0.77 ml on the other side, showing that histamine-induced hypersecretion is predominantly (>85%) the result of stimulation of sensory nerves and parasympathetic reflexes—and not

---

*   Department of Otology and Department of Allergy, Rigshospitalet, DK-2100 Copenhagen, Denmark.

the result of a direct histamine effect on glandular H_2 receptors. Corresponding figures for unilateral provocation with allergen were 1.59 and 1.17 ml, showing that also allergen induces rhinorrhea predominantly (>74%) by reflex activity [6].

When experimental challenge tests with histamine and with allergen are compared, it should be realized that a very high histamine dose (about 1 mg) is required in order to induce reproducible sneezing. This dosage is probably supraphysiological, as it corresponds to complete degranulation of a high number of mast cells (they contain 2–16 pg histamine each) [7]. Also, biochemical analyses of experimentally induced secretions indicate that a nasal histamine provocation test is artificial and poorly reflects what happens during natural allergen exposure. The concentration of albumin, a marker of plasma transudation, was considerably higher following provocation with histamine than with allergen and with metacholine [8].

Measurement of Histamine in Nasal Secretions

This topic is dealt with in detail by Bob Naclerio in another part of this book. I shall draw attention to some studies in which it was the disappointing result that the concentration of histamine in nasal secretions did not increase following allergen provocation [3, 9, 10]. Konno [11] found the same total amount of histamine in the two nasal cavities, following unilateral allergen provocation. These studies indicate that the measurement of histamine concentration and content in nasal secretions cannot be used to predict the role played by this mediator in allergic rhinitis—unless we assume that it does not play any role at all.

It seems necessary to use the wash-down technique of Naclerio [12] and remove "physiological histamine" from the nasal cavity before demonstrating any histamine-releasing effect of allergen or of any other stimuli. The role of the high physiological histamine concentration in the nose is unknown. One can wonder why we do not sneeze all the time, the median histamine concentration in a normal nose being 50 nmol/L [9].

Effect of Histamine Receptor Antagonists

A unilateral histamine challenge is inhibited by homolateral, and not by heterolateral, pretreatment with an H_1 antihistamine, showing that the antihistamine acts by a local mode of action in the mucous membrane and not by CNS activity [1]. The antihistamine inhibition of itching, sneezing, and hypersecretion is not due to a local analgesic or a parasympatholytic effect [13]. Therefore, an effect on sensory nerve H_1 receptors is the most likely mode of action, but, as mentioned earlier, these receptors have not yet been directly demonstrated.

An H_2 histamine receptor antagonist has no effect on histamine-induced itching, sneezing, and hypersecretion, while H_1 and H_2 antihistamines have added effect on blockage, suggesting the presence of both H_1 and H_2 receptors on nasal blood vessels [4].

H_1 antihistamines have a good effect on eye symptoms, nasal itching, sneezing, and hypersecretion in allergic rhinitis, while the effect on stuffiness is poor or absent [14, 15]. Consequently, antihistamines are more helpful in "sneezers" than in "blockers." Even nonallergic "sneezers" are often helped by an H_1 antihistamine [15], which is interesting, as it indicates either that the patients are exposed to undiscovered allergens or that histamine is a mediator of some cases of nonallergic rhinitis.

With regard to itching, sneezing, and watery hypersecretion in allergic rhinitis, Munch et al. [14] found the antihistamine dexchlorpheniramine maleate to be almost as effective as the steroid spray budesonide, and Wood [16] has recently reported an equal effect of the nonsedative antihistamine astemizole and of beclomethasone dipropionate spray. This is convincing evidence for histamine being by far the most important mediator of these allergic symptoms in the nose. Other biochemical mediators may contribute to chronic stuffiness and are probably responsible for allergen-induced nasal hyperreactivity.

References

1. Kirkegaard, J., C. Secher, P. Borum, and N. Mygind. 1983. Inhibition of histamine-induced nasal symptoms by the H_1 antihistamine chlorpheniramine. Br. J. Dis. Chest 77: 113–122.

2. Gronborg, H., P. Borum, and N. Mygind. 1986. Histamine and metacholine do not increase nasal reactivity. Clin. Allergy 16: 597–602.

3. Okuda, M. 1977. Mechanisms in nasal allergy, part 2. ORL Digest 39: 26.

4. Secher, C., J. Kirkegaard, P. Borum, A. Maansson, P. Osterhammel, and N. Mygind. 1982. Significance of H_1 and H_2 receptors in the human nose. J. Allergy Clin. Immunol. 70: 211–218.

5. Okuda, M., and N. Mygind. 1980. Pathophysiological basis for topical steroid treatment in the nose. In: Topical steroid treatment for asthma and rhinitis. N. Mygind and T. J. H. Clark, eds. London: Bailliere Tindall, pp. 22–33.

6. Konno, A., N. Terada, Y. Okamoto, and K. Togawa. 1987. The role of chemical mediators in nasal hyperreactivity in nasal allergy. J. Allergy Clin. Immunol. 79: 620–626.

7. Schulman, E. S., D. W. MacGlashan, Jr., R. P. Schleimer, S. P. Peters, A. Kagey-Sobotka, H. H. Newball, and L. M. Lichtenstein. 1983. Purified human basophils and mast cells: Current concepts of mediator release. Eur. J. Respir. Dis. 64 (Suppl. 128): 53–61.

8. Brofeldt, S., N. Mygind, C. H. Sorensen, A. S. Readman, and C. Marriott. 1986. Biochemical analysis of nasal secretions induced by methacholine, histamine and allergen provocation. Am. Rev. Respir. Dis. 133: 1138–1142.

9. Bisgaard, H., C. Robinson, F. Romeling, N. Mygind, M. Church, and S. T. Holgate. 1988. Leukotriene C4 and histamine in early allergic reaction in the nose. Allergy 43: 219–227.

10. Linder, A., K. Strandberg, and H. Deuschl. 1987. Histamine concentrations in nasal secretion and secretory activity in allergic rhinitis. Allergy 42: 126–134.

11. Konno, A., K. Togawa, and T. Fujiwara. 1983. The mechanisms involved in onset of allergic manifestations in the nose. Eur. J. Respir. Dis. 64 (Suppl. 128): 155–166.

12. Naclerio, R. M., D. Proud, A. Togias, N. F. Adkinson, Jr., D. A. Meyers, A. Kagey-Sobotka, M. Plaut, P. S. Norman, and L. M. Lichtenstein. 1985. Inflammatory mediators in late antigen-induced rhinitis. N. Engl. J. Med. 313: 65–69.

13. Kirkegaard, J., C. Secher, and N. Mygind. 1982. Effect of the H_1 antihistamine chlorpheniramine maleate on histamine-induced symptoms in the human conjunctiva. Allergy 37: 203–208.

14. Munch, E., M. Soborg, T. T. Norresleth, and N. Mygind. 1983. A comparative study of dexchlorpheniramine maleate sustained release tablets and budesonide nasal spray in seasonal allergic rhinitis. Allergy 38: 517–524.

15. Wihl, J.-A., B. N. Petersen, L. N. Petersen, G. Gundersen, K. Bresson, and N. Mygind. 1985. Effect of the nonsedative H_1-receptor antagonist astemizole in perennial allergic and nonallergic rhinitis. J. Allergy Clin. Immunol. 75: 720–727.

16. Wood, S. F. 1986. Oral antihistamine or nasal steroid in hay fever: A double-blind double-dummy comparative study of once daily oral astemizole vs twice daily nasal beclomethasone dipropionate. Clin. Allergy 16: 195–201.

Involvement of Different Cell Types in Allergic Rhinitis

Ulf Pipkorn*

Lately several new techniques have been devised for the non-traumatic harvesting of cells from the nasal mucosa in vivo in humans. These have been utilized in allergen challenge experiments as well as for the study of cellular changes occurring during natural allergen exposure. Following an allergen challenge, evidence of the activation of mast cells in the initiating part of the allergic response has been provided. This is then followed by an influx of granulocytes in a time relationship to a late-phase reaction, the most prominent finding being the increase in the number of eosinophilic granulocytes. Biochemical evidence has also been provided which shows that these cells are activated together with basophilic granulocytes also appearing during the late phase. Evidence of the participation of mast cells in hay fever during natural allergen exposure was provided through the demonstration of changes in the distribution of these cells, a change in intracellular histamine content and ultrastructural findings. In addition, seasonal allergen exposure was accompanied by a prominent increase in eosinophils on the surface of the nasal epithelium, an increase which correlated strongly to the degree of pollen exposure and symptoms experienced by the patients. Thus, human in vivo evidence of the active participation of mast cells and eosinophils also in the clinical disease of hay fever has been provided.

In recent years several new laboratory techniques for the monitoring of different parts of the response of the nasal mucosa to stimulatory events have been developed [1]. Such instruments have provided us with new opportunities for dissecting the pathophysiological events taking place within and upon the nasal mucous membrane as responses to allergen exposure. These include new techniques for the non-traumatic harvesting of cells from the nasal mucosa for quantitative and qualitative studies, techniques for measuring the release of inflammatory mediators, and techniques for monitoring different parts of the vascular response in terms of changes in the tone of different parts of the vasculature, as well as, changes in the "leakiness" of such vessels [7]. Through the combined use of such techniques during the last couple of years, we have obtained a considerable amount of human in vivo information as to the possible participation of different cell types in the pathogenesis of allergic rhinitis. Some information has been gathered in challenge studies, while other information has been acquired through the study of native disease, mostly hay fever during natural allergen exposure.

In vivo Human Evidence of the Active Engagement of a Certain Cell Type in Allergic Disease

The evidence given in the literature of the participation of a certain cell type in a specific disease in humans, like hay fever, is twofold. One type of evidence is the demonstration of a change in the number of cells and/or their distribution as part of the disease process [2–4; Figure 1); the other type of evidence demonstrates signs of activation, ultrastructural (Figure 2) or biochemical, of a certain cell type during the disease process [5–7]. The cellular changes or the signs of activation may be directly related to the symptoms experienced by the subjects. The biochemical data provided can be the demonstration of the release of a specific cell product such as histamine for mast cells/basophils [8], eosinophil cationic protein (ECP) or major basic protein (MBP) for eosinophils [3], or myeloperoxidase (MPO) for neutrophils [9]. The kinetics of the changes in cell number and their activation in vivo is another subject on which the data are largely

* ENT-Department, University Hospital, S-22185 Lund, Sweden.
  Supported by grants from the Swedish Medical Research Society (project No. 8803) and the Foundation of Torsten and Ragnar Söderberg.

237

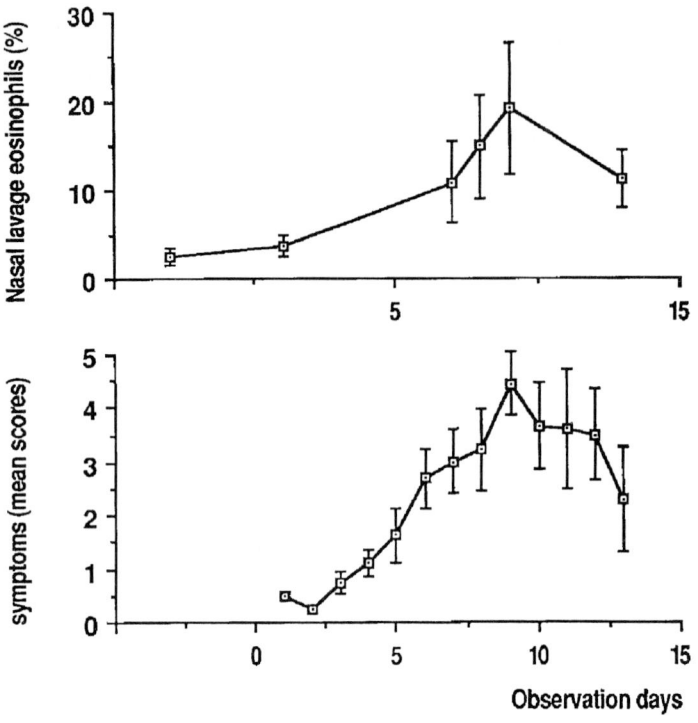

Figure 1. A composite graph showing the mean percentage in eosinophils of cells obtained by a nasal lavage in patients with allergic rhinitis. The graph demonstrates the results in specimens taken immediately prior to and at the beginning of the relevant pollen season. The lower half shows the mean nasal symptoms expressed as symptom scores for the same patients during the same period. Redrawn from [7].

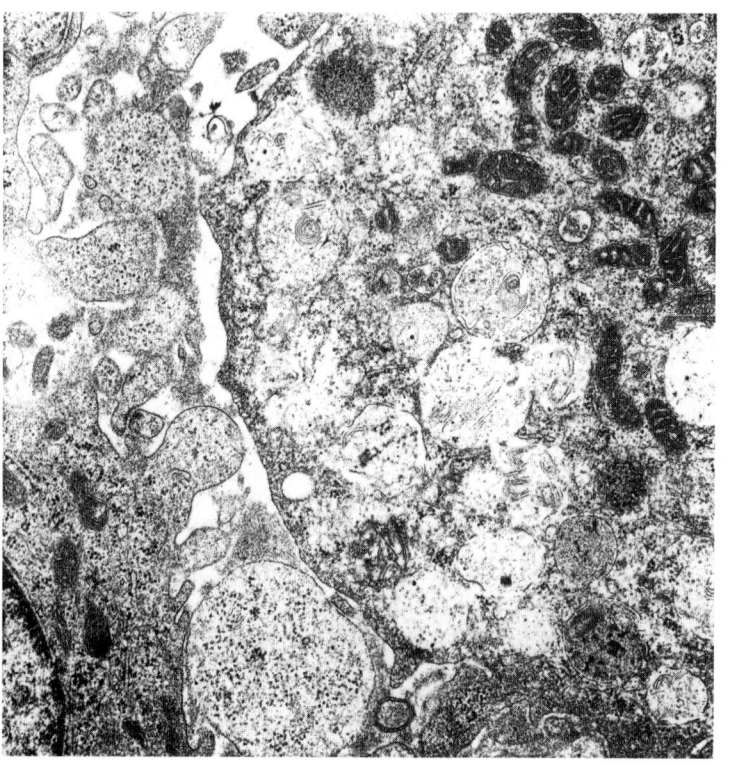

Figure 2. A higher power magnification electron micrograph of a mast cell obtained in a specimen taken during pollen exposure. Several signs of secretory activity, such as totally or partially empty mast cell granules and plasma membrane folds, are shown. Some contain a few scrolls and some show signs of fusion of membranes. Original magnification × 6000.

lacking. Some changes may be rapid, and these lend themselves to be demonstrated in short-term challenge experiments in the laboratory. Other changes appear to be slower and may only be demonstrated after repeated challenges or during prolonged natural allergen exposure. The role of the different cell types in hay fever is further complicated by the recent finding of a heterogeneity of the mast cell system also in humans. Like the rodent system, human mast cells in connective tissue differ in several functional and histochemical aspects from the mast cells in mucous membranes, such as in the nasal mucosa [4, 5, 10]. The mast cells in the nasal mucosa differ in their phenotypic expression of proteoglycans from the mast cells in the skin. This difference appears to be unrelated to the activation of these cells in hay fever during seasonal exposure, for example [10]. The interrelationship between the different cell types and the eventual causal relationship between changes in number and the activation of the cells and the symptoms and signs of disease are important issues which largely remains unanswered.

Experimental Allergen Challenge

After an appropriate allergen challenge of the upper airways, there is a rapid appearance of nasal symptoms that are generally ascribed to the triggering of the mast cells of the nasal mucosa with a subsequent release of inflammatory mediators, which are then in turn responsible for the generation of symptoms. It has also been shown in vivo in humans that a local challenge with allergen is associated with structural signs of mast-cell degranulation [11] as well as the appearance of mediators on the nasal mucosal surface that have a profile like those derived from isolated mast cells [12].

Early and Late Phases

In a significant proportion of patients this initial phase is followed after a couple of hours by a recurrence of symptoms—a late-phase reaction like the ones described in the skin and lower airways. This is associated with a local infiltration of the challenge site by inflammatory cells of vascular origin. Using the lavage approach for the harvesting of cells, it has been

possible to demonstrate such an increase in the number of inflammatory cells [2]. The most prominent finding is a specific increase in eosinophils with an associated local increase in the level of specific eosinophil derived proteins such as ECP and MBP [3]. An increase in the number of basophils accounts for part of the increase of inflammatory cells, although it is not as prominent as the increase in eosinophils. It should, however, be noted that there was no clear-cut relationship between these findings and the symptoms experienced by the subjects. On the basis of the profile of mediators harvested in the lavages during a late-phase reaction and on the basis of pharmacological evidence, it has been suggested that the basophil might play an active role in the generation of a late phase [13]. Thus, challenge experiments have demonstrated that the mast cells are activated in the initiation of the allergic reaction and that eosinophils and perhaps basophils play a role in the perpetuation of the inflammatory reaction of which the late phase is one part. It should, however, be pointed out that the relationship between such findings in experimental challenge studies and native disease is largely not understood.

Allergen-Induced Increase in Nasal Reactivity

One of the characteristics of the late phase of the lower airways is an increased responsiveness to unspecific and specific stimuli [14]. A similar feature can be found in the upper airways, although the correlation with the late phase remains to be clarified. This increase in responsiveness can be demonstrated in the laboratory in the majority of hay fever patients, but it has no clear-cut relationship to the size of the initiating allergic response [15]. The pathogenesis of this increased responsiveness is still unclarified, although some interesting aspects have been demonstrated. In this context it is also of interest to point out that this feature of the allergic response—increased responsiveness—is apparently not a general phenomenon of the allergic inflammation, but is limited to certain sites. Thus, immediate or late-phase dermal allergic reactions are not followed by an increase in local responsiveness to rechallenge with specific or unspecific agents [16]. On the contrary, the more likely response to dermal rechallenges is a decrease in reactivity. It has also been shown that the specific increase in responsiveness includes an increased generation of mediators, such as histamine, rather than an increase in responsiveness at the receptor level [8]. In terms of pathogenesis, it is conceivable that part of the change in responsiveness is due to changes in the barrier function of the mucous membrane. This might include elements of a changed effector cell distribution, some of which are more superficial and changes in the penetrability of the mucous membranes to macromolecules such as allergens. As has been previously pointed out, the most prominent cellular finding at the time when the increase in reactivity occurs is the specific increase in the number of eosinophils present on the surface of the nasal mucosa. It is interesting to speculate that the products of the activation of these cells may contribute to the increase in responsiveness by having a harmful effect on the nasal epithelium. It should be noted, however, that this must still be considered only as an interesting hypothesis.

Seasonal Disease

All challenge experiments are artificial situations which cannot mimic the continuous low-grade exposure occurring during natural exposure. Consequently, certain important events may well only be apparent during natural allergen exposure. One advantage of the human nose is that many of the techniques applied in the laboratory can also be applied effectively to monitor changes occurring at natural allergen exposure as well. Seasonal allergic rhinitis from pollen offers an opportunity to study the events taking place in and on the mucous membrane with knowledge of the initiating stimulus (pollen counts), and the symptoms experienced by the individual patient. A few such studies have been performed with the simultaneous monitoring of cellular as well as biochemical events [4–7].

Signs of Mast Cell Activation

Although challenge experiments and theoretical considerations point to the participation of the mast cell in the actual disease of hay fever, actual evidence is scarce. Using new tech-

niques for non-traumatic cell harvesting it has recently been possible to provide further evidence of the active involvement of mast cells in the pathogenesis of hay fever. Morphological studies have demonstrated a redistribution of mast cells from their normal habitat in the subepithelial layer toward the surface of the mucous membrane, with an increased proportion of these cells located intraepithelially during the pollen season [4–5]. Recently, further evidence of their active participation has been provided. It has been demonstrated that there is a change in the relationship between nasal mucosal mast cell density and histamine content from before to during the pollen season [6]. Before the pollen season there was a strong correlation between the mast-cell density and histamine content of the mucosa; a correlation which was not present during the pollen season thus indicating an extracellular pool of tissue histamine. It is interesting to note that the level of tissue histamine found during the pollen season in the nasal mucosa correlated strongly with the symptoms experienced by the patients. Further indications of the role of mast cells in the generation of the symptoms of hay fever were provided by the finding that there was a strong correlation between the number of mast cells on the surface of the epithelium immediately prior to the start of the pollen season and the nasal symptoms experienced later during the pollen season. Signs of secretory activity by the mast cells during natural allergen exposure were also provided by electron microscopy (Figure 2).

Participation of Eosinophils

The eosinophil is one cell type that consistently shows an increase locally following allergen challenge experiments. This is also true when it comes to natural allergen exposure. It was recently shown that there was a rapid increase in the proportion of eosinophils on the surface of the nasal mucosa from 2 to 20% at the start of the pollen season (Figure 1). Furthermore, this increase in number was strongly correlated to the degree of pollen exposure and symptoms experienced by the patients [7]. Although the presence of eosinophils during these conditions strongly indicates that these cells play an active role, the specific role of the eosinophils is still unexplained.

Conclusion

The upper airways offer an opportunity for continuous monitoring of allergic mucosal reactions, not only in the laboratory, but also during natural allergen exposure. Such studies will provide a further insight into the pathogenesis of allergic disease—an insight that might well be of a general nature and therefore also relevant to other parts of the airways.

References

1. Mygind, N., and U. Pipkorn. 1987. Allergic and vasomotor rhinitis; Pathophysiological aspects. Munksgaard, Copenhagen.

2. Bascom, R., U. Pipkorn, L. M. Lichtenstein, and R. M. Naclerio. 1988. The influx of inflammatory cells into nasal washings during the late response to antigen challenge: Effect of systemic corticosteroids. Am. Review of Respir. Dis., in press.

3. Bascom, R., U. Pipkorn, G. Gleich, L. M. Lichtenstein, and R. M. Naclerio. 1986. Effect of systemic steroids on eosinophils (EOS) and major basic protein (MBP) during nasal antigen challenge (abstract). J. Allergy Clin. Immunol. 77: 246.

4. Enerbäck, L., U. Pipkorn, and G. Granerus. 1986. Intraepithelial migration of nasal mucosal mast cells in hay fever. Int. Archs. Allergy appl. Immun. 80: 44.

5. Enerbäck, L., U. Pipkorn, and A. Olofsson. 1986. Intraeptithelial migration of nasal mucosal mast cells in hay fever: Ultrastructural observations. Int. Archs. Allergy appl. Immunol. 81: 289.

6. Pipkorn, U., G. Karlsson, and L. Enerbäck. 1988. Secretory activity of nasal mucosal mast cells and histamine release in hay fever. Int. Archs. Allergy appl. Immunol., in press.

7. Pipkorn, U., G. Karlsson, and L. Enerbäck. 1988. Cellular response of the human allergic nasal mucosa to natural allergen exposure. J. Allergy Clin. Immunol., in press.

8. Pipkorn, U., D. Proud, L. M. Lichtenstein, A. Kagey-Sobotka, P. S. Norman, and R. M. Naclerio. 1987. Inhibition of mediator release in allergic rhintis by pretreatment with topical glucocorticosteroids. N. Engl. J. Med. 316: 1506.

9. Linder, A., P. Venge, and H. Deuschl. 1987. Eosinophil cationic protein and myeloperoxidase in nasal secretion as markers of inflammation in allergic rhintis. Allergy 42: 583.

10. Pipkorn, U., G. Karlsson, and L. Enerbäck. 1988. Phenotypic expression of mast cells in the human nasal mucosa. Histochemical Journal, in press.

11. Gomez, E., O. J. Corrado, D. L. Baldwin, A. R. Swanston, and R. J. Davies. 1986. Direct in vivo evidence for mast cell degranulation during allergen-induced reactions in man. J. Allergy Clin. Immunol. 78: 637.

12. Naclerio, R. M., H. L Meier, A. Kagey-Sobotka, N. F. Adkinson Jr., D. A. Meyers, P. S. Norman, and L. M. Lichtenstein. 1983. Mediator release after nasal airway challenge with allergen. Am. Rev. Respir. Dis. 128: 597.

13. Cockcroft, D. W., R. E. Ruffin, J. Dolovich, and F. E.Hargreave. 1982. Allergen-induced increase in non allergic bronchial hyperreactivity. Clin. Allergy 7: 503.

14. Andersson, M., B. von Kogerer, P. Andersson, and U. Pipkorn. 1987. Allergen-induced nasal hyperresponsiveness appears unrelated to the size of the nasal and dermal immediate allergic reactions. Allergy 42: 631.

15. Andersson, M., and U. Pipkorn. 1988. Allergen-induced hyperreactivity is not a feature of dermal immediate allergic reactions—in contrast to reactions of airway mucosa. Clin. Allergy 18: 189.

Eustachian Tube Function and Allergy

*Philip Fireman**

The possibility that allergy contributes to ear disease, especially otitis media with effusion (OME) is not a new concept and its role has been suggested for years [1]. If a causal relationship between allergy and OME were established, then one would expect that antiallergic therapy would reduce the morbidity associated with the otitis. In addition, such therapy might be able to prevent the hearing loss and delay in verbal communication that has been suggested to result from persistence of fluid in the middle ear cavity. This presentation develops the concept that eustachian tube obstruction (ETO) contributes to the pathogenesis of OME. It also describes our recent studies, which have documented that ETO develops in allergic subjects after intranasal allergen or histamine provocation, and which supports our contention that allergic rhinitis is also a risk factor for middle ear disease.

Otitis media is a very common pediatric disease characterized by an acute or chronic inflammation of the middle ear mucosa frequently followed by the subsequent development of an effusion within the middle ear. This condition is called otitis media with effusion (OME). OME may be a recurrent or chronic condition and frequently is recognized as a sequelae of acute otitis media by visual otoscopy and tympanometry [2, 3, 4]. OME can also be diagnosed on routine examination as an occult condition, perhaps following a subclinical or protracted inflammation of the middle ear [3]. It most commonly occurs in infants and younger children under 4 years of age, but can be a problem in all age groups [4]. Many synonyms and pseudonyms have been used during the past 50 years to categorize OME, including *serous otitis media, secretory otitis media, mucoid otitis, "glue ear," nonsuppurative otitis media, catarrhal otitis, tubotympanic catarrh,* and *allergic otitis media.* These descriptive terms have created much confusion among allergists.

It is difficult to determine by history and visual inspection of the tympanic membrane the specific characteristics of the middle ear effusion. Without a diagnostic aspiration of the middle ear effusion one cannot ascertain if the fluid is serous, mucoid, purulent, nor can one identify its microbial characteristics. Since a diagnostic tympanocentesis is not currently recommended for most patients at the time of initial diagnosis, we prefer using the generic term: otitis media with effusion (OME). The other descriptive terms are not recommended at this time, since they may mislead the allergist in understanding the pathogenesis and potential etiology of the middle ear disease.

Pathophysiology

The pathogenesis of OME appears to be related in part to abnormal function of the eustachian tube (ET). Understanding the potential nature of this tubal dysfunction requires some familiarity with the anatomy and physiology of the upper airway constituted by the nasal cavity, nasopharynx, ET, middle ear, and mastoid air cells. The ET provides an anatomic communication between the nasopharynx and the middle ear, and is in a unique position to effect changes in the middle ear secondary to reactions in the nose. The ET and its relationship to the middle ear and the nasopharynx may be considered to be analogous in part to the bronchial tree and its relationship to the lung and nasopharynx. Thus, abnormal ET function may predispose the middle ear to infection, atelectasis, and effusion. In this regard, the ET like the bronchial airway serves several physiologic functions, *protection, drainage* and *ventilation: protection* from nasopharyngeal secretions, *drainage* into the nasopharynx of secretions produced within the middle ear, and *ventilation*

* Professor of Pediatrics, University of Pittsburgh School of Medicine; Director, Allergy, Immunology and Rheumatology, Children's Hospital of Pittsburgh, Pittsburgh, PA 15213.
  Supported by NIH Grant AI19262.
  Acknowledgements: The author acknowledges the contributions of his co-workers, Drs. Charles Bluestone, William Doyle, and David Skoner to their collaborative studies. The preparation of this manuscript by Carol Wagner is greatly appreciated.

of the middle ear to equilibrate air pressure in the middle ear with atmospheric pressure and to replenish oxygen that has been absorbed.

The normal ET is functionally collapsed at rest, with slight negative pressure existing in the middle ear. Active opening of the ET is accomplished by contraction of the tensor veli palatini muscle during swallowing. In normal tubal function, intermittent opening of the tube maintains near ambient pressures in the middle ear cavity. It is suspected that in cases in which active swallowings are inadequate to overcome tubal resistance, the tube remains persistently collapsed, and results in progressive negative middle ear pressure. This type of ventilation appears to be common in children, since moderate to high negative middle ear pressure have been identified by tympanometry in many who are apparently normal. However, periodic or persistently high negative pressure may be pathologic and has been associated with abnormal function of the ET. Persistent high negative middle ear pressure with severe retraction of the tympanic membrane has been termed *atelectasis* of the tympanic membrane-middle ear and result in acute otitis media [6]. If effective ventilation does not occur, because of persistent ETO, transudation of sterile MEE into the tympanum can result as a consequence of the constant absorption of oxygen by the middle ear epithelium. Since tubal opening could be possible in a middle ear with an effusion, aspiration of nasopharyngeal secretions might occur, thus creating the clinical condition in which persistent MEE and recurrent acute otitis media occur together.

Two types of ETO, either mechanical or functional, could result in acute or chronic OME. Table 1 shows a classification of common conditions associated with ETO.

Intrinsic mechanical obstruction may result from infection or allergy [7], whereas extrinsic obstruction may result from enlarged adenoids [10]. Experimentally, allergic rhinitis provoked in patients with a history of allergy has been

associated with the development of ETO [9]. This obstruction related to edema, and inflammation of the posterior nasopharynx could be both extrinsic and intrinsic. Persistent collapse of the ET during swallowing may result in functional obstruction, which appears to be related to increased tubal compliance, an inefficient active opening mechanism, or both [10]. Functional ETO is common in infants and younger children, since the amount and stiffness of the cartilage support of the ET are less than in older children and adults. Also, there appears to be marked age differences in the craniofacial base, which render the tensor veli palatini muscle less efficient before puberty.

Nasal obstruction may also be involved in the pathogenesis of OME. Swallowing when the nose is obstructed (inflammation or obstructive adenoids) creates a closed nasopharyngeal chamber. During swallowing, an initial positive nasopharyngeal air pressure is followed by a negative pressure phase within the closed system. The possible effect of these pressures on a pliant tube could be the following: With positive nasopharyngeal pressure, secretions might be insufflated into the middle ear, especially when the middle ear has a high negative pressure; with negative nasopharyngeal pressures, such a tube could be prevented from opening and functionally become further obstructed. This has been termed the "Toynbee phenomenon."

Eustachian Tube Function Testing

Eustachian tube function can also be evaluated following intranasal challenge by using either the pressure-swallow (9-step) test or the more recently describe sonotubometry, which can be performed within seconds of doing rhinomanometry with our computer-assisted technology. The 9-step test has been described in detail previously [4]. In this test, a tympanometer measures the pressure on the tympanic membrane in the external auditory canal. A pressure transducer is placed near the eardrum and baseline middle ear pressure is recorded. Slight positive pressure is applied by the tympanometer via the external auditory canal to the eardrum. This positive pressure creates negative pressure within the middle ear and causes a shift in the tympanometer readings. The patient is requested to swallow, and if ET function is normal, the tympanometer record-

Table 1. Classification of eustachian tube obstruction and associated symptoms.

Obstruction	Associated conditions
1. Mechanical	
a. Intrinsic	Infection, allergy
b. Extrinsic	Enlarged adenoids, allergy
2. Functional	Infancy, cleft palate

ings returns to the original baseline. Slight negative pressure is then applied to the eardrum with resultant positive pressure on the middle ear. Again, the patient is requested to swallow, and if tubal function is normal, the pressure readings by the tympanometer return to baseline. The normal ET is functionally collapsed at rest most of the time. Active opening of the ET during swallowing induces intermittent opening of the tube which maintains near ambient atmospheric pressure in the middle ear cavity. When active swallowings as described for the 9-step test are inadequate to overcome tubal resistance, the tube remains collapsed.

The principal advantages of using the sonotubometry equipment to test for ETO are that it does not require either a tympanic membrane perforation or the application of static pressure to the tympanic membrane. The sonotubometer used is a microcomputer-based device, developed and assembled in our laboratory. Sonotubometry evaluates tubal function on the basis of sound passage from the nose, through the ET. The speaker is equipped with a set of interchangeable tips through which the sound signal is introduced into the nose. Microphones in each external ear canal monitor the sound pressure level. When the ET opens, sound is transmitted to the microphone, and memory segments are displayed on an oscilloscope and can be recorded for analysis. For all stimuli, the duration and amplitude of the signal when displayed as a time function yield information with respect to the duration and extent of tubal opening. With tubal obstruction, decreased or no sound is transmitted. No change in the frequency spectrum following swallowing is interpreted as an inability to open the tube. The test sequence can then be repeated for sound introduced into the right nasal cavity. Maximum change in amplitude as well as the duration of tubal opening are recorded.

Etiology

OME is considered by many as a multifactorial disease process with several potential etiologies. Infection and ETO are the best understood etiologies. In addition, allergy and host defense defects may participate either directly or indirectly and thereby contribute to the OME.

Infectious Aspects

Bacteria have been cultured from 60% to 70% of middle ear effusions in children with acute otitis media and have been shown to be similar to those found in the nasopharynx. *Streptococcus pneumoniae* was cultured from approximately 30% and is the most common agent in all age groups. *Haemophilius influenzae,* non-typable, was found in about 20% of the ear effusions. In the past, the incidence of *Branhamella catarrhalis* has been about 5%, but as shown in the table, the incidence is now 12% and has been reported even higher by others [11]. The frequency of Group A beta-hemolytic streptococcus was 3%, and *Staphylococcus aureus* was present in less than 2%. Frequently, bouts of OME are preceded by a probable viral URI, and incidence of OME tracks the seasonal pattern of viral URI yet. Viruses have been infrequently cultured from middle aspirates of children who have acute otitis media, but viral antigens have been identified using immune assays in 10–20% of middle ear effusions [12, 13].

In association with the University of Virginia and the Gamble Institute of Cincinnati, we developed a human model utilizing experimental viral infection to delineate the pathophysiologic response of the nose, ET and middle ear to a viral URI. We have performed 5 challenge experiments with rhinovirus and one challenge experiment with each of Coxsackie A and Influenzae viruses. Similar test methods and protocols were used in all studies. The results showed that the pathophysiology induced by rhinovirus infection includes general malaise, decreased nasal patency, debilitated nasal clearance function, ET dysfunction, and abnormal middle ear pressures. Challenge results in an active infection rate of greater than 90% with over 70% developing a cold. Symptoms occur on the day following challenge, peak on days 3–5 and then decrease. Nasal congestion is decreased by day 2, peaks over days 3–8 and does not return to baseline until day 19. The frequencies of individuals with ETO and abnormal middle ear pressures increases on days 3–7 and then decreases to baseline. The frequency of individuals developing nasal congestion was 85%, 60%, and 60% for infection with rhinovirus, Coxsackie A, and Influenzae, respectively. Abnormal middle ear pressures were observed in 61%, 67%, and 50% of patients infected with Rhinovirus, Coxsackie A, and Influenzae, respectively.

Immunologic and Allergic Aspects

The potential for immune mechanisms to contribute to the pathogenesis of OME has been postulated by several studies which found many of the humoral and cellular immune response components in middle ear effusions [14–16]. That IgE-mediated allergic reactions participate in the pathogenesis of chronic OME has been suggested by clinical observations reporting a higher prevalence of chronic OME in allergic patients, but these studies were retrospective and lacked appropriate controls and experimental design [17]. The role of allergy in OME may involve one or more of the following mechanisms: (1) middle ear mucosa functioning as a target organ; (2) inflammatory swelling of the ET; (3) inflammatory obstruction of the nose and nasopharynx; or (4) reflux, insufflation, or aspiration of bacteria-laden allergic nasopharyngeal secretions into the middle ear cavity. The latter three mechanisms would be associated with abnormal function of the eustachian tube.

The chronically inflamed middle ear mucosa contains mast cells, lymphocytes as well as plasma cells, and has the potential of functioning as a "shock organ." This hypothesis has been frequently entertained in multiple anecdotes over the years especially of children with a history of gastrointestinal allergy to cow's milk. Unfortunately, there are no adequately controlled clinical studies to substantiate this theory. A few investigators have reported increased IgE levels in middle ear fluids from patients with chronic OME, but this has also not been substantiated. Bernstein and co-workers, in a study of children with chronic OME and documented respiratory allergy, could document IgE antibodies in middle ear effusions from only 7% of these patients [18]. Even though Skoner et al. in our laboratories found markedly elevated concentrations of histamine in middle ear fluids from most patients with chronic OME, convincing data have not yet been developed to prove that this increase in histamine has been elaborated by an allergic reaction [19].

Even though there is a lack of convincing evidence that allergy plays the primary role in the etiology of otitis media, there appears to be a relation between upper respiratory tract allergy and ETO. A prospective study of children with recurrent or chronic middle ear disease as well as functional ETO had more severe obstruction (mechanical) of the tube when an upper respiratory tract infection developed [5]. A similar relationship has been reported between upper respiratory tract allergy and ETO in a series of provocative intranasal allergen inhalation challenge studies by our group at the Children's Hospital of Pittsburgh. We studied adult volunteers who had a history of allergic rhinitis, normal tympanic membranes, and normal ET function prior to an intranasal challenge with the pollen to which they were allergic. All developed ETO along with the anticipated allergic rhinitis, but an effusion in the middle ear was not observed after this single allergen intranasal challenge [16]. This allergy-induced ETO has been shown to be allergen dose dependent, related to the magnitude of the allergen-specific serum IgE antibodies and persisted longer than the associated allergic rhinitis [23]. Recent observations suggest that IgE-mediated allergic rhinitis provoked by intranasal pollen challenge can be associated with both immediate (20 minutes) and late phase (4–8 hours) ETO [24]. This pathophysiology of the nose, nasopharynx, and ET has not only been provoked in patients with ragweed and grass pollen seasonal allergic rhinitis, but also in patients with house dust perennial allergic rhinitis following intranasal challenge with the house dust mite [25]. Monkeys that had been passively sensitized with high titer human anti-ragweed IgE sera also develop ETO following intranasal challenge with pollen [21, 26]. In both humans and monkeys, these brief episodes of allergy provoked ETO did not result in OME.

Our laboratory has also demonstrated in Rhesus monkeys that aerosolized intranasal histamine not only induced rhinitis, but also provoked ETO in a dose response that was more pronounced in juvenile than adult monkeys [27]. Skoner in our laboratory using a double-blind dose-response protocol documented a heightened responsiveness of the ET to histamine in allergic subjects [28, 29]. The efficacy of antihistamine decongestants in preventing antigen induced ETO has recently been shown in our laboratory [30].

From these studies, the following sequence of events is postulated in patients who have respiratory allergy and otitis media. Most likely, a basic ET dysfunction is present in certain infants and children whose tubal function becomes compromised in the presence of upper respiratory tract allergy similar to ETO caused by an upper respiratory tract infection. Upper respiratory tract allergy may cause some intrinsic as well as extrinsic mechanical obstruction in patients who have normal ET function, but their normal active opening mechanisms, i.e., tensor veli palatini muscle pull, is able to overcome the obstruction. Therefore, patients who have functional obstruction because of poor muscular opening would be at highest risk for developing sufficient mechanical obstruction to develop middle ear disease. Since many children as part of normal development have difficulty actively opening their ET, they are the population who probably are at risk for manifesting OME. If the ETO is minimal, the patient will have only signs and symptoms of ET dysfunction such as otalgia ("popping" and "snapping" sounds in the ear), mild hearing loss, tinnitus, or even vertigo. Many patients will experience these symptoms, but often they fluctuate and are present only during the worst periods of the patient's allergic rhinitis. Insufflation of nasopharyngeal secretions caused by allergic rhinitis could also be insufflated into the middle ear during noseblowing, jumping or diving into water when swimming, or in the infant who is crying or during closed-nose swallowing, i.e., the Toynbee phenomenon.

Allergic rhinitis severe enough to cause nasal obstruction could also induce middle ear disease because of the Toynbee phenomenon. If nasal obstruction exists, the nasopharyngeal pressures during closed-nose swallowing are first positive due to the elevation of the soft palate and closing off of the velopharyngeal space, followed by negative pressure when the soft palate is in a lower position. These pressures are similar to pressure changes that occur in the lower pharynx during physiologic swallowing. If the ET opens during the positive phase of closed-nose swallowing, allergic nasopharyngeal secretions could be insufflated into the middle ear resulting in otitis media. More likely, however, the ET is prevented from opening because of the high negative pressure developed in the nasopharynx during the second phase of closed-nose swallowing. This could cause ETO and negative middle ear pressure, which would be manifested by signs and symptoms of ET dysfunction including fluctuating or sustained otalgia, hearing loss, tinnitus, or vertigo. Atelectasis of the tympanic membrane-middle ear, or otitis media could develop. Under these circumstances it would be difficult for the patient to open the tube even after swallowing. Aspiration of allergic nasopharyngeal secretions in which bacteria were present could also be possible with this type of mechanisms.

Summary

At present there is no direct scientific proof in animals or humans that allergic rhinitis produces middle ear effusion, but the mechanism seems plausible. Likewise, there is no direct and conclusive evidence that upper respiratory tract allergy induces OME when there is a temporary provoked ET dysfunction. Nevertheless, our studies of allergic rhinitis patients who showed ETO following challenge with intranasal allergens document an allergic pathophysiology of the ET. OME developed 4 weeks after experimental surgical resection of a portion of the ET. It is our hypothesis that prolonged ETO is necessary for the manifestation of OME. Even though conclusive proof of this relationship is lacking, we suggest that allergic rhinitis is a risk factor in the pathogenesis of OME especially if there is partial ET dysfunction, especially in the young child. Future studies are needed in children to better define the proposed role of allergy in the pathophysiology of the ET and the pathogenesis of OME.

References

1. Welliver, R. C. 1987. Allergy and middle ear effusions: Fact or fiction. In: Immunology of the ear. J. M. Bernstein and P. L. Ogra, eds. New York: Raven Press.
2. Fiellau-Nkiolajsen, M. 1983. Tympanometry and secretory otitis media: Observations on diagnosis, epidemiology, treatment, and prevention in prospective cohort studies of three-year-old children. Acta Otolaryngol. 96 (Suppl. 394): 7.
3. Casselbrant, M. L., P. A. Okeowo, M. R. Flaherty et al. 1984. Prevalence and incidence of otitis media in a group of preschool children in the United States. In: Recent advances in otitis media with effusion. D. J. Lim, C. D. Bluestone

J. O. Klein, and J. D. Nelson, eds. Philadelphia: B.C. Decker.

4. Brownlee, P. C., W. R. DeLoache, C. C. Cowan, and H. P. Jackson. 1969. Otitis media in children: Incidence, treatment and prognosis in pediatric practice. J. Pediatr. 75: 636.

5. Bluestone, C. D., Q. C. Beery, and W. S. Andrus. 1974. Mechanics of the eustachian tube as it influences susceptibility to and persistence of middle ear effusions in children. Ann. Otol. Rhinol. Laryngol 83 (Suppl.): 27.

6. Bluestone, C. D., and Q. C. Beery. 1976. Concepts in the pathogenesis of middle ear effusions. Ann. Otol. Rhinol. Laryngol. 85 (Suppl.): 182.

7. Bluestone, C. D. 1983. Eustachian tube function: Physiology, pathophysiology and role of allergy in pathogenesis of otitis media. J. Allergy Clin. Immunol. 72: 242–251.

8. Bluestone, C. D., E. I. Cantekin, and Q. C. Beery. 1975. Certain effects of adenoidectomy on eustachian tube ventilatory function. Laryngoscope 85: 113.

9. Friedman, R. A., W. J. Doyle, M. L. Casselbrandt, C. D. Bluestone, and P. Fireman. 1983. Immunologic mediated eustachian tube obstruction: A double-blind crossover study. J. Allergy Clin. Immunol. 71: 442–447.

10. Bluestone, C. D., and W. J. Doyle (Eds.). 1985. Eustachian tube function: Physiology and role in otitis media. Ann. Otol Rhinol. Laryngol. 94 (Suppl. l20): 48–49.

11. Shurin, P. A., C. D. Marchant, C. H. Kim, G. F. Van Hare, C. E. Johnson, M. A. Tutihasi, and L. J. Knapp. 1983. Emergence of beta-lactamase producing strains of *Branhamella catarrhalis* as important agents of acute otitis media. Pediatr. Infect. Dis. 2: 34–38.

12. Sarkkinen, H., O. Ruuskanen, O. Meurman, H. Puhakka, E. Virolainen, and J. Eskola. 1985. Identification of respiratory virus antigens in middle ear fluids of children with acute otitis media. J Infect. Dis. 151(3): 444–448.

13. Chonmaitree, T., V. M. Howie, and A. L. Truant. 1986. Presence of respiratory viruses in middle ear fluid and nasal wash specimens from children with acute otitis media. Pediatrics 77(5)P: 698–702.

14. Bernstein, J. M., and P. Ogra. 1976. Mucosal immune system: Implication in otitis media with effusion. Ann Otol. Rhinol. Laryngol. 89(68): 362.

15. Veltri, R., and P. M. Sprinkle. 1976. Secretory otitis media, an immune complex disease. Ann Otol. Rhinol. Laryngol. 85 (suppl. 25): 135.

16. Bernstein, J. M., C. Szymanski, B. Albini et al. 1978. Lymphocyte subpopulations in otitis media with effusions. Pediatr. Res. 12: 786. (abstract)

17. Reisman, E. R., and J. Bernstein. 1975. Allergy and secretory otitis media. Pediatr. Clinics of North Am. 22: 251.

18. Bernstein, J. M., J. Lee, K. Cinby et al. 1983. Role of IgE mediated hypersensitivity in recurrent otitis media with effusion. Amer. J. Otol. 5: 66.

19. Skoner, D. P., P. K. Stillwagon, Casselbrandt, E. P. Tanner, W. J. Doyle, and P. Fireman. Inflammatory mediators in chronic otitis media with effusion. Arch Otolaryngol Head Neck Surgery, in press.

20. Miglets, A. 1973. The experimental production of allergic middle ear effusion. Laryngoscope 83: 1355.

2l. Doyle, W. J., T. Takahara, and P. Fireman. 1985. The role of allergy in the pathogenesis of otitis media with effusion. Arch. Otolaryngol. 111: 502–506.

22. Yamashita, T., N. Okozoki, and T. Kumuzawa. 1980. Relation between nasal and middle allergy. Ann. Otol. Rhinol. Laryngol 89 (Suppl. 68): 147.

23. Ackerman, M., R. Friedman, W. J. Doyle et al. 1984. Antigen induced ETO: A intranasal provocative challenge test. J. Allergy Clin. Immunol. 73: 604.

24. Fireman, P. 1988. Nasal provocation testing: An objective assessment for nasal and eustachian tube obstruction. J. Allergy Clin. Immunol. 81: 953–960.

25. Skoner, D. P., W. J. Doyle, A. Chamovitz, and P. Fireman. 1986. Eustachian tube obstruction after provocative intranasal challenge with house dust mite. Arch. Otolaryngol. 112: 840.

26. Doyle, W. J., R. Friedman, P. Fireman, and C. D. Bluestone. 1984. Eustachian tube obstruction after provocative nasal antigen challenge. Arch Otolaryngol. 110: 508–511.

27. Doyle, W. J., A. Ingram, and P. Fireman. 1985. Histamine-induced eustachian tube obstruction in monkeys. J. Allergy Clin. Immunol. 76: 551.

28. Walker, S. B., G. G. Shapiro, C. W. Bierman et al. 1985. Induction of eustachian tube dysfunction with histamine nasal provocation. J. Allergy Clin. Immunol. 76: 158.

29. Skoner, D. P., W. J. Doyle, and P. Fireman. 1987. Eustachian tube obstruction (ETO) after histamine nasal provocation: A double blind dose response study. J. Allergy Clin. Immunol. 79: 27–31.

30. Stillwagon, P.K., Doyle, W.J., and Fireman P. 1987. Effect of an antihistamine/decongestant on nasal and eustachian tube function following intranasal pollen challenge. Annals of Allergy 58: 442–446.

247

Perennial Allergic Conjunctivitis: The Nature of the Condition and Its Place in the Spectrum of Ocular Allergic Disease

*Roger J. Buckley**

Seasonal allergic conjunctivitis (SAC) is a very common component of the disease known as hay fever. In any affected individual, either the ocular or the nasal symptoms may predominate. The presumed mechanism of the disease is that air-borne allergenic particles are carried by or through the tear film to reach conjunctival mast cells previously coated by specific IgE. Mast cell degranulation then produces the characteristic conjunctival hyperaemia and oedema and the symptoms of itching and tearing. Also characteristic of SAC are the findings that the inflammatory mediators do not damage the corneal epithelium, and that there is no rise of histamine in the tears [1]. Presumably, the small quantities of histamine liberated are removed by endogenous histaminases; nevertheless, histamine instilled into the eye produces symptoms and signs indistinguishable from SAC. The significance of the reported contribution to the conjunctival microvascular permeability response of plasmin, produced not by the mast cell, but from plasminogen contained in the extracellular fluid of the challenged tissue [2] is not yet fully evaluated.

SAC is still the best attested example of an ocular allergic disease. The antigens initiating the disease have been characterised, specific antibody has been identified, an animal model of the disease has been made, and the disease has been produced in an unaffected human by passive sensitisation with serum from an affected individual [3].

Most of the textbooks of ocular immunopathology mention the existence of a perennial form of SAC, known as perennial allergic conjunctivitis (PAC), which is presumed to be caused by constantly present airborne allergens such as the house dust mite and animal danders. However, these accounts contain little or no information on the prevalence of this disease or on its diagnostic criteria. Recent work at Moorfields Eye Hospital in London has sought do address both of these matters [4].

Because both SAC and PAC are mild, non-sight-threatening diseases that usually respond readily to treatment prescribed by the general practitioner, or even to preparations bought "over the counter" by the patient, cases are rarely seen by the hospital-based ophthalmologist. For this reason, as we wished to study the characteristics of PAC and to estimate the prevalence of SAC and PAC, we arranged to examine patients presenting with ocular symptoms at a London Group General Practice. Here, nearly 14,000 patients were on the age, sex register of 7 general practitioners. For the clinical part of our study we also recruited patients presenting at an Allergy Clinic at Moorfields Eye Hospital.

Study Details

To enter the study, patients who had had conjunctival inflammation for not less than 3 weeks had to satisfy the following criteria:

History

At least 3 out of 4 following to be positive:

— perennial or seasonal symptoms

— a duration of symptoms of not less than 2 years

— the symptom of itch

— a personal and/or family history of atopic disease.

---

*   Moorfields Eye Hospital, London, England.

Clinical Signs

Limited to the following conjunctival signs:

– hyperaemia

– small papillae and/or follicles

– minimal cellular infiltrate

Clinical Investigations

At least one out of 4 following to be positive:

– one or more positive response(s) on intradermal skin prick testing to a panel of antigens including dusts, pollens, moulds, and foods

– eosinophils in conjunctival scrapes

– a raised tear IgE level

– a raised serum IgE level.

Summary of Results

Fourteen patients with PAC and 25 patients with SAC were identified on the basis of these criteria. There were no significant differences between the two groups in terms of age, age of onset, or length of history. The majority of patients in both groups had a personal history of atopic disease, but in both these were minorities who had no such history. There was an association with perennial rhinitis in 75% of the PAC patients, but in only 12% of the SAC group. None of the PAC patients had a family history of atopic disease, while this was the case in 28% of the SAC patients.

By definition, in PAC the symptoms occur year-round, but 79% of the patients reported seasonal exacerbations in addition. Symptoms were similar in both groups, but more severe in SAC. Clinical signs were also similar in PAC and SAC, being minimal in both. The almost normal clinical appearance of the ocular tissues is characteristic of these two conditions.

All patients had positive skin prick tests. The strongest responses were to dusts and pollens, the weakest to moulds and foods. The strongest response, assessed by weal size, was to pollens in the SAC group and to dusts in the PAC group. 71% of the PAC patients produced their strongest response to *Dermatophagoides pteronyssinus* (DPP); this was true also for only 4% of the SAC patients.

Eosinophils were present in the conjunctival scrapes of 43% of the PAC patients and in 25% of the SAC patients; the difference was not statistically significant.

The serum total IgE level falls below 125 IU/ml in 95% of normal adults [5]. This level was exceeded in 77% of PAC patients and in 71% of SAC patients, with the mean level significantly higher in the PAC group.

The tear total IgE was raised (i.e., above 0.5 IU/ml) in all patients but for one SAC patient.

DPP-specific IgE levels were raised in the serum of 89% of PAC patients and in 43% of SAC patients. The difference was not significant. Raised tear levels of DPP specific IgE occurred in 78% of patients with PAC and in none of those with SAC. These levels were higher than the corresponding serum levels, indicating that the immunoglobulin was locally produced by the eye.

Prevalence studies indicated an incidence for PAC in the population studied of 3.5:10,000 for a 3 month period. SAC was the commonest disease encountered among the patients seen at the Group General Practice; PAC was the eighth commonest.

Discussion

The study showed that the condition PAC could be diagnosed on the basis given. Patients had the same age range, length of history and symptoms as those with SAC. Total IgE levels in tears and serum were raised in both groups, and eosinophils were sometimes found in conjunctival scrapes. It appeared that house dust mite was responsible for PAC, while pollens caused SAC. DPP antigen-specific IgE was found in the tears of most PAC patients, but in no SAC patients.

PAC is a condition that shares many characteristics with SAC. It is less common, though still among the most commonly encountered eye diseases. Like SAC, it can be considered to be an immediate hypersensitivity phenomenon. There is a common association with perennial rhinitis.

PAC and SAC differ from vernal keratoconjunctivitis (VKC), atopic keratoconjunctivitis (AKC), and giant papillary conjunctivitis (GPC) in important respects. Signs are minimal, there being no clinical evidence of the chronic cellular infiltration and structural change which are characteristic of these other conditions. Corneal epithelial erosion and its sequel, which are the sight-threatening aspects of VKC and AKC, are not seen in either PAC or SAC.

PAC should now be recognised as a commonly encountered eye disease that can be defined by recommended diagnostic criteria. It is to be anticipated that perennial allergens other than DPP will be incriminated in other environments.

The treatment of PAC follows the same principles as the treatment of SAC. Antigen avoidance is impractical, as the responsible allergen(s) is/are perennial. Topical antihistamine use is unlikely to be lastingly successful, because of the development of tachyphylaxis and topical sensitisation reactions. The newer oral antihistamines, with their reduced sedative properties, may be useful, but they have not been systematically studied in this condition. Topical steroid preparations, with the high incidence of unwanted effects that they cause, should generally be avoided; if they are not, there is more potential damage to sight from the therapy than from the disease. Topical sodium cromoglycate in (2% eye drops twice to four times daily and/or 4% ointment once or twice daily) has been found to be effective and safe, in both PAC and SAC.

References

1. Allansmith, M. R. 1982. The eye and immunology. St. Louis: C. V. Mosby.
2. Salonen, E.-M., T. Tervo, E. Törmä et al. 1987. Plasmin in tear fluid of patients of corneal ulcers: basis for new therapy. Acta Ophthalmol. 65: 3–12.
3. Allansmith, M. R., and G. R. O'Connor. 1970. Immunoglobulins: structure, function and relation to the eye. Surv. Ophthalmol. 14: 367–402.
4. Dart, J. K. G., R. J. Buckley, M. Monnickendam, and J. Prasad. 1986. Perennial allergic conjunctivitis: definition, clinical characteristics and prevalence. Trans. Ophthalmol. Soc. UK. 105: 513–520.
5. Zetterstrom, O., and S. G. O. Johansson. 1981. IgE concentrations measured by PRIST in serum of healthy adults and in patients with respiratory allergy. Allergy 36: 537–547.

Sodium Cromoglycate in Tear Film Disease

Louis M.T. Collum, Maureen P. Hillery*, Anthony Benedict-Smith*,
Frank Kinsella*, Monique Hope-Ross*, William Power*, Barry Read***

Sodium cromoglycate (2%), in combination with hypromellose, was used in the management of tear film disorders. The patients were divided into two groups, involutional and immune. Each group was subdivided and treated with sodium cromoglycate in combination with hypromellose, or with hypromellose alone. The patients were allocated treatment on a randomised double-blind basis, and the effect of therapy was analysed at the end of a two-month period, using the Mann-Whitney U-Test. There was no difference in effect in the immune group, but in the involutional group the trend was in favour of the combination therapy, though the P value of 0.19 was not significant.

Tear film abnormalities are common in external eye disease clinics and may be due to abnormalities in any of the layers of the tears.

There are many conditions that affect tear production. There may be interference with the production of fat, as in patients with chronic inflammation of the eye lids. Abnormal or reduced fat allows more rapid evaporation and patients complain of ocular irritation, with dry spots, even though the eye may be wet. Disease of the goblet cells produces an upset in the mucous content of the tears. Mucous is necessary to ensure sufficient contact time of the tears with the conjunctiva and cornea and so prevents drying. Absence of mucous will therefore interfere with this contact time and patients experience symptoms, which may occur in the presence of a watery eye. Conditions that interfere with mucous production include inflammatory reactions in the conjunctiva, such as viral diseases, trachoma, or immune disorders, including rheumatoid arthritis.

The water content of the tears may be affected by disease of the lacrimal and accessory lacrimal glands including immune disorders and sarcoidosis. The water content is not as critical as the other constituents.

Abnormalities of any of these layers will therefore produce the symptoms of irritation, grittiness, redness, and mucous discharge. Therapy should be aimed at restoring the integrity of the tears by replacing the deficient component. Careful evaluation of the marginal strip, the pre-corneal film, the Schirmer test, Rose Bengal staining, and the patient's history will usually indicate which component is deficient. It is reasonable to suggest that all tear deficiencies will not respond to a single treatment, but that different medications may be indicated, depending on the component that is abnormal.

A possible therapeutic role for sodium cromoglycate in tear film disorders was suggested in 1985 [1]. This is the first paper that attempts to evaluate this possible effect. The basis for its use is that it appears to improve the overall tear film break up time by approximately 65%, which phenomenon is more marked in women than in men [2]. Because sodium cromoglycate is a water-binding molecule it may contribute to increased stability of the tear film. In addition, sodium cromoglycate is able to undergo thixotropic gelling in the presence of magnesium ions. Although the concentration of magnesium ions in the tears does not allow gelling, it is sufficient to increase the viscosity of the tears in the presence of sodium cromoglycate. It is known that the magnesium content of female tears is higher than that of males, and this is in keeping with the observation that there is a greater effect on the break-up time of the tear film in women.

There may, however, be another explanation for the effect of sodium cromoglycate in tear film disease. Degranulating mast cells are present in conjunctival biopsy specimens taken from patients with immune disease and it is possible that the drug may work by stabilising these cells, so reducing the release of substances which produce inflammation.

---

*   Royal Victoria Eye and Ear Hospital Dublin, Ireland. Royal College of Surgeons in Ireland.
**   Fisons Pharmaceuticals, Loughborough, Leicestershire, England.
Acknowledgement: The secretarial assistance was supplied by Mrs. P. Conn.

Materials and Methods

A clinical study was carried out in 101 patients with tear film disease. They were divided into two groups, involutional and immune. The involutional group consisted of patients who had no systemic or immune disorder, but did exhibit deficiencies in their tear film, as evidenced by reduced Schirmer test, staining with Rose Bengal of the conjunctiva and cornea, reduced marginal tear strip and reduced pre-corneal tear film with a short break up time. These patients had no other local eye disease. The second group consisted of those that had immune disease with auto antibodies in their blood and/or an abnormal immunophoretic pattern. Many of them had obvious systemic immune disease such as rheumatoid arthritis. Each group of patients was subdivided and allocated either 2% sodium cromoglycate in hypromellose or hypromellose alone, on a blind randomised basis. The appropriate regulatory and ethical approval was obtained and all patients gave informed consent. On the first visit a complete history was taken and the patient was evaluated, to see if he satisfied the criteria for inclusion in the study. The symptoms, namely, itching, pain, grittiness, tearing, and photophobia were assessed on a scale from 0–4 (0 = none, 4 = very severe). In addition, clinical signs such as keratopathy, conjunctival scarring, mucous strands, filaments, and meibomian gland disease were evaluated with a similar marking method. A Schirmer test was carried out, and the tear film break up time was evaluated. The presence or absence of debris in the tears was noted. A biopsy was taken, the patient started his treatment and was asked to return at 2 weeks, 4 weeks, 6 weeks, and 8 weeks. On each visit a full examination was carried out, but a further biopsy was not performed until the last visit.

Patients were withdrawn from the study if they experienced any side effect, or if their condition worsened at any time. A record was made of any side effects. Patients were given a score card to record their impressions of treatment. In addition, both the patients assessment of treatment and the clinicians assessment of the efficacy of the treatment were recorded on each visit. At the end of the 8-week period, the patients were commenced on standard medication. Using the Mann-Whitney U-Test, a statistical analysis of the results was carried out.

Results

There were 53 patients in the involutional group. The ages and male/female ratio in each sub-group were comparable. The number of females treated was much higher than that of males, there being 22 females and 4 males in the sodium cromoglycate group, and 22 females and 5 males in the hypromellose alone group. The duration of symptoms was comparable in both groups. Three patients were withdrawn from the sodium cromoglycate group because of possible lack of effect of treatment, while a similar number was withdrawn from the hypromellose group for the same reason. There appeared to be two adverse reactions in the hypromellose group, and one patient had a suspected adverse reaction in the sodium cromoglycate group. There was no statistical difference in these figures. Thirteen patients in the sodium cromoglycate group and 9 in the hypromellose group experienced some stinging after instillation. Signs and symptoms improved in both groups, but no statistically significant differences between the treatments were seen. In the opinion of patients that completed the study, good control was achieved in fourteen on sodium cromoglycate (70%) and in nine on hypromellose (46%). This corresponded to the clinician's opinion.

There were 50 patients in the immune group, comprising 35 females and 15 males, 24 of whom received sodium cromoglycate. The groups were comparable in relation to age, sex distribution, and duration of symptoms. Ten patients were withdrawn from the sodium cromoglycate group because of lack of effect, while 9 patients were withdrawn from the hypromellose group for similar reasons. No adverse reactions were recorded in either group. Fifteen patients in the sodium cromoglycate group and 16 patients in the hypromellose group completed the study. Signs and symptoms improved in both groups, but no statistically significant differences between the treatments were seen. In the patients' opinion, good control was achieved in 6 patients on sodium cromoglycate (40%) and in 9 patients on hypromellose (56%). This corresponded to the clinician's opinion.

Examination of the conjunctival biopsies showed that in the immune group there was significant mast cell activity.

Discussion

The results recorded in this study do not have statistical significance. There is, however, a trend in the involutional group in favour of sodium cromoglycate. Of those that completed the study, there was a 70% positive response in those having sodium cromoglycate, as against 46% in those having hypromellose. As there was no active immune or other inflammatory disease in these patients, the sodium cromoglycate combination effect is probably produced by increasing the viscosity of the tears.

There was no trend in favour of sodium cromoglycate in patients with immune disease. This is compatible with the fact that there was an active immunological response going on in the conjunctiva, involving immunoglobulins and lymphocytes though there was mast cell activity. Though there is some tissue uptake of ocular sodium cromoglycate [3, 4], which presumably had an effect on this mast cell activity, it is unlikely to have had a significant effect on the disease process, which is primarily immunoglobulin and lymphocyte mediated.

Though 101 patients commenced this study, only 70 patients completed the treatment, 31 in the immune group and 39 in the atrophic group. The ratio of females to males was in keeping with the greater incidence of immune disease in the former. As already indicated, there was a trend that suggested that sodium cromoglycate had a beneficial effect in the atrophic group. If more patients had completed the study, or if more patients had been included initially, it may have been possible to demonstrate a more definite trend in that direction. The problem with such patients, is that frequently their symptoms are not severe enough to motivate them to attend the number of times required.

Further work should be carried out on a larger number of patients, to establish whether the trend suggested is real and whether cromoglycate has a definite place to play in the management of tear film disease. Based on the outcome of this study, it is likely to be more helpful in involutional disease rather than where there is an active immune reaction in the conjunctiva.

References

1. Allansmith, M. R. 1985. In: The First Cromolyn Sodium in Ophthalmology Symposium. J. H. Lass, ed. Excerpta Medica. p. 35.
2. van Bijsterveld, O. P. 1983. Sodium cromoglycate (Opticrom) in chronic conjunctivitis and tear-film stabilisation. In: Allergic Eye Disease and Sodium Cromoglycate. Workshop Proceedings, Corsendock, Belgium. J. J. De Laey, ed. p. 31.
3. Lee, V. H. L., J. Swarbrick, R. E. Stratford Jr., K. W. Morimoto. 1983. Disposition of topically applied sodium cromoglycate in the albino rabbit eye. Journal of Pharmacy and Pharmacology 35: 445–450.
4. Nizami, R. M. 1981. Treatment of ragweed allergic conjunctivitis with 2% cromolyn solution in unit doses. Annals of Allergy 47: 5–7.

Influence of Environment on the Development of Allergies in Children

Bengt Björkstén, Gunnar Hattevig, N-I. Max Kjellman*

The impact of environmental risk factors is different in individuals with and without a genetic propensity to become sensitized. Tobacco smoke is the most important air pollutant that children are exposed to, but also other pollutants like NO_2, SO_2, and ozone seem to play a role in the development of allergy. Living in well-insulated buildings, particularly if smoking is allowed in the house, increases the risk for development of allergy. Infections with respiratory viruses and pertussis may also facilitate sensitization. Amount and time of exposure to allergen influence the rate of sensitization in children at risk of allergy development. Particularly the amount of exposure to house dust mites at different ages and early exposure to foreign food proteins, including small amounts present in human milk, household pets, and pollen appear to facilitate the sensitization to these allergens. Maternal avoidance of certain highly allergenic foods during the first three months of lactation appears to delay the onset of allergies in their babies.

Sensitization and subsequent allergic disease may develop in a child with an inherited susceptibility for IgE-mediated allergy when exposed to allergens. This is facilitated by various environmental factors. Several recent studies have clearly shown that the impact of such environmental risk factors is quite different in individuals with and without the genetically determined propensity to become sensitized. Clinical disease is therefore a consequence of an interplay between a genetic propensity for allergy, time and amount of exposure to sensitizing allergens and simultaneous exposure to nonspecific triggers that facilitate the sensitization. Since the genetic set-up of man has not changed appreciably over the last century, the apparent increase in the incidence of atopic diseases is most likely explained by environmental triggers, including life-style, housing conditions, foods, and environmental pollution.

There seem to be a period in early life during which the individual is particularly easily sensitized and conceivable is most vulnerable to environmental influences. In this review we therefore emphasize this period of life.

Exposure to Allergens

An individual must be exposed to the allergen in order to be sensitized against it and to develop symptoms of allergy. The sensitization is influenced by the amount and time of exposure and at what age the exposure takes place. Thus, a significantly increased risk for subsequent development of allergy to birch and grass pollen has been reported in Finnish children born in the spring [1]. Similar results have been reported for grass allergy in the U.K. [2] and for ragweed allergy in the United States [3]. This relation between season of birth and allergy development seems to be limited to children with a congenital propensity for allergy [4]. Similarly, early contact with animal ephitelia [5] and house dust mites [6] appear to influence the incidence of allergy.

Early feeding with foreign proteins has also been reported to be associated with an increased risk for allergic disease (reviewed in [7]). These observations prompted us to study the effects of maternal avoidance of allergenic foods such as eggs and cow's milk during the last trimester of pregnancy and during the first 3 months of lactation. The first study comprised 212 mothers who were randomized to diet or to a control group. The dietary manipulation had no effect on the incidence of allergy in the offspring through the first 18 months of life [8]. In a second study, 115 mothers were subject to dietary manipulation during the first

* Department of Pediatrics, Faculty of Health Sciences, University of Linköping, S- 58185 Linköping, Sweden.
Acknowledgements: The studies were supported by grants from the Swedish Medical Research Council (7510), the Swedish Board for Protection of the Environment, The County of Östergötland, Majblomman Fund, King Gustaf V 80-Years Anniversary Fund, The Expressen Prenatal Fund.

255

3 months of lactation. It was found that maternal avoidance of cow's milk and eggs delayed the onset of atopic dermatitis in babies with a high risk of allergy development [9]. This was defined as either a family history of allergy and/or cord blood IgE above 0.9 kU/l. The infants were all subject to accepted allergy-preventive measures, including avoidance of exposure to tobacco smoke and pets at home, and they were all either breast fed for at least three months or receive a casein hydrolysate formula (Nutramigen®). In addition, 65 of the mothers kept a diet, strictly avoiding eggs and cow's milk. The infants of diet mothers had a significantly lower rate of atopic dermatitis at 3 and 6 months. At 9 and 18 months there was still a non-significant trend toward less allergy. It was also found that sensitization, as indicated by the demonstration of IgE antibodies to foods, appeared later in the babies of mothers on diet. These studies clearly indicate that maternal avoidance of certain foods during the first months of lactation, but not during pregnancy, may delay the onset of allergy in their babies.

Non-Specific Triggers of Allergy

In addition to exposure to allergens, there are a number of environmental factors that facilitate sensitization to almost any allergen that the individual is exposed to (Table 1). Among these "adjuvant" factors, particularly air pollution and infections are usually mentioned, but there are also a number of other factors that should be considered.

Table 1. Environmental factors that possibly enhance sensitization to an allergen.

Tobacco smoke
Air pollution
Type of dwelling
Infection
Psychological factors
Pre- and perinatal medication and stress

Air Pollution

Tobacco smoke is the most important indoor air pollutant. In fact, the concentration of smoke in a room when someone is smoking far exceeds that caused by any emission from a polluting industry. There is now a confirmed clear relation between exposure to tobacco smoke and allergy. In children with parents who smoke at home, there is a significantly earlier onset and higher incidence of allergy and wheeze bronchitis as compared to children of non-smoking partners [11]. In a recent epidemiological survey of 5300 children in Sweden, we found that bronchial hyperreactivity and pollen allergy both were more common in children of parents who smoked at home [12]. This was particularly obvious in children living near a moderately air- polluting paper factory area compared to children in a forested area with no polluting industry, indicating that various sources of air pollution could be synergistic.

The effect of tobacco smoke on sensitization to allergens may be explained by a local effect on airways rather than a direct effect on the immune system. This is supported by our finding that smoking rats exposed to aerosolized antigen have higher IgE antibody responses than subcutaneously immunized animals and non-smoking aerosol immunized controls [13]. Other air pollutants like ozone, SO_2, and NO_2 all may increase serum IgE levels, at least in experimental animals [14].

Housing

Modern housing may be part of the explanation why allergy seems to be increasing in industrialized countries. Well-insulated building with poor ventilation may thus represent a risk factor for allergic sensitization. Various "sick buildings" characterized by damage due to dampness and indoor mold growth have become increasingly common as a consequence of improved insulation and energy saving. In an epidemiological survey of 5300 children, it was found that children living in homes with damage from dampness had a higher incidence of atopic disease and/or bronchial hyperreactivity [12] than children living in undamaged homes. For children living in houses with damage from dampness whose parents smoked at home there was a marked increase in allergic asthma and bronchial hyperreactivity as compared to children exposed to only one of these factors. It seems reasonable to explain the synergistic effects of exposure to tobacco smoke and damage from dampness by the fact that these houses are poorly ventilated and thus allow increased concentrations of air pollutants as well as allergens. The effect of these environmental conditions were most marked for children with a family history of asthma, supporting the notion that environmental influences only play an important role in individuals with a genetic susceptibility for allergic disease.

Infections

There are now several studies suggesting an association between upper respiratory infections and appearance of allergic disease. Possible explanations for these observations include that infectious agents may facilitate sensitization to environmental allergens, alter immune defence, act as adjuvants, or themselves act as allergens. It is well known from animal studies that *pertussis* bacteria are adjuvants for the induction of IgE antibody formation against various antigens [15]. There are also indications that this can be true in humans, suggesting the possibility that whooping cough may trigger allergy. This notion is further supported by the fact that whooping cough is often associated with a prolonged period of bronchial hyperreactivity. We have recently found that IgE antibodies against *pertussis* toxin are encountered in children and adults during whooping cough and in response to *pertussis* immunization [16]. The IgE antibody response was particularly pronounced after immunization with a vaccine containing $Al(OH)_3$ as adjuvant, supporting animal experiments in which alum is an excellent adjuvant for IgE antibody formation [17].

Psychological Factors

Less is known regarding the possible impact of psychological factors on the development of allergy in childhood. Animal studies and recent clinical observations indicate that stress may alter the immune response [18, 19]. Studies in our group have shown that families with a severely affected asthmatic child often demonstrate a rigid or chaotic interaction pattern as compared to families with children affected by another chronic disease, e.g., diabetes, and as compared to healthy children [20]. Family therapy for such families improved the severity of the asthma [21]. It is now known whether the particular interaction pattern commonly found in families of asthmatic children are consequences of the disease or whether they represent a primary factor that may increase the risk for asthma in an atopic individual born into the family. Prospective studies to assess this possibility are presently in progress.

Drugs

Drugs administered to women during pregnancy may have some immune regulatory activities. Progesterone has been suggested as significantly increasing cord blood IgE, but it does not seem to increase the risk for allergic disorders later in infancy and childhood [22]. In a double-blind placebo-controlled study of the β-adrenergic receptor-blocking agent metoprolol in pregnant women, it was found that children exposed *in utero* to a drug more often had elevated IgE levels in the cord blood and/or developed clinical allergy during the first four years of life than the children of placebo-treated control mothers [23]. If confirmed, this result lends support to animal studies showing that β-receptor blockade may increase and β-receptor stimulation lower IgE antibody levels.

Concluding Remarks

A number of factors associated with modern life-style in industrialized societies may in part explain the apparent increase in allergic diseases in children in such societies. But even if all these factors are taken together—less breast feeding, dietary changes, modern housing, exposure to tobacco smoke, air pollution, and perinatal stress—this cannot explain why allergy develops in many but not in all allergy-prone infants. Obviously, there is still a long way to go before we can adequately identify *all* environmental triggers of allergy.

References

1. Björkstén, F., I. Suoniemi, and V. Koski. 1980. Neonatal birch-pollen contact and subsequent allergy to birch pollen. Clin. Allergy 10: 581.
2. Morrison-Smith, J., and V. H. Springett. 1979. Atopic disease and month of birth. Clin. Allergy 9: 153.

3. Settipane, R. J., and G. W. Hagy. 1979. Effect of atmospheric pollen on the newborn. Rhode Island Med. J. 62: 477.

4. Croner, S., and N-I. M. Kjellman. 1986. Predictors of atopic disease: Cord blood IgE and month of birth. Allergy 41:68.

5. Suoniemi, I., F. Björkstén, and T. Haahtela. 1981. Dependence of immediate hypersensitivity in the adolescent period on factors encountered in infancy. Allergy 36: 263.

6. Rowntree, S., J. J. Cogswell, T. A. E. Platts-Mills, and E. B. Mitchell. 1985. Development of IgE and IgG antibodies to food and inhalant allergens in children at risk of allergic disease. Arch. Dis. Child. 60: 727.

7. Björkstén, B., and N-I. M. Kjellman. 1987. Perinatal factors influencing the development of allergy. Clin. Rev. Allergy 5: 339.

8. Fälth-Magnusson, K., and N-I. M. Kjellman. 1987. Development of atopic disease in babies whose mothers were on exclusion diet during pregnancy—a randomized study. J. Allergy Clin. Immunol. 80: 868.

9. Hattevig, G., B. Kjellman, N. Sigurs, B. Björkstén, and N-I. M. Kjellman. 1988. The effect of maternal avoidance of eggs, cow's milk and fish during lactation upon allergic manifestations in infants. Clin. Allergy, in press.

10. Liard, R., S. Perdrizet, and P. Retner. 1982. Wheezy bronchitis in infants and parents' smoking habits. Lancet i: 334.

11. Rantakallio, P. 1978. Relationship of maternal smoking to morbidity and mortality of the child up to the age of five. Acta Paediatr. Scand. 67: 621.

12. Andrae, S., O. Axelson, B. Björkstén, M. Fredriksson, N-I. M. Kjellman. 1988. Symptoms of bronchial hyperreactivity and asthma in relation to environmental factors. Arch. Dis. Child. 63: 473.

13. Zetterström, O., S. L. Nordvall, B. Björkstén, S. Ahlstedt, and M. Stehlander. 1985. Increased IgE antibody responses in rats exposed to tobacco smoke. J. Allergy Clin. Immunol. 75: 594.

14. Gershwin, J., J. E. Osebold, and Y. C. Zee. 1985. Immunoglobulin E-containing cells in mouse lungs following allergen inhalation and ozone exposure. Int. Arch. Allergy Appl. Immunol. 65: 266.

15. Pauwels, R., M. van der Straeten, B., Platteay, and H. Bazin. 1983. The non-specific enhancement of allergy. I. In vivo effects of *Bordetella pertussis* vaccine on IgE synthesis. Allergy 38: 239.

16. Hedenskog, S., B. Björkstén, M. Blennow, G. Granström, and M. Granström. 1988. Immunoglobulin E response to pertussis toxin in whooping cough after immunization with a whole cell and an acellular pertussis vaccine. Int. Arch. Allergy Appl. Immunol., in press.

17. Way, N. M., L. C. S. Maia, O. G. Hanson, and J. C. Lynch. 1971. Inhibition of homocytotropic antibody responses in adult inbred mice by previous feeding of the specific antigen. J. Allergy Clin. Immunol. 21: 11.

18. Haggerty, R. J. 1986. Stress and illness in children. Bull. N.Y. Acad. Med. 62: 707.

19. Jemmott, J. B., and S. E. Locke. 1984. Psychosocial factors, immunologic mediation and human susceptibility to infectious illnesses: How much do we know? Psychol. Bull. 95: 78.

20. Gustafsson, P. A., N-I. M. Kjellman, J. Ludvigsson, and M. Cederblad. 1987. Asthma and family interaction. Arch. Dis. Child. 62: 258.

21. Gustafsson, P. A., N-I. M. Kjellman, and M. Cederblad. 1986. Family therapy in the treatment of severe childhood asthma. J. Psychosom. Res. 30: 369.

22. Michel, J., J. Bousquet, Y. Coulomb, and M. Robinet-Lévy. 1981. Prediction of the high-allergic-risk newborn. In: Diagnosis and treatment of IgE-mediated diseases. S. G. O. Johansson, ed. Amsterdam- Oxford-Princeton: Excerpta Medica, p. 35.

23. Björkstén, B., O. Finnström, and K. Wichman. 1988. Intrauterine exposure to beta-adrenergic receptor blocking agent metoprolol and allergy. Int. Arch. Allergy Clin. Immunol., in press.

24. Homer, J. T., and W. A. Cain. 1979. Enhancement of IgE antibody formation in the rabbit by adrenergic antagonists. Int. Arch. Allergy Appl. Immunol. 59: 121.

Smoking and Allergy

John E. Salvaggio, Samuel B. Lehrer, Richard P. Stankus*

In recent years there has been increasing concern with regard to the quality of our environment and its resulting effects on health and well-being. This concern has prompted analysis of common, previously overlooked "pollutants." Tobacco smoke represents one such environmental agent, which has the potential for producing respiratory symptoms including the induction or aggravation of asthma.

Tobacco and its incineration products can also affect the immune system in several ways. As irritants or toxic agents they can interact with various cellular components of the host defense system altering the functional ability of these elements [1]; as potential antigens or allergens, they can interact with the immune system to induce specific antibody responses or specific immune responses, evidenced by production of antibodies, of different immunoglobulin class specificities [2]. They also possess the potential to effect production of cytokines and lymphokines by sensitized T cells and other cells of the mononuclear series.

Accordingly, this article focuses on the role of tobacco leaf and smoke products as antigens or allergens, and on the possible role of tobacco smoke exposure in the initiation or exacerbation of allergic respiratory disease.

Tobacco and the Immune System

The tobacco plant belongs to the botanical family *Solanaceae*. A wide range of foods including tomatoes, eggplants, potatoes, and green peppers are also members of this botanical family. Tobacco leaf extract is heterogeneous, containing many proteins plus bacterial and fungal contaminants and additives such as colophony, insecticide residues, and a large number of combustion products. Over 2,000 gaseous, semi-volatile, and particulate components have been detected in tobacco smoke [3]. There are two types of tobacco smoke: mainstream smoke, which is inhaled by the smoker, and sidestream smoke, emanating from the tip of a burning cigarette.

There were many studies of tobacco leaf antigens in the 1970s. Chu and co-workers demonstrated at least five carbohydrate-protein complexes in tobacco leaf with molecular weights ranging between 20,000 and 60,000 daltons which were immunogenic with experimental animals [4]. A study of Kreis and co-workers demonstrated tobacco-leaf components of relatively low molecular weight which were immunogenic in rabbits and gave positive precipitin reactions with human serum [5]. In another study, five tobacco plant proteins of widely different immunoelectrophoretic mobility were noted to exhibit the property of precipitating with human serum. Differences in antigenic activity were also noted among various tobacco-leaf extracts tested. Becker and co-workers, in a series of studies in 1976, demonstrated the presence of a glycoprotein in both tobacco-leaf and tobacco-smoke condensate [6]. This so-called tobacco glycoprotein (TGP) elicited positive wheal and flare skin reactions in humans, although the irritant threshold for the skin test reactions and the atopic status of the individuals tested were not defined [7].

TGP is a brown material rich in rutin or rutin-like polyphenol groups. It is distributed widely among members of the *Solanaceae* family and has a number of biologic activities and properties, including the ability to activate Hageman factor (thus possibly accelerating clotting processes); to serve as a mitogen for splenic peripheral blood and bone marrow lymphoid cells; to induce differentiation of spleen cells into antibody-producing cells; to inhibit complement activation via the classical pathway by binding C-2; to elicit homocytotrophic antibodies in the mouse; and to serve as a "T-independent" B-cell mitogen [1, 2, 8–10]. These biologic activities have led some to hypothesize that TGP might play an important role in the pathogenesis of atherosclerosis or

*   Tulane University School of Medicine, Department of Medicine, Section of Clinical Immunology and Allergy, 1700 Perdido Street, New Orleans, LA 70112, USA.

arteritis in humans or serve as an allergen or immunogen in the production of IgE-mediated respiratory disease. Conversely, other investigators believe that TGP may only represent a contaminant or artifact of separation from tobacco leaf [11].

More recently, tobacco leaf and smoke extracts have been shown to be highly immunogenic in experimental animal models. At least 37 different antigens have been detected in tobacco leaf by employing the technique of crossed immunoelectrophoresis [12]. Some of these are "allergens" as demonstrated by their capacity to react specifically with human anti-tobacco-leaf IgE antibodies by crossed radioimmunoelectrophoresis.

With regard to tobacco smoke, both stimulatory and inhibitory events have been reported on the immune system. Tobacco smoke has been shown to increase T and B cell ratios and to increase IgA-containing cells in lobar bronchi [13, 14]. Hypereosinophilia has been documented in a small number of cigarette smokers [15, 16], and increased levels of serum IgE and IgD have been demonstrated in "moderately heavy" cigarette smokers, while heavy cigarette smoking appears to result in a depression of these serum immunoglobulin levels [17–19]. Other demonstrable inhibitory effects of smoke and smoke-derived products on the immune system have included an impaired response to influenza virus in smoke-exposed experimental animals, impaired lymphocyte blastogenesis, impaired generation of antibody plaque-forming cells, and impaired IgG and IgM responses to certain administered antigens [20–25]. Thus, cigarette smoke and its products have been reported to both enhance and depress the immune response under different conditions in both experimental animals and humans.

Tobacco Smoke Hypersensitivity

There have been numerous studies of the possible role of hypersensitivity to tobacco smoke products in humans. Earlier animal model studies employing tobacco leaf suggested the development of a systemic antigen-antibody-induced arteritis. Based on these earlier observations, Harkavy speculated on the relationship between cigarette smoke and coronary artery disease in humans [26]. However, all of these studies employed tobacco-leaf extract. Many other uncontrolled or anecdotal observations have been made with regard to the possible role of tobacco smoke sensitivity in humans. These include the detection of positive wheal and erythema skin reactivity to tobacco-leaf extract in smoke-sensitive subjects [27] and the ability of tobacco smoke extract to stimulate lymphocytes [28]. In general, these studies have employed poorly defined patient populations and in many cases have been devoid of proper controls.

Conversely, evidence has been gathered against the role of tobacco-smoke hypersensitivity in smoke-sensitive individuals. Skin testing of smoke-sensitive subjects with tobacco-leaf extract in several large-scale studies has revealed no correlation between intensity of tobacco smoke sensitivity and skin reactivity [29, 30]. In other studies, techniques involving the use of both cigarette smoke and cigarette smoke suspended in human serum albumin have failed to detect antibody in the serum or bronchial secretions of smoke-sensitive individuals [31]. In addition, respiratory challenge with cigarette smoke in occupationally induced allergy to tobacco leaf has failed to produce significant declines of pulmonary function [32]. The above conflicting reports with their variations of study design stress the importance of obtaining more information through appropriately designed studies.

Immunologic Basis for Smoke Sensitivity

We have analyzed tobacco smoke and leaf extracts for ability to induce reaginic antibody and precipitating antibody production in the mouse and rabbit. Our studies employed several different sources of tobacco leaf and smoke "antigen." Among these were tobacco leaf extracted by homogenization in phosphate-buffered saline, smoke condensates prepared by homogenization in 4M urea, and smoke "extracts" obtained by passing cigarette smoke through solutions of either phosphate buffered saline or other extraction solvents containing various proteins followed by concentration and dialysis. All extracts of tobacco leaf contained antigens that stimulated a precipitating antibody response in rabbits, whereas most extracts of condensate and smoke failed to stimulate an antibody response [33, 34]. However, serum antibodies could be induced against either smoke condensate or smoke extract coupled to ovalbumin. Furthermore, several antisera from smoke immunized rabbits reacted with extracts of tobacco leaf.

Several strains of mice also produced reaginic antibody to extracts of tobacco leaf but not to smoke extract as demonstrable by the homologous 48-hour passive cutaneous anaphylaxis (PCA) reaction [34]. When mice were passively sensitized by intradermal inoculation with diluted serum samples from smoke-immunized animals followed by challenge with tobacco leaf extract, anti-tobacco-leaf reaginic antibody was demonstrated. Characterization of smoke extracts was undertaken employing standard immunochemical techniques including column chromatography (Bio Gel A), gel filtration, and immunodiffusion for reactivity of column fractions with smoke and leaf antisera. Results demonstrated that all antisera reacted with antigens corresponding to those eluted from a peak containing a molecular weight range of 150,000 daltons. Further fractionation of smoke extract on a Bio Gel A 0.5-M column demonstrated precipitating antigen in a peak with a molecular weight similar to that of ovalbumin. Further studies employing dialyzed and undialyzed smoke extract have suggested that small molecular weight dialyzable components in smoke extract (possibly haptens) may be important immunogens in tobacco smoke. The immunogens do not appear to be products of incineration since antisera to extracts of air passed through unlit cigarettes also react similarly to tobacco leaf extracts.

The allergenic potential of smoke immunogens in humans has been studied in 93 subjects, of whom 60 claimed sensitivity to tobacco smoke [35]. A significant number of individuals studied demonstrated positive immediate wheal and flare skin reactivity and RAST responses to tobacco-leaf antigen, but only small number responded to smoke antigens. Of importance was the fact that neither skin test or RAST reactivity to tobacco leaf and smoke antigens correlated with clinical tobacco smoke "sensitivity" or smoking history [35, 36]. Atopic individuals did, however, manifest significantly greater skin reactivity and RAST responses regardless of whether they were smokers, non-smokers, or ex-smokers. IgG-precipitating antibody responses were also detected in many of these test subjects, but they also did not correlate with either smoking history or clinical smoke sensitivity. Thus, these studies do not support a role for IgE-mediated hypersensitivity reactions to tobacco leaf or smoke antigens as a mechanism for subjective tobacco smoke "sensitivity" in humans.

In order to test the hypothesis that qualitative differences in IgE responses to tobacco leaf antigens might be related to smoke "sensitivity," tobacco leaf was analyzed for "allergens" by crossed radioimmunoelectrophoresis [12]. Sera demonstrating a positive RAST to tobacco leaf obtained from subjects reporting tobacco smoke sensitivity were compared with sera from non-sensitive subjects. Three of 37 tobacco leaf precipitins detectable by CIE were identified as "allergens" by virtue of their ability to bind IgE antibodies. However, sera from all test subjects reacted to at least one of these tobacco allergens and neither intensity or incidence of reactivity to these "allergens" correlated with smoking or clinical smoke sensitivity.

Challenge Studies with Tobacco Smoke

Much of the evidence linking passive cigarette smoke to exacerbations of asthma is anecdotal. Subjective data from early studies support a greater incidence of eye irritation, rhinorrhea, cough, wheezing, and pharyngeal irritation in allergic non-smoking subjects when compared with non-allergic non-smokers. Cough and wheezing on exposure to cigarette smoke has been reported to occur 2 to 4 times more frequently in allergic subjects compared to non-allergic individuals [37]. In a related study, wheezing following passive exposure to cigarettes was reported with more than twice the frequency in asthmatics when compared with non-asthmatics [38].

Objective challenge testing with tobacco smokes has yielded variable results. Shephard and colleagues studied 14 asthmatic subjects, who underwent 2-hour passive exposure to cigarette smoke. Thirty-six percent of their exposed subjects complained of wheezing and 46% of "chest tightness" [39]. However, measurements of declines in pulmonary function were insignificant, and dynamic lung volumes (FEV_1, $V_{max\ 50\%}$, VO, $V_{max\ 5\%}$, VC) were unaltered. This study is open to criticism, however, since all study subjects continued their usual bronchodilator and antiflammatory medications during the period of smoke challenge. Furthermore, few of these individuals claimed "clinical sensitivity" to cigarette smoke, and some had negative methacholine challenges.

In a second study, Dahms and co-workers studied 10 subjects with bronchial asthma and positive methacholine tests and 10 control subjects [40]. All were exposed to sidestream cigarette smoke for 1 hour in an environmental chamber. A significant linear decrease in pulmonary function was noted in the asthmatic subjects during the challenge procedure. FEV_1 decreased an average of 21%, $FEF_{25-75\%}$ decreased 19%, and FVC decreased 20% in the asthmatic group following 1 hour of exposure. No change in pulmonary function was noted in the control group following an identical challenge procedure.

Recently, Wiedemann and co-workers studied the acute effects of 1 hour of passive cigarette smoke exposure on pulmonary function and airways reactivity in 9 adult asthmatics [41]. Six of the 9 subjects had claimed aggravation of asthma by cigarette smoke. Tobacco smoke challenge produced no significant change in expiratory flow rates.

We designed a study of 21 adult asthmatic subjects who claimed exacerbation of asthma upon exposure to environmental smoke, had positive methacholine challenges, and were atopic as defined by broad patterns of immediate wheal and flare skin reactivity to common inhalant allergens [42]. A similar group of smoke-sensitive, nonasthmatic control subjects was also studied.

Subjects were asymptomatic and on no bronchodilators. They were challenged in a static inhalation chamber ($12 \times 7 \times 11$ ft.) in which a constant temperature of 21°C and a relative humidity of 50% were maintained. They were exposed for 2 hours to the cigarette particulate level produced by two ignited IR2F research cigarettes "smoked" via Borgwaldt fully automatic smoking machine ("low level" exposure) or 16 ignited 1R2F cigarettes ("high level" exposure). The level of cigarette smoke exposure during bronchial provocation challenge was quantitated by assessing carbon monoxide, nicotine, and total particulate levels in the chamber. Both mainstream and sidestream smoke were produced by this procedure. Airborne particulate levels were monitored with a sibata model T5H2 light-scattering aerosol indicator. Particulate target levels, as measured by this instrument, were 400, 800, and 1600 cpm. Carbon monoxide levels were monitored with a miran 1A gas infrared spectrophotometer and quantitation of airborne nicotine levels was based on a NIOSH manual and method.

Conjunctival irritation was experienced by all test subjects. Nasal congestion plus fronto-maxillary headache were also common. All subjects who experienced significant declines in FEV_1 also manifested cough and/or dyspnea. Seven of the 21 smoke challenge subjects—but none of the control group—demonstrated a significant (20%) decline in FEV_1. Peak expiratory flow rates and FVC demonstrated similar declines. No association was observed between severity of asthma and smoke-induced changes in lung function. Of the 7 responders, all but 2 responded only to the "high" level of cigarette exposure. Positive responses were easily reversed by administration of epinephrine and metaproterenol. Reproducibility of reactions was confirmed by elicitation of positive challenge tests in all responder subjects on subsequent days. Of importance was the fact that there was no association between positive wheal and flare skin reactivity or RAST activity to tobacco-leaf extract and the induction of a positive cigarette-smoke challenge. Collectively, these studies document a significant objective decline in pulmonary function in 33% of a population of smoke-sensitive asthmatics exposed to relatively "high-level" environmental tobacco smoke, but relatively little decline (9%) to a low level of environmental smoke. The data dissociate this effect from IgE-mediated tobacco-leaf and smoke hypersensitivity. It is obvious that considerable research remains to be done on the nature of tobacco-leaf and smoke antigens including TGP, and on their biologic activity in humans. In addition, the means by which tobacco incineration products and other "irritant" dusts produce minor nuisance conjunctival and nasal symptoms requires study. Among the many possibilities to be considered are possible nonspecific release of mast cell mediators by neuropeptides released from terminal nerve endings following exposure to such "irritants."

References

1. Choy, J. W., C. G. Becker, G. W. Siskind, and T. Francus. 1985. Effects of tobacco clycoprotein (TGP) on the immune system. I. TGP is a T-independent B cell mitogen for murine lymphoid cells. J. Immunol. 134: 3193–3198.
2. Becker, C. G., R. Levi, and J. Zavecz. 1978. Induction of IgE antibodies to antigen released from tobacco leaves and from cigarette smoke condensate. Am. J. Pathol. 96: 249.
3. Norman, V. 1977. An overview of the vapor phase, semivolatile and nonvolatile components of cigarette smoke. In: Tobacco Chemists Research Conference, Vol 30. Greensboro, North Carolina.
4. Chu, Y. M., R. C. Parlett, and G.L. Wright, Jr. 1970. A preliminary investigation of some immunologic aspects of tobacco use. Am. Rev. Respir. Dis. 102: 118.
5. Kreis, B., A. Peltier, S. Fournaud et al. 1970. Reaction depreciitation entre certains serums humains et des extraits solubles du tabac (Precipitation reaction between certain human sera and soluble tobacco extracts). Ann. Med. Inter. 121: 437.
6. Becker, C. G., T. Dublin, and H. P. Wiedemann. 1970. Hypersensitivity to tobacco antigen. Proc. Natl. Acad. Sci. 121: 437.
7. Becker, C. G., and T. Dubin. 1977. Activation of factor XII by tobacco glycoprotein. J. Exp. Med. 146: 457.
8. Becker, C. G., M. Van Harmant, and M. Wagner. 1981. Tobacco, cocoa, coffee, and ragweed crossreacting allergens that activate factor XII dependent pathways. Blood 58: 861.
9. Becker, C. G., and T. Dubin. 1977. Activation of Factor XII by tobacco glycoprotein. J. Exp. Med. 146: 457.
10. Firpo, A., M. J. Polley, and C. G. Becker. 1983. The effect of tobacco derived from products on the human complement system. Immunobiology 164: 318.
11. Stedman, R. L. 1978. Effect of smoking on nonsmokers. September 7 Hearing Before the Subcommittee on Tobacco of the Committee on Agriculture, House of Representatives, 95th Congress, Second Session, Serial No. 95-000, Washington, DC: U.S. Government Printing Office, pp. 82–97.
12. Lehrer, S. B., M. McCants, and J. E. Salvaggio. 1985. Analysis of tobacco leaf allergens by crossed radioimmunoelectrophoresis. Clin. Allergy 15: 616.
13. Soutar, C. A. 1976. Distribution of plasma cells and other cells containing immunoglobulin in the respiratory tract of normal man and class of immunoglobulin contained therein. Thorax 31: 158.
14. Warr, G. A., R. R. Martin, C. L. Holleman et al. 1976. Classification of bronchial lymphocytes from nonsmokers and smokers. Am. Rev. Respir. Dis. 113: 96.
15. Schoen, I., and M. Pizer. 1964. Eosinophilia apparently related to cigarette smoking. N. Engl. J. Med. 25: 1344.
16. Paintal, I. S., and R. J. Minina. 1975. Tobacco smoking—A probable cause of eosinophilia. Indian Pract. 5: 243.
17. Burrows, B., M. Haloneen, R. A. Barbee et al. 1981. The relationship of serum immunoglobulin E to cigarette smoking. Am. Rev. Respir. Dis. 124: 523.
18. Bonini, S. 1982. Smoking, IgE, and occupational allergy (letter). Br. Med. J. 284: 510.
19. Bahna, S. L., D. C. Heiner, and B. A. Myhre. 1983. Immunoglobulin E pattern in cigarette smokers. Allergy 38: 57.
20. Thomas, W. R., P. G. Holt, and D. Keast. 1974. Development of alterations in the primary immune response of mice by exposure to fresh cigarette smoke. Int. Arch. Allergy Appl. Immunol. 4: 481.
21. Mackenzie, J. S. 1976. The effect of cigarette smoke on influenza virus infection: A murine model system. Life Sci. 31: 409.
22. Roszman, T. L., L. H. Elliott, and A. S. Rogers. 1975. Suppression of lymphocyte function by products derived from cigarette smoke. Am. Rev. Respir. Dis. 4: 453.
23. Roszman, T. L. 1973. Effect of nicotine and water soluble condensate, from whole smoke in the in vitro secondary antibody response. Proceedings of the University of Kentucky Tobacco and Health Research Institute, Tobacco and Health Workshop Conference, Lexington, Kentucky. pp. 530–541.
24. Andersen, P., O. F. Pedersen, B. Back et al. 1982. Serum antibodies and immunoglobulins in smokers and nonsmokers. Clin. Exp. Immunol. 47: 467.
25. Roszman, T. L., and A. S. Rogers. 1973. The immunosuppressive potential of products derived from cigarette smoke. Am. Rev. Respir. Dis. 108: 1158.
26. Harkavy, J. 1968. Tobacco allergy in cardiovascular disease: A review. Ann. Allergy 26: 447.
27. Zussman, B. M. 1974. Tobacco sensitivity in the allergic population. J. Asthma Res. 11: 159.
28. Savel, H. 1970. Clinical hypersensitivity to cigarette smoke. Arch. Environ. Health 21: 146.
29. Speer, F. 1968. Tobacco and the nonsmoker. Arch. Environ. Health 16: 443.
30. Taylor, G. 1974. Tobacco smoke allergy—Does it exist? In: Environmental tobacco smoke effects on the nonsmoker. K. Rylaader, ed. Geneva: University of Geneva, p. 50.

31. McDougal, J. C., and G. J. Gleich. 1976. Tobacco allergy—Fact or fantasy. J. Allergy Clin. Immunol. 57: 237.

32. Gleich, C. J., P. W. Welsh, J. W. Yunginger et al. 1980. Allergy tobacco: An occupational hazard. N. Engl. J. Med. 302: 617.

33. Lehrer, S. B., M. R. Wilson, and J. E. Salvaggio. 1978. Immunogenic properties of tobacco smoke. J. Allergy Clin. Immunol. 62: 368.

34. Lehrer, S. B., M. R. Wilson, and J. E. Salvaggio. 1980. Immunogenicity of tobacco smoke components in rabbits and mice. Int. Arch. Allergy Appl. Immunol. 62: 16.

35. Lehrer, S. B., F. Barbandi, J. P. Taylor et al. 1984. Tobacco smoke "sensitivity"—Is there an immunological basis? J. Allergy Clin. Immunol. 73: 240.

36. Lehrer, S. B., M. R. Wilson, R. M. Karr et al. 1980. IgE antibody response of smokers, nonsmokers, and "smoke-sensitive" persons to tobacco leaf and smoke antigens. Am. Rev. Respir. Dis. 121: 168.

37. Speer, F. 1968. Tobacco and the nonsmoker. Health 16: 443.

38. Shephard, R. J., E. Ponsford, and R. LaBarre, P. K. 1979. Subjective reactions to passive cigarette smoke exposure. Effect of cigarette smoke on the eyes and airways. Int. Arch. Occup. Environ. Health, 43: 135.

39. Shephard, R. J., R. Collins, and I. Silverman. 1979. "Passive" exposure of asthmatic subjects to cigarette smoke. Environ. Res. 20: 392.

40. Dahms, I. E., J. F. Bolin, and R. G. Slavin. 1981. Passive smoking: Effects on bronchial asthma. Chest 80: 530.

41. Wiedemann, H. P., D. A. Mahler, J. Loke et al. 1986. Acute effects of passive smoking on lung function and airway reactivity in asthmatic subjects. Chest 89: 180.

42. Stankus, R. P., P. K. Menon, R. Rando et al. Cigarette smoke sensitive asthma: Challenge studies. J. Allergy Clin. Immunol., in press.

Allergy and Changing Environments—Industrial/Urban Pollution

Terumasa Miyamoto, Shigeru Takafuji, Shuji Suzuki, Kenji Tadokoro, Masaharu Muranaka*

The prevalence rate of allergic rhinitis and asthma has been increasing in Japan. To ascertain one of the causes, we studied in mice whether or not the adjuvant effect exists in diesel exhaust particles and suspended particle matters in IgE antibody production. IgE antibody production was enhanced when the mice were immunized with OA with these particles intraperitoneally and intranasally. From these results, it is possible to conclude that allergenic substances may combine with inhaled suspended particles on the surface of the human respiratory mucosa, and that the IgE antibody production may be subsequently enhanced, resulting in the increasing incidence of allergic diseases.

According to the Greek myth, Prometheus stole fire from Heaven. This is the origin of air pollution. Air pollution caused the acute episodes of respiratory disasters such as in Meuse Valley, Bergium, Donora, Pennsylvania, and London, where the excess of death and illness among susceptible populations with chronic respiratory and cardiac diseases were thought to be caused by the increased concentration of pollutants. Air pollution is a universal by-product of human occupational and domestic activity. The principal pollutants in the urban and industrial atmosphere arise from the industrial operations, automobiles, power production and space heating, incineration of wastes, etc. The gases that pollute the atmosphere can be listed by their sources of production. The gas combustion from motor vehicles gives rise to carbon monoxide (CO), nitrogen oxides (NO), and volatile hydrocarbons. The burning of coal and heavy oil for production of electrical energy or heating constitutes the principal source of sulfur dioxide (SO_2) and floating particles. Photochemical air pollution is a by-product of motor fuel combustion. The reaction between nitrogen dioxide and a variety of organic substances, notably hydro-

carbons in the presence of sunlight yields ozone (O_3), other oxidants and peroxy acetyl nitrite (PAN). It is well known that the high concentration of these chemical pollutants cause adverse effects, although the adverse effects of irritant gases on the respiratory system are related to concentration and duration of action. The effects of chemical or industrial pollutions have been reported in many papers and are well documented. Consequently, I like to limit my contribution mostly to the effect of floating particles.

Increase of Allergic Pollinosis in Japan

Before the end of the 2nd World War, cases of pollinosis did not exist in Japan, or if they existed, the number of cases were quite rare. In recent years, however, pollinosis has become a common allergic disease in Japan. Among these, Japanese cedar pollinosis has been the most common since it was first reported in 1964. It is, however, unreasonable to presume that airborne pollen has increased dramatically and accounts for the striking increase in pollinosis in Japan. The pollination period of Japanese cedar is usually in March and April, and over 90% of pollen during this period is Japanese cedar. In 1974, the incidence of pollinosis due to Japanese cedar pollen was less than 3.8%, but it went up to 5.8% in 1977, and 9.4% in 1981. This figure is still increasing further. Consequently, the prevalence studies of Japanese cedar pollinosis were performed by Ishizaki and coworkers [1] to determine the incidence of pollinosis in different areas of Nikko where there are many Japanese cedar trees. The sample was subdivided into 5 groups according to environmental differences:

---

*   Department of Medical and Physical Therapy, University of Tokyo, School of Medicine, Tokyo, Japan.

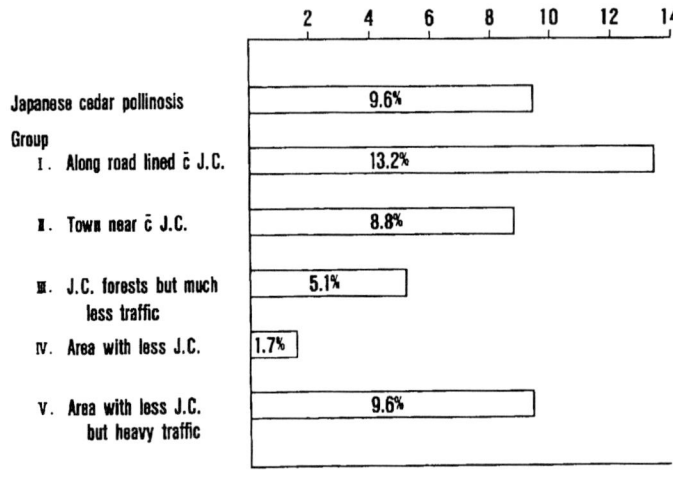

Figure 1. Incidences of Japanese cedar pollinosis patients in different environment.

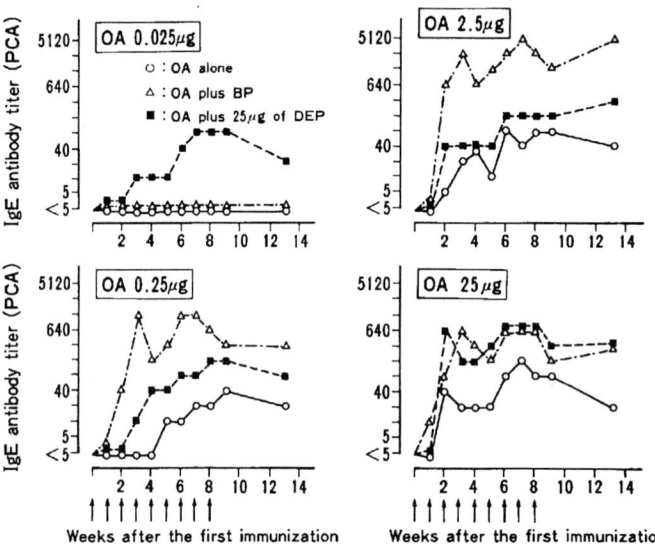

Figure 2. Anti-OA IgE antibody production in mice in response to weekly intranasal inoculation of OA alone, OA plus BP (Bordetella pertussis) or OA plus 25 µg of DEP (diesel exhaust particles).

— Group 1: those living within 200 m from inter-city roads, which are densely lined with old cedar trees and where traffic is heavy all day long.

— Group 2: those living in or near cedar forests.

— Group 3: those living in or near cedar forests, but where automobile traffic is much less.

— Group 4: those living in mountain areas with almost no cedar.

— Group 5: those living in town where Japanese cedar are much less but automobile traffic is heavy.

As shown in Figure 1, among people living in the area where Japanese cedar pollens are not so prevalent, the incidence of pollinosis is high if the area is heavily congested with traffic. Moreover, another study showed that the prevalence rate of allergic rhinitis among school children in districts with high levels of automobile exhaust was markedly higher compared to that in less polluted districts. The prevalence rate of allergic rhinitis was recently found to have reached 30% in children in some high-level districts. Not only allergic rhinitis, also the incidence of bronchial asthma has climbed 3 to 4 times during the last 30 years in

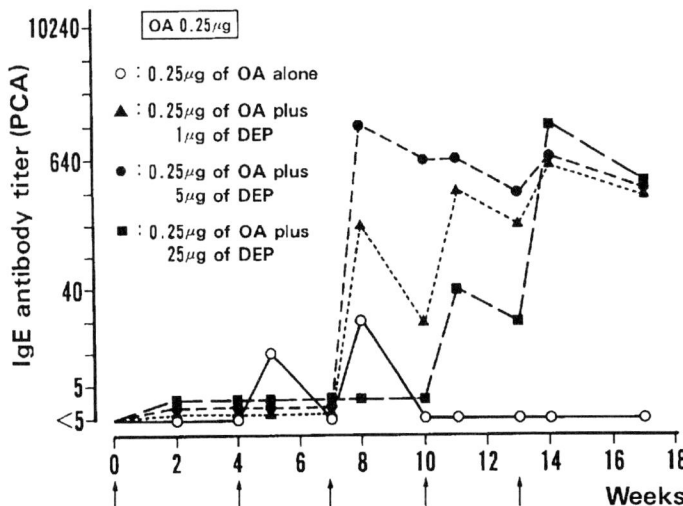

Figure 3. Effect of various doses of DEP (diesel exhaust particles) on the induction of anti-OA IgE antibody response in mice.

Japan. The incidence of asthma was higher along main roads where automobile traffic is heavy. These findings raised our attention to automobile exhaust as a possible cause of these higher incidence of allergic diseases.

Experiment Using Floating Particles

The number of diesel cars in Japan has increased rapidly from 20,000 in 1951 to 7,600,000 in 1988. The total number of automobiles is 53,000,000 in 1988. The number of cars is still increasing dramatically, and automobile exhaust has thus become one of the major causes of air pollution in Japanese urban districts. A striking increase in the prevalence rate of allergic pollinosis in districts in Japan having high levels of air pollutants has coincided with the rapid increase in the number of diesel cars being used. This fact attracted our attention to automobile exhaust as one of the possible causes of allergic rhinitis, and stimulated our interest in studying the effects of particles emitted from diesel cars on the production of IgE antibody.

Intraperitoneal Immunization with Diesel Exhaust Particles [2]

When 0.25 or 2.5 µg of ovalbumin (OA) mixed with 25 µg of diesel exhaust particles were injected repeatedly intraperitoneally into guinea pigs, IgE antibody production was enhanced in comparison with OA alone. Several additional experiments confirmed this. Therefore, we examined the adjuvant activity of diesel exhaust particles inoculated by the intranasal route, i.e., the natural route of entry.

Internasal Immunization with Diesel Exhaust Particles [3]

Groups of mice were inoculated intranasally once a week on nine occasions with 0.025, 0.25, 2.5, 25 µg of OA either alone or mixed with Bordetella pertussis (BP) or with 25 µg of diesel exhaust particles.

The magnitude of the anti-OA IgE antibody responses in mice immunized with OA plus 25 µg of diesel exhaust particles was greater than in mice immunized with OA without adjuvant. The magnitude of the responses was, however, less than that in mice immunized with OA plus BP (p<0.01) (Figure 2). Figure 3 illustrates the anti-OA IgE antibody responses in mice when the concentration of diesel exhaust particles mixed with 0.25 µg of OA was altered. Diesel exhaust particles had an enhancing effect on the anti-OA IgE antibody production, even at a small dose such as 1 µg inoculated intranasally with a 3-week interval.

From these results, it was also demonstrated that diesel exhaust particles had an enhancing effect on IgE antibody production by immunization via the respiratory tract.

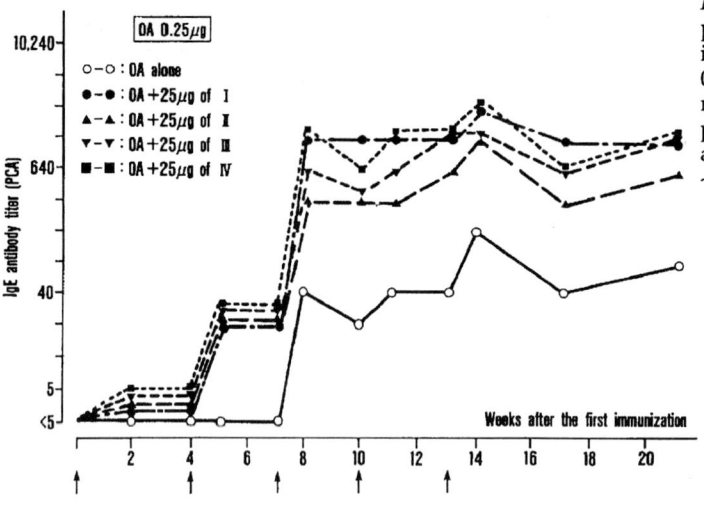

Figure 4. Anti-OA IgE antibody production in mice in response to intranasal administration of 0.25 μg of OA alone and OA mixed with 4 different size of suspended particle matters. I: 7.0 μ and larger, II: 3.3 ~ 7.0 μm, III: 2.0 ~ 3.3 μm, IV: 1.1 ~ 2.0 μm.

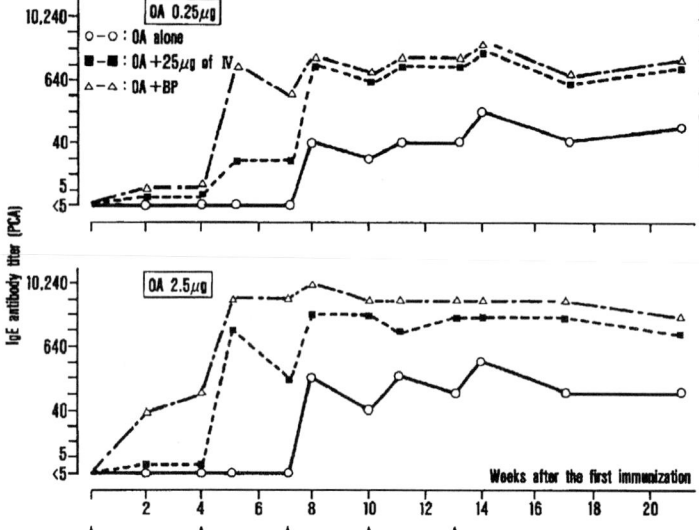

Figure 5. Anti-OA IgE antibody production in mice immunized with 0.25 μg or 2.5 μg of OA alone, OA mixed with small size of suspended particle matter (IV: 1.1 ~ 2.2 μm) and mixed with BP (*Bordetella pertussis*).

Immunization with Suspended Particles [4]

Since diesel exhaust particles have an adjuvant effect, we wondered whether suspended particles in the environmental atmosphere have an adjuvant activity for IgE antibody production. Suspended particles were collected according to the four different sizes by a high-volume air sampler. Namely, 7.0 μm and larger, 3.3. to 7.0 μm, 2.0 to 3.3 μm and less than 2.0 μm of size. Particles consisted mainly of carbon, calcium sulfate, quartz, calcite, rock salt, mica,

chlorite, cristobalite, and feldspat. The larger the size of particles, the more quartz, calcite, and rock salt. The smaller the size of particles, the more carbon and calcium sulfate. There was almost no difference in the quantity of mica, chlorite, cristobalite, or feldspar. The carbon content of the samples was 14.4%, 14.6%, 21.5%, and 37.3%, according to the size.

0.25 μg OA alone or OA mixed with 25 μg of four different sizes of particles in 25 μl of BBS were administered directly on the nostrils as drops to 5 groups of mice, and boosted 4 times. Anti-OA IgE antibody responses in mice immunized with OA mixed with particles was

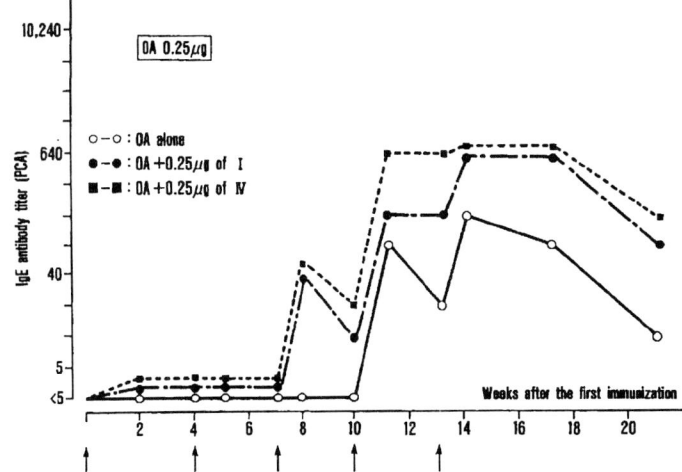

Figure 6. Anti-OA IgE antibody production in mice in response to intranasal administration of 0.25 μg of OA alone and OA mixed with large particle matters (I: 7.0 μm and larger) and small (IV: 1.1 ~ 2.2 μm).

greater than that of mice immunized with OA alone throughout the period of 21 weeks after the first immunization. There were no significant differences in IgE antibody responses in mice immunized with OA plus different size of particles.

Figure 5 illustrates the anti-OA IgE antibody responses to 0.25 or 2.5 μg of OA without adjuvant or mixed with 25 μg of small particles or with BP. Anti-OA IgE antibody responses immunized with OA plus particles was greater than than of mice immunized with the same doses of OA alone.

Figure 6 illustrates the anti-OA IgE antibody responses to intranasal administration of 0.25 μg of OA alone or mixed with 0.25 μg of large particles or with the same doses of small particles. Particles had an enhancing effect on the anti-OA IgE antibody production, even in a small dose such as 0.25 μg. There was no significant difference in the adjuvant activity between large and small suspended particles, however.

Summary

Our previous study had indicated that particles directly collected from exhaust of diesel cars had an adjuvant activity for the IgE antibody production in mice. Other various particles are also suspended in the atmosphere. Therefore, we examined the effect of suspended particles, which are kept buoyant in the atmosphere and inhaled into the human body, on the production of IgE antibody in mice. As a result, it was demonstrated that suspended particle matter has an enhancing effect on the IgE antibody production. The adjuvant activity of particles for the IgE antibody responses was demonstrated even when mice were administered a small dose of 0.25 μg. Suspended particle matter consists mostly of exhaust particles and soil dust in urban districts in Japan. In addition, it includes sea salt, tire wear, and secondary particles that have been created by chemical reactions in the atmosphere after being emitted as gaseous compounds.

In Japan, the concentration of suspended particle matter is calculated to be 40–90 μg/m^3 of air in general environments of urban districts, and 200–480 μg/m^3 of air in locations alongside busy roads. In our present study, we could not ascertain what component of suspended particle mainly exerted an enhancing effect.

In any case, it is possible that allergenic substances may combine with inhaled suspended particles on the surface of the human respiratory mucosa, and that the IgE antibody production may be subsequently enhanced. This may be one of the reasons why the incidence of allergic diseases has been increasing recently.

References

1. Ishizaki, T., K. Koizumi, R. Ikemori, Y. Ishiyama, and E. Kushibiki. 1987. Studies of prevalence of Japanese cedar pollinosis among the residents in a densely cultivated area. Ann. Allergy 58: 265.

2. Muranaka, M., S. Suzuki, K. Koizumi, S. Takafuji, T. Miyamoto, R. Ikemori, and H. Tokiwa. 1986. Adjuvant activity of diesel-exhaust particulates for the production of IgE antibody in mice. J. Allergy Clin. Immunol. 77: 616.

3. Takafuji, S., S. Suzuki, K. Koizumi, K. Tadokoro, T. Miyamoto, R. Ikemori, and M. Muranaka. 1987. Diesel-exhaust particulates inoculated by the intranasal route have an adjuvant activity for IgE production in mice. J. Allergy Clin. Immunol. 79: 639.

4. Takafuji, S., S. Suzuki, K. Koizumi, K. Tadokoro, T. Miyamoto, H. Ohasi, and M. Muranaka. Suspended particulate matter in the atmosphere has an adjuvant activity for IgE production in mice. Submitted for publication.

Correlation Between Air Pollution and Total IgE Serum Levels in Humans, and Studies on the IgE-Enhancing and Autoimmunizing Effects of Mercuric Chloride in Mice

Johannes Hallauer*, Claudia Spix**, Reinhard Dolgner**, Renate Stiller-Winkler*, Ernst Gleichmann**, Hans-Werner Schlipköter*/**

Epidemiologic studies were performed in groups of randomly selected subjects living in variously polluted areas of the state of North Rhine Westphalia (F.R.G.). The results of studies performed in three subsequent years revealed a positive correlation between the degree of outdoor air pollution and the total IgE concentration in serum.

Experiments in rodents indicate that, provided genetically susceptible strains are used, subtoxic doses of $HgCl_2$ can induce a marked increase in total serum IgE as well as the formation of various autoantibodies. As shown in the rat, these effects are due to an activation by $HgCl_2$ of T helper (TH) cells. Mice carrying the I-A^S haplotype and not expressing I-E proved to be highly susceptible to the immunostimulatory effect of $HgCl_2$. In addition to showing increased IgE serum levels, such mice produce IgG antinucleolar autoantibodies (ANolA) directed against a U3 snRNP termed fibrillarin.

Total IgE Serum Concentrations in Subjects from Areas with High and Low Air Pollution

In the state of North Rhine Westphalia, Federal Republic of Germany, densely populated and highly industrialized areas, such as the Rhine-Ruhr zones and the city of Cologne, contrast with rural areas in the degree of outdoor air pollution, which is regularly measured by the State Office for Immission Control. On the basis of these data, epidemiologic studies are performed for the Register of the Effects of the Clean Air Program established by the state government. In these studies, subjects living in the rural towns Borken and Dülmen, with relatively low pollutant concentrations, are compared with subjects living in areas with higher levels of atmospheric pollution.

In 1985, a pilot study was performed in which for the first time total IgE serum levels were determined [1]. During the period of March through May, 1985, blood samples were collected from 5–7-year-old children entering school. A total of 205 randomly selected children were studied: 77 children living in the reference areas of Borken and Dülmen, and 128 living in the industrial zones of Dortmund and Lünen located in the eastern part of the Rhine-Ruhr area. While there were no significant differences in the concentrations of SO_2, NO_2, and air-borne particulates between Borken and Dülmen on the one hand and Dortmund and Lünen on the other, dust fall in the center of Dortmund was twice as high as in Borken and Dülmen and by 50% higher than in the outerlying parts of the city. Social and anamnestic data of the children investigated were obtained by questionnaire. Serum IgE levels were determined by a commercial ELISA.

Independently of the place of residence, children with an anamnesis of hay fever had significantly higher geometrical mean values of total serum IgE. In the German children, the incidence of hay fever was about 3% and showed no significant dependency on the immissions considered. The highest mean values of IgE were found in the sera of children living in the inner-city area of Dortmund: Their IgE values were significantly higher than those of children living in all other districts mentioned

*   Institute of Hygiene of the University of Düsseldorf.
** Medical Institute of Environmental Hygiene at the University of Düsseldorf.
Supported in part by a grant of the program "Allergy and Environment" from the Federal Ministry of Research and Technology (BMFT), Bonn, Federal Republic of Germany.

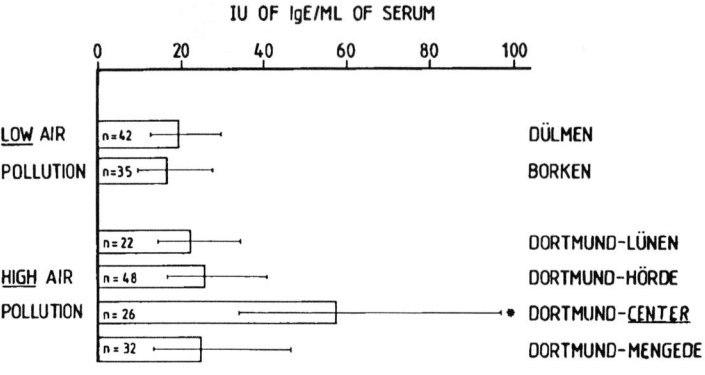

Figure 1. 1985: Mean geometric IgE levels (± coefficient of variation) in 205 randomly selected children entering school. $p < 0.05$.

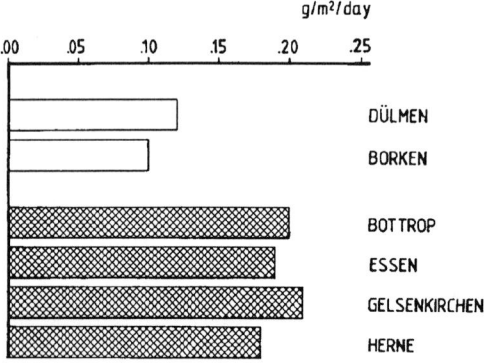

Figure 2. Mean dust fall values for at least two years (State Office for Air Quality Protection of Northrhine Westfalia, F.R.G.).

above, the lowest IgE values being found in the rural areas (Figure 1). Apart from hay fever, only the nationality of the children turned out to be a confounder because the IgE levels of German school children were lower than those of non-German children, who were mostly of Turkish origin. However, even after correcting for confounding with nationality the difference remained significant. Similar findings were made in a study performed in Spain [2].

In 1986, Borken and Dülmen served as reference areas for a similar study run in the cities of Bottrop, Essen, Gelsenkirchen, and Herne, all of which are located in the Central Ruhr area [3]. As shown in Figure 2, the long-term mean values of dust fall in Borken and Dülmen were lower than those measured in the four cities located in the Central Ruhr area. (It should be noted, however, that the actual mean values for the more heavily polluted areas are relatively low when compared with values

found in previous years.) The total group consisted of 1,393 (response rate = 67%) randomly selected German women born in 1931. In 1,033 of them, serum IgE levels were determined. In the analysis only smoking habits proved to be a significant confounding factor. Therefore, smokers were excluded from the final evaluation. Figure 3 shows the percentages of non-smoking women with serum IgE levels above 50 IU/ml in the two reference and the four index groups. These percentages were higher in the cities with relatively strong air pollution than in the areas of Borken and Dülmen, the difference being almost statistically significant ($p = 0.07$). Thus, there was evidence for a positive correlation between the degree of outdoor air pollution, as reflected by mean dust fall intensity and SO_2 concentration, and the proportion of subjects with elevated serum levels of IgE.

In 1987, German women, about 55 years of age and living in Borken (n = 230) and the city of Cologne (n = 220), were examined and compared as to their serum IgE levels [4]. Although evaluation of the results has not yet been completed, a conspicuous finding is that women living in the inner-city area of Cologne have much higher IgE levels than the women from all other areas studied, the peripheral districts of Cologne included. This result is reminiscent of the findings made in the 1985 pilot study (Figure 1). In both surveys, subjects living in the inner-city areas showed the highest IgE values. This effect might result from an increased concentration of car exhausts caused by the more intense automobile traffic in the centers of cities [cf. Miyamoto et al., this volume].

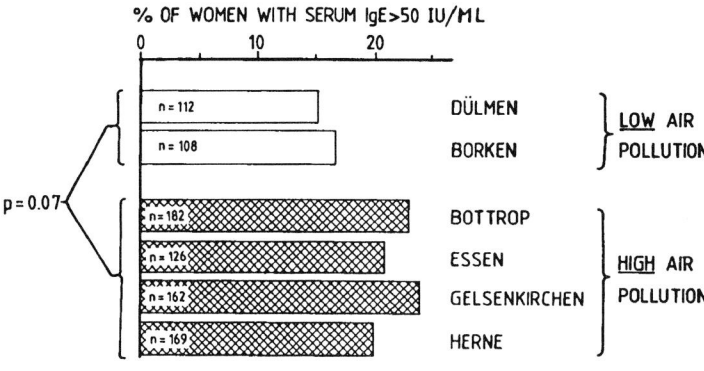

% OF WOMEN WITH SERUM IgE>50 IU/ML

Figure 3. 1986: Women born in 1931 (n = 859), excluding smokers.

IgE-Enhancing and Autoimmunizing Effects of Mercurials

In rats [5] and mice [Pietsch, Vohr, Degitz, & Gleichmann, submitted], non-toxic doses of mercurials, such as $HgCl_2$, are potent inducers of an increased IgE production. Moreover, addition of $HgCl_2$ to pokeweed-stimulated peripheral blood lymphocytes from non-atopic human donors induced a significant IgE production [6]. In view of these effects and the fact that mercury is an environmental pollutant, $HgCl_2$ can be considered as a model compound that allows to study the cellular and molecular mechanisms by which environmental chemicals may induce an increased IgE production. Studies in the rat [5] have established that the increased IgE production as well as all other immunopathological alterations inducible by $HgCl_2$ are initiated by an $HgCl_2$-induced activation of $CD4^+$ T cells. Two not mutually exclusive possibilities may account for this: First, $HgCl_2$ appears to exert a mitogen-like activity, and the resulting activation of $CD4^+$ T cells includes activation of TH cells that react against apparently unaltered self-MHC class-II molecules [5]; second, mercurials such as $HgCl_2$ are potent inducers of contact dermatitis which implies that they create epitopes seen by Hg^{2+}-specific $CD4^+$ T cells. Indeed, recent experiments from our laboratory indicate that the systemic exposure to $HgCl_2$ used for induction of increased IgE production in mice primes T cells specific for $HgCl_2$ as the nominal antigen [Muranyi et al., unpublished].

In both rats and mice, susceptibility to the IgE-enhancing effect of $HgCl_2$ is under strict genetic control in which MHC and non-MHC genes are involved [5, 7]. A striking abnormality in $H-2^s$ mice treated with $HgCl_2$ is the production of extremely high titers of IgG ANolA directed against a U3 snRNP termed fibrillarin. The same type of autoantibody is also seen in patients with idiopathic scleroderma [8]. Interestingly, expression of I-E, together with the I-As allele coding for susceptibility, "suppressed" formation of such autoantibodies [7].

References

1. Hallauer, J. F., U. Krämer, R. Stiller-Winkler, and R. Dolgner. 1987. Concentration of IgE in sera of children from residential areas with different air pollution (Abstract). Zbl. Bakt. Hyg. B 183: 432.
2. Berciano, F. A., M. Crespo, C. G. Bao, and F. V. Alvarez. 1987. Serum levels of total IgE in non-allergic children. Allergy 24: 276.
3. Hallauer, J. F., R. Stiller-Winkler, C. Spix, and R. Dolgner. 1988. IgE detection in epidemiological examination of women under the influence of immission factors (Abstract). Zbl. Bakt. Hyg. B 186: 449.
4. Stiller-Winkler, R., H. Idel, C. Spix, M. Risse, and H. Sidaoui. 1988. Protein profiles in sera of women in areas with a different degree of air pollution. Zbl. Bakt. Hyg. B, in press.
5. Druet, P., F. Hirsch, L. Pelletier, E. Druet, D. Baran, and C. Sapin. 1987. Mechanisms of chemical-induced glomerulonephritis. In Mechanisms of Cell Injury: Implications for Human Health. Dahlem Konferenzen. B. A. Fowler, ed. Chichester: John Wiley and Sons, Ltd., p. 153.
6. Kimata, H., K. Shinomiya, and H. Mikawa. 1983. Selective enhancement of human IgE production in vitro by synergy of pokeweed mitogen and mercuric chloride. Clin. exp. Immunol. 53: 183.

7. Gleichmann, E., M. Kavka, R. Stiller-Winkler, and J. Mirtschewa. 1988. Susceptibility to HgCl2-induced antinucleolar autoantibodies (ANolA) is determined by I-A, and concomitant expression of I-E seems to dampen it (Abstract). Immunobiology 178: 137.

8. Reuter, R., G. Tessars, H.-W. Vohr, E. Gleichmann, and R. Lührmann. 1988. Mercuric chloride induces autoantibodies against U3 small nuclear ribonucleoprotein in susceptible mice. Proc. Natl. Acad. Sci. USA, in press.

Aerobiology: Pollens

*J. Charpin**

This paper includes a review of methods used for atmospheric pollen studies and excludes all clinical facts concerning pollinosis.

Methods for Trapping Pollens

Studies of plants, made by a good botanist, are very important, but to obtain data, it is necessary to use air sampling. Different methods were have been used over the years. *Gravimetry* was created by Durham [1], whereby slides coated with glycerinated gel were protected between two steel discs. This was the only method used up to 1970. *Volumetric* methods use pumps oriented by a weather-cock and projecting known amounts of air on a slide [2] or an adhesive tape [3]. A tape lasts one week. This apparatus is used all over the world.

Cour's method [4, 5] exposes large pieces of gauze to the wind. It results in very rich analyses, but they are very time consuming to analyze. Leuschner's individual trap [6, 7], pinned to the coat lapel, gives individual complementary information.

All of these methods are described in detail in classical books on the subject [8, 9].

Calendars

These are very well known, both in Europe [10] and in the Unites States [9]. Small changes appear from time to time, as was the case for filaria [11] in the Mediterranean area, for colza [12], as for the migration of ragweed to and in Europe, which was signaled for the first time by P. Blamoutier [13], demonstrated largely by R. Touraine [14] and followed by M. Dechamp [15]. It was even seen in the sky of Marseille [16]. In the opposite direction, *Parieteria officinalis*, which is a great allergic offender in the Mediterranean area, has been observed in San Francisco [17].

Morphological Studies with Scanner

Almost all the well-known textbooks of palynology now include superb pictures of pollen grains obtained by scanner. On the other hand, Heslop Harrison [18] has studied the ultra-structural morphology of pollen grains. Recently, a very interesting group, the Interdisciplinary Program of Research on Environment (PIREN), was created in Europe. One of the topics of research chosen by the group was "pollen grains," and two recent programs of this group seem particularly promising: the possible identification by computer of the details of exine [19], another [20, 21] on correlations between details of exine and allergenic content of the grains.

Pollen Antigens

Identification of Pure Allergenic Fractions

Major work was undertaken during the last 20 years to isolate one or—more often—several allergenic fractions. Twenty years ago, King [22] and his group isolated antigen E from ragweed pollen (6% of total protein content and 90% of allergenic activity), then antigen K, antigen Ra3, Ra5, B.P.A.R. very similar to antigen E. For Ra5, the amino acids sequence is well known. Our group has isolated antigen P1 from plane-tree pollen [23]. Belin [24], then Apold [25], Ipsen and Lowenstein [26] isolated major allergens of birch pollen. B. David [27] with J. Peltre [28], through very specific techniques, obtained pure fractions of dactylis glomerata major allergen: Dac g 1.

In pollen grains we can also find lectines that are specific stimulants of lymphocytes [29] and many enzymes [30], even antagonists of allergens for dactylis.

* Department of Pneumology and Allergology, Hôpital Sainte-Marguerite, 13277 Marseille, France.

There are important discussions being held on pollens:

— Is it better to desensitize with pure fractions or with brut complex extract?

— Similarly, for standardization purposes, is it better to take very good extracts prepared in well-defined conditions, or to rely on the amount of some pure fractions?

How Do Allergens Go out of the Pollen's Grains?

This phenomenon has been well studied by Marsh [31] for grass pollens, by Anfosso-Capra [32] for plane-tree. It appears that major antigens go out more slowly than we would presume from the chronology of the clinical symptoms. This could mean that some minor allergens play a role in the beginning of the clinical phenomena.

Dosages of Pollen Allergens in the Atmosphere

Important recent works compared dosages of allergens with pollen counts [33–39]. Generally, a good correlation exists between the two figures, but curves of allergen dosages are often larger than the curves of pollen counts. It has been shown that the allergens come not only from pollen grains, but from other parts of the plant as well. We understand now why patients who are allergic to grass pollen sneeze when they cut the grass!

However, it will be more simple for a long time to count pollen grains than to dose the allergens, but these new facts seem very promising for the future.

How Do Pollen Allergens Enter the Bronchi?

This is a very controversial point, as it is difficult for particles of more than 10 μ diameter to enter the bronchi [40, 41]. Some authors showed that there are no pollen grains in the bronchi and parenchyma, but this was discussed by another group [42]. Now the discussions has lost part of its interest, because fragments of pollen grains, fragments of the plant

itself [43, 44, 45], and droplets of liquid carrying fragments of pollen grains may enter the bronchi.

It appeared too that fragments of pollen acting at larynx or pharynx level produce a allergenic reaction with a bronchial reflex [46, 47].

Conclusion

Pollen allergy is still the best model of reaginic phenomena.

References

1. Durham, O. C. 1946. A proposed standard method of gravity sampling, counting and volumetric interpolation of results. J. Allergy 1: 79.
2. Hirst, J. M. 1952. An automatic volumetric spore trap. Annals of Applied Biology 39: 257–265.
3. Burkard. Manufacturing Company Limited (Rickmansworth, Hertfordshire, England). Burkard "Seven-day recording volumetric spore trap."
4. Cour, P. 1974. Nouvelles techniques de détection des flux et des retombées polliniques: étude de la sédimentation des pollens déposés à la surface du sol. Pollen et Spores 16: 103.
5. Cour, P., Ch. Seignalet, L. Quet, Y. Decor, and F. B. Michel. 1975. Nouvelle méthode de recueil et d'examen du contenu sporopollinique de l'atmosphère. Rev. Fr. Allergol. 3: 15.
6. Leuschner, R. M., and G. Boehm. 1977. Individual pollen collector for use of hay fever patients in comparison with the Burkard Trap. Grana, 183–186.
7. Leuschner, R. M., and G. Boehm. 1979. Investigations with the "Individual Pollen Collector" and the "Burkard Trap" with reference to hay fever patients. J. Allergy Clin. Immunol. 9: 175–184.
8. Charpin, J., J. Aubert, M. Mallea, and F. Anfosso-Capra. 1986. Pneumallergènes polliniques du traité d'allergologie. Flammarion 2ème édition, 217–241.
9. Middleton, E., C. E. Reed, and E. F. Ellis. 1983. Allergy, principles and practice, chapter 53: Aerobiology and inhalant allergens. St. Louis: Mosby.
10. Charpin, J., R. Surinyach, and A. W. Frankland. 1980. Atlas of European allergenic pollens. Vaci, ed. Basel & Paris: Sandoz, pp. 80–81.
11. Michel, F. B., C. Seignalet, Y. Decor, J. P. Gaillard, L. Quet, and P. Cour. 1975. Calendrier pollinique de Montpellier réalisé par une méthode quantitative et sur ordinateur. Etude préliminaire. Rev. Fr. Allergol. 15: 185.

12. Faveret, C. 1976. La place de l'allergie au pollen de colza parmi les pollinoses de printemps. Rev. Fr. Allergol. 16: 91–95.

13. Blamoutier, P. 1955. La pollinose par Ambrosia observée depuis peu en France. Sem. Hôp. Paris 31: 1924.

14. Touraine, R., J. Charpin, J. Aubert, H. Charpin, J. Cornillon, M. Mallea, E. Guheo, and M. Renard. 1969. Le calendrier Pollinique de Lyon. Rev. Fr. Allergol. 9: 25.

15. Dechamp, C., and P. Cour. 1986. Pollen counts of ragweed and mugwort core collector in 1984 measured in 12 meteorological centers in the Rhône bassin and surrounding regions in France. Proceedings of the 3rd International Conference on Aerobiology, Basel, 437.

16. Charpin, H., M. Mallea et al. 1981. Les Ambrosiacées dans la région Marseillaise. Rev. Fr. Allergol. 21: 195–198.

17. Charpin, J., and H. Charpin. 1980. Parieteria Officinalis L. Allergy. Letter to the Editor. J. Allergy Clin. Immunol. 65: 80–81.

18. Heslop-Harrison, J. 1968. Pollen wall development. 161: 230–237.

19. Hideux, M., and M. C. Carbonnier-Jarreau. 1986. Information et palynologie: Méthodes d'aide à l'identification par micro-ordinateur des pollens de gramineae et perspectives. French-Swedish Symposium on Pollens of Cockfoot, Stockholm, p. 41.

20. Cerceau-Larrival, M.-Th. avec la collaboration technique de L. Derouet. 1986. Recherches biopalynologiques sur dactylis Glomerata L. French-Swedish Symposium on Pollens of Cockfoot, Stockholm, p. 13–18.

21. Cerceau-Larrival, M.-Th., and M. Hideux. 1986. Voyageuses du temps et de l'espace, les capsules à pollen. L'Univers du Vivant 13: 14–15.

22. King, T. P., P. Norman, and L. Lichtenstein. 1967. Isolation and characterization of allergens from ragweed pollen. Biochem. 6: 1992.

23. Anfosso, F., M. Soler, M. Mallea, and J. Charpin. 1977. Isolation and characterization in vitro of an allergen from plane-tree (*Platanus acerifolia*) pollen. Int. Archs. Allergy Appl. Immunol. 54: 481–486.

24. Belin, L. 1972. Separation and characterization of birch pollen antigens with special reference to the allergenic components. Int. Arch. Allergy Appl. Immunol. 42: 329.

25. Apold, J., E. Florvaag, and S. El Sayed. 1981. Comparative studies on tree-pollen allergens. I. Isolation and partial characterization of a major allergen from birch pollen (*Betula verrucosa*). Int. Arch. Allergy Appl. Immunol. 64: 439.

26. Ipsen, H. H., and H. Lowenstein. 1982. Immunochemical characterization of a crude aqueous extract and purified allergens of birch pollen (*Betula verrucosa*). J. Allergy Clin. Immunol. 37 (Suppl.): 41.

27. Mecheri, S., G. Peltre, and B. David. 1983. Inhibition of the passive cutaneous anaphylaxis reaction to dactylis glomerata pollen allergens by a purified component of this pollen. Immunology Letters 6: 257–263.

28. Peltre, G., M.-Th. Cerceau-Larrival, M. Hideux, M. Abadie, and B. David. Scanning and transmission electron microscopy related to immunochemical analysis of grass pollen. Grana 26: 158–170.

29. Anfosso, F. J., P. M. Guillard, and J. P. Charpin. 1983. Studies on a new lymphocyte mitogen from pollen aqueous extract: Induction of proliferation in human and rodent lymphocytes. Int. Archs. Allergy Appl. Immunol. 71: 6–14.

30. Bousquet, J., and F. B. Michel. 1979. Enzymes des pollens. In: Les pollinoses, Vol. 1. Fisons, ed. Paris.

31. Marsh, D., L. Belin, A. Bruce, L. Lichtenstein, and R. Hussain. 1981. Rapidly released allergens from short ragweed pollen. I. Kinetics of release of known allergens in relation to biologic activity. J. Allergy Clin. Immunol. 67: 206.

32. Anfosso, F., M. Soler, M. Mallea, and J. Charpin. 1977. Isolation and characterization in vitro of an allergen from plane-tree (*Platanus acerifolia*) pollen. Int. Archs. Allergy Appl. Immunol 54: 481–486.

33. Agarwal, M. K., J. W. Yunginger, M. C. Swanson, and C. E. Reed. 1981. An immunochemical method to measure atmospheric allergens. J. Allergy Clin. Immunol. 68: 194.

34. Agarwal, M. K., M. C. Swanson, C. E. Reed, and J. W. Yunginger. 1983. Immunochemical quantitation of airborne short ragweed, Alternia, antigen E, and Alt-I allergens: A two-year prospective study. J. Allergy Clin. Immunol. 72: 40–45.

35. Agarwal, M. K., M. C. Swanson, C. E. Reed, and J. W. Yunginger. 1984. Airborne ragweed allergens. Association with various particle sizes and short ragweed plant parts. J. Allergy Clin. Immunol 74: 587–693.

36. Fernandez-Caldas, E., E. O. Bandele, S. L. Dunnette, M. C. Swanson, and C. E. Reed. Rye grass group allergen content in leaves and stems from seven different grass species. In preparation.

37. Fernandez-Caldas, E., M. C. Swanson, J. Pravda, P. Welsh, J. W. Yunginger, and C. E. Reed. Immunochemical demonstration of red oak pollen aeroallergens outside the oak pollination season. In preparation.

38. Reed, C. E., M. C. Swanson, M. K. Agarwal, and J. W. Yunginger. 1985. Allergens that cause asthma identification and quantification. Chest (Suppl.) 87: 40–44.

39. Reed, C. E., M. C. Swanson, and J. W. Yunginger. 1986. Measurement of allergen con-

centration in the air as an aid in controlling exposure to aeroallergens. Environmental factors in allergic diseases. J. Allergy Clin. Immunol. 78: 1028–1030.

40. Soler, M., M. Mallea, M. Renard, H. Charpin, F. Montane, H. Izard, and G. Vallade. 1975. Le calendrier pollinique de Perpignan. Marseille Médical, 11.

41. Soler, M., M. Robert, F. Anfosso, and L. le Bouffant. 1977. Techniques d'emploi d'aérosols de pollen marqués en vue de l'étude de leur pénétration dans l'arbre bronchique. Bull. Europ. Physiopath. Resp. 13: 499.

42. Michel, F. B., J. P. Marty, L. Quet, and P. Cour. 1977. Penetration of inhaled pollen into the respiratory tract. Am. Rev. Resp. Dis. 115: 609.

43. Busse, W. W., C. E. Reed, and J. H. Hoehne. 1982. Where is the allergic reaction in ragweed asthma? J. Allergy Clin. Immunol. 50: 289–293.

44. Hirst, J. M. 1952. An automatic volumetric spore trap. Annals of Applied Biology, 39: 257–265.

45. Hyde, H. A., and K. F. Adams. 1958. An atlas of airborne pollen, Vol. 1. London: Macmillan.

46. Gold, W. M. 1973. Cholinergic pharmacology in asthma. In: Asthma, Vol. 1. K. F. Austen and L. M. Lichtenstein, eds. New York: Academic Press.

47. Orehek, J., P. Gaynard, Ch. Grimaud, and J. Charpin. 1975. Bronchoconstriction provoquée par inhalation d'allergène dans l'asthme: Effet antagoniste d'un anticholinergique de synthèse. Bull. Physio-Pathol. Resp. 11: 193.

The Role of Indoor Allergens in Asthma

Thomas A. E. Platts-Mills, Susan M. Pollart, Christina M. Luczynska,
Martin D. Chapman, Peter W. Heymann*

The high prevalence of positive skin tests to house dust among asthmatics was first recognized in 1921 [1]. Since then it has become clear that these positive skin tests can be attributed to many different constituents of house dust including animal dander, dust mites, fungi, insects (especially cockroaches), and rodent urine [2, 3, 4, 5]. In addition, the nature of some of the important proteins in house dust that induce IgE antibodies has been defined [4, 6, 7]. This has lead to the production of specific polyclonal and monoclonal (mAb)antibodies, which can be used to measure the levels of these foreign antigens in house dust [8–11]. Despite multiple reports on the prevalence of IgE antibodies to indoor allergens among clinic populations of asthmatics, and evidence that complete avoidance can lead to dramatic improvement including reversal of bronchial reactivity, there are still many physicians whose clinical practice does not recognize the important role of indoor allergens in perennial asthma. There appear to be several reasons for this:

— First, with the exception of cat allergic individuals, patients with asthma are generally not aware of the role that house dust plays in their asthma. This is particularly true for mite and cockroach allergic individuals, who often do not even appreciate that they are allergic.

— Until very recently the specific levels either of immediate hypersensitivity or of allergen exposure in houses that are associated with asthma have not been defined.

— Studies on reduction of allergen levels in houses have given conflicting results [11].

Levels of Exposure

Accurate standardizable assays of specific major allergens that are simple enough for wide-spread use have only recently become possible [11, 12]. However, these results can now be obtained in µg/g of dust with some confidence, both for the cat allergen (*Fel d* I) and mite allergens (*Der p* I and *Der f* I). The standards used are either International (e.g., the WHO standard for *D. pteronyssinus* NIBSC 82/518) [13] or national (the FDA standard for cat). Recent results using mAbs to the Group II allergens (*Der p* II and *Der f* II) have shown very widely different ratios of Group I to Group II allergens in commercial dust extracts, though in house dust the ratio is relatively stable at around 2:1 [7]. Although there are obvious reasons for wanting to measure airborne allergens the levels are generally very low (ng/m^3) and the results are critically dependent on disturbance [5, 9]. Thus, at present, it is really only possible to compare results and to propose standards (or risk levels) for allergens in floor dust [14].

Airborne Cat Allergen

Many cat-allergic individuals report the acute onset of symptoms including asthma on entering a house with a cat in it. By contrast, very few patients who are equally allergic to mite or cockroach proteins report rapid onset of symptoms on entering an "infested" house. This could be explained if exposure to mite allergens was gradual and involved inhaling relatively few "large" fecal particles which only become airborne during domestic disturbance [9]. The implication is that cat allergen may be airborne either continuously or in a different form. Previous studies on airborne cat allergen have supported this view but have been hampered by insensitive assays that required sampling of large volumes of air, or by relatively nonspecific assays [5, 15, 16]. Using a two-site mAb assay for *Fel d* I, sensitive to

*   Division of Allergy and Clinical Immunology, Box 225, Department of Medicine, University of Virginia, Charlottesville, VA 22908, USA.
    This work was supported by National Institutes of Health Grants No. A120565, A124261, and A124687.

≤0.5 ng, we were able to use different low volume air samplers that cause little or no disturbance of the room, i.e., a cascade impactor or a liquid impinger. Combining those results with studies on falling after artificial disturbance we can conclude the following:

— In most houses with cats, *Fel d* I remains airborne under conditions of no or minimal disturbance, and from 10–60% of the airborne *Fel d* I is associated with particles ≤2.5 μm in diameter.

— During domestic disturbance these particles can increase up to a level of 40 ng/m³, which is comparable to the levels produced by a nebulizer during bronchial provocation.

— The nature of the small particles carrying airborne *Fel d* I is not clear. However, the levels appear to be influenced not only by the presence of cats but by the quantity of soft furnishings (presumably acting as a reservoir) and also by air exchange rates. In an animal vivarium airborne *Fel d* I was almost all on large particles and this appears to relate both to the absence of furnishings and to a very high air exchange rate, i.e., 10–15 changes/hour compared to <0.5 changes/hour in domestic houses. Low exchange rates allow accumulation of small airborne particles which would otherwise be exhausted from the house.

The presence of small particles carrying cat allergen clearly accounts for these particles remaining airborne, and we presume also has specific relevance to the lung. The small particles would penetrate the lung better, and because of the extremely large number of particles of this size necessary to carry 10 ng (i.e., >10⁶), they would be expected to be distributed evenly over the bronchial walls. This is in complete contrast to natural exposure to mite allergens where the allergen is predominantly carried on fecal particles (≥10 μm diameter), and daily exposure may be as few as 100, of which 5–10% would be expected to enter the lungs [17].

Epidemiology of Acute Asthma: Emergency Room Studies

It is difficult to carry out epidemiological studies on asthma using clinic populations because referral patterns make it very difficult to match suitable controls and because of the very wide range of severity. On the other hand in population surveys where the "correct" control of population is available, it is often difficult to identify the severity of the patients since they are not seen at the time of exacerbations. In order to obtain a different approach to estimating the role of indoor allergens in asthma, we have studied patients presenting to an Emergency Room (ER) with acute asthma.

The rationale for studying the epidemiology of ER asthma visits includes:

— Patients are unselected and present at the time of an acute episode so that reversibility of obstruction can be documented.

— Approximately 2 million cases of asthma present to an ER in the USA each year and this rate appears to be increasing (National Center for Health Statistics).

— Non-asthmatic patients in the same ER represent an appropriate control group, i.e., same area and socioeconomic group.

— At present, routine treatment in most Emergency Rooms does not include any assessment of etiology.

We have carried out two studies of this kind, one in Virginia in a university hospital enrolling patients presenting year round [18]. The second study was in the ER of an Air Force hospital in Northern California enrolling patients during the spring "grass pollen season epidemic" [20]. In each study acute asthma patients were matched with controls and sera were assayed (by RAST) for IgE antibodies to dust mite, cockroach, cat, ragweed and rye grass pollen antigens. The RAST results were standardized relative to laboratory controls and an anti- mite serum pool (NIBSC 82/528) [13]. The unit of IgE antibody used has been shown to be equal to ~0.1 ng of IgE.

The University of Virginia ER study involved 102 patients with acute airway obstruction and 118 controls over the age range 16–76 years (Table 1). The results showed that the prevalence of >200 RAST units of IgE ab to one (or more) of these five allergens was increased significantly in patients less than 50 years old. This increased prevalence was significant for each of the three indoor allergens (Figure 1). Strikingly, the cat allergic and cockroach allergic patients were two separate socioeconomi-

Table 1. Elevated IgE antibody[1] as a risk factor for asthma.

A. *Patients <50 years old, University of Virginia ER [18]*

| | Prevalence of IgE ab | | Odds ratio (95% C1) | Population[4] attributable risk |
	Asthma	Control		
Five allergens[2]	42/67	12/81	9.7 (8.3–11.2)	56%
Indoor allergens[3]	35/67	8/81	9.8 (8.8–11.2)	47%

B. *IgE antibody to rye grass pollen in two studies [20]*

| | Prevalence of IgE ab[4] | | Odds ratio (95% C1) | Population[4] attributable risk |
	Asthma	Control		
Pollen season N. California	54/59	8/59	59.4	89%
August–December Virginia	6/55	6/52	0.94	<2%

Notes
[1] >200 RAST units of IgE antibody.
[2] Five allergens were mite, cat, cockroach, rye grass, and ragweed pollen.
[3] Indoor allergens were mite (*Dermatophagoides pteronyssinus*), cat, and cockroach.
[4] Calculation of population attributable risk assumes that these ER control populations reflect the population from which the asthmatic patients are drawn.

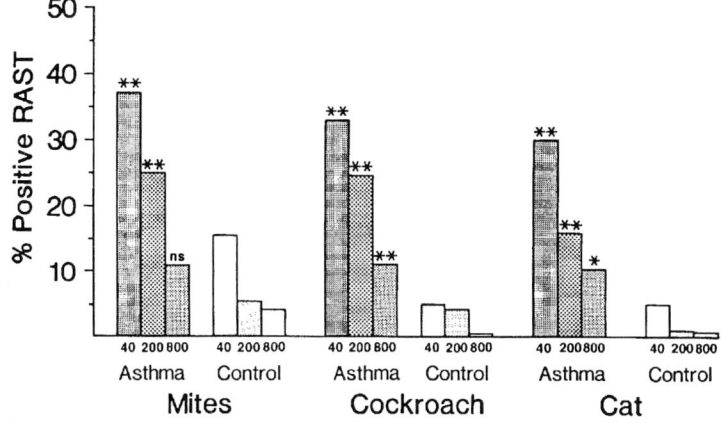

Figure 1. Prevalence of IgE ab to three indoor allergens in sera from 67 patients with asthma and 81 controls aged ≤50 years old presenting to an ER. Results were analyzed at three different levels of IgE ab, 40, 200 and 800 RAST units. (The unit ~0.1 ng) [18, 20]. Significant differences Chi[2] are indicated * = p<0.05 and ** = p<0.005. Reprinted from [18] by permission.

cally different populations. There was also a significant seasonal effect in that selectively mite allergic patients were more likely to present between August and December (the dust mite season in Virginia [21]), while grass pollen allergic patients presented predominantly in April-June.

In the second study at Travis Air Force Base almost all of the patients (54/59) had ≥200 units of IgE antibody to rye grass pollen. By contrast, the levels of IgE ab to cat and cock-roach allergens were no different in the control group than among the asthmatics. The results make it clear that the major factor correlating with asthma in Northern California during the grass pollen season was IgE antibody to rye grass pollen. Conversely, it appears that in this area where mite, cockroach, and cat allergens are generally low in the houses, IgE antibody to these indoor allergens was not an important factor.

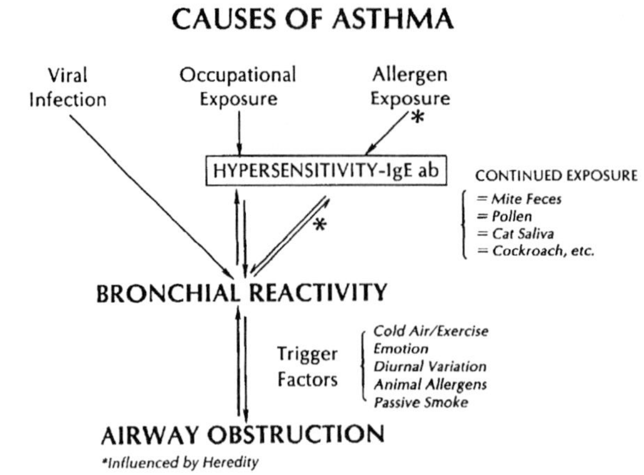

CAUSES OF ASTHMA

Figure 2. A diagram illustrating the ways in which different factors contribute to asthma. It is assumed that allergen exposure takes months or years to induce an immune response that includes IgE antibody (as well as IgG ab and T cells). The contribution of allergens to bronchial reactivity and lung inflammation may be rapid, i.e., hours but is probably more often a gradual process over days or weeks. Finally, the trigger factors are thought to act within a day, and allergens are thought to play less of a role than other factors as acute triggers.

Table 2. Provisional standards for levels of mites and mite allergens in houses that represent a risk for asthma.*

---

(1) Increased of sensitization, symptomatic asthma and increased bronchial reactivity:
➤ >2 µg *Der p* I (or *Der f* I)/g of dust (equivalent to 100 mites/g or 0.6 mg guanine/g)
(2) Increased risk of acute attacks of asthma:
➤ ≤10 µg *Der p* I (or *Der p* I)/g of dust (equivalent to 500 mites/g)

---

*Levels lower than 0.4 µg/g of dust are considered to be unlikely to cause symptoms or sensitization, while values between 0.4 µg and 2 µg are intermediate [14].

Population-Attributable Risk for IgE Antibodies in Relation to Acute Asthma

The prevalence of IgE antibodies among asthmatics in these two studies compared to the controls allows a simple calculation of odds ratio for disease [18, 20]. Making the assumption that the control population is representative of the overall population it is also possible to calculate a population attributable risk (Table 1). These results demonstrate that IgE antibodies are an important "risk factor" for acute asthma but do not establish causation. However, the seasonal differences, particularly the fact that IgE antibody to rye grass pollen is not a risk factor for asthma in the fall in Virginia, strongly suggest that IgE ab is primarily a risk factor for patients who are exposed to the relevant allergen. Our present view is that it is the combination of IgE anti-

body and exposure to a "significant level" of the relevant allergen that is the risk factor for asthma. There is nothing in the data that suggests a strict temporal relationship between exposure to allergens and these acute attacks. It seems more likely that exposure over a period of days or weeks prior to the ER visit is relevant in progressive "inflammation" of the lungs which leads to a situation where one of many non-specific "triggers" can precipitate an acute attack (Figure 2).

Justification for Proposing Risk Levels for Mite and Other Allergens

Without a defined level of allergen in houses to be regarded as a risk for asthma, it is very difficult to consider the size of the problem or to plan an appropriate course of action. No risk level is absolute, and at least part of the justification will be based on practical considerations. Thus, the normally accepted levels for cholesterol are those that can be achieved in a Western population, and the recommended "safe" level for radon is that which reasonably be achieved in North American houses. The values proposed for *Der p* I by a recent international workshop were based on a series of different studies (Table 2) [14]. In Denmark Jens Korsgaard reported that 100 mites/g of dust was a 7-fold risk factor for asthma [22]. In Australia, Woolcock and her colleagues showed that in a town where most dust samples contain >100 mites/g, dust mite allergy was strongly correlated with bronchial reactivity [23]. By contrast, in an inland town (Wagga Wagga) in which mites were rare mite allergy was not common among the bronchially reactive children [23]. In England, moving asthmatic patients from houses with a mean of 13.4 µg *Der p* I/g of dust to hospital rooms with <0.2 µg *Der p* I/g lead to both improvement in symptoms, reduced medication usage, and reduction in bronchial reactivity [24]. In Virginia, 17/19 mite allergic asthmatics presenting to clinic or ER with an exacerbation of their asthma were found to have >10 µg Group I allergen/g of dust in their houses [21].

Clearly, it is possible to define more than one risk level:

— the level that is a risk for developing sensitization to an allergen;

— the level that is a risk factor for disease in most sensitized individuals;

— the level to which an allergen needs to be reduced in order to achieve a given degree of symptomatic improvement.

None of these levels are absolute since the patients are individuals, and the levels that are relevant must also depend on the definition of sensitization. The question is: Are the levels proposed helpful, or should they be higher or lower? Studies reported to the ICACI conference from West Germany by Dr. Wahn and his group were very encouraging that these risk levels are indeed helpful [25].

While data for other allergens is scanty, it is already clear: that levels of cat allergen *Fel d* I are >10 µg/g in dust from houses with cats [10]; that grass pollen allergen is commonly at levels >10 µg/g dust in houses in Northern California during the grass pollen season [20]; and it appears likely that cockroach allergen is at levels >10 µg in houses of cockroach allergic asthmatic patients [Pollart, Platts-Mills and Chapman, unpublished results]. Obviously, it is unlikely that the risk levels are exactly the same, though it now seems possible that for many allergens the appropriate levels of major allergen are in the range of 1.0 µg/g to 10 µg/g dust.

Conclusions

It is now well established that allergens can contribute to bronchial reactivity [24, 26], and that prolonged allergen avoidance can lead to reduced bronchial reactivity [11, 24]. Further, analysis of airborne particle sizes provides a rationale for the fact that cat- allergic patients react rapidly in a house with a cat, while mite-allergic patients are often unaware of the role that house dust plays in their asthma. Because of this, histories are an unreliable way of identifying those individuals in whom dust mite or cockroach allergy contributes to their asthma. Nonetheless, the epidemiological results show clearly that IgE antibody to one or more or the major indoor allergens is an important risk factor for asthma exacerbations. The implication is that etiology should be investigated in all moderate or severe cases of asthma. In parallel with these developments we are increasingly recognizing specific levels of allergens in houses that are a risk for asthma. In recognizing risk levels it is clearly implied that levels "should be" decreased in the houses of allergic or asthmatic patients. The means of reducing mite allergen levels in houses are already reasonably well defined [11], however the use of acaricides is still in its infancy. At present several different acaricides (e.g., pirimiphos methyl, benzylbenzoate) or means of inactivating allergens (e.g., tannic acid) are undergoing trials. It is already possible to give specific advice to patients about reducing levels of mite allergen in their bedrooms, i.e., removing carpets, covering mattresses and hot washing of all bedding. Carpets, sofas and other upholstered furniture remain a problem.

Despite the introduction of many advances in the pharmacological management of asthma, the prevalence, morbidity, and mortality of the disease has been increasing in many parts of the developed world. It is possible that this increase reflects an increase in an etiological factor, and if so the most likely site for such an increase is indoors. Certainly there have been major changes in our houses that could have contributed to an increase in indoor allergens, e.g., central heating, fitted carpets, reduced ventilation and cool water detergents. Alternatively, it is possible that the widespread use of potent bronchodilators *without* reducing relevant allergen exposure has tended to increase the quantity of allergen that patients are inhaling. Whatever the truth is, it seems essential to take the etiology of perennial asthma seriously and to apply rigorous allergen avoidance wherever possible. We need to be able to measure levels of allergens in patients' houses and to outline specific practical measures for reducing both the sources and the airborne levels. The availability of simple sensitive assays for the major allergens in house dust means that the studies necessary to establish protocols for cleaning houses are now possible.

References

1. Kern, R. A. 1921. Dust sensitization in bronchial asthma. Med. Clin. North Am. 5: 751.
2. Voorhorst, R., F. Th. M. Spieksma, H. Varekamp, M. J. Leupen, and A. W. Lyklema. 1967. The house dust mite (*Dermatophagoides pteronyssinus*) and the allergens it produces: Identity with the house dust allergen. J. Allergy 39: 325.
3. Bernton, H. S., T. F. McMahon, and H. Brown. 1972. Cockroach asthma. Brit. J. Dis. Chest 66: 61.
4. Leiterman, K., and J. L. Ohman. 1984. Cat allergen 1: Biochemical, antigenic and allergenic properties. J. Allergy Clin. Immunol. 74: 147.
5. Swanson, M. C., M. K. Agarwal, and C. E. Reed. 1985. An immunochemical approach to indoor aeroallergen quantitation with a new volumetric air sampler: Studies with mite, roach, cat, mouse, and guinea pig antigens. J. Allergy. Clin. Immunol. 76: 724.
6. Chapman, M. D., and T. A. E. Platts-Mills. 1980. Purification and characterization of the major allergen from *Dermatophagoides pteronyssinus*-antigen P1. J. Immunol. 125: 587.
7. Heymann P. W., M. D. Chapman, R. C. Aalberse, J. W. Fox, T. A. E. Platts-Mills. 1988. Purification of *Der f* II and *Der f* III from pyroglyphid mites: Applications of monoclonal antibodies in structural and immunochemical analyses. J. Allergy Clin. Immunol., in press.
8. Chapman, M. D., W. M. Sutherland, and T. A. E. Platts-Mills. 1984. Recognition of two Dermatophagoides pteronyssinus-specific epitopes on antigen P1 using monoclonal antibodies: binding to each epitope can be inhibited by sera from dust mite-allergic patients. J. Immunol. 133: 2488.
9. Tovey, E. R., M. D. Chapman, C. W. Wells, and T. A. E. Platts-Mills. 1981. The distribution of dust mite allergen in the houses of patients with asthma. Am. Rev. Respir. Dis. 124: 630.
10. Chapman, M. D., R. C. Aalberse, M. J. Brown, and T. A. E. Platts-Mills. 1988. Monoclonal antibodies to the major feline allergen *Fel d* I. II. Single step affinity purification of *Fel d* I, N-Terminal sequence analysis, and development of a sensitive two-site immunoassay to assess *Fel d* I exposure. J. Immunol. 140: 812.
11. Platts-Mills, T. A. E., and M. D. Chapman. 1987. Dust mites: Immunology, allergic disease and environmental control. J. Allergy Clin. Immunol. 80: 755.
12. Chapman, M. D., P. W. Heymann, S. M. Pollart, and T. A. E. Platts-Mills. Allergen standardization using monoclonal antibodies to major allergens. In this volume.
13. Ford, A. W., F. C. Rawle, P. Lind, F. Th. M. Spieksma, H. Lowenstein, and T. A. E. Platts-Mills. 1985. Standardization of *Dermatophagoides pteronyssinus*: Assessment of potency and allergen content in ten coded extracts. Int. Arch. Allergy Appl. Immunol. 76: 58.
14. Platts-Mills, T. A. E., and A. L. de Weck. 1989. Dust mite allergens and asthma—A world wide problem. Report of an International Workshop Bad Kreuznach, F.R.G., September 1987. Bull WHO, in press.
15. Findley, S. R., E. Stotsky, K. Leiterman, Z. Hemody, and J. L. Ohman. 1983. Allergens detected in association with airborne particles capable of penetrating into the peripheral lung. Am. Rev. Respir. Dis. 128: 1008.
16. Van Metre, T. E., D. G. Marsh, N. F. Adkinson, J. E. Fish, A. Kagey-Sobotka, P. S. Norman, E. B. Radden, and G. L. Rosenberg. 1986. Dose of cat (*Felis domesticus*) allergen 1 (*Fel d* I) that induces asthma. J. Allergy Clin. Immunol. 78: 62.
17. Platts-Mills, T. A. E., P. W. Heymann, M. D. Chapman, E. B. Mitchell, M. L. Hayden, and S. R. Wilkins. 1986. Immunologic triggers in asthma. In: Proceedings of the XII International Congress of Allergology and Clinical Immunology. C.E. Reed, ed. St. Louis: Mosby, p. 214.
18. Pollart, S. M., M. D. Chapman, G. P. Fiocco, G. Rose, and T. A. E. Platts-Mills. 1989. Epidemiology of acute asthma: IgE antibodies to common inhalant allergens as a risk factor for Emergency Room visits. J. Allergy Clin. Immunol., in press.
19. Reid, M. J., R. B. Moss, Y. P. Hsu, J. M. Kwasnicki, T. M. Commerford, and B. L. Nelson. 1986. Seasonal asthma in northern California: Allergic causes and efficacy of immunotherapy. J. Allergy Clin. Immunol. 78: 590.
20. Pollart, S., M. Reid, M. Brown, M. Kwasnicki, J. Fling, M. Chapman, and T. A. E. Platts-Mills. 1988. Epidemiology of emergency room asthma in Northern California: Association with IgE antibody to rye grass pollen. J. Allergy Clin. Immunol. 82: 224.
21. Platts-Mills, T. A. E., M. L. Hayden, M. D. Chapman, and S. R. Wilkins. 1986. Seasonal variation in dust mite and grass pollen allergens in dust from the houses of patients with asthma. J. Allergy Clin. Immunol. 79: 781.
22. Korsgaard, J. 1983. Mite asthma and residency: A case-control study on the impact of exposure to house dust mites in dwellings. Am. Rev. Respir. Dis. 128.

23. Green, W. F., A. J. Woolcock, M. Stuckey, C. Sedgwick, and S. R. Leeder. 1986. House dust mites and skin tests in different Australian localities. Aust. NZ J. Med. 16: 639.

24. Platts-Mills, T. A. E., E. R. Tovey, E. B. Mitchell, H. Moszoro, P. Nock, and S. R. Wilkins. 1982. Reduction of bronchial hyperreactivity during prolonged allergen avoidance. Lancet 2: 675.

25. Chur, V., G. Falkenhorst, P. Hermannsdorfer, S. Lau, and U. Wahn. 1988. Studies on the influ-ence of mite allergen exposure on sensitization and bronchial hyperreactivity of atopic children. N. Eng. Reg. Allergy Proc. 9: 295.

26. Cartier, A., N. C. Thomson, P. A. Frith, M. Roberts, and F. E. Hargreave. 1982. Allergen-induced increase in bronchial responsiveness to histamine: relationship to the late asthmatic response and change in airway caliber. J. Allergy Clin. Immunol. 70: 170.

Air-Conditioning and Allergic Diseases

*Claude Molina**

Allergic building-related illnesses fall into three main categories: rhinitis or asthma, hypersensitivity pneumonitis, and humidifier fever. These diseases must be differentiated from infectious diseases and from the Building Sickness Syndrome. A large number of allergens may be responsible for these allergic symptoms, but other factors may be taken into account: physical, chemical, and psychological factors. These problems must be recognized not only by allergists who have to provide for their prevention and treatment, but also by architects, engineers, buildings experts, the designers of large tower blocks, and air-conditioning specialists.

At a time when outdoor pollution in large towns and cities seems to be on the decrease (except in cases of accident) as a result of the measures taken to control domestic heating and the emissions of industrial smoke and car exhaust fumes, the problem of indoor air quality is becoming a matter of concern.

Town-dwellers spend less than an hour a day (0.7 hour) outside; the rest of the time they are at home, at work, or in some means of transport.

Since the 1970s and the oil crisis, energy-saving measures have led to insufficient ventilation of rooms and the use of synthetic insulating materials which emit various chemical substances, resulting in an increased concentration of household pollutants and the appearances of a wide variety of disorders.

In 1970, following the observations of Banaszak et al., the attention of the medical profession was drawn to a number of manifestations of alveolitis among employees working in air-conditioned offices. The allergic nature of these disorders was suggested by the discovery of precipitating antibodies in the serum and thermophilic actinomycetes in air-conditioning systems and in the indoor air. These thermophilic actinomycetes being the same as those found in moldy hay in agriculture, we were led to conclude that the human race cannot escape its fate, since it has abandoned rural living in favor of the urban civilization, where it now finds exactly the same pathogens.

"Air-conditioner disease" was therefore classified as a type of allergic alveolitis which are becoming more and more numerous—said to be a veritable Pandora's box—and are described anecdotally in literature. It is similar to "humidifier fever," which has been described both in homes (De Weck; Patterson et al.; Burke et al.) and in industrial situations where cold water spray humidification systems become heavily contaminated with microorganisms.

In Philadelphia, in 1976, there was an outbreak of a hitherto unknown infectious disease: Legionnaire's Disease. This serious illness, which primarily affects the lungs, was caused by a previously unidentified bacteria that had probably developed in the air-conditioning system of a Philadelphia hotel where the members of the Legion of Veterans of the American Army were meeting. It was given the name *Legionella*.

By extension, Legionnaire's Disease and its more benign homologue, Pontiac Fever, are also considered to be sicknesses due to air-conditioning systems. They are, in fact, nothing of the kind, but rather a contamination of the incoming air by *Legionella* organisms caused by vapor drift from contaminated cooling towers, located near the air-conditioning system. Several epidemics have been noted scattered virtually over the entire globe, associated with a significant mortality.

Finally, apart from these allergic and infectious disorders, company doctors are confronted daily with a number of complaints from individuals who work in air-conditioned atmospheres, complaints concerning mucous membranes of eyes, nose, and throat as well as headache and lethargy. These symptoms appear to be benign and related to the building in which the individuals work.

They are generally observed in modern buildings with air-conditioning systems and artificial lighting. Some authors call these dis-

---

* Professeur de Clinique Pneumologique à l'Université, Chef de Service, Hôpital Sabourin, B.P. 125, 63020 Clermont Ferrand Cedex, France.

orders the "sick building syndrome," others the "building sickness syndrome." In the United States they speak of the "tight building syndrome," while in France some have suggested the name "maladie des gratte-ciel" (skyscraper disease) or "maladie des batiments malsains"; in Canada (Quebec) it is called "maladie des tours à bureaux," in Denmark "indoor climate illness" has been suggested.

Extent of the Problem

This is a worldwide problem because air-conditioning is used in many different situations for the purpose of comfort, safety, and even noise abatement, not only in large blocks of flats or individual dwellings in hot countries (for example, detached houses, hospitals, hotels, department stores, city office blocks, museums, and libraries containing valuable documents), but also in numerous industries in which humidification is indispensable, such as printing and high-tech industries such as electronics, data processing, and magnetic tape manufacture.

There are, therefore, millions of people living or working on premises where the ventilation is regulated and where use is made of air-conditioning systems.

The current literature suggests that 20–30% of office employees regularly experience symptoms, which probably reduces their working efficiency; and that up to 30% of new and refurbished buildings throughout the world may be affected by these different syndromes (WHO 1983 and 1986 a).

Symptomatology

Paradoxically, allergic patients who should do better in an air-conditioned environment which protects them against dust and particules are often affected by many troubles.

Allergic building-related illnesses fall into three main categories:

— Asthma or rhinitis

— Hypersensitivity pneumonitis (extrinsic allergic alveolitis)

— Humidifier fever.

Asthma, Rhinitis

In general, allergic responses of the upper and lower respiratory tracts occur secondarily to the inhalation of allergens in poorly maintained buildings where the cold water spray humidifiers have become contaminated by micro-organisms. Bronchial asthma in a family has been described, as caused by a simple home humidifier contaminated by *Rhodotorula* spores (Solomon) and also in a factory situation where print workers developed asthma due to heavy microbial contamination of a central cold water spray humidifier (Finnegan et al). The features are those of any form of occupational asthma with increasing asthmatic symptoms over the working week, improving on days away from work, over weekends, and holidays.

Hypersensitivity Pneumonitis

This is the most serious form of allergic response which may be related to buildings. It occurs when heat-exchange systems become contaminated, usually by thermophilic actinomycetes (for example, micropolyspora faeni). The number of cases reported in the literature has been small, occurring both in air-conditioned office blocks in the center of cities (Fink) and also in air-conditioned homes. The principal symptoms, which occur some hours after exposure, include fever, malaise, and breathlessness. A great loss of weight may be an accompanying feature.

On auscultation of the lungs late inspiratory crackles are generally present, and chest X-ray reveals a micronodular infiltrate. Pulmonary function tests are abnormal. The classical pattern is that of a restrictive lung defect with impaired gas transfer.

Serological tests usually show the presence of precipitating antibodies to the causative allergen. Bronchial provocation studies may be used to confirm the diagnosis.

Occasionally, lung biopsy is necessary to establish the diagnosis. The characteristic historical changes are of a histiocytic cellular infiltration with giant cell and granuloma formation.

Humidifier Fever or "Monday Fever"

This condition was first described in 1956 by Pestalozzi. He described an outbreak of systemic and respiratory symptoms in a group of workers in a carpentry shop. Symptoms occur on the first day of the working week, a similar periodicity to byssinosis, developing over the second half of the working shift or in the evening after leaving the workplace. Although exposure continues at work, symptoms improve progressively over the working week and subsequent weekend, recurring again on the first day back at work after a weekend or holiday. The symptoms of humidifier fever are "flu-like," lethargy, myalgia, arthralgia, headache, and fever. In more severe cases these symptoms are associated with coughing and breathlessness. They resolve over a 12-hour period, and the individual is usually able to work normally the following day.

Physical examination at the height of the reaction reveals the presence of late inspiratory crackles on auscultation, and lung function shows a restrictive defect with impaired gas transfer. Lung function is normal between attacks. In all cases the chest radiograph is normal.

Immunological investigations almost always reveal the presence of precipitating antibodies to antigen extracted from the humidifiers.

Bronchial provocation tests with water from the humidifier usually reproduce the symptoms and physiological changes in affected individuals but not in control subjects.

The cause or causes of humidifier fever are not known. Outbreaks nearly always occur when humidifiers have become heavily contaminated by microorganisms. A number of different causes have been postulated including *Naegleria gruberi*, *Acanthamoeba polyphaga*, *Bacillus subtilis*, *Aureobasidium pullulans* and endotoxin. All of these suggested causes are based on serological investigations. At the present time, none has been proved to be the cause by provocation studies.

Diagnosis

Other causes of building-related illnesses should be excluded:

Infections

Bacterial

The most serious infection associated with air-conditioning systems is that caused by *Legionella pneumophila*. Individuals are infected by vapor drip containing this bacteria from contaminated cooling towers. This may occur in the streets in the vicinity of the cooling tower or inside buildings when water droplets are drawn into the building via the air-conditioning system. Legionnaire's disease has not been described as a result of contaminated cold water spray humidifiers.

Fungal

Infections caused by the fungal species *Aspergillus* have been described as a result of contaminated incoming air to buildings and due to contamination of duct work. This is a particular problem in hospitals, affecting old and immunocompromised patients. Good maintenance procedures and appropriate filters prevent outbreaks of this type of disease.

Viral

An epidemic infection of measles has been described in which the mode of spread appeared to be via the air-conditioning system. It is not known whether such systems have a role in the spread of upper respiratory tract infections in buildings.

Building Sickness Syndromes (B.S.S.)

The symptomatology of this syndrome is extremely varied, but 5 different classes of symptoms are encountered:

— Respiratory manifestations: The symptoms most frequently observed are a feeling of irritation and dryness of the nasal and pharyngeal mucosae. There may also be obstructive rhinitis with or without nasal discharge (Caillaud).

— Ocular manifestations

— Cutaneous manifestations

— Odor and taste complaints

— Neuropsychic manifestations.

Overall there is a feeling of discomfort.

It is important to note that in our own survey *atopic* subjects (presenting personal or family antecedents, skin tests proving positive to common inhalation allergens, high serum concentration of IgE) seem to have a particular predisposition toward manifestations of building sickness syndrome, in statistically significant way (Caillaud). Atopic subjects may, therefore, be considered to be veritable "sentinels" of pollution.

Further, the other characteristics of the syndrome may be summarized as follows: predominance in women, benignity, disappearance on leaving work, and reappearance on return to work.

How to Conduct Building-Associated Investigations

In the presence of such building-related illnesses, a detailed two-stage assessment should be drawn up:

1. Qualitative Assessment

— Both of the *disorders found* (by questionnaires, interviews), provided that there is a sufficiently large number of symptomatic patients; and

— of the main *physical, chemical,* and *biological parameters* of the establishment concerned and of the air-conditioning system.

Physical factors we must take into account:

— temperature, relative humidity (which has to be kept below 70% to avoid the risk of rapid multiplication of microbes), air velocity, artificial light, vibrations, noises.

Chemical factors: environmental *tobacco smoke* is by far the most important source of pollution.

It is well known that tobacco smoke can also act as an allergen (Lehrer) affecting the bronchial or alveolar immune defence mechanisms (Molina). As a rule smoking should be prohibited in air-conditioned working environments.

Formaldehyde: The presence of formaldehyde results from the use of wood-based products (like particle board, plywood), urea- formaldehyde foam for insulation, and a variety of other products, mainly used for disinfection, cleaning, and painting. It has been suggested that this might be the cause of allergic disorders including asthma. In fact, concentrations in the ambient atmosphere of buildings are rarely sufficient to cause symptoms.

Volatile organic compounds: Whether they come from building materials, furniture, household maintenance products (waxes, detergents, insecticides), products of personal hygiene (cosmetics), do-it-yourself goods (resins), office materials (photocopier ink), or ETS, these compounds may affect the respiratory system and are also the source of more or less disagreeable odors.

Biocides: Biocides are currently used in most cold water spray humidifiers to control microbial growth. These products are highly irritant in concentrated form; when dispersed in the indoor atmosphere, at low concentrations, they may cause mucous membrane irritation in susceptible individuals.

Odors: Many gas and vapors give rise to odor, which may be a disturbing factor.

Questionnaire

Here, there are a number of distortions or bias factors to be avoided, resulting from a poor selection of the population to be studied. This is why the *data collection* method has to be accurate. The only valid data are those collected either by self- questionnaire or by interviews conducted by trained investigators (S. Perdrizet).

Finally, in the epidemiological approach, the role of a suspected pathogenic factor has to be confirmed by studying the effects of its *exclusion*.

Quantitative Assessment

If the problem cannot be solved by simple measures, quantitative methods have to be used.

— From the medical angle, by using exploratory tests of respiratory function, either of the upper tract (rhinomanometry) or of the bronchi and the parenchyma (spirometry, flow-volume curve, etc.). Simple methods like testing with the peak flowmeter at the workplace or even portable rhinomanometers which are easy to use several times a day may also be applied.

— As regards the *objective* criteria relation to buildings to be surveyed, variables to be taken into account:

1. the physical parameters of the building

2. the effectiveness of the ventilation.

So, whether it is a case of a finished building or especially one which is under construction, consultation between building experts, engineers, and also doctors on design, siting, air-conditioning and ventilation is absolutely essential today.

General Technical Recommendations

These recommendations primarily concern the central installations of large blocks and not individual installations.

In principle, the allergic pathology must be connected with dust and particles that have escaped from filters and carriers of more or less specific antigens.

For the *siting* of air-conditioning systems, it is sufficient for the air-cooling towers to be located where their effluent is not sucked in again by the fans of the conditioning plant and redistributed throughout the building with the conditioned air.

Regarding *humidification*, which is an essential stage, the recommendations have to be very strict: Dry steam should be used wherever possible since it contains less bacterial or mycological contamination. When water is produced, it must not be allowed to stagnate; there must be easy access to the installation ducts.

The *filters* have two essential purposes: to protect the components and to stop the dust that may harbor bacteria or allergens. Prefiltration is a necessary upstream of the air treatment chain, while more effective filtration should be provided downstream to ensure that the air is of a quality appropriate to the use being made of the room. The choice of filter is therefore particularly important. A good filter must have a high efficiency for particles of 1 µm at least, the correct filtration material must be used (fine glass fiber), and a large-area fine filter must be selected in order to cut operating costs. Finally, filters must be placed as near as possible to the source to be guarded (e.g., a hospital operating theater).

As regards the *design* of equipment and *construction* itself, there should be detailed and statutory recommendations concerning exterior air intakes, filtration and air coolers, humidifiers, and silencers.

Installation monitoring and *maintenance* can begin immediately on receipt of the installations. The pre-startup assessment must include a particle count, and the maintenance contract must specify the frequency of services and the required qualifications of technicians.

Finally, the medical law aspect must not be forgotten, since the users of premises in which employees have contracted an illness are going to lay the blame first and foremost on the installers. In France, in particular, allergic manifestations are to be found in a table of occupational diseases among employees working in air-conditioned buildings where air-conditioning systems are not regularly serviced and maintained.

Cost-Effectiveness

As the WHO has pointed out in the document on Indoor Air Quality research (WHO 1986 b), the effort to save energy will continue in the coming years in most countries, and this will lead to increasing problems in buildings, if those responsible do not have a clear idea that energy economy is not the unique parameter to deal with in evaluating costs.

A recent working document of the European Parliament on Indoor Air Quality quoted a comparative evaluation of the possible realistic cost reduction in the heating and ventilation of a large building on one side and of a 1% additional absenteeism among the employees on the other side. Under the hypotheses assumed for the calculation, the cost of the latter is roughly 100 times greater than the money saved through energy savings. Moreover, the absenteeism attributed to allergic building-related illnesses is probably much greater than 1%.

Suggested Reading

References to this topic may be found in *Air Conditioner Diseases*, Claude Molina (Ed.). Paris: INSERM, 1985.

Environmental Allergy and/or Clinical Ecology

*Abba I. Terr**

Clinical ecology is a form of medical practice which proposes the existence of an "environmental illness" in which the patient has multiple food and environmental chemical sensitivities. The diagnosis is usually made on patients with long-standing multiple symptomatology with no defining objective physical findings or laboratory abnormalities. The principal diagnostic test is provocation-neutralization, a procedure lacking scientific validity.

Treatment by avoidance of numerous foods and environmental chemicals, symptom-neutralization by sublingual or subcutaneous injection of food and chemical extracts, and antifungal medications for "Candida hypersensitivity syndrome" has not been shown to be efficacious by properly controlled clinical studies. Proponents of clinical ecology should subject their theories and methods to critical appraisal through accepted scientific and clinical study.

Clinical ecology evolved from the practice of allergy. Beginning about 40 years ago, a small group of allergists proposed that allergy to foods causes a variety of physical and psychological illnesses and are responsible for symptoms involving the musculoskeletal system, joints, and gastrointestinal tract, as well as a host of nonspecific complaints, in patients who often have no objective physical signs. To this movement was later added the concept that environmental chemicals, both natural and synthetic, are implicated as a cause of these symptoms. The practice that is based on these ideas became known as clinical ecology [1–3]. Today hundreds of physicians from a number of different medical specialties have joined the ranks of clinical ecology, which they consider to be a form of alternative or complementary medicine.

The clinical ecology theories of disease differ from the original allergy concept. It has been postulated that these patients suffer from failure of the human species to adapt to synthetic chemicals [4]. One theory proposes that symptoms represent the exhaustion of normal homeostasis, caused by ingestion of foods and inhalation of chemicals. Another theory is based on the concept that these environmental substances are toxic to the human immune system, specifically interfering with the function of T lymphocytes in the regulation of the immune response. Clinical ecology theories include certain unique concepts, such as a maximum total body load of antigen, masked food hypersensitivity, and a spreading phenomenon [3].

Environmental Illness

The practice of clinical ecology centers on a diagnosis of "environmental illness," which has also been called ecologic illness, chemical hypersensitivity syndrome, total allergy syndrome, and 20th-century disease. According to the journal *Clinical Ecology*, "ecologic illness is a polysymptomatic, multisystem chronic disorder manifested by adverse reactions to environmental excitants, as they are modified by individual susceptibility in terms of specific adaptations. The excitants are present in air, water, drugs, and our habitats." Although "environmental illness" is perceived as a specific disease, the diagnosis is applied to patients having a wide variety of clinical symptoms [5]. In some cases, the diagnosis is used to describe patients with a single problem, such as asthma, migraine headaches, premenstrual syndrome, arthralgias, or recurrent abdominal pain, although most often it is applied to patients with multiple long-standing symptoms that defy a circumscribed physical illness. It is also used as a diagnosis for patients with bizarre conversion reactions, anxiety and depression, or psychosomatic illness. Some patients are asymptomatic. No specific physical abnormality or laboratory abnormality is required for diagnosis.

---
* Stanford University, Stanford, CA, USA.

Diagnostic Methods

Because of the lack of a characteristic history or pathognomonic physical sign or laboratory test, clinical ecologists use a diagnostic procedure known as provocation-neutralization. This procedure involves the testing of the patient by sublingual or intracutaneous application of environmental substances to elicit subjective symptoms within a 10-minute time period. The substances most commonly tested in this way are food extracts; chemicals such as phenol, formaldehyde, and ethanol; inhalant allergen extracts; hormones; autocoids such as histamine and serotonin; and even saline or water. Immediately after each sublingual test drop or intracutaneous test injection, the patient records any and all symptoms for a period of 10 minutes. The test is regarded as positive if any symptom appears, regardless of whether or not the same symptom is present in the history of the illness. Published reports of provocation-neutralization testing yield widely conflicting results [6–8]. To date, there has not been a definitive study of this procedure. Those studies reported so far are based on subjects with varying clinical manifestations, and different testing methods have been used with differing criteria for a positive test. Many of the studies lack placebo controls, and very few include normal control subjects for comparison. In all of the published reports, statistical analyses have been absent or inappropriate. Therefore, no scientific basis can be offered at this time for provocation-neutralization testing as practiced by clinical ecologists [7, 8].

In the United States, there are several Environmental Control Units in which patients are subjected to airborne exposure to chemicals in testing booths. Unlike bronchial provocation testing in asthma, a positive test for environmental illness is designated by the appearance of self-reported symptoms only. There are no published reports of controlled studies of this method of testing.

Some clinical ecologists are now using the measurement of serum immunoglobulins, complement components, blood level of lymphocyte subsets, and blood or tissue level of pesticides as a supplement to provocation-neutralization in diagnosis. Although the current clinical ecology theory is based on several immunologic models that suggest that disease can be caused by the toxic effect of environmental chemicals on the immune system, allergic sensitivity to these chemicals, or a combination of these two proposed effects, it is not clear what abnormalities in immunologic parameters are supposed to indicate the presence of environmental illness. The few published reports show a variable and often conflicting set of abnormalities of dubious clinical significance, since these reports lack proper controls or evidence of reproducibility [9].

Clinical Ecology Treatment Methods

The two principal methods of treatment advocated by clinical ecologists are avoidance therapy and neutralization therapy [1–3]. Avoidance of foods believed to cause or aggravate illness is accomplished by rotary diversified diet, which is based on the belief that multiple food "sensitivities" occur in this illness. Avoidance of all food additives is recommended. Avoidance of environmental synthetic chemicals and even some natural chemicals is a universal feature of clinical ecology treatment, though the degree of avoidance varies with the enthusiasm of the patient and physician. Most commonly, patients eliminate scented household products, synthetic fabrics and plastics, and pesticides. They generally try to limit exposure to air pollutants, gasoline fumes, and vehicle exhaust fumes. In the United States, several isolated rural communities have been established for those patients deemed unsuitable for the urban environment.

Neutralization therapy is achieved by self-administered sublingual or subcutaneous injections of food and chemical extracts. Patients are advised to administer these substances either before anticipated exposure to an environmental chemical or food, or they may take a neutralizing treatment after exposure to relieve symptoms. None of these forms of treatment—either singly or in combination—have been evaluated in properly controlled studies to determine efficacy or potential adverse effects, although clinical ecologists and their patients claim that these method are successful.

Clinical ecologists of the recommend megadose vitamin therapy, mineral or amino acid supplements, and antioxidants such as vitamin E, on the rationale that these treatments strengthen the immune system and enhance immune responses. Experimental or clinical evidence to support this premise has yet to be presented.

Drug therapy is generally condemned as a form of chemical exposure, although oxygen, mineral salts, and antifungal drugs are frequently prescribed.

Candida Hypersensitivity Syndrome

In recent years "environmental illness" has been linked causally with the yeast *Candida albicans* normally resident in the microflora of the gastrointestinal and female genito-urinary mucus membranes [10, 11]. Many persons with no clinical evidence of Candida infection and no evidence of defective local or systemic natural or acquired immunity, pregnancy, diabetes mellitus, endocrine diseases, or medications known to cause opportunistic candidiasis are said to suffer an illness known as "Candida hypersensitivity syndrome." The syndrome is otherwise indistinguishable from "environmental illness." Clinical ecologists credit *Candida albicans* as a cause of behavioral and emotional diseases and of a variety of physical illnesses and symptomatic states. Individuals who have ever received antibiotics, corticosteroids, birth control pills, or have ever been pregnant, even in the remote past, are said to be susceptible to this syndrome. Diagnosis is made by history and not by diagnostic testing. The recommended treatment is avoidance of sugar, yeast, and mold in the diet, and the use of a rotary diversified diet. Nystatin, ketaconazole, cyprylic acid, and vitamin and mineral supplements are recommended. This syndrome is reminiscent of the concept of "autointoxication" that was popular 50 years ago. In the opinion of some practitioners in that era, the bacterial component of the normal intestinal flora was considered to cause numerous physical and psychological disabilities.

Conclusion

Physicians who are engaged in primary medical care and specialists in allergy and immunology encounter patients with a diagnosis of "environmental illness," "Candida hypersensitivity syndrome," "chemical hypersensitivity," and "total allergy." In order to properly evaluate and manage these patients, it is important to conduct an independent thorough examination of the clinical findings to rule out the presence of other diseases. Many patients with these diagnoses have underlying personality features or frank psychological illness that may explain their somatic complaint [12, 13]. Others will be found to have undiagnosed diseases related to the environment [5]. The clinical ecology concept of an "environmental illness," however, often leads to a restricted and isolated lifestyle that has yet to be shown to eliminate symptoms or improve the sense of well-being [5]. Proponents of clinical ecology need to appraise their theories and methods more critically, since there is insufficient scientific support to endorse their concepts or their clinical methods [14].

References

1. Randolph, T. G. 1962. Human ecology and susceptibility to the chemical environment. Springfield, IL: C.C. Thomas.
2. Dickey, L. D. 1976. Clinical ecology. Springfield, IL: C.C. Thomas.
3. Bell, I. R. 1982. Clinical ecology: A new medical approach to environmental illness. Bolinas, CA: Common Knowledge Press.
4. Randolph, T. G. 1956. The specific adaptation syndrome, J. Lab. Clin. Med. 48: 934.
5. Terr, A. I. 1986. Environmental illness: A clinical review of 50 cases. Arch. Intern. Med. 146: 145–149.
6. Van Metre, T. E. 1983. Critique of controversial and unproven procedures for diagnosis and therapy of allergic disease. Pediat. Clin. North Amer. 30: 807–817.
7. American Academy of Allergy and Immunology. 1981. Position statements—Controversial techniques. J. Allergy Clin. Immunol 67: 333–338.
8. California Medical Association Scientific Board Task Force on Clinical Ecology. 1986. Clinical ecology—A critical appraisal. West. J. Med. 144: 239–245.
9. Terr, A. I. 1987, "Multiple chemical sensitivities": Immunologic critique of clinical ecology theories and practice. Occupational Medicine State of the Art Reviews 2: 683–694.
10. Crook, W. G. 1984. The yeast connection: A medical breakthrough (2nd ed.). Jackson, TN: Professional Books.

11. American Academy of Allergy and Immunology. 1986. Position statements—Candida hypersensitivity syndrome. J. Allergy Clin. Immunol. 78: 271–273.

12. Brodsky, C. M. 1983. "Allergic to everything": A medical subculture. Psychosomatics 24: 731–742.

13. Stewart, D. E., and J. Raskin. 1985. Psychiatric assessment of patients with "20th century disease" ("total allergy syndrome"). Can. Med. Assoc. J. 133: 1001–1003.

14. American Academy of Allergy and Immunology. 1986. Position statements—Clinical ecology. J. Allergy Clin. Immunol. 78: 269–270.

Maternal Food Intake During Pregnancy and Lactation: Effect on High Allergy Risk Infants

N.-I. Max Kjellman, Karin Fälth-Magnusson, Gunnar Hattevig,
Bengt Björkstén*

The immune interplay between mother and foetus/infant was studied in three groups of high allergy risk families. Total elimination of cow's milk and egg as compared to normal intake of these nutrients during the three last months of pregnancy had no significant effect on the development of allergy and atopic disease to 3 1/2 years of age. Increased intake of the same foods increased food antibody concentrations in the pregnant mother but had no influence on the children. High IgG antibody concentrations neonatally did not offer protection against atopic disease. In contrast, elimination of egg, milk and fish during the first 3 months of lactation delayed food sensitization and atopic disease in the infant. Maternal diet during lactation, but not during pregnancy, may be considered, provided that the diet is surveyed by a dietitian.

Allergy preventive measures with emphasis on early infant feeding have been discussed for the past 50 years, since the demonstration by Grulee and Sanford that bottle-fed infants developed atopic disease 7 times more often than breast-fed infants [1]. Several recent recommendations include dietary restrictions to the nursing mother and even elimination of basic nutrients during pregnancy in high allergy risk families [2, 3, 4]. Before maternal dietary restrictions are included in an allergy prevention program, possible negative as well as positive effects of such restrictions should, however, be thoroughly evaluated.

There are several problems in evaluating published studies regarding the effect of allergy preventive measures, especially when it comes to the evaluation of early infant feeding. There is still no agreement on the allergy preventive effect of breast feeding (summarized in [5]). Studies in this field were for many reasons not randomized, and they are thus subject to a considerable degree of self selection bias. Evaluation was not blinded, and retrospective information was often accepted. Feeding at the maternity ward (often = cow's milk formula) was only rarely recorded.

IgE antibodies against milk and egg have been demonstrated, although rarely in newborn infants, indicating that sensitization can occur during pregnancy (summarized in [6]). Allergens, IgG (but not IgE) antibodies, cells and various mediators are transferred through placenta. They may modulate the foetal immune response [6].

Sensitization is, however, much more common during the first months of life than during pregnancy [7]. It has been demonstrated, that maternal food contents are present in the breast milk [8]. Furthermore, infant symptoms may disappear with maternal avoidance of a certain food and reappear when the food is reintroduced into her diet [7, 8].

The effect of a maternal elimination diet during lactation and pregnancy has not previously been evaluated separately. Hence, we started two separate studies with randomized maternal food intake during pregnancy and lactation. The immune interplay between mother and her foetus/child as well as the development of allergy and atopic disease in infancy has been reported previously [9, 10, 11) and is briefly summarized here. In addition, some unpublished results are also included.

Maternal Diet during Pregnancy

The personal and family history of allergy was carefully recorded in all pregnant women in

*   Department of Pediatrics, Faculty of Health Sciences and University Hospital, Linköping, Sweden, S-581 85 Linköping, Sweden.
Acknowledgements: Financial support by the Swedish Medical Research Council (grant no. 7510), the Medical Research Fund of the County of Östergötland, King Gustaf Vth 80-Year-Anniversary Fund, the First of May Flower Annual Campaign for Children's Health, Konsul Th. Berg Foundation, Riksförbundet mot Astma-Allergi and the Expressen Perinatal Research Fund is gratefully acknowledged.

295

three Swedish cities over a period of 18 months. Mothers-to-be were addressed during mid-pregnancy provided they were expecting babies with a family history of obvious atopic disease in at least one member of the family. In most of the mothers the history was confirmed by records and tests including Phadiatop (Pharmacia Diagnostics, Uppsala, Sweden) and skin prick tests (SPT) using standardized extracts.

In *Study A*, 212 mothers were randomized either to an elimination diet during pregnancy, starting in week 28 and ending at delivery, or to normal food intake [9, 10]. The elimination group had to exclude all cows milk and egg, and they were offered supplementation with a casein hydrolysate (Nutramigen®) and calcium phosphate tablets. There diet was carefully surveyed by a dietitian. 180 infants completed the whole study to the age of 18 months. Additional information is now also available regarding the children in study A at 3.5 years of age. *Study B* comprised 163 pregnant atopic women who were similarly randomized either to a high intake of milk (at least one liter a day) and egg or to a low intake of these nutrients (no "visible" egg or milk) from week 28 [10].

The infants in both studies were blindly evaluated at 18 months of age. Blood was drawn from the mothers in week 25 and at delivery, from the cord blood of the newborns and at 6 weeks, 6 months, and 18 months of age. Breast milk samples were collected during the first week.

IgE antibodies to cow's milk and egg were analyzed with a modified RAST technique, allowing the detection of low antibody concentrations (cut-off 0.12 PRU). Food antibodies of the IgG, IgA, and IgM classes were analyzed with ELISA. SPT was performed with food allergens, mites, molds, animal dander, and pollens.

Maternal weight gain was significantly lower during pregnancy in mothers who had eliminated cow's milk and egg as compared to mothers on normal food intake but no significant group difference was found regarding birth weights [9]. Food antibodies in maternal serum were highly influenced by maternal intake [11]. They decreased significantly more with no intake of milk and egg than with a low intake of these foods and increased significantly with a high intake of milk and egg. On the other hand, neonatal food antibody concentrations seemed virtually uninfluenced by maternal food intake, and the concentrations were usually higher than in the corresponding maternal sera at delivery.

High concentrations of food specific IgG, IgA, or IgM antibodies in maternal serum or in cord blood did not seem to protect against the development of atopic disease during infancy [10] in contrast to what has been suggested by others [12].

Similarly, food antibody concentrations in colostral samples were lower than in the corresponding serum samples, and no significant difference was found between the breast milk of mothers who during pregnancy had been on an elimination diet and that of the control group [Fälth-Magnusson et al., manuscript in preparation].

More importantly, none of more than 200 risk infants had IgE antibodies to cow's milk or egg in cord blood [10]. Sixteen percent of the children in study A were sensitized to egg during the first year despite the intention not to deliberately give them egg before 12 months of age [9]. There was no significant difference in egg sensitization between the two diet groups (with no intake or normal maternal intake during pregnancy). Eight percent of the infants had proven egg allergy and no significant group difference was found in this respect.

A positive egg skin prick test was more common at 6 months of age in a subgroup of children completely breast fed to three months of age (16%) as compared to a group fed breast supplemented with Nutramigen from an early age (4%; p < 0.01) [Fälth-Magnusson et al., manuscript in preparation]. The type of maternal food intake during pregnancy in study A did not seem to influence the development of atopic disease (mostly atopic dermatitis) to 18 months (Table 1) nor to 3 1/2 years of age, when 35% of children in both groups had prevalent atopic disease.

Preliminary results from the follow-up at 18 months of age of the children in study B indicate no protective effect from high maternal food intake during pregnancy [Lilja et al., manuscript in preparation]. The development of atopic disease and food allergy during infancy was quite similar in the group with a high maternal intake of milk and egg during pregnancy (23%) and in the group where mothers had avoided all "visible" egg and milk during pregnancy (19%).

Table 1. Atopic diseases (in % of 171 babies) before 18 months of age in relation to maternal food intake during the last 3 months of pregnancy (adapted from 9). Diet = avoidance of all cow's milk and egg. No significant group difference was found.

	Diet	Non-diet
Number	76	95
Atopic eczema	46.1	35.8
Bronchial asthma	9.2	8.4
Allergic rhinitis	3.9	0

Influence of Maternal Food Intake during Lactation

The importance of maternal food intake during lactation has been investigated in another prospective, study (*Study C*) with matched groups in 115 allergy risk infants [13]. After normal food intake during pregnancy, one group of nursing mothers completely avoided cow's milk, egg and fish during the first 3 months of lactation with the help of a dietitian, while the control group had normal amounts of these nutrients.

At 3 and 6 months of age, infants of mothers who were on elimination diet showed significantly less atopic dermatitis than the control group (Table 2). At 9 months, the experimental group showed less severe eczema. At 12 and 18 months there was still a statistically nonsignificant trend in favor of the elimination diet. Similarly, IgE antibodies to foods were significantly less common in infants of mothers on diet at 3 months but not at 6 and 9 months. Thus, maternal allergen avoidance seems to delay, but not prevent appearance of infant allergy. This study tallies partly with results from Chandra's group [4], where significantly less atopic disease occurred in breast-fed allergy risk infants as compared to bottle-fed risk babies, but only in a subgroup where the mothers had been on a diet during lactation (and during pregnancy). Food allergen present in most normal breast milk samples may explain the lack of allergy protection from breast feeding reported in many studies [5].

Discussion and Conclusions

From these and other studies it may be concluded that dietary restrictions during late pregnancy do *not* reduce the risk for allergy/atopic disease during early infancy. As food manipulation may impose a risk for suboptimal nutrition we only recommend pregnant women to abstain from smoking [14, 15] and discourage them from trying a diet unless required for their own well-being. Increased intake of allergenic food, although supported by animal experiments [16], did not appear rewarding in pregnant women.

High allergy risk families who want to delay the onset of symptoms and reduce their severity during early infancy should be guided and surveyed by a dietitian if the mothers want to keep an elimination diet during lactation.

Table 2. Atopic dermatitis (accumulated incidence in %) before 18 months of age in 115 infants in relation to maternal food intake during the first 3 months of lactation [Hattevig et al., manuscript in preparation].

	Age (months)				
	3	6	9	12	18
Diet group	3.1	10.8	16.9	23.1	26.2
Non-diet group	22.0	28.0	30.0	38.0	40.0
p	<0.01	<0.05	n.s.	n.s.	n.s.

References

1. Grulee, C., and H. N Sanford. 1936. The influence of breast and artificial feeding on infantile eczema. J. Pediatr. 9: 223–225.
2. Businco, L., A. Cantani, and G. Bruno. 1987. Prevention of atopy: results of long-term (7 months to 8 years) follow-up. Ann. Allergy 59 (part II): 183–186.
3. Zeiger, R. S., S. Heller, M. Mellon, R. O'Connor, and R. N. Hamburger. 1986. Effectiveness of dietary manipulation in the prevention of food allergy in infants. J. Allergy Clin. Immunol. 78: 224–238.
4. Chandra, R. K., S. Puri, C. Suraya, and P. S. Cheema. 1986. Influence of maternal food antigen avoidance during pregnancy and lactation on incidence of atopic eczema in infants. Clin. Allergy 16: 563–569.
5. Michel, F. B., J. Bousquet, A. Dannæus, R. N. Hamburger, J. A. Bellanti, M. L. Businco, and J. Soothill. 1986. Preventive measures in early childhood allergy. J. Allergy Clin. Immunol. 78: 1022–1027.
6. Björkstén, B., and N.-I. M. Kjellman. 1987. Perinatal factors influencing the development of allergy. Clin Rev Allergy 5: 339–347.

7. Gerrard, J. W. 1979. Allergy in breast fed babies to ingredients in breast milk. Ann. Allergy 42: 69–71.
8. Cant, A., R. A. Marsden, and P. A. Kilshaw. 1985. Egg and cow's milk hypersensitivity in exclusively breast fed infants with eczema, and detection of egg protein in breast milk. Brit. Med. J. 291: 932–935.
9. Fälth-Magnusson, K., and N.-I. M. Kjellman. 1987. Development of atopic disease in babies whose mothers were on exclusion diet during pregnancy—A randomized study. J. Allergy Clin. Immunol. 80: 968–975.
10. Fälth-Magnusson, K., N.-I. M. Kjellman, and K.-E. Magnusson. 1988. Antibodies IgG, IgA and IgM to food antigens during the first 18 months of life in relation to feeding and atopic disease. J. Allergy Clin. Immunol. 81: 743–749.
11. Lilja, G., A. Dannæus, K. Fälth-Magnusson, V. Graff-Lonnevig, S. G..O. Johansson, N.-I. M. Kjellman, and H. Öhman. 1988. Immune response of the atopic woman and foetus: effects of high- and low-dose food allergen intake during late pregnancy. Clin. Allergy 18: 131–142.
12. Casimir, G., B. Gossart, H. L. Vis, and J. Duchateau. 1985. Antibody against betalactoglobulin (IgG) and cow's milk allergy. J. Allergy Clin. Immunol. 75: 206.
13. Hattevig, G., B. Kjellman, N. Sigurs, B. Björkstén, and N.-I. M. Kjellman. Maternal avoidance of eggs, cow's milk and fish during lactation. Clin. Exp. Allergy, in press.
14. Rantakallio, P. 1978. Relationship of maternal smoking to morbidity and mortality of the child up to the age of five. Acta Paediatr. Scand. 67: 621–631.
15. Andræ, S., O. Axelsson, B. Björkstén, M. Fredriksson, and N.-I. M. Kjellman. 1988. Symptoms of bronchial hyperreactivity and asthma in relation to environmental factors. Arch. Dis. Child. 63: 473–478.
16. Jarrett, E. E., and E. Hall. 1984. The development of IgE-suppressive immunocompetence in young animals: Influence of exposure to antigen in the presence and absence of maternal immunity. Immunology 53: 365–373.

Antigen Specific IgG, IgG₄, and IgE Antibodies: Measurement in Pregnant Mothers, Their Cord Blood, and Their Children

Yoji Iikura, Kenichi Akimoto, Akira Akazawa, Kazuo Nonomura, Tadashi Uekusa, Hirohisa Saito, Akira Kawakita, Donald C. Reason, Motohiro Ebisawa, and Toshikazu Nagakura*

In this paper we present the evaluation of specific IgG antibody in allergic disease in childhood and the specific antibody levels in the pregnant mother's blood, cord blood, and infant's blood.

According to our recent study of children aged 2–12, the prevalence of asthma in Japan is 6.8% [1]. This number is almost seven times that of 15 years ago in non-air-polluted areas of Japan. Since there is a strong tendency for atopic dermatitis to develop into bronchial asthma, we should consider this condition not only as dermatitis, but also as part of the total circle in allergy.

The patient who suffers from allergic disease is very difficult to cure completely, and so our prime concern has been to determine the best method for preventing allergic disease. If we are to prevent allergic disease in the newborn infant, we have to determine the pregnant woman's allergic status, because human fetal cells are known to produce IgE antibodies from the eleventh week of gestation [2].

Some papers have reported that skin test positivity has been demonstrated in newborn babies [3], but in many infants, skin test, RAST, and clinical symptoms did not correlate [4]. From these results we assume that if we study only IgE antibody in infants, we may miss some antigens that influence the infants allergic condition.

Recently, we studied specific IgG antibody in allergic patients. From our results we concluded that specific IgG antibody titer was a useful parameter to follow when using the elimination of specific foods as therapy in infant atopic dermatitis [4].

Subjects and Methods

Comparison of specific antibody levels in pregnant women's blood and cord blood: Blood was taken from 150 women 7–8 months pregnant, and the serum was stored at –40 °C. Cord blood was collected from the same mothers at delivery. Serum IgE measurement was done by a highly sensitive radioimmunoassay method (Daiichi Radio Isotope, Tokyo). This method is sensitive to 0.3 U/ml. RAST was performed using a commercial kit (Pharmacia). Specific IgG and IgG4 antibody levels were determined by enzyme-linked immunosorbent assay with polyethylene plates.

Premature infants specific IgG antibody production study: Forty premature infants, body weight from 594–2350 g, were followed until full-term period. Blood samples from these babies were drawn at delivery time, one week after, one month after, and full-term period.

Results

1) There was *no correlation* between the mother's total IgE and cord blood IgE in 150 paired cases.

2) *Correlation between mother's specific IgG antibodies and mother's specific IgG4 antibodies:* There was good correlation between mother's specific IgG and IgG4 antibodies specific for egg white (Figure 1).

3) *Cord blood specific IgG antibody:* The levels of IgG4 antibody specific for egg, milk and mite (*Dermatophagoides farinae*) antigens were significantly higher in the cord blood of women

* Department of Allergy and Clinical Immunology, National Children's Medical Research Center, 3-35-31 Taishido, Setagaya-ku, Tokyo 154, Japan.

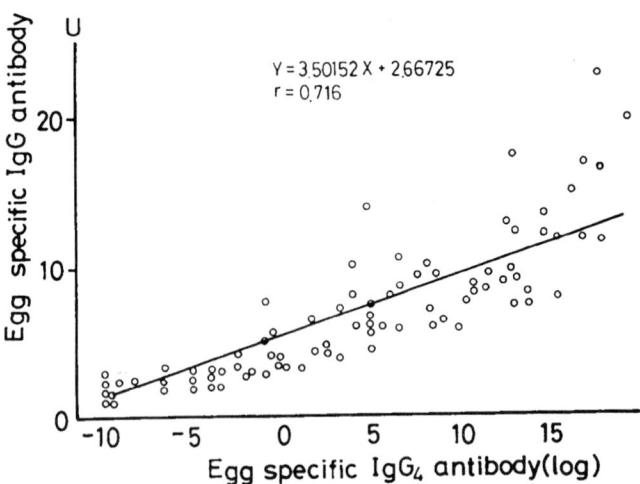

Figure 1. Correlation between mother's egg specific IgG and IgG4 antibodies.

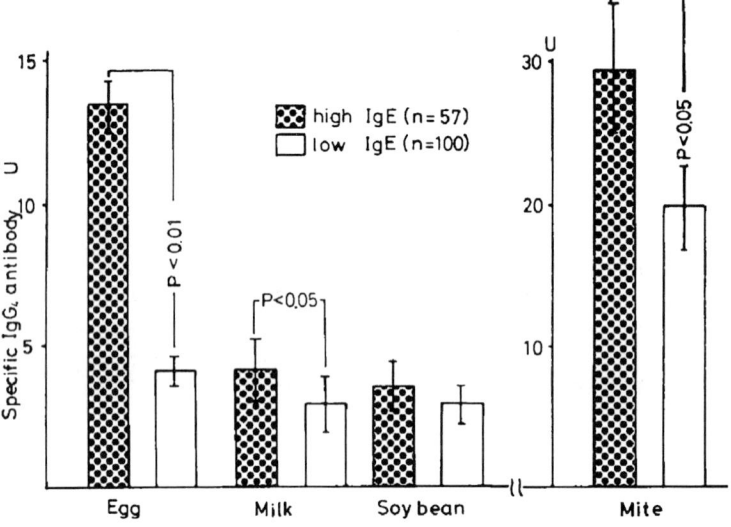

Figure 2. Cord blood specific IgG4 antibody. Comparison between maternal high and low IgE values.

with elevated total IgE compared to women whose IgE levels were low (Figure 2).

4) *Milk-specific IgG antibody and mother's milk intake during pregnancy:* The cord blood of mothers who took over 200 ml of milk per day showed a statistically higher level of specific IgG milk antibody than those who eliminated milk (Figure 3).

5) *Cord blood total IgE and cord blood specific IgG antibody:* The cord blood of the high total IgE group showed a statistically higher level of specific IgG milk antibody than the low total IgE group (p < 0.01).

6) *Relationship between clinical symptoms and egg specific IgG antibodies in infants:* Infants with high egg specific IgG antibody levels in cord blood were statistically more prone to develop allergic disease (mainly atopic dermatitis) (Table 1).

7) *Total IgE and specific IgG antibodies in premature infants:* Total IgE levels were low at birth, but increased significantly over one month. IgG antibody specific for cow's milk antigen was increased significantly at one month and full-term period. This antibody increase tends to correlate with high IgE values.

From these data, cow's milk antigen is pre-

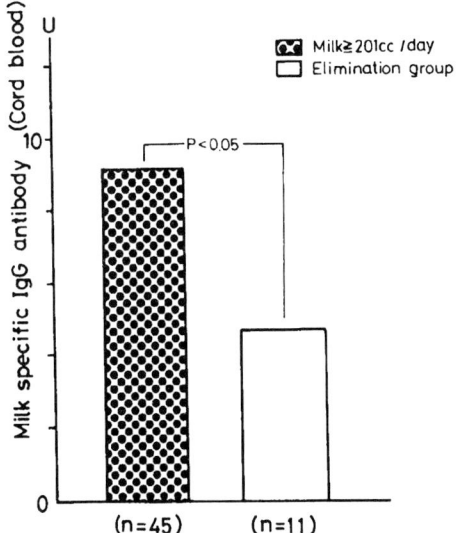

Figure 3. Milk specific IgG antibody in cord blood. Comparison between mothers who took over 200 ml of milk per day and milk elimination group.

Table 1. Relationship between clinical symptoms and egg-specific IgG antibodies in infants.

Clinical symptoms	Egg IgG (U)		
	≥30	<10	Total
Positive	10	15	25
Negative	5	42	47
Total number	15	57	72

p<0.01

sumed to be one of the factors leading to total IgE increase (Table 2).

Infants with a family history of allergy tended to display high levels of IgG antibody specific for antigens in cow's milk.

Discussion

We found that the pregnant women's daily life-style influenced specific IgG production in the fetus, and that in premature babies an increase in IgE correlated with IgG antibody production specific for milk antigens.

In general, when talking about allergic dis-ease, serum IgE levels and specific IgE antibod-ies are very important parameters to measure when evaluating the allergic condition. Neonatal serum IgE concentration gives us a good indication of the possibility of future atopic disease [5, 6].

For this reason, cord blood and newborn in-fant IgE studies are very important in under-standing the development of allergic disease. But it is not easy to detect specific IgE antibody in cord blood and newborn infants, because of the low IgE level during this period.

Atopic dermatitis is one of the main allergic disorders in young infants, and in some cases the patient's clinical condition improved after breastfeeding was stopped. But there were many cases in which specific milk and egg IgE antibody could not be detected. This type of complex evidence is common in the daily clini-

Table 2. Changes in total IgE and specific IgG after delivery in premature baby.

	At delivery	7 days	1 month	Full term (20–111 days after delivery)
Body weight	594–2350 g			
IgE	40	27	33**	35**
<0.3 (IU/ml)	82%	93	30	23
0.31–1.0	15%	7	21	26
>1.1	3%	0	49	51
Specific IgG	24	23	21	20
egg white	4.5	3.8	1.9	1.5*
(U/ml)	(0.2–13.8)	(0.2–11.0)	(0.3–8.5)	(0.3–4.0)
milk	4.4	3.5	33.3**	47.7**
	(0.3–19.6)	(0.3–14.0)	(0.4–100.0)	(0.4–100.0)

IgE level evaluated by χ^2; specific IgG evaluated by Wilcoxon analysis
*p<0.05 (compared with levels at delivery)
**p<0.01 (compared with levels at delivery)

cal care of newborn infants with atopic dermatitis. Therefore, we studied specific IgG and total IgE levels in the cord blood and the newborn infant.

The important thing is whether or not specific IgG or IgG4 antibody is correlated to allergic disease [7]. Here, our data suggest that high specific IgG antibody in the cord blood is related to the infant's allergic disease.

This theory contradicts the former concept of specific IgG antibody in allergic disease [8], in which the specific IgG antibody is considered a blocking antibody.

If specific IgG antibody is a blocking antibody, then high antibody levels should be beneficial for patients with allergic disease. There is a paper on food specific IgG antibody which correlates with severe anemia and chronic bronchitis and is associated with a markedly elevated level of IgG specific for cow's milk protein [9].

There are many types of food allergy reactions in young infants. One of these, atopic dermatitis, is not solely an immediate reaction. Hill et al. [10] reported high levels of IgE antibodies to cow milk in both immediate and delayed type reaction patients. Fallstrom et al. [11] also reported that elevated levels of IgE antibodies to cow milk in patients with slow onset of reactions. There are many different reports about food allergy in the clinical literature, but it is impossible to correlate specific IgE and clinical symptom in all food allergy patients.

Many physicians have examined specific IgE antibody levels in young allergic patients by using RAST and advised the patient's family that the test was negative, suggesting that if the RAST is negative food elimination is not necessary. However, as our study showed [4], IgE is not always detected in every allergic condition.

In our premature baby study, high levels of specific IgG antibody seem to correlate with IgE production. This evidence is important in understanding the development of human allergy. It is important to consider the history of allergy in the family when evaluating the children's allergic condition. But it may be that some food or other antigen is capable of stimulating the B-cell to initiate specific IgG antibody production, and then this antibody influences the allergic condition.

Although the function of specific IgG antibody is still unclear, high specific IgG antibody is one of the parameters to be considered when eliminating food or other antigens.

Many pediatric allergists are interested in the prevention of allergy and advise pregnant mothers about their daily lifestyle. At this point, pregnant mothers are often told not to consume egg and milk in late pregnancy, but this theory is also unreliable [12].

From our data we conclude that cord blood specific IgG antibody measurement is important in determining the newborn babies' allergic status. The operation room is very busy at delivery time, but we must have access to cord blood to further our clinical studies. In my clinic, we check not only specific IgE antibody, but also IgG antibody in those who show symptoms of allergy. IgG is also a useful indicator of allergic status.

References

1. Inoue, K., T. Ohtani, Y. Iikura, M. Arai, N. Kitami, and H. Inui. 1983. Clinical epidemiology of bronchial asthma in children report. Jap. J. Allergology. 32: 138–148.
2. Miller, D. L., T. Hirvonen, and D. Gitlin. 1973. Synthesis of IgE by the human conceptus. J. Allergy Clin. Immunol. 52: 182–188.
3. Kaufman, H. 1971. Allergy in the newborn: Skin test reactions confirmed by the Prausnitz-Küstner test at birth. Clinical Allergy 1: 363–367.
4. Iikura, Y., T. Nagakura, K. Akimoto, J. Iwahara, and T. Uekusa. 1987. Study of specific IgE, IgG and IgG4 antibody to egg white, milk, and soybean in children with atopic dermatitis. Jap. J. Allergology 36: 921–930.
5. Vandenplas, Y., and Sacre, L. 1986. Influence of neonatal serum IgE concentration, family history and diet on the incidence of cow's milk allergy. Eur. J. Pediatr. 145: 493–495.
6. Croner, S., N.-I. M. Kjellman, B. Eriksson, and A. Roth. 1982. IgE screening in 1701 newborn infants and the development of atopic disease during infancy. Archives of Disease in Childhood 57: 364–368.
7. Akimoto, K., A. Akazawa, and Y. Iikura. 1987. Clinical research of antigen specific IgE, IgG and IgG4 antibodies both in the serum of pregnant mothers and in their cord blood. Jap. J. Ped. Allergy and Clin. Immunol. 1: 40–45.
8. Creticos, P. S., T. E. Van Meter, and M. R. Mardiney. 1984. Dose response of IgE and IgG antibodies during ragweed immunotherapy. J. Allergy Clin. Immunol. 73: 94–104.

9. Cohen, G. A., G. Hartman, R. N. Hamburger, and R. D. O'Conner. 1985. Severe anemia and chronic bronchitis associated with a markedly elevated specific IgG to cow's milk protein. Ann. Allergy. 55: 38–40.

10. Hill, D. J., M. A. Fier, M. J. Shelton, and E. S. Hosking. 1986. Manifestations of milk allergy in infancy: Clinical and immunologic findings. J. Pediatr. 109: 270–276.

11. Fallstrom, S. P., Ahlstedt, S., and L. A. Hanson. 1978. Specific antibodies in infants with gastrointestinal intolerance to cow's milk protein. Arch. Allergy Immunol. 56: 97–103.

12. Falth-Magnusson, K., and N.-I. M. Kjellman. 1987. Development of atopic disease in babies whose mothers were receiving exclusion diet during pregnancy—A randomized study. J. Allergy Clin. Immunol. 80: 869–875.

Viral Infections and the Possible Role of Molecular Mimicry in Allergy

Oscar L. Frick*

Respiratory tract viral infections act as triggers for attacks of asthma and has been documented for the last 20 years. The two definitive studies were by McIntosh et al. [1] and Minor et al. [2]. In the McIntosh study, viral culture or rising antibody titers of proven respiratory viral infections, especially respiratory syncytial virus and parainfluenza, occurred in 42% (58/139) wheezing episodes in 32 preschool asthmatic children. Similarly, proven viral respiratory infections, especially rhinovirus and influenza A, precipitated wheezing attacks in 39% (24/61) in 16 school-age (3–11 years) non-atopic asthmatic children. Furthermore, in Henderson's study [3], proven *Mycoplasma pneumoniae* and other respiratory viruses were responsible for 21% of wheezing attacks in a wider age-range of children.

Suggested mechanisms for virus infections causing asthmatic attacks have involved viral-induced denudation (stripping off) of the respiratory epithelium to expose irritant cough receptors that induce a vagal reflex bronchoconstriction. Partial loss of the epithelial barrier would also facilitate increased allergen absorption to trigger subepithelial mast cells to release mediators. Furthermore, loss of epithelium would decrease the amount of epithelial relaxing factor or relaxin available to counteract or relieve bronchoconstriction. Busse [4] has beautifully demonstrated an impaired β-adrenergic responsiveness in neutrophils' release of granular contents such as β-glucuronidase in the presence of viruses or interferon. Viral infections blocked β-adrenergic responsiveness causing autonomic imbalance in bronchial smooth muscles and mast cells. Ragweed-induced mediator release from sensitized human basophils was markedly augmented by viruses or interferon in the medium [5]. These asthma-triggering aspects of viral respiratory infections are so well-known that we shall elaborate no further on this important theme.

However, I would like to turn to the possibility that viral infections affect cells of the respiratory and gastrointestinal tracts and the immune system that may have special effects in allergic individuals, such effects on β-adrenergic receptors, intestinal mucosa, and lymphocytes making IgE antibodies.

Molecular biology techniques are proving of great help in defining specific viral proteins and polypeptides, and by the use of suitable mutant strains, the diverse functions of these viral components are being elucidated. Viral infections require the virus to enter the host and multiply in the host tissues, spread from the site of entry into adjacent tissues or disseminate in blood or lymph to distant tissues, possibly with a special tropism for a particular viral strain, and finally overcome the host's defenses. The reoviruses have been especially useful as a prototype model virus for such studies [6].

Reoviruses or "respiratory enteric orphan virus" inhabit the respiratory and intestinal tracts, but the early ones identified caused no disease. The special reovirus-ring or orbivirus causes Colorado tick fever in campers and lumbermen from wood ticks, *Dermacenter andersoni*; it causes a 3–6 day fever, severe muscle pain in back and legs, and retroorbital pain and headache. Much more common are the wheel-like rotaviruses, which are the major cause of infectious infantile diarrhea and responsible annually for thousands of deaths in infants in Third World countries, such as in the current Bangladesh post-flood disaster. Ubiquitous in every species of domestic animal, it causes diarrhea or "scours" in the young. Five human serotypes have been identified, two of which occur also in dogs and pigs. In children, rotaviruses cause vomiting, then diarrhea, dehydration, and finally death if lost fluids are not replaced.

Reovirus infections occur in children and are almost universal; 80% have anti-reovirus anti-

---

*   University of California, San Francisco, Department of Pediatrics, San Francisco, CA, USA.

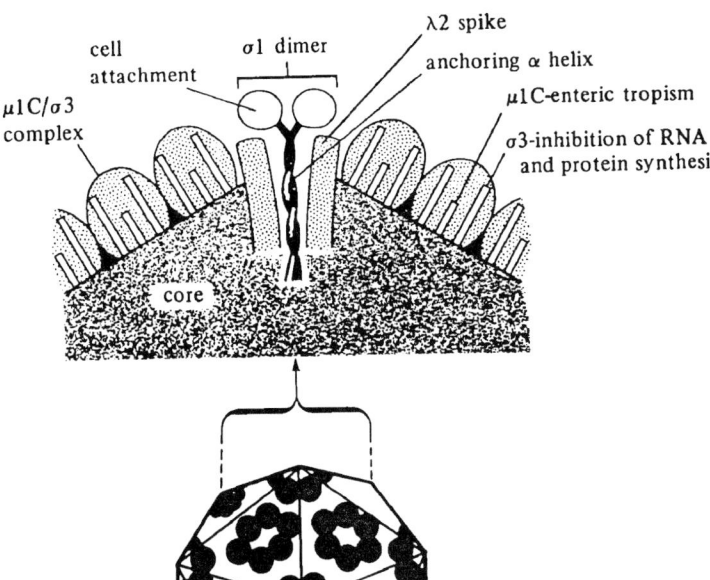

Figure 1. The location in the reovirus capsid of the poly-peptides that play major roles in virulence. σ1 is located at the vertices of the icosahedron and consists of two components: a globular dimer at the surface, which is responsible for hemagglutination and cell attachment, and an α-helical region that anchors the hemagglutinin by interaction with the λ2 spike protein, μ1c and σ3 are associated with each other on the surfaces of the icosahedral capsid. (Modified from R. Basel-Duby et al. and reprinted by permission from *Nature* (London) 1985, 314: 421.)

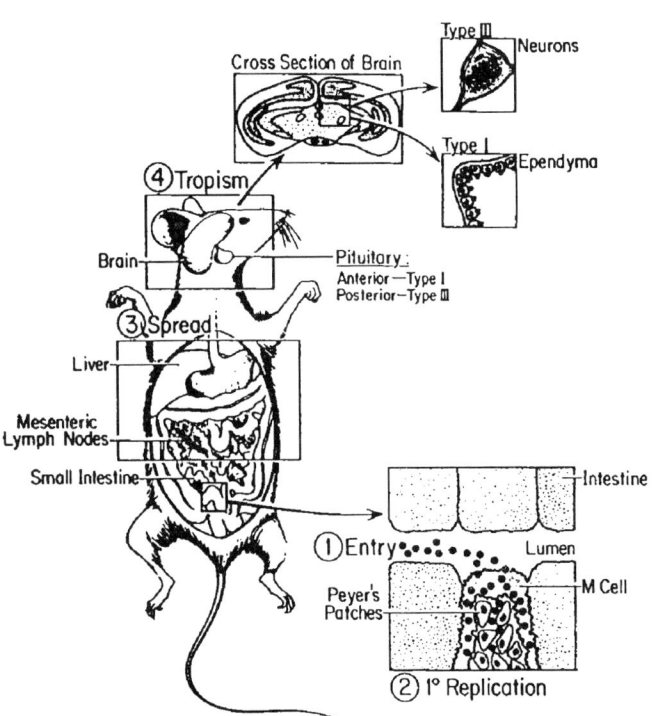

Figure 2. Stages of reovirus infection. Reovirus enters the mouse host through the gastrointestinal tract, penetrates the intestinal epithelium through Peyer's patches, and spreads to the brain. Type 1 reovirus is localized in ependymal cells, and type 3 reovirus in neuronal cells. (Reprinted by permission from A. H. Sharpe and B. N. Fields (1985). *New England Journal of Medicine*, 321: 486.)

bodies by age 16. They cause mild respiratory and gastrointestinal infections, and perhaps biliary atresia in neonates [7], but few or no clinical symptoms in adults. There are three serotypes: reovirus types 1, 2, 3 with important molecular differences, especially in newborn mice which can be infected by all three serotypes. Type 1 causes hydrocephalus and type 3 causes acute and fatal encephalitis [6].

Reoviruses are double-stranded RNA spherical virions 60–80 nm that consist of two icosahedral capsids and a core [8]. The double-stranded RNA genome has 10 segments grouped in large (L 1, 2, 3), medium (M 1, 2, 3), and small (S 1, 2, 3, 4) sizes. Each RNA segment transcribes a different polypeptide or protein also grouped into large (lambda 1, 2, 3), medium (mu 1, 2, 3), and small (sigma 1, 2, 3, 4), which appear sequentially, sigmas first at 2–4 h to peak at 4–6 h, then mu, and finally lambda in the mature viral genome RNA. The products of these reovirus genes have been isolated and their functions determined by studying reassortment viral mutants.

Three genes (S 1, M 2, and S 4) (Figure 1) code for polypeptides on the outer capsid, each of which has a part in determining virulence: gene S 1 codes for sigma 1 or hemagglutinin responsible for attachment and cell tropism; gene M 2 codes for protein ulc, which determines sensitivity or resistance to chymotrypsin and growth in intestine, while gene S 4 codes for peptide sigma 3 that inhibits host RNA and protein synthesis to permit viral latency. Specific attenuated mutants exhibit various specific functional changes, such as persistent long term infection secondary to changes in sigma 3; decreased capacity to grow in intestine from changes in ulc and also loss of T-suppressor cell stimulation; and changes in sigma 1 causes loss of neurovirulence and altered antibodies and cytotoxic lymphocyte (CTL) responses of host lymphocytes.

The stages of reovirus pathogenesis (Figure 2) are determined by these genes and polypeptides. Reovirus in young mice enters through M-cells of Peyer's patches in intestine and spreads via mesenteric lymph nodes, then spreads further via circulating lymphocytes to the brain and pituitary gland. In the brain, reovirus type 1 attaches to ependymal cells causing hydrocephalus, and type 3 goes to neurons to cause encephalitis and death. Type 1 goes to anterior pituitary, while type 3 goes to posterior pituitary [6].

In newborn mice fed reoviruses, type 1 crosses the intestinal mucosa via the M-cells of Peyer's patches and grow well in intestinal tissues, whereas type 3 does not grow well. The ability of reovirus type 1 to grow depends upon its M 2 gene encoding for ulc capsid polypeptide which confers resistance to chymotrypsin which is abundant in the upper ileum. Type 1 grows well in in vitro cultures, in the presence of chymotrypsin, whereas type 3 loses its infectivity; type 3 apparently has a different M 2 gene and product. Rotaviruses localize in intestinal cells causing local inflammation and diarrhea. Reoviruses do not localize, but spread from Peyer's patches to mesenteric nodes via lymphocytes. The S 1 gene coding for sigma 1 hemagglutinin determines

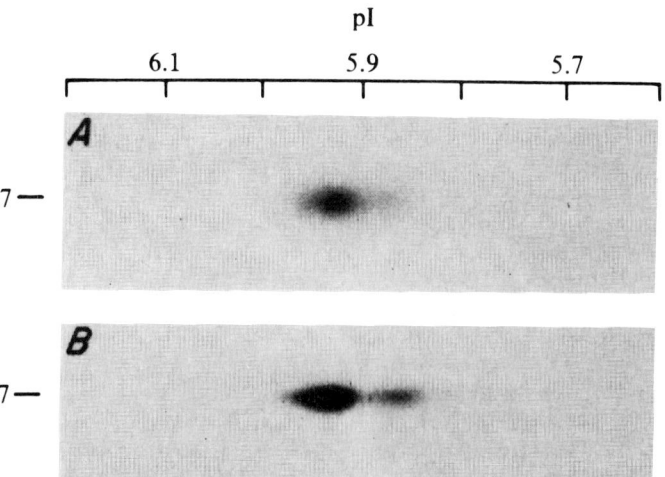

pl

Figure 3. Two-dimensional gel electrophoresis of immunoprecipitated reovirus type 3 receptor and β-adrenergic receptor. (A) Reovirus receptor isolated from murine thymoma R 1.1 cells, (B) β-adrenergic receptor affinity-purified from calf lung. Both receptors show a molecular mass of 67 KDa and a PI of 5.8–6.0. (Reprinted by permission from M. S. Co et al. (1985). *Proc. Natl. Acad. Sci. USA* 82: 5315.)

the ability of both types 1 and 3 reoviruses to spread to mesenteric nodes and subsequent spread by lymphocytes to the central nervous system (CNS). Measles, poliomyelitis, and adenoviruses also disseminate from lymph nodes to distant tissue sites via lymphocytes and macrophages.

In CNS, the S 1 gene of type 3 reovirus makes sigma 1 polypeptide which selects neurons as target cells causing acute and fatal encephalitis in newborn mice. Type 1 reovirus has tropism for ependymal cells by its S 1 gene encoding for sigma 1 polypeptide to cause hydrocephalus. Similarly, in pituitary gland, reoviruses types 1 and 3 affect anterior and posterior lobes, respectively. Type 1 directed by its sigma 1 peptide infects the anterior pituitary growth-hormone-producing cells to cause a runting syndrome [9]. Furthermore, Type 1 S 1 gene in SJL/3 mice causes poly-autoantibody formation to insulin in pancreas resulting in diabetes mellitus and other polyendocrinopathies. This sigma 1 peptide causes recognition and binding to cell surface receptors.

The type 3 reovirus 67 kd receptor glycoprotein has been isolated, cloned, and sequenced [10]. This was done by raising an anti-anti-hemagglutinin idiotype (Ab 2) antibody that substituted for the reovirus type 3 itself. Reovirus type 3 does not bind to cytotoxic T-cells, but prefers suppressor T-cells,. and loss of suppressor signals may lead to virus-induced overproduction of autoantibodies. Therefore, the single S 1 segment coding for sigma 1 determines type 3 specificity for neurons, T-cells, post-pituitary cells, and other non-immune cells, so that this single epitope sigma 1 peptide is responsible for cell tropism, disease pattern, and receptor recognition of reovirus.

Molecular mimicry by viruses is an intriguing concept proposed by Oldstone [11] that may bear upon expression of allergic reactions or even possibly on immune regulation, especially of the IgE antibody system. The most familiar example is HIV (AIDS virus) that binds to T4 protein receptor of T-helper lymphocytes and interferes with the immunologic functions and destroys such T-helper cells. Co et al. [12] demonstrated a physicochemical and functional identity between the β_2-adrenergic receptors in calf lung cells and purified receptors for reovirus type 3 from mouse thymus cell line (Figure 3, Table 1).

Table 1. Binding of ^{125}I-labeled reovirus and β-adrenergic receptors to anti-idiotypic antibodies.

Receptor	Anti-idiotype cpm	Normal Ig, cpm
Reovirus	3530	121
β-adrenergic	3018	250

Lysate from surface-labeled R1.1 cells and labeled affinity-purified β-adrenergic receptor from calf lung were each incubated with 10 μg of anti-idiotypic antibodies or normal immunoglobulins for 2 h at room temperature. The immune complexes were recovered subsequently by Sepharose-protein A and washed extensively. The beads were then assayed for radioactivity in a γ counter. Reprinted by permission from [12].

They also isolated and purified β-adrenergic receptors from calf lung epithelial cells' solubilized membrane by acebutolol affinity column and elution with alprenolol and further purified by HPLC. Such isolated β-adrenergic receptors bound [125I] iodohydroxybenzylpindolol (IHYP) in a dose/response manner. This binding was inhibited 90% by 1 mM isoproterenol (30' at 37°C).

The anti-idiotype antibody, substituting for reovirus 3, bound equally well to the purified reovirus receptor and the purified β-adrenergic receptor, whereas with normal rabbit immunoglobulin, only background binding occurred. On two-dimensional gel electrophoresis immunoprecipitation, both receptors showed identical patterns with 67 Kd and pI 5.8–6.0. After partial trypsin-digestion, both proteins fragmented to give a major 50 Kd band and two minor bands at 57 Kd and 25 Kd showing essentially identical structures. Finally, ^{125}I-HYP bound to the immunoprecipitated reovirus receptor, and this binding too was inhibited 90% if pretreated with 1 mM isoproterenol to the same degree that isolated purified β-adrenergic receptor bound ^{125}I-HYP and was inhibited by isoproterenol.

The pathophysiologic consequences of this molecular mimicry of reovirus and β-agonist binding is under investigation, so one can only speculate at this point in terms of its possible implication in asthma. Reoviruses could either (1) occupy the β-adrenergic receptors completely and prevent adenylated cyclase activity in increasing the muscle relaxing cAMP, thus, exacerbating asthma; or (2) reovirus could substitute for the β-adrenergic agonist and increase cAMP for muscle relaxation or possibly block the initial cyclic AMP-dependent protein kinase activation for IgE-dependent receptor mediator release. Furthermore, it is quite conceivable that molecular mimicry by certain viruses might affect IgE high affinity receptor I (Fcε-R I) on mast cells directly, or upon the IgE-low affinity receptors (Fcε-R II) in regulatory T-lymphocytes, monocytes, and eosinophils. While reoviruses are uncommon, the closely related rotavirus-induced infantile diarrhea is very common and could, conceivably, trigger asthma and mediator release or increased IgE antibody production in susceptible infants.

In this context, one could speculate that if rotaviruses have a similar molecular mimicry sequence of its receptor to β-adrenergic receptor, stimulation of β-adrenergic receptors by rotaviruses in the intestine could stimulate adenylate cyclase to produce large amounts of cyclic AMP in the intestinal mucosa, thus, simulating the action of cholera toxin [13] in producing a profuse diarrhea, dehydration, and death in infants.

Reoviruses also alter host cells. Type 3 through its sigma 1 peptide inhibits cellular DNA synthesis in mouse L cells. Type 2 reovirus through its S 4 gene inhibits the cells' RNA and protein synthesis [6]. The 3 reovirus types alter cytoskeleton by disrupting and reorganizing the vimentin subclass of intermediate filaments, but sparing microtubules and microfilaments [14]. Reovirus inclusion-bearing monkey kidney CV-1 cells have disrupted intermediate filament organization with vimentin antibody staining within the viral inclusions. At the EM level, these inclusions had kinky vimentin filaments. This disruption of intermediate filaments by reovirus may be related to the virus' ability to inhibit host protein synthesis via its sigma 3 polypeptide. The reovirus then reorganizes vimentin filaments forming unique viral structures of the "viral factory." The intermediate filaments are also involved in the distribution of mitochondria, which in reovirus infected cells are aggregated around the nucleus and occasionally at the cell surface. This suggests that the intermediate filament's vimentin may play a major role in replication and assembly of reoviruses.

In a probably similar manner, Carson et al. [15] showed that a number of human respiratory viruses cause an acute microtubule disorganization in cilia in the nasal epithelium of children with URIs. In a child with influenza Type B, this shows additions to the central pair of microtubules with disorganization in direction of ciliary beating patterns. In an Adenovirus type 1 infection, there were additional peripheral microtubules. These abnormal ciliary patterns occurred in acute viral infections, but returned to normal in 6–10 weeks post-infection. Respiratory viruses responsible for these ciliary disruptions included influenza A and B, parainfluenzae, adenovirus, respiratory syncytial virus (RSV), and herpes simplex. Whether such acquired ciliary defects persist with chronic respiratory viral infections is still an open question.

Returning again to reovirus genomes, the L 1 gene codes for large 140 kd lambda 2 core protein which has a surface spike adjacent to sigma 1 protein [6]. Reoviruses are generally lytic viruses, but in mouse L-cells cultures, mutants generated by the L 2 gene, which is part of the viral core transcriptase, initiate the S 4 gene and its 34 kd sigma 3 product to inhibit the host cell's RNA and protein synthesis which causes persistent infection; this is probably maintained through the sigma 1 gene and its receptor binding function.

In summary of this reovirus model, the 10 separate genomal double-stranded RNA segments determine: the ability of the virus to penetrate intestinal mucosa via M cells and survive in chymotrypsin by ulc protein; cell tropism via S 1 gene and sigma 1 protein for neurons or ependymal cells in CNS or anterior or posterior pituitary and T-suppressor cells, later resulting in autoantibody produced polyendocrinopathies, such as diabetes, and cytoskeletal changes; and finally via L 2 gene - core lambda 2 protein induces S 4 gene to establish persistent non-lytic infection. In a similar manner, genomes and gene products of other viruses are being cloned, sequenced, and polypeptides are analyzed for molecular mimicry.

About a decade ago, we [16] reported on a prospective study of infants born into high allergic risk families and found that viral respiratory infections, especially RSV and parainfluenza, immediately preceded the onset of IgE-allergic antibody sensitization to environmental and dietary antigens and allergic symptoms, as in this child. Subsequently, we [17] were able to confirm that viral infections followed by antigen exposure in puppies lead to IgE antibody formation while non-infected littermates made no IgE antibodies. Later these dogs had airway hyperreactivity and late phase reactions after pollen inhalation (18).

Firer at al. [19] took our lead in trying to document past rotaviral infections in children with cow's milk allergy. they were unable to find elevated anti-rotavirus antibodies in children with immediate IgE reactions to cow's milk challenge. However, children with delayed onset 1–24 h "non-IgE reactions" to cow's milk did have significantly higher titers of rotavirus antibodies; they suggested that rotavirus infection causes major damage to the intestinal mucosa leading to increased permeability and increased absorption of milk proteins to stimulate IgM and IgA antibodies which upon subsequent challenge with milk caused late onset milk-induced gastroenteropathy. However, 5/15 of their immediate milk challenge positive children did have elevated rotavirus antibodies and elevated IgE antibodies to cow's milk;2 had the highest IgE antibodies to milk, so that rotavirus infections could still play a role in IgE sensitization.

Celiac disease symptoms are aggravated by ingestion of wheat gluten fraction, A-gliadin [19]. The ElB protein of Adenovirus Ad-12 shares an 8 amino acid sequence with A-gliadin and antibodies directed against ElB cross-react with A-gliadin. In celiac patients, 89% carried Ad-12 vs 17% in controls, but not closely related Ad-18 or ECHO 11. This suggests that Adeno Ad-12 infection might sensitize the patient who forms IgA antibodies, and that, subsequently, these react with the recognized octapeptide in A-gliadin—thus, another example of viral molecular mimicry.

Respiratory syncytial virus genome and its cloned viral genes and their products are being isolated. Like reoviruses, the single-stranded RNA-RSV genome codes for at least 10 proteins [20]. The two best studied are two envelope glycoproteins of 90 kd and 70 kd. The 90 kd G glycoprotein is heavily glycosylated and acts as attachment protein to initiate RSV infection. The 70 kd fusion F protein mediates penetration of the virus and causes cell-to-cell spread via syncytia formation. Young infants 1–8 months of age had poor responses to F fusion protein and could not neutralize them [21], but they had good IgG antibodies to G-protein, presumably passively from the mother. This may account for the susceptibility of young infants to the syncytial spreading of RSV caused by F proteins. These and other RSV proteins are being studied in order to develop live attenuated vaccines.

Chronic low-grade viral infections have been associated with marked coincidence with atopy. Most notable is chronic infectious mononucleosis syndrome with serologic evidence of chronic active EBV infection associated with chronic fatigue and lassitude. The role of EBV in this syndrome is still not established; some suggest that other viruses may be involved. However, there is a high incidence of atopic symptoms in such patients [22]. Recently, Szczeklik [23] has proposed a hypothesis that aspirin-induced asthma is a viral disease. He suggests that in response to a viral infection, even long after initial exposure, the body responds with viral-specific cytotoxic T-lymphocytes. However, their activity is suppressed by alveolar macrophages that produce PGE2. Aspirin and other cyclo-oxygenase analgesics block PGE2 production that permits these CTLs to attack the virus-infected respiratory epithelial target cells. In this process, lysosomal enzymes, mediators, and toxic oxygen radicals precipitate asthmatic attacks. In such patients, asthma is persistent due to chronic viral infection.

In summary, molecular biologic technology is helping to define specific viral components with function. The reovirus model prototype may be useful in defining actions, especially molecular mimicry for normal physiologic components, such as the β-adrenergic receptor and immune regulatory lymphocytes which have important implications for understanding pathophysiology of asthma and atopy.

References

1. McIntosh K., E. F. Ellis, L. S. Hoffman et al. 1973. The association of viral   in young asthmatic children. J. Pediatr. 82: 578.
2. Minor, T. E., E. D. Dick, A. N. DeMeo et al. 1974. Viruses as precipitants of asthmatic attacks in children. J.A.M.A. 227: 292.
3. Henderson, F. W., W. A. Clyde,Jr., A. M. Collier A.M. et al. 1979. The etiology and epidemiologic spectrum of bronchiolitis in pediatric practice. J. Pediatr. 95: 183.

309

4. Busse, W. W. 1977. Decreased granulocyte response to isoproterenol in asthma during upper respiratory infections. Am. Rev. Respir. Dis. 115: 783.

5. Ida, S., J. J. Hooks, R. P. Siraganian, and A. L. Notkins. 1977. Enhancement of IgE mediated histamine release from human blood basophil by viruses: Role of interferon. J. Exp. Med. 145: 892.

6. Sharpe, A. H., and B. N. Fields. 1985. Pathogenesis of viral infections: Basic concepts derived from the reovirus model. N. Engl. J. Med. 312: 486.

7. Bangaru, B., R. Morecki, J. H. Glaser et al. 1980. Comparative studies of biliary atresia in the human newborn and reovirus-induced cholangitis in weanling mice. Lab. Invest. 43: 456.

8. White, D. O., and F. J. Fenner. Viral genetics and evolution. In: Medical Virology. New York: Academic Press, p. 91.

9. Onodera, T., A. Toniolo, U. R. Ray et al. 1981. Virus-induced diabetes mellitus. XX. Polyendocrinopathy and autoimmunity. J. Exp. Med. 153: 1457.

10. Co, M. S., G. N. Gaulton, B. N.Fields, and M. I. Greene. 1985. Isolation and biochemical characterization of the mammalian reovirus type 3 cell-surface receptor. Proc. Natl. Acad. Sci. USA 82: 1494.

11. Oldstone, M. B. A., and A. L. Notkins. 1986. Molecular mimicry.In: Concepts in viral pathogenesis II. New York: Springer-Verlag, p. 198. and ibid. 1987. Molecular mimicry and autoimmune disease. Cell 50: 819.

12. Co, M. S., G. N. Gaulton, A. Tominaga et al. 1985. Structural similarities between the mammalian B-adrenergic and reovirus type 3 receptors. Proc. Natl. Acad. Sci. USA 82: 5315.

13. Gilman, A. G. 1987. G proteins: Transducers of receptor-generated signals. Ann. Rev. Biochem. 56: 615.

14. Sharpe, A. H., L. B. Chen, and B. N. Fields. 1982. The interaction of mammalian reoviruses with the cytoskeleton of monkey kidney CV-1 cells. Virology 120: 399.

15. Carson, J. L.,A. M. Collier, S. H. Shih-Chin. 1985. Acquired ciliary defects in nasal epithelium of children with acute viral upper respiratory infections. N. Engl. J. Med. 312: 463.

16. Frick, O. L., D. F. German, and J. Mills. 1979. Development of allergy in children: Association with virus infections. J. Allergy Clin. Immunol. 63: 228.

17. Frick, O. L., and D. L. Brooks. 1984. Immunoglobulin E antibodies to pollen in dogs augmented in dogs by virus vaccines. Am. J. Vet Res. 44:.440.

18. Chung, K. F., A. B. Becker, S. C. Lazarus et al. 1985. Antigen-induced airway hyperresponsiveness and pulmonary inflammation in allergic dogs. J. Appl. Physiol. 58: 1347.

19. Firer, M. A., C. S. Hosking, and D. J. Hill. 1988. Possible role for rotavirus in the development of cow's milk enteropathy in infants. Clin. Allergy 18: 53.

20. Kagnoff, M. F., R. K. Austin, J. J. Hubert et al. 1984. Possible role for a human adenovirus in the pathogenesis of celiac disease. J. Exp. Med. 160: 1544.

21. Murphy, B. R., D. W. Alling, M. H. Snyder et al. 1986. Effect of age and preexisting antibody on serum antibody response of infants and children to the F and G glycoproteins during respiratory syncytial virus infection. J. Clin. Microbiol. 24: 894.

22. Olson, G. B., M. N. Kanaan, G. M. Gersuk et al. 1986. Correlation between allergy and persistent Epstein-Barr virus infections in chronic-active Epstein-Barr virus-infected patients. J. Allergy Clin. Immunol. 78: 308.

23. Szczeklik, A. 1988. Aspirin-induced asthma as a viral disease. Clin. Allergy 18: 15.

An Integrative View of Cells and Mediators in Skin

*Georg Stingl**

Bone marrow-derived antigen-presenting cells residing in the epidermis (= Langerhans cells), keratinocytes, epidermal (and dermal) T cells, and draining peripheral lymph nodes have been proposed by Streilein to form collectively an integrated system of skin-associated lymphoid tissues (SALT) which provide the skin with unique immune surveillance mechanisms [46]. While in the past the primary research goal was to explore the phenotypic and functional properties of the various constituents of SALT, major emphasis is now given to the elucidation of the mutual influences between the various (immune) cells of the epidermis and the skin in general. It is likely that the adequate functioning of each of the subpopulations is dependent upon a delicately balanced signal exchange between them. Disturbance of this equilibrium by exogenous (e.g., physicochemical agents, microorganisms) and/or endogenous (e.g., neoantigens) noxious agents may result either in the initiation of effective host defense mechanisms ultimately leading to the elimination of the pathogen or, alternatively, in the functional impairment of the epidermal immune system, resulting in the uncontrolled spread of infectious and/or neoplastic processes affecting the skin.

When, in the not-so-distant past, the skin was discussed in the context of immunological reactions, it was generally viewed as a target for immune-mediated injury. Recent advances have radically changed this concept of an exclusively passive role in immune-mediated reactions, in that there is now ample evidence that the skin, in particular the epidermis, functions not only as a physicochemical, but also as an immunological barrier by initiating immune responses against both exogenous pathogens and neoantigens generated in this tissue itself. The generation of the immune response is dependent on three major requirements [1]:

— accessory cells that are capable of antigen uptake and processing (which frequently requires antigen degradation and association with histocompatibility antigens) followed by the presentation of the antigen to lymphocyte;

— T cells that proliferate in response to antigenic signals mostly, though not necessarily, delivered by antigen-presenting cells;

— cytokines that are either part of or amplify such signals.

The epidermis contains all these elements, and we now have good evidence that they are operative both in in vitro models and in vivo. The present review therefore focuses on this issue and singles out antigen-presenting Langerhans cells, some of the immune modulatory cytokines produced by keratinocytes, and a population of intraepidermal T lymphocytes. The attempt is made to integrate this knowledge into the concept of the epidermis as an immune organ.

Langerhans Cells

Langerhans cells (LC) are dendritic cells of bone marrow derivation that reside mainly within stratified squamous epithelia, but have also been shown to occur in mesenchymal tissues such as the dermis and lymph nodes [2]. In the epidermis, they are usually located at a suprabasal level and constitute approximately 3–4% of all epidermal cells. LC visualization at the light microscopic level requires the use of appropriate histochemical and/or immuno-labeling techniques (Figure 1a, Table 1). Ultrastructurally, LC display unique trilaminar cytoplasmic organelles (Birbeck granules) that allow their identification.

* Division of Cutaneous Immunobiology, Department of Dermatology I, University of Vienna Medical School, Vienna, Austria.
This work was supported in part by a grant from the Bürgermeisterfonds der Stadt Wien. *Acknowledgement:* I thank Mrs. Renate Kopp for carefully typing this manuscript.

311

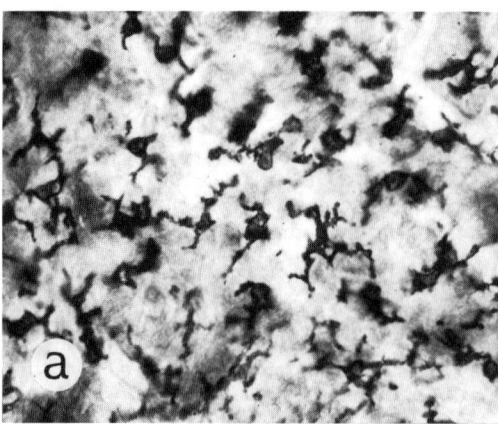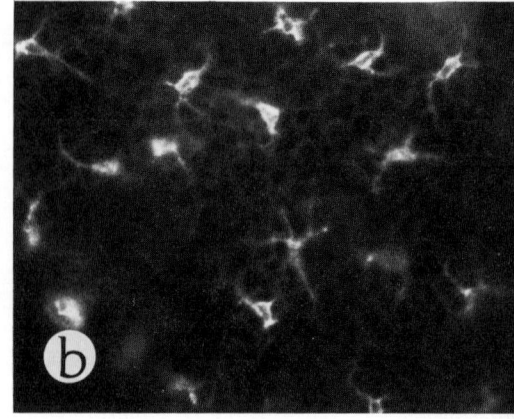

Figure 1. Visualization of bone marrow-derived dendritic epidermal cells within sheet preparations of murine epidermis. (a) Langerhans cells demonstrated histochemically by the ADPase technique. (b) Thy-1$^+$ dendritic epidermal cells demonstrated by using an anti-Thy-1 monoclonal antibody in an indirect immunofluorescence technique.

Adenosine tri(d9)phosphatase	Fc-IgG receptors	
Nonspecific esterase	Receptors for complement components	
	CD1a antigens (man)	
Birbeck granules		
CD45 antigen (= common leukocyte antigen)	CD4 antigens (man)	
MHC class I antigens	F4/80 antigens (mouse)	
MHC class II antigens	NLDC-145 antigens (mouse)	

Table 1. Phenotypic features of resident epidermal Langerhans cells.

LC as Immunocytes

LC carry receptors for the Fc portion of IgG and for complement components and display a number of other phenotypic markers characteristic of "established" immune cells [3] (Table 1). From a functional viewpoint, the expression of major histocompatibility complex (MHC)-induced alloantigens by LC is of utmost importance.

Whereas all epidermal cell populations (with the possible exception of melanocytes) bear class I alloantigens, LC are the only cells in normal epidermis that synthesize and express class II (Ia) alloantigens [3]. These are encoded for by immune response genes of the I region of the MHC which control the capacity to respond to certain defined synthetic antigens, proteins, and alloantigens. In humans, they are encoded for by the HLA-DR/-DQ/-DP loci, in the mouse by the I-A/-E subregion of the I region genes. The crucial importance of these antigens for the antigen-presenting capacity of

LC is discussed further below.

It should be emphasized that the phenotype of LC is not a stable trait, but rather depends upon their state of maturation and differentiation. This issue has been best investigated in the mouse system, though preliminary evidence indicates that human LC also undergo phenotypic changes during their life cycle.

Although murine LC enter the epidermis at day 16 to 17 of gestation, it is not until birth that at least some of them start to express class II antigens; this process is not completed until the second week of life [4]. In the adult animal, resident murine LC share many phenotypic features with mononuclear phagocytes (MP), but, on the other hand, also display certain characteristics of non-lymphoid dendritic cells (DC), which are known to be potent stimulators of both naive and sensitized T cells [5]. MP-like features of resident LC include the expression of Fc-IgG and complement receptors, adenosine triphosphatase (ATP-ase) and esterase activity and the reactivity with the monoclonal antibody F4/80, which is thought to be a selective marker for murine MP [6]. In contrast to MP and in common with DC, LC have a dendritic shape, adhere poorly to glass or plastic surfaces, lack the capacity of avid phagocytosis, and react with the monoclonal antibody NLDC-145 considered to be a marker for DC [7]. On the basis of these findings, it is tempting to speculate about an ontogenetic link between MP and DC, with LC being the bridge. When LC are monitored in epidermal cell cultures, profound changes are observed in the LC phenotype already 24 to 48 h after isolation of epidermal cells. While their MP-like features as well as their Birbeck granules gradually disappear, their class II and also class I antigenic density dramatically increases [8]; thus, cultured LC greatly resemble cells of the DC system. Recent evidence exists that granulocyte/macrophage colony-stimulating factor (GM-CSF) and interleukin 1 (IL-1) are, at least partly, responsible for the changes LC undergo in tissue culture [9]. Interestingly enough, keratinocytes have been shown to be a source of both cytokines [3, 10].

In vitro Functions of LC

It has long been established that antigen recognition by resting T lymphocytes requires an initial interaction of these antigens with an MP-like cell, and that the functional interaction between antigen-exposed MP and T lymphocyte, which finally results in marked T cell activation, is regulated by gene products encoded for by the I region of the MHC [11]. This functional property of MP is known as antigen-presentation function. It appears that antigen presentation is not a function confined to MP, but rather a feature of many Ia-bearing cells, e.g., DC and B lymphocytes.

Using strategies similar to those successfully employed to elucidate the T cell-activating properties of MP, several groups of investigators have clearly shown that epidermal cells can promote antigen-specific activation of sensitized and resting T cells, and that this functional property of epidermal cells is critically linked to the presence of Ia-bearing LC [3, 8, 12, 13, 14, 15]. Owing to the lack of appropriate techniques for Lc purification, it could not be decided for quite some time whether the antigen presentation function of LC-containing epidermal cells resided in the LC population alone or required the presence of other epidermal cells. Recent experiments by Inaba et al. [16] have addressed this issue and showed that LC purified from freshly isolated epidermal cell suspensions were potent stimulators of primed, but not of resting T cells. In contrast, LC purified from 72 h-cultured epidermal cells (thus having been exposed to keratinocyte-derived GM-CSF and IL-1) evoked a vigorous immune response in both primed and resting T cells and, thus functionally resembled nonlymphoid DC. Although it is not clear from these in vitro experiments whether freshly isolated or cultured LC are more representative of the in vivo functions of resident LC, it can be speculated that a transition similar phenotypically and functionally to that of freshly isolated to cultured LC does actually occur in vivo. Following this reasoning, macrophage-like resident LC take up antigen and start to migrate to the regional lymphoid tissues. During this journey, they might change their surface marker repertoire to become DC and, as such, stimulate resting T cells upon arrival in the lymph node. Although speculative, this concept is supported by the demonstration of increased numbers of veiled cells (DC-like cells) in the afferent lymphatics after epicutaneous sensitization [17].

Another important functional property of LC was disclosed by the finding that LC containing no foreign antigens (alloantigens, haptens) on their surface can trigger the generation of cytotoxic T cells against antigenic moieties on cells that, by themselves are unable to induce activation of resting purified T cells [18]. This may indicate that LC play a key role in the generation of a protective effector T cell response toward a variety of antigens (alloantigens, haptens, differentiation antigens, neoantigens, and tumor antigens) expressed on their epidermal symbionts, namely, keratinocytes and melanocytes.

In vivo Functions of LC

The above discussion has clearly shown that the LC-dependent in vitro functions of epidermal cells known so far affect primarily the afferent limb of the immune response. It is thus reasonable to assume that the major in vivo function of LC is to provide the principal sensitizing signal in skin-induced immune responses.

Immune surveillance function: The epidermis, as the outer-most barrier of the host against the environment, is continuously exposed to a variety of potentially injurious agents, some of which are antigenic. The generation of T cell-dependent immune responses against these exogenous antigens as well as against antigens newly generated within the skin is an effective mechanism to maintain the homeostasis of the host. It is conceivable that LC account for the effective presentation of microbial and tumor-associated antigens (expressed either on LC or on other epidermal symbionts) and thus play a crucial role in the prevention of the spread of microorganisms infecting the skin and also in the elimination of neoplastic clones within the epidermis.

Quantitative and qualitative impairment of the epidermal LC population by ultraviolet radiation [19, 20] or by the human immunodeficiency virus [21, 22] therefore allows the escape of microorganisms and neoplastic cells from detection by the immune system. This results in the devastating spread of mucocutaneous infections (particularly viral and fungal) and in the uncontrolled growth of neoplasms.

It is likely that their role in immune surveillance is the most important biological function of LC. In addition, they appear to be of critical importance in the induction of skin allograft rejection [23, 24] and contact hypersensitivity [25, 26], and probably also in the pathogenesis of various other skin diseases the discussion of which would exceed the scope of this review.

Keratinocytes

Keratinocytes represent the bulk of the epidermal cells and differentiate to form the protective horny layer of the skin surface. It is now clear that these keratinizing cells produce and secrete mediators of both the inflammatory and the immune response including arachidonic acid metabolites and cytokines. Table 2 summarizes the most important keratinocyte-derived cytokines identified so far, including IL-1, contra-IL-1, interleukin 6 (IL-6), the hematopoietic colony-stimulating factors interleukin 3 (IL-3) and GM-CSF, and certain factors governing the growth of both epithelial and

Table 2. Important keratinocyte-derived cytokines (growth factors).

	Reference
Interleukin 1 (IL-1)	10, 27, 28
Contra-IL-1	29
Interleukin 3 (IL-3)	30
Granulocyte/macrophage colony-stimulating factor (GM-CSF)	31
Interleukin 6 (IL-6)	32, 33, 34
Transforming growth factor-alpha (TGF-α)	35
Transforming growth factor-beta (TGF-β)	36
Basic fibroblast growth factor (bFGF)	37

mesenchymal cells such as transforming growth factors (TGF) α and β and basic fibroblast growth factor (BFGF). In order to understand the putative role of keratinocyte cytokines (a) in maintaining the homeostasis of skin (local effects) and even of the entire host organism (system effects), and (b) in the pathogenesis of a large number of inflammatory and immunological skin diseases, it must be kept in mind that —with the possible exception of IL-1—most of these factors are apparently not produced constitutively, but only after the delivering of certain stimuli (e.g., ultraviolet radiation, injury, phorbel ester, cytokines, etc; [10]). Thus, it will be essential to correlate cytokine gene expression in keratinocytes in vivo with localized and/or systemic pathophysiological reaction patterns. These studies will also enable us to assess the mode of action of certain therapeutic regimens (e.g., corticosteroids, retinoids, cyclosporin A, photo-(chemo)therapy) frequently used for the treatment of inflammatory/immunological skin diseases.

Epidermal T Lymphocytes

In the past 2 years, evidence has accumulated that the normal mammalian epidermis harbors a lymphocyte population. These lymphocytes are almost exclusively T lymphocytes as defined by the surface expression of CD3-associated T cell antigen receptors (TCR). To date, two major types of TCR have been identified:

— α/β heterodimers—these are expressed on most peripheral T cells and recognize the nominal antigen in conjunction with MHC-encoded antigens [38];

— γ/δ heterodimers—these are present on early fetal thymocytes and on a minor fraction of adult thymocytes and peripheral blood lymphocytes [39, 40]. Although the occurrence of signal transduction via CD3-TCR γ/δ has been described under experimental conditions, the physiological ligand of this type of TCR is yet unknown.

Murine Epidermal T Lymphocytes

The mouse epidermis harbors a population of basally located CD3$^+$ cells which are Th-1$^+$/asialo-GM-1$^+$/CD5$^-$/CD4$^-$/CD8$^-$/Ia$^-$, highly dendritic in shape, and appear to exclusively express CD3-associated disulfide-linked TCR α/β heterodimers (Figure 1b) [41, 42, 43, 44]. These cells have been referred to as Thy-1$^+$ dendritic epidermal cells (Thy-1$^+$ DEC) or, more recently, as dendritic epidermal T cells (DETC). It appears that the heterogeneity of their TCR repertoire is rather limited and most closely resembles that of day 15 fetal thymocytes [45]. The functional role of these DETC has not yet been clarified, but some evidence exists that administration of an antigen in the context of DETC results in the generation of antigen-specific suppressor cell circuits [26].

Human Epidermal T Lymphocytes

Although several investigators have searched for the human equivalent to the murine DETC, no comparable population has been documented to date in humans. The human epidermis does harbor a population of TCR γ/δ-bearing lymphocytes, but they comprise only a minor subset of intraepidermal T cells, which are predominantly CD1$^-$/CD8$^+$/CD2$^+$/CD3$^+$ with TCR α/β heterodimers. Intraepidermal human T cells are primarily located within the basal layer of the epidermis and the acrosyringial epithelium; their highest density is encountered within the plantar epidermis [Foster et al., in preparation]. Attempts are currently being made to isolate and propagate these cells, which will enable us to define their activation state, their TCR repertoire, and, finally, their functional role in immune responses affecting the skin.

References

1. Nossal, G. J. V. 1987. Current concepts: Immunology. The basic components of the immune system. N. Engl. J. Med. 316: 1320.
2. Wolff, K. 1972. The Langerhans cell. In: Current problems in dermatology, Vol. 4. Basel: Karger, p. 79.
3. Stingl, G., C. Hauser, E. Tschachler, V. Groh, and K. Wolff. 1989. Immune functions of epidermal cells. In: Immune mechanisms in cutaneous disease. D. A. Norris, ed. New York: Marcel Dekker.
4. Romani, N., G. Schuler, and P. Fritsch. 1986. Ontogeny of Ia$^+$ and Thy-1$^+$ leukocytes of murine epidermis. J. Invest. Dermatol. 86: 129.
5. Steinman, R. M., G. Schuler, N. Romani, and G. Kaplan. 1987. Dendritic cells. In: Atlas of blood cells: Function and pathology. D. Zucker-Franklin, M. F. Greaves, C. E. Grossi, A. M. Marmont, eds. Philadelphia: Lea & Febiger, p. 359.
6. Hume, D. A., A. P. Robinson, G. G. MacPherson, and S. Gordon. 1983. The mononuclear phagocyte system of the mouse defined by immunohistochemical localization of antigen F4/80. Relationship between macrophages, Langerhans cells, reticular cells, and dendritic cells in lymphoid and hematopoietic organs. J. Exp. Med. 158: 1522.
7. Kraal, G., M. Breel., M. Janse, and G. Bruin. 1986. Langerhans cells, veiled cells, and interdigitating cells in the mouse recognized by a monoclonal antibody. J. Exp. Med. 163: 981.
8. Schuler, G., and R. M. Steinman. 1985. Murine epidermal Langerhans cells mature into potent immunostimulatory dendritic cells in vitro. J. Exp. Med. 161: 526.
9. Heufler, C., F. Koch, and G. Schuler. 1987. Granulocyte-macrophage colony-stimulating factor and interleukin-1 mediate the maturation of murine epidermal Langerhans cells into potent immunostimulatory dendritic cells. J. Exp. Med. 167: 700.
10. Kupper, T. S. 1988. Interleukin 1 and other human keratinocyte cytokines: Molecular and functional characterization. In: Advances in dermatology, Vol. 3. J. P. Callen, M. V. Dahl, L. E. Golitz, L. A. Schachner, and S. J. Stegman, eds. Chicago-London-Boca Raton: Year Book Medical Publ., p. 293.
11. Shevach, E. M. 1984. Macrophages and other accessory cells. In: Fundamental immunology. W. E. Paul, ed. New York: Raven Press, p. 71.
12. Stingl, G., S. I. Katz, L. Clement, I. Green, and E. M. Shevach. 1978. Immunologic functions of Ia-

bearing epidermal Langerhans cells. J. Immunol. 121: 2005.

13. Braathen, L. R., and E. Thorsby. 1980. Studies on human epidermal Langerhans cells. I. Allo-activating and antigen-presenting capacity. Scand. J. Immunol. 11: 401.

14. Faure, M., A. Frappaz, D. Schmitt, C. Dezutter-Dambuyant, and J. Thivolet. 1984. Role of HLA-DR-bearing Langerhans and epidermal indeterminate cells in the in vitro generation of allo-reactive cytotoxic T cells in man. Cell. Immunol. 83: 271.

15. Hauser, C., and S. I. Katz. 1988. Activation and expansion of hapten- and protein-specific T helper cells from nonsensitized mice. Proc. Natl. Acad. Sci. USA 85: 5625.

16. Inaba, K., G. Schuler, M. D. Witmer, J. Valinsky, B. Atassi, and R. M. Steinman. 1986. Immunologic properties of purified epidermal Langerhans cells. Distinct requirements for stimulation of unprimed and sensitized T lymphocytes. J. Exp. Med. 164: 605.

17. Hoefsmit, E. C. M., A. M. Duivestijn, and E. W. A. Kamperdijk. 1982. Relation between Langerhans cells, veiled cells, and interdigitating cells. Immunobiology 161: 255.

18. Steiner, G., K. Wolff, H. Pehamberger, and G. Stingl. 1985. Epidermal cells as accessory cells in the generation of allo-reactive and hapten-specific cytotoxic T. lymphocyte (CTL) responses. J. Immunol. 134: 736.

19. Bergstresser, P. R. 1986. Ultraviolet B. radiation induces "local" immunosuppression. In: Curr. Probl. Derm. (Therapeutic photomedicine), Vol. 15. H. Hönigsmann and G. Stingl, eds. Basel: Karger, p. 205.

20. Stingl, L. A., D. N. Sauder, M. Iijima, K. Wolff, H. Pehamberger, and G. Stingl. 1983. Mechanism of UV-B-induced impairment of the antigen-presenting capacity of murine epidermal cells. J. Immunol. 130: 1586.

21. Belsito, D. V., M. R. Sanchez, R. L. Baer, F. Valentine, and G. J. Thorbecke. 1984. Reduced Langerhans' cells Ia antigen and ATPase activity in patients with the acquired immunodeficiency syndrome. N. Engl. J. Med. 310: 1279.

22. Tschachler, E., V. Groh, M. Popovic, D. L. Mann, K. Konrad, B. Safai, L. Eron, F. diMarzo Veronese, K. Wolff, and G. Stingl. 1987. Epidermal Langerhans cells—A target for HTLV-III/LAV infection. J. Invest. Dermatol. 88: 233.

23. Streilein, J. W., G. B. Toews, and P. R. Bergstresser. 1979. Corneal allografts fail to express Ia antigens. Nature 282: 326.

24. Auböck, J., E. Irschick, N. Romani, P. Kompatscher, R. Höpfl, M. Herold, G. Schuler, M. Bauer, Ch. Huber, and P. Fritsch. 1988. Rejection, after a slightly prolonged survival time, of Langerhans cell-free allogeneic cultured epidermis for wound coverage in humans. Transplantation 45: 730.

25. Toews, G. B., P. R. Bergstresser, and J. W. Streilein. 1980. Epidermal Langerhans cell density determines whether contact hypersensitivity or unresponsiveness follows skin painting with DNFB. J. Immunol. 124: 445.

26. Sullivan, S., P. R. Bergstresser, R. E. Tigelaar, and J. W. Streilein. 1986. Induction and regulation of contact hypersensitivity by resident, bone marrow-derived dendritic epidermal cells: Langerhans cells and Thy-1[+] epidermal cells. J. Immunol. 137: 2460.

27. Sauder, D. N., C. S. Carter, S. I. Katz, and J. J. Oppenheim. 1982. Epidermal cell production of thymocyte activating factor (ETAF). J. Invest. Dermatol. 79: 34.

28. Luger, T. A., B. M. Stadler, B. M. Luger, B. J. Mathieson, M. Mage, J. A. Schmidt, and J. J. Oppenheim. 1982. Murine epidermal cell-derived thymocyte activating factor resembles murine interleukin 1. J. Immunol. 128: 2147.

29. Schwarz, T., A. Urbanska, F. Gschnait, and T. A. Luger. 1987. UV-irradiated epidermal cells produce a specific inhibitor of interleukin 1 activity. J. Immunol. 138: 1457.

30. Luger, T. A., U. Wirth, and A. Köck. 1985. Epidermal cells synthesize a cytokine with interleukin 3-like properties. J. Immunol. 134: 915.

31. Kupper, T. S., F. Lee, D. Coleman, J. Chodakewitz, P. Flood, and M. Horowitz. 1988. Keratinocyte derived T-cell growth factor (KTGF) is identical to granulocyte macrophage colony stimulating factor (GM-CSF). J. Invest. Dermatol. 91: 185.

32. Köck, A., T. Luger, and J. Ansel. 1988. Expression of IL-6 in human epidermoid carcinoma cells. Clin. Res. 36: 377A.

33. Kupper, T., L. May, N. Birchall, and P. Sehgal. 1988. Keratinocytes produce interleukin 6, a cytokine which can provide a 2nd signal in the activation of T cells. Clin. Res. 36: 665A.

34. Yamada, H., T. Matsuda, M. Harada, T. Hirano, T. Kishimoto, and T. Tezuka. 1988. Keratinocytes produce BSF-2 (interleukin 6). Clin. Res. 36: 706A.

35. Coffey, R. J. Jr., R. Derynck, J. N. Wilcox, T. S. Bringman, A. S. Goustin, H. L. Moses, and M. R. Pittelkow. 1987. Production and auto-induction of transforming growth factor-α in human keratinocytes. Nature 328: 817.

36. Akhurst, R. J., F. Fee, and A. Balmain. 1988. Localized production of TGF-β mRNA in tumor promoter-stimulated mouse epidermis. Nature 331: 363.

37. Langdon, R. C., R. Halabon, and J. McGuire. 1988. Cultured human keratinocytes produce mRNA for basic fibroblast growth factor (bFGF). Clin. Res. 36: 666A.

316

38. Marrack, P., and J. Kappler. 1986. The antigen-specific, major histocompatibility complex, restricted receptor on T cells. Adv. Immunol. 38: 1.

39. Brenner, M. B., J. McLean, D. P. Dialynas, J. L. Strominger, J. A. Smith, F. L. Owen, J. G. Sdieman, S. Ip, F. Rosen, and M. S. Krangel. 1986. Identification of a putative second T-cell receptor. Nature 322: 145.

40. Pardoll, D. M., A. M. Kruisbeeck, B. J. Fowlkes, J. E. Coligan, and R. H. Schwartz. 1987. The unfolding story of T cell receptor γ. FASEB J. 1: 103.

41. Romani, N., G. Stingl, E. Tschachler, M. D. Witmer, R. M. Steinman, E. M. Shevach, and G. Schuler. 1985. The Thy-1-bearing cell of murine epidermis: A leukocyte distinct from Langerhans cells and perhaps related to NK cells. J. Exp. Med. 161: 1368.

42. Stingl, G., F. Koning, H. Yamada, W. M. Yokoyama, E. Tschachler, J. A. Bluestone, G. Steiner, L. E. Samelson, A. M. Lew, J. E. Coligan, and E. M. Shevach. 1987. Thy-1[+] dendritic epidermal cells express T3 antigen and the T cell receptor γ chain. Proc. Natl. Acad. Sci. USA 84: 4586.

43. Bonyhady, M., A. Weiss, P. W. Tucker, R. E. Tigelaar, and J. P. Allison. 1987. Delta is the C_x-gene product in the γ/δ antigen receptor of dendritic epidermal cells. Nature 330: 574.

44. Steiner, G., F. Koning, A. Elbe, E. Tschachler, W. M. Yokoyama, E. M. Shevach, G. Stingl, and J. E. Coligan. 1988. Characterization of T cell receptors on resident murine dendritic epidermal T cells. Europ. J. Immunol. 18: 1323.

45. Havran, W. L., and J. P. Allison. 1988. Developmentally ordered appearance of thymocyte expressing different T-cell antigen receptors. Nature 335: 443.

46. Streilein, J. W. 1983. Skin-associated lymphoid tissues (SALT): Origin and functions. J. Invest. Dermatol. 80: 12s.

T Cell Subsets that Act in Sequence to Mediate Delayed-Type Hypersensitivity

Philip W. Askenase, Jean Claude Ameisen, Wulf R. Herzog*

Elicitation of delayed-type hypersensitivity (DTH) in mice requires an early local release of serotonin (5-HT) to induce vasoactivity and to activate recruited effector T cells via stimulation of serotonin-2 receptors ($5-HT_2R$) that are present on both the endothelial cells and on the effector T cells. A unique DTH-initiating T cell, which is relatively thymic independent and triple negative (CD4−, CD8−, CD3−), and which releases circulating, IgE-like, antigen-specific factors, is responsible for sensitizing 5-HT-containing cells like mast cells, and perhaps platelets, and therefore mediates the required, early (2 h), antigen-specific local release of 5-HT. This leads to local extravascular recruitment *and* activation of classical, lymphokine-producing, Ag/MHC-Class II-restricted, Th-1/inflammatory, $CD3^+$, $CD4^+$, late-acting (24 h) DTH effector T cells.

DTH reactions are in vivo examples of T cell-mediated immunity. We have shown that DTH is due to the sequential action of two different T cells [1–7] (Figure 1). A DTH-initiating T cell produces an antigen-specific T cell factor (TCF) that mediates an early (2 h), immediate hypersensitivity-like phase of DTH by sensitizing tissues for release of the vasoactive mediator 5-HT. In picryl chloride (PCl) contact sensitivity, PCl-factor (PCl-F) is the prototype factor, and in oxazolone contact sensitivity oxazolone-factor (OX-F) is analogous. The 5-HT mediated vasoactivity induced by PCl-F/OX-F following antigen challenge allows local recruitment of the late-acting, DTH effector T cell that is $CD4^+$, has antigen/MHC-Class II-restricted α:β T cell receptors, and locally releases inflammatory lymphokines that recruit nonspecific bone marrow-derived effector cells to constitute the DTH infiltrate. DTH correlates with host resistance to many microorganisms and with acquired resistance to some tumors. Thus, immune resistance depends in part on the ability of antigen-specific, lymphokine-producing, inflammatory $CD4^+$ T cells to recruit non-specific effector cells to tissue sites of invasion. Absence of DTH recruitment by $CD4^+$ T cells is a major cause of opportunistic infections in AIDS. Studies in model systems indicate that the concept of two sequential T cell activities in DTH pertains to five important areas: (1) contact sensitivity; (2) Tuberculin (PPD) sensitivity; (3) immune resistance to some tumors; (4) immune hypersensitivity to helminthic parasites; and (5) autoimmunity. Thus, DTH-initiating T cells are involved in a broad range of biologically relevant reactions.

1. *A requirement for initiating T cells to locally recruit late-acting T cells has been demonstrated in several other systems:* In PPD-specific DTH, PPD-pulsed macrophages act as antigen-presenting cells for induction of non-MHC-restricted initiating T cells, while PPD-pulsed splenic dendritic cells selectively induce MHC-restricted late-acting T cells [8]; DTH footpad responses to tumor cells in sensitized mice show a biphasic pattern, with a T cell-dependent early, 2 h initiating phase and a late, 24 h inflammatory component, similar to that found in contact sensitivity [9–11]. In a well-characterized, UV-induced tumor system, it has been shown that a cultured line of tumor-specific T cells that contains a mixture of late-acting $CD4^+$ DTH T cells and $CD8^+$ cytotoxic T cells is unable to transfer tumor resistance alone, but synergizes with small numbers of early-acting, DTH-initiating T cells to prevent tumor growth [10]. Results in another system suggested that antigen(tumor)-specific T cell factors play a role in initiation of immune inflammatory responses to tumors, leading to DTH responses that recruit macrophages which are cytotoxic to the tumor cells [11]. In studies of intestinal

*   Section of Allergy & Clinical Immunology, Department of Medicine, Yale University School of Medicine, New Haven, CT 06510, USA.
     Supported in part by NIH grants (AI-12211, CA-29606), and a Pfizer Grant; and by a Burroughs-Wellcome Fellowship from the Asthma and Allergy Foundation of America, to J.C.A. Wulf R. Herzog is supported by the Deutsche Forschungsgemeinschaft.

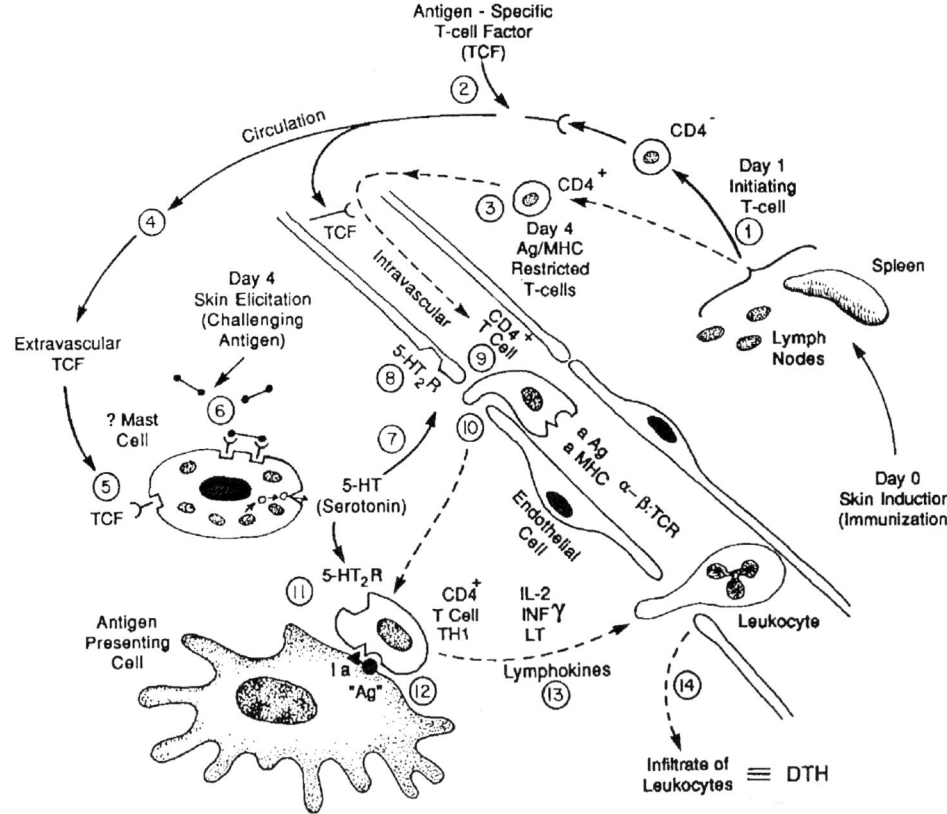

Figure 1. The DTH cascade.

inflammation in mice infected with the helminth *Trichinella spiralis*, a T cell-derived, trinchinella-specific, DTH-initiating factor has been described. Findings are consistent with the hypothesis that a DTH-initiating T cell is involved in the inflammatory events that lead to an infiltrate rich in mucosal mast cells and eosinophils. A role for DTH-initiating T cells has been suggested in experimental allergic encephalomyelitis (EAE) of rats [12]. EAE-mediating T cell lines are able to transfer DTH with both an early and late component and drugs that influence mast cells or 5-HT interfere with the elicitation of EAE following T cell transfer. In rats with type II collagen arthritis, and in mycobacterial adjutant-induced arthritis, an arthrogenic factor binds the antigen (type II collagen), and initiates a cellular immune reaction in the synovium that is accompanied by mast cell degranulation [13].

2. *Mechanisms of DTH initiation (Figure 1):* DTH-initiating T cells, unlike DTH-inflammatory T cells, do not need to recirculate nor be present at the site of a DTH reaction. Initiator T cells are found in the lymph nodes and spleen within one day of sensitization [1–3], and act by elaborating an antigen-specific factor that circulates [6] and passively sensitizes peripheral tissues. These DTH-initiating factors bind specific antigen and thus can be purified with antigen affinity columns [4–6]. Although these factors have biologic activities like IgE, they have been clearly separated from IgE by a variety of criteria [4–7, 14–16]. Prior to local challenge to elicit DTH, cells containing the vasoactive amine 5-HT, such as mast cells [3, 6, 7, 14–21], and perhaps platelets [19, 22], are sensitized with PCl-F or OX-F, etc., via specific surface receptors for a "constant region" isotype-like portion of the factor [14]. Early (within 2 h) after local antigen challenge, the factor

binds antigen and the sensitized cells release 5-HT [7, 9, 15, 17, 18] that interacts with specific 5-HT receptors on local venules. This causes activation of the endothelium and formation of gaps between endothelial cells that allow circulating, CD4$^+$, late-acting DTH-effector T cells to enter into the tissues to interact with processed antigen + MHC/Class II molecules on the surface of local antigen presenting cells. Then these recruited T cells produce an inflammatory profile of lymphokines that recruits local accumulation of circulating, non-specific, bone marrow-derived leukocytes to constitute the classical, late 24–48 h perivascular infiltrate that characterizes DTH (Figure 1).

3. *Release of 3H-5-HT by mast cells sensitized with PCl-F or IgE* [15]. Murine peritoneal mast cells from normal animals were purified and incubated in vitro with ^{3}H-5-HT, which is taken up into their storage granules, and simultaneously were sensitized with PCl-F (which is TNP-specific), or monoclonal anti-TNP IgE antibody. After washing, they were challenged in vitro with antigen (TNP-BSA), which caused 5-HT release in both cases. PCl-F dependent 5-HT release, like IgE-dependent release, required phosphatidyl serine and was antigen specific. It was shown that a monoclonal antibody (called 14-30) directed against a serologic determinant found on several antigen-specific T cell factors [6], could stimulate PCl-F or OX-F dependent release of 5-HT. It was concluded:

1) that PCL-F and OX-F were antigen specific T cell factors of the same "isotype";

2) that this putative isotypic constant region interacted with specific receptors on mast cells and,

3) that 14-30 bound a determinant of this common isotypic portion of the factors, allowing cross linking and release of 5-HT.

To rule out that IgE contamination was responsible for 5-HT release, it was shown that reduction and alkylation, which destroyed the ability of IgE to interact with Fc-ε on receptors, did not affect the ability of PCl-F to link to its binding site on mast cells and mediate release of 5-HT. Experiments also were performed to determine whether antibody-linked affinity columns could distinguish the mast cell sensitizing 5-HT release activity of PCl-F. Monoclonal anti-TNP IgE or PCl-F were applied to

affinity columns linked with either 14-30 antibody or with rabbit anti-IgE. The effluent and eluate fractions were collected, dialyzed, and used to sensitize mast cells. The 5-HT release activity of PCl-F for mast cells was retained by, and eluted from the 14-30 column, but passed through the anti-IgE column. Conversely, the 5-HT release activity of IgE was retained by and could be eluted from the anti-IgE column, but was found in the filtrate of the 14-30 column. These results indicated that PCl-F does not contain IgE antibody, and that the monoclonal antibody 14-30 can specifically bind to the mast cell sensitizing factor PCl-F, but not to IgE antibody.

The mast cells from normal animals employed above were already coated with IgE that was acquired in vivo. Thus, experiments were conducted to determine whether PCl-F-induced release of 5-HT was dependent on this endogenous coating of IgE. Mast cells were treated with lactic acid to remove IgE, then were sensitized with IgE, or with PCl-F, and then were challenged. Acid treatment removed 60–70% of IgE as reflected by the ability to release 5-HT with anti-IgE. The acid-treated cells were not impaired since they could be sensitized again with IgE, resulting in full restoration of 5-HT release by anti-IgE. Importantly, acid stripping, which significantly depleted surface IgE, had no effect on the ability of PCl-F to sensitize mast cells for 5-HT release. We concluded that PCl-F-induced release of 5-HT from mast cells was not dependent on the presence of IgE.

4. *Simulation of the early 2 h component of DTH following local challenge with 14-30 monoclonal anti-factor antibody.* The antigen-specific T-cell factor PCl-F mediates initiation of murine DTH. Initiating ear swelling reactions are elicited 2 h after local challenge with the antigen (PCl) in actively PCl contact sensitized mice [1, 3], and in naive mice receiving PCl-F transfers [4–7]. We investigated whether 14-30 could elicit 2 h ear swelling reactions in vivo. Mice challenged locally with 14-30 antibody four days after PCl sensitization, as well as mice that received PCl-F, elicited 2 h ear swelling reactions. 14-30 also could elicit 2 h *but not* 24 h ear swelling reactions in recipients of immune cells of *either* PCl or OX specificity. Taken together, these results indicate that the interaction of PCl-F with 14-30 antibody, to cause mast cells to release 5-HT in vitro corresponds to the in vivo, early, 2 h initiation of DTH. Furthermore, elicitation of 2 h *but not* 24 h reactions by local challenge with 14-30, in recipients of either OX or PCl immune cells, suggests that a common "isotypic" portion of in vivo-produced antigen-specific T cell factors are involved in the 2 h reactions, *but not* in the 24 h component of CS, which only was elicited by specific antigens and is due to CD4$^+$, lymphokine-producing T cells.

5. *Characteristics of DTH-initiating T cells.* Results with polyclonal T cells from actively sensitized mice indicate that this is a distinct T cell subset that is clearly separable from the late-acting, classical DTH-T cell. The DTH-initiating T cell is a unique, relatively thymic-independent T cell that produces an antigen-binding T cell factor that may serve as a non-MHC-restricted receptor on these cells. The surface phenotype of this T cell is Thy1$^+$, Ly1$^+$, CD4$^-$, CD8$^-$, and interestingly CD3$^-$. In contrast to the DTH-initiating T cells, the late-acting DTH effector T cells are CD4$^+$, produce nonspecific inflammatory lymphokines, and have surface CD3-linked antigen/MHC-restricted, α:β surface receptors. Thus, our recent results demonstrate:

— that adult athymic nude mice, which lack CD4$^+$ inflammatory T cells, but have CD4$^-$ T cells, are able to produce antigen-binding T cell factors of the type that initiate DTH;

— that the surface phenotype of PCl-F/OX-F-producing T cells in CBA mice is Thy1$^+$, Ly1$^+$, CD4$^-$, CD8$^-$, and CD3$^-$;

— that selecting for this phenotype we have derived an in vitro line that produces an antigen-specific DTH-initiating factor, and have isolated an antigen-specific DTH-initiating clone with the surface phenotype: Thy1$^+$, Ly1$^+$, CD4$^-$, CD8$^-$, CD3$^-$, PCl-F$^+$.

6. *The late component of DTH is also 5-HT dependent.* 5-HT is a vasoactive amine that in many species is stored by platelets. In mice 5-HT is also stored by mast cells. In murine DTH, an early vasoactive component is T cell mediated and dependent on local release of 5-HT. This early component of DTH is required for subsequent elicitation of the late, 24 h component of DTH that is due to local recruitment of DTH effector T cells. We have found recently that

the late component of DTH is *also* 5-HT dependent. Administration of a single I.V. bolus of ketanserin (0.16 mg/kg), a selective serotonin-2 receptor (5-HT2R) antagonist, before or, importantly 2–6 h *after* the early vasoactive phase of DTH, inhibits 24 h DTH in actively sensitized mice. In addition, lymphoid cells from sensitized mice that were treated in vivo with 5-HT2R antagonists were inhibited in their ability to transfer DTH reactivity to adoptive recipients, suggesting a direct effect of the 5-HT2R antagonist on DTH T cells. Furthermore, in vitro treatment of purified T cells from sensitized mice with 10^{-7} to 10^{-9} M of the 5HT2R antagonists methysergide, ketanserin, ritanserin, or LY 53857, followed by 3 washings, inhibited their ability to transfer DTH. This inhibition was not related to any leaking of drug into the recipient, nor to the induction of suppressive mechanisms, as shown by cotransfer experiments of 5-HT2R antagonist-treated vs untreated sensitized cells. 5-HT2R selectivity of drug inhibition was suggested by the absence of effect of an alpha-adrenergic receptor antagonist.

7. *The locus of action of 5-HT2R antagonists is on late-acting (24 hr) DTH effector cells, but not the early-acting (2 h) DTH-initiating T cells.* 5-HT2R antagonists could affect T cell function at one or more steps in the DTH cascade. The fact that I.V. injection of 5-HT2R antagonists inhibited 24 h DTH when given after the 2 h early component, suggested that the locus of action of 5-HT2R antagonists on lymphocytes acting in DTH was on the late-acting T cells. However, these experiments left open the possibility that early-acting DTH-initiating T cells also could be affected by 5-HT2R antagonists. To test for this possibility, 4-day DTH effector cells were incubated in vitro with 5-HT2R antagonists and then were adoptively transferred I.V. to naive recipients. It was found that the late component of DTH was inhibited by in vitro incubation of the cells with the 5-HT2R antagonists ketanserin or ritanserin, while the 2 h ear swelling activity that is mediated by the early-acting, DTH-initiating T cells was not inhibited.

An important finding was that preincubation of DTH T cells with a 5-HT2R *agonist* prevented subsequent inhibition by a serotonin *antagonist*. This finding suggested that activation of functional 5-HT2R on late-acting T cells is required in vivo for their mediation of the 24 h inflammatory aspects of DTH. The fact that *local* adoptive transfer of DTH also was inhibited when immune cells were incubated in vitro with 5-HT2R antagonists suggests that events occurring subsequent to local extravascular recruitment of lymphokine-producing T cells are dependent on a positive signal provided by an endogenous 5-HT2R ligand.

These results suggest that, in addition to early vascular effects of 5-HT in DTH, functional 5-H2R receptors on late-acting DTH effector T cells must be activated, possibly after these cells are recruited locally. Perhaps this permits antigen/MHC-restricted activation and lymphokine synthesis to produce the inflammatory component of DTH. The possible sources of local 5-HT include mast cells and platelets, but it is possible that an endogenous ligand of 5-HT2R other than 5-HT is involved. The finding of functional 5-HT2R on T cells may mean that newly employed 5-HT2R antagonists, although given for neuropsychiatric and hypertensive illnesses, may possess unanticipated immunomodulatory properties.

References

1. Van Loveren H., and P. W. Askenase. 1984. Delayed-type hypersensitivity is mediated by a sequence of two different T cell activities. J. Immunol. 133: 2397.

2. Van Loveren H., K. Kato, R. Meade, D. R. Green, M. Horowitz, W. Ptak, and P. W. Askenase. 1984. Characterization of two different Lyl[+] T cell populations that mediate delayed-type hypersensitivity. J. Immunol. 133: 2402.

3. Van Loveren, H., R. Meade, and P. W. Askenase. 1983. An early component of delayed-type hypersensitivity mediated by T cells and mast cells. J. Exp. Med. 157: 1604.

4. Ptak, W., P. W. Askenase, R. W. Rosenstein, and R. K. Gershon. 1982. Transfer of an antigen specific immediate hypersensitivity-like reaction with an antigen binding factor produced by T cells. Proc. Nat. Acad. Sci. USA. 79: 1969.

5. Askenase, P. W., R. W. Rosenstein, and W. Ptak. 1983. T cells produce an antigen binding factor with in vivo activity analogous to IgE antibody. J. Exp. Med. 157: 862.

6. Van Loveren, H, R. E. Ratzlaff, K. Kato, R. Meade, R. T. Fergueson, G. M. Iverson, C. A. Janeway, and P. W. Askenase. 1986. Immune serum from mice contact sensitized with picryl chloride contains an antigen-specific T cell factor that transfers immediate cutaneous reactivity. Eur. J. Immunol. 16: 1203.

7. Van Loveren, H., S. Kraeuter-Kops, and P. W. Askenase. 1984. Different mechanisms of release of vasoactive amines by mast cells occur in T cell-dependent compared to IgE-dependent cutaneous hypersensitivity responses. Eur. J. Immunol. 14: 40.

8. Mukherjee, S., Katz, D. R., and Rook, G. A. W. 1986. Differing role of dendritic cells and macrophages in the induction of delayed-type hypersensitivity responses to PPD. Immunol., 59: 229.

9. Van Loveren, H., Den Otter, W., Meade, R., Terheggen, P. M. A., and Askenase, P. W. 1985. A role for mast cells and the vasoactive amine serotonin in T cell dependent immunity to tumors. J. Immunol. 134: 1292

10. Trail, J. 1988. Early-acting delayed-type hypersensitivity T cells cooperate with cultured effector cells in tumor rejection. Cancer Research, in press.

11. Van Loveren, H., DeWeger, R. A., Garssen, J., Los, G., and Askenase, P. W. 1988. Impairment of allograft tumor immunity by isotype-like suppression of antigen-specific T cell factors. Transplantation, in press.

12. Hinrichs, D., Dietsch, G., and Wagner, C. 1987. The role of mast cells in the development of allergic encephalomyelitis. Immune Regulation of Characterized Polypeptides. Alan R. Liss, Inc., p. 641.

13. Helfgott, S. M., Kieval, R. I., Breedveld, F. C., Brahn, E., Young, C. T., Dysesium-Trentham, R, and Trentham, D.E. 1988. Detection of arthritogenic factor in adjuvant arthritis. J. Immunol 140: 1838.

14. Kraeuter-Kops, S., Ratzlaff, R. E., Meade, R., Iverson, G. M. and Askenase, P. W. 1986. Interaction of antigen-specific T cell factors with unique "receptors" on the surface of mast cells: demonstration in vitro by an indirect rosetting technique. J. Immunol. 136: 4515.

15. Meade, R., Van Loveren, H., Parmentier, H., Iverson, G. M. and Askenase, P.W. 1988. The antigen-binding T cell factor PCl-F sensitizes mast cells for in vitro release of serotonin: Comparison with monoclonal IgE antibody. J. Immunol., in press.

16. Kraeuter-Kops, S., Van Loveren, H., Rosenstein, R. W., Ptak, W., and Askenase, P. W. 1984. Mast cell activation and vascular alterations in immediate hypersensitivity-like reactions induced by a T cell-derived antigen binding factor. Lab. Invest. 50: 421.

17. Gershon, R. K., Askenase, P. W., and Gershon, M. 1975. Requirement for vasoactive amines in the production of the skin reactions of delayed-type hypersensitivity. J. Exp. Med. 142: 732.

18. Askenase, P. W., Bursztajn, S., Gershon, M. D., and Gershon, R. K.1980. T cell dependent mast cell degranulation and release of serotonin in murine delayed-type hypersensitivity. J. Exp. Med. 152: 1358.

19. Askenase, P. W., Van Loveren, H., Kraeuter-Kops, S., Ron, Yl, Meade, R., Theoharides, T.C., Nordlund, J.J., Scovern, H., Gershon, M.D., and Ptak, W. 1983. Defective elicitation of delayed-type hypersensitivity in W/W^v and S1/S1^d mast cell deficient mice J. Immunol. 131: 2687.

20. Miyachi, Y., Imamura, S., Tokura, Y., and Taki-gawa, M. 1986. Mechanisms of contact photo-sensitivity in mice. VII diminished elicitation by reserpine and defective expression in mast cell-deficient mice. J. Invest. Derm. 87: 38.

21. Kerdel, F. A., Belsito, D. V., Scotto-Chinnici, R., and Soter, N. A. 1987. Mast cell participation during the elicitation of murine allergic contact hypersensitivity. J. Invest. Derm. 88: 686.

22. Galli, S. J., and Hammel, I. 1984. Unequivocal delayed hypersensitivity in mast cell deficient and beige mice. Science 226: 710.

The Role of Epidermal Cytokines During the Pathogenesis of Allergic Skin Diseases

Thomas A. Luger*

The skin was recently discovered as a site for the initiation of immune responses. Among the immunocompetent cells of the epidermis, keratinocytes have been identified as a potent source of immunoregulatory cytokines. A network of interacting cytokines appears to be crucial for the regulation of immunity and inflammation including hypersensitivity reactions. Therefore, through the production of activating factors such as interleukin-1, interleukin-6, and colony-stimulating factors as well as suppressor factors, including contra-interleukin-1 and transforming growth factors, epidermal cells may contribute positive and negative signals during the pathogenesis of allergic disease.

The clinical manifestations of allergic disorders are related to the distinct biological effects of several mediators of immunity and inflammation which act as messengers between primary target cells and secondary effector cells. The physiochemical characteristics, mechanisms of generation and release as well as pathophysiological effects of these biological activities provide a molecular and cellular basis for understanding allergic diseases. In addition to the "classical" mediators of hypersensitivity recently described, soluble molecules termed lymphokines have been recognized as playing a crucial role in the regulation of many aspects of hypersensitivity reactions [1, 2]. Lymphokines are glycoproteins that regulate the growth and differentiation of cells involved in immunity, inflammation, and hematopoiesis which originally were thought to be released only by lymphocytes and to interact selectively on immunocompetent cells. Because it is now clear that neither the production nor the effects of these mediators are restricted to cells of the immune system, the term cytokine was introduced to define this group of molecules [3].

The concept of the epidermis as a site for the initiation of immune response has only arisen over the past decade. There is strong evidence that three types of epidermal cells (EC) have immune functions. Dendritic bone marrow-derived cells such as Langerhans cells are potent stimulators of many types of T cell responses [4]. In the mouse epidermis, the recently discovered dendritic Thy-1 cells belongs to the T-cell family [5]. Moreover, keratinocytes, which represent the majority of epidermal cells, have been shown to produce a variety of cytokines regulating the growth and differentiation of immune and non-immune cells (Table 1) [3]. Accordingly, keratinocytes synthesize and release interleukin's (IL) such as IL-1α, IL-1β, and IL-6, colony-stimulating factors (CSF), tumor necrosis factor, and several growth factors. Other cytokines, which are in the process of being characterized as keratinocyte products, include differentiation factors, chemotactic mediators, and suppressor factors.

Table 1. Cytokines produced by keratinocytes.

Interleukin-1 α and β
Interleukin-6 (BSF2, IFNβ2)
Colony-stimulating factors (CSF)
    Interleukin 3 (multi-CSF)
    Granulocyte-macrophage CSF
    Granulocyte-CSF
    Macrophage-CSF (CSF1)
Thymopoietin
Interferon α and β
Tumor necrosis factor α
Monocyte-derived neutrophil-activating peptide (MONAP)
    Mononuclear cell-derived neutrophil chemotactic factor
Epidermal cell lymphocyte chemotactic factor
Epidermal cell lymphocyte differentiation factor
Epidermal cell suppressor factor
Epidermal cell-contra-IL-1
Transforming growth factor α and β
Platelet-derived growth factor
Basic fibroblast growth factor

* Department of Dermatology II and LBI-DVS, Laboratory for Cell Biology, University of Vienna, Vienna, Austria. This work was supported by the "Medizinisch-Wissenschaftlichen Fond des Bürgermeisters der Bundeshauptstadt Wien" and the "Jubiläumsfonds der Österreichischen Nationalbank." The author wishes to thank Ms. M. Bednar for her secretarial assistance.

The biochemical and molecular characteristics of epidermal cytokines as well as their biological functions recently have been reviewed [3]. Therefore, the following focuses only on epidermal cytokines in view of their regulatory functions in the pathogenesis of allergic diseases.

EC Cytokines Involved in Immediate-Type Hypersensitivity Reactions

Immediate type of hypersensitivity (Type I) occurs when biologically active mediators are released upon antigen induction from mast cells or basophilic leukocytes sensitized with a specific IgE antibody. The resulting IgE-mediated acute inflammatory reactions are manifested as asthma, hay fever, rhinitis, urticaria, and some drug as well as occupational allergies. Specific IgE bound to IgE receptors on basophils or mast cells can be crosslinked by allergens leading to degranulation. Mediators released by these cells include preformed mediators such as histamine and newly synthesized factors such as prostaglandins, leukotrienes, platelet-activating factor, chemotactic factors, and slow-reacting substance of anaphylaxis. In addition to mast cell activation via crosslinking of

Fc receptors, other stimuli such as breakdown products of complement activation (C3a, C5a), cytokines (IL-3), calcium ionophers, certain drugs, and ACTH are capable of activating mast cells directly [2].

It recently became evident that cytokines also are capable of modulating growth and differentiation of effector cells involved in immediate-type reactions such as mast cells, basophils, T- and B-lymphocytes. Type I allergic reactions may be regulated at the level of IgE synthesis by B-cells or the interaction of IgE with high-affinity Fc receptors on mast cells and basophils. Mostly T-cell-derived cytokines such as IL-3, IL-4, and IL-5 appear to play an important role in this regulator circuit [1]. Moreover, mediators produced by various cells including keratinocytes such as IL-1, IL-3, IL-6, and GM-CSF may have some additional costimulatory effects by enhancing B-cell growth and differentiation as well as the production of T- and B-cell-activating cytokines such as IL-2, IL-3, IL-4, IL-5, and IFN [1, 6]. In the mouse system, IL-3 is also known to be produced by keratinocytes and, in concert with IL-4, to stimulate the growth of mast cells [4, 7]. In the human system, IL-3 and a recently described T-cell-derived basophil-promoting activity have been shown to stimulate basophils and mast cells [8]. In both systems, IL-4 stimu-

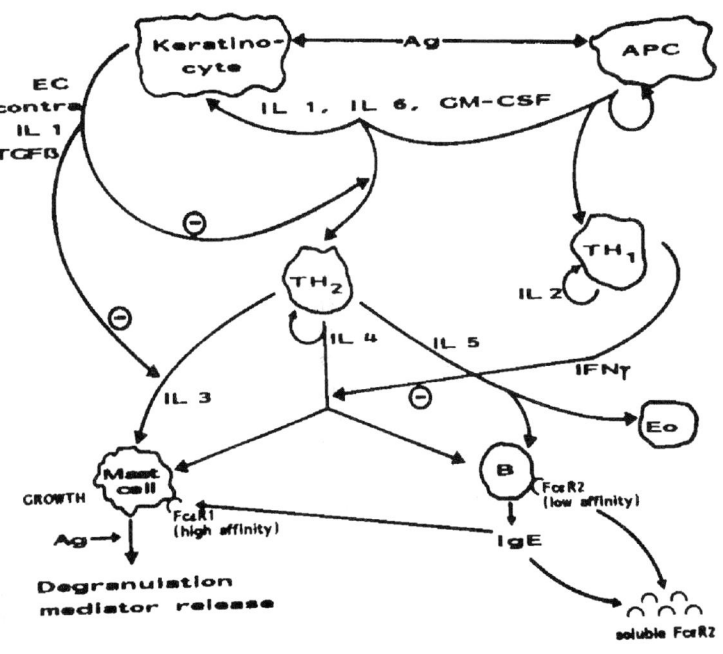

Figure 1. Possible role of cytokines in the regulation of IgE-mediated allergic response in the skin.

lates IgE production as well as the expression of a low-affinity Fc receptor on B-cells, monocytes, and epidermal Langerhans cells [1]. According to recent data, an increased release of soluble Fc R may also be required for IL-4- and IL5-mediated IgE production. In addition to its role in IgE and IgA synthesis, IL-5 also stimulates proliferation of eosinophils, although the function of eosinophils in this regulatory network is unclear [1, 6]. An inhibitory effect on IL-4-induced IgE synthesis and Fc R expression has been demonstrated for IFN-β produced by T-cells [1]. Transforming growth factor-β, which upon stimulation is produced by keratinocytes, has been shown to block IL-3 activity [9] (Figure 1). Moreover, the role of T-cell-derived IgE potentiating or suppressing factors remains to be determined [10].

These findings indicate that the inflammatory response induced by foreign antigens is highly regulated by a network of positive and negative cytokines (Figure 1). Since keratinocytes produce B-cell-costimulating mediators such as IL-1 and IL-6, but also inhibitors including EC-contra-IL-1, a potent inhibitor of IL-1 activity and transforming growth factor-β, they may represent a crucial part in the regulatory pathways of immediate-type hypersensitivity.

EC Cytokines Involved in Delayed-Type Hypersensitivity Reactions

Within the epidermis several dendritic cells belonging to the immune system have been described. Langerhans cells are bone-marrow-derived major histocompatibility complex (MHC) class II antigen expressing and Fc as well as C3 receptor-bearing leukocytes which are known to play an important role in the induction of delayed and contact hypersensitivity to haptens [4]. There is evidence for a similarity between epidermal Langerhans cells and splenic dendritic cells according to their surface antigen expression and their capacity to present antigen and thus to promote the activation of T-cells [11]. For the activation of T-cells, several signals provided by accessory cells are required including the expression of MHC class II antigens on the cell surface, processing of antigen and production of cytokines

such as IL-1 and IL-6 [12]. These signals induce T-cells to produce growth factors like IL-2 and to express IL-2 receptors. Because of their capacity to release these cytokines, keratinocytes may function as accessory cells. However, keratinocytes also may downregulate T-cell activation via the production of EC-contra-IL-1 [13]. Moreover, EC-contra-IL-1 is closely related to EC-suppressor factor (EC-SF), which is also released by keratinocytes upon UV-B irradiation and blocks the induction of CHS [14, 15]. The findings of keratinocytes producing both stimulators and inhibitors of T-cell activation indicate that depending on the trigger sensitization or tolerance induction may originate in the skin. There is also evidence that keratinocyte-derived cytokines may regulate T-cell activation via modulating Langerhans cell function. Accordingly, Langerhans cells in the presence of keratinocyte-derived GM-CSF and IL-1 mature into potent antigen-presenting cells and tumor necrosis factor-α (TNFα), which also is produced by keratinocytes and appears to be a growth signal for Langerhans cells [3, 11].

There is recent evidence from several studies for the existence of two major phenotypes of CD4[+] lymphocytes, each one having a distinct role in immunity. Inflammatory CD4[+] T-cells (Th1) mediate killing and delayed-type hypersensitivity reactions, whereas helper CD4[+] T-cells (Th2) provide help to B-lymphocytes [16]. In addition to their distinct functions, they also vary in their growth factor requirements as well as cytokine secretion patterns. Inflammatory T-cells produce IL-2, GM-CSF, and IFN-γ and proliferate in response to IL-2. Helper T-cells release IL-3, IL-4, and GM-CSF and proliferate in response to IL-4 and IL-1. Contact hypersensitivity reactions are characterized by an intense MHC class II antigen expression on keratinocytes probably because of IFN-γ production by dermal Th1 cells. Therefore, by expressing class II antigen and by releasing IL-1 and GM-CSF, keratinocytes may further enhance T-cell-mediated responses (Figure 2). In contrast, keratinocytes in atopic lesions usually do not express MHC class II antigens, and an increased number of mast cells and elevations of IgE are commonly found. Thus, the T-cell involved in atopic dermatitis primarily may be a helper CD4[+] T-cell secreting IL-4 a potent activator of B-cells and IgE production as well as Fc R expression.

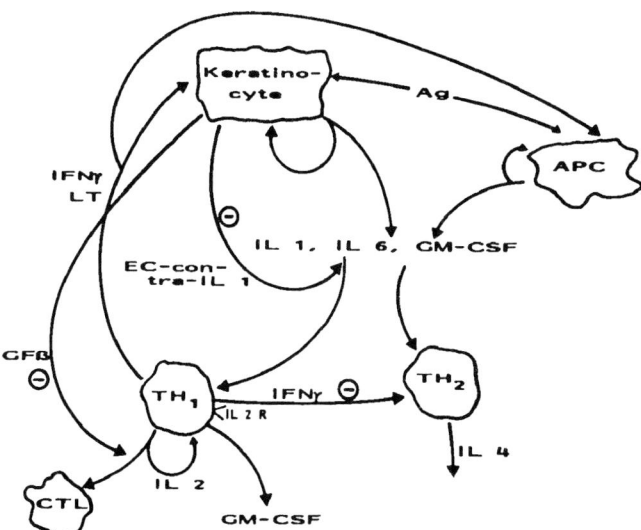

Figure 2. Possible role of cytokines in T-cell activation in the skin.

Concluding Remarks

Keratinocytes are important constituents of the immune system via their capacity to produce cytokines. Although most keratinocyte-derived cytokines only have been characterized in in vitro systems and no causative role of a cytokine has been established in any disease, altered synthesis and release of these soluble mediators by epidermal cells may contribute to certain disease states. Moreover, there is evidence for a network of interacting cytokines maintaining a proper balance, which has so far only partially been discovered. These observations illustrate that cytokines produced by epidermal cells may indeed be involved in immediate-type as well as delayed-type hypersensitivity by directly or indirectly affecting functions of effector cells such as mast cells, basophils, monocytes, and lymphocytes. Future investigations are needed to elucidate the cytokine cascade and to clarify the role of EC cytokines in allergic diseases. This subsequently may enable us to apply directly certain cytokines or to mediate selectively EC cytokine production in the therapy of allergic diseases.

References

1. Miyajima, A., S. Miyatake, J. Schreurs, J. DeVries, N. Arai, T. Yokota, and K. Arai. 1988. Coordinate regulation of immune and inflammatory responses by T-cell derived lymphokines. FASEB J. 2: 2462.
2. Stadler, B. M., and A. L. de Weck. 1984. Role of lymphokines in immediate type allergy. In: Immunopathology, Vol. 7. Heidelberg: Springer-Verlag, p. 415.
3. Luger, T. A., and T. Schwarz. 1988. Epidermal cytokines. In: Skin immune system. J. D. Bos, ed. Boca Raton, FL: CRC Press, in press.
4. Stingl, G., K. Tamaki, and S. I. Katz. 1980. Origin and function of epidermal Langerhans cells. Immunol. Rev. 53: 149.
5. Stingl, G., K. C. Gunter, E. Tschachler, H. Yamada, R. I. Lechler, W. M. Yokomyama, G. Steiner, R. N. Germain, and E. M. Shevach. 1987. Thy-1[+] dendritic epidermal cells belong to the T-cell lineage. Proc. Natl. Acad. Sci. USA 84: 2430.
6. O'Garra, A., S. Umland, T. DeFrance, and J. Christiansen. 1988. B-cell factors are pleiotropic. Immunol. Today 9: 45.
7. Luger, T. A., U. Wirth, and A. Köck. 1986. Epidermal cells synthesize a cytokine with interleukin 3-like properties. J. Immunol. 134: 915.
8. Stadler, B. M., and K. Hirai. 1988. Human growth factor for metachromatically staining cells. In: Lymphokines, Vol. 15. J. W. Schrader, ed. New York: Academic Press, p. 341.
9. Ruscetti, F., G. Sing, L. Ellingsworth, S. Ruscetti, and J. Keller. 1988. Transforming growth factor β: A selective growth inhibitor for hematopoietic progenitor cells. In: Monokines and other non-lymphocytic cytokines. M. C. Powanda, J. J. Oppenhiem, M. J. Kluger, and C. A. Dinarello, eds. New York: Alan R. Liss, p. 307.

10. Iwata, M., M. Akasaki, P. Jardieu, and K. Ishizaka. 1987. Role of glycosylation inhibiting factor (GIF), a phospholipase inhibiting protein, in the generation of antigen specific suppressor cells. In: Molecular basis of lymphokine action. D. R. Webb, C. W. Pirce, and S. Cohen, eds. Clifton: Humana Press, p. 21.

11. Heufler, C., F. Koch, and G. Schuler. 1988. Granulocyte/macrophage colony-stimulating factor and interleukin 1 mediate the maturation of murine epidermal Langerhans cells into potent immunostimulator dendritic cells. J. Exp. Med. 167: 700.

12. Krutmann, J., R. Kirnbauer, T. Schwarz, L. T. May, P. B. Sehal, and T. A. Luger. 1988. Interleukin 6: A novel accessory cell signal involved in human T-lymphocyte activation. J. Immunol., in press.

13. Krutmann, J., T. Schwarz, R. Kirnbauer, A. Urbanski, and T. A. Luger. 1988. Epidermal cell-contra-interleukin 1 inhibits human accessory cell function by specifically blocking IL 1 activity. Arch. Derm. Res., in press.

14. Schwarz, T., A. Urbanska, F. Gschnait, and T. A. Luger. 1986. Inhibition of the induction of contact hypersensitivity by a UV-mediated epidermal cytokine. J. Invest. Dermatol. 87: 289.

15. Schwarz, T., A. Urbanska, F. Gschnait, and T. A. Luger. 1987. UV-irradiated epidermal cells produce a specific inhibitor of interleukin-1 activity. J. Immunol. 138: 1457.

16. Bottomly, K. 1988. A functional dichotomy in CD4[+] T-lymphocytes. Immunol. Today 9: 268.

Langerhans Cells Activate T Helper Cells for both Contact Sensitivity and IgE Synthesis: A Model for Cutaneous Allergic Reactions

*Conrad Hauser and Jean H. Saurat**

Exposure of the skin to antigens or haptens can result in various immunological responses. For example, the exposure of the skin of atopics to various environmental antigens may result in IgE-mediated immediate type urticaria or angioedema. In other subjects the exposure of the skin to antigens such as certain metal ions and other small reactive molecules leads to a delayed-type dermatitis, i.e., allergic contact eczema. Advances in immunological and dermatological research in the last few years have given considerable insight into mechanisms leading to IgE-mediated immediate type skin reactions and delayed-type contact sensitivity reactions.

Langerhans Cells Are Cutaneous Antigen Presenting Cells [1]

Langerhans cells (LC) are intraepidermal, dendritically shaped, bone- marrow-derived leucocytes. They are located in the suprabasal layer and form—by virtue of their dendrites—a contiguous intraepidermal network. In situ, they can be stained by the ATPase reaction. Though their immunolabeling profile (MHC class II$^+$, Fcγ-receptor$^+$, C3bi receptor+, F4/80$^+$(mouse)) brings them into vicinity of monocytes-macrophages, they are poorly phagocytic and do not adhere to glass or plastic surfaces. In addition, they bear markers found on cells of the T lineage such as CD1a, (T6, human), T1a (mouse), CD4 (T4, human), and, as recently reported, CD3 (T3, human). In vitro, epidermal cell suspensions have been able to stimulate allogeneic and—in the presence of the appropriate antigen—syngeneic T cells from sensitized individuals. Elimination of MHC class II positive cells from the epidermal cell suspension abrogated the T cell responses. Since in normal epidermal cell suspension only LC express MHC class II antigens, the T cell stimulatory capacity of epidermal cells was attributed to LC. Only recently, highly purified LC populations have been shown to subserve the above-cited functions. Murine Langerhans cells have been shown to undergo a dramatic phenotypic change in short-term whole epidermal cell cultures. They no longer express the F4/80 marker and lose receptors for the Fc fragment of IgG; rather, they increase in size, become more highly dendritic, express large amounts of surface MHC class II antigens, and become potent stimulators in vitro of allogeneic small resting T cells and increase their stimulatory capacity for T cell clones by 20–50 times compared to freshly prepared LC.

The above-mentioned phenotypical transition can be induced by granulocyte- macrophage colony-stimulating factor together with interleukin 1. Both lymphokines can be produced by keratinocytes. Cultured LC therefore resemble spleen-cell-derived dendritic cells in terms of surface markers and function. Dendritic cells are regarded as one of the antigen presenting cell for primary T cell responses.

Langerhans Cells Activate Small Resting T Helper Cells in an Antigen- Specific Manner

In our recent studies [1] on the T helper cell activating capacity of cultured LC, we found that, when modified with a hapten, cultured LC are capable of stimulating a *primary* proliferative response in small resting T helper cell populations from nonsensitized mice. Upon restimulation with hapten-modified spleen cells, the T helper cell population primed in vitro

*   Clinique de Dermatologie, Hôpital Cantonal Universitaire, CH-1211 Geneva 4, Switzerland.
     Supported in part by a grant from the Schweizerische Stiftung für Medizinisch-Biologische Stipendien and from the Schweizerischer Nationalfonds zur Förderung der wissenschaftlichen Forschung No. ???.

with cultured LC responded in a hapten-specific fashion. Repeated stimulation of these T helper cell population led to the establishment of hapten-specific T helper cell lines. Using cultured LC and a similar in vitro sensitization technique, it was also possible to obtain T helper cell populations specific to soluble protein antigens and alloantigens. This demonstrates that cultured LC are capable to activate small resting T helper cells in an antigen-specific manner. The in vitro sensitizing capacity of cultured LC might be useful for adoptive immunotherapy of specific T cell populations.

However, less is known about the capacity of LC to activate cytotoxic T cells. Although LC act as accessory cells for the generation of cytotoxic T cells [1], it is presently unknown whether LC are able to directly activate cytotoxic T cells and to stimulate their proliferation.

T Helper Cells Grown with Hapten-Modified LC Produce IL4 and Stimulate IgE Synthesis

Mosmann et al. have recently shown that, within cloned T helper cell lines, a heterogeneity exists with regard to lymphokine production [2, 3]. Type 1 T helper clones produce interleukin 2 (IL-2), interferon-γ (IFN-γ) lymphotoxin, whereas type 2 T helper cells secrete interleukin 4 (IL-4) and interleukin 5 as respectively exclusive lymphokines. Type 1, but not type 2, T helper cells have been described as being able to act as effector cells for delayed in time hypersensitivity reactions [4]. IFN-γ presumably produced by type 1 T helper cells seems to be the major effector lymphokine since administration of monoclonal antibodies to IFN-γ was able abrogate the delayed type hypersensitivity reactions. However, IL-4, a lymphokine produced by type 2 T helper cells, is capable to stimulate IgE synthesis in LPS stimulated B cell blasts [6].

The analysis of conditioned media from our LC activated T helper cells was performed with a T cell growth factor dependent cell line (CTLL), which responds to both IL-2 and IL-4. CTLL growth-promoting activity produced by our T helper cells in primary culture was inhibited by monoclonal antibodies to IL-2 but not to IL-4 [7]. However, when we analyzed the conditioned media of *long-term T helper cell lines*, (>5 cycles of stimulation with cultured

LC), we found only CTLL growth promoting activity which was inhibited by a monoclonal antibody to IL-4 [7].

Furthermore, these T helper cell lines used IL-4 as autorine growth factor and showed typical activation requirements of type 2 helper cells, i.e., they proliferated in response to IL-1 and concanavalin A. All long-term cell lines generated with cultured LC showed features of type 2 helper cells. To analyze whether these type 2 cells would be capable of stimulating IgE synthesis in small resting B cells—as predicted from the "B cell + LPS + IL-4" model—we incubated our hapten-specific T helper lines with small resting B cells modified with either the relevant or an irrelevant hapten. After 6 days, we measured IgE synthesis in the conditioned media by ELISA: IgE production was observed in cultures containing the relevant T-B cell combination, but not in cultures with the irrelevant T-B cell combination [7]. This experiment showed clearly that type 2 helper cells can activate small resting B cells to produce IgE under cognate conditions. Production of IgE was inhibited by a monoclonal antibody to IL-4 but not by an isotype matched control antibody. This indicates that the production of IL-4 by the T helper cells is crucial for the IgE production of the B cells.

LC Express Low Activity Fc IgE Receptors upon IL4 Stimulation

But the production of IL-4 by T helper cells can have further consequences. IL-4 has been described as inducing the expression of low affinity Fc IgE receptors (CD23) on monocytes-macrophages. Since LC share many features with the monocyte-macrophage lineage, we wondered whether LC would express CD23 after stimulation with IL-4. Indeed, CD23 expression can be observed in human LC after incubation with IL-4 [9]. This observation is important in the context of atopic dermatitis, because IgE has been observed on the surface of LC in lesional skin of atopic dermatitis patients [10]. Since the histological and immunohistological picture of atopic dermatitis lesions resembles rather a T cell-mediated, delayed-type hypersensitivity reaction than an IgE-mediated, immediate-type reaction, it is conceivable that a local T helper cell response to chronic exposure of environmental antigens is main-

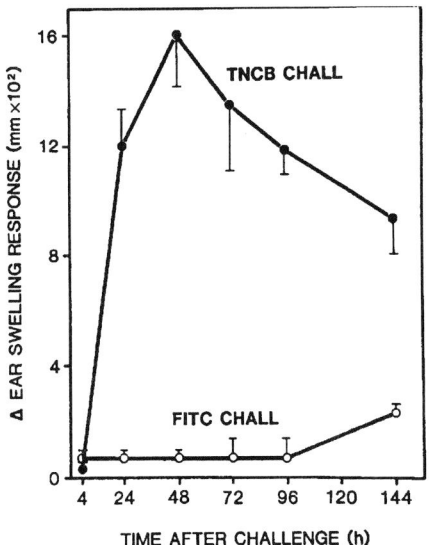

Figure 1. T cells purified from nonsensitized Balb/c mice were incubated with cultured LC which were modified with trinitrobenzenesulfonic acid (TNP). After 5 d recombinant human IL-2 was added. After 10 d the cells were washed and injected into the lateral tail vein of nonsensitized Balb/c recipient animals. The mice were immediately challenged on the ear with either trinitrochlorobenzene (TNCB) or fluorescein isothiocyanate (FITC). Δ Ear-swelling responses were assessed at the indicated time after challenge.

tained by LC. It is possible that the resulting IL-4 production leads to increased IgE synthesis and IgE receptor expression. The armoring of LC with cytophilic IgE in turn might enhance the local antigen presenting function of LC. Finally, it should be mentioned that IgE alone has been described to induce delayed-type reactions in the skin [11].

LC Induce Effector Cells of Contact Hypersensitivity

In primary cultures our T helper cells activated in vitro with LC resembled type 1 cells; since type 1 cells have been reported to induce delayed type hypersensitivity reactions after adoptive transfer, we expanded in recombinant IL-2 T cell blasts obtained from primary stimulation cultures. These cells were then injected into the lateral tail vein of syngeneic recipient mice. The mice were immediately challenged with the relevant or the irrelevant

hapten. After 24 hours ear swelling responses in recipient mice were assessed. Mice challenged with the relevant hapten showed ear swelling whereas mice challenged with the irrelevant hapten showed no ear swelling. Maximal ear swelling was observed after 24–48 h (Figure 1). Thus, this is the first demonstration that Langerhans cells are capable to directly induce effector cells of contact sensitivity.

LC, therefore, seem to activate mainly type 1 helper cells in early stimulation whereas repeated (> 4×) stimulation leads to activation of type 2 cells. A switch of type 1 to type 2 cells or selection of a few type 2 cells with loss of type 1 cells could explain these results. Whether the LC plays a role in such a switch or selection is unknown.

References

1. Stingl, G., C. Hauser, E. Tschachler, V. Groh, and K. Wolff. 1988. Immune functions of epidermal cells. In: Immunodermatology. D. Norris, ed. New York: Marcel Dekker, in press.
2. Hauser, C., and S. I. Katz. Activation and expansion of hapten- and protein-specific T helper cells from nonsensitized mice. Proc. Natl. Acad. Sci. USA, in press.
3. Mosmann, T. R., H. Cherwinski, M. W. Bond, M. A. Giedlin, and R. L. Coffman. 1986. Two types of murine helper T cell clone. I. Definition according to profiles of lymphokine activities and secreted proteins. J. Immunol. 136: 2348.
4. Cherwinski, H. M., J. H. Schumacher, K. D. Brown, and T. R. Mosmann. 1987. Two types of mouse helper T cell clone. III. Further differences in lymphokine synthesis between Th1 and Th2 clones revealed by RNA hybridization, functionally monospecific bioassays, and monoclonal antibodies. J. Exp. Med. 166: 1229.
5. Cher, D. J., and T. R. Mosmann. 1987. Two types of murine helper T cell clone. II. Delayed-type hypersensitivity is mediated by Th1 clones. J. Immunol. 138: 3688.
6. Mosmann, T. R. 1988. Annual Meeting of the Swiss Society of Allergology and Immunology.
7. Coffman, R. L., J. Ohara, M. W. Bond, J. Carty, A. Zlotnik, and W. E. Paul. 1986. B cell stimulatory factor-1 enhances the IgE response of lipopolysaccharide activated B cells. J. Immunol. 136: 4538.
8. Hauser, C., C. M. Snapper, J. Ohara, W. E. Paul, and S. I. Katz. T helper cells grown with hapten-modified cultured Langerhans cells produce interleukin 4 and stimulate IgE production by B cells. Submitted.

9. Biber T. 1988. ESDR-Meeting, Munich (presentation No. 98).

10. Bruynzeel-Koomen, C., D. F. van Wichen, J. Toonstra, L. Berrens, and P. L. B. Bruynzeel. 1986. The presence of IgE molecules on epidermal Langerhans cells in patients with atopic dermatitis. Arch. Dermatol. Res. 278: 199.

11. Ray, M. C., M. D. Tharp, T. J. Sullivan, and R. E. Tigelaar. 1983. Contact hypersensitivity reactions to dinitrofluorobenzene mediated by monoclonal IgE anti-DNP antibodies. J. Immunol. 131: 1096.

Recent Advances in Molecular Aspects of Allergic Contact Dermatitis and Skin Tolerance

*Claude Benezra**

Stereospecifity of allergic contact dermatitis is observed when chiral centers are close to the site of protein attachment such as beta-substituted alpha-methylen-gamma-butyrolactone. With gamma-substituted derivatives no specificity was observed. Skin tolerance can be induced in guinea pigs by using hapten derivatives: double-headed haptens, hydrosoluble derivations, or properly substituted allergens such as 5-methyl-pentadecylcatechol. The two main topics of this review will be specificity of molecular recognition of allergic contact dermatitis (ACD) and some aspects of skin tolerance.

Specificity of Molecular Recognition of ACD

The specificity of recognition of a given hapten lies in the T-cell receptors.

Enantiomers are compounds with a chemical structure the relationship of which is the same as the one existing between a subject and his mirror image. Alice in Wonderland, when going through the mirror, should have her heart on the right side, her liver on the left. The two Alices, the real one and the image, are *not superimposable*. Examples of enantiomers are known in ACD. Thus, in nature two usnic acids, two frullanolides, do occur. Most of the time, only *one* enantiomer exists in nature. This is the case for tulipalin B, one of the allergens of tulip; we have synthesized its mirror image (-)-tulipalin B. Both tulipalins are equally good sensitizers in guinea pigs, and there are no cross reactions between them [1].

Mitchell and Shibata [2] have shown that their patients only reacted to d-usnic acid. There was no reaction to its nonsuperimpos-

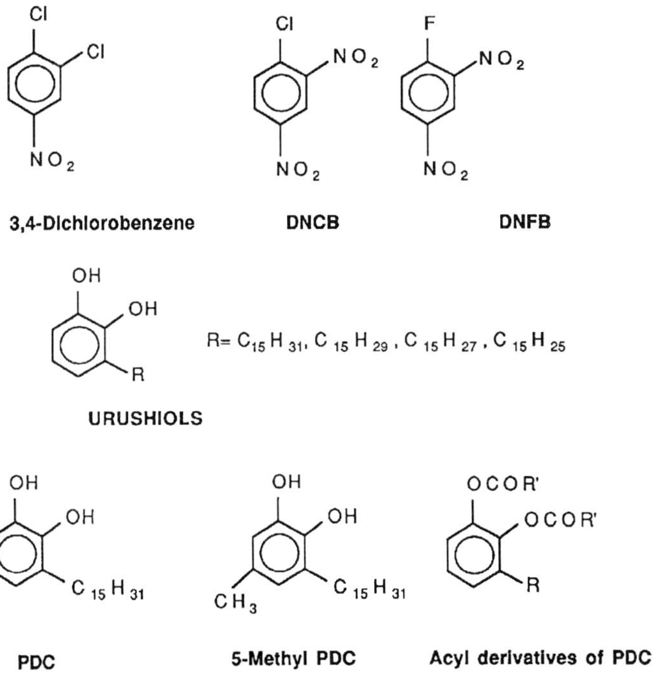

Figure 1. Chemical compounds referred to in this article.

3,4-Dichlorobenzene   DNCB   DNFB

URUSHIOLS   R= $C_{15}H_{31}$, $C_{15}H_{29}$, $C_{15}H_{27}$, $C_{15}H_{25}$

PDC   5-Methyl PDC   Acyl derivatives of PDC

*   Université Louis Pasteur, Strasbourg, France.

333

able mirror image or *enantiomer*, 1-usnic acid. This shows the specificity of ACD to usnic acid enontiomers or *enantiospecificity*. Later, Salo et al. [3] showed that lichen pickers in Finland reacted to one usnic acid, to its enantiomer, or even to both of them. Reaction to either one of the usnic acid enantiomers or to *both* of them is certainly a case of multiple concomitant sensitization.

The position of the chiral center (i.e., the source of asymmetry) is not indifferent to show enantiospecificity. Thus, when we sensitized two groups of guinea pigs to gamma-methyl-alpha-methylene-gamma-butyrolactone and its (-)-enantiomer, the two groups reacted to both enantiomers: no enantiospecificity was observed [4]. However, we were able to sensitize guinea pigs to both enantiomers of a sesquiterpene lactone, (+)- and (-)-frullanolides and show that complete enantiospecificity existed [5]. Beta-substituted alpha-methylene-gamma-butyrolactones also showed total enantiospecificity: (+)-tulipalin B (beta-hydroxy-substituted lactone)-sensitized guinea pigs did not react to (-)-tulipalin B sensitized ones [1]. A possible interpretation is that the closer the chiral center is to the center of attack by a nucleophilic protein, the higher is the specificity recognition. In other words, when the source of asymmetry is in the beta position, enantiospecificity is observed, whereas when it is in the position gamma (and therefore further away), no specificity exists. This is summarized in Figure 1.

These results give a firm stand to the hypothesis of antigen formation by a chemical reaction between a carrier (protein) and a hapten.

Skin Tolerance

Tolerance to cutaneous haptens was demonstrated as early as 1946 by Chase [6]: Prior feeding of animals with dinitrochlorobenzene (DNCB) prevented them from becoming sensitized to this hapten. An intravenous injection of sodium dinitrobenzenesulfonate (DNSBSO3Na) also prevented further sensitization to DNCB [7].

These two examples illustrate the way of experimentally immune tolerance. This occurs when:

— the hapten is introduced into the organism by a route different from the regular sensiti-

zation route (epicutaneous or intradermal);

— a hapten derivative is introduced either by a route different from the regular sensitization route or by the same route.

Hapten processing by cells is essential in leading either to sensitization or tolerance. One cell plays a particularly important role in ACD: the Langerhans cell. When some of its functions are impaired by chemical or physico-chemical means, it can lead to either sensitization or tolerance. Thus, when DNFB was painted on an 8 cm^2 area on the shaved skin of a guinea pig and 24 h later a second hapten, urushiol (present in poison ivy and poison oak) was deposited on the same area, induction to the second hapten was observed [8]. When the Langerhans cells were intact, sensitization was induced to DNFB; 24 h later the number of "ATPase positive" Langerhans cells dropped dramatically. Painting urushiol on this same surface resulted in tolerance to the latter. "ATPase positive" cells, therefore, seem necessary to process haptens.

Hapten derivatives have been used to induce tolerance to the corresponding hapten:

— esterified derivatives of pentadecylcatechol or PDC [9]

— dipeptide derivatives of sesquiterpene lactones [Stampf et al., unpublished results];

— dichloronitrobenzene induced tolerance to DNCB;

— 5-methylpentadecylcatechol (5-Me-PDC) induced tolerance to urushiol, allergens from poison ivy and poison oak in both mice [10] and guinea pigs [11].

Conclusions

It has been demonstrated that molecular recognition in allergic contact dermatitis is *enantiospecific*, i.e., enantiomeric haptens could be distinguished by T-cell receptors.

Concerning immune tolerance, derivatization of allergens, or transformation of Langerhans cell, receptors have successfully made model animals (mice and guinea pigs) tolerant to further sensitization. This tolerance has been shown to be specific.

References

1. Papageorgiou, C., J. L. Stampf, and C. Benezra. 1988. Allergic contact dermatitis to tulips: An example of enantiospecificity. Arch. Dermatol. Res. 280: 5–7.

2. Mitchel, J. C., and S. Shibata, 1969. Immunological activity of some substances derived from lichenized fungi. J. Invest. Derm. 52: 517–520.

3. Salo, H., M. Hannuksela, and B. M. Hausen. 1981. Lichen pickers dermatitis (*Cladonia alpestris* (L) Rab.) Contact Dermatitis 7: 9–13.

4. Barbier, P., and C. Benezra. 1982. Allergenic alpha-methylene-gamma-butyrolactone. Stereospecific synthesis of (+)- and (-)-gamma-methyl-alpha-methylene-gamma-butyrolactone. A study of the specificity of (+)- and (-)-enantiomer in inducing ACD. J. Med. Chem. 25: 943–946.

5. Barbier, P., and C. Benezra. 1982. Stereospecificity of allergic contact dermatitis induced by two natural enantiomers, (+)- and (-)-frullanolides, in guinea pigs. Naturwissenschaften 62: 296–297.

6. Chase, M. W. 1946. Inhibition of experimental drug allergy by prior feeding of the sensitizing agent. Proceedings Soc. Exp. Biol. and Med. 61: 257–259.

7. Polak, L. 1980. Immunological aspects of contact sensitivity. An experimental study. Monographs in Allergy, vol. 15, p. 7.

8. Hanau, D., J. L. Stampf, M. Fabre, E. Grosshans, and C. Benezra. 1985. Induction of tolerance to urushiol by epicutaneous application of this hapten on dinitrofluorobenzene-treated skin. J. Invest. Dermatol. 85: 9–11.

9. Watson, E. S., J. C. Murphy, C. W. Waller, and M. A. Elsohly. 1981. Immunologic studies on poisonous Anacardiacae. I: Production of tolerance and desensitization to poison ivy and oak urushiols using esterified urushiol derivatives in guinea pigs. J. Invest. Dermatol. 76: 164–170.

10. Dunn, I. S., D. J. Liberato, J. Castagnoli, Jr., and V. S. Byers. 1982. Contact sensitivity to urushiol: Role of covalent bond formation. Cell Immunol. 74: 220–233.

11. Stampf, J. L., C. Benezra, V. S. Byers, and H. Castagnoli Jr. 1986. Induction of tolerance to poison ivy urushiol in the guinea pig by epicutaneous application of the structural analog 5-Methyl-3-n-pentadecylcatechol. J. Invest. Dermatol. 86: 535–538.

IgE and the Pathogenesis of Atopic Eczema

Rebecca H. Buckley*

Atopic dermatitis is an excellent model for studying (1) late-phase IgE-mediated reactions, (2) host defense factors needed for protection against certain viral agents and staphylococci, and (3) human IgE regulation. Patients with allergic eczema have the highest serum IgE concentrations of any atopic disorder. Oral exposure to foods or prolonged topical application of dust mite allergens to lightly abraded skin in sensitive patients both result in lesions resembling those of atopic dermatitis, consistent with a late-phase IgE-mediated reaction. Susceptibility of such patients to herpes virus infections and their markedly elevated serum IgE concentrations have both suggested abnormal T cell function, but delineation of the precise defect or defects has thus far not been possible. Recent studies from the author's laboratory have shown that small quantities of recombinant human interleukin 4 (rhIL-4) can stimulate synthesis of substantial quantities of IgE by human blood mononuclear cells (MNC) in a reproducible and dose-dependent manner. This system for inducing IgE synthesis in vitro makes possible for the first time a careful dissection of the role of various cells and cytokines in the regulation of human IgE synthesis. Such information will be of great value in delineating at a cellular and molecular level the causative differences between humans (such as eczema patients) who produce excessive quantities of IgE and those who do not. Once such differences are identified, this information could lead to major therapeutic advances for IgE-mediated allergic diseases.

Soon after it was noted that patients with asthma and hay fever manifest an immediate wheal and flare reaction when skin tested with extracts of environmental substances, the word atopic came to be used in referring to the pruritic dermatitis seen in many such individuals [1]. Intriguingly, higher serum IgE concentrations have been found in patients with allergic eczema than in any other atopic disorder [2]. Indeed, among atopic patients' sera evaluated for specific IgE antibodies by the radioallergosorbent test (RAST), those from patients with atopic dermatitis gave both the highest number of positive RASTs and the most strongly positive reactions [3]. In addition, serum IgE concentrations have been noted to drop precipitously following intervals as brief as two years after remission or healing of allergic eczema [4] and much more rapidly in patients who have eliminated foods identified in controlled challenges to cause exacerbations of their eczema [5]. All of this implicates a relationship between IgE antibodies and atopic dermatitis. However, the mononuclear character of the dermal cellular infiltrate in eczema skin lesions [6] and the seemingly poor correlation of skin-testing results with clinical sensitivity have led many to doubt a role for IgE in the pathogenesis of atopic eczema. Results of double-blind, placebo-controlled food challenges in children with atopic dermatitis have, nevertheless, demonstrated that immediate hypersensitivity reactions induced by ingestion of foods to which the patients are sensitive can provoke cutaneous pruritus and erythema, which lead to scratching and subsequent eczematoid lesions [5]. Mast cells, which bear Type I or high avidity Fc receptors for IgE, are found in increased number in tissue sections from areas of chronic lichenified atopic eczema skin [6]. Since prick and intradermal tests eliciting immediate hypersensitivity reactions in the skin rarely if ever evolve into eczematoid lesions, it had always been assumed that such reactions had not role in the pathogenesis of eczema. It is now appreciated, however, that immediate reactions mediated by IgE may be followed by late-phase cutaneous reactions both in humans and in rodents [7]. Such late-phase reactions are characterized at 8 hours by a mixed cellular infiltrate consisting of eosinophils, lymphocytes, basophils, and neutrophils—with lymphocytes predominating—and, thereafter, by a mononuclear round cell infiltrate. Similar inflammatory histology has been noted in biopsies of eczema patients' normal skin which had been gently abraded,

*   Duke University School of Medicine, P.O. Box 2898, Durham, North Carolina 27710.
    Supported by an NIH Asthma and Allergic Diseases Center grant, P50 AI12026.

then patch-tested for 48 hours with aqueous allergen extracts known to elicit IgE-mediated responses in them [8]. Moreover, the positive reactions were characterized grossly by confluent papular erythema, edema, and exudation, similar to eczema lesions. Thus, there is evidence that IgE antibody-antigen reactions can lead to late-phase cutaneous reactions resembling atopic eczema. Constituents of IgE-mediated reactions which could contribute to the inflammatory lesion seen in eczema include

— products of arachidonic acid metabolism, particularly leukotriene B$_4$, which is highly chemotactic for a variety of cells;

— eosinophil major basic protein (MBP), known to be capable of damaging intestinal, spleen, and skin cells [9].

It is generally agreed that lesions of atopic dermatitis are preceded by intense pruritus, and eczema is known as "the itch that rashes" [2]. When itching occurs as a consequence of histamine release during the immediate reaction, it is possible that trauma and tissue damage induced by scratching could be compounded by release of substance P and/or eosinophil MBP. The resultant inflammatory reaction, plus the cellular infiltrate elicited by extruded mast cell granular enzymes, could thus account for the histology seen in biopsies of eczema skin.

The above-noted association of allergic eczema with excessive IgE antibody production, plus data accumulated over the past two decades implicating a fundamental role for T cells in both the initiation and regulation of IgE synthesis in rodents, have triggered interest in cellular immunity in patients with atopic dermatitis [10]. Since manipulation of the immune response in low IgE responder mice by treatments known to abrogate suppressor T cell function led to enhanced and persistent IgE antibody formation, the hypothesis was made that high IgE responder mice were genetically deficient in such a cellular control mechanism. Similarly, it has been postulated that humans with excessive IgE antibody formation—like high IgE responder mice—may be deficient in non-antigen-specific, IgE-isotype-specific regulatory T cells. However, evidence to date that excessive IgE production in humans is due to faulty immunoregulation is still primarily circumstantial. Increased IgE production has been detected with high frequency in some primary immunodeficiency syndrome characterized by partial but not complete deficiencies in T-cell function [11]. In addition, a number of studies have been published to suggest that cell-mediated immunity (CMI) may be depressed in patients with atopic dermatitis. It has long been known that eczema patients have a heightened susceptibility to infections with herpes simplex, vaccinia, and molluscum contagiosum viruses. One of the first suggestions that CMI is depressed in atopic dermatitis was reported in 1937 by Rostenberg and Sulzberger, who found a low incidence of positive patch tests to common contact sensitizers among eczema patients in testing a large number of patients with verious dermatologic disorders [12]. Palacios et al. [13] in 1966 and Jones et al. [14] in 1973 found that patients with allergic eczema were less readily sensitized with dinitrochlorobenzene and to Rhus extract, respectively, than were normals. In 1975, McGeady and the author conducted studies of immune function in 21 patients with atopic eczema [15]. All 15 patients with active lesions, whether localized or generalized, had marked delayed cutaneous anergy to the ubiquitous antigens candida and streptokinase-streptodornase, whereas those with nearly healed eczema had positive delayed skin tests to one or both antigens. In in vitro studies of lymphocyte responsiveness to mitogens and of Con A-induced suppressor cell activity, no differences were found between the activities of eczema patients' and normal controls' blood lymphocytes. Using monoclonal antibodies to T cell surface antigens, Leung et al. [16] conducted a study in which they reported finding a statistically lower percentage of cells of the suppressor/cytotoxic (CD8) phenotype. In functional studies, they also reported significantly decreased cell-mediated lympholysis (CML) by eczema patients' cells during mixed lymphocyte culture, as compared to that by normal controls' cells. Their finding of a decreased percentage of cells of the suppressor/cytotoxic (CD8) phenotype could not be confirmed by others. In addition, cytofluorographic studies by the author of blood lymphocytes from over 30 patients with atopic dermatitis, using monoclonal antibodies recognizing most T lymphocytes (CD3) and those with the helper (CD4) and suppressor (CD8) phenotypes, also failed to reveal values significantly different from normal. Since the experimental work in lower species points to a deficiency of isotype-specific T suppressor cells in animals with augmented IgE antibody production, it is unlikely that that kind of deficiency would be reflected in general tests of T-cell function.

Attempts to examine directly whether excessive IgE production in patients with atopic eczema is due to faulty T cell immunoregulation have been difficult because of the inability to conduct experiments with cells from lymphoid organs or in human subjects in vivo. In vitro studies of human IgE synthesis by B cells in the only readily accessible tissue, i.e., blood, have been hampered by the following factors:

— the failure of pokeweed mitogen (PWM) and other polyclonal B cell activators to stimulate IgE synthesis [17, 18];

— frequent failure of investigators to control adequately for preformed IgE which often exceeds the picogram quantities of "spontaneously synthesized" IgE in most reports;

— the variable sensitivity, specificity, and precision of immunoassays for quantifying the very low amount of IgE in cell culture supernatants, with reproducible sensitivity only at IgE concentrations greater than 0.5 ng/ml.

Although factors structurally analogous to rodent IgE binding factors which either potentiate or suppress IgE synthesis have been reported to be produced by human T cells, demonstration of biologic effects of such factors has been difficult because of these problems [19]. After a different non-IgE binding molecule (i.e., B cell stimulatory factor 1 or IL-4) was reported to stimulate the synthesis of microgram quantities of IgE in rodents, a structurally similar human molecule was identified through recombinant DNA technology [20]. IL-4 is a 15–20 kd glycoprotein produced by activated T cells and mast cells. It is known to have multiple effects on murine B cells including induction of the expression of the low affinity or Type II Fcε receptor (CD23) and stimulation of IgE and IgG1 secretion by LPS-stimulated B cells. It is also a growth factor for murine T, B, and mast cells, and its receptors are found on numerous cells of hematopoietic lineage. Human recombinant IL-4 (rhIL-4) has been shown to promote the growth of human T cells and pre-activated B cells and to promote the growth of human T cells and pre-activated B cells and to promote the appearance of CD23

on human B cells. However, until recently, only very small amounts of IgE and/or IgG had been detected in cultures of human B cells stimulated with rhIL-4. Recently, the author and her associates found that the addition of very small quantities (0.312 ng/ml or greater) of rhIL-4 to unfractionated human blood mononuclear cells (MNC) or to enriched B cells plus fresh or cloned T cells under the conditions of our culture system resulted consistently in the production of substantial quantities of IgE, some exceeding 200 ng/ml, or 10-fold greater than those reported in previous in vitro studies of human IgE synthesis. IgG synthesis was also induced, but unlike murine IL-4, there was no preferential stimulation of any IgG subclass. Time-course studies revealed that synthesis of both IgE and IgG began at around 9 days and peaked at 18 days of culture. Studies with purified populations of T and B cells have thus far indicated a requirement for the physical presence of T cells for this effect of rhIL-4. However, cell proliferation (either T or B) does not appear to be necessary for rhIL-4-induced human IgE synthesis. Both atopic and non-atopic B cells have been induced by rhIL-4 to synthesize IgE and IgG, and this effect of rhIL-4 is completely abrogated by the presence of PWM. Thus, for the first time there now exists a reproducibly positive system for inducing human IgE synthesis in vitro, opening the door to a careful dissection of the roles of various cells and cytokines in the regulation of human IgE synthesis. This information will obviously be of great value in delineating at a cellular and molecular level the differences between humans (such as those with atopic eczema) who produce excessive quantities of IgE and those who do not. Once such differences can be pinpointed, this information could lead to major therapeutic advances for IgE-mediated diseases.

References

1. Atherton, D. J. 1981. Allergy and atopic eczema, I and II. Clin. Exp. Dermatol. 6: 191, 317.
2. Kaplan, A. P., R. H. Buckley, and K. P. Mathews. 1987. Allergic skin disorders. In: Primer on allergic and immunologic diseases (2nd ed.). R. F. Lockey, ed. J. Am. Med. Assoc 258: 2900.
3. Hoffman, D. R., F. Y. Yamamoto, B. Sellar et al. 1975. Specific IgE antibodies in atopic eczema. J. Allerg. Clin. Immunol. 55: 256.

4. Johansson, S. G. O., and L. Juhlin. 1970. Immunoglobulin E in "healed" atopic dermatitis and after treatment with corticosteroids and azathioprine. Brit. J. Derm. 82: 10.

5. Sampson, H. A. 1983. Role of immediate food hypersensitivity in the pathogenesis of atopic dermatitis. J. Allergy Clin. Immunol. 71: 473.

6. Mihm, M. C. Jr., N. A. Soter, H.F. Dvorak et al. 1976. The structure of normal skin and the morphology of atopic eczema. J. Invest. Dermatol. 67: 305.

7. Atkins, P. C., and B. Zweiman. 1987. The IgE-mediated late-phase skin response—unraveling the enigma. J. Allergy Clin. Immunol. 79: 12.

8. Mitchell, E. B., J. Crow, M. D. Chapman et al. 1982. Basophils in allergen-induced patch test sites in atopic dermatitis. Lancet i: 127.

9. Butterworth, A. E., and J. R. David. 1981. Eosinophil function. New Engl. J. Med. 304: 154.

10. Tada, T. 1975. Regulation of reaginic antibody formation in animals. Prog. Allergy 19: 122.

11. Buckley, R. H. 1988. Immunologic deficiency and allergic diseases. In: Allergy: Principles and practice, Voo. 1. E. Middleton, C. E. Reed, and E. F. Ellis, eds. St. Louis: C. V. Mosby, p. 295.

12. Rostenberg, A., and M. B. Sulzberger. 1937. Some results of patch tests. Arch. Dermatol. Syph. 35: 433.

13. Palacios, J., E. W. Fuller, and W. K. Blaylock. 1966. Immunological capabilities of patients with atopic dermatitis. J. Invest. Dermatol. 47: 484.

14. Jones, H. E., C. W. Lewis, and S. L. McMarlin. 1973. Allergic contact sensitivity in atopic dermatitis. Arch. Dermatol. 107: 217.

15. McGeady, S. J., and R. H. Buckley. 1975. Depression of cell-mediated immunity in atopic eczema. J. Allergy Clin. Immunol. 56: 393.

16. Leung, D. Y. M., A. R. Rhodes, and R. S. Geha. 1981. Enumeration of T cells subsets in atopic dermatitis using monoclonal antibodies. J. Allergy Clin. Immunol. 67: 450.

17. Fiser, P. M., and R. H. Buckley. 1979. Human IgE biosynthesis in vitro: Studies with atopic and normal blood mononuclear cells and subpopulations. J. Immunol. 123: 1788:

18. Sampson, H. A., and R. H. Buckley. 1981. Human IgE synthesis in vitro: A reassessment. J. Immunol. 127: 829.

19. Ishizaka, K. 1988. IgE-binding factors and regulation of the IgE antibody response. Ann. Rev. Immunol. 6: 513.

20. Paul, W. E., and J. Ohara. 1987. B-cell stimulatory factor-1/interleukin 4. Ann. Rev. Immunol. 5: 429.

Pathogenic Role of Food Hypersensitivity in Atopic Dermatitis

*Hugh A. Sampson**

Food hypersensitivity plays a significant pathogenic role in many patients (especially children) with atopic dermatitis. Although a variety of immunologic mechanisms may be involved, IgE-mediated hypersensitivity reactions are most clearly documented. The pathogenic role of "classical" and potential IgE-mediated reactions to food allergens in the eczematous skin lesions of atopic dermatitis are discussed.

A variety of non-immunologic and immunologic factors contribute to the cutaneous pruritus and secondary trauma central to the development of eczematous skin lesions in atopic dermatitis [1]. While several different immunologic mechanisms may play a pathogenic role in this disorder, this review will focus on known and potential pathogenic pathways involving IgE molecules. Utilizing double-blind placebo-controlled oral food challenges (DBPCFC) conducted in a controlled environment, we have demonstrated clinically significant reactions to foods in approximately 50% of a select referral population of children with severe atopic dermatitis [2, 3]. Burks [4], using a similar DBPCFC protocol, found a 35% reaction rate to foods in a population of children with atopic dermatitis presenting to a university dermatology and allergy clinic. Appropriate diagnosis and exclusion of foods eliciting reactions by DBPCFC resulted in significant symptomatic improvement in children with atopic dermatitis and food allergy compared to children not adhering to their diet or in children with no demonstrable food hypersensitivity [3].

Food hypersensitivity has been investigated in 210 patients with atopic dermatitis. Two hundred thirty-five DBPCFC's have been interpreted as positive; 75% involved cutaneous symptoms, 45% involved gastrointestinal symptoms, and 25% respiratory symptoms. Cutaneous symptoms generally developed abruptly within 10–120 minutes of initiating the challenge, consisted of a pruritic erythematous morbilliform rash, and commonly involved predilection sites. As symptoms began to subside, many children became drowsy and fell asleep for 1–2 hours, and some were noted to develop a slight rise in temperature. Upon awakening, symptoms usually appeared fully resolved (2–3 hours post-challenge), but pruritus and a less distinct erythematous macular rash not infrequently developed 4–6 hours later and lasted for several hours.

Although Walzer [5] clearly demonstrated the rapidity with which food allergens can penetrate the gut barrier and reach sensitized cutaneous mast cells, the role of IgE-mediated food hypersensitivity in the pathogenesis of atopic dermatitis has been doubted for years. In view of our studies and others, it seems likely that several immunologic reactions involving IgE play a pathogenic role in atopic dermatitis. Both clinical and laboratory evidence suggest that classical immediate and late-phase IgE-mediated food reactions occur in atopic dermatitis. As published previously [6], only children experiencing a positive DBPCFC developed a rise in plasma histamine, from a mean of 196 ± 80 pg/ml to 1055 ± 356 pg/ml ($P < 0.001$), whereas children having no symptoms to a food antigen or placebo had no change in plasma histamine. To determine whether food antigen-antibody complex formation could account for complement activation and subsequent mast cell/basophil activation, C3a desArg and C5a desArg were measured prior to DBPCFC and immediately, 15 minutes, and 30 minutes after the development

* Johns Hopkins University Medical School, Johns Hopkins Hospital, 600 N. Wolfe Street, Baltimore, Maryland 21205, USA.
Supported by grant AI24439 and AI00830 from the National Institute of Allergy and Infectious Diseases, and by grants RR-30 and RR-00052 from the General Clinical Research Centers Program of the Division of Research Resources, National Institutes of Health. Data was managed and analyzed with CLINFO. Dr. Sampson is a recipient of the Allergic Diseases Academic Award, NIH.

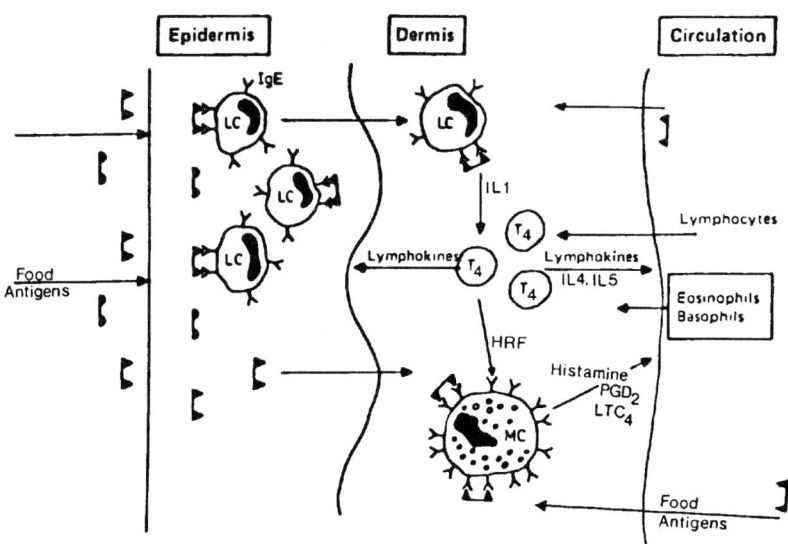

Figure 1. Food antigens may reach cutaneous immunoreactive cells via the circulation following ingestion or via penetration of the epidermal layer following contact. IgE-coated mast cells and Langerhans cells may become activated setting in motion the release of various mediators and recruitment of inflammatory cells.

of clinical symptoms. There was no change in C3a levels, and C5a remained undetectable throughout [7]. To determine whether circulating basophils were activated and accounting for the rise in plasma histamine, venous blood samples obtained before DBPCFC, and 15 minutes and 30 minutes after development of clinical symptoms were analyzed for basophil number, total histamine content of a leukocyte preparation, and unstimulated (spontaneous) histamine release in vitro [8]. There was no difference in basophil number, total histamine content, or unstimulated histamine release at any time point. Taken together, it would appear that early cutaneous symptoms secondary to food challenges are the result of IgE-mediated mast cell activation. Since circulating histamine is catabolized so rapidly, and since many patients experienced only cutaneous symptoms, it is most likely that the rise in plasma histamine predominantly reflected cutaneous mast cell histamine release.

As now appreciated with other atopic disorders, the late-phase IgE-mediated response is probably a major pathogenic factor in atopic dermatitis. During the late-phase response, neutrophils and eosinophils infiltrate the inflammatory site 4–8 hours after the initial reaction, and mononuclear round cells (lymphocytes and monocytes) predominantly after 24–48 hours [9]. Biopsy specimens of atopic dermatitis lesions generally demonstrate an ab-

sence of eosinophils and a heavy mononuclear cell infiltrate. However, in a study with Leiferman et al. [10], evidence of previous eosinophil infiltration was demonstrated by the presence of eosinophil major basic protein (MBP). MBP, a cytolytic protein secreted almost exclusively by eosinophils, was selectively deposited in eczematous lesions and not in normal appearing skin of patients with atopic dermatitis. Two food-allergic patients who experienced resolution of cutaneous symptoms while maintaining an appropriate allergen avoidance diet underwent repeat DBPCFCs in a subsequent study [7]. Early pruritic morbilliform rashes again developed following the challenges. Skin biopsies were obtained at lesional sites 4 and 14 hours later; both revealed eosinophil infiltration and early deposition of MBP. These findings correlate with the late development of pruritus and erythematous rashes seen following many positive DBPCFC and demonstrate physiologic activation of the IgE-mediated late-phase reaction.

In contrast to non-atopics, atopic individuals develop marked eosinophilotactic activity following the injection of allergen or platelet-activating factor (PAF) acether into the skin [11]. Once present in the skin, the eosinophil is capable of releasing a variety of mediators which could contribute to the eczematous changes: MBP is toxic to several cell types and can induce histamine release from mast cells; eosino-

341

phil-derived neurotoxin is capable of demyelinating nerves and may be responsible for demyelinated nerve endings seen in eczematous skin lesions; and PAF and LTC4, both are capable of promoting inflammation and edema in the skin.

Recent studies suggest that IgE-mediated contact hypersensitivity may contribute to eczematous skin lesions in atopic dermatitis. Mitchell et al. [12] demonstrated the development of eczematous skin lesions and increase in skin mast cells following the repeated application of mite antigen to lightly abraded skin of sensitized individuals. Adinoff et al. [13] had similar findings following the application (for 48 hours) of a variety of aeroallergens to normal appearing skin of sensitized patients. Given the eating styles of most young infants, it is not uncommon to have extensive application of various foods to the hands, arms, face, and neck. Many parents report the development of erythematous, pruritic skin lesions following their child's contact with certain foods. It is likely that contact, as well as ingestion of certain food allergens, contributes to eczematous skin lesions.

It seems likely that a variety of other immunologic reactions involving IgE are active in atopic dermatitis. Food-allergic patients with atopic dermatitis were found to have high "spontaneous" basophil histamine release (BHR) in vitro and "spontaneous" generation of histamine-releasing factor (HRF) from peripheral blood mononuclear cells cultured 24 h in vitro (submitted for publication). HRF was shown to activate cells through surface-bound IgE molecules. Once the appropriate food allergen was excluded from the diet and skin symptoms largely improved, "spontaneous" BHR normalized and "spontaneous" generation of HRF disappeared. Food allergen-induced production of HRF in vivo could account for the increased basophil releasability reported in some patients with atopic dermatitis [14] and lead to a state of "cutaneous hyperreactivity," similar to that seen in the airway of patients with atopic asthma.

Recent studies have demonstrated the presence of IgE on Langerhans' cells (LC) only in patients with atopic dermatitis [15]. As depicted in Figure 1, food allergen also could induce LC activation with release of IL-1 and various arachidonic acid metabolites. In turn, local lymphocytes could be activated to release HRF, IL-4, IL-5, and other lymphokines. IL-4 may serve as a local growth factor for mast cells, and promotes differentiation of FcE-bearing B cells and IgE synthesis; IL-5 is a chemoattractant for eosinophils and promotes their differentiation [16]. Some lines of evidence suggest a central pathogenic role for IgE-bearing LCs: LC numbers are markedly increased in skin lesions of atopic dermatitis, UV-B therapy (which selectively inactivates LCs) is an effective form of therapy for atopic dermatitis, and many children experiencing symptoms following a DBPCFC develop drowsiness and mild temperature elevation (IL-1 effects). It is likely that a complex interaction of immunologic pathways contribute to the inflammation and histologic changes seen in atopic dermatitis.

Present evidence clearly implicates a pathogenic role for food hypersensitivity in a significant number of children with atopic dermatitis. While several immunologic pathways may be involved in the development of eczematous lesions, our research and this review has focused on potential IgE-mediated mechanisms. Classical IgE-mediated "immediate" and "late-phase" hypersensitivity responses are clearly involved in some patients. However, with the finding of "spontaneously" generated HRF in food allergic patients and the presence of IgE-bearing LCs, it seems highly likely that the repertoire of IgE-mediated hypersensitivity responses is much greater than originally appreciated. Whether the IgE molecule is critical for the activation and response of the various cells to which it binds remains to be established. The further study of food hypersensitivity in patients with atopic dermatitis may help elucidate the full role of IgE in hypersensitivity disorders.

References

1. Hanifin, J. M. 1988. Atopic dermatitis. In: Allergy: Principles and practice. E. Middleton, C. E. Reed, E. F. Ellis, N. F. Adkinson, and J. W. Yunginger, eds. St. Louis: C. V. Mosby, p. 1403–28.
2. Sampson, H. A. 1983. Role of immediate food hypersensitivity in the pathogenesis of atopic dermatitis. J. Allergy Clin. Immunol. 71: 473.
3. Sampson, H. A. 1985. Food hypersensitivity and atopic dermatitis: Evaluation of 113 patients. J Pediatr. 107: 669.

4. Burks, A. W., S. B. Mallory, L. W. Williams, and M. A. Shirrell. 1988. Atopic dermatitis: Clinical relevance of food hypersensitivity reactions. J. Pediatr. 113: 447.

5. Wilson, S. J., and M. Walzer. 1935. Absorption of undigested proteins in human beings: The absorption of unaltered egg protein in infants. Am. J. Dis. Child. 50: 49.

6. Sampson, H. A., and P. L. Jolie. 1984. Increased plasma histamine concentrations after food challenges in children with atopic dermatitis. New Engl. J. Med. 311: 372.

7. Sampson, H. A. 1988. Role of food allergy and mediator release in atopic dermatitis. J. Allergy Clin. Immunol. 81: 635.

8. Sampson, H. A., and K. Broadbent. 1987. "Spontaneous" basophil histamine release and histamine-releasing factor in patients with atopic dermatitis and food hypersensitivity. J. Allergy Clin. Immunol. 79: 241.

9. Lemanske, R. F., and M. A. Kaliner. 1988. Late-phase allergic reactions. In: Allergy: Principles and practice. E. Middleton, C. E. Reed, E. F. Ellis, N. F. Adkinson, and J. W. Yunginger, eds. St. Louis: C. V. Mosby, p. 224–246.

10. Leiferman, K. M., S. J. Ackerman, H. A. Sampson et al. 1985. Dermal deposition of eosinophil granule major basic protein in atopic dermatitis. New Engl. J. Med. 313: 282.

11. Henocq, E., and B. B. Vargaftig. 1988. Skin eosinophilia in atopic patients. J. Allergy Clin. Immunol. 81: 691.

12. Mitchell, E. B., J. Crow, G. Williams, and T. A. E. Platts-Mills. 1986. Increase in skin mast cells following chronic house dust mite exposure. Br. J. Dermatol. 114:65.

13. Adinoff, A. D., P. Tellez, R. A. F. Clark. 1988. Atopic dermatitis and aeroallergen contact sensitivity. J. Allergy Clin. Immunol. 81: 736.

14. Marone, R. Giugliano, G. Lembo, and F. Ayala. 1986. Human basophil releasability. II. Changes in basophil releasability in patients with atopic dermatitis. J. Invest. Dermatol. 87: 19.

15. Bruynzeel-Koomen, C., D. F. van Wichen, J. Toonstra et al. 1986. Presence of IgE molecules on epidermal Langerhans cells in patients with atopic dermatitis. Arch. Dermatol. Res. 278: 199.

16. O'Gara, S. Umland, T. DeFrance, and J. Christiansen. 1988. "B-cell factors" are pleiotropic. Immunol. Today 9: 45.

Influence of Mountain Climate on Immune Parameters in Atopic Dermatitis, Psoriasis and Controls

Brunello Wüthrich*, Helen Joller- Jemelka**, Peter Grob**, Peter Späth***, Dieter Hasler****, Peter Braun****

In patients with atopic dermatitis (AD) n = 37), psoriasis (P) (n = 11), and in controls (C) (n = 11) from the Department for Dermatology and Allergy of the Zurich High Mountain Clinic Clavadel (1600 m altitude), extensive immune parameters, such as serum immunoglobulins (IgE, IgA, IgM, IgG, and IgG-subclasses), specific IgE (RAST) against nine common allergens (in AD alone), immune complexes, complement concentrations and complement functions as well as α_1-antitrypsin, neopterin, β_2-microglobulin and soluble interleukin-2 receptors (sIL-2R) were investigated at admission (A) and at discharge (D) (on the average 36 days as inpatient). The severity of the skin manifestations in the AD-patients were quantified precisely.

A measurable influence of mountain climate on the humoral immune parameters could not be confirmed statistically, although the skin conditions of the AD- and P-patients improved significantly. The serum sIL-2R in AD-patients at A was, at 907 IU/ml (normal range 0–477 IU/ml), significantly elevated in comparison to P-patients with 339 IU/ml (p < 0.005) and dropped significantly (p < 0.05) down to 670 IU/ml at D. The measurement of sIL-2R could be a marker for the activity of the atopic skin disease.

Despite the advances in modern therapy of skin diseases, climatic therapy, either at the sea or in the high mountains, still retains its established value, particularly with respect to atopic dermatitis (AD) and the non-pustular forms of psoriasis (P) [1, 2]. 70–80% of AD-patients on systemic or local steroid treatment are able to discontinue this medication during their stay in high mountain areas [1]. Climatic therapy consists of changing the environment, heliotherapy, invigoration, and recovering together with an appropriate medical care. The positive effect seems to persist for several months following the climatotherapy. This can be assessed by the prolongation of the intervals between relapses [1]. While the influence of the mountain climate on the autonomic nervous system [3], on endocrine functions [4], and on skin reactivity (intracutaneous injection of vasoactive mediators, such as histamine, bradykinin, acethylcholin, serotinin, and prostaglandins E_1, E_2, and $F1\alpha$) has been relatively well investigated [5–9], little is known about its influence on the immune system [10]. One explanation of the climatic benefit in allergic respiratory diseases is the removal of some allergens from the atmosphere, especially house dust mites [11].

The present study was undertaken in order to investigate a possible influence of the high mountain climate on the immune system in patients with AD, P, and in controls (C).

Patients and Methods

37 patients (19 females and 18 males, age range 14–60 years) with a diagnosis of AD, according to the the definition of Hanifin and Rajka [12], were evaluated on admission (A) to the Zurich High Mountain Clinic of Clavadel-Davos (1,600 m altitude) and at discharge (D). The duration of the stay for the patients averaged 37.4 days (range 19–54 days). The severity of the course of the disease (degree I–V) and of the skin manifestations were quantified (score 1–5) according to our previous classification at A and D [13, 14].

---

*   Allergy Station, Department of Dermatology, University Hospital, Basel, Switzerland.
**   Institute of Immunology, Department of Medicine, University Hospital Zurich, Switzerland.
***   Central Laboratory, Blood Transfusion Service SRC, Bern, Switzerland.
****Zurich High Mountain Clinic, Clavadel-Davos, Switzerland.

16 patients (4 females and 12 males, age range 15–46 years) with psoriasis vulgaris (one with arthropathy) served as one (P) and 11 patients with different, mainly respiratory diseases, but without any skin manifestation, as a second control group (C). The duration of the stay in the clinic was comparable in both control groups: P 36 days with a range of 20–57 days, and C 35.4 days with a range of 22–45 days.

Serum and plasma samples were obtained from all the patients at A and D and then stored in aliquots at –70° until testing in the different laboratories.

Measurement of Total Serum IgE Levels and Specific IgE

The total IgE was determined with a competitive binding radioimmunoassay (Quanticlone, Kallestad), performed as recommended by the manufacturer. All sera of the AD-patients were tested for specific IgE by the radioallergosorbent test (Phadebas RAST, Pharmacia) using timothy grass pollen, birch pollen, mugwort pollen, house dust (Hollister-Stier), house dust mite (*Dermatophagoides pteronyssinus*), candica albicans, egg white, cow's milk, and wheat flour discs. Results were expressed in RAST classes 0 (negative) to 1–4 (positive).

Measurement of Immunoglobulins and Other Plasma Proteins

The quantitative determination of the immunoglobulins IgG, IgA, and IgM and α_1-Antitrypsin was performed with automatized laser-nephelometry by using a Behring Nephelo meter-Analyzer (Behringwerke, Marburg, FRG). The quantitation of β-2- Microglobulin was determined by using an Elisa Test Kit (Enzygnost β-2-M Elisa, Behringwerke, Marburg, FRG). The quantitation of the IgG-subclasses (1, 2, 3, 4) was determined with a sandwich-enzymimmunoassay by using monoclonal antibodies anti-human G_1—Clone IL512, anti-human G_2—Clone GOM 1, anti-human G_3—Clone ZG4, and anti-human G_4—Clone RJ 4 (Seward Laboratory, Bedford, England) and biotin-marked monospecific anti- human IgG antisera (Vector Laboratories, Inc., USA).

The determination of interleukin-2 receptors, α-interferon and γ-interferon was performed by using commercially available test kits: CELLFREE IL-2R Enzymimmunoassay (T-Cell Sciences, Cambridge, USA), ALPHA-INTERFERON RIA (Abbott Laboratories, North Chicago, USA), GAMMA INTERFERON (CENTOCOR, Malvern, PA, USA).

Measurement of Immune Complexes, Complement Concentrations and Complement Functions

Concentrations of all components of complement were assessed except Factor D and S-protein. Individual levels of complement components were measured either by radial immunodiffusion [15] or nephelometry [16] using monospecific antisera. Results were expressed relative to a pool of 150 healthy blood donors in percent or as g/l, respectively. Titration of functional total complement (CH50) was performed according to standard laboratory technique using a micromethod [17].

Functional alternative pathway of complement (APH50) was assessed at physiological ionic strength in presence of 8 mmol/l EGTA and 2 mmol/l Mg++ [18, 19]. Circulating immune complexes were measured as C1q- binding activity of serum [20]. Functional C1-inhibitor (INH) was assessed by three different methods. One method directly measures interaction of C1-INH with its natural substrate, the subcomponent C1r of the first complement component, C1, at physiological concentrations of C1r and C1-INH [21]. The two other methods are based on inhibition by C1-INH of amidolytic activity of exogenous C1s (C1-esterase) added to the sample to be tested. The rate of cleavage of two different nonphysiologic chromogenic substrates by C1s was followed. Both methods were performed using commercially available test kits (Behringwerke, Marburg, FRG, and Immuno, Vienna, Austria, respectively).

Statistical Calculations

Statistical analyses were made on arithmetic or geometric mean values (± SD) using the Student's test to compare the mean values at A and D for each group, using a Hewlett-Packard calculator.

Results

The overall skin conditions of the AD patients improved from score 3.16 at A to score 1.51 at D on average (Table 1). On the basis of case history and allergological investigations, the AD-patients could be further subdivided into the two "extrinsic" (high IgE levels, positive RAST, positive skin tests of the immediate type) (n = 28) and "intrinsic" (without any specific IgE sensitizations to inhalants and/or foods) (n = 9) [22, 23].

Table 1. Severity in the course of the atopic dermatitis (degree) and of the skin conditions (score) at admission (A) and at discharge (D) (x = score on average).

Severity of course Degree	n	Severity of skin conditions (score)					
		A	n		D		n
I	0	0	:	0	0	:	3
II	3	1	:	1	1	:	18
III	9	2	:	8	2	:	10
IV	19*	3	:	14	3	:	6
V	6*	5	:	2	5	:	0

*Degrees IV and V together = 68%.

Figures 1a and 1b show the geometric mean values of serum IgE with the corresponding standard deviation (± SD) on admission (A) and discharge (D) in patients with AD, P, and in controls (C), respectively, in the "extrinsic" and "intrinsic" type of AD. As expected, statistical differences could be found only between the AD group and P and C, respectively, or between the "extrinsic" and the "intrinsic" type of AD. The IgE levels did not show significant changes at A and D. Furthermore, the RAST score for each allergen and the average of the sum of the scores remained unchanged (Table 2).

The mean levels of the immunoglobulins IgA, IgM, IgG, and of α_1-Antitrypsin were within the normal ranges and remained uninfluenced by the altitude (Table 3.).

Figure 1. (a) Geometric serum IgE levels in atopic dermatitis, psoriasis and controls at admission (A) and at discharge (D). (b) Serum IgE levels in extrinsic and intrinsic type atopic dermatitis.

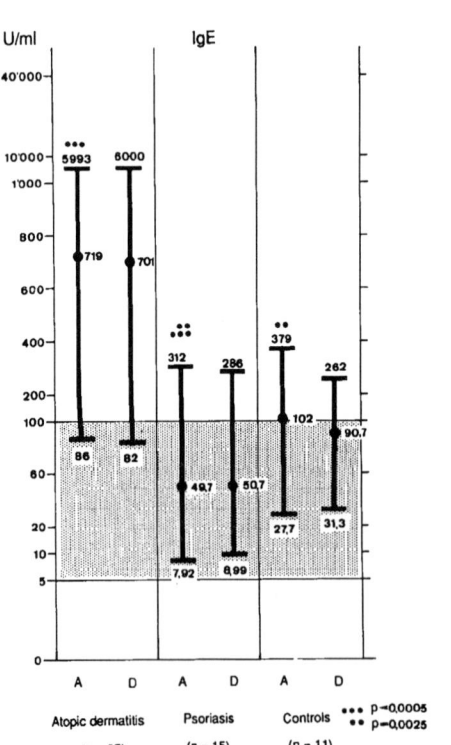

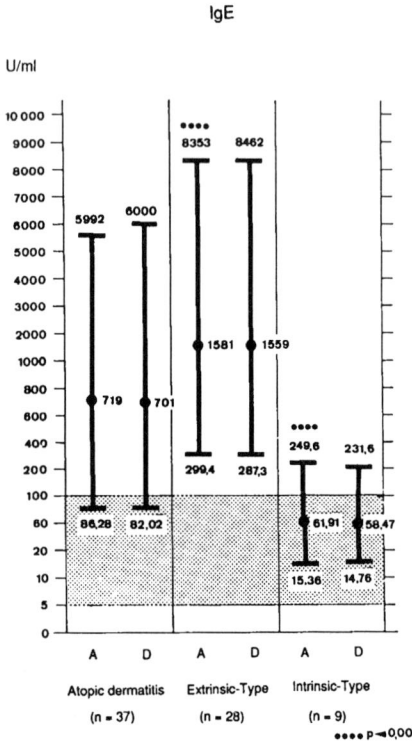

Table 2. RAST-patients at admission (A) and at discharge (D) in the group of patients with atopic dermatitis of "extrinsic" type (n=28*).

| | Positivity** | | Score | |
	n	%	A	D
Timothy	24	86	2.78	2.75
Birch	18	64	1.53	1.61
Mugworth	19	68	1.35	1.39
House dust	20	71	1.89	1.78
House dust mite	16	57	1.75	1.82
Candida alb.	16	57	1.32	1.28
Egg white	8	28	0.50	0.64
Cow's milk	9	32	0.57	0.51
Wheat flour	16	57	1.00	1.00
Average of sum of the scores			1.41	1.42

*In 9 AD-patients, the RASTs as well as the skin tests of the immediate type were negative.

The levels of the IgG subclasses, expressed as percentages of the total IgG, are depicted in Figures 2 a–d. At A, the arithmetic mean level of IgG_4 was the only value found above the normal range: 44.4% of the AD-patients presented elevated IgG4 levels (>5.9%) versus only 18.7% of the P-patients (Table 4). However, in 8 cases (29.6%), the IgG_4 levels were diminished (<2.5%), and in 4 cases they could not be determined (<1%). The comparison of IgG_4 levels at A and D in individual AD-patients revealed generally lower levels at D (Figure 3). The results of extensive determinations of circulating immune complexes, concentrations of individual complement components and complement functions for AD-patients are shown in Table 5. In Table 6 one finds the statistical analyses (p values) for the comparison of the three patient groups at A.

Table 3. Levels of immunoglobulins IgA, IgM, IgG, and α_1-antitrypsin in atopic dermatitis, psoriasis, and controls at admission (A) and at discharge (D).

| | | Atopic dermatitis n = 37 | | Psoriasis n = 16 | | Controls n = 11 | |
		A	D	A	D	A	D
gA (mg/ml)	$\bar{y}$	2.22	2.26	2.34	2.08	2.59	2.39
(normal range: 0.7–4.4	+1SD	3.17	3.24	3.80	3.38	4.00	4.08
	−1SD	1.55	1.58	1.44	1.27	1.67	1.41
IgM (mg/ml)	$\bar{y}$	1.17	1.18	1.09	1.16	1.29	1.30
(normal range: 0.4–2.6	+1SD	1.97	1.99	1.74	1.85	2.37	2.66
	−1SD	0.69	0.71	0.69	0.73	0.70	0.64
IgG (mg/ml)	$\bar{y}$	12.71	13.12	11.73	11.30	12.24	12.20
(normal range: 7.0–19.0)	+1SD	16.47	17.12	14.29	14.15	15.43	15.56
	−1SD	9.81	10.06	9.63	9.03	9.71	9.57
α_1-antitrypsin (mg/ml)	$\bar{x}$	2.29	2.27	2.14	2.05	2.09	2.17
(normal range: 1.9–3.5)	±1SD	0.47	0.38	0.36	0.28	0.23	0.40

$\bar{y}$ = geometric means, $\bar{x}$ = arithmetic means, SD = standard deviation
t-test: no statistically significant differences were found between values at A and at D in each patient groups or between the three groups of patients, respectively.

Table 4. IgG_4 levels in atopic dermatitis and in psoriasis at admission (A) and at discharge (D).

| IgG_4 | Atopic dermatitis (n=27) | | Psoriasis (n=16) | |
	A	D	A	D
Elevated >5.9%	12 (44.4%)	11 (40.8%)	3 (18.7%)	3 (18.7%)
Normal 2.5–5.9	7 (25.9%)	8 (29.6%)	10 (62.5%)	10 (62.5%)
Diminished <2.5%	8 (29.6%)	8 (29.6%)	3 (18.7%)	3 (18.7%)

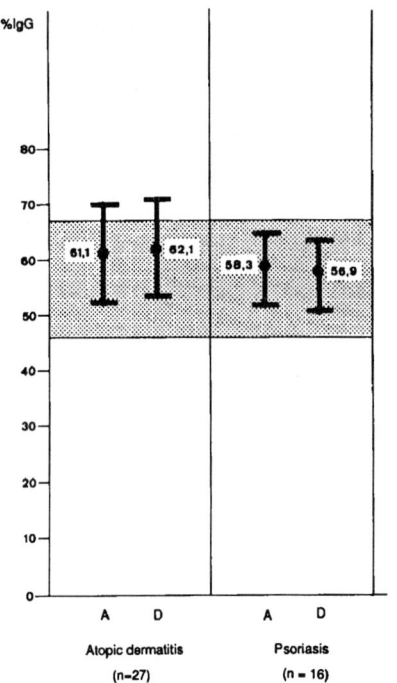

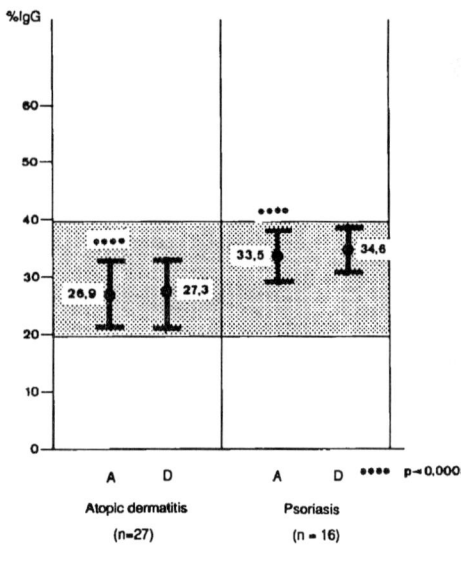

Figure 2 a–d. Levels of IgG subclasses (1–4) in atopic dermatitis and in psoriasis at admission (A) and at discharge (D).

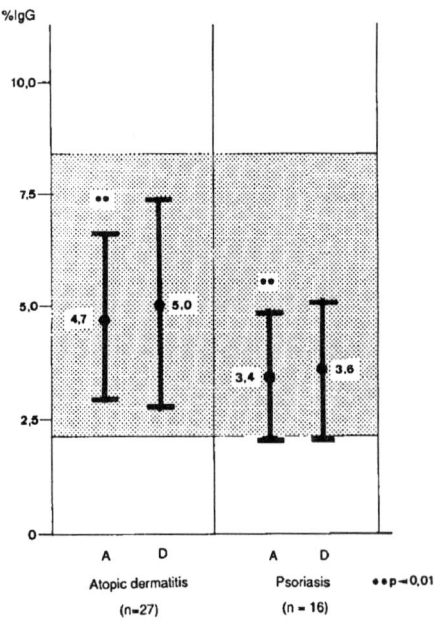

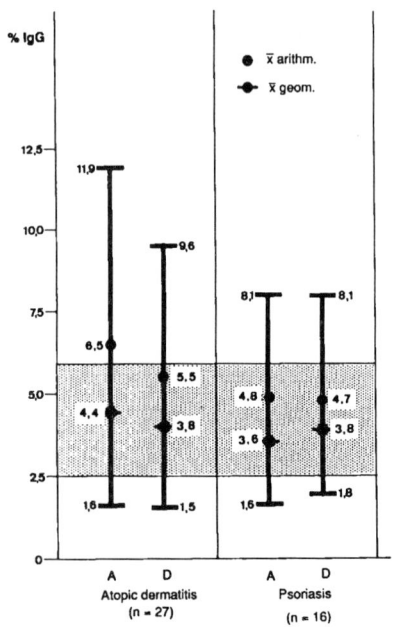

348

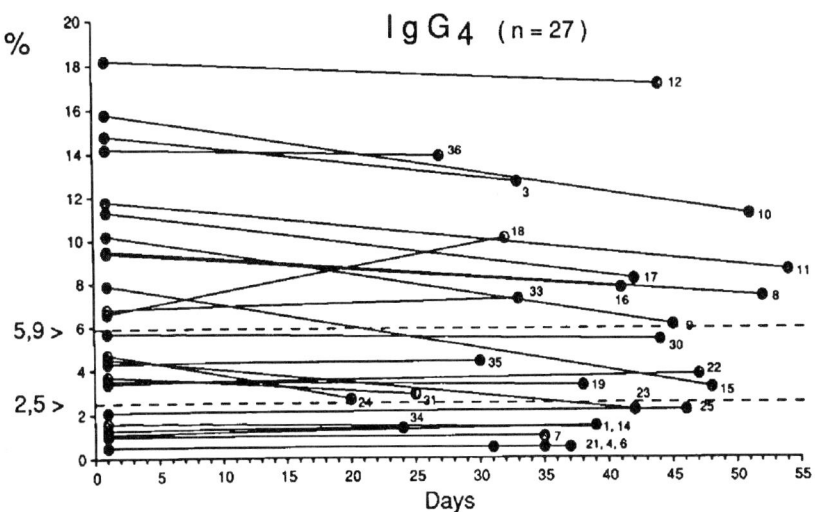

Figure 3. Individual levels of IgG₄ in atopic dermatitis at admission (A) and at discharge (D).

Table 5. Arithmetic values (x ± 1SD) of immune complexes, complement factors and complement functions in atopic dermatitis patients (n=37) at admission (A) and at discharge (D).

	Normal values	$\bar{x}$ ± 1SD	
		A	D
C1q-binding activity (%)	<5	0.72 ± 0.98	0.95 ± 1.23
C1q (g/l)	0.10–0.25	0.17 ± 0.02	0.16 ± 0.03
C1r (%)	75–125	106 ± 20	105 ± 18
C1s (%)	70–125	111 ± 20	109 ± 19
C2 (%)	67–125	104 ± 29	98 ± 19
C3 D, G (%)	<15	6 ± 2	6 ± 2
C3 (C3c) (g/l)	0.75–1.4	1 ± 0.33	0.24 ± 0.08
C5 (%)	68–122	110 ± 23	105 ± 25
C6 (%)	68–126	111 ± 25	107 ± 25
C7 (%)	68–132	95 ± 27	98 ±34
C8 (%)	70–120	102 ± 25	102 ± 24
C9 (%)	52–122	124 ± 40	123 ± 42
Factor B (%)	60–140	108 ± 29	105 ± 24
Factor P (Properdin) (%)	60–135	98 ±14*	90 ± 15*
C1-INH (g/l)	0.11–0.26	0.20 ± 0.04	0.19 ± 0.05
C4-BP (%)	8–137	111 ± 33	110 ± 27
Factor H (%)	60–130	113 ± 26	110 ± 20
Factor I (%)	60–135	109 ± 22	108 ± 20
C1-INH (C1r) (%)	70–135	101 ± 9	99 ±
C1-INH (Behringwerke) (%)	70–130	66 ± 18	78 ± 19
C1-INH (Immuno) (%)	80–125	84 ±17	62 ± 16
CH50 (μ/ml)	300–510	417 ± 84	410 ± 79
APH 50 (μ/ml)	25–55	44 ± 10	40 ± 10

*p = 0.012
**p = 0.05

Table 6. Results (P) of statistical analysis (t-test) of the values of immune complexes, complement factors, and complement functions between the three patient groups at admission (A).

	AD/P	AD/C	P/C
C1q-binding activity	0.05	0.05	n.s.
C1q (g/l)	n.s.	n.s.	n.s.
C1r (%)	n.s.	n.s.	n.s.
C1s (%)	n.s.	0.05	n.s.
C2 (%)	n.s.	n.s.	n.s.
C3 D,G (%)	n.s.	n.s.	n.s.
C3 (C3c) (g/l)	n.s.	n.s.	0.025
C4 (g/l)	n.s.	n.s.	n.s.
C5 (%)	n.s.	n.s.	n.s.
C6 (%)	n.s.	n.s.	n.s.
C7 (%)	n.s.	n.s.	n.s.
C8 (%)	n.s.	n.s.	n.s.
C9 (%)	n.s.	n.s.	n.s.
Factor B (%)	n.s.	n.s.	n.s.
Factor P (Properdin) (%)	n.s.	n.s.	0.05
C1-INH (g/l)	n.s.	n.s.	n.s.
C4-BP (%)	n.s.	n.s.	0.05
Factor H (%)	0.025	n.s.	n.s.
Factor I (%)	n.s.	n.s.	n.s.
C1-INH (C1r) (%)	n.s.	n.s.	n.s.
C1-INH (Behringwerke) (%)	0.005	0.005	n.s.
C1-INH (Immuno) (%)	n.s.	n.s.	n.s.
CH50 (μ/ml)	n.s.	n.s.	n.s.
APH50 (μ/ml)	n.s.	n.s.	0.05

Figure 4. Mean levels of soluble interleukin-2 receptors in atopic dermatitis and psoriasis at admission (A) and at discharge (D).

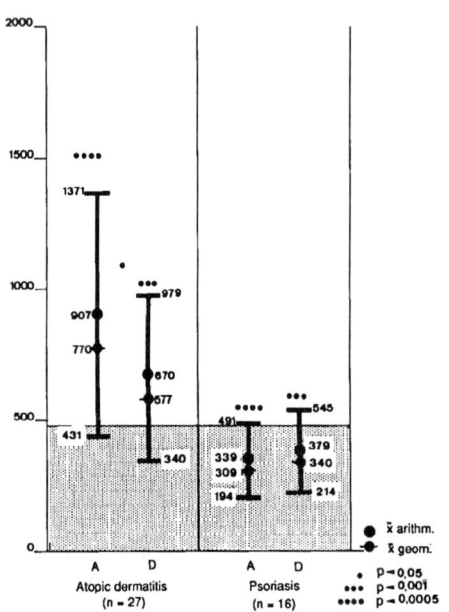

In none of the sera from patients suffering from AD (and in controls) was an elevated C1q-binding activity found, while in only one patient with psoriasis was this binding activity found to be above the upper limit of normal (>5% C_{1q} recipitated).

Mean plasma levels of all components of complement as well as the total complement hemolytic and the hemolytic activity of the alternative pathway of complement were found within the normal range at A and at D for all three groups of patients. In the AD-patients, the only concentration significantly different at A and at D was for properdin, a protein of the alternative pathway of complement.

The only highly significant difference at A between patients with AD and P or AD and C was for C1-INH function when assessed by chromogenic substrate (commercial kit, Immuno). Mean functional level in AD-patients was below the lower level of the normal range and normalized during the high mountain stay.

α- and γ-interferon activity could not be measured in any sera of the AD- and P-patients; the mean values of neopterin and β_2-microglobulin were in the normal ranges. Only in 2 AD-patients and in 1 P-patient was neopterin increased (>2.5 mg/ml), probably in coincidence with intercurrent viral diseases.

Finally, the mean values of soluble interleukin-2 receptors (sIL-2R), the distribution of the elevated and the normal values and the individual levels of the 27 AD-patients are presented in Figure 4 and Table 7, respectively. These figures clearly indicate that the serum concentrations of sIL-2R was significantly elevated in AD- in comparison to P-patients and dropped significantly at D.

Discussion

A measurable influence of the mountain climate on the humoral immune function could not be observed during an average stay of 36 days in any group, though the skin conditions of the AD- and P- patients improved signifi-

Table 7. Levels of soluble interleukin-2 receptors in atopic dermatitis and in psoriasis at admission (A) and at discharge (D).

Soluble interleukin-2 receptors	Atopic dermatitis (n=27)		Psoriasis (n=16)	
	A	D	A	D
Elevated (>477 µ/ml)	21 (77.7%)	15 (55.5%)	4 (25.0%)	4 (25.0%)
Normal (≤477 µ/ml)	6 (22.2%)	12 (44.4)	12 (75.0%)	12 (75.0%)

cantly. Like others, we did not find any significant changes in the immunoglobulins before and after climatotherapy [7, 11, 13].

In this study we could confirm the presence of elevated serum IgE levels in AD [13, 14], but there are some cases of AD without increased IgE levels and without allergen-specific IgE against inhalants or food either in the skin tests or in RAST analysis. Such patients belong to the "intrinsic" type of AD [22, 23], and the lack of an IgE sensitization indicates no pathogenetic significance of IgE at least for a subgroup of AD. Although IgG4 were slightly elevated on the average, the arithmetic mean values of the IgG4 were above the normal range at A, and they were diminished in 8 cases. Since it was recently shown that IgG4 does not sensitize normal basophils [24], and there are reports identifying IgG4 as being a protective, allergen-blocking antibody [25, 26], IgG4 unlikely plays a role in the pathogenesis of AD. In a previous study we have shown that elevated IgG4 is probably associated with the accompanying respiratory diseases [27].

There are conflicting reports concerning complement and circulating immune complexes in AD, but most studies indicate no significant correlation of these parameters with grade of severity of the skin manifestations [28–33]. In this study, concentrations of almost all of the complement proteins and several of the complement functions were assessed in three different groups of patients. We found no significant influence of high mountain climate on complement concentrations or functions in either group of patient, except for properdin concentration in the AD-patients. The most striking differences at A between the AD and the other groups of patients were found for C1-INH function when assessed by chromogenic substrate (commercial kit, Immuno). When C1-INH function was assessed with two other tests, no such difference became apparent. When results of the two methods based on the same principle (chromogenic substrates) were compared (commercial kits, Immuno vs.

Behring), changes of C1-INH functions during the high mountain stay proved to be of opposite directions. This questions the quality of C1-INH functional assessment by chromogenic substrates.

We observed significantly elevated serum levels of sIL-2R in the Ad-patients, which almost fell toward normal at D. We believe that the reduction in the sIL-2R levels observed in the AD-patients during the stay reflects the improvement of the skin conditions and not a climate effect. IL-2R is the protein that mediates the action of interleukin-2 , a T cell growth hormone. When T lymphocytes are stimulated by a challenge to the immune system and begin to proliferate, more molecules of IL-2R are expressed on the cell's plasma membrane and a soluble IL-2R is released in proportion to its rate of synthesis [28]. Levels of sIL-2R have been show to be raised in a number of pathological conditions accompanied by T-cell activation or in immunopathies, such as in certain lymphomas and leukemias [28, 29], in transplant recipients experiencing rejection episodes [30], in persons with viral infections such as acquired immune deficiency syndrome (AIDS), and in certain autoimmune diseases [31]. Our elevated sIL-2R levels suggest that the T-cell immune system is activated in AD, and that this activation may be of pathogenetic significance. The serum levels of the sIL-2R may reflect the situation in the dermis, so that the measurement of the sIL-2R could be a marker for the activity of the atopic skin disease. Further studies of the cellular immune function, especially in the "intrinsic" type of AD, are in progress.

References

1. Kneist, W., and J. Rakoski. 1987. Neurodermitis atopica—Klimatherapie im Hochgebirge. Allergologie 10: 531.
2. Pürschel, W. 1987. Neurodermitis atopica—Klimabehandlung am Meer. Allergologie 10: 526.
3. Huegin, F., J. Keith, F. Verzar, and H. Wirz. 1956.

Änderungen der vegetativ-autonomen Erregbarkeit im Höhenklima. Schweiz. med. Wschr. 22: 650.

4. von Deschwanden, J., K. Schram, and J. C. Thams. 1968. In: Der Mensch im Klima der Alpen. Bern/Stuttgart: Hans Huber Verlag.

5. Borelli, S., and S. Chlebarov. 1966. Änderung der Histamine-Reagibilität der Haut nach Hochgebirgs-Klimabehandlung. Münch. med. Wschr. 108: 592.

6. Borelli, S., P. Michailov, and C. Ene-Popescu. 1967. Die Veränderungen der allergisch-mediatorischen Reaktivität bei Neurodermitis-constitutionalis-Kranken nach Höhenklimatherapie. Hautarzt 10: 456.

7. Ferencikova, J., and J. Kolesar. 1979. Einfluß der klimatischen Behandlung auf das Komplementniveau und auf einige Lysosomenzyme im Serum von Patienten mit Asthma bronchiale. Allergie u. Immunol. 25: 197.

8. Michailov, P., N. Berowa, N. Tsankov et al. 1983. Der Einfluß der Hochgebirgsklimatherapie auf die Hautreaktivität gegenüber den Prostaglandinen E_1, E_2 und $Fl\alpha$ bei allergischen Dermatosen. Dermatol. Monatsschr. 169: 305.

9. Pürschel, W., O. Pahl, and A. Aljounied. 1982. Fluvographische Untersuchungen bei Neurodermitis während Klimatherapie an der Nordsee. Z. Hautkr. 57: 38.

10. Hoesli, F. 1948. Untersuchungen über den Einfluß des Höhenklimas auf allergische Reaktionsvorgänge. Dermatologica 96: 151.

11. Vervloet, D., A. Penau, H. Razzouk et al. 1982. Altitude and house dust mites. J. Allergy clin. Immunol. 69: 290.

12. Hanifin, J. M., and G. Rajka. 1980. Diagnostic features of atopic dermatitis. Acta derm. venereol. (Suppl.) 92: 44.

13. Wüthrich, B. 1975. Zur Immunpathologie der Neurodermitis constitutionalis. Eine klinisch-immunologische Studie mit besonderer Berücksichtigung der Immunglobulin E und der spezifischen Reagine im zeitlichen Verlauf. Bern/Stuttgart/Wien: Hans Huber Verlag.

14. Wüthrich, B. 1978. Serum IgE in atopic dermatitis. Clin. Allergy 8: 241.

15. Mancini, G., O. A. Carbonara, and J. F. Heremans. 1965. Immunochemical quantification of antigens by single radial immunodiffusion. Immunochemistry 2: 235.

16. Alper, C. A. 1974. Plasma protein measurements as diagnostic aid. N. Engl. J. Med. 291: 287.

17. Mayer, M. M. 1972. Complement and complement fixation. In: Experimental immunochemistry (2nd ed.). E. A. Kabat and M. M. Mayer, eds. Springfield, IL: C.C. Thomas, p. 133.

18. Platts-Mills, T. A. E., and K. Ishizaka. 1974. Activation of the alternative pathway of human complement by rabbit cells. J. Immun. 110: 348.

19. Joiner, K. A., A. Hawiger, and J. A. Gelfand. 1983. A study of optimal reaction conditions for an assay of the human alternative pathway. American Journal of Clinical Pathology 79: 65.

20. Späth, P., A. Corvetta, U. U. Nydegger et al. 1983. An extended C1q-binding assay using lactoperoxidase- and chloramine-T- iodinated C1q. Immediate distinction between immune-aggregate-mediated and non-immune aggregate-mediated C1q binding. Scand. J. Immunol. 18: 319.

21. Späth, P., B. Wüthrich, and R. Bütler. 1984. Quantification of C1-inhibitor functional activities by immunodiffusion assay in plasma of patients with hereditary angioedema—Evidence of a functionally critical level of C-inhibitor concentration. Complement 1: 147.

22. Boner, A. L., I. Antolini, M. Zambellini et al. 1985. Preliminary report on histamine release. Circulating immune complexes and complement activation in children with atopic dermatitis after oral challenge with mild and egg antigens. Ann. Allergy 54: 442.

23. Trindade, J. C., M. L. Palma-Carlos, A. G. Palma-Carlos et al. 1978. IgE and complement in allergic children. Allergol. et Immunopathol. VI: 519.

24. Ferguson, A. C., and F. A. Salinas. 1984. Elevated IgG immune complexes in children with atopic eczema. J. Allergy clin. Immunol. 74: 678.

25. Kapp, A., H. Wokalek, and E. Schöpf. 1985. Involvement of complement in psoriasis and atopic dermatitis—Measurement of C3a and C5a, C3, C4 and C1 inactivator. Arch. Dermatol. Res. 277: 359.

26. Kapp, A., A. Kemper, E. Schöpf, and H. Deicher. 1986. Detection of circulating immune complexes in patients with atopic dermatitis and psoriasis. Acta Derm. Vener. (Stockh.) 66: 121.

27. Ring, J., T. Senter, R. C. Coronell et al. 1979. Plasma complement and histamine changes in atopic dermatitis. J. Dermatol. 100: 521.

28. Robb, R. J. 1984. Interleukin 2: The molecule and its function. Immunology Today 5: 203.

29. Nelson, D. L. 1986. Soluble interleukin-2 receptors. Analysis in normal individuals and in certain disease states. Fed. Proc. 45: 377.

30. Wagner, D. K., J. Kiwannka, B. K. Edwards et al. 1987. Serum interleukin-2 receptor levels in patients with undifferentiated and lymphoblastic lymphomas. Correlation with survival. J. Clin. Oncology 5: 1262.

31. Colvin, R. B., T. C. Fuller, L. MacKeen et al. 1987. Plasma interleukin-2 receptor levels in renal allograft recipients. Clin. Immunol. Immunopathol. 43: 273.

32. Reddy, M. M., and H. M. Grieco. 1988. Elevated soluble interleukin-2 receptor levels in serum of human immunodeficiency virus infected populations. Aids Research and Human Retroviruses. 4: 115.

Intolerance to Food and Food Additives

Maurice H. Lessof*, Robert D. Murdoch*, Ian Pollock**, Elspeth Young***

Epidemiology

There are many difficulties in identifying adverse reactions to food and food additives, not least because of the difference between popular concepts about food allergy and the results of objective tests. Out of 18,582 people who answered a questionnaire about reactions to food or food additives [1], 15.6% thought they had symptoms caused by foods and 7.4% thought the same about food additives. In this particular study, a clinical assessment was carried out on 1,223 people in order to ascertain whether food additives could be shown to cause the reactions attributed to them. Only 132 had recurring symptoms which justified the use of a challenge procedure with additive-containing capsules in a double-blind trial, and there was thus a substantial difference between the large number of individuals who believed they had a problem and those who were thought to merit further investigation. Of the 84 who eventually attended for challenge, only 3 had a reproducible reaction, suggesting an overall prevalence of the order of 0.026%.

Questionnaire-based studies are not without their problems. Kerr [2] asked questions about 18 food-associated symptoms of which three (chest tightness, burning, numbness) were thought to be characteristically caused by the flavouring enhancer monosodium glutamate. Of the 6.6% who, on these criteria, were suspected of having a possible intolerance to glutamate, 31% replied to a second questionnaire by stating that they had adverse effects related to restaurant food. Two further questionnaires were then designed which avoided the use of leading questions [3]. The positive response rate to these further questionnaires was much lower at 1.8% and 2.3%.

Diagnostic Difficulties

The reliability of an epidemiological study depends ultimately on the accuracy of its diagnostic methods. Since food intolerance can result from a number of different mechanisms and may present in many ways, no single laboratory test could be expected to identify all sufferers. The most acceptable criterion is therefore the occurrence of reproducible symptoms after blind challenge, and a positive result might indicate one of a number of disparate conditions. Such results might be due to toxic effects of preservatives such as metabisulphite, resulting in asthma. By a very different mechanism, the pharmacological effects of caffeine may cause tachycardia, tremor, and the irritable bowel syndrome, while nitrites in meat can cause vasodilation and flushing. The metabolic effects of enzyme deficiencies can lead to alcohol intolerance and an antabuse-like effect in those who are deficient in aldehyde dehydrogenase, or to the irritable bowel effects of milk in those who are deficient in lactase. Angioedema and eczema can occur in those with IgE-mediated sensitivity to egg or some other food. More complex immunological reactions can occur in coeliac disease, in response to gluten. Furthermore, each of these reactions may be subject to the potentiating effects of exercise, stress, or the numerous local tissue factors which determine target organ susceptibility.

The variability of food intolerant symptoms has made it difficult to accept that a single negative challenge procedure is sufficient to exclude the diagnosis. Patients who have immunoglobin E (IgE) antibodies to foods may fail to react on some occasions but have severe or even dangerous reactions if they take exercise after eating [4, 5]. It has also been noted that, even in subjects with tartrazine reactions diagnosed by double-blind testing [6], there may be difficulty in reproducing challenge test

*   United Medical and Dental Schools, Guy's Campus, London, SE1 9RT, England.
** The Cardiothoracic Institute, Brompton Hospital, London, SW3 6HP, England.
*** Wycombe General Hospital, High Wycombe, Bucks.

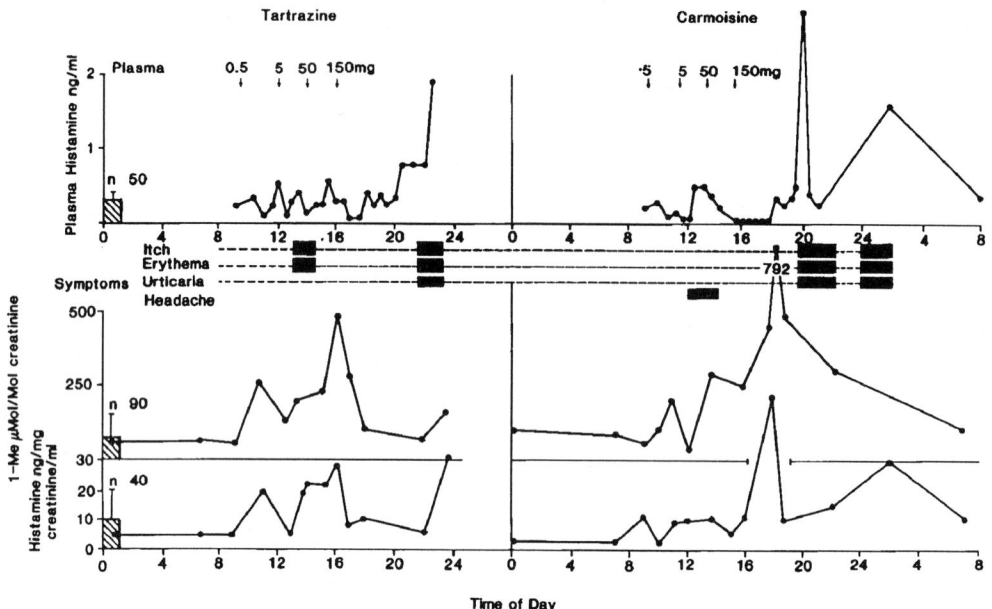

Figure 1. Consecutive daily challenges with tartrazine and carmoisine given at regular time periods (⇓). Clinical symptoms include urticaria, itch, erythema, and headache. Mediator measurements include plasma histamine, urinary 1Methyl-histamine (1Me), and histamine. (Prostaglandin 6-keto Flα, Thromboxane B$_2$ and Prostaglandin E$_2$ measurements showed similar changes to histamine—not shown).

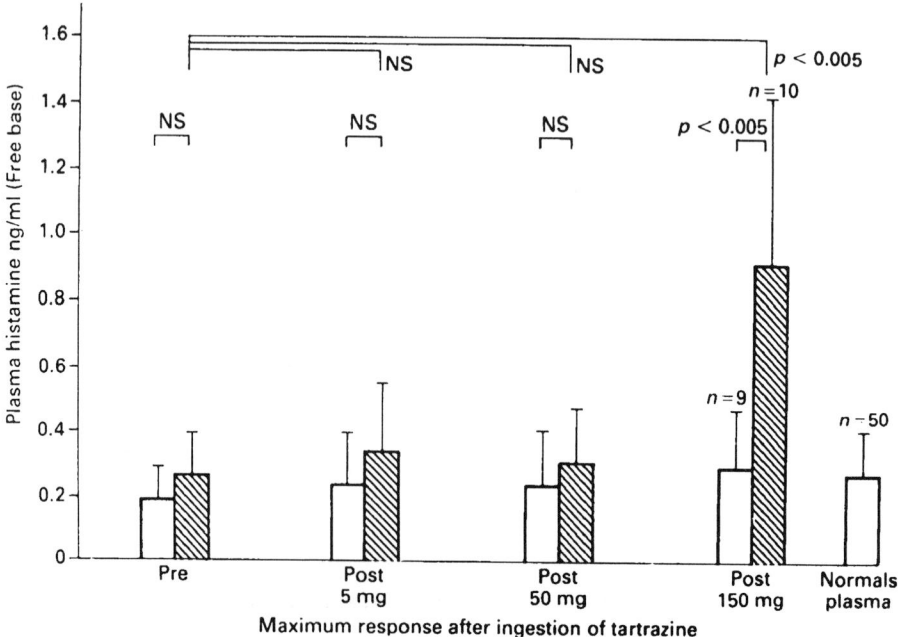

Figure 2. Maximum plasma histamine levels (mean ± SEM) in 10 symptomless volunteers following ingestion of tartrazine (shaded) or placebo (unshaded) in a double-blind study. (Reproduced from *Journal of Royal College of Physicians*, 21 (1987), 237–266.)

results consistently. In part this is because the patient's reactivity may not persist indefinitely. A recent study by Pollock and Warner [7] has highlighted the transient nature of most cases of food additive intolerance in children. If a direct pharmacological effect is involved, it is also possible that there are other influences such as variations in the rate of absorption of small molecules, for example during intestinal infections [8].

Because of the difficulty in defining a clinical endpoint for challenge tests and because of their relative insensitivity, attempts have been made to supplement the clinical findings by measuring IgE antibodies to foods and by measuring the release of inflammatory mediators. One outcome has been the demonstration that "pseudo-allergic" reactions, including urticaria and asthma, are frequently present without evidence of an IgE response or of any other immunological mechanism. We have demonstrated the release of histamine and arachidonic acid metabolites in food additive-induced urticaria, without any evidence of an

allergic mechanism [9] (Figure 1) and have also shown that high doses (150 mg) of tartrazine can induce histamine release in healthy subjects [10] (Figure 2).

The clinical response to histamine release can vary considerably, however. Our healthy volunteers who swallowed tartrazine had substantial rises in plasma histamine level, but had no clinical symptoms. We have since demonstrated, by means of histamine infusion studies, that atopic subjects develop symptoms at significantly lower levels of blood histamine than do healthy controls. Interestingly, the infusion of relatively small amounts of histamine in urticarial subjects was sufficient to raise the blood level significantly and, after infusion, the half life of circulating histamine was significantly prolonged (Figure 3). Other evidence indicates that at least some patients with this condition may have abnormally low levels of the histamine metabolising enzyme diamine oxidase (Figure 4). Since we have also found that some patients with aspirin-induced urticaria have low levels of aspirin esterase [11],

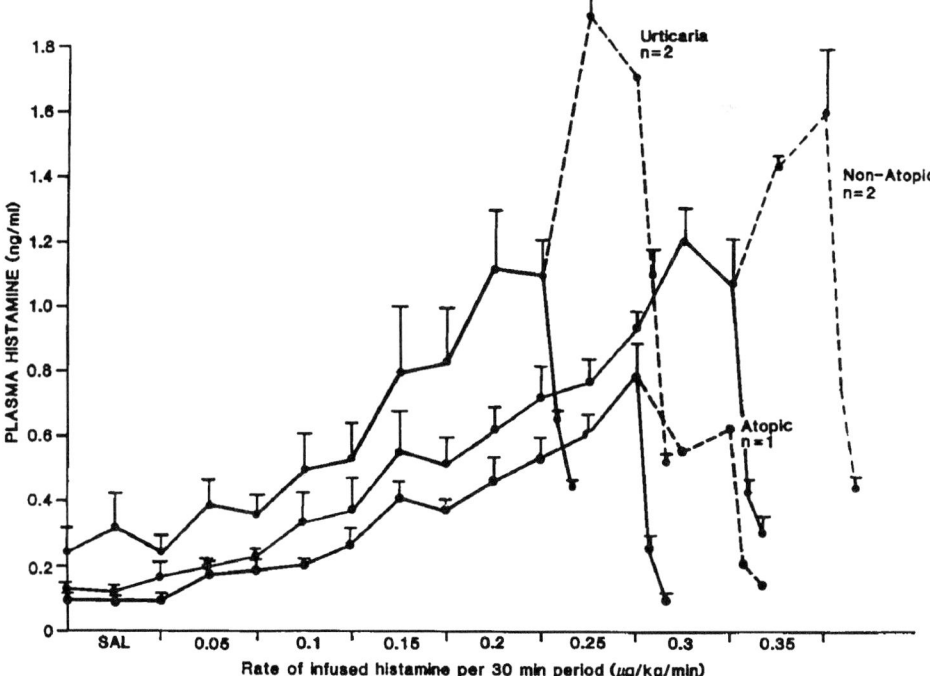

Figure 3. Circulating plasma histamine levels (ng/ml) in 5 nonatopic, atopic, and urticarial subjects following the infusion of histamine over 30-min periods, in sequentially increasing dosage rates from 0.05–0.35 µg/kg/min. The dotted line indicates the levels of histamine achieved in those few (excluded from statistical analysis) who tolerated a higher histamine infusion rate than the others in the same group.

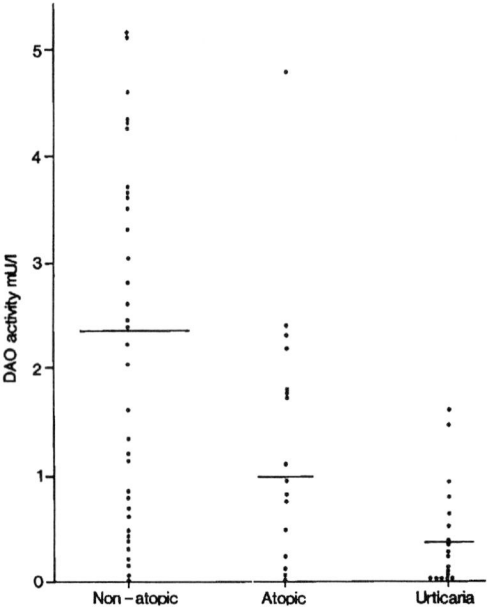

Figure 4. Serum diamine oxidase levels (mU/l) in groups of nonatopic, atopic and urticarial subjects.

we may be dealing with examples of an apparently homogeneous clinical manifestation that can be caused by different mechanisms. The corollary is that there may be other clinical manifestations which appear to be "allergic", but which are also due to enzyme deficiencies.

The most important implication of these studies is that measurement of mediator release may add a more sensitive method for evaluating challenge tests than a purely clinical assessment. Since mediator release is not dependent on a single mechanism, it also had advantages over methods which are based on the assessment of IgE-mediated hypersensitivity.

It should be accepted that our laboratory findings may not always reflect the clinical response of the individual. In some cases the release of inflammatory mediators provides a more sensitive method of detecting a subclinical response to a food challenge in an individual with a clear past history of adverse reactions to the food in question. In other cases, as in the tartrazine-induced release of histamine in healthy subjects, it remains to be established whether our findings can be said to demonstrate a pharmacological effect at the chosen dose level. This is not a purely hypothetical

question. Although the challenge dose given in our tartrazine study was substantially higher than the 50 mg which is regarded as a maximum daily intake, it does not provide the tenfold safety factor which is usually recommended. Further studies are therefore indicated to determine the validity of plasma histamine measurements as an indicator of an adverse effect.

Other approaches that have been used include the measurement of histamine release from washed leukocytes in vitro after the addition of food additives [12]. In our hands this method has failed to distinguish between healthy subjects, those with atopy, and those with idiopathic or food additive-induced urticaria. The possibilities for the development of an in vitro test have not yet been fully explored.

References

1. Young, E., S. Patel, M. Stoneham, M., R. Rona, & J. D. Wilkinson. 1987. The prevalence of reaction to food additives in a survey population. J. Roy. Coll. Phys. 21: 241.
2. Kerr, G. R., M. Wu-Lee, M. El-Lozy, R. McGandy, & F. J. Stare. 1977. Objectivity of food symptomatology surveys. J. Amer. Diet. Assoc. 71: 263.
3. Kerr, G. R., M. Wu-Lee, M. El-Lozy, R. McGandy, & F. J. Stare. 1979. Food symptomatology questionnaires: Risks of demand-bias questions and population-biased surveys. In Glutamic acid: Advances in biochemistry and physiology. L. J. Filer, S. Garatlini et al., eds. Raven Press, New York, p. 375.
4. Maulitz, R. M., D. S. Pratt, & A. L. Schocket. 1979. Exercise induced anaphylactic reaction to shellfish. J. Allergy. Clin. Immunol. 63: 633.
5. Kidd III, J. M., S. H. Cohen, A. J. Sosman, & J. N. Fink. 1983. Food dependent exercise-induced anaphylaxis. J. Allergy Clin. Immunol. 71: 407.
6. Gibson, A., & R. Clancy, R. 1980. Management of chronic idiopathic urticaria by the identification and exclusion of dietary factors. Clin. Allergy. 10: 699.
7. Pollock, I., & J. O. Warner. 1987. A follow-up study of childhood food additive intolerance. J. Roy. Coll. Phys. 21: 248.
8. Noone, C., I. S. Menzies, J. E. Banatvala, & J. W. Scopes. 1986. Intestinal permeability and lactose hydrolysis in human rotaviral gastroenteritis assessed simultaneously by non-invasive differential sugar permeation. Eur. J. Clin Invest. 16: 217.
9. Murdoch, R. D., I. Pollock, E. Young, & M. H.

Lessof. 1987. Food additive-induced urticaria: studies of mediator release during provocation tests. J. Roy. Coll. Phys. 21: 262.

10. Murdoch, R. D., I. Pollock, & S. Naeem. 1987. Tartrazine induced histamine release in vivo in normal subjects. J. Roy. Coll. Phys. 21: 257.

11. Williams, F. M., S. I. Asad, M. H. Lessof, & M. D. Rawlins. 1987. Plasma esterase activity in patients with aspirin-sensitive asthma or urticaria. Eur J. Clin. Pharmacol. 33: 387.

12. Murdoch, R. D., M. H. Lessof, I. Pollock, & E. Young. 1987. Effects of food additives on leukocyte histamine release in normal and urticaria subjects. J. Roy. Coll. Phys. 21: 251.

The Natural History of Adverse Food Reactions

*S. Allan Bock and F. M. Atkins**

Within the last decade, a number of studies have begun to appear which examine the question of the longitudinal course or natural history of adverse reactions to foods. These studies have shown that some foods are tolerated after a few months (egg, milk, soy, wheat), while allergy to others (peanut, nuts) may persist for years, perhaps indefinitely.

Longitudinal Studies in Children with Positive Double-Blind, Placebo-Controlled Food Challenges (DBPCFC)

A 1982 study [1] examined children who had previously been proved to have symptomatic sensitivity (allergy) to food by DBPCFC food challenge. Seventy-five children were studied one to seven years after their original food challenge reaction. There had been 105 positive DBPCFC in these 75 children. Reactions still occurred during ingestion with 43 (41%) of the foods originally causing reactions. Reactions no longer occurred and the problem seemed to be "outgrown" for 31 (30%) of the previously positive food reactions. Challenges were not performed and the food was assiduously avoided for the remaining 30%. Foods most likely to have stopped producing reactions were egg, milk, and soy. The foods most like to continue to produce symptoms upon ingestion were peanuts, fish, and other nuts (although the numbers were small for the latter two foods). A recently completed study [2] reexamined some of the same subjects and added others to evaluate the natural history of peanut allergy. One hundred fourteen children underwent DBPCFC to peanut over a period of 12 years, and 46 of these youngsters had a positive DBPCFC. Of the 32 located for continuing evaluation, 16 had experienced symptoms due to an accidental ingestion of peanut in the preceding year and an additional 8 subjects within the preceding 5 years. Only 8 of these subjects had managed to completely avoid ingestion of peanut. The reactions ranged from mild cutaneous symptoms to severe systemic symptoms. In both of these studies, each youngster with a positive DBPCFC had a positive skin test performed as described [1]. Taken together, these studies support the conclusion that some foods are more likely to stop producing reactions (egg, milk, soy) than others (peanut). Further longitudinal studies are needed to expand this experience and, especially, to add other foods to one list or the other.

Natural History of Anaphylactic Reactions to Foods

Anecdotal reports of the loss of life-threatening reactivity to food ingestion and pressure from the parents of these children led us to examine extremely carefully the loss of anaphylactic reactivity in 9 children over a period of years [3]. At present, 8 of 9 of these youngsters are able to tolerate the offending food in usual portions or at least small quantities without precipitating frightening symptoms. The ninth patient continues to have significant systemic symptoms during the accidental ingestion of milk, the offending food. In this study, the offending foods were milk, egg, and soy. It is important to note that each of these children was quite young when the initial reaction occurred. This study was important for several reasons. First, it confirmed the anecdotal impression that life-threatening reactions to foods can disappear to be "outgrown." Second, the mechanism in each of these youngsters was highly likely to be an IgE-initiated reaction as demonstrated by the presence of a positive skin test to the offending food and, in some cases, positive RAST or leukocyte histamine release. Third, it demonstrated that careful challenges could be accomplished under observation in anaphylactically sensitive subjects without producing severe systemic symptoms such as laryngospasm or circulatory collapse. This approach seemed far

---

* Department of Pediatrics, National Jewish Center for Immunology and Respiratory Medicine; Department of Pediatrics, University of Colorado School of Medicine, Denver, Colorado.

preferable to haphazard or accidental ingestion of these foods. Fourth, the study demonstrated perhaps more vividly than the other longitudinal study the progressive nature of loss of reactivity; that is, the loss of reactivity followed a dose-response relationship such that progressively larger amounts of the offending food could be introduced into the diet over a period of time. Fifth, despite the loss of clinical reactivity over time, the skin test to the extract of food under study continued to be positive long after the food could be safely ingested.

An important note about these studies is that in addition to being prospectively performed, they began with confirmation of the original history by DBPCFC, i.e., it was established with certainty that the patient had the purported problem at the start. Thus, the data were not inflated or distorted by inclusion of patients whose history of adverse food reaction was not accurate. In order to acquire accurate information in the absence of an unequivocal laboratory test, DBPCFC should be considered the "golden standard." The ethics and propriety of repeated longitudinal challenge require careful consideration; however, the frequency of accidental ingestion encourages the use of carefully controlled and supervised challenges to ascertain the clinical persistence of food reaction.

The Natural History of Adverse Reactions to Food in the First Three Years of Life

The studies described above involved a highly atopic population of youngsters whose history of food sensitivity was confirmed prior to their inclusion in their longitudinal studies. This study [4] involved a group of normal children who were not selected for the presence of atopic symptoms in themselves or in their families. The 501 children in this study were consecutive births into a large pediatric practice. Of the 501 children enrolled, 480 were followed prospectively from birth until each had his/her third birthday. The mothers of these children were consulted regularly about their child's diet and particularly about any adverse reaction to food which was suspected or observed. These observations were pursued using blinded or in some cases open food challenges all under observation. A number of interesting observations emerged from this study. First, 208 of 480 (43%) children had some symptom that was suspected of being triggered by a food. Second, a wide range of foods was incriminated. Most commonly mentioned were cow's mild and fruit or fruit juice. Third, 80% of the initial complaints occurred during the first year of life, with the number of new foods incriminated diminishing during the second and third years of life. Fourth, the duration of symptoms which could be described was surprisingly brief. The vast majority of reactions disappeared within a few months. Fifth, the number of foods producing blind-challenge-confirmed reactions was small and included milk (11), peanut (3), soy (2), and egg (1). Foods observed to produce symptoms during open challenge included mild (14), egg (2), soy (2), peanut (1), wheat (1), corn (1), and rice (1). Ninety-six reactions to foods (other than fruit or fruit juice) could not be reproduced. Of 75 youngsters with histories of adverse reaction to fruit or fruit juice, 56 were reproduced during open challenge. Sixth, although not all children in whom it would have been appropriate were skin tested, a minority of those with convincing reactions could be shown to have a positive skin reaction to an extract of the incriminated food. Excluding fruit, seven adverse reactions to food were accompanied by a positive skin test, 10 confirmed reactions were accompanied by a negative skin test, and 11 probable food reactions were associated with negative skin tests. Seventh, although open food challenges were utilized in this study, their primary purpose should be to refute vague histories of symptoms associated with food ingestion. The DBPCFC should continue to be regarded as the "Gold Standard" for the objective confirmation of histories of adverse reactions to foods.

Review of the Literature

Dannaeus and Johansson [5] reported, in 1979, on a group of 47 children with adverse reactions to cow's mild and other foods who were then followed up for four years. Most children in the study tolerated increased amounts of milk as the study progressed. It was observed that no children exhibited an increased sensitivity to mild as time passed. Also of note was the finding that children with lower antibody levels tolerated milk ingestion sooner than those with higher levels. In 1981, Dannaeus and Inganäs [6] described 82 children with adverse reactions to foods followed two to five years. At the time of reevaluation, more than half of the children (those with asthma and atopic dermatitis) exhibited a reduction in symptoms or complete tolerance when the previously offending food was ingested. Of particular interest was the observation that sensitivity to fish and nuts seemed more likely to persist with age than clinical reactivity to other foods. Jakobsson and Lindberg [7] reported on 20 children with adverse reactions to milk. Longitudinally performed challenges indicated a progressive increase in tolerance to milk over a period of time in 12 of the children.

Ford and Taylor [8] performed an excellent study of egg allergy using a prospective design and DBPCFC with 25 children. Between 2 and 2 1/2 years following the initial evaluation, 11 of 25 children were found to tolerate egg without symptoms. Sampson [9] has also repeated DBPCFC in some of his challenge-positive atopic dermatitis subjects, and found that some of them are progressively losing their clinical reactivity to foods.

In 1987, Hattevig et al. [10] reported the continuing evaluation of a group of children originally described in a 1984 paper [11]. Six of the 13 children with adverse reactions to foods could tolerate the food upon ingestion. Of note is the finding that some of the children clinically able to ingest a food which previously caused symptoms continued to demonstrate significant titers of IgE to the food. Businco et al. [12] followed 41 infants whose chronic diarrhea was attributed to milk ingestion. Over a period of seven years the majority was able to tolerate the reintroduction of milk into the diet. Another more detailed review of this subject was recently published by Eggleston [13] and should be of interest to the reader.

It seems apparent from the cited studies that a great deal of the adverse food reactions seen by clinicians occur in children. The trend in well over half of these children is for them to lose their clinical reactivity even though they may retain their immunologic reactivity as detected by skin tests or RAST. A number of considerations should play a role in future studies in this area now that the foundation has been established. First, diagnoses should always be confirmed by DBPCFC. In fact, a major weakness of some of the cited studies is the lack of objective confirmation of patient histories by DBPCFC. Second, longitudinal studies for the understanding and clarification of the natural history of adverse food reactions are distinctly preferable to cross-sectional studies. Third, when it is ethically permissible to perform repeated challenges over a long period of time, they should be DBPCFC. Finally, the biochemical mechanism whereby the clinical reactivity is lost despite the maintenance of immunologic reactivity needs to be elucidated.

References

1. Bock, S. A. 1982. The natural history of food sensitivity. J. Allergy Clin. Immunol. 69: 173.
2. Bock, S. A. 1988. The natural history of peanut allergy. J. Allergy Clin. Immunol. 81: 188 (Abstract). Submitted.
3. Bock, S. A. 1985. Natural history of severe reactions to food in young children. J. Pediatr. 107: 676.
4. Bock, S. A. 1987. Prospective appraisal of complaints of adverse reactions to foods in children during the first 3 years of life. Pediatrics 79: 683.
5. Dannaeus, A., and S. G. O. Johansson. 1979. A follow-up study of infants with adverse reactions to cow's milk. Acta Paediatr. Scand. 68: 377.
6. Dannaeus, A., and M. Inganäs. 1981. A follow-up study of children with food allergy. Clinical course in relation to serum IgE- and IgG-antibody levels to milk, egg and fish. Clinical Allergy 11: 533.
7. Jakobsson, I., and T. Lindberg. 1979. A prospective study of cow's milk protein intolerance in Swedish infants. Acta Paediatr. Scand. 68: 853.
8. Ford, R. P. K., and B. Taylor. 1982. Natural history of egg hypersensitivity. Arch. Dis. Child. 57: 649.
9. Sampson, H. A. 1988. The role of food allergy and mediator release in atopic dermatitis. J. Allergy Clin. Immunol. 81: 635.
10. Hattevig, G., B. Kjellman, and B. Björkstén. 1987. Clinical symptoms and IgE responses to common food proteins and inhalants in the first 7 years of life. Clin. Allergy 17: 571.
11. Hattevig, G., B. Kjellman, S. G. O. Johansson, and B. Björkstén. 1984. Clinical symptoms and IgE responses to common proteins in atopic and healthy children. Clin. Allergy 14: 551.
12. Businco, L., N. Benincori, A. Cantani, L. Tacconi, and A. Picarazzi. 1985. Chronic diarrhea due to cow's milk allergy. A 4 to 10 year follow-up study. Ann. Allergy 55: 844.
13. Eggleston, P. A. 1987. Prospective studies in the natural history of food allergy. Ann. Allergy 59 (Part II): 179.

Eosinophilic Gastroenteritis from Severe Food Allergy

*Kyung-Up Min and Dean D. Metcalfe**

Eosinophilic gastroenteritis (EG) is characterized by peripheral eosinophilia, eosinophilic infiltration of the bowel wall, and gastrointestinal symptoms. The sites of involvement include the esophagus, stomach, small intestine, and colon. Approximately one-half of the cases have allergic features and are related to food allergy. In the remainder of patients, EG is a disease of unknown etiology. Contrary to the complexity of the etiology, the treatment is simple and consists of steroid therapy and/or an elimination diet. The prognosis is good and fatality is exceptional.

Since the first description by Kaijser in 1937 [1], over 100 cases of the eosinophilic gastroenteritis (EG) have been reported. The variable terminology describing this entity has included pyloric hypertrophy with eosinophilic infiltration, gastric lesion of Loeffler's syndrome, gastric granuloma with eosinophilic infiltration, eosinophilic granuloma, infiltrative eosinophilic gastritis, and eosinophilic (allergic) gastroenteritis. This disorder is characterized by peripheral eosinophilia, eosinophilic infiltration of the bowel and diverse clinical manifestations according to the involved anatomic sites. This article presents an overview of the pathological and clinical features of EG, with an emphasis on food-induced cases.

Etiology and Pathogenesis

The cause of most cases of EG is unknown, although an allergic or immunologic mechanism seems most likely. Atopic disorders, such as childhood food sensitivities, eczema, allergic rhinitis, bronchial asthma, and a therapeutic response to steroids are common in patients with EG [2]. Moreover, many patients have an elevated serum IgE and positive radioallergosorbent tests (RAST) for specific IgE antibodies to food antigens [3]. These results correlate with positive skin tests and symptomatic re-

sponses to these food substances [4]. In addition, mononuclear cells containing IgE have been identified in the lamina propria of the large intestine [5]. In this study, the number of IgE containing cells and eosinophils fell after an elimination diet, which was accompanied by symptomatic improvement.

All patients with EG, however, are not atopic, and all cases cannot be explained by food allergy. Less than one-half of all patients have findings consistent with atopy [6]. Many patients show no personal or family history of allergy, no adverse reactions to foods, no positive skin tests for food allergens, and no elevation in serum IgE. Even in patients with suspected food allergies, sequential withdrawal of various food substances may fail to provide amelioration of symptoms, and there may be a poor correlation between the results of skin tests to specific food antigens and the results of an elimination diet. In addition, there are some patients who show no abnormality following extensive immunological studies, including serum immunoglobulins, complement levels, lymphocyte quantitation, and lymphocyte responses to nonspecific mitogens [2].

A number of other pathologic processes, including viral infections, parasitic infestations, and malignancies, have been considered as an explanation for EG in patients without obvious food allergies. Viral infections have been proposed because of the observation that EG may follow viral gastroenteritis. A history of flu-like symptoms, laboratory data including viral cultures, serologies, gastric histology showing inclusion bodies, and a spontaneous remissions in a few weeks, are consistent with this hypothesis. Several patients have had evidence of infection withcytomegalovirus [7] or parainfluenza virus [8]. Interestingly, it has been reported that certain viral infections may provoke allergic reactions by preferentially depressing IgE T-suppressor cells, thereby

* Mast Cell Physiology Section, Laboratory of Clinical Investigation, National Institute of Allergy and Infectious Diseases, National Institutes of Health, Bethesda, MD, 20892, USA.

allowing T-helper cells to stimulate IgE production [9]. Moreover, the increased absorption of antigen through mucosa damaged by a viral infection may stimulate immune responses. Parasite infestation is often associated with peripheral eosinophilia and eosinophilic infiltrations [10]. Eosinophilic infiltrations in the gut wall have been reported and may be the result of parasite infestation, although this possibility has been eliminated in most cases. The association of massive eosinophilia with nonhematopoietic malignancy is described. EG has been reported in a patient with ovarian malignancy with regression of eosinophilic gastritis after resection of this tumor [11]. Other diseases associated with EG include scleroderma, polymyositis, dermatomyositis and polyarteritis nodosa [12]. The mechanisms behind such associations are poorly understood, but the gastrointestinal disease may foretell the development of these diseases, sometimes by several years.

Classification and Clinical Manifestations

Rational classification of a disease is best developed out of an understanding of its etiology and pathogenesis. Lacking a precise knowledge of these aspects in EG, any attempt to classify this disorder will not be conclusive. The first classification proposed for EG was based on the pathologic and clinical picture derived from a study of the literature as well as their own patients [13]. They defined two major classes: class I, diffuse eosinophilic gastroenteritis, in which the gut wall is diffusely infiltrated by eosinophils and peripheral eosinophilia is prominent; and class II, circumscribed eosinophil infiltrated granuloma, in which there is a circumscribed granuloma, taking the form of either a pseudo tumor or a polyp, massively infiltrated by eosinophils but unassociated with peripheral eosinophilia. There has been much confusion about the terminology indicating the latter entity. Recently, inflammatory fibroid polyp was proposed for the polypoid group of class II to avoid confusion with eosinophilic granuloma of bone (histiocytosis X) [14]. The classification has been further refined, subdividing diffuse eosinophilic gastroenteritis (class I) into three types (Table 1), linking the clinical manifestations

Table 1. Clinical manifestations of diffuse eosinophilic gastroenteritis related to the depth of the maximal disease process.

Type	Predominant involvement	Manifestations
I	Mucosal	Abdominal pain, nausea, vomiting, iron deficiency anemia, diarrhea, growth retardation, weight loss, fecal blood loss
II	Muscular	Abdominal pain, nausea, vomiting, weight loss, early satiety
III	Serosal	Abdominal pain, nausea, vomiting, diarrhea, ascites

and the depth of the maximal disease process [6]. Type I is predominant mucosal disease characterized by fecal blood loss, iron deficiency anemia, protein-losing enteropathy, and/or malabsorption syndrome. Type II is predominantly a muscle layer disease with obstructive symptoms due to thickening and rigidity of the gut. Type III is predominantly a serosal disease with eosinophilic ascites. More than one site may be involved in a given patient.

Patients with mucosal involvement (the most frequent type of the three patterns) commonly have histories of atopic disease, as do members of their families [15–17]. Some of these patients can identify specific foods that precipitate their symptoms [4]. The total serum IgE level may be elevated [15, 17], and specific IgE to food antigen has been detected in their serum. Specific food challenge has been shown to produce gastrointestinal symptoms with a histologic change in the gut mucosa [18, 19]. Elimination diets have often resolved the clinical manifestations. These findings strongly suggest that mucosal eosinophilic gastroenteritis may be an IgE-mediated disease with specific foods acting as the inciting antigens. In contrast to patients with disease of the mucosa, those with predominantly muscularis disease lack specific food sensitivity and have normal IgE levels [4]. Other than eosinophilia, there is no evidence of a hypersensitivity phenomenon in this disorder. Approximately 10% of the reported cases of eosinophilic gastroenteritis have been of serosal type [20]. These patients with serosal involvement usually have some degree of mucosal disease. The patients may have a history of allergy, elevated IgE levels, peripheral eosinophilia, and respond to steroid therapy. These findings suggest the possibility of an allergic etiology. In EG involving the mucosa, muscle, or serosa, any segment may be involved from esophagus to rectum, although the most common sites are the gastric antrum and proximal small bowel. Colonic or esophageal involvement, isolated or combined, are being recognized with increasing frequency, suggesting the designation of this disease as gastroenteritis is too limiting [21].

In addition to a classification based upon the region of involvement, others have separated disease based on etiology. An analysis of children who showed eosinophilic infiltration of the stomach and small intestine, peripheral eosinophilia, iron deficiency anemia secondary to fecal blood loss, and protein-losing enteropathy revealed two distinct groups [22]. The first group had a transient milk-sensitive enteropathy. They presented in the first year of life, and exhibited symptoms that remitted on withdrawal of milk from the diet, and was apparently not associated with IgE-mediated immediate hypersensitivity. In contrast, the second group with eosinophilic gastroenteropathy presented with chronic disease that had its onset later in childhood. In these patients, there was an association with other atopic diseases, a markedly increased serum IgE, specific IgE to food antigens, and positive skin tests. And dietary manipulations prevented ana-phylactic reactions precipitated by foods, but did not influence gastrointestinal symptoms. Steroid therapy was required to establish a remission.

Colitis and proctitis induced by milk protein and other food allergens have been reported [21]. In the isolated form of colitis or proctitis, these disorders usually occur in early childhood, with most cases under 6 months of age. Common features include bloody diarrhea, a history of other allergic diseases in the child or the family, peripheral eosinophilia, an elevated serum IgE, specific IgE antibodies, positive skin tests to food antigens, and resolution of symptoms on an appropriate elimination diet.

Radiological Findings

There is no pathognomonic radiological finding in EG [23]. In mucosal disease, the stomach exhibits mucosal thickening similar to hypertrophic gastritis or Menetrier's disease. With further thickening of the folds, a polypoid gastritis or a discrete polyp may be observed. The changes in the small bowel may be striking and consist of patchy thickening and distortion of the folds, spasm, irritability, and increased secretions, more prominent in the jejunum. The thickened folds may produce a nodular configuration along the contour of the bowel. Colonic changes are unusual and may simulate inflammatory bowel disease. In the muscular type, changes in the stomach are usually limited to the antrum, producing a radiological appearance of hypertrophic pyloric stenosis. When muscular thickening is diffuse, an appearance simulating scirrhous sarcinoma may be produced. The small bowel may also show changes consistent with muscle involvement. If EG involves only the serosa, radiological findings will be those of ascites.

Diagnosis

The diagnosis of EG is not difficult if the histology of the bowel wall reveals eosinophilic infiltration in a patient with peripheral eosinophilia and characteristic clinical symptoms. The pertinent clinical setting may include a personal and family history of atopic disease, and characteristic gastrointestinal symptoms. Iron deficiency anemia, hypoproteinemia, and an increased IgE level may be present. The ESR is usually normal. Food-specific IgE antibodies may be detected in the serum, and the patient may show positive skin tests to food antigens. Symptoms may be related to exposure to specific foods. Challenge with a suspected food may provoke a severe exacerbation of symptoms and should not routinely be performed, although under carefully controlled conditions, food challenge may aid in diagnosis.

The histologic diagnosis may be made by mucosal biopsy in patients with mucosal disease, but patients with infiltration of deeper layers may require full thickness biopsies. Alterations of the gastric antrum are more constant and profound, suggesting biopsy of this site is the most sensitive and discriminating for diagnosis, even when gastric involvement is not suspected linically [21]. The intestinal lesions are often patchy and multiple biopsies may be required [17].

363

Treatment and Prognosis

The ideal treatment of EG is to identify and remove the food allergens from the diet that cause disease. Unfortunately, this is only rarely successful. A trial of an elimination diet is thus justified, especially in those patients with atopy. Substances known or suspected by the patient to exacerbate symptoms should be rigidly excluded. In the absence of a clinically suspected food sensitivity, trial elimination diets can be based upon results of skin testing and RAST. Steroids are successfully used in patients with EG who fail to respond to elimination diets. The dosages employed range from 20 to 40 mg of prednisone daily. The response is usually prompt. occasionally patients require continuous administration of low dosage steroids to control symptoms. Cromolyn sodium and ketotifen have been used in some patients, but with no consistent effect. However, such trials are reasonable as these drugs have negligible side effects [18]. Some patients with food hypersensitivities may have anaphylactic episodes following exposure to certain foods. These patients must be identified and instructed to avoid these incriminated foods. Such individuals should be prepared to self-administer adrenalin if a systemic reaction should occur following inadvertent exposure. Surgery should be reserved for those who present with obstructive symptoms, bowel perforation, or uncertain diagnosis. It is possible that bowel obstruction can be managed with steroids if detected early [2]. A few patients have shown a persistent remission of EG after surgical excision of the involved bowel segment [24]. The long-term prognosis for patients with EG is reasonable. Most patients experiencing recrudescence of symptoms can be managed by dietary manipulation or a short course of steroid therapy. Fatal cases are very rare and usually due to bowel perforation [25] or other associated diseases.

References

1. Kaijer, R. 1937. Zur Kenntnis der allergischen Affektionen des Verdauungskanals von Standpunkt des Chirurgen aus. Arch. Klin. Chir. 188: 36.
2. Caldwell, J. H., H. S. Mekhjian, P. E. Hurtubise, and F. M. Beman. 1978. Eosinophilic gastroenteritis with obstruction—Immunological studies of seven patients. Gastroenterology 4: 825.
3. Elkon, K. B., R. Sher, and H. C. Seftel. 1977. Immunological studies of eosinophilic gastroenteritis and treatment with disodium cromoglycate and beclomethasone dipropionate. S. Afr. Med. J. 52: 838.
4. Caldwell, J. H., J. I. Tennenbaum, and H. Bronstein. 1975. Serum IgE in eosinophilic gastroenteritis. Response to intestinal challenge in two cases. N. Engl. J. Med. 292: 1388.
5. Jenkins, H. R., J. R. Pincott, J. F. Soothill, P. J. Milla, and J. T. Harries. 1984. Food allergy: The major cause of infantile colitis. Arch. Dis. Child. 59: 326.
6. Klein, N. C., R. L. Hargrove, M. H. Sleisenger, and G. H. Jeffries. 1970. Eosinophilic gastroenteritis. Medicine (Baltimore) 49: 299.
7. Stillman, A. E., O. Sieber, U. Manthei, and J. Pinnas. 1981. Transient protein-losing enteropathy and enlarged gastric rugae in childhood. Am. J. Dis. Child. 135: 29.
8. Herskovic, T., H. M. Spiro, and J. D. Gryboski. 1968. Acute transient gastrointestinal protein loss. Pediatrics 41: 818.
9. Frick, O. L., D. F. German, and J. Mills. 1979. Development of allergy in children: 1. Association with virus infections. J. Allergy Clin. Immunol. 63: 228.
10. Hesdorffer, C. S. 1982. Eosinophilic gastro-enteritis—A complication of schistosomiasis and peripheral eosinophilia? S. Afr. Med. J. 61: 591.
11. Reshef, R., J. Manaster, E. Ezekiel, H. Suprun, and E. Manor. 1987. Malignant tumor masquerading as eosinophilic gastroenteritis. Isr. J. Med. Sci. 23: 281.
12. De Schryver-Kecskemeti, K., and R. E. Clouse. 1984. A previously unrecognized subgroup of "eosinophilic gastroenteritis"—Association with connective tissue diseases. Am. J. Surg. Pathol. 8: 171.
13. Ureles, A. L., T. Alschibaja, D. Lodico, and S. J. Stabins. 1961. Idiopathic eosinophilic infiltration of the gastrointestinal tract, diffuse and circumscribed—A proposed classification and review of the literature, with two additional cases. Am. J. Med. 30: 899.
14. Blackshaw, A. J., and D. A. Levison. 1986. Eosinophilic infiltrates of the gastrointestinal tract. J. Clin. Pathol. 39: 1.
15. Caldwell, J. H., H. M. Sharma, P. E. Hurtubise, and D. L. Colwell. 1979. Eosinophilic gastroenteritis in extreme allergy—Immunopathological comparison with nonallergic gastrointestinal disease. Gastroenterology 77: 560.
16. Lucak, B. K., C. Sansaricq, S. E. Snyderman, M. A. Greco, E. P. Fazzini, and G. R. Bazaz. 1982. Disseminated ulcerations in allergic eosinophilic gastroenterocolitis. Am. J. Gastroenterol. 7: 248.

17. Katz, A. J., H. Goldman, and R. J. Grand. 1977. Gastric mucosal biopsy in eosinophilic (allergic) gastroenteritis. Gastroenterology 73: 705.
18. Greenberger, N. J., J. I. Tennenbaum, and R. D. Ruppert. 1967. Protein-losing enteropathy associated with gastrointestinal allergy. Am. J. Med. 43: 777.
19. Shiner, M., J. Ballard, C. G. D. Brook, and S. Herman. 1975. Intestinal biopsy in the diagnosis of cow's milk protein intolerance without acute symptoms. Lancet i: 1060.
20. Harmon, W. A., and C. A. Helman. 1981. Eosinophilic gastroenteritis and ascites. J. Clin. Gastroenterol. 3: 371.
21. Goldman, H., and R. Proujansky. 1986. Allergic proctitis and gastroenteritis in children—Clinical and mucosal biopsy features in 53 cases. Am.

J. Surg. Pathol. 10: 75.
22. Katz, A. J., F. J. Twarog, R. S. Zeiger, and Z. M. Falchuk. 1984. Milk-sensitive and eosinophilic gastroenteropathy: Similar clinical features with contrasting mechanisms and clinical course. J. Allergy Clin. Immunol. 74: 72.
23. Marshak, R. H., A. Lindner, D. Maklansky, and A. Gelb. 1981. Eosinophilic gastroenteritis. JAMA 245: 1677.
24. Lysey, J., and A. Eid. 1986. Eosinophilic gastroenteritis with small bowel perforation. J. Clin. Gastroenterol. 8: 694.
25. Felt-Bersma, R. J. F., S. G. M. Meuwissen, and D. van Velzen. 1984. Perforation of the small intestine due to eosinophilic gastroenteritis. Am. J. Gastroenterol. 79: 442.

365

Immunotherapy—Past, Present, and Future

*Philip S. Norman**

Immunotherapy with allergenic extracts continues to be a mainstay of the clinical practice of allergy and the subject of continuing studies of efficacy and mechanism. Controlled clinical studies of immunotherapy in ragweed hay fever demonstrate that: (1) clinical results depend on adequate dose, with small doses having a poor rate of success or being totally ineffective [1, 2]; (2) relapse may occur once booster injections are discontinued [3]; and (3) results are specific, being effective only for the allergen(s) being administered and ineffective for excluded allergens [4, 5]. These results depended on performing studies which compare a treatment regimen with either placebo treatment or another regimen as controls. Groups of patients large enough to obtain statistically valid comparisons of the results of symptom diaries collected during natural exposure continue to be required in clinical studies.

Immunologically, a variety of changes have been demonstrated that may in part be responsible for the relief of allergic symptoms. Among these changes are (1) a rise in serum IgG "blocking" antibodies [6, 7, 8]; (2) a suppression in the usual seasonal rise in IgE antibodies which follows environmental exposure and a slow decline during several years in the level of specific IgE antibodies (although complete disappearance is rare) [9,10]; (3) an increase in blocking IgA and IgG antibodies in secretions [11,12]; (4) reduced basophil reactivity and sensitivity to allergens (as determined by in vitro leukocyte histamine release studies) [8, 13]; (5) an increase in allergen-specific suppressor cells [14, 15, 16]; and (6) reduced in vitro lymphocyte proliferation and production of lymphokines in response to allergens [17, 18].

Correlations between immunologic change and clinical results have been difficult to establish. The only immunologic response that shows any relationship to clinical improvement has been the serum IgG antibody response [2, 19]. In general, those patients who have higher titers of specific anti-ragweed IgG have more favorable clinical responses, and those who have low levels of IgG antibody have less favorable clinical responses, though there are clear exceptions to such a general rule. Studies of IgG subclass show that the initial response is usually a combination of IgG1 and IgG4, but that, with continued immunotherapy, circulating antibodies are almost entirely IgG4 by one year [20,21]. IgG4 antibodies are functionally monovalent and do not make precipitates with antigen or fix complement [22]. Hence, they appear to be the appropriate class of antibodies for blocking. Nevertheless, no clear relationship between the development of IgG4 antibodies and the success or failure of immunotherapy has emerged [23].

Antibodies in secretions may be ideally placed to interfere with mucosal reactions between allergens and mediator containing cells, but are present in vanishingly small amounts and so far have shown little correlation with clinical improvement [11, 12].

Factors not immediately subject to analysis may complicate the observation of any underlying relationship between antibodies and clinical improvement. For example:

— Actual exposure differs according the the microclimate the patient occupies.

— Patients vary in their tendency to report symptoms as severe.

— Allergies not treated for also cause symptoms.

— The several allergenic proteins in a species of an allergen such as ragweed contribute to symptoms in varying degrees from patient to patient.

The first three of these could not be controlled for by any testing technique that depends on natural exposure and the patients' perceptions of their disease. A quantitative challenge

*   Department of Medicine, Division of Clinical Immunology, The Johns Hopkins University School of Medicine at The Good Samaritan Hospital, 5601 Loch Raven Boulevard, Baltimore, Maryland 21239.
    Supported by Grants AI 04866 and AI 10304 from the National Institutes of Health, Bethesda, Maryland.

followed by measurements of physiological response or mediators released allows the observer to bypass both the subjective nature of symptom reporting and interference from other environmental allergens.

Challenges to the mucosae of the eyes, nose, and bronchi have often been used in the study of immunotherapy for respiratory and ocular allergies and have regularly demonstrated efficacy. The original study of Noon in 1911 involved ocular challenge with grass extract. Responses were reduced after a preseasonal course of injections of the grass extract [24]. In ragweed hay fever, the concentration of ragweed extract instilled into the nose required to elicit symptoms was increased several fold after immunotherapy [25]. Several controlled studies using bronchoprovocation with aerosols of allergenic extract indicate diminution of the physiologic pulmonary response after immunotherapy [26, 27, 28, 29].

A more recent method of nasal challenge developed by Naclerio et al. in our laboratory employs mucosal exposure to either whole pollen or pollen extracts followed by measurement of mediators appearing in nasal secretions [30]. The mediators found in immediate reactions to date include histamine, prostaglandin (Pg) D2, TAME- esterases [30], kinins [31], PgE, 6-ketoPgF2a, and peptide leukotrienes [32]. TAME-esterase activity in nasal secretions measures mainly a plasma kallikrein-α2-macroglobulin complex but also a mast cell tryptase [33]. This measurement is more sensitive than histamine and PGD2 to the effects of challenge and probably reflects the multiplier effect that comes from mast-cell mediators secondarily stimulating kallikrein production. Furthermore, there is an outpouring of serum proteins as indicated by increased amounts of serum albumin. These proteins include kininogen, thus providing the substrate for kinin conversion [34]. Mediators and proteins appear within minutes after challenge at a time when sneezing and other symptoms are at a maximum and disappear in 10—30 minutes after challenge is discontinued [30].

To determine whether specific immunotherapy alters in vivo mediator release, Creticos et al. compared 27 untreated highly sensitive ragweed-allergic subjects with 12 similarly sensitive patients receiving long-term immunotherapy with ragweed extract (median dose = 6 µg Amb a I [RW AgE]). The two groups were equally sensitive by skin tests and basophil histamine release. Patients on immunotherapy required larger threshold pollen doses not only to provoke sneezing but also to elicit release of TAME-esterase, PgD2 and histamine. At any given dose, the treated groups also released less mediator. The

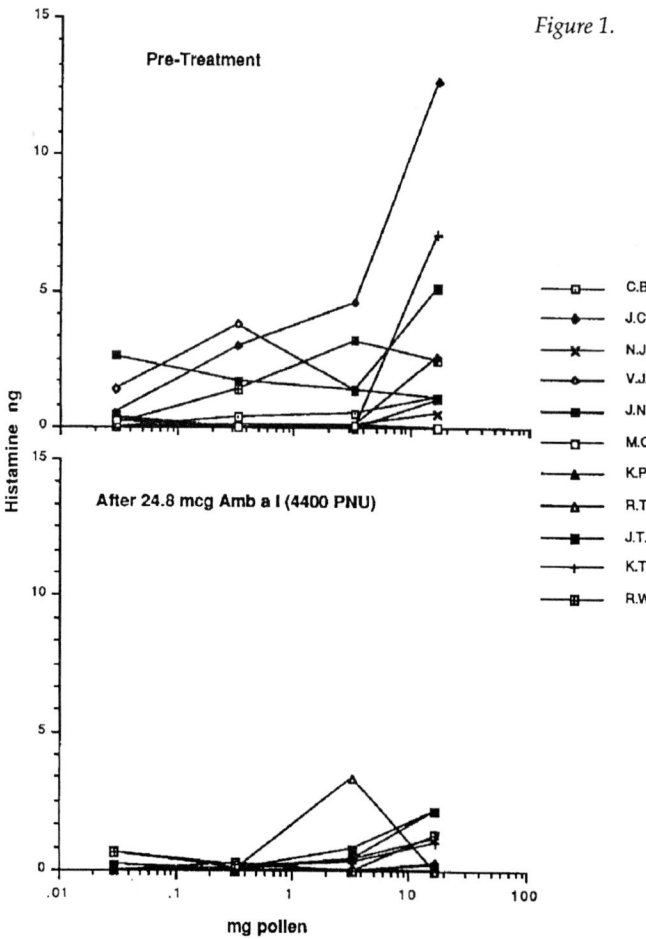

Figure 1.

C.B.
J.C.
N.J.
V.J.
J.N.
M.O.
K.P.
R.T.
J.T.
K.T.
R.W.

thresholds for both mediator release and sneezing required a pollen challenge dose in most treated patients higher than typically encountered in natural exposure. The pollen challenges are in excess of natural exposure, but do demonstrate that reactivity has not been completely ablated, at least by this dose of immunotherapy [35].

In a prospective study, patients starting immunotherapy with whole ragweed extract were challenged serially over many months and showed increasing thresholds for mediator release as the therapeutic dose was raised. Figure 1 shows curves of the appearance of histamine in nasal secretions during graded challenges in 11 patients before treatment and after a course of immunotherapy culminating in a 4,400 PNU dose of extract equivalent 24.8 µg of the major allergen of ragweed, antigen E (Amb a I in the new nomenclature). After a low dose of 0.6 µg of Amb a I, there was no detectable change in the response to challenge, but at the dose of 12.4 µg per injection, many of the patients failed to release any histamine, and those that do required very high doses of pollen of around 500,000 grains (data not shown). Raising the dose to 24.8 µg seemed to add little more. Similar data were obtained with measurements of TAME-esterase in the secretions. Such data place the optimum dose somewhere higher than 0.6 µg of the major allergen, and we hope to perform more studies with intermediate doses to narrow down the range of optimum dose.

Attempts to correlate these changes in challenge responses with antibody responses were unsuccessful and indicate that measurement of serum antibody responses have little predictive value in assessing results in a single patient.

A more complete view of the pathogenesis of allergic reactions emphasizes that there is more to clinical reactions than a transient release of short-acting mediators resulting in evanescent manifestations. IgE-mediated allergic reactions are not necessarily immediate and short lived. In the skin, nasal passages, and lower airways, challenges often lead not only to immediate responses, but a subsequent "late-phase" reaction starting 3 to 11 hours after exposure which may be quite prolonged in time [36]. In the skin, IgE antibodies are clearly necessary to such a reaction and recent evidence in the lung and the nose links these reaction to a secondary release of many of the same mediators which appear in the immediate reaction [37]. For instance, a nasal challenge study by Naclerio et al. shows a second wave of symptoms and mediator release 3 to 11 hours after the initial challenge. The mediators found include histamine, TAME-esterase, and kinins, but curiously prostaglandin D_2 is never found. The absence of PgD_2 raises the possibility of a different cellular source for the second wave of mediators as a second challenge 11 hours after the first will, in contrast, result in the prompt appearance of PgD_2 along with the other mediators [38].

It seems likely that the late-phase reaction is just as important in the pathogenesis of allergic disease as the early reaction. For instance, asthmatic attacks are uncommonly immediate, but rather take hours or days to develop and clear up completely only after days or weeks of treatment. Nasal disease can show the same pattern. Furthermore, corticosteroids the most effective drug for these condition ablate the late phase more readily than the early phase [39]. An antigen bronchoprovocation model in rabbits provides both an early- and a late-phase reaction if neonatal rabbits that make only IgE antibodies are immunized with an allergen. If IgG antibody is transfused or induced by secondary immunization when the rabbit is more mature, the late but not the early IgE mediated bronchial response to challenge is ablated [40].

In humans several studies indicate that immunotherapy changes the late-phase reaction to bronchial challenge more than it changes the immediate reaction. Using Alternaria, the same antigen that was employed in the animal studies, Metzger challenged sensitive asthmatic patients before and after high-dose immunotherapy (> 100,000 PNU). After immunotherapy the acute response was not changed but the late reaction was decreased by about 70% [41]. In a controlled trial of immunotherapy with D. pteronyssinus, Warner found that the immediate response to antigen challenge was unchanged, while the late response was lost in half of the patients. Furthermore, the children who failed to manifest the delayed response had the best clinical outcome [28]. In addition, Pienkowski et al. found that patients who have received immunotherapy for allergic rhinitis have much smaller late skin responses to antigen than untreated control patients even though the early skin responses are the same [42].

A recent study in our laboratory by Il-iopoulis et al. in matched treated and placebo ragweed sensitive patients treated at a maintenance dose of approximately 2.0 µg Amb a I confirmed the reduction in late phase skin responses in patients on immunotherapy for ragweed, but found no preferential effect on the late phase mediator response to nasal challenge. Reductions in late phase response occurred in those patients who had a preceding reduction in acute response. Evaluation of the effect of immunotherapy on the late phase response was complicated by the fact that only about half of the patients had a late-phase increase of mediators in nasal secretions. If one looks only at the patients who had a pre-treatment late-phase mediator response, it is significantly less in the treated patients than the placebo patients. On the other hand, the post-challenge increase of inflammatory cells (neutrophils, eosinophils, Alcian blue positive cells—presumably basophils—and mononuclear cells) in nasal secretions was a more regular phenomenon than mediator release. Immunotherapy was highly effective in reducing the eosinophil and basophil response, but had little effect on the neutrophil and mononuclear response in patients on immunotherapy in comparison to untreated controls [43].

What dose of extract is required for optimum efficacy of immunotherapy is a constant topic for discussion. Although improved standardization of extracts will help to collect data on this important subject, a certain number of efficacy studies have employed extracts standardized in a way that allows comparison. As newer units based on biological activity have been introduced only recently, the only method that offers a common denominator in a sufficient number of studies is the measurement of one or more major allergens in the extract. Table 1 summarizes data on four classes of allergens, showing (where available) both the largest single dose and the cumulative annual dose in terms of the mcg of major allergen. In several early studies, only the cumulative dose was available. For insect venom, it has been established that a maximum dose of

Table 1. Doses of allergens proved to be effective in immunotherapy.

Maximum Dose	Range	Cumulative dose*	Range	Unit	Ref
Ragweed					
No data		6.5	0.13–17	AgE (*Amb a* I)	47
No data		24	2.7–67.5	AgE	1
9.4	1.7–18.8	70	16.4–252	AgE	48
4.7	0.4–28.1	17.1	2.? 147	AgE (clustered schedule)	48
11.1	3.7–46.8	84.9	18.1–351.1	AgE	49
6	1.2–18.6	No data		AgE**	35
12.4	None	No data		AgE**	50
Grass					
18.6	No data	34.8	7.2–99	Rye Gp I (*Lol p* I)	51
18	12.9–20.4	118.2	59.4–152.1	Ag19*** (*Phl p* VI)	52
36	25.8–40.8	236.4	118.8–304.2	Ag 25 (*Phl p* V)	
Cat					
No data		3.4	1.7–4.7	Cat 1 (*Fel d* I)	27
No data		10.9	0.24–24.8	Cat 1	53
No data		41	13–65	Cat 1	54
15.1	9–23	231	18–579	Cat 1	55
Insects					
12	None	No data		Honey Bee PLA (*Api m* I)	56, 44
2.9	None	No data		WF Hornet Ag 5 (*Dol m* V)	
3.4	None	No data		YF Hornet Ag 5 (*Dol a* V)	
4.6	None	No data		Yellow Jacket Ag 5 (*Ves g* V)	

*In µg major allergen in the extract
**Challenge study
***Two major antigens measured in one extract

100 μg of whole venom from each of four species is regularly effective in preventing anaphylaxis. The venom figures represent the content of major allergen in this amount of venom from the calculations of King [44].

From both clinical and immunologic evidence, it seems likely that the maximum or the final dose is the more meaningful than a cumulative annual dose. From the data in this table, the maximum dose is remarkably similar for a variety of allergens, lying somewhere between just under 5 μg and 20 μg. It should be noted that most of these studies were designed to describe the maximum tolerated dose, so that the lower figures may be more appropriate as a guide to a safe but effective dose. Two studies with ragweed indicate that doses of less than 1 μg AgE equivalent are not measurably effective by present clinical or challenge methods [45, 46]. As any of the biologically determined units can usually be estimated by determination of a major allergen, these numbers provide a rough guide to the target dosage in an immunotherapy regimen. As the relationship between units biologically determined and the content of major allergen is worked out, it should be possible to describe accurately a target dose which is likely to be effective for a number of allergens.

References

1. Norman, P. S., W. L. Winkenwerder, and L. M. Lichtenstein. 1968. Immunotherapy of hay fever with ragweed antigen E: Comparisons with whole pollen extract and placebos. J. Allergy 42: 93.
2. Lichtenstein, L. M., P. S. Norman, and W. L. Winkenwerder. 1971. A single year of immunotherapy for ragweed hay fever: Immunologic and clinical studies. Ann. Intern. Med. 75: 663.
3. Norman, P. S. 1974. Specific therapy in allergy. Pro (With Reservations). Med. Clin. North America 58: 230.
4. Lowell, F. C., and W. Franklin. 1965. A double-blind study of the effectiveness and specificity of injection therapy in ragweed hay fever. N. Engl. J. Med. 273: 675.
5. Norman, P. S., and L. M. Lichtenstein. 1978. The clinical and immunologic specificity of immunotherapy. J. Allergy Clin. Immunol. 61: 370.
6. Cooke, R. A., J. H. Barnard, S. Hebald, and A. Stull. 1935. Serological evidence of immunity with coexisting sensitization in a type of human allergy (hay fever). J. Exp. Med. 62: 733.
7. Loveless, M. H. 1943. Immunological studies of pollinosis: IV. The relationship between thermostable antibody in the circulation and clinical immunity. J. Immunol. 47: 165.
8. Lichtenstein, L. M., P. S. Norman, W. L. Winkenwerder, and A. G. Osler. 1966. In vitro studies of human ragweed allergy: Changes in cellular and humoral activity associated with specific desensitization. J. Clin. Invest. 45: 1126.
9. Lichtenstein, L. M., K. Ishizaka, P. S. Norman, A. K. Sobotka, and B. M. Hill. 1973. IgE antibody measurements in ragweed hay fever: Relationship to clinical severity and the results of immunotherapy. J. Clin. Invest. 52: 472.
10. Gleich, G. J., G. L. Jacob, J. W. Yunginger, and L. L. Henderson. 1977. Measurement of the absolute levels of IgE antibodies in patients with ragweed hay fever: Effect of immunotherapy on seasonal changes and relationship to IgG antibodies. J. Allergy Clin. Immunol. 60: 188.
11. Platts-Mills, T. A. E., R. K. Von Maur, K. Ishizaka, P. S. Norman, and L. M. Lichtenstein. 1976. IgA and IgG anti-ragweed antibodies in nasal secretions. J. Clin. Invest. 57: 1041.
12. Platts-Mills, T. A. E. 1979. Local production of IgG, IgA, and IgE antibodies in grass pollen hay fever. J. Immunol. 122: 2218.
13. Sadan, N., M. B. Rhyne, E. D. Mellits, E. O. Goldstein, D. A. Levy, and L. M. Lichtenstein. 1969. Immunotherapy of pollinosis in children: Investigation of the immunologic basis of clinical improvement. N. Engl. J. Med. 280: 623.
14. Nagoya, H. 1985. Induction of antigen-specific suppressor cells in patients with hayfever receiving immunotherapy. J. Allergy Clin. Immunol. 75: 388.
15. Tamir, R., J. M. Castracane, and R. E. Rocklin. 1987. Generation of suppressor cells in atopic patients during immunotherapy that modulate IgE synthesis. J. Allergy Clin. Immunol. 79: 591.
16. Rocklin, R. E., A. L. Sheffer, D. K. Greineder, and K. L. Melmon. 1980. Generation of antigen-specific suppressor cells during allergy desensitization. N. Engl. J. Med. 302: 1213.
17. Rocklin, R. E., H. Pence, H. Kaplan, and R. Evans. 1974. Cell-mediated immune response of ragweed-sensitive patients to ragweed antigen E: In vitro lymphocyte transformation and elaboration of lymphocyte mediators. J. Clin. Invest. 53: 735.
18. Evans, R., H. Pence, H. Kaplan, and R. E. Rocklin. 1976. The effect of immunotherapy on humoral and cellular responses in ragweed hayfever. J. Clin. Invest. 57: 1378.
19. Lichtenstein, L. M., P. S. Norman, and W. L. Winkenwerder. 1968. Clinical and in vitro studies on the role of immunotherapy in ragweed hay fever. Am. J. Med. 44: 514.

20. Devey, M. E., D. V. Wilson, and A. W. Wheeler. 1976. The IgG subclass of antibodies to grass pollen allergens produced in hay fever patients during hyposensitization. Clin. Allergy 6: 227.

21. Aalberse, R. C., R. van der Gaag, and J. van Leeuwen. 1983. Serologic aspects of IgG4 antibodies. I. Prolonged immunization results in an IgG4-restricted response. J. Immunol. 130: 722.

22. van der Zee, J. S., P. van Swieten, and R. C. Aalberse. 1986. Serologic aspects of IgG4 antibodies. II. IgG4 antibodies form small, nonprecipitating Immune Complexes due to functional monovalency. J. Immunol. 137: 3566.

23. Malling, H.-J. and R. Djurup. 1988. Diagnosis and immunotherapy of mold allergy VII. IgG subclass response and relation to the clinical efficacy of immunotherapy with Cladosporium. Allergy 413: 60.

24. Noon, L. 1911. Prophylactic inoculation against hay fever. Lancet 1: 1572.

25. Feinberg, S. M., R. A. Stier, and W. C. Grater. 1952. A suggested quantitative evaluation of the degree of sensitivity of patients with ragweed pollinosis. J. Allergy 23: 387.

26. Åas, K. 1971. Hyposensitization in house dust allergy asthma: A double-blind controlled study with evaluation of the effect on bronchial sensitivity to house dust. Acta. Pediat. Scand. 60: 264.

27. Taylor, W. W., J. L. Ohman, and F. C. Lowell. 1978. Immunotherapy in cat-induced asthma: Double-blind trial with evaluation of bronchial responses to cat allergen and histamine. J. Allergy Clin. Immunol. 61: 283.

28. Warner, J. D., J. F. Price, J. F. Soothill, and E. N. Hey. 1978. Controlled trial of hyposensitization to Dermatophagoides pteronyssinus in children with asthma. Lancet 2: 912.

29. Sundin, B., G. Lilja, V. Graff-Lonevig, G. Hedlin, H. Heilborn, K. Norrlind, K. O. Pegelow, and H. Løwenstein. 1986. Immunotherapy with partially purified and standardized animal dander extracts. I. Clinical results from a double-blind study on patients with animal dander asthma. J. Allergy Clin. Immunol. 77: 478.

30. Naclerio, R. M., H. L. Meier, A. Kagey-Sobotka, N. F. Adkinson Jr., D. A. Meyers, P. S. Norman, and L. M. Lichtenstein. 1983. Mediator release after nasal airway challenge with allergen. Am. Rev. Respir. Dis. 128: 597.

31. Proud, D., A. Togias, R. M. Naclerio, S. A. Crush, P. S. Norman, and L. M. Lichtenstein. 1983. Kinins are generated in vivo following nasal airway challenge of allergic individuals with allergen. J. Clin. Invest. 72: 1678.

32. Creticos, P. S., S. P. Peters, N. F. Adkinson Jr., R. M. Naclerio, E. C. Hayes, P. S. Norman, and L. M. Lichtenstein. 1984. Peptide leukotriene release after antigen challenge in patients sensitive to ragweed. N. Engl. J. Med. 310: 1626.

33. Baumgarten, C. R., R. C. Nichols, R. M. Naclerio, L. M. Lichtenstein, P. S. Norman, and D. Proud. 1986. Plasma kallikrein during experimentally-induced allergic rhinitis: Role in kinin formation and contribution to TAME-esterase activity in nasal secretions. J. Immunol. 137: 977.

34. Baumgarten, C. R., A. G. Togias, R. M. Naclerio, L. M. Lichtenstein, P. S. Norman, and D. Proud. 1985. Influx of kininogens into nasal secretions after antigen challenge of allergic individuals. J. Clin. Invest. 76: 191.

35. Creticos, P. S., N. F. Adkinson Jr., A. Kagey-Sobotka, D. Proud, H. L. Meier, R. M. Naclerio, L. M. Lichtenstein, and P. S. Norman. 1985. Nasal challenge with ragweed pollen in hay fever patients: Effect of immunotherapy. J. Clin. Invest. 76: 2247.

36. Herxheimer, H. 1952. The late bronchial reaction in induced asthma. Int. Arch. Allergy Appl. Immunol. 3: 323.

37. Solley, G. O., G. J. Gleich, R. E. Jordon, and A. L. Schroeter. 1976. The late phase of the immediate wheal and flare skin reaction: Its dependence upon IgE antibodies. J. Clin. Invest. 58: 408.

38. Naclerio, R. M., D. Proud, A. Togias, N. F. Adkinson Jr., D. A. Meyers, A. Kagey-Sobotka, M. Plaut, P. S. Norman, and L. M. Lichtenstein. 1985. Inflammatory mediators in late antigen-induced rhinitis. New Engl. J. Med. 313: 65.

39. Pipkorn, U., D. Proud, L. M. Lichtenstein, R. P. Schleimer, S. P. Peters, N. F. Adkinson Jr., A. Kagey-Sobotka, P. S. Norman, and R. M. Naclerio. 1987. Effect of short-term systemic glucocorticoid treatment on human nasal mediator release after antigen challenge. J. Clin. Invest. 80: 957.

40. Shampain, M. P., B. L. Behrens, G. L. Larsen, and P. M. Henson. 1982. An animal model of late pulmonary responses to Alternaria challenge. Am. Rev. Respir. Dis. 126: 493.

41. Metzger, W. J., B. A. Donnelly, and H. B. Richardson. 1983. Modification of late asthmatic responses (LAR) during immunotherapy for Alternaria-induced asthma. J. Allergy Clin. Immunol. 71: 119.

42. Pienkowski, M. M., P. S. Norman, and L. M. Lichtenstein. 1985. Suppression of late-phase skin reactions by immunotherapy with ragweed extract. J. Allergy Clin. Immunol. 76: 729.

43. Iliopolous, O., D. Proud, A. Kagey-Sobotka, P. S. Creticos, P. S. Norman, L. M. Lichtenstein, and R. M. Naclerio. 1988. Effects of immunotherapy on early and late reactions to nasal challenge. J. Allergy Clin. Immunol. 81: 291.

44. King, T. P., A. K. Sobotka, A. Alagon, L. Kochumian, and L. M. Lichtenstein. 1978. Protein allergens of white-faced Hornet, yellow hornet, and yellow jacket venoms. Biochemistry 17: 5165.

45. Creticos, P. S., D. G. Marsh, N. F. Adkinson Jr., D. Proud, R. M. Naclerio, A. Kagey-Sobotka, L. M. Lichtenstein, and P. S. Norman PS. 1984. Evaluation by nasal pollen challenge of immunotherapy with rapidly released ragweed allergens. J. Allergy Clin. Immunol. 73: 141.

46. Creticos, P. S., D. G. Marsh, N. F. Adkinson Jr., D. Proud, R. M. Naclerio, A. Kagey-Sobotka, L. M. Lichtenstein, and P. S. Norman. 1984. Evaluation by nasal pollen challenge of immunotherapy with rapidly released ragweed allergens. J. Allergy Clin. Immunol. 73: 141.

47. Norman, P. S., and L. M. Lichtenstein. 1978. Comparisons of alum-precipitated and unprecipitated aqueous ragweed pollen extracts in the treatment of hay fever. J. Allergy Clin. Immunol. 61: 384.

48. Van Metre, T. E. Jr., N. F. Adkinson Jr., F. J. Amodio, A. Kagey-Sobotka, L. M. Lichtenstein, M. R. Mardiney Jr., P. S. Norman, and G. L. Rosenberg. 1982. A comparison of immunotherapy schedules for injection treatment of ragweed pollen hay fever. J. Allergy Clin. Immunol. 69: 181.

49. Van Metre, T. E. Jr., N. F. Adkinson Jr., F. J. Amodio, L. M. Lichtenstein, M. R. Mardiney Jr, P. S. Norman, G. L. Rosenberg, A. K. Sobotka, and M. D. Valentine. 1980. A comparative study of the effectiveness of the Rinkel method and the current standard method of immunotherapy for ragweed pollen hay fever. J. Allergy Clin. Immunol. 66: 500.

50. Creticos, P. S., D. G. Marsh, N. F. Adkinson Jr., D. Proud, R. M. Naclerio, A. Kagey-Sobotka, L. M. Lichtenstein, and P. S. Norman. 1984. Evaluation by nasal pollen challenge of immunotherapy with rapidly released ragweed allergens. J. Allergy Clin. Immunol. 73: 141.

51. Moss, R. B., Y.-P. Hsu, J. M. Kwasnicki, M. M. Sullivan, and M. J. Reid. 1987. Isotypic and antigenic restriction of the blocking antibody response to rye grass pollen: Correlation of rye group I antigen-specific IgG1 with clinical response. J. Allergy Clin. Immunol. 79: 387.

52. Østerballe, O. 1982. Immunotherapy with grass pollen allergens. Clinical results from a prospective 3-year double blind study. Allergy 37: 379.

53. Ohman, J. L. Jr., S. R. Findlay, and K. M. Leitermann. 1984. Immunotherapy in cat-induced asthma. Double-blind trial with evaluation of in vivo and in vitro responses. J. Allergy Clin. Immunol. 74: 230.

54. Sundin, B., G. Lilja, V. Graff-Lonevig, G. Hedlin, H. Heilborn, K. Norrlind, K.-O.Pegelow, and H. Løwenstein. 1986. Immunotherapy with partially purified and standardized animal dander extracts. I. Clinical results from a double-blind study on patients with animal dander asthma. J. Allergy Clin. Immunol. 77: 478.

55. Van Metre, T. E. Unpublished data.

56. Hunt, K. J., A. K. Sobotka, F. J. Amodio, M. D. Valentine, A. W. Benton, and L. M. Lichtenstein. 1978. A controlled trial of immunotherapy in insect hypersensitivity. N. Engl. J. Med. 299: 257.

Allergen Immunotherapy: Advances in Treatment and Mechanisms

Roy Patterson, Leslie C. Grammer, Martha A. Shaughnessy*

Allergen immunotherapy is the injection of un- avoidable inhalant allergens to patients with IgE- mediated respiratory allergy. With proper use, it is safe, effective, and the only available method of immunomodulation of these diseases. Effectiveness is dependent on proper total dose of antigen, and the most likely immunologic mechanism depends upon enhanced protective IgG antibody response, although individual IgG immune responses may not correlate with symptomatic improvement. Improved immunotherapy, which is safer, more cost effective, and available for all inhalant antigens is a goal for governmental programs and the health care and pharmaceutical industries. The theoretical basis of polymerized allergens—reduced allergenicity with retained immunogenicity—meets the criteria for improved therapy.

In this review we discuss the definition of allergen immunotherapy (IT), its safety, indications for use, efficacy, and current methodology as background information for new therapeutic advances in IT.

Definitions

IT is the administration of gradually increasing doses of extracts of unavoidable inhalant allergens to individuals with IgE-mediated respiratory allergy. This therapy is not desensitization, which is best defined as the rapid administration of increasing doses of antigen in an attempt to neutralize IgE antibody. This is a procedure with significant risk and is performed in order to administer essential therapeutic agents such as penicillin. The characteristics of IT, as commonly used, are listed in Table 1. Further detailed discussions can be found in standard textbooks of allergy [2–5]. The therapy is most clearly demonstrated as effective in controlled studies with pollen allergens in pollen induced rhinitis. In addition,

Table 1. Summary statements on current IT as generally used.

1. Consists of injections of small and then increasing doses of unavoidable inhalant antigens for IgE-mediated respiratory disease.
2. With proper diagnosis it is effective most probably through enhanced production of protective IgG antibody and, with prolonged therapy, decreased IgE antibody in some cases.
3. It is generally safe when managed by appropriately trained physicians, but the risk of fatal anaphylaxis is present.
4. It should not be confused with various unproven technique which vary from ineffective to possibly hazardous [1].
5. It is time consuming and expensive.

there are studies demonstrating effectiveness in mold spore and dust-mite allergy, and IT is considered by many to be of therapeutic value in IgE-triggered inhalant asthma.

A summary of theoretical and practical methods of modifying IgE mediated disease by modulation of the immune system or its reactions is shown in Table 2. All of these methods have been or are being studied in humans except pharmacologic destruction or suppression of production of IgE antibody. Although the latter therapy is an ideal goal, there would have to be no interference with other protective products of the immune system, and achievement of this goal within three decades is unlikely. Modified allergens is the final type of therapy listed in Table 2. The rationale for modified IT is that if standard IT is effective but time-consuming and expensive, modified allergens might maintain benefit while reducing frequency of IT and duration of therapy. The primary goals in the development of modified allergens have been to slow absorption of allergens, to alter allergens to form allergoids, or to form conjugates with the goal of inhib-

*   Section of Allergy-Immunology, Department of Medicine, Northwestern University Medical School, Chicago, Illinois 60611.
Supported by the Ernest S. Bazley Grant and USPHS Asthma and Allergic Diseases Center Grant AI 11403.

Table 2. Theoretical methods and mechanisms of immunologic control or termination of IgE-mediated disease.

Method	Mechanism	Status
Desensitization	Neutralization of IgE antibody by high doses of antigen	Very high risk of anaphylaxis. Indicated only in rare emergencies
Pharmacologic inhibition or termination of IgE antibody production	Possible in theory; must be accomplished without interference with IgG, IgA or IgM production	Theoretical only
Inhibition of binding of IgE to mast cells and basophils	Polypeptide reportedly can inhibit IgE binding by blocking Fc receptor site	Conflicting results
Allergen immunotherapy as currently used and as described in text and Table 1	Most probably the result of enhanced production of protective IgG antibody	With proper diagnosis and indications is effective; problems in use are expense, treatment duration and risk
Modified allergens: Polymerized allergens used as a primary example	Most probably the result of enhanced production of protective IgG antibody	Demonstrated significant decrease in symptom-medication scores, induction of IgG response, and sharply reduced treatment duration [4]

iting specific IgE production. Varying degrees of success have been reported in animal models and in man. These methods have recently been reviewed [4, 6, 7].

Polymerized Allergens

A model system of modified allergens is reviewed briefly in order to demonstrate that improved IT is an achievable goal in theory and in practice. The hypothesis is that polymers of monomeric allergens would be less allergenic therapeutic agents for IT because they would be less able than monomeric allergens, on a weight basis, to stimulate mast-cell mediator release through mast-cell-bound IgE. By contrast, they would induce protective IgG antibody equally well as monomeric allergens on a weight basis. Over a 12-year period these theoretical concepts were tested in a variety of studies and were upheld. The studies in animals and humans showed reduced allergenicity and retained immunogenicity. Safety and reduction in symptom-medication scores using a 12–15-week injection schedule were demonstrated in multiple clinical trials. The therapy obviously works for weeds and grasses and should be effective for other polymers. Polymerized venoms, mold spore antigen, dust mite, and even cat and dog danders could provide a spectrum of therapeutic IT suitable for the individual therapeutic needs of patients.

The Role of Industry and Government

Recognizing that IT is successful as a treatment modality is important. The goal of government and industry should be to foster, develop, and offer new IT products to the large patient population with IgE-mediated respiratory diseases. This is the only improved manner in which these prevalent diseases with complications can be controlled using immunomodulation.

References

1. American Academy of Allergy and Immunology. 1986. Position paper: Unproven procedures for diagnosis and treatment of allergic and immunologic diseases. J. Allergy Clin. Im-

munol. 78: 275.

2. Norman, P. S., and L. M. Lichtenstein. 1978. Allergic rhinitis. In: Immunological diseases, Vol. 2. M. Samter, ed. Philadelphia, PA: Little Brown, p. 839.

3. Parker, C. W. 1980. Asthma and rhinitis. In: Clinical immunology, Vol. 2. C.W. Parker, ed. Philadelphia, PA: W.B. Saunders, p. 1429.

4. Van Metre, T. E., and N. F. Adkinson. 1988. Immunotherapy for aeroallergen disease. In: Allergy: Principles and practice, Vol. 2. E. Middleton, C. E. Reed, E. F. Ellis, N. F. Adkinson, and J. W. Yunginger, eds. St. Louis, MO: C.V. Mosby, p. 1327.

5. Grammer, L. C. 1985. Principles of immunologic management of allergic diseases due to extrinsic antigens. In: Allergic diseases: Diagnosis and management. R. Patterson, ed. Phildelphia, PA: J.B. Lippincott, p. 358.

6. Lee, T. M., L. C. Grammer, and M. A. Shaughnessy. 1986. Modified antigens in the treatment of allergic disease. In: The year in immunology. H. J. Wedner, ed. Basel: S. Karger, p. 338.

7. Grammer, L. C., M. A. Shaughnessy, and R. Patterson. 1985. Modified forms of allergen immunotherapy. J. Allergy Clin. Immunol. 76: 397.

The Value of Specific Immunotherapy in the Treatment of Allergic Diseases

*Jean Bousquet, Philippe Godard, François-B. Michel**

Though specific immunotherapy has been used for more than 75 years, it is still a matter of controversy since many allergen extracts are unsatisfactory and injections of high-quality extracts may lead to severe systemic reactions. Recent improvement in the pharmacological treatment of allergic diseases has led to improved efficacy and reduced side effects. It is therefore important to characterize patients who should be treated by immunological treatment. Specific immunotherapy is effective in the treatment of rhino-conjunctivitis and asthma due to pollens and house dust mites and can be used in selected patients. Venom immunotherapy is highly effective and represents the only available treatment. Mold or animal dander immunotherapy was found to be effective in highly selected patients using standardized allergen extracts, but results obtained cannot be extended to treatments done in clinical practice. Finally, immunotherapy with totally uncharacterized allergens such as house dust, *Candida albicans*, or bacterial extracts must not be done any more.

Specific immunotherapy (SIT) was introduced in 1911 for the treatment of pollinosis and is one of the most common treatments in children and adolescents in many parts of the world. Nevertheless, it is a highly controversial treatment. In the 1970s many doctors and patients questioned its efficacy, since the quality of many extracts used was far from optimal [1]. Within the past 15 years considerable progress has been made, and SIT is effective under optimal conditions including a demonstrated IgE mediated disease, a high-quality extract and proper dose, and a correct indication [2]. However, the introduction of standardized extracts made SIT dangerous, and fatalities have been observed leading to the almost complete withdrawal of SIT in some countries, including the UK [3]. Finally, the pharmacologic treatment of allergy was also improved, especially by the introduction of nonsedative antihistamines. It is therefore important to compare the risk/benefit ratio of SIT and pharmacotherapy before starting allergen injections.

Efficacy

The efficacy of SIT is now widely documented in optimally designed controlled trials for allergen species including hymenoptera venoms, pollen, and mites.

Hymenoptera Venom Immunotherapy

Immunotherapy with venoms protects over 90% of allergic individuals, though SIT with honey bee venom appears to be less effective than that of vespid venoms [4]. One of the problems of venom SIT is its duration. Recent data showed that (1) after 5 years of treatment most patients can stop SIT whatever the results of skin tests and/or specific IgE are [5], and (2) over 50% of vespid venom allergic individuals and 35% of honey bee venom-sensitive patients have negative skin tests and RAST after 3 years of treatment [6]. These recent studies indicate that venom SIT is no longer a life-span treatment. Moreover, SIT cannot be replaced by any other treatment in venom allergy.

Pollen Allergy

Immunotherapy with grass and ragweed pollen extracts has been largely studied [7, 8]. In rhino-conjunctivitis, it was observed that SIT decreased symptoms and medications during the pollen season [9–12], and nasal or conjunctival challenges confirmed the efficacy of SIT [8, 13, 14]. In pollen-induced asthma, the results of SIT were equivocal until the past 5 years, but many recent studies found that SIT is at least as effective as in rhino-conjunctivitis (Figure 1) [10, 12].

* Clinique des Maladies Respiratoires, Centre Hospitalier Universitaire, 34059 Montpellier Cedex, France.
This paper was supported in part by a Grant of the INSERM (Paris), No. 86-2-15-5-E.

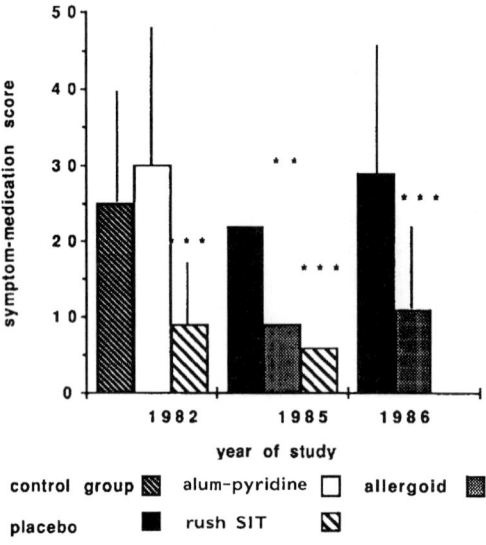

Figure 1. Efficacy of specific immunotherapy with different grass pollen extracts in the treatment of pollen-induced asthma. *p<0.01, **p<0.005. From [10, 12, 14].

The comparison between pharmacotherapy and SIT is missing for most pollen species. Using nasal challenges with orchard grass pollens, we compared the efficacy of terfenadine, a widely used nonsedative antihistamine and rush IT with a standardized orchard grass pollen extract in a double-blind, placebo-controlled study. We preferred to use pollen grains during the challenge procedure since this method is closer to natural pollen exposure, and testing patients with the same extract as that used for the treatment might introduce a bias into the study. It was observed that both treatments were significantly more effective than placebo, but SIT was significantly ($p<0.015$, Mann-Whitney U test) more effective than terfenadine (Figure 2). Moreover, SIT is both efficient in nasal and bronchial symptoms, whereas antihistamines only have a small effect in asthma.

Only few studies have been carried out with *Parietaria*, Betulaceae, and mountain cedar pollens [15]. In most cases, SIT resulted in a significant improvement of patients, though these trials should be confirmed. With other pollen species, data are lacking, and it is postulated that SIT is effective. But proper studies have to be done. In patients with multiple pollen sensitivities, SIT may be less effective [17].

House Dust Mites

Immunotherapy in house dust mite asthma is also effective. Bronchial challenge with mites extracts performed before and after SIT clearly shows the efficacy of the treatment [17, 18], but the relative importance of allergic factors and airways inflammation should be considered before starting SIT. The sustained allergic reaction in the bronchi of mite allergic asthmatics leads to a severe inflammation and bronchial hyperactivity. After a natural course of two or three decades, many patients present an irre-

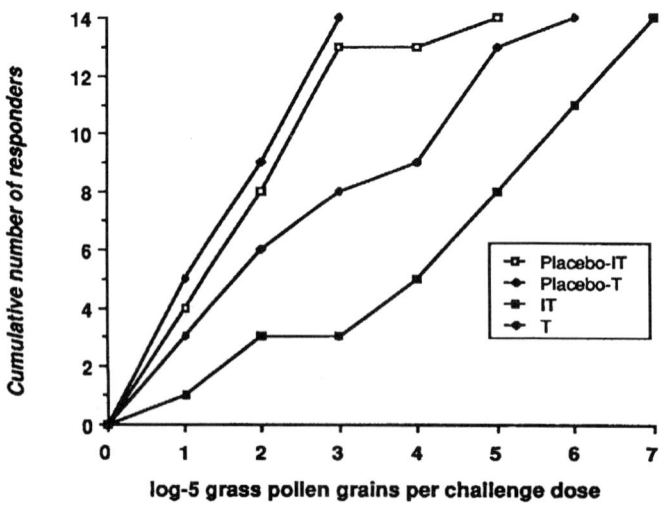

Figure 2. Results of nasal challenge with orchard grass pollen grains in patients receiving placebo (IT: immunotherapy group; T: terfenadine group) or active treatment (IT: immunotherapy group; T: terfenadine group). Placebo-IT/placebo: p = NS; placebo-IT/IT: p<0.001; placebo-T/T: p<0.01; IT/T: p<0.015. Statistical analysis by nonparametric tests.

versible airways obstruction and the response to SIT is usually poor. It was therefore observed that (1) children respond more favorably to mite SIT than adults, (2) patients with an irreversible airways obstruction are rarely improved by SIT, and (3) the more severe the asthma, the worse the improvement [19]. Moreover, although it may be postulated that the treatment of one of the components of asthma may improve the course of the disease, patients with multiple sensitivities or presenting both a mite sensitivity and nonallergic triggers (aspirin intolerance or chronic sinusitis) are not improved by mite SIT. In mite-rhinitis, SIT was only effective when the treatment was done with standardized extracts [20].

Animal Danders

Specific immunotherapy was proposed in animal dander allergy and results are not completely clear. Results of provocative challenges have found that allergen injections reduce the bronchial sensitivity to allergen, but symptoms were not always decreased in patients living with animals [21–23].

Molds

Only pilot studies have as yet been started with molds, and interesting results have been produced. Using standardized extracts of high quality, it was observed that SIT with either *Cladosporium* [24, 25], or *Alternaria* [Horst &

Bousquet, submitted] resulted in a decrease in skin test, nasal, and/or conjunctival sensitivities. Symptoms and medications were not decreased in studies with *Cladosporium* since most treated patients were sensitized to many mold species. On the other hand, in a recent study in patients only allergic to *Alternaria*, we found that, in the actively treated group, (1) symptoms and medications were significantly reduced (Figure 3), (2) the mean threshold dose inducing a positive nasal challenge was significantly increased, and (3) skin tests were decreased [Horst & Bousquet, submitted]. However, very few patients are only sensitized to a single mold species, and most commercially available extracts are unstandardized, so that it is not possible to extend these results to mold SIT done in clinical practice.

Other Extracts

Immunotherapy with house dust, *Candida albicans*, or bacterial vaccines was largely used in the past but it is no longer advisable. Some anecdotal data gave the impression that foods or occupational allergens might be used to treat patients, but these extracts should be restricted to controlled trials [2].

Side Effects

In October 1986, the Committee on Safety of Medicines of the United Kingdom published a paper stating that immunotherapy was a

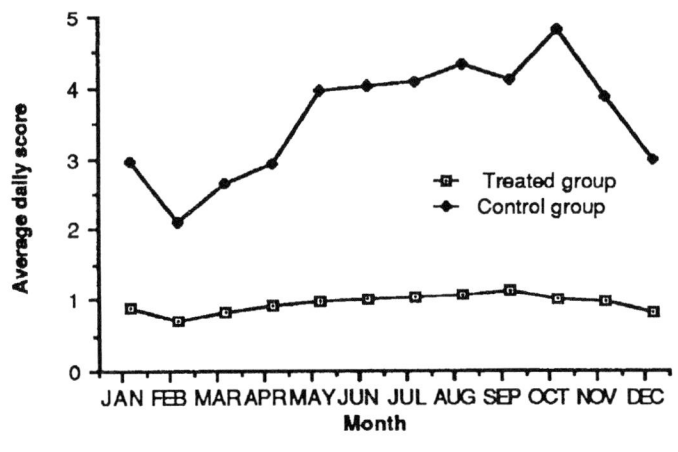

Figure 3. Average daily symptom-medication score for each month of the year. From Horst & Bousquet, submitted.

Table 1. Comparison between immunotherapy and the pharmacologic treatment of allergic diseases.

	Venom allergy	Pollen rhinitis mild	Pollen rhinitis severe	Pollen asthma	Mite asthma
Efficacy					
IT	high	high	usually good	high	none to high
drugs	none*	high	usually fair	high	fair to high
Side effects					
IT	possibly severe	possibly severe		possibly severe	possibly severe
drugs		none to mild		none to mild	none to severe
Duration					
IT	3–5 yr	3 yr–life span		3 yr–life span	3 yr–life span
drugs		life span		life span	life span
Cost of health care					
IT	expensive	expensive		expensive	expensive
drugs		lower cost		lower cost	may be expensive

* no preventive drugs, adrenaline may not be given early enough to cure anaphylaxis
IT = immunotherapy

dangerous treatment, should only be performed when full cardio-respiratory resuscitation equipment is available, and that the patient should be kept for 2 hours afterwards under the supervision of a physician [3]. The analysis of death certificates of recent fatal cases indicates clearly that (1) recent potent extracts are more dangerous than previous ones, and (2) patients presenting with allergic asthma are more prone to develop life-threatening systemic reactions [3, 26–28]. Systemic reactions occur frequently with rush SIT with either pollens [8, 10, 11], animal danders [21, 22], mites [20, 27], or molds [24, 25]. It is possible that rush SIT protocols expose patients to a higher incidence of systemic reactions [29], but this may be related to the use of standardized extracts. Polymerized high molecular weight extracts were shown to give less systemic side effects and may be of great value in the future [12, 20].

Since life-threatening reactions are not rare with high-quality extracts, before any injection, patients should be monitored carefully and the treatment delayed if the patient presents any symptom of asthma or infection. Injections should only be given under the close supervision of a trained physician, in settings in which anaphylactic reactions can be immediately corrected. The patient should be followed for up to at least 30 minutes after the shot. Systemic reactions occurring after allergen injection should be regarded as possibly serious and adrenaline (and oxygen therapy) should be immediately administered if necessary [2].

Indications

Double-blind, controlled studies have therefore confirmed the efficacy of SIT but pharmacologic treatment is also available for the treatment of allergic diseases. This was improved in recent years since it is more effective and side effects have been significantly decreased, so that before starting SIT the relative efficacy, risk, duration, and cost of immunologic and pharmacologic treatments should be carefully compared (Table 1).

For indications other than venoms, SIT should only be started when serious attempts at allergen avoidance have been made. Before starting immunotherapy, each patient should be carefully informed of the risks, duration, and effectiveness of this treatment; patient cooperation and compliance to the treatment are absolutely required before starting it. The specific indications have been extensively studied. It is commonly accepted that immunotherapy is indicated in severe pollinosis, especially when asthma complicates rhinoconjunctivitis, in mite allergy (though severe asthmatic patients should be excluded due to possible untoward side reactions) and in life-threatening reactions to hymenoptera venoms. This form of treatment may be started in some selected cases of animal dander allergy but allergen avoidance is favored. Mold extracts might be used in the future, but, at present, high-quality extracts are merely unavailable in practice.

Conclusions

Specific immunotherapy may be used in several situations, but its value depends on the indication, the allergen extract, the protocol, and the dose. This latter point is of great importance since it was observed that the Rinkel regimen [31] was not better than placebo. However, very high doses of standardized allergen extracts lead to systemic reactions, so that an "optimal" dose combining efficacy and safety has to be defined for all allergen extracts.

References

1. Lichtenstein, L. M. 1978. An evaluation of the role of immunotherapy in asthma. Am. Rev. Respir. Dis. 117: 191–197.
2. Malling, H. J. et al. 1988. Specific immunotherapy. Position paper of the European Academy of Allergy and Clinical Immunology. Allergy 6 (Suppl.): 1–33.
3. Committee on Safety of Medicine. 1986. Desensitizing vaccines. Br. Med. J. 193: 948.
4. Bousquet, J., U. R. Müller, S. Dreborg, R. Jarish, H. J. Malling, H. Mosbech et al. 1987. Immunotherapy with hymenoptera venoms. Allergy 42: 707–720.
5. Golden, D. B. K., A. Kagey Sobotka, K. A. Kwiterovich, M. D. Valentine, and L. M. Lichtenstein. 1988. Immunologic response to sequential stings after stopping venom immunotherapy in adults. J. Allergy Clin. Immunol. 81: 201.
6. Bousquet, J., D. Knani, G. Velasquez, J. L. Ménardo, L. Guilloux, and F. B. Michel. 1989. Follow-up of 200 hymenoptera venom allergic patients over 3 years. J. Allergy Clin. Immunol., in press.
7. Norman, P. S. 1981. Immunotherapy. Prog. Allergy 32: 318–355.
8. Osterballe, O. 1982. Nasal and skin sensitivity during immunotherapy with two major allergens 19, 25, and partially purified pollen extract of timothy grass. Allergy 37: 169–177.
9. Juniper, E. F., J. O'Connor, R. S. Roberts, S. Evans, F. E. Hargreave, and J. Dolovich. 1986. Polyethylene glycol-modified ragweed extract: Comparison of two treatment regimens. J. Allergy Clin. Immunol. 78: 851–856.
10. Bousquet, J., B. Guérin, A. Dotte, H. Dhivert, F. Djoukhadar, and F. B. Michel. 1985. Comparison between rush immunotherapy with a standardized allergen and an alum adjuved pyridine extracted material in grass pollen allergy. Clin. Allergy 15: 179–194.
11. Bousquet, J., A. Hejjaoui, W. Skassa-Brociek, B. Guérin, H. Maasch, H. Dhivert, and F. B. Michel. 1987. Double-blind placebo controlled immunotherapy with mixed grass pollen allergoids. I. Rush immunotherapy with allergoids and standardized orchard grass pollen. J. Allergy Clin. Immunol. 80: 591–598.
12. Bousquet, J., H. Maasch, A. Hejjaoui et al. 1988. Double-blind placebo controlled immunotherapy with mixed grass pollen allergoids. III. Comparison with an unfractionated allergoid, a fractionated allergoid and a standardized orchard grass pollen extract in rhinitis, conjunctivitis and asthma. J. Allergy Clin. Immunol., in press.
13. Bousquet, J. B. Martinot, H. J. Maasch et al. 1988. Double-blind placebo controlled immunotherapy with mixed grass pollen allergoids. II. Comparison between parameters assessing the efficacy of immunotherapy. J. Allergy Clin. Immunol., in press.
14. Bousquet, J., E. Franck, M. Soussana, R. Wahl, H. Maasch, and F. B. Michel. 1987. Comparison of parameters assessing the efficacy of immunotherapy with allergoid in grass pollenosis. Int. Archs. Allergy Appl. Immun. 77: 542–545.
15. Pence, H. L., D. Q. Mitchell, R. L. Greely, B. R. Pudegraff, and H. A. Selfridge. 1976. Immunotherapy for mountain cedar immunotherapy. A double blind controlled study. J. Allergy Clin. Immunol. 58: 39–50.
16. Chanal, I., J. Bousquet, B. Lebel, and F. B. Michel. 1988. Efficacy of rush immunotherapy with grass or multiple pollen species assessed by nasal challenge. J. Allergy Clin. Immunol. 88: 261.
17. Bousquet, J., P. Calcayrac, B. Guérin et al. 1985. Immunotherapy with a standardized *Dermatophagoides pteronyssinus* extract. I. In vivo and in vitro parameters after a short course of treatment. J. Allergy Clin. Immunol. 76: 734–744.
18. Warner, J. O., J. F. Price, J. F. Soothill et al. 1978. Controlled trial of hyposensitization to *Dermatophagoides pteronyssinus* in children with asthma. Lancet II: 912–916.
19. Bousquet, J., A. Hejjaoui, A. M. Clauzel et al. 1989. Specific immunotherapy with a standardized *Dermatophagoides pteronyssinus* extract. II Prediction of efficacy of immunotherapy. J. Allergy Clin. Immunol., in press.
20. Ewan, P., M. M. Alexander, C. Snape, P. W. Ind, B. Agrell, and S. Dreborg. 1988. Effective hyposensitization in allergic rhinitis using a potent partially purified extract of house dust mite. Clin. Allergy 18: 501–508.

21. Sundin, B. G. Lilja, V. Graff-Lonnevig et al. 1986. Immunotherapy with partially purified and standardized animal dander extracts. I. Clinical results from a double-blind study on patients with animal dander asthma. J. Allergy Clin. Immunol. 77: 478–487.

22. Ohman, J. L., S. R. Findlay, and K. M. Leitermann. 1984. Immunotherapy in cat-induced asthma. Double-blind trial with evaluation of in vivo and in vitro responses. J. Allergy Clin. Immunol. 74: 230–239.

23. Valovirta, E., M. Viander, A. Koivikko, T. Vanto, and L. Ingeman 1986. Immunotherapy in allergy to dog. Immunologic and clinical findings of a double-blind study. Allergy 57: 173–179.

24. Dreborg, S., B. Agrell, T. Foucard, N. I. M. Kjellman, A. Koivikko, and S. Nilsson. 1986. A double-blind, multicenter immunotherapy trial in children using a purified and standardized *Cladosporium herbarum* preparation. I. Clinical results. Allergy 41: 131–140.

25. Malling, H. J., S. Dreborg, and B. Weeke. 1986. Diagnosis and immunotherapy of mould allergy. V. Clinical efficacy and side effects of immunotherapy with *Cladosporium herbarum*. Allergy 41: 507–519.

26. Lockey, R. F., L. M. Benedict, P. C. Turkeltaub, and S. C. Bukantz. 1987. Fatalities from immunotherapy (IT) and skin testing. J. Allergy Clin. Immunol. 79: 660–677.

27. Norman, P. S. 1987. Fatal misadventures. J. Allergy Clin. Immunol. 79: 572–573.

28. Bousquet, J., A. Hejjaoui, H. Dhivert, A. M. Clauzel, and F. B. Michel. 1989. Specific immunotherapy with a standardized *Dermatophagoides pteronyssinus* extract. III. Systemic reactions during the rush protocol in patients suffering from asthma. J. Allergy Clin. Immunol., in press.

29. Vervloet, D., E. Khairallal, A. Arnaud, and J. Charpin. 1980. A prospective national study of the safety of immunotherapy. Clin. Allergy 10: 59–64.

30. Patterson, R., and I. M. Suszko. 1974. Polymerized ragweed antigen E: III. Differences in immune response to three molecular weight ranges of monomer and plymer. J. Immunol. 112: 1855–1860.

31. Van Metre, T. E., N. F. Adkinson Jr., F. J. Amodio et al., 198 al., 1980. A comparative study of the effectiveness of the Rinkel method and the current standard method of immunotherapy for ragweed pollen hay fever. J. Allergy Clin. Immunol. 66: 500–513.

Follow Up of Patients on Immunotherapy

*Ulrich R. Müller**

Primary goals of the follow-up of patients on IT are to monitor for efficacy and for safety of the treatment. National and European guidelines for safety monitoring are available. The most reliable parameters for efficacy monitoring are provocation tests and—in controlled trials—symptom medication scores. Other in vitro or in vivo tests have to be evaluated in direct relation to treatment success or failure as indicated by these two parameters.

The efficacy of immunotherapy for the treatment of IgE-mediated allergic disease is well documented in controlled prospective trials, especially for allergic rhinitis due to pollen and for systemic allergic reactions following *Hymenoptera* stings [1, 2, 3]. For optimal success of immunotherapy, a treatment course of at least three years is considered necessary. A large proportion of patients, however, does not complete these recommended three years of immunotherapy, most often because of an inadequate follow-up of the patient. Insufficient initial information about immunotherapy, which should be both oral and written [2], is another cause for dropouts, while circumstances like pregnancy, intercurrent disease, etc., account for only a minority of these failures.

Goals of the Follow-up

The primary goals of a correct follow-up of a patient on immunotherapy are (1) to judge its efficacy (*efficacy monitoring*) and as a consequence to decide about modifications of this treatment and finally also about its duration; (2) to optimize its safety (*safety monitoring*). This includes a questionnaire completed by the treating physician before each injection; correct dosage, application, and storage of extracts; observation of the patient for at least 30 minutes after each injection in the presence of the treating physician; and correct emergency treatment in case of side effects. Many national guidelines on safety measures are available.

The recently published position paper of the European Academy of Allergy and Clinical Immunology provides European directions [2]. It is preferable that the follow-up lie in the hands of a trained allergist. Where this is not possible, the treatment by the general practitioner should be supervised by an allergist during at least yearly evaluations.

Efficacy Monitoring

This can be done by (1) clinical observation of the patient, (2) clinical tests, and (3) laboratory tests.

Clinical Observation

The clinical observation includes the evaluation of the patient by the patient and by the physician: Does the patient feel better than during the last pollen season or before starting immunotherapy in the case of perennial allergies? Has the patient's condition improved according to clinical examination? What about days off work, visits to emergency stations, hospitalisations for his asthma? Of course, both patient self-evaluation and the physician's evaluation may be subject to considerable bias. Results of incidental reexposure are valuable especially in *Hymenoptera* sting allergy, when field stings by the culprit insect occur, more rarely also in inhalatory allergies, e.g., due to animal dander or to occupational allergens.

Symptom medication scores are very valuable parameters in clinical trials [2], where groups of patients on different treatments are compared. In the individual patient this method is laborious and of limited value: Comparison to pretreatment symptoms is questionable because of the year-to-year and day-to-day variation of the allergen concentration in the air. Relevant control groups are usually not available.

* Medical Division, Zieglerspital, Bern, Switzerland.

Clinical Tests

These comprise nonspecific methods like pulmonary function tests including daily peak flow measurements and estimation of nonspecific reactivity to histamine, metacholine or cold air in bronchial asthma. Repeated single measurements of pulmonary function may not be very reliable because of the considerable spontaneous variation during disease. Regarding nonspecific bronchial hyperreactivity, some authors find a decrease during immunotherapy, others an increase [2].

Specific clinical tests comprise skin tests and provocation tests. Skin test reactivity initially increases during immunotherapy [3], but with a prolonged course of effective treatment decreases below pretreatment values as a rule. In order to get comparable results over time, parallel-line skin test assay should be used [4]. This test is laborious but rather reliable regarding prediction of efficacy. The late-phase skin reaction to high allergen doses given intracutaneously is strongly suppressed during successful ragweed immunotherapy [5].

Allergen provocation tests are probably the most reliable parameter for efficacy monitoring, at least when performed in the shock organ [2]. Such tests should be done in all controlled clinical trials on immunotherapy. Provocation tests, especially bronchial provocation tests, are, however, not without risk and are therefore rejected by many authors for routine follow-up of patients on immunotherapy. In bronchial provocation tests, the allergen dose used to induce a significant drop in FEV_1 or peak flow usually increases during successful IT [6]. The sting challenge is thought to be the gold standard to evaluate efficacy of venom immunotherapy in *Hymenoptera* sting allergy [7]. If it is performed in patients on venom immunotherapy under controlled clinical conditions with an intravenous infusion running and intensive care facilities available, it bares minimal risk for the patient.

Table 1 shows results from 123 patients challenged during venom immunotherapy. They seem considerably more favorable in yellow jacket than in honey bee venom-treated patients. This difference probably results from the fact that a sting challenge is less reliable when performed with vespids. Vespids in contrast to bees use their sting apparatus daily in order to kill prey animals and also may squirt their venom without actually stinging when threatened. Thus, the amount of venom delivered by a vespid sting is less constant [8].

In vitro Tests

These include estimation of allergen-specific antibodies in serum or secretions and cellular tests such as leucocyte histamine release (LHR), basophile degranulation test (BDT), and the platelet activation test (PAT). Commercial kits are now available for LHR and BDT. According to several studies, the cellular sensitivity measured by these tests decreased during immunotherapy [9, 10, 11]. Thus far, however, convincing data showing correlation of these changes to clinical efficacy are largely lacking.

Serum antibodies have been studied more thoroughly in this respect. Allergen-specific IgE, after an initial rise, usually decrease over prolonged immunotherapy [3]. Low or undetectable serum IgE antibodies to *Hymenoptera* venoms have been proposed as a criterion for discontinuation of venom immunotherapy [8, 12]. Others have tried to correlate an initial IgE increase to particular pollen allergens to treatment success [2]. We have been unable to predict efficacy of bee venom immunotherapy from changes in venom-specific IgE antibodies (Figure 1). No significant differences of venom-specific IgE obtained before treatment and before challenge could be observed between reactors and nonreactors to the challenge.

Allergen-specific IgE increase during immunotherapy with potent allergen extracts [2, 3] and remain elevated throughout the treatment. A protective effect of passive immunization with bee keeper gammaglobulins has been demonstrated in several studies [8, 13]. However, in the individual patient, even on bee

Table 1. Sting challenge in 126 patients on venom immunotherapy.

Immunotherapy with	No. of patients	Reaction to sting challenge (%) Local only	Systemic
Honey bee venom	98	79 (79)	21 (21)
Vespula (sp) venom	28	27 (96)	1 (4)

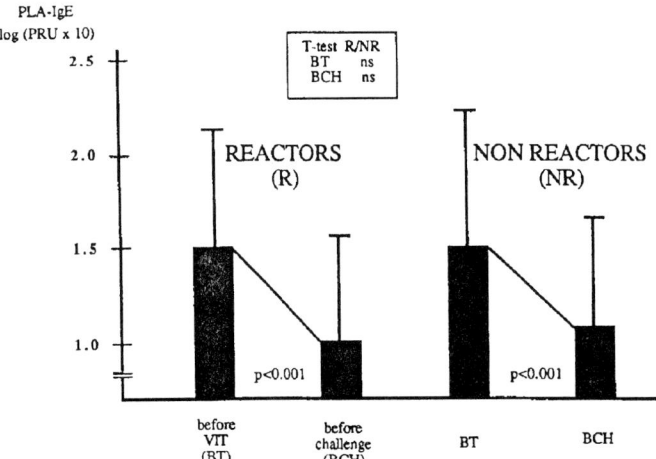

Figure 1. PLA-IgE before treatment and before challenge in 67 bee venom allergic patients on venom immunotherapy.

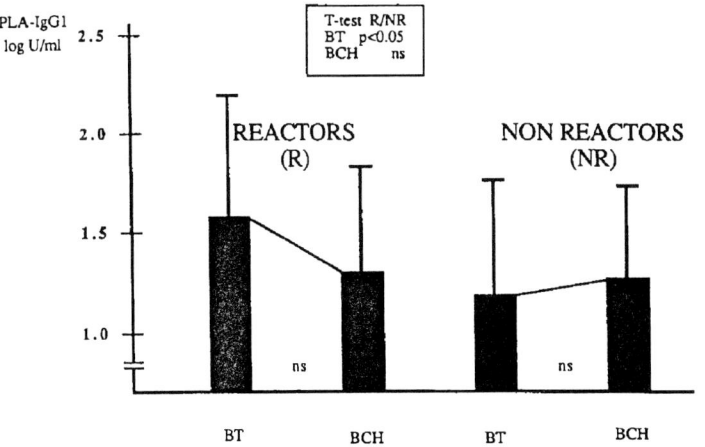

Figure 2. PLA-IgG1 before treatment and before challenge in 67 bee venom allergic patients on venom immunotherapy.

venom immunotherapy, specific serum IgG antibodies do not predict protection reliably [8].

Aalberse [14] has observed an increase of bee venom-specific IgG1 antibodies during the initial phase of bee keeping and of bee venom immunotherapy, while in long-standing bee keepers and in patients on protracted bee venom immunotherapy the IgG4 response was predominant. Unfortunately, neither of these IgG subclass antibodies is predictive of treatment success in the individual patient, when studied in relation to the results of a sting challenge (Figures 2, 3). In the total group of patients, a high IgG4 response is even correlated to an unfavorable clinical result. Similar results regarding allergen-specific IgG4 antibodies

have been reported for pollen allergies [2].

Estimation of allergen specific IgG, IgA, and IgE antibodies in nasal secretions during immunotherapy for allergic rhinitis is not correlated to treatment success either [2].

Any change of allergen-specific antibody in serum or secretions observed during immunotherapy may thus indicate immunostimulation induced by this treatment but not protection.

Conclusions

The most valuable parameters for efficacy monitoring during immunotherapy are provocation tests, especially the sting challenge, and symptom medication scores, the latter, of

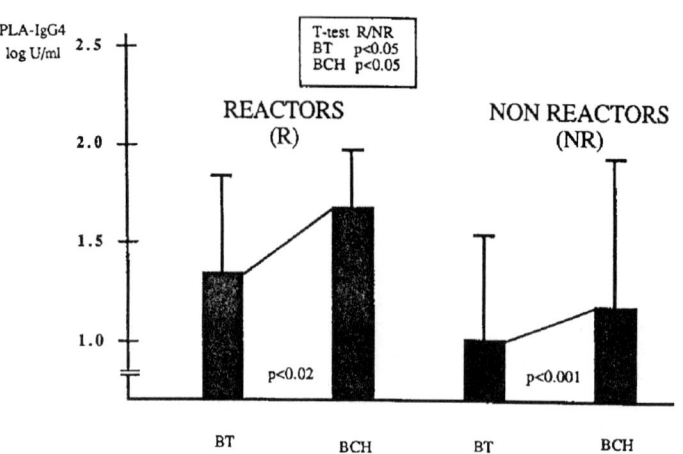

Figure 3. PLA-IgG$_4$ before treatment and before challenge in 67 bee venom allergic patients on venom immunotherapy.

course, only in clinical trials where adequate control groups are available.

The predictive value of any other clinical or in vitro test must be judged in direct relation to treatment success or failure, as indicated by provocation tests or—in controlled trials—by symptom medication scores. Under these circumstances no other parameter so far has been documented as a reliable predictor for the efficacy of immunotherapy. Some, like LHR, PAT, and modifications of skin test procedures, have not been evaluated sufficiently to this day.

In clinical practice, efficacy monitoring will have to rely mainly on clinical observation and skin testing. Where available, provocation tests are recommended. Serum antibody estimations may have some significance as indicators that the extract used is immunologically active.

References

1. Aas, K. 1982. Adequate clinical trials of immunotherapy. Allergy 37: 1–14.
2. Immunotherapy Subcommittee, European Academy of Allergology and Clinical Immunology. 1988. Immunotherapy, position paper. H. J. Malling (ed.). Allergy 43 (Suppl. 6): 1–33.
3. Müller, U. 1983. Immuntherapie allergischer Krankheiten: Gegenwart und Zukunft. Schweiz. med. Wschr. 113: 1982–1988.
4. Dreborg, S. 1987. The skin prick test. Linköping University. Medical Dissertation. Linköping.
5. Pienkowski, M. M., P. S. Norman, and L. M. Lichtenstein. 1985. Suppression of late-phase skin reactions by immunotherapy with ragweed extract. J. Allergy Clin. Immunol. 76: 729–734.
6. Sundin, B., G. Lilja, V. Graff-Lonnevig, G. Hedlin, H. Heilborn, K. Norrelind, K.-O. Pegelow, and H. Lowenstein. 1986. Immunotherapy with partially purified and standardized animal dander extracts. 77: 478–487.
7. Urbanek, R., Karitzky, and J. Forster. 1978. Die Hyposensibilisierungsbehandlung mit reinem Bienengift. Dtsch. med. Wschr. 103: 1656–1660.
8. Müller, U. R. 1988. Insektenstichallergie. Klinik, Diagnostik und Therapie. Gustav Fischer Verlag: Stuttgart.
9. Nüsslein, H. G., and H. W. Baenkler. 1985. Spontaneous loss of hypersensitivity in patients allergic to bee or wasp stings. Ann. Allergy 54: 516–520.
10. Mumcuoglu, Y., and F. Wortmann. 1980. Modified basophil degranulation test in diagnosis of bee and wasp sting allergies. Allergy 35: 335–340.
11. Tsicopoulos, A., A. B. Tonnel, B. Wallaert, M. Joseph, J. C. Ameisen et al. 1988. Decrease of IgE-dependent platelet activation in *Hymenoptera* hypersensitivity after specific rush desensitization. Clin. exp. Immunol. 71: 433–438.
12. Randolph, C. C., and R. E. Reisman 1986. Evaluation of decline in serum venom-specific IgE as a criterion for stopping venom immunotherapy. J. Allergy Clin. Immunol. 77: 823–827.
13. Lessof, M. H., A. K. Sobotka, and L. M. Lichtenstein. 1977. Effects of passive antibody in bee venom anaphylaxis. John Hopk. Med. J. 142: 1–7.
14. Aalberse, R. C., R. van der Gaag, and J. Leeuwen. 1983. Serologic aspects of IgG4 antibodies. I. Prolonged immunization results in an IgG4-restricted response. J. Immunol. 130: 722–726.

Reduction of Side Effects of Specific Immunotherapy

R. Jarisch*, M. Götz**, R. Sidl*, A. Stable*, J. Zajc*, A. Wechsler-Fördös*

In an initial study (Study I), 884 patients with allergic rhinitis, bronchial asthma, and insect venom allergy undergoing specific immunotherapy (ALK) were investigated. A total of 14,141 injections were administered. At least 30 minutes prior to injection, one tablet of 6 mg chlorpheniraminmaleat (Polaramin®), later on astemizol (Hismanal® or terfenadine (Triludan®) was given. The number of systemic reactions was 0.5%, thus markedly below comparable studies [2, 3]. This was statistically significant (p<0.001–0.05) according to local systemic reactions or pollen and house dust-mite allergens. Despite a diminished number of side effects, all possible reactions were retained. Thus, the so-called early warning symptoms were not suppressed.

A follow-up study (Study II), done with 3,857 injections, investigated the effect of reduction of maximal dosage. In comparison to Study I a reduction of serious systemic side effects (29/14,141) to 0/3,857) was observed. This difference is statistically significant (p<0.01). The number of mild systemic reactions remained equal. Thus, a shift of serious systemic side effects toward mild reactions had occurred, and mild reactions were shifted to local or absent side effects. Study III demonstrates a further reduction of local and systemic side effects if the starting dose was reduced (1/10 dilution) from 12% to 4%. Antihistamine premedication prior to injection, commencement of immunotherapy in 1/10 dilution (reduction of mild systemic reactions), reduction of maximal dosage to 50,000 SQ-U/ml (reduction of severe systemic reactions) are thus recommended.

A change of efficacy of specific immunotherapy has not been observed to date. The present success rate is 82% (reduction of symptoms between 70% and 100%).

To date specific immunotherapy of allergic diseases is the only treatment acting on the presumably defective immune system. However, reports of severe systemic side effects of specific immunotherapy cause anxiety in numerous physicians and limit the use of this treatment.

We demonstrated the safety of specific immunotherapy in a large number of patients by premedication with antihistamines. An additional goal of this study was the question whether an increased risk of side effects to certain allergens exist (Table 1) and whether an increase of side effects attributable to certain dosages. This was to be the basis for newly established dosage guidelines leading to further reduction of side effects.

Material and Methods

The indication for specific immunotherapy was based on a clear-cut history frequently accompanied by a complaint diary, a positive skin-prick testing, and positive RAST. Patients were requested to take one tablet of 6 mg chlorpheniraminmaleat (Polaramin®) 30 minutes at the latest prior to injection; later on astemizol or terfenadine were used in the morning and/or a half hour prior to injection. Regular usage was monitored continuously. Dosages followed guidelines of ALK, with adjustment to individual requirements of patients. In dubious cases no injection or low-dose treatment was carried out. Vaccines were from ALK and SQ preparations were used whenever available; only depot preparations were used.

A total of more than 25,000 injections administered on our premises were analyzed. Injections performed outside were not included. When problems related to immunotherapy were observed, the GP was not involved and such patients were kept under our own constant surveillance. The study also included reactions occurring after hours at home, based on reports by patients.

* Dermatolog.-pediatric Allergy Clinic, Franz Jonaspl. 8, A-1210 Vienna, Austria.
** University Children's Hospital, Währingergürtel, A-1090 Vienna, Austria.

Erythema, swelling, severe swelling, local urticaria, and itching were considered as local side effects. Mild systemic reactions were based on the following symptoms: conjunctivitis, sneezing, rhinitis, swelling of lips and throat, generalized itch, urticaria, vascular problems without lowering of blood pressure. Serious systemic reactions were based on the following symptoms: joint and muscle pain, generalized diffuse erythema, serious shortness of breath, tachycardia.

In a further study (Study II), an assessment of the reduction of systemic side effects, predicted on the basis of the initial study, by limitation of the maximal dosage to 50,000 SQ-U/ml could actually be achieved. For this purpose, 3,857 injections in patients with antihistamine premedication were analyzed; reduction of immunotherapy dosage to 50,000 SQ-U/ml was done in addition in all cases.

Study III investigated the advantage of the use of a 1/10 dilution of vial I.

Results

The relative potency of allergens eliciting marked systemic reactions is shown in Table 1. Results demonstrate a tenfold higher potency of bee venom compared to pollen.

The results of Study I are given in Tables 2 and 3, demonstrating a reduction of local and systemic side effects between 32% and 48%. All results are statistically significant between $p<0.01$ and $p<0.05$.

The results of Study II are given in Table 4. Although 8 serious systemic reactions were expected, none occurred. This difference is statistically significant. The incidence of mild systemic reactions between Study I and Study II was not different. This means that a shift from serious systemic reactions to mild systemic reactions and from mild systemic reactions to no reactions took place.

Results of Study III are given in Table 5. The data show a reduction of all kinds of side effects from 12% to 4%. We found an increase of mild systemic reactions, however, especially when the first injection of strength 0 was given. Evaluation of symptoms showed that most of the reported symptoms could not be seen objectively (like itch in the eyes and the nose, etc.). We therefore believe that this increase in mild systemic reactions is rather related to psychological reasons than to clear-cut side effects.

Table 1. Frequency of allergens eliciting marked systemic reactions.

1. Bee venom	1%
2. Wasp venom	0.7%
3. Mites	0.63%
4. Alternaria	0.47%
5. Pollen	0.13%

Table 2. Immunotherapy with pollen extracts (ALK). Comparison of side effects with and without antihistamine premedication.

	Litvin et al. (1986) without antihist.	Jarisch et al. (1988) with antihist.
Number of injections	4242	9853
Systemic side effects	29	42 (p<0.05)

Table 3. Immunotherapy with house dust mite (ALK). Comparison of side effects with and without antihistamine premedication.

	Persson (1986) without antihist.	Jarisch et al. (1988) with antihist.
Number of injections	1146	2226
Local side effects	276	362 (p<0.001)
Systemic side effects	20	16 (p<0.01)

Table 4. Mild and systemic side effects in patients with immunotherapy. Study I: Antihistamine premedication, dosage as recommended = maximal dosage of 100,000 SQ-U/ml. Study II: Antihistamine premedication, maximal dosage 50,000 SQ-U/ml.

	Mild systemic reactions	Serious systemic reactions
Study I (n=14,141)	48 (0.34%)*	29 (0.2%)**
Study II (n=3,857)	17 (0.44%)*	0 **

* not significant
** p<0.01

Table 5. Comparison of frequency of side effects at start of immunotherapy. Group A: commencement with strength 0+1 (n=2322); Group B: commencement with strength I (n=5567).

	Pollen allergens		Mite allergens		Total pollen, mite and insect venom allergens	
Number of injections	A	B	A	B	A	B
	n=804	n=2142	n=325	n=551	n=1193	n=2874
Side effects	in %		in %		in %	
Erythema	0.8	11	0	10	0.5	10
Swelling	0.1	1	0	0.4	0.1	0.7
Serious swelling	0.1	0.1	0	0	0.1	0.1
Urticaria, local itch	0	0.1	0.3	0.4	0.1	0.2
Mild systemic side effects	3.1	0.7	2.2	0.7	2.8	0.7
Serious side effects	0	0.1	0	0.4	0	0.1
Total	4.1	12.0	2.5	11.9	3.6	11.8

Discussion

Publication of deaths in immunotherapy and the large number of unpublished serious systemic reactions require assessment of treatment leading to clear-cut reduction of side effects.

Since allergic patients are injected with an allergen against which they are intolerant, each injection could in fact lead to hypersensitivity. It is all the most astonishing that 47% of our patients had no side effects during the whole course of a two-year immunotherapy, and that 12,314 out of 14,141 injections were tolerated without complaints (Study I). This has to be seen in the context that all of our patients received antihistamine premedication.

The number of systemic side effects found in Study I of 0.5% on average (mild and serious reactions) from all allergens is clearly below figures given in the literature (Litvin: 0.7%; Persson: 1.7%). Study I shows in comparison to other international assessments with a similar design [2, 3] (though without antihistamine premedication) that the side effects can be statistically significantly lowered (p<0.001, 0.01, and 0.05).

The primary goal of Study was thus the demonstration of possible reduction of side effects. The extent of the reduction is considerable and varies according to local or systemic reactions as well as according to allergens (grass pollen or house dust mite) between 32% and 58%.

Two further consequences of Study I were limitation of maximal dosage to 50,000 SQ-U/ml (Study II) and initiation of immunotherapy with a 1/10 dilution step (Study III).

Thus, reduction of the maximal dosage to 50,000 SQ-U/ml was subsequently done in Study II. We analyzed close to 4000 injections and were gratified to show a marked reduction of severe systemic side effects, which could not be demonstrated in a single case in 3857 injections! We therefore assume that a shift of severe systemic side effects toward mild side effects and from mild to local or no side effects was achieved. Statistical analysis verified the prognosticated reduction as actually achievable (p<0.01; Fischer's exact test).

As can be seen in Table 5, an impressive reduction of side effects from 12% to 4% or less was seen following the introduction of a predilution 1/10 of vial I. Serious systemic side effects in the beginning were not seen at all. Thus, antihistamine premedication and introduction of an extra dilution strength does not lead to camouflaging of the warning symptoms of an anaphylactic reaction. All results demonstrated that possible side effects are still to be seen—however, in a greatly reduced number. The effect that presently no serious systemic side effects were observed does not exclude the necessity of the awareness of this problem.

In conclusion, we are convinced that in general immunotherapy in the hands of an experienced unit is a safe procedure. As has been shown by reduction of high dosages, through introduction of premedication and an additional starter dilution, possible risks of side effects of immunotherapy can be eliminated. It seems reasonable to expect the possibility of less successful treatment of a very small number of patients in view of an overall decrease of side effects of immunotherapy.

References

1. Jarisch, R., M. Götz, R. Sidl, A. Stabel, J. Zajc, and A. Wechsler-Fördös. 1988. Reduction of side effects of specific immunotherapy by premedication with antihistamines and reduction of maximal dosage to 50,000 SQ-U/ml. In: Regulatory control and standardization of allergenic extracts. Int. Paul Ehrlich Seminar, Stuttgart 82. New York: Fischer Verlag, pp. 163–175.

2. Litvin, E., Rosendahl, and A. E. Lassen. 1985. Hyposensitization with Alutard-SQ in atopic children. A retrospective evaluation after three years of experience (abstract). Annual Meeting of the European Academy of Allergology and Clinical Immunology, Stockholm, June 2–5, p. 166.

3. Persson, G. 1986. Immunotherapy with house dust mite. Personal communication.

Changes in Skin and Mucosa Sensitivity Correlated with Specific IgE- and IgG-Subclass Antibodies in Hyposensitized Patients

R. Urbanek and M. Collet*

Since the beginning of the century, immunotherapy has increasingly been used in the management of grass pollen allergy. The efficacy of subcutaneous administration of grass pollen extracts has repeatedly been demonstrated in controlled double-blind studies [4, 5, 6, 8]. Although many clinicians are convinced of the efficacy of such treatment, objective parameters with predictive value are lacking.

As a model a perennial hyposensitization treatment over 2 years was performed in 18 pollen-allergic patients and controlled with standardized in vivo and in vitro procedures. The aim of the study was to find out which diagnostic or follow-up criterium is of the highest predictive value and enables us to monitor a successful allergen immunotherapy.

Patients and Methods

Eighteen children and young adults (14 children aged 7–14 years, 4 adults aged 20–30 years) with a positive history of seasonal rhinoconjunctivitis were admitted into the study. The selection for therapy was provided by allergen titration in skin-prick test, conjunctival provocation test, and by the estimation of specific IgE, IgG, and IgG-subclass (IgG_1, IgG_4) antibodies. An identical standardized and purified grass pollen extract (Scherax, ALK, Denmark) was used. All patients were investigated before the therapy and in five prospective intervals during the next 2 years. The study was carried out between Autumn 1985 and October 1987. Diary cards were handed out for the recording of symptoms and medication intake during the season. Additionally, standardized interviews for the assessment of subjective improvement were performed by a non-involved medical person.

In vivo Tests

In vivo testing was performed employing a lyophylized standardized grass pollen extract graded according to the Scandinavian Allergic Association from 0.01–10.0 HEP. Reference solutions were histamine (1 mg/ml) for skin-prick test and 0.9% NaCl solution for conjunctival provocation test. Skin-prick tests were performed in duplicates, and the mean of the maximal weal diameter for each allergen concentration was expressed as an index in relation to the weal diameter of histamine.

Conjunctival provocation test was performed by administering a drop of 0.9% NaCl in the conjunctival sack of the left eye. The lowest concentration of the allergen solution (0.035 HEP) was applied in the conjunctival sack of the right eye, and if no reaction occurred within 10 minutes, the next concentration of the test solution was applied in the left eye. Conjunctival provocation test was regarded as positive if conjunctival congestion and itching of the exposed eye occurred. The highest used dose was 10.0 HEP [3].

In vitro Tests

Specific IgE antibodies were analyzed using the Radio-Allergo-Sorbent-Test (RAST) as described elsewhere [1]. An Enzyme-Linked-Immuno-Sorbent-Test (ELISA) was employed [7] to measure specific IgG and IgG-subclass antibodies.

Symptom and Medication Records

Patients or their parents were instructed to judge daily symptoms according to an identical pattern (0–3 points/day) and to record

---

*   Universitäts-Kinderklinik, Mathildenstraße 1, D-7800 Freiburg, Federal Republic of Germany.

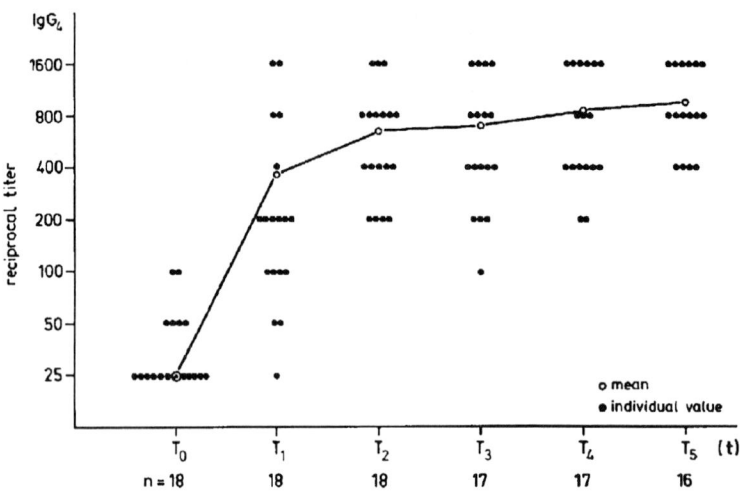

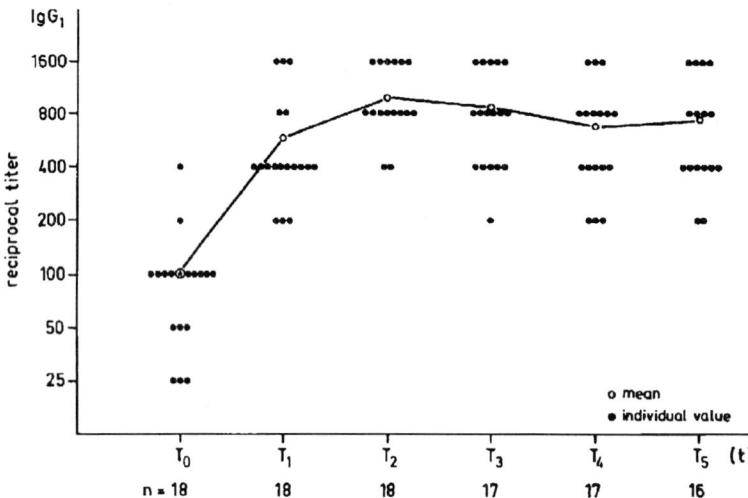

Figures 1 and 2. Specific IgG1 and IgG4 antibodies to grass pollen in hyposensitized patients. T_0 = before therapy, T_{1-5} = during therapy. There is a significant increase of both antibodies in all treated patients with no correlation to subjective assessment of therapeutic efficacy.

them in the dairy card. They were also asked to record daily medication intake.

At the end of the treatment, the patient's assessment of the effect was recorded in a standardized interview.

Statistics

Student t-test was employed to analyze skin-prick test and IgE/IgG antibodies. Wilcoxon test was used to calculate conjunctival provocation test differences.

Results

All but two patients tolerated the standardized hyposensitization treatment well. However, the maintenance dose of 10 HEP was achieved in all persons pre-seasonally before the second control investigation.

In vivo Tests

In all individuals, a reduction of cutaneous sensitivity already in the pre-seasonal period reached a statistical significance ($p \leq 0.001$). The most pronounced changes in the weal diameter offered the higher allergen-extract concentration of 1.0 HEP, 10.0 HEP, respectively. During the maintenance therapy, reduced skin sensitivity persisted. However, the further decrease in cutaneous sensitivity or a complete disappearance was not achieved in any single patient.

According to the skin-test results, also the conjunctival sensitivity decreased. The decrease was slightly delayed and achieved the maximum after 1 year of treatment. During the maintenance therapy there were no further significant changes. As in the skin test, also in the eye the once decreased sensitivity persisted but never disappeared. On the average, a reduction of one log step in the conjunctival reactivity was achieved.

In vitro Tests

In the pre-seasonal period a significant increase of specific IgE antibodies was noted. The rise of IgE was more marked during the first season. The co-seasonal increase in the second year was blunted.

During the first 3 months of allergen immunotherapy, a highly significant increase in specific IgG, IgG_1, and IgG_4 antibodies was observed ($p \leq 0.001$). The elevated IgG and IgG-subclass levels persisted during the whole treatment period (Figures 1 and 2).

Regarding the quantitative relationship between IgG and IgE antibodies (IgG/IgE ratio), a significant increase was noted simultaneously with the IgG rise.

Symptom and Medication Scores and Subjective Assessment

Although all patients registered an improvement of seasonal symptoms, we were not able to differentiate between less or more symptomatic patients on the basis of skin-prick test, conjunctival provocation test, or IgG/IgE ratio.

Discussion

Although allergen-specific immunotherapy was introduced into clinical practice at the beginning of this century, treatment has remained essentially unchanged from its empirical origin. Above all changes in the serological variables during hyposensitization, including antigen-specific declines in immediate cutaneous reactivity, levels of serum IgE antibodies, blunting of seasonal rises in specific IgE and increases of specific IgG or IgG-subclass levels are reported as a consequence of a successful immunotherapy [2, 4]. We can confirm that all the mentioned procedures are reliable diagnostic methods for detection of specific sensitization or immunization—though neither the in vivo nor the in vitro parameters correlate well with the patient's assessment of suffering.

For the objective proof of treatment results, in vivo and in vitro tests were carried out throughout the investigation. Skin-prick test and conjunctival provocation tests proved to be safe, easy to perform, and yielded reproducible results. Although in our study a successful allergen immunotherapy was associated with significant changes of skin and conjunctival sensitivity, we were not able, on the basis of these in vivo results, to differentiate between less or more suffering patients. Similar experience was obtained regarding the results of immunologic investigations. Specific IgE, IgG, and IgG-subclass response showed an intercorrelated increase as a response to allergen administration. Specific IgE depression was not decisively influenced by specific IgG or IgG-subclass levels. On the contrary, there was the tendency, however not significant, that patients with high IgE response also developed a high IgG or IgG-subclass antibody level. This suggests that there are similar immunoregulatory controls operating for IgE and IgG production. We could not confirm an earlier suggestion that specific IgG/IgE ratio is of greater value than single isotype antibody assays in efficacy assessment of immunotherapy. Furthermore, specific IgG antibodies provide information on immunogenic response to allergen immunotherapy as isotypic estimations of specific IgG_1 and specific IgG_4 measurements do.

We conclude that a patient's history and assessment of allergic symptoms cannot be replaced by a diagnostic test. In our experience, there is no single diagnostic or follow-up procedure with a superior predictive value. Finally, only the synopsis of in vivo and in vitro results enables us to estimate the decrease and changes of a patient's reactivity to allergens.

References

1. Berg, T., H. Bennich, and S. G. Johannsson. 1971. In-vitro diagnosis of atopic allergy. Int. Arch. Allergy 40: 770–776.

2. Creticos, P. S., T. E. van Metre, M. R. Mardiney, G. L. Rosenberg, P. H. S. Norman, and N. F. Adkinson Jr. 1984. Dose response of IgE and IgG antibodies during ragweed immunotherapy. J. Allergy Clin. Immunol. 73: 94–104.

3. Möller, C. H., B. Björksten, G. Nisson, and S. Dreborg. 1984. The precision of the conjunctival provocation test. Allergy 39: 37–41.

4. Ortolani, C., E. Pastorello, R. B. Moss, Y. Hsu, M. Restuccia, G. Joppolo, A. Miadonna, U. Cornelli, G. Halpern, and C. Zanussi. 1984. Grass pollen immunotherapy: A single year double blind, placebo-controlled study in patients with grass pollen-induced asthma and rhinitis. J. Allergy Clin. Immunol. 72: 283–290.

5. Osterballe, O. 1980. Immunotherapy in hayfever with two major allergens 19, 25 and partially purified extract of timothy grass pollen. Allergy 35: 473–489.

6. Patterson, R., L. C., Grammer, and M. A. Shaughnessy. 1985. Immunotherapy: Parameters of assessment. J. Allergy Clin. Immunol. 76: 394–397.

7. Urbanek, R., H. J. Maasch, W. Geissler, W. Kuhn, and J. Blumberg. 1987. Untersuchungen der spezifischen IgE- und IgG-Antikörper bei Pollen Allergikern: Gekreuzte Radio-Immuno-Elektrophorese (CRIE), Radio-Allergo-Sorbent-Test (RAST) und Enzym-Immun-Test (ELISA) unter Immuntherapie. Allergologie 10: 203–207.

8. Weyer, A., C. Doinel, M. Debbia, C. L'Heriter, L. Rivat, J. Le Mao, C. Hirth, and B. David. 1981. Grass pollen hyposensitization versus placebo therapy. Allergy 36: 319–328.

New Trends in Immunological Diagnosis

*Alain L. de Weck**

New trends in the development of serological immunoassays and of cellular assays for diagnosis in allergy and clinical immunology are briefly reviewed.

Progress in immunological technologies during the past decade have been spectacular. Diagnostic tests using immunological techniques have also invaded many fields of human activities beyond medicine. This paper reviews briefly some of the trends and perspectives in the development of serological and cellular tests which may be relevant for the diagnostic of allergic diseases.

New Trends in Serological Diagnosis

Serological immunological tests essentially rely upon the interaction of antigens and antibodies, be it for the detection of antibodies in serum or other body fluids, be it for the detection in the same fluids of antigens against which the investigator possesses some specific antibody. Most of the technology on which the development of immunology relied for over a century, such as precipitation or agglutination tests, is on its way out, although such assays are still widely used in areas such as blood group serology and microbiological serology. In most serological tests of later generations, the procedure used for labeling antibody or antigen, and the label by which immunological interactions may be followed, are the elements distinguishing the various types of tests (Table 1). The currently dominating radioimmunoassays (RIA) and enzyme-linked immuno assays (ELISA) may be increasingly replaced by practical and sensitive markers, such as fluorescence, metallic labels (gold), or chemoluminescence.

In the development of new serological tests, requirements and goals to be achieved are slightly different according to the person who sets them up. For the marketing salesman, for

Table 1. Labels used for serological immunoassays.

RadioImmunoAssay (RIA)
ELISA
Fluorescence (FIA)
"Metallic" labels (lanthanium, gold)
Chemoluminescence

example, it seems to become increasingly desirable to propose fast immunological tests that yield an answer in 10 minutes or less. Tests should be performed if possible on whole blood with no additional dilution step or manipulation. The test should be "fool- and idiotproof," with no special skills required, thus enabling also the development of home diagnostic tests. However, in a number of conditions requiring immunological tests, such as pregnancy or HIV infection, it may, from ethical and medical point of views, be seriously questioned whether such tests should be made available to a wider public at all.

For the clinical immunologist, the first requirements should be that the test be clinically relevant. The test should be reproducible with a small variation coefficient and few dubious results. When needed, a precise quantitation should be achievable with a minimum of manipulation, calculation, and investment into expensive instruments. The test should be simple and cheap, provide the maximum diagnosis information for the least work, and the least money.

In large laboratories with a sizeable routine load, some other criteria apply as well. Tests should be amenable to the largest possible degree of automation with the least possible personnel and manual work required. The handling of multiple samples should be foolproof, with little sample error. The costs per test unit should also be kept as low as possible.

Obviously, a number of these requirements may be contradictory; therefore, most of the immunological tests as used in daily practice are the result of some compromises.

*   Institute of Clinical Immunology, Inselspital, 3010 Bern, Switzerland.

It should be recognized that there are some inherent limitations to immunological reactions. The rate of such reactions is relatively slow and is determined by antibody affinity within a rather narrow range. The partners in the reaction, that is, antigen and antibody, are often present in unequal concentration, hence difficulties in achieving saturation or steady state levels. In most instances, the reagents have to be added successively and include washing steps for reproducible results, thus leading to a multistep procedure. Finally, there are many interfering substances in whole blood or serum which may affect antigen-antibody reactions.

In recent years, the majority of serological immunoassays have been based on solid-phase

Table 2. Solid-phase supports (for antigen or antibody).

Glass (tube, slide)
Plastic (tube, microtiter plate, bead)
Paper pad or disk, covalent binding
Absorbing membrane (nitrocellulose and similar)
Covalent binding membrane
Absorbing pad or foam

---

technology, where one of the reactants, either antigen or antibody, is bound to a solid-phase support. The types of solid phase currently used are summarized in Table 2. In allergy research, the detection of IgE antibodies in so-called RAST-type assays has for a long time been performed exclusively with paper disks as physical support. New trends are appearing based on solid phases that may be able to absorb and present larger amounts of antigen. A new system developed by Pharmacia [1] uses caps loaded with an absorbing foam, which obviously permits one to absorb and present markedly more antigen. Even then, however, the kinetics of the antigen-antibody reaction still require several minutes to reach a saturation point. Another type of solid support becoming increasingly popular are various types of membranes, using antigen-loaded strips, as in the Immunodot or DAST assays [2, 3]. Because of their larger absorbing capacity for antigen, these new types of support enable better discrimination and quantitation of allergen-specific IgE antibodies in the higher clinical ranges without having to perform additional serum sample dilutions. The presence of an-

tigen on flat solid phases also permits distribution of several antigens on the same surface, thereby enabling multiple assays and results with a single manipulation.

Cellular Assays

T lymphocytes occupy a central position in immunological reactions and in immunologically mediated diseases. Accordingly, assays directed to the study of lymphocyte activation and functions would be expected to yield a number of important diagnostic information. One severe limitation, however, is that only peripheral blood lymphocytes are easily accessible; these may not always reflect immunological events occurring at the local organ or tissue level. Among cellular immunological tests, the lymphocyte proliferation or ^{3}H-thymidine uptake assays have occupied a central and almost lonely place during the past 15 years. This, however, is rapidly changing.

Besides the determination of lymphocyte subpopulations based on monoclonal antibodies and protein membrane markers (the so-called CD antigens), a number of new assays are emerging and are potentially amenable to large-scale routine performance. Such assays are summarized in Table 3. I wish here to present briefly some new cellular assays that have been established by our group and that have potential not only for pathophysiological research but also for routine investigations in allergic diseases.

Quantitative kinetic microfluorometry is based on a video imaging stem, enabling analysis of immunological and biochemical phenomena at the single cell level [4]. Several types

Table 3. Determination of lymphocyte activation and functions.

Proliferation (^{3}H-thymidine incorporatin in DNA)
Membrane activation antigens and receptor expression (cytoflurometry)
Lymphokine production
—biological assay (proliferation cell line)
—biological assay (interferon, O_2 burst generated by TNF and others)
—immunoassay (monoclonal antibodies against LK)
—gene expression and mRNA synthesis
    –at the population level (Northern plot)
    –at the single cell level (in situ hybridization)

---

of cells, such as lymphocytes, blood basophils, macrophages, neutrophils, or platelets have been investigated with this technology. The origins of cells studied may be cell lines, peripheral blood, bronchial lavage, nasal lavage, or skin windows. The technology appears to be readily applicable also to biopsy inprints and possibly to periodontal lavage fluid. These days we are experiencing an explosion in the number of fluorescent markers available for assessing intracellular calcium influx or mobilization, intracellular oxidation, protease activity, pH membrane potential, etc. [5]. The use of fluorescent ligands for receptor studies also enables new insights. Immunological and biochemical investigations at the single cell level are opening a new dimension in diagnosis. This technology permits the assessment of individual cells in a mixed population, without need for prior purification. A very small number of cells is required to obtain significant results, and this may reveal new ways for the study of local inflammation. One of the main results obtained hitherto in such studies has been the realization how important functional heterogeneity is in a cell population. Subpopulations of cells, which up to now had been considered functionally in a global way, indeed possess a large degree of functional microheterogeneity.

A similar development has occurred in *chemoluminescence microscopy*, which also enables assessment of the production of oxygen radicals at the single cell level [6]. Although requiring a very much greater level of sensitivity than fluorescent assays, the chemoluminescence assay has already permitted detection of functional microheterogeneity in neutrophils as well as development of some new applications in the field of drug allergy. The number and practical applications of chemoluminescent markers have also been steadily increasing. It may well be visualized that this technology may become applicable not only in the field of immunology, but also—using suitable labeled DNA or RNA probes—to single-cell analysis in molecular biology.

A potentially useful development for routine diagnosis based on chemoluminescent techniques has been the development in our group of a *chemoluminescence multiwell analyzer* [7], also based on a videoimaging system. In this machine, the chemoluminescence emanating from 192 microtiterplate wells can be assessed and quantitated simultaneously, enabling not only simultaneous handling of a large number of samples, but also the choice of various kinetic parameters at will. In the study of lymphokine functions, the purification of lymphokines from complex mixtures, and the detection of lymphocyte activation in supernatants of lymphocyte culture, this machine has already rendered very valuable services. It has the potential of replacing lymphocyte proliferation assays by ^{3}H-thymidine.

Impact of Molecular Biological Technology on Allergy and Immunology Diagnosis

There is little doubt that molecular biological techniques, which after all, like antigen-antibody reactions, are also based on the specificity of hybridization interactions, will play an increasing role in allergy diagnosis in the future. In particular in the field of cellular immunology and analysis of lymphokine production, molecular biological tools have already become indispensable. Besides the quantitative assessment of mRNA synthesis for lymphokine and lymphokine receptors, which can be standardized in the form of Northern blot or dot blot assays [8], the application of in situ hybridization techniques for detection of lymphokine mRNA synthesis promises to reveal interesting insights, in particular in the regulation of IgE synthesis in humans. A comparison between results obtained at the whole population level or at the single cell level has revealed that the production of the one or the other lymphokine is the result of full production by a small number of cells rather than small-scale production by the whole cell population [9].

With increasing sensitivity and also with a degree of specificity which in many instances markedly supersedes that of immunological assays, molecular biological assays may also become the diagnostic technology of the 21st century in the field of allergy and clinical immunology.

I hope I have been able to show you in these few considerations that also in the field of allergy diagnosis there are exciting developments ahead of us. They will enable us to better understand the pathophysiology of allergic disease and to more accurately establish diagnostic parameters for our patients.

References

1. Pharmacia (Uppsala). Introduction to the CAP System. ICACI Montreux, 1988.
2. Derer, M. M., S. Miescher, B. Johansson, H. Frost, and J. Gordon. 1984. Application of the immunobinding assay to allergy diagnosis. J. Allergy Clin. Immunol. 74: 85–92.
3. Hong, C. S., B. M. Stadler, M. Wälti, and A. L. de Weck. 1986. Dot immunobinding assay with monoclonal anti-IgE antibodies for the detection and quantitation of human IgE. J. Immunol. Methods 95: 195–202.
4. de Weck, A. L., and R. Fritzsche. 1989. Immunopharmacology at the single cell level. A new approach to the study of allergic inflammation. Allergy and Clinical Immunology News, 1(1): 13–17.
5. Bioprobes, Molecular Probes Inc., Eugene, OR, No. 8, June 1988.
6. Fritzsche, R., and A. L. de Weck. 1988. Chemiluminescence microscopy reveals functional heterogeneity in single neutrophils undergoing oxygen burst. Eur. J. Immunol. 18: 817–821.
7. Maly, F. E., A. Urwyler, H. P. Rolli, C. A. Dahinden, and A. L. de Weck. 1988. A single photon imaging system for the simultaneous quantitation of luminescent emissions from multiple samples. Analytical Biochemistry 168: 462–469.
8. Gauchat, J. F., C. Walker, A. L. de Weck, and B. M. Stadler. 1986. Relation of supernatant IL-2 to steady state levels of IL-2 mRNA. Lymphokine Res. 5: 43–47.
9. Qiu, G., J. F. Gauchat, U. Wirthmüller, A. L. de Weck, and B. M. Stadler. 1988. Lymphokine production by human peripheral blood lymphocytes: Analysis by in situ hybridisation. Lymphokine Research, in press.

Allergen Standardization: Use of International Standards

Henning Løwenstein*

Under the auspices of the IUIS a number of standards for allergenic extracts have been developed to enable standardization of allergenic extracts. So far standards of short ragweed pollen, timothy grass pollen, the house dust mite—*D. pteronyssinus*—and birch pollen have all been approved by the WHO as international standards. A further four extracts have approval at WHO pending, two are still in the process of being developed, and a further five extracts are planned. Although now available, these standards are still not in real use, neither by national legal authorities nor by manufacturers. This paper argues for use of these standards to label all corresponding allergenic extracts for content of major allergens which can be performed practically independently of methods and reagents used.

The purpose of allergen standardization was to obtain safer and more efficient extracts for specific diagnosis and treatment of the allergic patient. In order to obtain this, the International Union of Immunological Societies (IUIS) decided, in consultation with the WHO, to coordinate the international level on a permanent basis in the field of allergen standardization. The goals were (1) to generate and make available to investigators, manufacturers, and control authorities allergen reference preparations (with assigned arbitrary international units), standards and reagents; (2) to develop and publicize on the basis of the appropriate collaborative trials, tests enabling assessment of (a) allergenic activity and (b) composition and content of important allergenic molecules; (3) to provide an international collaborative framework for immunochemical allergen research [1].

The first of these goals—the generation of international standards of allergenic extracts—has been achieved to some degree, and a number of these standards have been approved by WHO. During their development, they have been shown to be workable standards. However, they are still not in real use as international standards for both technical and political reasons. This presentation discusses these problems and proposes the practical use of the developed international standards (IS).

Background

Allergenic extracts are complex mixtures of antigenic components. The number of these components varies greatly from one allergen source to another. Generally, we are able to detect a number of components between 15 and 80 with the methods used today, but there might be many more components represented in too small amounts to be detected. The number of components visualized is usually lowest for hair and dander extracts, greater for mite and pollen extracts, and largest for mold extracts.

The allergenic patients reveal individual responses against potential allergens—regarding both intensity and specificity. This has been shown in a great number of investigations, and it gives us the statistical basis for demonstrating that some of the components are more significant as allergens than others because they most often bind IgE from a selected allergic population.

Thus, we are faced with the situation that there are a great many different components that are able to bind IgE, and patients respond quite individually against these components. Since our problem is to control extracts in a manner that ensures that they fulfill their purpose as both diagnostic preparations able to detect all the allergenic patients and as preparations effective when used for hyposensitization, we have to ensure through our control that all essential components are included.

Logically, the optimal situation would be to control for all the individual components in an allergenic extract. However, this would not be realistic, and this control has therefore to be

---

*   Director of R & D, ALK Laboratories, and Associate Professor, Bøge Allé 10, DK-2970 Hørsholm Denmark.

399

reduced to cover—from the allergic point of view—only the most important constituents. Another principle to be used for standardization could be a measurement of the total allergenic activity (potency), but this is just a contribution from all the individual components and will be heavily dependent upon the method and reagents used.

Standards

A number of international standards of allergenic extracts have been developed and approved by the WHO. These are short ragweed pollen [2], timothy grass pollen [3], house dust mite *D. pteronyssinus* [4] and birch pollen [5]. Standards for dog hair and dander [6], the mould *Alternaria alternata* [7], bermuda grass pollen [8], and rye grass pollen [9] have also been developed, and their approval by WHO is pending. Further under development are extracts of cat hair and dander and the house dust mite *D. farinae*. Finally, it is planned to further develop standards of mugwort pollen, Paritaria pollen, olive pollen, oak pollen, and the mould *Cladosporium herbarum*. The approved standards are all presently available through the NIBSC in England.

Common to these international standards are that they are representative of the extracts of the various allergen sources. In order to obtain these, some general specifications for the standards were agreed upon before their development. These are, briefly [10]:

— Cultivated allergen sources must be grown in non-allergenic culture medium. The final extract must be demonstrated to be free of allergenic components due to the culture medium. These requirements also include an identification of the source material by, for example, microscopy. They might also include immunochemical investigations for irrelevant allergenic components suspected to be included in the final extract.

— The standard should be obtained by aqueous extraction and performed under such conditions that all allergenic molecules are present in unchanged, native form in the standard. Further, it was required that the standard during its preparation should not lose more than 20% of its native allergenic activity as measured by various relevant tests.

— The obtained standard must be useful for various in vitro tests.

— The standard must be comparable with the majority of existing allergenic extracts on the market, but should not be outstandingly good or poor. The biological activity should also be demonstrable, either by skin testing or histamine release assay.

— Of each standard there should be at least 3–4,000 sealed glass ampules, each containing 1–5 mg freeze dried material.

— In the standards a specified number of antigens, allergens, and proteins should be demonstrable. For those allergen sources for which the necessary information was available, a certain amount of the most important allergenic constituents relative to the dry weight material was required.

The philosophy of the international standards is that they should be comparable with that material to which individuals are exposed when the allergens are extracted in vivo on the human mucosa. This assumes that the extractions are performed on relevant material (i.e., pollen and not the whole plant). It also assumes that the extractions are performed by methods that do not influence the native confirmation of the allergens. Furthermore, the extracted material should contain all potential allergens (i.e., any components that might give rise to any allergen in any individual). It is also one of the assumptions that international standards should not contain irrelevant allergenic material (i.e., allergenic material that, under natural conditions, would not have been found in that allergen source). Finally, the natural ratio between the allergenic molecules should be retained after the preparation of the standards and be comparable with that of natural extraction on the human mucosa.

The standards have all undergone an international collaborative study, which includes that the standard, together with other extracts of the same source to be compared with, was analyzed by a minimum number of different laboratories in a minimum number of different countries by any version of any methods using any relevant reagents. The results of these collaborative studies, which were all performed in a blind coded system and analyzed according to the WHO rules for development of standards, all proved to be workable standards. For all these standards each ampule has arbitrarily been assigned 100000 International Units, which applies for both potency and any individual components. The standards are, of course, not perfect, and they are not expected to be the very best for specific diagnosis or immunotherapy; rather, they should make it possible to standardize allergenic extracts from the same source. How they will be used depends on the various national control authorities, but the intention for their use has been clearly formulated by the IUIS Subcommittee on Allergen Standardization.

Recommended Use of Standards

The variation of quality of allergenic extracts is tremendous from one allergen manufacturer to another. A great number of studies has shown large variability in antigenic composition from case to case [11, 12, 13]. Most often, however, the extracts contain the major allergenic constituents. Also the potency level of the highest concentration available from a producer varies greatly from one manufacturer to another. Consequently, there must be huge differences in the ratios between the allergenic molecules from extracts from one producer to another. Finally, in some cases commercial extracts have included irrelevant material or denatured material.

Today, there are no data available which describe the optimal allergenic extract. Consequently, the allergen standardization group decided that the developed standards had to be used as a yardstick, meaning something to be compared with in any respect including both potency (total allergenic activity) by and the concentration of individual constituents such as defined major allergens. This also means that it should not be used as a blueprint—as something to be identical with or similar to in any respect including potency or concentration of individual constituents. This decision is partly a political one, since it generally corresponds with the policy of the use of the other WHO standards, and also due to the fact that very little is known about what should be called the optimal allergenic extract. This decision, however, does have some practical implications such as the difficulty in using them for measurement of potency, which in reality is only possible to measure provided extracts to be compared have nearly the same composition and also require the same version of methods and the same reagents requirements, which only partly corresponds to the way the WHO standards are generally used. The yardstick principle requires, however, greater flexibility on the part of the various national legal authorities in control of allergenic extracts for quality and potency. As the situation is today, some countries require specific tests to be performed using developed reagents and protocols. This is in principle a blueprint requirement, and those legal authorities define what they understand as optimal allergenic extracts. On the other hand, other countries accept— within some limitations—control of potency and quality performed with methods proposed by the manufacturer, using their own protocols and reagents. These countries may be open for the acceptance of the yardstick principle for standardization.

As stated above, two major principles exist for standardization methods of allergenic extracts: measurement of the potency or measurement of the concentration of the individual constituents. Potency is measured by means of methods such as RAST inhibition, ELISA inhibition, histamine release, quantitative skin test, etc.; these have in common that they all use human IgE as a reagent, thereby being dependent on the group of patients selected for the test or the combination of patients whose sera are included in the used serum pool. Thus, this measurement is dependent on the reagent used, and to some degree, also on the version of method used. Furthermore, for extracts that differ significantly from each other in composition, such potency measurement cannot be performed statistically validly.

Measurements of concentration of a selected number of allergenic constituents can be performed with methods such as single radio immunodiffusion, ELISA technique, CIE/CRIE, rocket immunoelectrophoresis, using various radio or enzyme immunoassays in various combinations of polyspecific or polyclonal monospecific or monoclonal antibodies. Common to these is that they are only dependent on the performed identification of the selected allergenic molecule but not on the various reagents used.

As a consequence, and also because no one seems to be willing to define or even agree upon a common optimal allergenic extract, the Immunotherapy Subcommittee of the European Academy of Allergology and Clinical Immunology recommend use of the international standards as reference for individual constituents only. This means that the developed international standards can be used according to the yardstick principle. It also means that only those parameters that can be compared will in fact be compared. It avoids confusion by having the same numbers (units) of extracts from different manufacturers which are of different compositions and therefore are not comparable, and it allows the legal authorities to control the manufacturers' products for content of selected allergenic constituents as well as the ratio between them from batch to batch—which is indirectly a measurement of the potency. The level of potency, however, has to be measured independently, and might be settled by an in-house standard by the various producers, for example, by quantitative skin testing and subsequent control of future batches by other in vitro biological methods for measurement of potency.

Our general knowledge of important allergenic constituents within important allergenic extracts increases rapidly. We are in the situation that many of these constituents are sequenced, some are already cloned, and many monospecific reagents, whether mono or polyclonal, have been developed. All this information will greatly facilitate the use of the international standards as references for individual components in produced allergenic extracts.

References

1. Løwenstein, H. 1983. Report on behalf of the International Union of Immunological Societies (IUIS) allergen standardization committee. Stuttgart: Gustav Fischer Verlag, 41–48.
2. Helm, R. M., B. A. Gauerke, H. Baer, H. Løwenstein, A. Ford, D. A. Levy, P. S. Norman, and J.W. Yunginger. 1984. Production and testing of an international reference standard of short ragweed pollen extract. J. Allergy Clin. Immunol. 73: 790–800.
3. Gjesing, B., L. Jäger, D. G. Marsh, and H. Løwenstein. 1985. The international collaborative study establishing the first international standard for timothy (*Phleum pratense*) grass pollen allergenic extract. J. Allergy Clin. Immunol. 75: 258–267.
4. Ford, A., V. Seagroatt, T. A. E. Platts-Mills, and H. Løwenstein. 1985. A collaborative study on the first international standard of *Dermatophagoides pteronyssinus* (house dust mite) extract. J. Allergy Clin. Immunol. 75: 676–686.
5. Arntzen, F. C., T. W. Wilhelmsen, H. Løwenstein, B. Gjesing, H. J. Maasch, R. Strömberg, R. Einarsson, A. Backman, S. Mkinen-Kiljunen, and A. Ford. 1988. The international collaborative study on the first international standard of birch (*Betula verrucosa*) pollen extract. J. Allergy Clin. Immunol., in press.
6. Nedergaard Larsen, J. A. Ford, B. Gjesing, D. Levy, B. Petrunov, L. Silvestri, and H. Løwenstein. 1988. The collaborative study of the first international standard of a dog, *Canis domesticus*, hair/dander extract. J. Allergy Clin. Immunol., in press.
7. Helm, R. M., D. L. Squillace, L. Aukrush, S. M. Borch, H. Baer, R. K. Bush, H. Løwenstein, R. Znamirowski, W. Nitchuk, and J. W. Yunginger. 1987. Production of an international reference standard Alternaria extract. Int. Arch. Allergy appl. Immun. 82: 178–189.
8. Baer, H., M. C. Anderson, R. M. Helm, J. W. Yunginger, H. Løwenstein, B. Gjesing, W. White, G. Douglass, P. Reiman Phillips, M. Schumacher, B. Hewitt, B. G. Guerin, J. Charpin, J. Carreira, M. Lombardero, A. K. M. Ekramodoullah, F. Kisil, and R. Einarsson. 1986. The preparation and testing of the proposed International Reference (IRP) Bermuda grass (*Cynodon dactylon*)-pollen extract. J. Allergy Clin. Immunol. 78: 624–631.
9. Stewart, G. A., K. J. Turner, B. A. Baldo, A. W. Cripps, A. Ford, V. Seagroatt, H. Løwenstein, and A. K. M. Ekramoddoullah. 1988. Standardization of rye-grass pollen (*Lolium perenne*) extract. Int. Archs. Allergy appl. Immun. 86: 9–18.
10. Løwenstein, H. 1987. Selection of reference preparation. IUIS reference preparation criteria. Stuttgart: Gustav Fischer Verlag, 75–78.
11. Løwenstein, H., P. Lind, and B. Weeke. 1985. Identification and clinical significance of allergenic molecules of cat origin. A part of the DAS 76 study. Allergy 40: 430–441.
12. Ford, A., F. C. Rawle, P. Lind, F. T. M. Spieksma, H. Løwenstein, and T. A. E. Platts-Mills. 1985. Standardization of *Dermatophagoides pteronyssinus*: Assessment of potency and allergen content in ten coded extracts. Int. Archs. Allergy appl. Immun. 76: 58–67.
13. Ingemann, L., H. Formgren, H. Løwenstein, and H. Ipsen. 1985. The use of a reference allergenic extract in the evaluation of allergen products. Allergy 40: 273–281.

In vitro Methods for Standardization of Allergenic Extracts

*John W. Yunginger**

Allergenic extracts are complex mixtures, of which allergens constitute only a small proportion. Allergen standardization programs are designed to ensure maximum potency and to minimize lot-to-lot variation in the composition of diagnostic and therapeutic extracts. Standardization efforts have been advanced by the more widespread availability of reference extracts and the development of in vitro tests such as RAST inhibition, polyacrylamide gel electrophoresis, thin layer isoelectrofocusing, and crossed immunoelectrophoresis.

The goals of allergen standardization are to ensure the lot-to-lot consistency of allergenic extracts and to quantitate the relative potency of allergenic extracts. Standardization requires that reference preparations be available and used as calibrators of allergenic potency. Such reference preparations are available from national regulatory agencies or from the World Health Organization [1].

Protein Assay

Attempts have been made to standardize allergenic extracts for diagnostic and therapeutic use for over 50 years, beginning with the measurement of protein in the extract by phosphotungstic acid precipitation. [2] Because allergens may constitute only a small proportion of the total protein in an extract, however, it was not surprising that the protein content was subsequently shown to be a poor correlate of in vivo potency. During the past decade, a number of improved in vitro standardization procedures have evolved and are being used with increasing frequency.

Radioallergosorbent Test (RAST)

In the RAST procedure, allergens are adsorbed or covalently bound to a solid phase support, which is initially allowed to react with pooled sera containing IgE antibodies that have been collected from allergic individuals. IgE antibodies, as well as antibodies of the other immunoglobulin classes, react with the allergen present on the solid-phase support and form allergen-antibody complexes. IgE antibodies directed against allergens other than those on the solid phase support, as well as other serum components, are washed away at the end of the first step of the reaction.

In the second step of the RAST, the washed solid phase allergen-antibody complexes are reacted with radioiodinated affinity chromatography-purified antibody to human IgE. The purified anti-IgE binds to the IgE on the surface of the solid-phase complex. After washing to remove unbound anti-IgE, the radioactivity associated with the complex is measured in a gamma scintillation counter. The quantity of radioactivity bound is related to the quantity of IgE antibody present in the serum pool tested.

As usually performed, the RAST is an assay for IgE antibody. However, the test can also be modified for measurement of allergens [3]. This is done by introducing varying quantities of soluble allergenic extracts as inhibitors in the first stage of the RAST. Dose-response inhibition curves can be constructed from various test extracts and compared to the dose-response curve of some allergenic standard extract having a defined potency. In this method, the potency of the extract depends on the spectrum of IgE antibodies present in the serum pool, as well as the display of allergens on the solid phase reagent. It is important to include sera from as many sensitive individuals as possible in the serum pool, to ensure that IgE antibodies to both major and minor allergens are represented. Also, it is important that the solid phase allergen preparation display both major and minor allergens, preferably in the same ratio as they exist in the fluid phase extract.

*   Allergic Diseases Research Laboratory, Mayo Clinic and Foundation, and the Department of Pediatrics, Mayo Medical School, Rochester, MN 55905. Supported in part by NIH Contract AI-72621.

There are many advantages of the RAST inhibition assay for standardization of allergenic extracts. The solid-phase allergens are quite stable during storage, and the IgE antibody pools used in the assay can be stored indefinitely when lyophilized. Also, virtually any allergenic extract can be standardized, provided it can be bound to the solid-phase support. Lastly, the procedure can be used to standardize even those extracts in which the allergenic components have not been isolated and characterized. A complete description of the technical details of RAST assays have been published [4]. For several different allergens, RAST inhibition estimates of potency have correlated well with results of endpoint skin test titrations in sensitive individuals.

Polyacrylamide Gel Electrophoresis

Most macromolecular components in allergenic extracts are electrically charged and can therefore be characterized by their rate of movement in an electric field. Most studies have been conducted by polyacrylamide gel electrophoresis (PAGE). The molecular weights of protein allergens can be determined by measuring their mobility in polyacrylamide gels containing sodium dodecyl sulfate (SDS-PAGE) [5]. Each SDS-PAGE assay is usually run with a mixture of calibration proteins of known molecular weight.

Components separated by SDS-PAGE can be examined for their ability to bind IgE antibody by Western blotting. The separated components are passively or electrophoretically blotted onto nitrocellulose paper, which is subsequently washed in albumin-containing buffer, then incubated sequentially with IgE antibody-containing sera and radiolabeled anti-IgE. The washed nitrocellulose strip is then incubated with X-ray film to produce an autoradiograph. If Western blots are performed using sera from individual allergic patients, varying patterns of radiostaining will be observed, reflecting the differing abilities of individuals to respond to the various components in an allergen extract.

Thin-Layer Isoelectric Focusing (TLIEF)

Allergenic extracts can also be characterized qualitatively by TLIEF in polyacrylamide gels [6]. This technique separates the components of an extract on the basis of their isoelectric points. After electrofocusing, the gel is stained, and the intensity of the stain is proportional to the amount of protein at a given isoelectric point. While TLIEF is not a quantitative procedure, it provides a "fingerprint" pattern that is useful to compare one lot of extract to another or to a reference extract, and to identify degradation components or contaminants in allergenic extracts. It is important to realize that two or more proteins with distinct isoelectric points may possess identical allergenic determinants and therefore be immunologically identical. Put differently, a highly purified allergen may produce several bands when tested by TLIEF.

The separated components in a TLIEF gel can be electrophoretically blotted onto nitrocellulose paper and sequentially reacted with IgE antibodies and radiolabeled anti-IgE, as in Western blotting [7]. This procedure is known as blotted radioimmunoelectrophoresis (BRIEF) and is useful to distinguish which protein-stained bands represent allergenic components.

Crossed Immunoelectrophoresis (CIE)

In the CIE technique, the components of an allergenic extract are separated electrophoretically in a agarose gel [8]. The separated components are then electrophoresed at right angles to the first electrophoresis into a gel containing rabbit antibodies to the allergen extract in question. Every component to which a corresponding antibody is present produces a precipitation arc whose area is correlated to the amount of that component. These antigen-antibody precipitin arcs can be stained with Coomassie blue directly to visualize the bands, or unstained gels can be sequentially incubated with human IgE antibody and radiolabeled anti-IgE to prepare autoradiographs. The latter technique is called crossed radioimmunoelectrophoresis (CRIE).

Although proponents of CIE claim that it is a quantitative technique for measuring the content of allergens in an extract, some limitations are present. The procedure requires purified concentrated rabbit IgG to develop the precipitates, and there is the potential for variability in animals to recognize certain antigens. Also, in several different allergen systems, radio-stained CRIE bands are present which do not correspond to Coomassie stained protein bands, indicating that humans can recognize allergens in the extract that are not antigenic to rabbits.

Leukocyte Histamine Release

Allergenic extracts can be standardized by their ability to trigger release of histamine from sensitized basophils [9] Peripheral blood leukocytes are isolated from sensitized persons and mixed in vitro with varying quantities of allergen. The histamine released as a consequence of the interaction of allergen with basophil-fixed IgE antibody is measured by photofluorometric or radioenzymatic procedures. Although an automated system for the histamine release assay has been reported [10], the usefulness of this assay is limited by the requirement for fresh blood cells and by the fact that approximately 15% of individuals have leukocytes that fail to release histamine in vitro, even when challenged with anti-IgE.

Purified Allergens

In some instances, allergens have been isolated from crude extracts and purified to homogeneity. When such purified antigens are available, their concentration in extracts can be determined using radial immunodiffusion. Precipitating antibody is raised in rabbits or other animals by injection of the purified allergen. This animal antibody is then incorporated into agarose gel. When crude or purified allergens are subsequently introduced into wells cut in the agarose and allowed to diffuse, a precipitin ring is formed around the well; the diameter of the ring is directly proportional to the quantity of purified allergen in the sample. This procedure has been used to measure the amount of *Amb a* I (antigen E) in short ragweed extracts [11]. Short ragweed extracts marketed for sale in the United States are required to contain a minimum quantity of Amb a I (>135 micrograms/ml in a 1:10 w:v extract).

Insect venoms contain a number of enzymes, including phospholipase A, hyaluronidase, and acid phosphatase [12]. In vitro assays for these enzyme activities can therefore be used to characterize and standardize venom extracts. Venom sac extracts marketed for sale in the United States are standardized based on their hyaluronidase content.

References

1. Helm, R. M., M. B. Gauerke, H. Baer, H. Løwenstein, H., A. Ford, D. A. Levy, P. S. Norman, and J. W. Yunginger. 1984. Production and testing of an international reference standard of short ragweed pollen extract. J. Allergy Clin. Immunol. 73: 790.
2. Stull, A., R. A. Cooke, and J. Tennant. 1933. The allergen content of pollen extracts. Its determination and its deterioration. J. Allergy 4: 455.
3. Gleich, G. J., J. B. Larson, R. T. Jones, and H. Baer. 1974. Measurement of the potency of allergy extracts by their inhibitory capacities in the radioallergosorbent test. J. Allergy Clin. Immunol. 53: 158.
4. Adolphson, C. R., G. J. Gleich, and J. W. Yunginger. 1986. Standardization of allergens. In: Manual of clinical laboratory immunology (3rd ed.). N. R. Rose, H. Friedman, and J. L. Fahey, eds. Washington, DC: American Society for Microbiology, pp. 652–659.
5. Weber, K., and M. Osborn. 1969. The reliability of molecular weight determinations by dodecyl sulfate-polyacrylamide gel electrophoresis. J. Biol. Chem. 244: 4406.
6. Varga, J. M., and M. Ceska. 1972. Characterization of allergen extracts by gel isoelectrofocusing and radioimmunosorbent allergen assay. J. Allergy Clin. Immunol. 49: 274.
7. Baer, H., and M. C. Anderson. 1988. Allergenic extracts. I. Sources, preparation, and in vitro standardization. In: Allergy principles and practice (3rd ed.). E. Middleton, Jr., C. E. Reed, E. F. Ellis, N. F. Adkinson, Jr., and J. W. Yunginger, eds. St. Louis: Mosby, pp. 373–388.
8. Løwenstein, H. 1978. Quantitative immunoelectrophoretic methods: A tool for the analysis and isolation of allergens. Prog. Allergy 25: 1.
9. May, C. D., M. Lyman, R. Alberto, and J. Cheng. 1970. Procedures for immunochemical study of histamine release from leukocytes with small volume of blood. J. Allergy 46: 12.
10. Siraganian, R. P., and W. A. Hook. 1986. Hista-

mine release and assay methods for the study of human allergy. In: Manual of clinical laboratory immunology (3rd ed.). N. R. Rose, H. Friedman, and J. L. Fahey, eds. Washington, DC: American Society for Microbiology, pp. 675–684.

11. Baer, H., H. Godfrey, C. J. Maloney, P. S. Nor-man, and L. M. Lichtenstein. 1970. The potency and antigen E content of commercially prepared ragweed extracts. J. Allergy 45: 317.

12. Levine, M. I., and R. F. Lockey (eds.). 1986. Monograph on insect allergy (2nd ed.). Pittsburgh, PA: Dave Lambert Associates.

Allergen Standardization Using Monoclonal Antibodies to Major Allergens

Martin D. Chapman, Peter W. Heymann, Susan M. Pollart,
*Thomas A. E. Platts-Mills**

This paper briefly outlines recent progress in the production of allergen specific monoclonal antibodies and the applications of these antibodies in allergen standardization.

At the XII International Congress (Washington, DC, 1985), both Drs. de Weck and Baldo proposed that monoclonal antibodies (mAb) would play an important role in the investigation of allergic disease, and, indeed, over the past 3 years, there has been significant progress in the use of mAb in allergy research. The main advance in terms of allergen standardization has been the production of mAb to a series of major allergens (e.g., from dust mite, cat dander, and grass, ragweed, and other pollens) and the use of these mAb for allergen quantitation, purification, and epitope analysis [1, 2]. The rationale for assessing the potency of allergen extracts by measuring major allergens is that these reagents are, by definition, a major cause of IgE antibody responses; they are well defined immunochemically; and they can be precisely quantified in absolute units (µg of protein). These objective measurements can be accurately compared from year to year and also allow direct comparison of allergen levels in different extracts. The advantages of using mAb, as compared to polyclonal antibodies or human serum pools, for allergen standardization are outlined in Table 1. The specificity and reproducibility of mAb is ideal for long term use, and the development of mAb immunoassays has made it much easier to maintain consistent allergen measurements.

Panels of mAb have now been produced against several major allergens, including *Fel d* I, *Lol p* I, *Amb a* I, *Par j* I and the Group I and Group II dust mite allergens [3–12]. Improved standardization can be achieved primarily through using these reagents for aller-

Table 1. Advantages of using monoclonal antibodies in allergen standardization.

1. Their specificity can be accurately defined and remains constant, i.e., can be consistently be reproduced over several years.
2. They can readily be produced in gram quantities.
3. Simple monoclonal immunoassays can be used to measure individual allergens in an extract. These assays are:
   a) highly sensitive (ng range)
   b) do no require purified allergen
   c) technically straightforward and suitable for testing large numbers of samples.
4. Once the specificity of a monoclonal antibody has been defined, the monoclonal serves as the primary reagent for identifying the allergen.

gen identification and purification and in immunoassays. Single-step mAb affinity chromatography techniques have been developed for purifying major mite, cat, and pollen allergens. These techniques can be used to purify mg amounts of allergen and are particularly useful when the source material is heterogeneous or in short supply. For example, it is difficult to obtain sufficient cat allergen from manufacturers to purify *Fel d* I using conventional techniques. However, we have been able to purify *Fel d* I direct from house dust extracts containing high levels of this allergen using mAb chromatography [3]. Similar techniques have been developed for the Group I and Group II mite allergens [12] and for some pollen allergens [5, 8, 9]. The production of mAb is increasingly becoming the first step in allergen identification. We recently identified a major cockroach allergen using mAb 10A6 and used this mAb in an ELISA assay for the allergen, even though the allergen identified by the mAb has not yet been fully purified. This approach is also being

* Division of Allergy and Clinical Immunology, Department of Medicine, University of Virginia, Charlottesville, VA 22908, USA.
This work was supported by National Institutes of Health Grants A120565, A124261, and A124687.

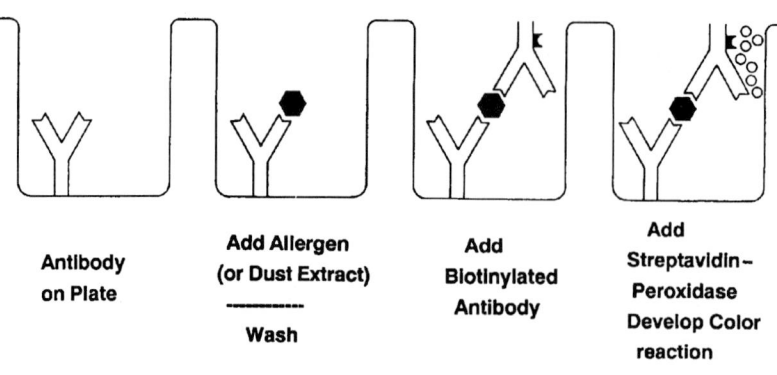

Figure 1. Monoclonal antibody-based ELISA ffor allergens.

| Antibody on Plate | Add Allergen (or Dust Extract) ---------- Wash | Add Biotinylated Antibody | Add Streptavidin– Peroxidase Develop Color reaction |

Table 2. Monoclonal immunoassays for common allergens in house dust*.

Allergen	Solid phase Mab	Second antibody	Reference standards	Assay
Der p I	5H8	4C1	NISC 82/518 UVA 87/03	RIA, ELISA
Der f I	6A8	4C1	OBRR E1-Df UVA 87/02	RIA, ELISA
Group II	7A1	6D6	*Der f* II	RIA
Fel d I	6F9	3E4	OBRR Cat E3	RIA, ELISA
Cockroach	10A6	Rabbit IgG ab	UVA cockroach	RIA

*Most mAb raised against *Der p* I or *Der f* I are "species specific" and separate assays are used for each allergen. The mAb to *Der p* II and *Der f* II are fully cross-reactive, and a single assay can be used for both allergens. The UVA reference mite extracts have been substandardized against the WHO/IUIS *D. pteronyssinus* International Reference Preparation (NIBSC 82/518).

applied to the isolation of fungal allergens. Thus the use of mAb purification techniques provides investigators with a much better "handle" on the allergen and makes it easier to confirm the identity of allergens isolated in different laboratories.

For most allergens, mAb with different epitope specificities have been produced and pairs of mAb directed against nonoverlapping epitopes have been used to develop two site immunoassays (Figure 1). The mAb and reference standards currently used in assays in our laboratory are shown in Table 2. Similar assays for mite, cat, and pollen allergens have also been developed in other laboratories [4, 11]. Using these assays, allergists can be provided with precise information about the quantities of specific allergens present in extracts used for diagnosis and treatment and can more easily compare extracts from different companies. Allergen manufacturers can also use these assays to monitor "in-house" quality control and to pro-

duce more consistent and reliable extracts. Comparisons of commercial extracts using mAb assay have shown that *Fel d* I levels in cat dander/epithelium extracts may vary by as much as 300 fold, and that some house dust extracts contain more *Fel d* I than cat extracts [3].

While major allergen measurements are generally accepted as giving a good guide to "overall" potency (e.g., by RAST inhibition) in cat or pollen extracts, their use in assessing mite extracts has been controversial (see [2, 13]). The apparent problem with mite stem from the use of two different source materials (whole mite culture or isolated mite bodies) for extract preparation, and the presence of two major allergens in different proportions in each type of extract. Measurements of Group I mite allergens correlate well with total potency in assays of whole culture extracts, but may underestimate the potency of mite body extracts. The recent development of a mAb assay for the

Group II allergens [12] has enabled us to compare levels of these two groups of major allergens in different mite extracts. In commercial extracts, levels of Group I and Group II allergens are reasonably consistent (range from 5–100 µg/ml and 1–40 µg/ml, respectively). However, the Group I:Group II ratio in these extracts varied by up to 350 fold (from 0.1–35:1). The ratio in the WHO/IUIS *D. pteronyssinus* reference was 35:1, and it is now clear that the low level of Group II allergen in this extract explains why this appeared to be a weak extract on RAST inhibition, when compared with whole body mite extracts, which usually have about a 1:1 ratio.

The important feature of mAb assays is that they provide objective data upon which decisions about standardization can be based. For example, the clinical significance of having mite extracts with different Group I:Group II allergen ratios is not yet clear; however, the use of mAb assays will make it possible to compare mite extracts with different allergen levels in clinical studies. The mAb assays for "indoor" allergens are also being used extensively to monitor allergen exposure in patients houses and its relationship to the development of clinical symptoms, especially asthma (see article by Platts-Mills in these proceedings). This makes it possible for the allergist to use information on the same allergens in extracts used for diagnosis and treatment and to compare them with allergen levels to which patients are exposed at home. A good example of this is the current National Institute of Health trial of mite immunotherapy in asthma, in which the extracts are being monitored by mAb assays to establish doses of specific allergens used for treatment and allergen levels inside patients homes are being compared with symptom scores, immunologic changes, medication, and response to treatment.

References

1. Chapman, M. D. 1988. Allergen specific monoclonal antibodies: New tools for the management of allergic disease. Allergy 43 (5): 7.
2. Platts-Mills, T. A. E., and M. D. Chapman. 1987. Dust mites: Immunology, allergic disease, and environmental control. J. Allergy Clin. Immunol. 80: 755.
3. Chapman, M. D., M. Brown, J. Van Leeuwen, R. C. Aalberse, and T. A. E. Platts-Mills. 1988. Monoclonal antibodies to the major feline allergen Fel d I. I. J. Immunol. 140: 818.
4. Lombardero, M., J. Carreira, and O. Duffort. 1988. Monoclonal antibody based radioimmunoassay for the quantitation of the main cat allergen (Fel d I or Cat-1). J. Immunol. Meths. 108: 71.
5. Kahn, C. R., and D. G. Marsh. 1986. Monoclonal antibodies to the major Lolium perenne (rye grass) pollen allergen Lol p I (Rye I). Mol. Immunol. 23: 1281.
6. Bose, R., E. S. Rector, J. Fisher, R. Taronno, and G. Delespesse. 1986. Production and characterization of mouse monoclonal antibodies to allergenic epitopes on Lol p I (Rye I). Immunology 59: 309.
7. Esch, R. E., and D. G. Klapper. 1987. Cross-reactive and unique grass Group I antigenic determinants defined by monoclonal antibodies. J. Allergy Clin. Immunol. 79: 489.
8. Ekramoddoullah, A., F. T. Kisil, R. T. Cook, and A. H. Sehon. 1987. Recognition of a site of a Kentucky Blue Grass pollen allergen by antibodies in the sera of allergic and non-atopic humans and a murine monoclonal antibody. J. Immunol. 138: 1739.
9. Corbi, A. L., C. Ley, F. Sanchez-Madrid, and J. Carreira. 1985. Isolation of the major IgE binding protein from Parietaria judaica pollen using monoclonal antibodies. Mol. Immunol. 22: 1081.
10. Chapman, M. D., P. W. Heymann, and T. A. E. Platts-Mills. 1987. Epitope mapping of two major inhalant allergens, Der p I and Der f I, from mites of the genus Dermatophagoides. J. Immunol. 139: 1479.
11. Lind, P., O. C. Hansen, and N. Horn. 1988. The binding of mouse hybridoma and human IgE antibodies to the major fecal allergen, Der p I, of Dermatophagoides pteronyssinus. J. Immunol. 140: 4256.
12. Heymann, P. W., M. D. Chapman, J. Fox, R. C. Aalberse, and T. A. E. Platts-Mills. 1989. Antigenic and structural analysis of Group II allergens (Der p II and Der f II) from house dust mites (Dermatophagoides spp.). J. Allergy Clin. Immunol., in press.
13. Tovey, E. R., and B. A. Baldo. 1987. Comparison by electroblotting of IgE binding components in extracts of house dust mite bodies and spent mite culture. J. Allergy Clin. Immunol. 79: 93.

Monoclonal Antibodies in Identification and Standardization of Allergens

*Lothar Jäger, Christian Diener, Wolf-Dieter Müller, and Gerhard Schlenvoigt**

Monoclonal antibodies (mabs) introduce new qualities into allergology because of their homogeneity, their identical production for unlimited time, and their availability in adequate amounts. Through mabs in the analysis of allergens, distinct epitopes could be identified—both IgE binding as well as cross-reacting between molecules from the same or different species. This capability can be used in standardization, circumventing the unpredictable influences of different pooled sera. This is presently possible in sensitization by a single allergen or mixtures containing immunodominant and/or cross-reacting structures. In other cases detailed information concerning the role of so-called minor allergens is necessary. Further applications are, for example, purification of allergens and quantification of natural exposure—besides their use in basic research.

The efforts to identify allergens and to standardize the allergic potential date back to the turn of the century. The most advanced approach at present are the recommendations of the Subcommittee on Allergen Standardization of the IUIS/WHO. They use conventional immunological techniques and International Standards as "yardsticks." What role do monoclonal antibodies play in this field? I shall restrict my presentation to two aspects:

— identification of allergens including the analysis of epitopes;

— standardization.

Identification of Allergens and Epitopes

Allergen-Specific Monoclonal Antibodies

Monoclonal antibodies (mabs) usually are derived from immunized rodents. Each antibody recognizes a distinct pattern of the antigen used for immunization. The advantages of mabs are their homogeneity, their identical production for almost unlimited time, and their availability in adequate amounts. The decisive quality of any mab is determined by the role of the epitope it recognizes.

We started to produce mabs for pollen allergens using timothy (*Phleum pratense*). The result of a typical fusion is shown in Figure 1. The mabs 1C4 and 1G2 would be useful to determine the content of timothy in mixed grass pollen. But this is no clinically relevant prob-lem, as the sensitization is not species-specific. The broad reactivity of the mabs 3H10 and 4D3 arises from their binding to widely distributed carbohydrate moieties. The most interesting mab from this fusion is D11 binding to all extracts from grass pollen investigated so far. By CRIE of extracts from timothy, it could be shown that this mab binds to major allergens. The number of mabs binding to allergens is steadily increasing. An international database for these mabs has been established at the Royal North Shore Hospital Sydney, Australia.

Epitope Mapping

Mabs are valuable tools in experimental immunology for analyzing antigens. By inhibition reactions up to 4 epitopes have been identified on several allergens.

IgE Binding Epitopes

Especially interesting are those investigations searching for IgE binding epitopes. The identification of the IgE binding (and inducing) structure could

— improve our insight into the mechanisms of sensitization,

---

* Department of Clinical Immunology, Friedrich Schiller University, Humboldtstrasse 3, DDR-6900 Jena, German Democratic Republic

Monoclonal antibodies

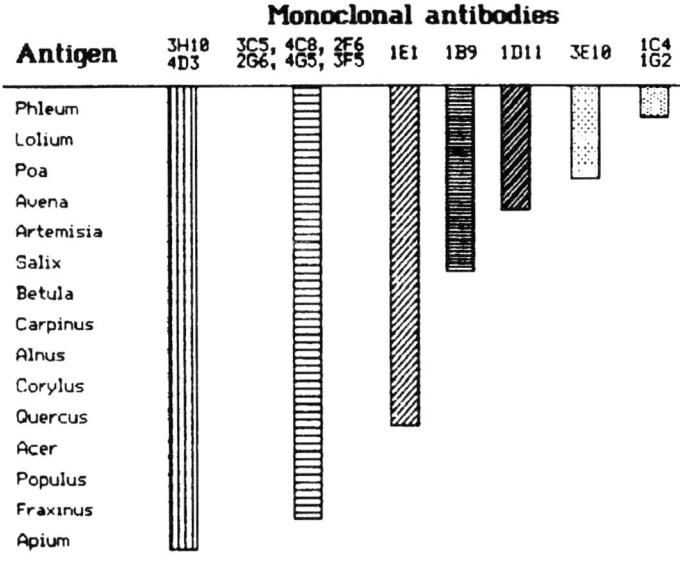

Figure 1. Spectrum of monoclonal antibodies derived from timothy-immunized mice.

Figure 2. Evaluation of IgE-binding epitopes (for details, see text).

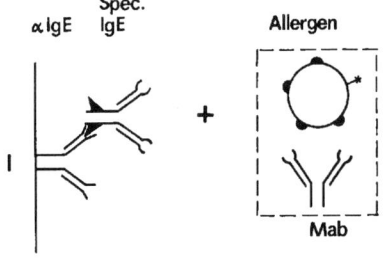

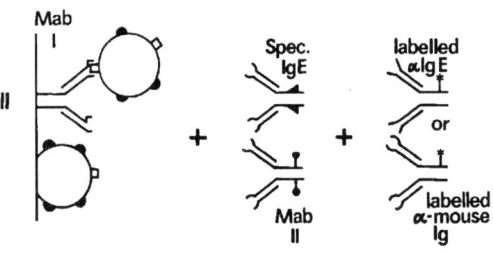

— solve the riddle of the mechanisms underlying immunotherapy,

— offer possibilities to synthesize antigens for diagnosis as well as for therapy.

The interference between mabs and IgE-ab is usually analyzed by sandwich assays (Figure 2). In the first variant, the IgE-ab is bound to the solid phase. By adding a mixture of mabs and labeled allergen, the competition of both ab can be evaluated. In the second variant, the allergen is bound to the solid phase—either directly or by means of an allergen-specific mab I. The solid phase thus prepared is incubated with a mixture of the mab II to be evaluated with varying amounts of IgE-containing sera vice versa. Their binding can be determined by adequately labeled antisera.

Surprisingly, most murine mabs do not interfere with human IgE. The interpretation of these negative results, however, must be cautious, as concentrations and affinities of the different populations of antibodies (abs) play an important role. Moreover, it could be that one binding site for IgE has been blocked by the mab, whereas those with different structures remain accessible. The reverse evaluation, therefore, is more conclusive. Our mab D11 did not interfere significantly. Similar results have been reported by Mazur et al. [12] for their mab to chironomidae. Contrary to the species-specific mabs in Chapman's experiments, there was a significant but limited interference between the mab to the cross-reacting structure of Der p I and human IgE-ab (mean inhibition 38%) [2]. Olson and Klapper [14] in their investigations in ragweed allergy provided evidence that the combination of mabs to two different binding sites increases the inhibition up to 80%. At least two binding sites have

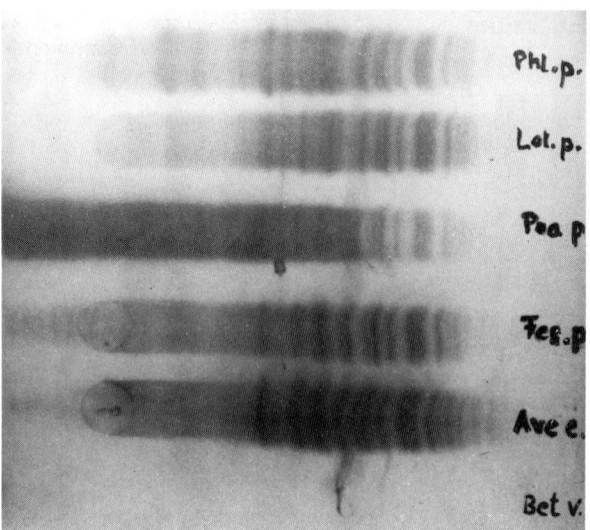

Phl. p.

Lol. p.

Poa p

Fes. p

Ave e.

Bet v.

Figure 3. Immunoblots of extracts from selected pollen using mab D11.

been identified on Lol p IV and Fer d I [8, 10]. Sera from different patients seem to differ in their binding preferences. Because of the polyclonality of the sera obtained from patients, such statements, however, are difficult to substantiate.

Cross-Reacting Epitopes

(a) *Cross-reactivity within the same species.* Using CRIE mab D11 binds at least to three different allergens. After purification by means of affinity chromatography, three fractions could be identified as Phl p V, VI and VII. Even higher (>10) is the number of fractions binding D11 after IEF. Their Mr ranges from 14 to 37 K. Haas et al. [6] identified all seven major allergens from timothy with a single mab. The mab of Lauzurica et al. [9] binds to two major allergens of olive—besides other fractions.

(b) *Cross-reacting epitopes in other species.* We could demonstrate that the global binding of mab D11 to other pollen identified by means of EIA is distributed to different fractions (Figure 3)—always including IgE-binding ones. Especially remarkable is that those fractions purified by means of affinity chromatography are able to absorb >90% of the total pollen-specific IgE-ab from a pooled serum from hayfever patients. All these results predispose this mab for standardization.

Similar results have been reported by Ekramodoullah et al. [5] starting from *Poa pratensis*—both concerning the cross-reactivity within the species as well as across species barriers.

This has been confirmed for several other grass pollens too [1, 6, 8, 13, 15]. These experiences can explain that patients with hayfever possess IgE-ab binding to pollen to which they have never been exposed before. Analogous cross-reactivities have been identified in parietaria [4], chironomides [12], and mites [11].

Although the information available up to now does not allow generalizations, it can be supposed that the number of IgE-binding epitopes is smaller than the number of allergens identified by means of CRIE or blotting procedures. The phenomena of "major" and "minor" allergens could be well explained by certain dissimilarities between the epitopes influencing the affinity of ab-binding.

Standardization

Standardization is indispensable for any improvement of diagnosis and immunotherapy in allergic diseases. The present tendency—backed by the IUIS/WHO—is to create international reference preparations to be used as "yardsticks" for national control authorities as well as producers. Such comparisons using RAST inhibition critically depend on the composition of IgE-abs in the serum pool used. CIE is similarly influenced by the specificity of the serum raised in animals. Comparison by skin test is biased by the population of patients tested. Can mabs help to circumvent these problems? The advantage of mabs depends on

412

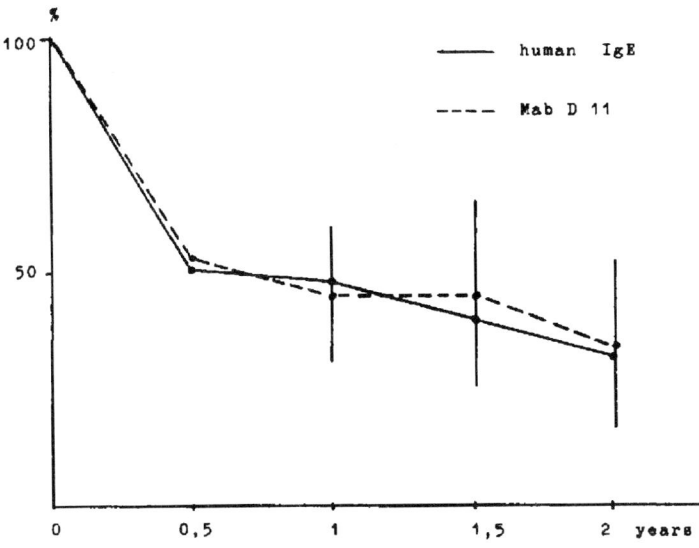

Figure 4. Evaluation of the stability of aluminium hydroxide-adsorbed pollenextract by pooled serum and mab D11.

the composition of the allergen to be analyzed. Different situations can be envisaged.

— *Situation A:* There is a single allergen only, maybe with a single epitope, e.g., a drug or another chemical compound. In principle, mabs would be advantageous if there were no alternative and more simple chemical reactions.

— *Situation B:* The allergenic potency in principle depends on a single (or a few) major allergen(s). This situation is covered in another paper.

— *Situation C:* The composition of the extract is more complex. However, there are cross-reactivities between the dominant allergens. This is the situation in allergies to grass pollen. As already demonstrated, our mab D11 binds to most major allergens of the pollen species investigated till now. We used this mab successfully, for example, to evaluate the binding of allergen to the adsorbate, to analyze degradation processes (Figure 4), to compare the allergenic potency of different extracts from Lolium within the IUIS/WHO collaborating study. An analogous situation seems to exist in house dust allergy—at least for the sensitization by house dust mites. Heyman et al. [7] demonstrated that 80–95% of patients with this allergy possess ab to cross-reacting structures of *Der. farinae* and *Der. pteronyssinus.* The same group [3] reported excellent correlations between the

combined determination of Der p I/Der f I and the cross-reacting P1Eq.

In these cases the application of adequate mabs can improve standardization by avoiding the problems of polyclonal sera or pooled sera, and by guaranteeing identical situations all over the world and for almost unlimited time. The application of a cocktail of mabs binding to the same allergen will increase the reproducibility.

The problems, however, are must more complicated in situations where a natural mixture of allergens induces quite different patterns of sensitization by non-cross-reacting allergens. Of course, it would be possible to develop a cocktail of mabs that are able to identify all allergens. As they are of varying importance in the individual patients, the global content of allergens determined in such a way would not be very meaningful. By investigating an adequate sample of patients, the quantitative contribution of the different allergens could be evaluated. But it would be a cumbersome procedure to develop an adequate composed mixture of mabs. We urgently need much more information on the real importance of those structures we call "minor" allergens—whether they can really induce symptoms independent of the "major" allergens. Without doubt such situations may exist. On the other hand, there are cross-reactions even between major allergens. We moved from the level of conventional extracts to the level of allergenic molecules.

The heterogeneity on this level, however, still has to be identified.

In spite of these limitations and uncertainties, we are convinced that the application of mabs will improve standardization of most clinically relevant allergens. Mabs already have begun to change our approaches to identification, analysis, and standardization of allergens. Taking into account their application in purification, in quantifying natural exposure—for example, in epidemiological investigations—there is no doubt that they improve clinical practice. Moreover, they will open up new possibilities in basic research.

References

1. Bose, R., A. K. M., Ekramoddoullah, F. T. Kisil, and A. H. Sehon. 1988. Human and murine antibodies to rye grass pollen allergen Lol p IV share a common idiotype. Immunology 63: 579.
2. Chapman, M. D., P. W. Heymann, and T. A. E. Platts-Mills. 1987. Epitope mapping of two major inhalant allergens, Der p I and Der f I, from mites of the genus *dermatophagoides*. J. Immunol. 139: 1479.
3. Chapman, M. D., P. W. Heymann, S. R. Wilkins, M. J. Brown, and T. A. E. Platts-Mills. 1987. Monoclonal immunoassays for major dust mite *(Dermatophagoides)* allergens, Der p I and Der f I, and quantitative analysis of the allergen content of mite and house dust extracts. J. Allergy Clin. Immunol. 80: 184.
4. Corbi, A. L., C. Cortes, J. Bousquet, A. Basomba, A. Cistero, J. Garcia-Selles, G. D'Amato, and J. Carreira. 1985. Allergenic cross-reactivity among pollens of *Urticaceae*. Int. Arch. Allergy appl. Immunol. 77: 377.
5. Ekramoddoullah, A. K. M., F. T. Kisil, and A. H. Sehon. 1986. Partial characterization of an antigenic site of high molecular weight basic antigen, a ryegrass pollen allergen, using a monoclonal antibody. Molec. Immunol. 23: 111.
6. Haas, H., W.-M. Becker, H. J. Maasch, and M. Schlaak. 1986. Analysis of allergen components

in grass pollen extracts using immunoblotting. Int. Arch. Allergy appl. Immunol. 79: 434.
7. Heymann, P. W., M. D. Champan, and T. A. E. Platts-Mills. 1986. Antigen Der f I from the dust mite *Dermatophagoides farinae*: Structural comparison with Der p I from *Dermatophagoides pteronyssinus* and epitope specificity of murine IgG and human IgE antibodies. J. Immunol. 137: 2841.
8. Jaggi, K. S., A. K. M. Ekramoddoullah, F. T. Kisil, J. M. M. Dzuba-Fischer, E. S. Rector, and A. H. Sehon. 1988. Identification of two distinct allergenic sites of a rye grass pollen allergen, Lol p IV (abstr.). J. Allergy Clin. Immunol. 81: 307.
9. Lauzurica, P., C. Gurbindo, N. Maruri, B. Galocha, R. Diaz, J. Gonzalez, R. Garcia, and C. Lahoz. 1988. Olive *(Olea europae)* pollen allergens. I. Immunochemical characterization by immunoblotting, CRIE and immunodetection by a monoclonal antibody. Molec. Immunol. 25: 329.
10. Li, Y., and M. D. Chapman. 1988. Epitope mapping of the major feline salivary allergen, Fel d I (abstr.). J. Allergy Clin. Immunol. 81: 308.
11. Lind, P., O. C. Hansen, and N. Horn. 1988. The binding of mouse hypridoma and human IgE to the major fecal allergen, Der p I, of *Dermatophagoides pteronyssinus*. J. Immunol. 140: 4256.
12. Mazur, G., W.-M. Becker, and X. Baur. 1987. Epitope mapping of major insect allergens (chironomid hemoglobins) with monoclonal antibodies. J. Allergy Clin. Immunol. 80: 876.
13. Mecheri, S., G. Peltre, A. Weyer, and B. David. 1985. Production of a monoclonal antibody against a major allergen on *Dactylis glomerata* pollen (Dg1). Ann. Inst. Pasteur 136C: 195.
14. Olson, J. R., and D. G. Klapper. 1986. Two major human allergenic sites on ragweed pollen allergen antigen E identified by using monoclonal antibodies. J. Immunol. 136: 2109.
15. Singh, M. B., and R. B. Knox. 1985. Grass pollen allergens. Antigenic relationships detected using monoclonal antibodies and dot blotting immunoassay. Int. Arch. Allergy appl. Immunol. 78: 300.

In vitro Diagnosis of Atopic Allergy

S. G. O. Johansson*

Quantitative determination of IgE and IgE antibody in serum are well-established methods in the diagnostic work up of a possible allergic patient. In the first step, the atopic state of the patient is established. An elevated serum level of IgE or a positive Phadiatop test, which has a sensitivity above 90% for inhalant allergy, is highly indicative of atopy. A total IgE determination is the only in vitro test for atopy that is independent of the allergen specificity of the sensitization. It is therefore useful in allergy to foods and rare allergens, e.g., occupational allergy.

Recently, the Pharmacia CAP System was developed. Clinical studies have shown that about 10% more relevant allergies are detected than by RAST. Some studies report a correlation between IgE antibody concentration as measured by the CAP-System and severity of disease, findings that should be further studied.

The presence of an active principle, later called reagin, present in the serum of persons with allergy and capable of mediating immediate hypersensitivity reactions, was suggested in 1921 when Prausnitz and Kustner performed their classic experiment of passively sensitizing human skin with serum from an allergic person. It was not until the late 1960s, however, that the nature of the reagin was revealed and the fifth immunoglobulin class, IgE, was officially recognized [1].

The Diagnosis of Atopy

A basic characteristic of an individual suffering from classic allergy is the atopic constitution. An atopic individual has a genetically determined tendency to develop IgE antibodies in response to contact with naturally occurring protein antigens in low concentration, and such as person is prone to develop allergic diseases such as asthma, rhinoconjunctivitis, urticaria, atopic dermatitis, and anaphylactic reactions. The genetic background is complex, and an atopic person is therefore best identified via immune response: an increased total IgE level or an IgE sensitization to a common, naturally occurring allergen. The diagnosis of atopy should be the first step in the medical work up of a patient with hypersensitivity symptoms, because only in atopic allergy can a specific sensitizing factor be detected and specific hyposensitization therapy be expected to be effective.

IgE Levels in Serum

The usefulness of IgE determination in clinical practice was first suggested by a study on IgE in serum from patients with asthma [2]. Patients with atopic allergy such as asthma, hay fever, eczema, urticaria, and anaphylactic reactions often have elevated serum concentrations of IgE [3]. The more intensive the allergen exposure, the higher the total IgE concentration, and variations of up to two- to three-fold have been seen in patients with hay fever during the pollen season. Thus, the IgE level is correlated to the degree of immune stimulation—not only the degree of allergen exposure but also the number of allergens to which the patient is allergic—and to the severity of the patient's symptoms. Also, an IgE determination is the only test for atopy that is independent of the allergen specificity of the sensitization.

The specificity of a test for IgE in the diagnosis of atopy is influenced by the fact that high IgE concentrations are regularly found, not only in patients with atopic disorders, but also in patients with parasitic infestations [4]. Much less pronounced influence on IgE production is exerted by bacterial and viral infections. In mononucleosis, such an increase in non-antibody-specific IgE is regularly seen. Usually, viral-induced IgE is polyclonal, but specific IgE

* Department of Clinical Immunology, Karolinska Hospital, S-10401 Stockholm, Sweden.
Acknowledgements: This work was supported by grants from the Swedish Medical Research Council (grant 16X–105), the Swedish Work Environment Fund and the Swedish National Association against Heart and Chest Diseases.

antibodies have been reported to antigens of, for example, respiratory syncytial virus, rubella, pertussis, and others.

Specific Sensitization as an Indication of Atopy

Since an atopic individual is capable of producing IgE-antibodies to naturally occurring inhalant allergens, the diagnosis of atopy could be based on the detection of such a sensitization. Skin test panels of common allergens is one approach but recently an in vitro test has become available which is very useful in this context. Phadiatop® (Pharmacia Diagnostics AB, Uppsala, Sweden) is a RAST disc to which common inhalant allergens can be detected in one test. When Phadiatop was compared to case history and skin and provocation tests, a sensitivity and specificity of more than 90% for detection of inhalent atopy in adults was found [5]. However, since the test does not detect food allergy, it is not so useful in very young infants. Also, in certain occupational environments workers exposed to high concentrations of unique allergens might become sensitized although their atopy is of such a low grade that they have not produced IgE antibodies to common allergens.

Allergen Specific Diagnosis

Methodological Aspects

The radioallergosorbent test, RAST, was described by Wide et al. [6] as a technique for determining IgE antibody in serum. It was suggested that RAST be used as an in vitro diagnostic test for atopic allergy. Extensive investigations all over the world have confirmed this prediction.

Several reagents are of critical importance for the quality of the RAST test. One is the solid matrix used for the allergen. The matrix should have a high protein-binding capacity, the protein allergen should be covalently linked to the matrix, and the nonspecific trapping of IgE should be minimal. The quality of the allergen preparation is also important, but with use of the RAST test it is possible to obtain reproducible allergen preparations. There should be

an excess of allergen on the solid phrase which will lead to optimal sensitivity of the RAST test.

Certain allergen extracts, such as bacterial preparations, might contain substances that bind IgE or anti-IgE in a non-allergen-antibody fashion. Protein A from *Staphylococcus aureus* is one example [7]. Thus, detection of IgE binding to RAST discs coated with bacterial extracts does not necessarily prove the presence of an IgE antibody. Similar problems may arise when extracts of certain vegetable containing lectins are used.

The specificity of the anti-IgE antibody used in RAST is also of great importance. In our experience the highest sensitivity is obtained with an anti-IgE having Dϵ2 specificity.

Recently, a new method for quantitative determination of IgE antibody was reported—the Pharmacia CAP System (Pharmacia Diagnostics AB, Uppsala, Sweden) based on the RAST principle. The solid phase consists of a flexible hydrophilic carrier polymer encased in a capsule. The cellulose derivative of the carrier is CNBr-activated, and its protein binding capacity is very high—at least three times that of a corresponding filter paper disc and approximately 50 times that of a passively coated plastic surface. The micro environment of the capsule allows rapid kinetics, and the technique has the potential of incubation times in the order of minutes. The high protein-binding capacity ensures that every allergen can be presented in allergen excess and therefore expression of the IgE antibody concentration in kU of IgE is meaningful.

The usefulness of the CAP-System for allergy diagnosis based on a quantitative measurement of IgE antibody in serum was recently evaluated [8]. The correlation between the results obtained with the new system and with Phadebas RAST (Pharmacia Diagnostics AB, Uppsala, Sweden) was very good, but the new test was more sensitive. Of the 6838 tests compared the CAP-System was positive in 564 tests (8%) in which RAST was negative. Of these, 470 occurred in patients that were classified as allergic. The results of such a comparison obtained in one of the studies is illustrated in Figure 1. Most of the 470 tests were significant for the symptoms of the patient present at the time of the investigation but in some cases no obvious correlation was noticed. Further studies should be performed to evaluate the precise

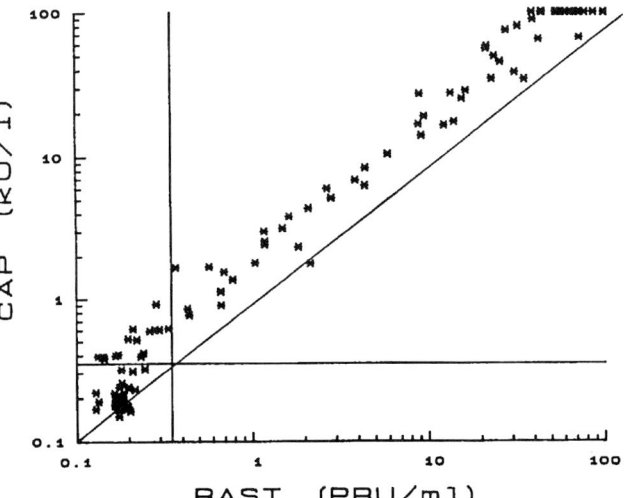

Figure 1. The relation between IgE antibody levels to timothy allergen as measured by RAST and the Pharmacia CAP System. Data from [8].

Table 1. Some new, well-documented, mainly airborne allergens, many of which are important occupational allergens now available in RAST.

Animals	*Occupational*	*Miscellaneous*
Hamster	Castor bean	Barn dust mites
Mouse	Green coffee bean	—Acarus siro
Rat	Isocyanates	—Lepidoglyphus destructor
Rabbit	—TDI	—Tyrophagus putrescentiae
Budgerigar	—MDI	—Glycyphagus domesticus
Chicken	—HDI	House dust mites
Duck	Phthalic anhydride	—Euroglyphus maynei
Goose	Trimellitic anhydride	Other insects
	Formaldehyde	—Cockroach
Drugs	Silk	—Mosquitos
Insulin	Weeping willow	—Trogoderma
Ispaghula laxative	Latex	—Chironomus
		Silverfish

clinical importance of an IgE-sensitization in relation to the natural history of the allergic disease.

Several studies reported a correlation between the concentration of IgE antibodies as measured by the CAP-System and the severity of the allergic disease [8], thus confirming early observations [9]. There seems to be a relationship between the sum of IgE antibodies specific to various allergens and the degree of involvement of mucosal membranes in respiratory allergic diseases. It is possible that a quantitative value of the IgE sensitization is a useful parameter for the evaluation of the allergic inflammation of an allergic disease. If this is found to be the case in further studies, information on the concentration of IgE antibody in circulation will be useful not only for the diagnosis of an atopic allergy as such, but also be one important factor in the evaluation of the allergic inflammation.

RAST in Allergy Diagnosis

Already in the first study of the RAST test it was found that patients with clinically relevant atopic allergies were RAST positive. This finding led to several hundreds of studies on the value of RAST in allergy diagnosis and this test is now a well established routine diagnostic procedure all over the world. Several hundreds of allergens have been applied successfully in RAST; some inhalant allergens mainly occurring in occupational environments are presented in the Table 1.

417

Allergy to the house dust mite (*Dermatophagoides pteronyssinus* and *D. farinae*) is a well-known and great clinical problem. However, also several species of storage mites have been suspected to be allergenic. About 50,000 species of mites have been described. The three most commonly found in barn dust in Europe and Asia are *Lepidoglyphus destructor*, *Acarus siro*, and *Tyrophagus putrescentiae*. In a study of farmers on the Swedish island of Gotland in the Baltic Sea, the prevalence of allergy to storage mites among all farmers was 6.2% and among atopic farmers 37.8% [10]. *Lepidoglyphus destructor* was the species that most often gave a positive RAST. No significant cross-reaction was found in RAST inhibition studies between *L. destructor* and *G. domesticus* on one hand and *D. pteronyssinus* on the other [11]. The major allergens of *L. destructor* were found to have molecular weights in the order of 16,000–18,000 daltons using SDS-PAGE and immunoblotting [12]. The house dust mite *Euroglyphus maynei* was also found to be a common cause of asthma and rhinitis among the farmers on Gotland. The prevalence of allergy to *E. maynei* among all farmers was 4.5% compared to 5.2% for allergy to *D. pteronyssinus* [13].

In addition to allergy to classic airborne allergens, atopic individuals may develop allergy to very special allergens to which they are exposed in certain environments. A typical example is occupational asthma and rhinitis. Since the allergen load in an occupational setting often is high also persons with a low degree of atopy might react. Examples of occupational inhalant allergens are given in the table. Under very special circumstances an individual might be exposed to an allergenic substance by injection. A hymenoptera sting is a classic example, but low molecular weight compounds, such as ethylene oxide and formaldehyde, leaking from plastic tubings after sterilization is another, quite common allergy. Prevalence figures for IgE-mediated, RAST-positive allergy to ethylene oxide among patients undergoing chronic haemodialysis or plasma donors are as high as 10–20%. Similar figures were reported for allergy to formaldehyde when this chemical was used for sterilization. Most cases with asthma reacting to formaldehyde probably are hyperreactive, but formaldehyde has been reported to be an occupational allergen probably sensitizing by inhalation.

References

1. Bennich, H., K. Ishizaka, S. G. O. Johansson, D. S. Rowe, D. R. Stanworth, and W. D. Terry. 1968. Immunoglobulin E. A new class of human immunoglobulin. Bull. Wld. Hlth. Org. 38: 151.

2. Johansson, S. G. O. 1967. Raised levels of a new immunoglobulin class (IgND) in asthma. Lancet II: 951.

3. Johansson, S. G. O., H. Bennich, and T. Berg. 1972. The clinical significance of IgE. Prog. Clin. Immunol. 1: 157.

4. Johansson, S. G. O., T. Mellbin, and B. Wahlquist. 1968. Immunoglobulin levels in Ethiopian preschool children with special reference to high concentrations of immunoglobulin E (IgND). Lancet ii: 1118.

5. Duc, J., R. Peitrequin, and A. Pécoud. 1988. Value of a new screening test for respiratory allergy. Allergy 43: 332.

6. Wide, L., H. Bennich, and S. G. O. Johansson. 1967. Diagnosis of allergy by an in vitro test for allergen antibodies. Lancet ii: 105.

7. Johansson, S. G. O., and M. Inganäs. 1978. Interaction of polyclonal human IgE with protein-A from *Taphylococcus aureus*. Immunol. Rev. 41: 248.

8. Johansson, S. G. O. (Eds.). 1988. Clinical Workshop. IgE antibodies and the Pharmacia CAP System in allergy diagnosis. Sputnic AB Projects, Stockholm, Sweden.

9. Norman, P. S., L. M. Lichtenstein, and K. Ishizaka. 1973. Comparisons of specific IgE antibodies, leukocyte sensitivity by histamine release, direct skin test, and symptoms in hay fever. In: Mechanisms in allergy—Reagin-mediated hypersensitivity. L. Goodfriend, A. H. Sehon, and R. P. Orange, eds. New York: Marcel Dekker, p. 151.

10. van Hage-Hamsten, M., S. G. O. Johansson, S. Höglund, P. Tull, A. Wirén, and O. Zetterström. 1985. Storage mite allergy is common in a farming population. Clinical Allergy 15: 555.

11. van Hage-Hamsten, M., S. G. O. Johansson, E. Johansson, and A. Wirén. 1987. Lack of allergenic cross-reactivity between storage mites and Dermatophagoides pteronyssinus. Clinical Allergy 17: 23.

12. Johansson, E., M. van Hage-Hamsten, and S. G. O. Johansson. 1988. The prevalence of allergy and IgE antibodies to inhalant allergens in Swedish school-children. Acta Ped. Scand. 75: 349.

13. van Hage-Hamsten, M., and Johansson, S. G. O. 1988. Clinical significance and allergenic cross-reactivity and other non-pyroglyphid and pyroglyphid mites. J. Allergy Clin. Immunol., in press.

Crossreactivity of IgE Antibodies

*Rob C. Aalberse**

A steadily increasing number of crossreactivities of IgE antibodies are becoming apparent. Many of these are quite unexpected. These crossreactions have practical implications for the diagnosis and treatment of IgE-mediated disease. From a more theoretical point of view, these crossreactions are interesting because they might provide a mechanism for the induction of IgE antibodies via crossreactive priming. Two examples are discussed in more detail: (1) sensitization toward potato with a possibly causal relation to the development of IgE antibodies to grass pollen; (2) sensitization toward pork with a possibly causal relation to the development of IgE antibodies to cat dander.

Examples of Crossreactivity

The existence of crossreactive IgE antibodies to a wide variety of allergens is well established now (e.g., [1–14] and references in those papers). Examples are:

— chicken egg yolk—caged bird serum proteins [6, 11]. Perhaps not completely unexpected, but yet with clearcut practical implications: egg yolk sensitivity without egg white sensitivity in an adult strongly suggests an allergy toward caged birds. This might be an example of an inhalant allergen inducing an allergy toward foods [6].

— birch—apple [5, 8, 9]. Here again the history of these cross-allergies suggest that the inhalant allergen upon prolonged allergen provocation induces the food allergy. Apart from apples many stony fruits like cherries and apricots are involved.

— grass—potato/tomato [3, 5, 13]. This will be discussed in more detail later on.

— weeds—celery [10]. In this situation the food

sensitivity may be severe. A relation with spices is possible [12].

— caddisfly (inhalant insect allergen)–crab and other shellfish [4].

— pork—cat [14]. This is another example that will be discussed in more detail below.

Mechanistic Questions and Implications

An intriguing question is whether IgE antibodies are more crossreactive than other isotypes. If the answer were "Yes," the obvious question would be: "Why?" It might indicate that there would be less affinity maturation in the IgE response and/or a preference for conserved epitopes by lack of evolutionary pressure. Another possibility would be that the induction of IgE antibodies would be facilitated by crossreactive priming (see below).

Another problem posed by crossreactivity between allergens is whether mast cell triggering can be accomplished. I will take the birch—apple crossreactivity as an example, assuming that this starts with a specific (i.e., non-crossreactive) birch pollen allergy. Upon continuing pollen stimulation, IgE antibodies against other epitopes will develop, some of which will be crossreactive with an epitope on an apple antigen. Assuming that the apple antigen is a single-chain molecule, one would expect at least two crossreactive epitopes recognized by two different crossreactive IgE antibodies in patients with apple sensitivity. Since some patients have no apple-specific IgE at all, one would predict that there are some patients with just one crossreactive IgE antibody; these patients would be crossreactive in a serologic test (RAST) but not in a bioassay (skin test,

* Central Laboratory of the Netherlands Red Cross Blood Transfusion Service and Laboratory for Clinical and Experimental Immunology, University of Amsterdam, NL-1006 Amsterdam, The Netherlands.
Acknowledgements: Many of the experimental results on which the ideas presented in this overview are based or were obtained by former or present co-workers at the CLB: M. Aalbers, A. M. van den Bosch, P. G. Calkhoven, P. Kant, V. L. Koshte, O. Pos, R. van Ree, S. O. Stapel, A. W van Toorenenbergen and J. S. van der Zee. Clinical support for these investigations was provided by R. W. Griffioen, S. L. Kagen, J. C. van Nierop, H. D. Oei, A. P. Oranje P. P. M. Schilte and J. L. Yntema. Financial support was provided by the Netherlands Asthma Foundation, grant 83.26.

basophil test). We did not identify such a patient as yet.

Concepts for discussion: (1) Crossreactive priming and (2) the Trojan horse.

1. *Crossreactive priming.* The hypothesis is that prior immunization with an antigen induces an enhanced immune responsiveness toward a crossreactive antigen. The resulting antibodies are not necessarily crossreactive.

2. *Trojan Horse.* The postulate is that sensitization toward one allergen may enhance the response toward other antigens present on the same particle. This hypothesis is an extension of the "gatekeeper"-hypothesis [15]. The overall effect would be that an IgE-allergen interaction at a mucosal membrane may "open the gates" for other allergens that happen to be near, i.e., originated from the same allergen-carrying particle. Examples of such "Trojan Horses" are: a pollen grain, a mite decal pellet, and a cat skin flake.

These two concepts might be relevant for understanding the generation of a complex IgE response. The hypothesis is that this is a two-step process:

1. response toward a *primary allergen,* facilitated by crossreactive priming;

2. response toward *secondary allergens,* facilitated by "Trojan Horse"-effect.

One example illustrating how a complex IgE response to grass pollen might develop is the case of potato/tomato sensitivity in children with grass pollinosis [5] and particularly in children that will subsequently develop grass pollinosis [13]. The first sensitization would be against foods. Crossreactive IgE antibodies would develop. Upon contact between this crossreactive IgE and a pollen grain in the airway mucosa, other antigen from the pollen grain would enter the site of the local allergic reaction and IgE antibodies against these other, non-crossreactive components would develop.

Another example is that of the development of an IgE response to the cat allergen Fel d I (Cat1) in children with pork sensitivity [14]. The Fel d I molecule itself is not particularly crossreactive; only reactivity with other feline species has been found (H. de Groot, personal communication). However, a marked crossreactivity was found between cat serum and pig serum, especially in young children. We iden-

tified 4 children with a transient IgE response to cat serum who subsequently developed IgE antibodies to Fel d I. A transient IgE response is typical for a food response. In these children we found a transient IgE response to pork and pig serum (but not beef or bovine serum). By RAST-inhibition we found that pork serum inhibited the cat-serum RAST. In this case the crossreactive antibodies to pig serum proteins, by crossreaction with cat serum proteins present on the cat skin flake, would have "opened the gates" for Fel d I. Interestingly, mouse ascites was also found to crossreact with these IgE antibodies.

References

1. Aalberse, R. C., V. Koshte, and J. G. J. Clemens. 1981. Cross-reactions between vegetable foods, pollen and bee venom due to IgE antibodies to a ubiquitous carbohydrate determinant. Int. Archs. Allergy appl. Immun. 66 (Suppl. 1): 259–260.

2. Aalberse, R. C., V. Koshte, & J. G. J. Clemens. 1981. Immunoglobulin E antibodies that crossreact with vegetable foods, pollen, and Hymenoptera venom. J. Allergy Clin. Immunol. 68: 356–364.

3. Aalberse, R. C., P. Kant, & V. Koshte. 1983. Unexpected cross-reactions of human IgE antibodies. In Recent developments in RAST and other solid-phase immunoassay systems. D.M. Kemeny and M.H. Lessof, eds. Excerpta Medica Amsterdam, pp. 17–25.

4. Koshte, V. L., S. L. Kagen, & R. C. Aalberse. 1988. Crossreactivity of IgE antibodies to Caddisfly with arthropoda and mollusca. J. Allergy Clin. Immunol., in press.

5. Calkhoven, P. G., M. Aalbers, V. L. Koshte, O. Pos, H. D. Oei, & R. C. Aalberse. 1987. Cross-reactivity among birch pollen, vegetables and fruits as detected by IgE antibodies is due to at least three distinct cross-reactive structures. Allergy 42: 382–390.

6. De Maat-Bleeker, F., A. G. van Dijk, & L. Berrens. 1985. Allergy to egg yolk possibly induced by sensitization to bird serum antigens. Ann. Allergy 54: 245–248.

7. De Martino, M., E. Novembre, G. Cozza, A. de Marco, P. Bonazza, & A. Vierrucci. 1988. Sensitivity to tomato and peanut allergens in children monosensitized to grass pollen. Allergy 43: 206–213.

8. Eriksson, N. H. Formgren, & E. Svenonius 1982. Food hypersensitivity in patients with pollen allergy. Allergy 37: 437–443.

9. Lahti, A., F. Bjorksten, & M. Hannuksela. 1980. Allergy to birch pollen and apple,and cross-reactivity of the allergens studied with the RAST. Allergy 35: 297–300.
10. Pauli, G., J. C. Bessot, A. Dietemann-Molard, P. A. Braun, & R. Thierry. 1985. Celery sensitivity: Clinical and immunological correlations with pollen allergy. Clin. Allergy 15: 273–279.
11. Van Toorenenbergen, A. W., R. Gerth van Wijk, G. van Dooremalen, & P. H. Dieges. 1985. Immunoglobulin E antibodies against budgerigar and canary feathers. Int. Arch. Allergy Appl. Immunol. 77: 433–437.
12. Van Toorenenbergen, A. W., & P. H. Dieges. 1987. Demonstration of spice-specific IgE in patients with suspected food allergies. J. Allergy Clin. Immunol. 79: 108–113.
13. Calkhoven, P. G., M. Aalbers, V. L. Koshte, R. van Ree, & R. C. Aalberse. Does sensitization by crossreacting antigens in foods predispose to the development of IgE antibodies to grass pollen. In preparation.
14. Stapel, S. O., P. G. Calkhoven, M. Aalbers, & R. C. Aalberse. Induction of IgE antibodies to cat allergens by pork. In preparation.
15. Steinberg, P. K. Ishizaka, & P. S. Norman. 1974. Possible role of IgE-mediated reaction in immunity. J. Allergy 54: 359–366.

421

Improved Immuno-Detection Methods in Allergy Diagnosis

B. David, G. Peltre, J. P. Dandeu, J. Rabillon, X. Desvaux*

Several immunochemical techniques are now available to detect and quantify IgE-specific antibodies, based upon radioimmunoassays [1] or enzymoimmunoassays [2]. Other techniques were developed to study the allergen (and/or antigen) heterogeneity in complex crude extracts responsible for immediate-type hypersensitivity in humans and also to characterize allergenic molecules. First, we show one application of the use of the immunoprint technique and then present another approach using the combination of crossed immunoelectrophoretic methods.

The Nitrocellulose Immunoprint Technique

Our technique is based upon agarose isoelectric focusing (IEF) with a transfer to nitrocellulose (NC) sheet by pressure blotting [3].

Materials and Methods

Allergenic Extracts

A grass pollen soluble extract was obtained by stirring 50 mg of *D. glomerata* pollen from our own production, suspended in 450 µl of distilled water for 1 h at room temperature. A mite soluble extract was obtained from a whole mite culture of *D. farinae* as previously described for *D. pteronyssinus* crude extract [4], lyophilized, and dissolved in distilled water to a protein content of 50 mg/ml. The *D. glomerata* and *D. farinae* extracts were centrifuged for 5 min at 9000 g just before use.

Patient Selection

Anti-*D. glomerata* sera were obtained from *D. glomerata*-pollen-sensitive patients whose radioallergosorbent tests (RAST, Pharmacia) were of class IV, with total IgE levels less than 200 IU/ml. Anti-*D. farinae* sera were obtained from *D. farinae*-sensitive patients with different RAST class values and total IgE levels less than 400 IU/ml.

Agarose Isoelectrofocusing

IEF on thin agarose gels was performed as described by Peltre et al. [3] in a mixture of carrier ampholytes ranging from pH 3 to 10. Two percent Servalyt pH 3 to 7 carrier ampholytes (Serva), were used for IEF of the *D. farinae* extract. Extracts (200 µl) were applied on the gel at 2 cm from the anode parallel to the electrodes (10 cm × 10 cm gel). The IEF separation was performed at 4 °C at a constant power of 4 W for 90 min. Then, the separated components were transferred onto the nitrocellulose membranes.

Cyanogen Bromide (CNBr) Activated Sheets

Previously, a technique was described to activate the nitrocellulose membranes (a-NC) [5]. Ten g of CNBr (Merck) were dissolved, under a hood in 600 ml of distilled water at room temperature. Under constant stirring and pH monitoring, two NC sheets were immersed in the CNBr solution and 20 ml of 1 N NaHCO$_3$ solution. Two other sheets were immersed in the CNBr solution and 20 ml of 1 N NaOH added. This procedure was repeated for a total of sixteen sheets. The a-NC sheets were washed 3 times in 5 mM NaHCO$_3$, dehydrated by blotting between filter papers, dried overnight at 37 °C and stored in sealed plastic bags at –20 °C.

Activated-Nitrocellulose Immunoprints

A print of the agarose gel was taken on a nitrocellulose (a-NC) sheet by blotting and pressing. The a-NC sheet was finally dried 15 minutes under a fan in order to bind efficiently the

---

*   Department of Immuno-Allergy, Institut Pasteur, Paris, France.

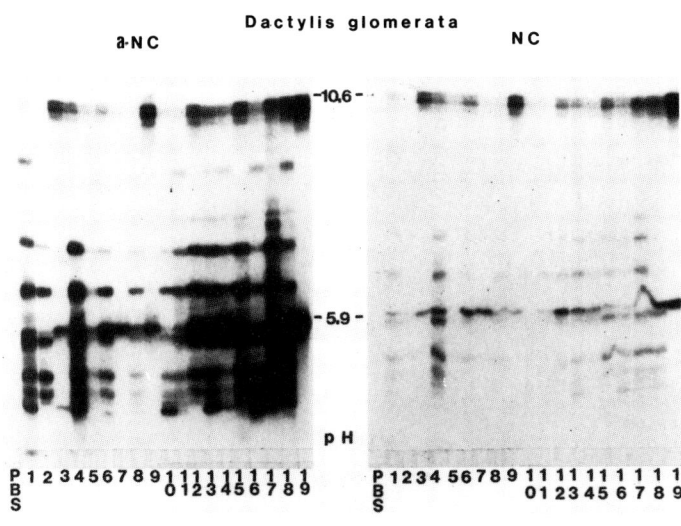

Dactylis glomerata

a-NC

NC

pH

P 1 2 3 4 5 6 7 8 9 1 1 1 1 1 1 1 1 1 1
B   0 1 2 3 4 5 6 7 8 9
S

P 1 2 3 4 5 6 7 8 9 1 1 1 1 1 1 1 1 1 1
B   0 1 2 3 4 5 6 7 8 9
S

Figure 1. Autoradiography of *D. glomerata* allergen IEF patterns after transfer onto NC and a-NC membranes.

allergens onto the a-NC. The a-NC print was then cut into strips. The strips were removed from the dried agarose gel by soaking in saturation solution (1% BSA or 5% defatted dry milk), 0.1% Tween 20 in phosphate buffered saline (PBS) pH 7.4 for 1 h at 45 °C. Each strip was incubated overnight with 100 µl of individual patient serum diluted 1/10 in PBS, 0.1% Tween 20, 1% BSA at room temperature. After incubation, the strips were washed three times in saline-0.1% Tween 20. All the antibodies detections were made at room temperature.

a) *IgE detection:* The strips were incubated with 20,000 cpm/strip of ^{125}I rabbit labelled anti-IgE (Pharmacia), for 2 h, washed three times in saline 0.1% Tween 20, dried, and then submitted to autoradiography for 5 days at – 70 °C in one cassette with an intensifier screen.

b) *IgA and IgM detection:* The strips were incubated with peroxydase-labeled sheep anti-IgA or anti-IgM (Diagnostic Pasteur) 1/1000 in PBS, 0.1% Tween 20, 1% BSA for 1 h, washed four times in saline-0.1% Tween 20, and detected by diamino benzidine (DAB) (Sigma): 10 mg in 20 ml phosphate buffer 0.1 M, pH 7.4, 30 µl of 30% H_2O_2.

c) *IgG subclasses detection:* The strips were incubated with monoclonal antibodies from mouse (anti IgG1, IgG3, IgG4, Unipath) and anti IgG2 (BioMakoor), 1/1000 in PBS, 0.1% Tween 20, 1% BSA for 1 h, washed and incubated with a second antibody (peroxydase

labeled rabbit anti-mouse globulin (Dakopatt), 1/500 in PBS, 0.1% Tween 20, 1% BSA. After washing, the detection was performed with DAB staining.

Results

To illustrate the use of the immunoprint technique, we analyzed allergens from a grass pollen *D. glomerata*. Bound radioactivity counts and immunoprinting patterns (Figure 1) clearly show a higher recognition of the allergens by anti-*D. glomerata* IgE when the transfer had been performed on activated nitrocellulose (a-NC) membranes than on native NC membranes. The intensity of the allergen bands detected on the native NC strips was generally enhanced on the a-NC membranes and, in addition, new allergen bands appeared. Detection of the allergens around pI 10.6 was not as strongly enhanced as the less basic allergens. The enhancement of bound radioactivity depended upon the sera employed, ranging from 25 cpm (serum 5) to 650 cpm (serum 17). For some sera (10 and 11) no specific radioactivity was found on the native NC membranes as compared with the negative controls, while a fair amount of radioactivity was bound onto the a-NC membranes.

With the same immunoprint technique used for the detection of the *D. glomerata* allergens, a few positive immunoprint patterns with mite *D. farinae* allergen bands were observed after

423

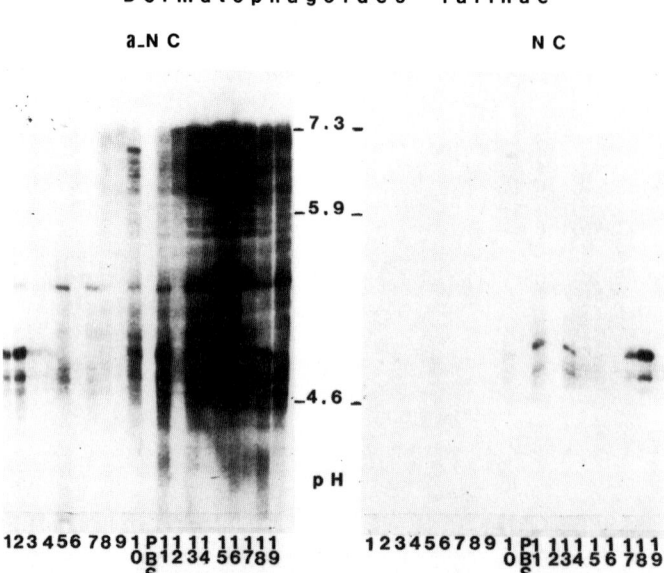

Dermatophagoïdes farinae

a_N C   NC

Figure 2. Autoradiography of *D. farinae* allergen IEF patterns after transfer onto NC and a-NC membranes.

transfer on native NC membranes (Figure 2). In comparison with crossed radioimmunoelectrophoresis or SAS-PAGE, this technique was not considered optimal. Allergens already detected on native NC were stained darker on the a-NC, whereas many sera showed a positive immunoprint pattern, including sera of RAST class II. Some allergens not detectable on native NC were detected on a-NC pI between 4.6 and 7.3. A new allergen at pI 5.4, which was not detected on native NC could be recognized on a-NC by sera from 12 of the 19 patients. The detection of these allergens may be due to the fact that owing to hydrophilic properties they are not bound to native NC membrane whereas on the a-NC membranes they might be covalently linked. In some cases, e.g., serum 6, neither allergen nor bound radioactivity could be detected, even on a-NC because the *D. farinae* extract was dissolved in distilled water to be suitable for IEF, and some of the less soluble allergens may not have been solubilized under these conditions. So, the a-NC membranes offer great potential for immunoprint techniques because of their improved binding capacities (up to 10 times) in comparison with untreated native NC membranes.

This improved native blotting technique was also used to study the specificity of different classes of antibodies present in the patients sera. The specificity of IgE and IgG4 antibodies was compared in 10 patients selected and

IgE   IgG4

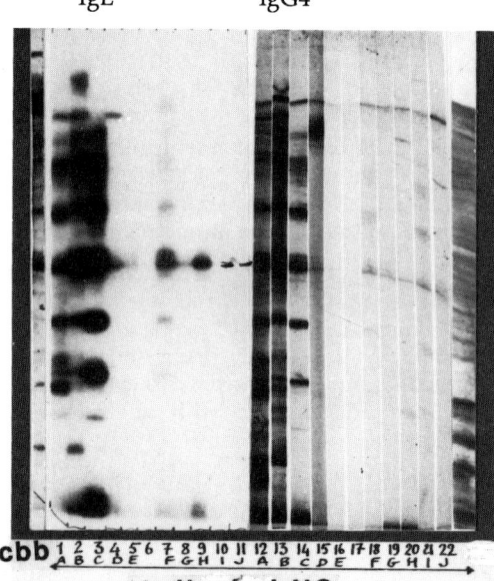

Activated NC

Figure 3. Comparison between IgE and IgG4 antigen spectra. A, B, C, D, E, F, G, H, I, J: Individual sera; cbb: Coomassie brilliant blue staining of pollen components; pbs: control (sera 6 and 17).

ordered following the decreasing heterogeneity of the grass pollen allergens recognized by these antibodies (Figure 3). Concerning the comparison between IgE and IgG4 antigen spectra, there is a noticeable similarity of these two antigen spectra. Most of the pollen components recognized by IgE are also detected by IgG4. The antigen spectra obtained with IgG1, IgG2, and IgG3 showed not obvious relationship with the allergen spectrum. Furthermore, a very high heterogeneity was observed in the antigens detected by the IgA and IgM classes of our patients, with no clear relationship to their allergen spectra.

Identification of Allergenic Components Using Crossed Immuno-Electrophoresis (CIE), Crossed Line Immuno-Electrophoresis (CLIE), and Crossed Radio Immuno-Electrophoresis (CRIE)

The combination of CIE, CLIE, and CRIE methods provide for the possibility of immunodetection of allergenic components for individual patients as does immunoprint technique. This new test is named IDALI-test [6].

Material and Methods

Allergenic Extracts of *D. Farinae* and Patient Selection

(See Material and Methods in Immunoprint Technique)

Rabbits Antibodies Against Whole Mite Crude Extract (WMCE) of *D. Farinae*

Sera were prepared according to a successful method previously described to obtain high antibody titer against WMFE [7].

Immunochemical Methods

CIE, CLIE, and CRIE were performed as previously described by Axelsen but using a Gelbond film (F.M.C., Rockland, U.S.A.) instead of a glass plate [8].

Methodology

In order to study individual sensitization to the different allergenic constituents of WMCE of

D. farinae, the IDALI test was performed as follows:

a) A crossed immuno-electrophoresis was carried out with *D. farinae* rabbit IgG and with the crude *D. farinae* mite extract of which 920 µg (W/V) were previously submitted to electrophoresis in the first dimension (Figure 4 a).

b) A crossed line immuno-electrophoresis (the right part of which is lengthened by a line immuno-electrophoresis) was performed under the same conditions as those described for the CIE. The intermediate gel contained 540 µg/cm^2 of *D. farinae* mite extract for the whole plate (Figure 4 b).

c) The narrow strips were cut and each of them was incubated overnight with 50 µl of a human patient serum, at room temperature. After incubation, the strips were washed three times in saline. Then the strips were incubated with 50 µl of ^{125}I rabbit labelled anti-IgE (Pharmacia) overnight, washed three times in saline, 1% BSA, dried and submitted to autoradiography for 48 h at –70°C in one cassette with an intensifier screen, as described for CRIE [7] (Figure 4 c).

Results (Figure 4 c)

First, there was no reaction with control sera from nonallergic patients nor from patients sensitized to different allergen, e.g., grass pollen. Secondly, in a group of mite sensitive patients, radiolabeling greatly differed for each allergenic constituent. The minimal number of allergen bands recognized are three major allergens. The sensitivity of the IDALI test is such that even RAST class II patients can be analyzed. Nevertheless, in almost every case the highest intensity was observed for the major allergen Der f 1. Moreover, the radiolabeling may be quantified with a densitometer.

In conclusion, potential uses of the immunoprint technique and the IDALI test allow for studying the immune response to one or several allergenic components during the patient treatment, either by drugs, or by hyposensitization. The interest of these techniques is not to put it in place of classical radioimmunoassays or enzymoimmunoassays for in vitro diagnosis in allergic diseases but to bring another approach in the clinical study of allergic patients.

425

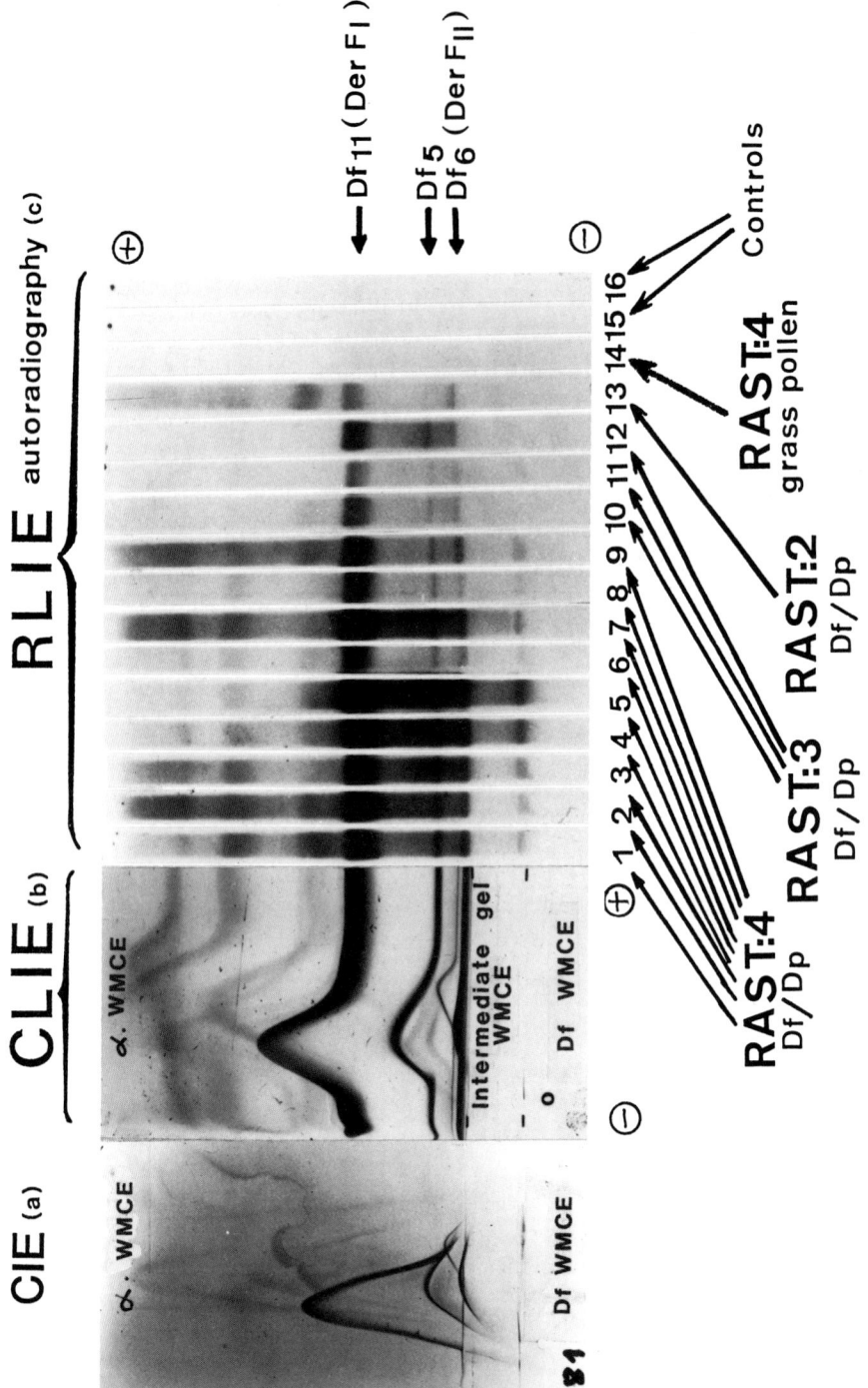

Figure 4. (a) CIE and (b) CLIE: *D. farinae* (WMCE) precipitates with specific rabbit antibodies (α-WMCE) arcs and lines are revealed by Coomassie Blue staining. (c) RLIE: IDALI performed on 13 mite sensitive patients sera. DF: *D. farinae;* Dp: *D. pteronyssinus;* RLIE: Radio Line Immuno Electrophoresis.

By means of these techniques, it is possible to type patients following heterogeneity of the allergens they recognized and select different phenotypes. Phenotypes restricted to only one allergen recognized are very important for a future research. Have these patients common genes in the Major Histocompatibility Complex, responsible for their sensitivity to this allergen?

References

1. Wide, L., H. Bennich, and S. G. O. Johansson. 1967. Diagnosis of allergy by an in vitro test for allergen antibodies. Lancet ii: 1105.

2. Guesdon, J. L., B. David, and J. Lapeyre. 1978. Magnetic enzyme immunoassay of anti-grass pollen specific IgE in human sera. Clin. Exp. Immunol. 33: 430.

3. Peltre, G., J. Lapeyre, and B. David. 1982. Heterogeneity of grass pollen allergens (*Dactylis glomerata*) recognized by IgE antibodies in human patients sera by a new nitrocellulose immunoprint technique. Immunol. Lett. 5: 127.

4. Le Mao, J. 1978. Evaluation de l'activité allergénique de préparations de *Dermatophagoides pteronyssinus* par dosage radio immunologique des antigènes extraits. Ann. Immunol. (Inst. Pasteur, Paris) 129C: 63.

5. Ceska, M., and U. Lundkvist. 1972. A new and simple radioimmunoassay method for the determination of IgE. Immunochemistry 9: 1021.

6. Rabillon, J., J. P. Dandeu, and B. David. 1987. Immuno-detection of individual allergens. J. Allergy Clin. Immunol. (abstract) 79(1): 32.

7. Le Mao, J., J. P. Dandeu, J. Rabillon, M. Lux, and B. David. 1983. Comparison of antigenic and allergenic composition of two partially purified extracts from *Dermatophagoides pteronyssinus* mite cultures. J. Allergy Clin. Immunol. 71(6): 588.

8. Axelsen, N. H., J. Kroll, and B. Weeke. 1973. A manual of quantitative immuno-electrophoresis. Methods and Applications. Suppl. 1 of Scandinavian J. Immunol.

427

Optimal Use of in vitro Diagnostic Tests in Clinical Allergy

*Alain R. Pécoud**

The practicing allergist is increasingly confronted with newer commercialized assays for the diagnosis of allergy. This short review describes some of the recently developed tests, either for the determination of specific IgE or for the measurement of histamine release. It also emphasizes the quality control that the practitioner should always require from the manufacturers. A correct interpretation of the results might, however, be the most crucial step in the allergy diagnosis: Since many subjects are sensitized to various allergens without presenting an actual disease, the primary task of the allergist is to establish the link between the in vivo/in vitro diagnosis of hypersensitivity and the patient's disease.

During the last years, a series of new assays for the in vitro diagnosis of allergy have been developed, commercialized, and proposed to the family physician or to the practicing allergist. This includes new screening tests for atopy, technically improved assays for specific IgE and new systems for the routine determination of histamine release. This short review intends to put this exuberant growth in perspective and emphasizes the need for a correct interpretation of the results.

Screening Tests for Atopy

The idea that the detection, in one single test, of specific IgEs for a small number of frequently diagnosed allergens could provide a rapid and easy way to screen the patients suffering from respiratory allergy dates back to 1978, when Merrett et al. showed that a multi-RAST with *Dermatophagoides pteronyssinus*, grass pollen, and cat dander could identify a high proportion of the allergic population [1]. What was found in UK was also true in the USA when ragweed was added in the multi-RAST system [2].

A commercially available assay (Phadiatop TM, Pharmacia, Sweden) was then tested in a series of studies performed in many European countries [3, 4, 5]. The test proved to be highly specific in predicting allergy to inhalants (virtually no false positive) and reasonably sensitive (about 15–20% false negative, when compared to results of skin tests). The latter observation could be expected since allergy screening with Phadiatop is based on the presence of specific IgE in serum. Indeed, numerous studies have shown that RAST is generally less sensitive than skin tests [6, 7, 8]. Nevertheless, in our study as in others, Phadiatop proved to be a better predictor of allergy than the total IgE level used so far for this purpose (Table 1) [5].

The primary care physician, who should be the main user of an allergy screening test, may be helped therefore by a positive Phadiatop when having to decide which patient to refer to a specialist for a more extensive allergy work-up. When the Phadiatop result is negative, however, the physician must be well aware of the limitations of this assay in order to use correctly the information it provides. First, the test investigates allergy to inhalants exclusively and does not give any information about food, hymenoptera and drug allergy. Second, the choice of allergens in the test makes it possible to miss some rarely diagnosed allergens such as those encountered in professional diseases. Third, as mentioned above, the clinician should not forget that Phadiatop is negative in 10–15% of patients who have nevertheless positive skin prick tests (SPT) for some well-characterized allergens.

New Assays for Specific IgE

In recent years, the development of assays for specific IgE did not bring spectacular breakthroughs, but rather resulted in some technical

---

* Division of Allergy and Clinical Immunology, Department of Medicine, Centre Hospitalier Universitaire Vaudois, CH-1011 Lausanne, Switzerland.

Table 1. Prediction of allergy in 100 adult patients (p.) suffering from rhinitis and/or asthma*: comparison of total IgE and Phadiatop.

a) Allergic patients

Definition of allergy	No. of patients	% patients with	
		IgE>100	pos. Phadiatop
with 1 pos. SPT	74	61	85
with 1 pos. RAST	67	64	94
with 1 pos. SPT+RAST	65	66	94

b) Non-allergic patients

with 15 neg. SPT and RAST	33	6	0

*All tested with 15 SPT/RAST for frequently diagnosed allergens (pollens, mites, epithelia, molds).

Table 2. Determination of specific IgE in 145 patients: comparison of Phadebas IgE RAST® (R) and Pharmacia CAP systems (C).

	No. of			
	Concording results		Discording results	
Allergen	R+/C+	R-/C-	R+/C-	R-/C+
d. pteronyssinus	23	104	0	18
cat	31	109	0	5
dog	14	121	1	9
horse	15	105	2	21
orchard grass	55	86	0	4
birch	24	114	0	7
mugwort	19	111	2	13
ribwort	18	107	0	20
Total	119	857	5	97
%	17.2	74.0	0.4	8.4

improvements applied to the original RAST system [9]. A great effort has been made by manufacturers toward a miniaturization of the assays by using microtiter plates instead of tubes, replacing radioactivity by spectrophotometric, fluorometric, or chemiluminescence reading. Some companies have even tried to bring the complete set into the doctor's office. An extreme of this tendency is represented by the "test strips" now available with which specific IgE can be detected in less than two hours by the physician reading color changes on a paper strip.

Confronted with the multitude of these assays, the practitioner should remain highly concerned about the quality controls of each test proposed; for each one should know figures concerning the specificity and the sensitivity of the test, compared to the results of established methods such as SPT, provocation tests, or RAST already in use. Negative controls such as serum from cord blood or from nonallergic subjects should also be tested. All these data should be gathered by several independent laboratories. This should avoid such highly discordant results reported in the past with some assays [10].

Another development of the RAST technology is represented by the improvement of assays to be used by large laboratories handling a great number of samples. One novel automatized system has been recently developed and will be available soon: the Pharmacia CAP system (Pharmacia, Uppsala, Sweden). In this assay, a new solid phase is used which allows greater binding of allergens. To detect the bound IgE, a mixture of enzyme labeled monoclonal and polyclonal anti-IgE antibodies is used and a shorter handling time is obtained by fluorometric reading. The CAP system has been tested recently in 12 laboratories, including our own. As summarized in Table 2, our data suggest that the CAP system is more sensitive than the presently available Phadebas RAST. This is shown with each of the 8 allergens tested. Similar findings have been reported independently by the other investigators.

Whenever some increase in the sensitivity of a diagnostic test is claimed, one should be concerned by a decrease in specificity. Indeed, when results of the CAP system were compared to those of SPT performed with standardized allergens, we found a higher number of positive CAP results when the SPT were negative: 10% with the CAP instead of 4% with the Phadebas RAST. However, more than 95% of these "apparently false positive" results were found in patients clearly allergic, as judged by the positive results of SPT and

Phadebas RAST for other allergens. In addition, only three "borderline" positive results were found out of 240 tests (1.2%) performed in sera that should not contain any specific IgE: cord blood and serum obtained from nonallergic normal volunteers, as defined by the absence of disease, 15 negative skin prick tests, and RAST. Further studies are needed to determine the clinical significance of the positive CAP results, particularly in patients with negative SPT.

Another novel and quite different approach to the routine in vitro diagnostic is currently proposed to the clinician under the form of a new, simple assay for histamine release [11, 12]. Measurement of histamine after triggering basophils or mast cells with allergen has been used for many years as a research tool, but only recently have some technical improvements allowed the development of an assay suitable for the routine diagnostic. It is now possible to use a very small specimen of whole blood (50 μl) instead of isolated cells, and a new rapid and reliable histamine assay is now available. Studies are now in progress comparing the results of these tests to those obtained by the determination of specific IgE. In theory, an assay based on histamine release should be closer to the clinical situation than a test measuring specific IgE since (a) it could diagnose non IgE-mediated reactions and (b) it could take in account the cell responsiveness ("releasability") to the allergen stimulation. This hypothesis is not verified so far, and both tests seem to have their own drawbacks. It has been shown, for instance, that the basophil histamine release induced by mite or grass pollen is impaired in about 10% of patients clearly allergic to these allergens [13, 14].

Importance of Interpreting the Results of Allergy Diagnosis

Whatever the advantages and limits of the method chosen, the most important clinical step, by far, resides in the correct interpretation of the results.

It has been shown in many countries that, depending on the allergen tested, between 10% and 50% of an unselected population have some positive skin tests [15]. In contrast, epidemiologic surveys have shown that allergic diseases (asthma, rhinitis, etc.) are clearly less frequent [16]. There is, therefore, some epidemiological evidence that many subjects have positive diagnostic tests (SPT or RAST) without suffering from any overt disease; this is sometimes called "latent allergy." This discrepancy is found very often by the practicing allergist and even more often by the clinical investigator who is searching for a control group of non allergic subjects.

Some of the subjects with positive skin test (and/or RAST) without any disease have suffered from contact with this allergen in the past. It is well known that hay fever, for instance, can improve or disappear, whereas SPT and RAST remain positive for a longer period of time. On the other hand, allergy is sometimes truly "latent" since, as shown by Hagy et al., healthy subjects with positive SPT are at higher risk to develop clinical allergy in the future [17]. But some of these subjects have never been and will never be sick. There is, therefore, a gap between the ability to mount an IgE immune response and a disease, and this gap is not understood so far. A likely explanation could reside in the degree of "nonspecific" hyperreactivity of the nasal or bronchial mucosae, although the tests presently available for investigating the degree of hyperreactivity (metacholin or histamine challenge) do not allow a good discrimination between active and "latent" allergy, whether performed in the bronchi or in the nose. Recently, a novel and fascinating approach has been proposed by Dr. Lichtenstein's group, when it was suggested that the IgE of the "clinically responder" (IgE+) could be different from the IgE of the "nonresponder." It might well be that several different conditions have to coincide in the same individual to fill the gap between the allergic reaction and the disease; this has been suggested by Crimi et al., who could precisely predict the severity of a bronchial obstruction (early phase or late phase) after a challenge with house dust mite by using a score combining the degree of skin reactivity to mite, the amount of mite specific IgE, the base line FEV1 and the degree of non specific bronchial reactivity [19].

For the time being, there is no better way to interpret correctly the results of the in vivo or in vitro tests than to take a careful case history, based on a good knowledge of the patient's environment. Indeed the provocation tests fail sometimes to establish the relevance of the al-

Table 3. Correlation between SPT, RAST and provocation tests in 88 patients with rhinitis and/or asthma (allergen: D. pteronyssinus, Pharmalgen).

No. of patients	SPT result* class	mean diameter of wheal	RAST** class	Provocation test positive	negative
52	≥+++	129%	≥++	52	0
18	++	61%	0	10	8
18	0	0%	0	0	18

*performed with 100,000 BU/ml; +++ = reaction induced by 0.1% histamine (100%)
**Phadezym IgE RAST

the new CAP system tends to question this general rule. In addition, in many countries, SPT remain by far the least expensive diagnostic method of allergy. It is logical, therefore, to propose that an allergy work-up start with skin testing. Under these conditions, the in vitro assay investigating either specific IgE or histamine release are indicated as a confirmation test for selected, important allergens. It must be remembered, however, that more and more allergens are now available only in the in vitro assays and are not available for skin testing.

But, whatever the diagnostic method used, allergy will remain one important example in medicine where the results of any test must always be confronted with a careful history and an accurate clinical appreciation of the patient.

lergen diagnosed, because they do not mimic perfectly the natural exposure of the patients: During the challenge, the allergen is usually presented in solution (and not carried by solid particles) and in quantities that can exceed by large natural exposure [20]. In addition, provocation tests should be used with caution in the routine diagnostic, owing to the long-lasting increase in nasal or bronchial hyperreactivity they can induce [21].

The diagnostic methods available now do not permit one to discriminate completely between "clinically relevant" allergens and those of a "latent allergy"; it must be remembered though that some degree of correlation exists between the level of specific IgE and the intensity of disease. The practitioner knows that very high levels of specific IgE are sometimes but rarely found in healthy subjects. We investigated 80 patients suffering from asthma and rhinitis using a standardized mite extract (Pharmalgen) in order to correlate the intensity of the SPT/RAST to the results of a bronchial or nasal provocation test with this extract. As shown in Table 3, all patients with at least a 3+ skin reaction to HDM had a positive RAST and had a positive provocation test. In contrast, patients who had a skin test of smaller intensity had a negative RAST, and 50% of them were found negative in a provocation test. We conclude that the presence of a positive RAST indicates a higher degree of allergy which is therefore more likely to interfere (but not always) with the patient's health.

Conclusion

So far, most of the in vitro tests have been found less sensitive than skin testing, although

References

1. Merrett, J., and T. G. Merrett. 1978. RAST atopy screen. Clin. Allergy 8: 235.
2. Ownby, D. R., J. A. Anderson, G. L. Jacobs, and H. A. Hamburger. 1984. Development and comparative evaluation of a multiple-antigen RAST as a screening test for inhalant allergy. J. Allergy Clin. Immunol. 73: 466.
3. Merrett, J., and T. G. Merrett. 1987. Phadiatop—A novel IgE antibody screening test. Clin. Allergy 17: 409.
4. Gustafsson, D., and D. Danielsson. 1988. In vitro diagnosis of atopic allergy in children. A comparison between total IgE, conventional RAST and a new multi-RAST (Phadiatop®). Allergy 43: 105.
5. Duc, J., R. Peitrequin, and A. Pécoud. 1988. Value of a new screening test for respiratory allergy. Allergy 43: 332.
6. Aas, K., and S. G. O. Johansson. 1971. The radio allergo sorbent test in the in vitro diagnosis of multiple reagenic allergy. J. Allergy Clin. Immunol. 48: 134.
7. Eriksson, N. E., S. Ahlstedt, and L. Belin. 1976. Diagnosis of reagenic allergy with house dust, animal dander and pollen allergens in adult patients. I. A comparison between RAST, skin tests and provocation tests. 1976. Int. Arch. Allergy appl. Immunology 52: 335.

8. Pécoud, A., M. Ochsner, H. Arrendal, and P. C. Frei. 1982. Improvement of the radio-allegrosorbent test (RAST) sensitivity by using an antibody specific for the determinant D 2. Clin. Allergy 12: 75.

9. Wide, L., H. Bennich, and S. G. O. Johansson. 1967. Diagnosis of allergy by an in vitro test for allergen antibodies. Lancet ii: 1105.

10. Pécoud, A., R. Peitrequin, J. Fasel, and P. C. Frei. 1986. Comparison of two assays for the determination of specific IgE in serum of atopic and nonatopic subjects: The Allergenetics FAST® and the Phadezym RAST®. Allergy 41: 243.

11. Stahl Skov, P., S. Norn, and B. Weeke. 1984. Histamine release and pathological states. A new method for detecting histamine release. Agents Action 14: 414.

12. Stahl Skov., P., H. Mosbeck, S. Norn, and B. Weeke. 1985. Sensitive glass microfiber-based histamine analysis for allergy testing in washed blood cells. Allergy 40: 213.

13. Mosbeck, H., A. Dirksen, F. Maden, P. Stahl Skov, and B. Weeke. House dust mite asthma. Correlation between allergen sensitivity in various organs. 1987. Allergy 42: 456.

14. Stahl Skov, P., S. Norn, B. Weeke, and H. Nolte. 1987. Impaired basophil histamine release from allergic patients. Agents Actions 20: 303.

15. Barbee, R. A., W. Kaltenborn, M. D. Lebowitz, B. Burrows. 1987. Longitudinal changes in allergen skin test reactivity in a community population sample. J. Allergy Clin. Immunol. 79: 16.

16. Montgomery Smith, J. 1978. Epidemiology and natural history of asthma, allergic rhinitis and atopic dermatitis (eczema). In "Allergy, Principles and Practice" Vol. 2. E. Middleton Jr., C. R. Reed, E. F. Ellis, eds. C. V. Mosby Company, p. 633.

17. Hagy, G. W., and G. A. Settipane. 1976. Risk factors for developing asthma and allergic rhinitis. A seven years follow-up study of college students. J. Allergy Clin. Immunol. 58: 330.

18. Lichtenstein, L. M. 1988. Histamine-releasing factors and IgE heterogeneity. J. Allergy Clin. Immunol. 81: 814.

19. Crimi, E., V. Brusasco, E. Losurdo, and P. Crimi. 1986. Predictive accuracy of late asthmatic reaction to Dermatophagoides pteronyssinus. J. Allergy Clin. Immunol. 78: 908.

20. Platts-Mills, T. A. E., and M. D. Chapman. 1987. Dust mites: immunology, allergic disease, and environmental control. J. Allergy Clin. Immunol. 80: 755.

21. Cockroft, D. W., R. E. Ruffin, J. Dolovitch, and F. E. Hargreave. 1977. Allergen-induced increase in non-allergic bronchial reactivity. Clin. Allergy 7: 502.

Monitoring Mediators in the Diagnosis of Allergic Inflammation

Steffan Ahlstedt*

Allergic diseases are normally diagnosed with the help of IgE and IgG antibodies. When such antibodies are not present in the circulation, e.g., in food intolerance, the diagnostic tools have been limited. In such cases challenges can be performed, although the objective determination of the the outcome of such challenge has not been obvious. Objective measures of therapy and therapy monitoring have also been uncertain. This article describes substances released during allergy and allergy-like inflammations and discusses their use for differential and specific diagnosis as well as for therapy monitoring.

Allergic diseases manifest themselves as immune hyperreactivity to certain agents and may thus be regarded as a result of immune dysfunction. Consequently, atopic disease is characterized by an overproduction of IgE antibodies—the only molecules whose presence has been well established as correlating with clinical disease. When the IgE antibodies are cell fixed, they mediate the release of mediators by reacting with the specific allergen. The cells, i.e., basophils, mast cells, and eosinophils, are also stimulated to differentiate and become activated by immune T cell derived factors. Other allergy-like conditions are not linked with the overproduction of IgE antibodies, but with other proteins such as IgG antibodies, complement and other inflammation-mediating peptides. The various allergy-like conditions need to be distinguished from each other. Today, objective monitoring of the development of disease and of therapy is not commonly done. Here, we focus on the possibilities of differential diagnosis of atopic allergy and allergy-like conditions as well on the monitoring of the progress and therapy of such diseases. This can be achieved by determination of the various immune substances, mediators, and cell-derived signal substances released during the immune-mediated inflammatory reaction. Different products can be measured for different lengths of time in the circulation, and thus they can be used differently in the diagnosis.

Levels of Diagnosis

It is crucial to distinguish between atopy mediated inflammations from other inflammations, e.g., viral and bacterial infections. The latter can be determined by measurements of neopterin [7] and C-reactive protein, respectively. Thus, dependent on exposure to antigen, IgG antibodies require months to a year before a change can be seen, IgE antibodies at least months, IgA antibodies weeks to months. The regulating factors for antibody formation and cells can take weeks before changed levels are reached, whereas the cell-derived inflammation driving peptides like eosinophil cationic protein and tryptase as well as monocyte markers like neopterin change within hours. The levels of histamine and prostaglandin change within minutes. Leukotrienes are very short lived and complicated to determine routinely. This points to the importance of differential diagnosis, which then can be followed up with specific diagnosis, as outlined in Figure 1.

Differential Diagnosis

Atopy is manifested by IgE production to a variety of antigens, and can very effectively be determined with special allergen-coupled discs in RAST.

Determination of factors regulating the synthesis of IgE may give additional information since the IgE synthesis is so crucial for the manifestation of anaphylactic type reactions. Thus, products released in vivo regulating the IgE formation, e.g., IL-4 [5], may be possible to use for differential diagnosis, although this has to be established.

---

*   Department of Allergy and Immunology, Pharmacia Diagnostics, Uppsala, and Department of Clinical Immunology, University of Gothenburg, Sweden.

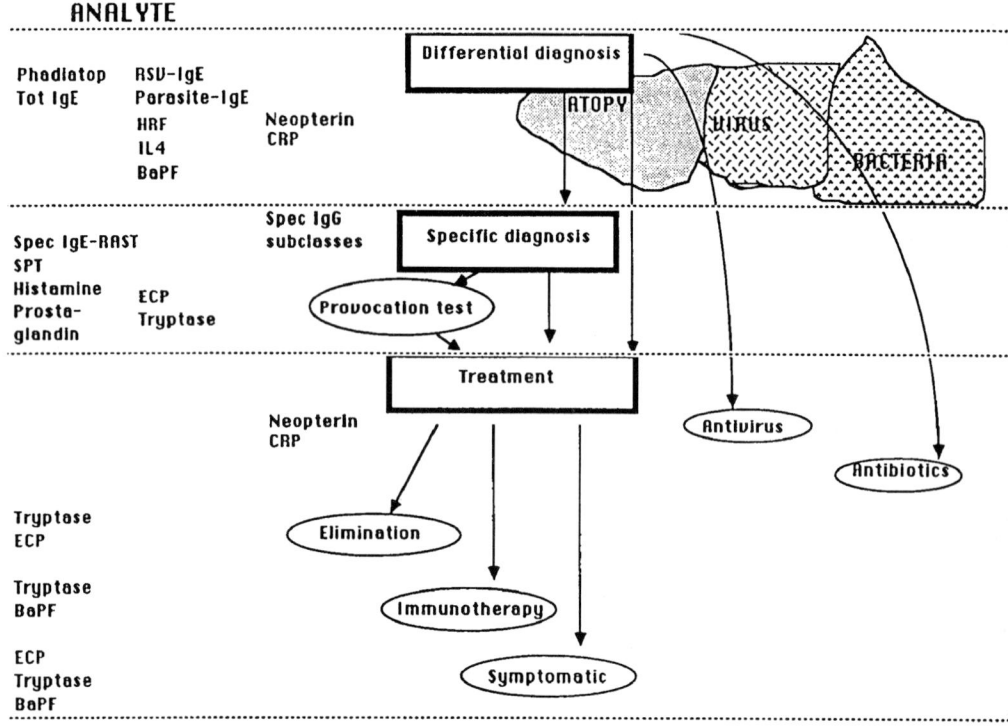

Figure 1. Theoretical consideration of the use of various analysis methods as diagnostic tools.

Differential cell counts of especially basophils and eosinophils have long been used in the diagnosis of atopic disease. In atopic individuals, the numbers of basophilic leukocytes can be used to determine exposure to the causative allergen. Recently, it was shown that the absolute and relative numbers of basophils were elevated in subjects with symptoms of allergic rhinitis compared to non-atopic subjects [8, 20].

Furthermore, counting progenitors of basophils, mast cells, and eosinophils may be useful in determining the allergic state in atopic patients. This response seems to be driven by cell growth promoting factors specific for each cell type. The cell growth factors are produced by a variety of human cells in response to antigen and possibly more from atopic than from nonatopic patients [17]. Our recent results revealed that patients with ongoing reactions could be distinguished from those without such reactions by determination of basophil-propagating factor together with eosinophil counts [2]. The techniques used must, however, be further developed before any clear clinical conclusions can be drawn.

Other mediators to be determined as a consequence of the triggering of mast cells and basophils are histamine and tryptase. Histamine levels are easily quantified in the bronchial fluid of patients with an ongoing asthmatic reaction [6, 12]. This type of mediator is not specific to allergic disease, but rather reflects the activity of ongoing inflammation. Thus, the histamine levels in the lungs of subjects with asthma were not elevated in cases with mild and stable disease, whereas patients with an ongoing allergic reaction and also those with alveolitis and fibrotic lung disease showed elevated levels of histamine [19].

Determinations of mast cell products like tryptase in patients who experienced corresponding anaphylactic reactions after specific allergens seem promising. As for histamine, this type of mediator release is not specific to atopic disease, and in patients with systemic mastocytosis the tryptase levels in plasma were linearly related to those of histamine. Certain specificity to disease can be seen, however, since no elevations were found in patients presenting with myocardial disease or sepsis [21].

Prostaglandin D is also a product of the human mast cell and is released from human pulmonary mast cells during IgE-dependent activation in asthmatic patients. In man PGD2 is selectively metabolized to 9-α-11β-PGF2, with a half life of 4 h in plasma. The metabolite is easily assayed in the urine of patients with activated mast cells [9]. The relative usefulness of histamine, tryptase, and prostaglandin is not yet established, although all three have certain potentials [25]. Tryptase may be advantageous because of its longer half life when testing blood, whereas histamine and prostaglandin with short half lives in circulation have the advantage of being determined in urine.

In patients with asthma, eosinophils occur frequently, although the levels of eosinophil cationic protein have not always been found to be elevated. Thus, some patients with intrinsic asthma have shown very low levels of eosinophil cationic protein, despite pronounced eosinophilia [22]. Eosinophil cationic protein is not specific to IgE mediated allergy. In patients developing acute respiratory distress syndrome the eosinophil cationic protein level seems to be a prognostic marker, together with some of the complement split products [11].

Other mediators also seem to give information about the inflammatory process. The time course of appearance and disappearance of the kininogens, kinins and albumin have been found to be highly correlated [3, 16].

A new possibility of monitoring inflammation progress might be products that affect the release of the mediators from the cells, such as histamine-releasing factor. Whether this can be used for differential diagnosis is yet unexplored, but it has been observed that lymphocytes from patients with intrinsic asthma spontaneously produced this cytokine [1].

Thus, it seems that IgE and IgE modulating substances will tell us about atopy, whereas histamine, prostaglandin, and substances like histamine releasing factor will give us information on the activity of the inflammatory process.

Specific Diagnosis

The use of specific IgE antibodies has been extensively discussed during this congress and is not included in this paper.

Together with IgE antibodies, IgG antibodies can be used in the diagnosis of allergic bronchopulmonary aspergillosis [13].IgA and IgG antibodies against β-lactoglobulin and gliadin are markers of gastrointestinal inflammation in children with cow's milk protein intolerance and celiac disease. The highest levels of IgA β-lactoglobulin antibodies have been found in patients with untreated celiac disease, whereas celiac patients in remission exhibit considerably ablylower antibody levels [14]. Particularly the IgA antibodies can be used for diagnostic purposes. Since elevated IgA β-lactoglobulin antibody levels occur in both patients with celiac disease and delayed-onset cow's milk protein intolerance, such antibodies might only reflect an immunologically triggered gastrointestinal tract, and they must be interpreted in view of other possible reasons for such inflammation.

Allergy Provocations

It is important to have objective measures of provocations. During provocation several mediators may be released. Histamine has been determined in serum, secretion and urine subsequent to challenge in patients with atopic allergy [12, 18, 21, 25].

The concentration of eosinophil cationic protein has been found to be significantly correlated with the strength of the challenge reaction one day after the challenge. Challenge may induce a transient decrease of eosinophil cationic protein in the presence of high eosinophilia in patients with allergic bronchial asthma [15].

Eosinophil cationic protein is not restricted to IgE-mediated allergic reactions only, and it can also be used as a marker of inflammation in conditions other than allergy. Patients with coeliac disease exhibit increased levels of eosinophil cationic protain in their serum upon challenge. Patients with rheumatoid arthritis also exhibited increased serum levels of eosinophil cationic protein [10].

In disease affecting the connective tissue, hyaluronate and type III propeptide can be assayed in bronchoalveolar lavage fluids like in patients with allergic alveolitis [4].

Therapy Monitoring

In certain instances, it can be of importance to monitor the efficacy of therapy. Immunotherapy of allergic patients with rhinoconjunctivitis and wheezing during the birch season has been found to decrease both the bronchial response to histamine and the levels of eosinophil cationic protein. The levels of eosinophil cationic protein increased during the season in untreated patients but not in the treated ones [23].

The levels of histamine, TAME-esterase activity (tryptase), and kinins in nasal fluid have been found related to symptoms at challenge in patients with allergic rhinitis. In one study, treatment with histamine synthesis inhibitor induced a 60% reduction in histamine levels in the lavage fluids before and after antigen challenge, as well as a reduction in the main urinary histamine metabolite. In contrast, the levels of kinins and TAME-esterase activity (tryptase) were not significantly reduced [18].

Intranasal corticosteroid therapy resulted in a significant decrease in the levels of mediators from different cells, like the eosinophil cationic protein concentration during the pollen season. In one study, the mediators from neutrophilic leukocytes like myeloperoxidase were about 10 times higher than that of eosinophil cationic protein, although the changes in myeloperoxidase were non-significant throughout the observation period [15].

In another study, several parameters were related using multiple regression analysis of the levels of eosinophil granule proteins in serum after allergen challenge of asthmatic patients and the effects of anti-asthmatic medication. The results showed that eosinophil protein X was the only independent variable significantly related to the late asthmatic reaction, whereas those of the eosinophil cationic protein and blood eosinophils were not [23].

Conclusion

The present information reveal good possibilities to develop packages of markers for differential diagnosis, specific diagnosis, and therapy monitoring of inflammatory conditions with allergic and allergy-like etiology.

References

1. Alam, R., P. Kuna, J. Rozniecki, and B. Kuzminska. 1987. The magnitude of the spontaneous production of histamine-releasing factor (HRF) by lymphocytes in vitro correlated with the state of bronchial hyperreactivity in patients with asthma. J. Allergy Clin. Immunol. 79: 103.
2. Almlöf I., A. Ulfgren, K. Nilsson, S. Ahlstedt, and P. Matsson. 1988. Induction of basophil propagation in the prebasophilic cell line KU-812 by conditioned media from cultured blood cells from allergic and non-allergic individuals. J. Allergy Clin. Immunol., in press.
3. Baumgarten, C. R., R. M. Naclerio, L. M. Lichtenstein, P. S. Norman, and D. Proud. 1988. Generation of kinins in vivo during allergic rhinitis. Atemw.-Lungenkrkh. 14: 74.
4. Bjermer L., A. Engström-Laurent, R. Lundgren, and R. Hällgren. 1987. Hyaluronic acid and procollagen III peptide in bronchoalveolar lavage fluid as indicators of lung disease activity in Farmer's lung. Br. Med. J. 295: 803.
5. Bonnefoy J. Y., T. Defrance, C. Peronne, C. Menetrier, F. Rousset, J. Pene, J. E. DeVries, and J. Banchreau. 1988. Human recombinant interleukin 4 induces normal B cells to produce CD23/IgE-binding factor analogous to that spontaneously released by lymphoblastoid B cell lines. Eur. J. Immunol. 18: 117.
6. Casale, T. B., D. Wood, H. B. Richerson, S. Trapp, W. J. Metzger, D. Zavala, and G. W. Hunninghake. 1987. Elevated bronchoalveolar lavage fluid histamine levels in allergic asthmatics are associated with methacholine bronchial hyperresponsiveness. J. Clin. Invest. 79: 1197.
7. Fuchs, D., G. Granditsch, A. Hausen, G. Reibnegger, and H. Wachter. 1983. Urinary neopterin excretion in coeliac disease. Lancet: 463.
8. Hirsch, S. R., and J. H. Kalbfleisch. 1976. Circulating basophils in normal subjects and in subjects with hay fever. J. Allergy Clin. Immunol. 58: 676.
9. Holgate, S. T. 1987. Contribution of inflammatory mediators to the immediate asthmatic reaction. Am. Rev. Respir. Dis. 135: 57.
10. Hällgren, R., N. Feltelius, K. Svenson, and P. Venge. 1985. Eosinophil involvement in rheumatoid arthritis as reflected by elevated serum levels of eosinophil cationic protein. Clin. exp. Immunol. 59: 539.
11. Hällgren, R., T. Samuelsson, P. Venge, and J. Modig. 1987. Eosinophil activation in the lung is related to lung damage in adult respiratory distress syndrome. Am. Rev. Respir. Dis. 135: 639.
12. Kinsella, M., H. Salari, H. Chan, K. S. Tse, and M. Chan-Yeung. 1987. Plasma histamine after methacholine, allergen, and aspirin challenges.

J. Asthma 24: 327.

13. Lam, S., H. Chan, J. C. LeRiche, M. Chan-Yeung, and H. Salari. 1988. Release of leukotrienes in patients with bronchial asthma. J. Allergy Clin. Immunol. 81: 711.

14. Lee, T. M., P. A. Greenberger, R. Patterson, M. Roberts, and J. L. Liotta. 1987. Stage V (fibrotic) allergic bronchopulmonary aspergillosis. Arch. Intern. Med. 147: 319.

15. Lindberg, T., L.-Å. Nilsson, S. Borulf, S. P. Fällström, U. Jansson, L. Stenhammar, and G. Stinzing. 1985. Serum IgA and IgG gliadin antibodies and small intestinal mucosal damage in children. J. Pediatric Gastroenterology and Nutrition 4: 917.

16. Linder, A., P. Venge, and H. Deuschl. 1987. Eosinophil cationic protein and myeloperoxidase in nasal secretion as markers of inflammation in allergic rhinitis. Allergy 42: 583.

17. Metzger, W. J., G. W. Hunninghake, and H. B. Richerson. 1985. Late asthmatic responses: Inquiry into mechanisms and significance. Clin. Rev. Allergy 3: 145.

18. Otsuka, H., J. Dolovich, D. Befus, J. Bienenstock, and J. Denburg. 1986. Peripheral blood basophils, basophil progenitors and nasal metachromatic cells in allergic rhinitis. Am. Rev. respir. Dis. 133: 757.

19. Pipkorn, U., G. Granerus, D. Proud, A. Kagey-Sobotka, P. S. Norman, L. M. Lichtenstein, and R. M. Naclerio. 1987. The effect of a histamine synthesis inhibitor on the immediate nasal allergic reaction. Allergy 42: 496.

20. Rankin, J. A., M. Kaliner, and H. Y. Reynolds. 1987. Histamine levels in bronchoalveolar lavage from patients with asthma, sarcoidosis, and idiopathic pulmonary fibrosis. J. Allergy Clin. Immunol. 79: 371.

21. Reilly, K. M., P. L. Yap, J. Dawes, R. S. C. Barnetson, F. MacKenzie, and T. L. Allan, T.L. 1987. Circulating basophil counts in atopic individuals. Int. Archs. Allergy appl. Immun. 84: 424.

22. Schwartz, L. B. 1987. Mediators of human mast cells and human mast cell subsets. Annals of Allergy. 58: 226.

23. Venge, P., L. Håkansson, and C. G. B. Peterson. 1987. Eosinophil activation in allergic disease. Int. Archs. Allergy appl. Immun. 82: 333.

24. Venge P., R. Dahl, and C. G. B. Peterson. 1988. Eosinophil granule proteins in serum after challenge of asthmatic patients and the effects of anti-asthmatic medication. Int. Archs. Allergy appl. Immun., in press.

25. Walden S. M., D. Proud, R. Bascom, L. M. Lichtenstein, A. Kagey-Sobotka, N. F. Adkinson, and R. M. Naclerio. 1988. Experimentally induced nasal allergic responses. J. Allergy Clin. Immunol. 81: 940.

Relative Immunogenicity of β-Lactam Antibiotics

*N. Franklin Adkinson, Jr.**

The relative immunogenicity of β-lactam antibiotics is difficult to determine directly in humans because of differential prior exposure. To explore the relative sensitizing capacity of three classes of β-lactam antibiotics (penicillins, cephalosporins, and monobactams), we undertook antibiotic dosing studies of naive rabbits. Sera were assayed for major determinant IgG antibody using radioimmuno-precipitation and I^{125}-HSA drug conjugates. Based on a limited series of studies, the relative immunogenicity among β-lactam molecules appears to vary over at least two orders of magnitude. Aztreonam (a prototype monobactam) and cefadroxil and cephalexin (oral cephalosporins) are about 10-fold less immunogenic than benzylpenicillin and cephalothin. Despite an identical side-chain, ceftazidime (3rd generation cephalosporin) is at least 10-fold less immunogenic than aztreonam. Factors determining intrinsic immunogenicity of these structurally related compounds are presently unknown.

We reported a number of years ago that the immunogenicity of penicillins was not invariable despite the universal haptenization of serum albumin under physiologic conditions. Only 40–60% of human subjects receiving ≥2 g of penicillin daily for at least 10 days made a detectable penicilloyl IgG antibody response [1]. Relative immunogenicity among β-lactam molecules is difficult to study directly in humans because of differential prior exposure. This is particularly true when considering third-generation cephalosporins, monobactams, and penicillin analogs that have come into widespread usage only recently. We have therefore developed an animal model using naive rabbits to study the relative immunogenicity of β-lactam compounds. The strategy employed is to screen outbred colonies of rabbits for penicilloyl IgG antibody, and then eliminate any responders on the presumption that they have previously encountered β-lactam molecules. The remaining group of "naive animals" can then be used to establish the relative sensitizing potential of various β-lactam drugs.

Table 1. Relative immunogenicity of some β-lactams antibiotics in a rabbit model.

	Index
Benzylpenicillin	1
Cephalothin	.41, .90
Aztreonam	.10
Cefadroxil	.08
Cephalexin	.07
Ceftazidime	.004

We have now applied this model to the study of six β-lactam antibiotics with interesting results.

Materials and Methods

Protocol

In the first experiment, outbred Texas white rabbits of mean weight 8.1 ± 1.1 kg were used. One hundred male and 100 female rabbits were screened for benzylpenilloyl IgG (BPO-IgG) antibody; 23 males and 25 females were eliminated as prior responders. In a second experiment, juvenile New Zealand white rabbits, 3–4 kg in weight, were used with a similar prevalence of prior responders. The remaining "naive" animals were randomized into four treatment groups. Each treatment group received 100 mg/day of the test antibiotic for 5 days per week for 3 weeks. After a 2-week rest, a second 2-week course at the same dose was given. Bleedings were taken before each weekly treatment course.

Assays for β-Lactam IgG Antibody

Radioimmuno-precipitation assays were developed using goat anti-rabbit γ-globulin and the immunizing antibiotic coupled by mild alkaline hydrolysis to I^{125}-labelled HSA [2]. Previously prepared rabbit antiserum against

* Johns Hopkins University School of Medicine, Good Samaritan Hospital, Baltimore, MD, USA.

each major determinant was used for standardization. For each bleed, the ratio of cpm bound in the test bleed to cpm bound with the autologous pre-immunization bleed was calculated. If this ratio was greater than the upper 99% confidence limit for all pre-treatment bleeds, the response was considered positive. Drug-specific IgG antibody was quantitated on the final bleeds for each animal by interpolation from a benzylpenicilloyl-IgG standard references curve previously calibrated by saturation analysis in ng/ml units [2]. Multiple dilutions were evaluated for each test serum with good agreement (CVs < 20%), indicating parallel dilution curves.

Results

For the first experiment, rabbits receiving penicillin or cephalothin behaved almost identically, manifesting an early response to a near maximum 65% response rate after a 3-week course of therapy. Secondary treatment courses (weeks 4 and 5) did not further boost the response rate. In marked contrast, the aztreonam and ceftazidime treatment rabbits had a response rate of <10% at 3 weeks. Two additional weeks of treatment increased the aztreonam response rate to 13%. Only one of 36 ceftazidime-treated rabbits had a detectable IgG response at the end of the study.

The final bleed from each responding rabbit was evaluated quantitatively for IgG antibody content. The threshold for all assays was about 20 ng/ml. The geometric mean antibody response for penicillin-treated rabbits was 264 ng/ml (n=25). The mean antibody concentration for cephalothin-treated animals was similar (126 ng/ml; n=13). The five aztreonam responders had an average of 111 ng/ml IgG, while the single ceftazidime responder had 26 ng/ml IgG antibody.

The second experiment was performed using juvenile New Zealand white rabbits. The results with penicillin and cephalothin-treated rabbits were again similar, but the response rate was somewhat higher (78–79% at 3 weeks), and the secondary treatment course (weeks 4 and 5) boosted the response rate to greater than 95% for both groups. In contrast, cefadroxil and cephalexin groups had less than 12% responders after 3 weeks of therapy. However, the response rate for both was boosted to about 70% by the end of week 5. Quantitatively, the average penicilloyl concentrations for IgG responders was 186 ± 26; n=45. The cephalothin-treatment group was quite similar (176 ± 24; n=43). The cefadroxil-treated group had substantially less antibody (22 ± 2.1; n=21). The three cephalexin responders had an average of 18 ± 0.9 ng/ml at the end of week 5.

An immunogenicity index was calculated by multiplying the maximum response rate for each antibiotic times the average drug-specific IgG concentration from the responder animals. In each case this product was nomalized to the penicillin index in each experiment. The immunogenicity indices for each of the six β-lactam compounds studied in these two experiments is shown in Table 1. Benzylpenicillin and cephalothin had comparable immunogenicity. Aztreonam, cefadroxil, and cephalexin had indices that were on the order of 10-fold less immunogenic than penicillin and cephalothin. Finally, ceftazidime was more than 100-fold less immunogenic than benzylpenicillin. It is noteworthy that aztreonam and ceftazidime had markedly different immunogenicity indexes despite identical aminothiazolyl side-chains. Ceftazidime had a bicyclic cephalosporanic acid nucleus, while aztreonam is the prototype monobactam.

Discussion

There is a widely held clinical impression that the newer β-lactam antibiotics, especially third generation cephalosporins and the recently introduced monobactam aztreonam, elicit allergic reactions much less frequently than the penicillins and early cephalosporins. One possible explanation is that cumulative exposure, especially regarding repeated courses of therapy, is likely to be much greater with the older β-lactam antibiotics, and that this differential exposure over time is responsible for the higher rates of allergic reactivity among penicillins and early cephalosporins. The data presented here suggest that an alternative hypothesis needs to be considered: that β-lactam molecules may differ in their intrinsic immunogenic potential—and that by at least two orders of magnitude judging from our limited data.

Our studies to date do not permit any firm conclusions to be drawn about the relationship of β-lactam structure to immunogenicity index.

Cephalosporins with the same nucleus but very different side-chains (e.g., cephalothin and ceftazidime) be 100-fold apart in immunogenicity. Conversely, aztreonam and ceftazidime differ markedly in their immunogenicity despite identical side-chains. A much larger series of compounds will need to be studied before conclusions can be drawn about whether one class of β-lactam molecules is in general weaker in immunogenicity than another.

One would also have difficulty explaining these rather dramatic differences in intrinsic immunogenicity on the basis of the chemical properties of the molecules such as their acylation rates. It is known that spontaneous acylation rates for conjugation of β-lactams to protein backbones do vary somewhat as a function of nuclear and side-chain conformation. However, the spread of acylation rates under physiologic conditions is well within one order of magnitude and is therefore considerably more limited than the range of immunogenicity itself. Dr. Sullivan has presented preliminary data to suggest that deacylation rates may vary widely among patients and are in general slower among patients with histories of allergic reactions [3]. This new idea deserves further study as both acylation and deacylation rates may potentially contribute to intrinsic immunogenicity insofar as they vary substantially among β-lactam molecules.

This brings us to a final question of considerable importance. How relevant are these immunogenicity data obtained in rabbits for human subjects? Two observations are noteworthy in this regard. First, the rate of penicilloyl responders in our rabbit studes closely parallels the 40–60% response rate we had previously observed in human subjects receiving at least 2 g of penicillin daily for 10 days or more. Whether higher doses or more prolonged courses of therapy can increase the response rate substantially in patient populations as it did for juvenile rabbits in our second study remains to be determined.

Ultimately, however, the question of relative immunogenicity must be addressed head on in humans. The issue of differential of prior exposure is an important consideration that cannot be overlooked. But the effect of any prior exposure to a particular β-lactam molecule can be reduced if not overcome entirely by comparing multiple courses of therapy. We hope to exploit this strategy in clinical studies in Scandinavia where standard practice is to provide prophylactic β-lactam therapy every 3 to 4 months to cystic fibrosis patients to prevent recurrent pseudomonas infections. A variety of semisynthetic penicillins, cephalosporins, and more recently aztreonam are being used for this purpose. Studies of the relative immunogenicity of these antibiotics are now underway in these populations and should yield in time some relevant information about relative immunogenicity to β-lactam molecules in humans.

If additional work in this area confirms the wide spectrum of immunogenicity among β-lactam molecules, investigation will clearly be needed to establish the biological and/or chemical basis of these remarkable differences.

References

1. Adkinson, N. F., Jr., and B. Wheeler. 1983. Risk factors for IgE-dependent reactions to penicillin. In: XI International Congress of Allergology and Clinical Immunology. J. W. Kerr and M. A. Ganderton, eds. London: MacMillan, pp. 55–59.
2. Adkinson, N. F., Jr., A. K. Sobotka, and L. M. Lichtenstein. 1979. Evaluation of the quantity and affinity of human IgG "blocking antibodies." J. Immunol. 122: 965–972.
3. Sullivan, T. J. 1988. Dehaptenation of albumin substituted with benzylpenicillin G determinants. J. Allergy Clin. Immunol. 81: 222 (abstract).

T Cell Reactivity to Drugs

*Werner J. Pichler**

T-cells play a key role in the generation of an immune response, as they provide help for Ig-synthesis as well as for the maturation of effector cells. Which function of T cells or which T cell subset is promoted depends on the manner in which antigen is presented for recognition by T cells [1].

Drugs are an interesting example of how variable the immune reactions to one substance can be and how many clinical symptoms can become manifest in allergic individuals. Most drugs, by virtue of their small size, are haptens, and are thus classified as incomplete antigens. If they themselves are reactive or if reactive metabolites are generated, they can bind to cell membranes, or alternatively they may bind and antigenically modify soluble proteins. It is likely that, depending on the soluble or corpuscular carrier, a different type of immune reaction will be mounted, resulting in distinct clinical symptoms.

During the last years, we have attempted to better understand the drug allergic reactions by analyzing T-cell-mediated reactions to drugs [2, 3]. We chose penicillin as an example, because this drug binds as hapten to various proteins, because nonreactive compounds are available, and because allergic reactions are relatively frequent [4]. We tried both to analyze which T cell subset is mainly stimulated and to what penicillin-carrier complex the T cell reactivity is directed.

Materials and Methods

Patients for study were selected from our outpatient clinic on the basis of a history of penicillin allergy (mainly exanthematous reactions), and as previous investigations had revealed a positive lymphocyte transformation test (LTT) to penicillin G. The allergic event had occurred at least half a year ago and in most instances had happened over 2 years previously.

The lymphocyte transformation test was performed as described [2, 3]. Penicillin, penicillin-conjugates, and penicillin-modified autologous cells were used as stimulans. Autologous cells were modified by incubating them in 1 mg/ml Penicillin G for 16 h, followed by a 30-min incubation in 25 µg/ml mitomycin C, to render the cells metabolically inactive. The cells were extensively washed to remove unbound penicillin G and mitomycin C. The cultures were performed for 5–6 days and 3H-thymidine uptake was measured. The stimulation index was calculated by the formula cpm + antigen/cpm – antigen.

The analysis of in vitro activated cells was performed using either pyronin Y staining or phycoerythrin-labeled anti-IL-2 receptor antibodies [5, 6]. Using a second FITC-labeled anti-CD3, CD4, CD8, or Leu8 antibody, the percentage of double-labeled cells was analyzed in a flow cytometer. As additional antigens tetanus toxoid (TT 0.2–.4 LfU/ml), purified protein derivative (PPD 0.1–10 µg/ml) and influenza virus, strain HK H3N2, or EB virus, strain B95-8, was used. In the virus cultures, peak proliferation occurred between day 8 to 11.

Results

Lymphocytes of patients with various, mainly exanthematous allergic reactions to β-lactam antibiotics can develop a strong proliferative response to penicillin G in in vitro cultures. Of similar magnitude was the proliferation observed if autologous, penicillin G-modified cells were used as stimulators (Table 1). Without modification by penicillin G, the (unseparated) autologous cells were not stimulatory. Addition of nonreactive penicillin salts (α-ethyl- or α-methyl-benzyl-penicilloate) was unable to elicit a proliferative response (data not shown).

If soluble penicillin G conjugates like benzylpenicilloyl-polylysin (BPO-PL) or benzylpenicilloyl-albumin (BPO-HSA) were added, no or

* Institute of Clinical Immunology, Inselspital, CH-3010 Bern, Switzerland

Table 1. Comparison of lymphocyte proliferation induced by penicillin (LTT) or autologous pencillin-modified cells.

Patients	Allergic reaction*	LTT Pen G 1000 µg/ml	Autologous MLC with Pen G modif. cells
I.S.	U,E	8.9	3.8
W.B.	E	3.8	1.5
M.B.	E	21.5	26.0
U.B.	AS	10.9	6.2
H.Z.	E,U	8.4	4.4
M.S.	AS,E	16.0	3.2
Mean SI:		11.5	7.5

*U = Urticaria, E = Exanthema,
AS = Anaphylactic shock

Table 2. Pencillin G., but not BPO-HSA, PBO-PL, BPO-HEX are potent stimulators of Pen G-specific T cells.

Patients Allergic reaction*	M.P. E	H.J. U,E	F.L. U,A	U.B. AS	Z.H. AS
Control (cpm × 10³)	1.3	0.4	0.7	0.7	
PenG 1000 µg/ml	24.5	13.3	11.4	35.7	47.8
BPO-HSA**	3.3	2.9	3.9	0.9	0.8
BPO-PL	1.5	2.9	4.0	28.1	1.3
BPO₂-HEX	1.7	3.6	1.8	0.9	0.6
BPO-PL skin test	+	+	+	+	+

*U = Urticaria, E = Exanthema, AS = Anaphylactic shock, A = Asthma
**BPO-HSA = benyzlpenicilloyl-human serum albumin, BPO-PL = benzylpenicilloyl-poly-L-lysine, BPO-HEX = benzylpenicilloyl-diaminohexane

Table 3. Percentage of activated (Pyronin Y^+) cells expressing the phenotype*.

	CD4	CD8	Leu8
Pen G**	88	16	69
PPD	94	9	10
TT	93	7	35
EB-virus	94	8	55
Infl. A virus	85	15	71

*Mean values of different donors and of 2–4 experiments. Culture for 5–11 days. Data calculated by following formula:
% pyronin Y^+ plus mcl Ab+ cells / % pyronin Y^+ cells.
24–56% of the cells were activated (Pyronin Y^+/3H-Thymidine incorpation was between 40,000–200,000 cpm).
**Data of optimal concentration/culture.

that purpose we activated T cell with PPD, TT, and influenza or EB-virus. After 5–11 days, a strong proliferative response was seen, which allowed us to analyze the activated cells by pyronin Y staining and simultaneous labeling with monoclonal antibody to CD3, CD4, CD8, and Leu8. The latter antibody dissects the CD4 subset into inducer cells for cytotoxic/suppressor cells ($CD4^+$, $Leu8^+$) and helper cells for antibody production ($CD4^+$, $Leu8^-$). As shown in Table 3, the soluble antigens TT and PPD activated mainly $CD4^+$ $Leu8^-$ cells, and only very few $CD8^+$ cells. In contrast, penicillin G as well as the virus infected cultures activated mainly $CD4^+$ $Leu8^+$ cells and also some $CD8^+$ cells.

Discussion

Patients with allergic skin reactions to penicillin G and other β-lactam antibiotics can develop a strong T cell activation and proliferation in vitro to β-lactam antibiotics. This T cell activation is directed to penicillin modified cell membranes for the following reasons:

only a weak proliferative response was seen. Only one patient's lymphocytes were strongly activated by BPO-PL. Taken together, these data suggest that the majority of penicillin-sensitized lymphocytes in allergic individuals is reacting to membrane-bound penicillin, and that penicillin G in a reactive form has to be added to the cultures in order that this membrane modification occurs.

If T cells react with membrane bound penicillin only, one may expect that a specific T cell subset is activated. We therefore analyzed the phenotype of the reactive T cells stimulated with soluble or membrane-bound antigens. For

1. Autologous cells, modified by pre-incubation in media containing 1 mg/ml penicillin G were stimulatory, while unmodified autologous cells did not induce a proliferative response.

2. Nonreactive penicillin compounds, unable to bind to cell membranes, were not stimulatory.

3. Soluble penicillin conjugates like BPO-HSA were in most instances not stimulatory.

4. The reactive T cell subset was mainly of the $CD4^+$ $Leu8^+$ phenotype (also inducer cells for suppressor/cytotoxic cells). Also $CD8^+$ cells were stimulated. This pattern of T cell reactivity is phenotypically identical to the T-cell activation induced by virus-infected cells, which is also directed to autologous modified cells, as viral proteins are presented in association with MHC antigens [8]. It is clearly distinct from the T-cell subset activation elicited by soluble antigens ($CD4^+$, $Leu8^-$).

The patients studied were recruited because they had a high proliferative response in the LTT. Most of them had mainly an exanthematous skin reaction, in addition to some other allergic symptoms. Whether the phenomena described are only relevant for a certain type of allergic reaction (exanthema) is at present unclear and requires further investigation.

The data, specifically the similarity of reactive T cells using penicillin G or viruses as stimulans, is interesting with regard to the frequent coincidence of allergic reactions during acute viral infections. For example, about 90% of persons receiving ampicillin during an acute EB-virus infection develop an exanthematous skin reaction and possibly additional allergic symptoms. We suggest that this coincidence may be due to the fact that the viral infection results in an activation of $CD4^+$, $Leu8^+$, and also $CD8^+$ cells, and that this preactivation lowers the threshold of activating the same T cell subsets by β-lactam antibiotics. That means that $CD4^+$, $Leu8^+$, and $CD8^+$ cells were activated by EB-virus infected cells [9]; and because the lymphokines required for this activation were already secreted, an allergic reaction to penicillin G is far easier elicited.

In addition, it is possible that the exanthematous skin reaction during viral or allergic reactions are morphologically so similar, because they are due to the same immunological reactions.

References

1. Meuer, S. C., S. F. Schlossmann, and E. L. Reinherz. 1982. Clonal analyses of human cytotoxic T lymphocytes: T4$^+$ and T8$^+$ effector T cells recognize products of different major histocompatibility complex regions. Proc. Natl. Acad. Sci. USA 79: 4395.

2. Koponen, M., W. J. Pichler, and A. L. de Weck. 1986. T cell reactivity to penicillin: Phenotypic analysis of in vitro activated cell subsets. J. Allergy Clin. Immunol. 78: 645.

3. Bell, S. J. D., and W. J. Pichler. Penicillin allergic patients react to penicillin-modified "self." Allergy, in press.

4. de Weck, A. L., and H. Bundgaard. 1983. Allergic reactions to drugs. Springer-Verlag, Berlin.

5. Shapiro, M. H. 1981. Flow cytometric estimation of DNA and RNA content in intact cells stained with Hoechst 33342 and pyronin Y. Cytometry 2: 143.

6. Walker, C., W. J Pichler, and A. L. de Weck. 1986. Different T cell subset stimulation by IgG1 or IgG2a anti T3 antibodies. Immunobiol. 171: 424.

7. Damle, N. K., N. Mohagheghpour, and E. G. Engleman. 1984. Soluble antigen-primed inducer T cells activate antigen specific suppressor T cells in the absence of antigen pulsed accessory cells: Phenotypic definition of suppressor-inducer and suppressor-effector cells. J. Immunol. 132: 644.

8. Biddison, W. E., G. M. Shearer, and S. Shaw. 1981. Influenza virus-specific cytotoxic T cells are restricted by multiple HLA-A-3-related self antigens: evidence for recognition of distinct self structures in conjunction with different foreign antigens. J. Immunol. 127: 2231.

9. Tosato, G., J. Magrath, I. Koski, W. Dooley, and M. Blaese. 1979. Activation of suppressor T-cells during Epstein-Barr virus induced infectious mononucleosis. N. Engl. J. Med. 301: 1133.

Immediate-Type Allergy and General Anesthesia

*D. Vervloet, M. Pradal, D. Charpin, F. Lagier, J. Birnbaum, J. Charpin**

The first conclusive evidence of a hypersensitivity reaction was reported in 1952 [1] following a standard dose of thiopental. Up to this time, many researchers did not believe in the reality of such reactions. However, the number of anaphylactic, or anaphylactoid, reactions occurring during general anesthesia appears to be increasing. The exact frequency of such complications is difficult to ascertain, but Fisher claims that the incidence in Australia rose from 1 in 28,000 anesthesias in 1970 to 1 in 5,000 in 1981. For Germany and the Netherlands, Langrehr et al. [2] estimated the incidence to be 1 in 600, whereas for France Laxenaire et al. reported 1 in 1,500. Recently a French national study comprising 200,000 general anesthesias indicated that one severe accident occurred for every 4,500 anesthesias. Despite appropriate treatment, about 6% of the patients who suffered such reactions died [3]. The increasing number of reports is probably due to a greater awareness of this problem. Muscle relaxants are responsible for half of the adverse reactions occurring during general anesthesia.

Primary Drugs Involved

Tables 1 and 2 show the primary drugs involved and the incidence of allergic or anaphylactoid reactions for each of them.

Hypnotics

Hypnotics are induction agents belonging either to the group of barbiturates or to the group of nonbarbiturates.

Among the barbiturates, thiopentone is the known best. Published reports of reactions are few, but the number being investigated is increasing. Estimates of reaction incidence are notoriously difficult and seem to vary between 1/23,000 and 1/36,000. Methohexital and thi-

Table 1. Primary drugs involved.

Hypnotics	– Barbiturates: Thiopentone
	– Nonbarbiturates: Propanidid, Propofol, Althesin, Etomidate
Narcotics	– Codeine, Fentanyl
	– Meperidine, Morphine
Neuroleptics Diazepam	Droperidol
Muscle relaxants	Gallamine, Suxamethonium, Alloferine, Pancuronium, Vecuronium, Atracurium
Plasma volume expanders	Dextrans, Gelatins

Table 2.

Neuroleptics	exceptional
Diazepam	exceptional if no cremophor EL
Muscle relaxants	1/4500
Plasma volume expanders	
	Dextran 1/1000
	Fluid gelatins 1/1000

amylal have been implicated in rare reactions. Propanidid, althesin, and propofol resulted in many adverse reactions that are known to be due to the solvent cremophor EL. Althesin is no longer used, and for propofol another lipid solvent is now utilized. Etomidate can induce some episodes of cutaneous and gastrointestinal side effects but very few anaphylactoid reactions.

Narcotics

"Pseudoallergic" or anaphylactoid reactions have been estimated to occur as frequently as one in every 400–1,000 anesthetics. However, true anaphylactic reactions are exceptional. As will be discussed later, clinical reactions are related to the histamine releaser properties of some narcotics.

*   Clinique des Maladies Respiratoires et Allergiques, Hôpital Sainte-Marguerite, B.P. 29, 13277 Marseille Cedex 9, France.

Neuroleptics

Accidents with droperidol were reported but are exceptional.

Diazepam

Reports of general reactions after injections of diazepam were reported with an overall incidence of 1/1,000 when the drug was mixed with cremophor EL. However, diazepam without cremophor EL is very safe and used largely without allergic or pseudoallergic side effects.

Muscle Relaxants

Muscle relaxants seem to be responsible for more than 50% of adverse reactions occurring during general anesthesia. The following muscle relaxants are predominantly implicated: D-tubocurarine, alcuronium, gallamine suxamethonium, pancuronium vecuronium, and more recently atracurium. Alcuronium is mostly involved in Australia, whereas in France anaphylactic shocks are rather provoked by suxamethonium. The incidence of reactions seems to be near 1/4,500.

Plasma Volume Expanders

With the increasing use of folloid plasma substitutes (divided into three groups: dextrans, modified fluid gelatins produced by animal collagen hydrolysis, and hydroxyethyl starch produced by acid hydrolysis of corn and soybeans after hydroxyethyl coupling), reports of adverse reactions to these colloids have appeared more frequently. In a multicenter prospective trial, 69 cases of anaphylactoid reactions were observed among 200,906 infusions of colloid plasma substitutes. The frequency of severe reactions (shock, cardiac, and/or respiratory arrest) was 0.003% for plasma protein solutions, 0.006% for hydroxyethyl starch, 0.008% for dextran, and 0.038% for gelatin solutions [4].

The frequency of all allergic or pseudoallergic reactions seems to be around 1/1,000. In a recent paper, a prospective study of dextran-induced anaphylactoid reactions in 5,745 gynecological and obstetric patients who received dextran 70 solution intravenously while undergoing major surgery revealed 8 patients who had grade I or II reactions, and 7 who had grade III or IV. The incidence of severe reactions was 1/833 patients treated [5].

Clinical Symptoms

The clinical diagnosis of severe anaphylactoid reactions has always depended on the presence of several manifestations affecting different organs. As shown in Table 3 from a study done in Nancy on more than 200 patients with anaphylactoid reactions, tachycardia, vascular collapse, and cutaneous signs were the most frequent ones encountered [6].

Table 3. Clinical symptoms (French experience with 200 patients). From [6].

Circulatory collapse	92%
Tachycardia	94%
Skin symptoms	79%
Bradycardia	6%
Arrhythmia	4%
Cardiac arrest	14%
Bronchospasm	39%

In a series of 41 patients who had developed an anaphylactic reaction after injection of muscle relaxants, urticaria was observed 20 times, bronchospasm 13, collapse 38. The outcome of these allergic reactions was dependent mainly on the severity of the cardiovascular consequences and the precise clinical management of shock, i.e., the administration of plasma substitutes, oxygen, and adrenalin. Cardiac arrest was common and may have been precipitated by severe bronchospasm or prolonged collapse [7].

Risk Factors

The role of atopy or allergy in predisposing a patient to an anaphylactic incident during general anesthesia is still being debated. British, Australian, and French epidemiological studies have reported evidence correlating allergic asthma, drug allergy, or atopy with complication during anesthesia. However, in none of these series was atopy or allergy precisely defined, nor were total IgE levels and skin tests to common inhalant allergens systematically performed. Furthermore, the control population was not matched to the patient population in terms of sex, age, and social conditions, and no distinction was made regarding the anesthetic agents used (i.e., muscle relaxants, thiopentone, althesin, propanidid, etc.). Thus, we performed a case-control study comparing the distribution of various clinical and biologic signs of atopy. The case group included 32 patients with a history of anaphylactic reactions to suxamethonium, the most commonly used muscle relaxant. The control group included 128 subjects, matched to the case group according to age, gender, and socioeconomic status. The case group consisted mainly of young and middle-aged women. Distribution of symptoms suggestive of atopy and of skin tests and specific IgE to common aeroallergens was similar in both groups. In contrast, total serum IgE level was much higher in the case group, suggesting the presence of specific IgE against suxamethonium or other drugs [8]. Some French authors have stressed other predisposing factors such as spasmophilia, increased reactivity to histamine, and overanxiety. In most publications, the incidence of adverse reactions to muscle relaxants was higher in women. This observation has not yet been satisfactorily explained and raises the problem of genetic factors and/or sensitization.

Mechanisms of Reactions

Thiopentone

Although the underlying mechanism(s) of these reactions is unclear, the chemical features indicate that at least some may be true type I hypersensitivity responses. Positive immediate skin tests were found in some cases, and the presence of IgE antibodies against different molecules of barbiturates as thiopentone, pentobarbitone, phenobarbitone, barbitone, and methohexital was demonstrated with some crossreactivities [9]. On a structure activity basis, it appears that the thiopentone reactive IgE antibodies recognize the barbiturate ring. The size and the composition of the side chain alkyl groups R1 and R2 are also important for recognition. The sulphur atoms of thiopentone seems also to be important for recognition by the IgE antibody molecule since the other four barbiturate drugs (which contain instead an

oxygen atom) were considerably weaker inhibitors.

Nonbarbiturate Drugs

The majority of the reactions due to propanidid, althesin, or propofol implicated the presence of cremophor EL. Cremophor EL is a polyoxyethylated caster oil and a complexed mixture of compounds used as a solvent for several drugs that are poorly soluble in aqueous media. Mechanisms can involve classical or alternative complement pathway and nonspecific histamine release. In this case, skin tests are usually negative. Nowadays, propofol no longer contains cremophor EL, which was replaced by another lipid solvent (from egg and soja lipids). This new preparation of propofol seems to be safe, with little or no histamine-releasing properties [10].

Narcotics

Narcotic analgesics are capable of releasing histamine both in vitro and in vivo in animals as well as in humans. This histamine release is thought not to represent a true allergic response, but rather the ability of these basic drugs to act directly in some unknown manner upon the blood and tissue cells to release histamine. Recently, Flacke et al. [11], in a double-blind study in humans, showed clearly that meperidine and morphine are substances that give nonspecific histamine release in vivo. On the other hand, fentanyl and sufentanyl are poor histamine releasers. Furthermore, clinical symptoms appeared only in people with in vivo histamine release. Two cases of true allergic reactions were reported, one involving meperidine [12] and presence of specific IgE antibodies and one demonstrating specific positive immediate skin test to fentanyl [13].

Muscle Relaxants

Skin testing with muscle relaxants is not only a reliable method of detecting allergy, it also provides great insight into the underlying mechanisms. Patients can be extremely sensitive; we recorded positive skin tests for some patients with doses of suxamethonium as small as

0.01 μg/ml. In formal volunteers, doses 10 to 10^5 times higher were necessary to obtain positive skin tests. Crossreactivity between muscle relaxants and especially between suxamethonium and gallamine has been reported by several authors. Such crossreactivity is due to the presence of ammonium ions in the molecules (see below). The reproducibility of positive or negative skin tests with muscle relaxant after 1 to 4 years indicates that these tests are worthwhile [14]. Finally, while there is no doubt as to the usefulness of skin tests for diagnostic purpose [15], their predictive value is uncertain. The presence of IgE antibodies was suggested by passive transfer tests and leukocyte histamine release. Direct evidence for the presence of IgE antibodies was supplied by an Australian group that, by covalently coupling alcuronium and d-tubocurarine, found high concentrations of drug reactive IgE antibodies in some subjects who were hypersensitive to these muscle relaxants [16]. Assays using choline coupled to activated sepharose have also been developed for the detection of IgE antibodies reactive to suxamethonium. Results of direct binding and inhibition experiments as well as correlations with clinical findings demonstrate that these assays can be effective for the detection of IgE antibodies to the drugs. Furthermore, leukocytes from patients can release their histamine content specifically in the presence of muscle relaxants. The role of quaternary ammonium ions in mediating allergic reactions suggested by previous findings was confirmed by subsequent experiments. Notably, it has been shown that synthesized diammonium salts with various chain lengths according to the formula $(CH_3)_3$ $N+-(CH_2)_n$ $-N+(CH_3)_3$ (n=2, 4, 6, 8) can specially inhibit the in vitro binding of IgE antibodies to choline sepharose in the same way as suxamethonium. The length of the chain linking the ammonium groups seems to play an important role. In fact, when the length was 4 Å, no significant histamine release could be obtained, and the optimal length appeared to be >6 Å. Flexibility of the chain linking the hapten determinants may play an important role in the bridging of two IgE molecules on the membrane of target cells [17]. In some instances, allergy to muscle relaxants does not involve N+ alone and may be related to the presence of IgE directed against some additional determinants [personal unpublished data].

Plasma Volume Expanders

In humans, however, dextran in its clinically used form is not a potent histamine releaser. Histamine is probably not the only mediator of anaphylactoid reactions, although recent publications of Lorenz and co-workers suggest a contributory role of histamine on the basis of plasma histamine measurements in patients and volunteers after dextran infusion. A possible role of serotonin release from platelets by interaction with dextran-antidextran immune complexes has also been proposed. Macromolecular contaminants, which have been found in some batches of dextran, do not seem to play a role in initiating reactions, neither does direct activation of the complement system by the alternative pathway, as was suggested on the basis of animal experiments and human studies in vitro. On the contrary, complement activation by the classical pathway has been demonstrated. Participation of an IgE-mediated reaction has been ruled out by extensive radioallergosorbent test and passive cutaneous anaphylaxis studies. There is a correlation between titers of antidextran antibodies in sera of patients with dextran-induced anaphylactic reactions prior to the eliciting dextran infusion and severity of anaphylactic reactions. Antibodies from the IgG class seem to be involved. Immunoreaction can be due to crossreactivity between dextrans and bacterial polysaccharides from gastrointestinal flora. Prevention of the accidents by monovalent hapten injection (10 to 20 ml) given intravenously over 1 to 2 minutes immediately before the first infusion of dextran was described [18].

Histamine is probably the predominant mediator of the anaphylactoid reactions observed after fluid gelatins infusions especially with urea-linked gelatins. Since purification procedures were improved with a reduction in the amount of free diisocyanate in the supernatant the frequency of anaphylactoid reactions to this new polygeline has been reduced. True allergic reactions may also occur in some cases with specific histamine release in vitro and specific positive skin tests [19].

Conclusions

Allergists must be aware of the possible severe anaphylactic or anaphylactoid reactions during general anesthesia. Muscle relaxants seem to be greatly involved at least in some countries. In this case, diagnosis can be done easily by skin tests and mechanisms are IgE mediated. For other anesthetics, diagnosis can be more difficult. However, the better knowledge of the relationship between structure of the drugs and adverse reactions (for instance, the role of the sulphur atom of barbiturates, the role of rigidity of the muscle relaxant chain, the role of cremophor) can be the best way to decrease the accidents and to obtain safer drugs. Finally, anaphylactic shock during surgery may be due to some other factors than anesthetics. As an example, some anaphylactic reactions because of an allergy to latex gloves have been reported in some patients [20].

References

1. Evans, F., and J. Gould. 1952. Relation between sensitivity to thiopentone, sulphonamides and sunlight. Br. Med. J. 1: 417.
2. Vervloet, D. 1985. Allergy to muscle relaxants and related compounds. Clinical Allergy. 15: 501–508.
3. Hatton, F., L. Tiret, L. Maujol, P. N'Dove, G. Vourch, J. M. Desmonts, J. C. Otteni, and P. Scherpereel. 1983. Enquête épidémiologique sur les anesthésies. Ann. Fr. Anesth. Réanim. 2: 333–385.
4. Ring, J., and K. Messmer. 1977. Incidence and severity of anaphylactoid reactions to colloid volume substitutes. Lancet 1: 466.
5. Paull, J. 1987. A prospective study of Dextran-induced anaphylactoid reactions in 5745 patients. Aneasth. Intens. Care 15: 163–167.
6. Laxenaire, M. C., D. A. Moneret-Vautrin, and D. Vervloet. 1985. The French experience of anaphylactoid reactions. In: Anaphylactoid reactions in anesthesia in international anesthesiology clinics. D. J. Sage, ed. 23, No. 3: 145–160.
7. Vervloet, D., E. Nizankowska, A. Arnaud, M. Senft, and J. Charpin. 1983. Adverse reactions to suxamethonium and other muscle relaxants under general anesthesia. J. Allergy Clin. Immunol. 6: 552–559.
8. Charpin, D., M. Benzarti, Y. Hemon, M. Senft, M. Alazia, A. Arnaud, D. Vervloet, and J. Char-

pin. 1988. Atopy and anaphylactic reactions to suxamethonium. J. Allergy and Clin. Immunol., in press.
9. Harle, D. G., B. A. Baldo, M. A. Smal, P. Wajon, and M. M. Fisher. 1986. Detection of thiopentone-reactive IgE antibodies following anaphylactoid reactions during anesthesia. Clinical Allergy 16: 493–498.
10. Laxenaire, M. C., J. L. Gueant, and J. B. Bois. 1987. Histaminolibération et porpofol. Journées Méditerranéennes d'anesthésie-réanimation, ed. Annette. 91–99.
11. Flacke, J. W., W. E. Flacke, B. C. Bloor, A. P. Van Etten, and B. J. Kripke. 1987. Histamine release by four narcotics: A double-blind study in humans. Anesth. Analg. 66: 723–730.
12. Levy, J. H., and M. A. Rockoff. 1982. Anaphylaxis to Meperidine. Anesth. Analg. 61, 3: 301–303.
13. Bennett, M. J., L. K. Anderson, J. C. McMillan, J. M. Ebertz, J. M. Hanifin, and C. A. Hirshman. 1986. Anaphylactic reaction during anaesthesia associated with positive intradermal skin test to fentanyl. Can. Anaesth. Soc. J. 33, 1: 75–78.
14. Didier, A., M. Benzarti, M. Senft, D. Charpin, F. Lagier, J. Charpin, and D. Vervloet. 1987. Allergy to suxamethonium: Persisting abnormalities in skin tests, specific IgE antibodies and leucocyte histamine release. Clinical Allergy 17: 385–392.
15. Leynadier, F., M Sansarricq, J. M. Didier, and J. Dry. 1987. Prick tests in the diagnosis of anaphylaxis to general anesthetics. Br. J. Anaesth. 59: 683–689.
16. Baldo, B. A., and M. Fisher. 1983. Substituted ammonium ions as allergenic determinant in drug allergy. Nature 306: 262–264.
17. Didier, A., D. Cador, P. Bongrand, R. Furstoss, P. Fourneron, M. Senft, D. Philip-Joet, D. Charpin, J. Charpin, and D. Vervloet. 1987. Role of the quaternary ammonium ion determinants in allergy to muscle relaxants. J. Allergy Clin. Immunol. 79: 578–584.
18. Ring, J. 1985. Anaphylactoid reactions to plasma substitutes. In: Anaphylactoid reactions in anesthesia in international anesthesiology clinics. D. J. Sage, ed. 23, 3: 67–95.
19. Vervloet, D., M. Senft, P. Dugue, A. Arnaud, and J. Charpin. 1983. Anaphylactic reactions to modified fluid gelatins. J. Allergy Clin. Immunol. 71, 6: 535–540.
20. Pecquet, C., F. Leynadier, and J. Dry. 1988. Hypersensibilité immédiate au latex. Med. et Hyg. 46: 967–968.

Anaphylactic Reactions to Muscle Relaxants

D. A. Moneret-Vautrin*, M. C. Laxenaire**, J. L. Gueant***

Muscle relaxants are substances used by anesthetists in order to obtain relaxed striated and smooth muscles for surgical or intubation purposes. The most commonly used are suxamethonium, alcuronium, gallamine, pancuronium, vecuronium, atracurium. D-tubocurarine, metocurine, decamethonium, and fazadinium are not used in France [10]. Pharmacological activity is linked to the presence of quaternary ammonium ions.

Epidemiology

The frequency of anaphylactic reactions (AR) during general anesthesia (GA) varies from country to country and with the substances used; the rate is about 1 case per 1500 [17]. The death rate in these cases would seem to be about 6% [15]. Muscle relaxants are responsible for 51% of these reactions [3]. Twenty-two cases were reported between 1957 and 1972, and there have been hundreds since then [8, 16, 21, 28]. The first publications underlined the role of suxamethonium and alcuronium, and more recent ones concerned the risks of using pancuronium, vecuronium, and atracurium [20, 26, 27].

Historical Background

Nonspecific histamine release was long thought to account for anaphylactic reactions to muscle relaxants, given their molecular structure [25] and in the light of numerous studies proving the frequency of this nonspecific histamine release in all subjects at the normal doses [4–7]. D-tubocurarine and atracurium result in the greatest histamine release; on the other hand, pancuronium and vecuronium are very safe. According to Galletly, the neuromuscular/histamine-releasing safety margin is the ratio of cutaneous histamine-releasing concentration to the concentration that produces 95% paralysis. This ratio is 4 for D-tubocurarine and atracurium, 88 for alcuronium, and over 300 for pancuronium and vecuronium [11]. However, as early as 1967, the possibility of a real anaphylactic reaction is considered, thanks to the positivity of a Prausnitz-Küstner test [16].

IgE-Dependent Anaphylaxis

Veritable anaphylaxis has been highly suspected because of the positive reactions at very low concentrations which are non-histamine-releasing and reproducible long after the accident [8, 21, 22, 30].

The IgE nature of the incriminated antibodies has also been postulated from results obtained with the Prausnitz-Küstner tests, human basophil degranulation tests, studies of leucocyte histamine release, soon completed by the inhibition of leukocyte histamine release using basophils, which are previously desensitized by anti-IgE [21, 29, 31].

The existence of specific IgE has been demonstrated by Baldo by a radio-immunological technique using a sepharose-alcuronium complex [1]. The Australian team has also more recently proved the existence of specific IgE for other muscle relaxants, coupled with a solid-phase carrier: D-tubocurarine, or choline and triethylcholine, fixed on the activated sepharose, accounting for specific IgE to suxamethonium and gallamine [2–14]. A complementary study has been published [12].

The epitope of muscle relaxants involves quaternary ammonium ion. This is shown by the inhibitory effect of soluble muscle relaxants on the level of specific IgE (from patient sera) which are adsorbed on the solid-drug phase. Other substances of varied chemical structures including a quaternary ammonium, such as neostigmine, promethazine, trimetaphan, morphine demonstrated also such an inhibitory effect [1].

*   Service de Médecine D. Immuno-allergologie—CHU Brabois Vandoeuvre-les-Nancy 54500, France.
**   Département d'Anesthésie—Hôpital Central, Nancy 54000, France.
*** Unité Inserm 115—Laboratoire de Biochimie—UER Médecine Vandoeuvre-les-Nancy 54500, France.

The binding of specific IgE molecules by quaternary ammonium ions has been recently confirmed by results obtained using a solid phase: an analogue of choline (with a quaternary ammonium ion) coupled to sepharose with a good and reproducible yield. The sera of patients having suffered an anaphylactic shock and whose RIA to alcuronium or choline was positive showed a high incidence of positivity (Figure 1). Incubation of the sera with the incriminated muscle relaxant provoked a strong inhibition. This technique is more sensitive and more easily reproducible than those requiring the coupling of a muscle relaxant to activated epoxy sepharose [13].

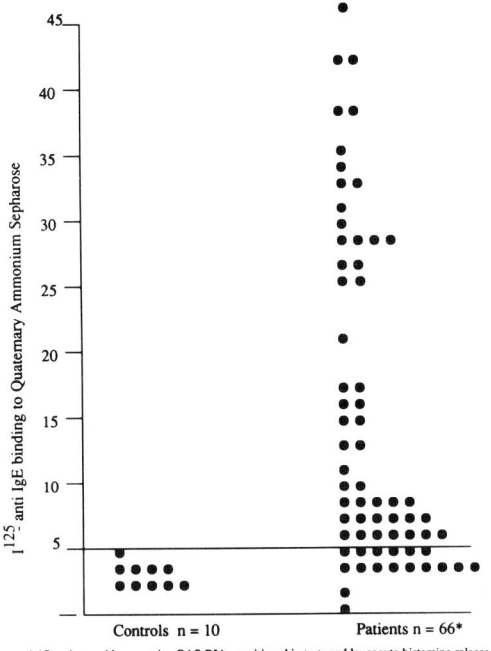

Figure 1. Radioimmunoassay with a quaternary ammonium hydrated gel of sepharose.

IgE-dependent histamine release raises the question of the bridging of two antibody molecules. This bridging demands certain conditions such as divalence and distance between the epitopes of an antigenic determinant [18]. The molecules of curarizing agents are divalent except for gallamine, which is trivalent, and vecuronium, which is monovalent. The latter, however, contains tertiary nitrogen and multimolecular substances in solution and could

provide a multivalent structure. Vecuronium might perhaps constitute plurivalent oligomers. The distance between the quaternary ammonium epitopes is 10.7 A for D-tubocurarine, 11.1 A for pancuronium, and 11.6 A for suxamethonium. Leucocyte histamine release can be obtained using leucocytes from sensitized patients with ammonium salts of variable lengths when the distance between epitopes is over 6.2 A. The structure of the molecule also plays a role: Rigid molecules (pancuronium) are considered less active in linking than flexible ones (suxamethonium) [6].

Six tests of different sensitivity are presently available for diagnosing anaphylaxis to muscle relaxants. A comparative study of 27 patients showed that ID and prick tests are both highly sensitive (96.3%), followed by QAS-RIA (87%), LHR (70%), RIA for muscle relaxants fixed on sepharose (37%), and HBDT (26%). These last two tests are not longer carried out in Nancy.

Three Points of Present Interest

At present, interest is focused on tracing anaphylaxis, preventing cross anaphylaxis by choosing a nonreactive muscle relaxant, and using a monovalent hapten to prevent anaphylaxis.

The *reproducibility of IDRs*, years after the shock, has led to the idea of screening hypersensitivity to muscle relaxants. However, dilutions weaker than 1/1000 present the risk of nonspecific reactions [8, 22, 29].

Prick tests carried out on the anterior part of the forearm with commercial solutions of muscle relaxants were recently proposed [19–23]. The correlation with IDRs is excellent; they are equally sensitive (over 95%) and absolutely specific, except for atracurium. They are also reproducible.

Skin reactivity is different when tested by epidermal and intradermal reactions. Usually, the prick test needs a 100–1000-fold higher concentration of the drug than the IDR to get similar results. For example, the positivity of a prick test with an undiluted muscle relaxant often corresponds to a positive IDR at a dilution of 1/1000. If the sensitization is moderate with a positive IDR at a dilution of 1/100, the prick test can be falsely negative. To lower this risk, a prick test should be carried out with all muscle relaxants in undiluted form to screen a

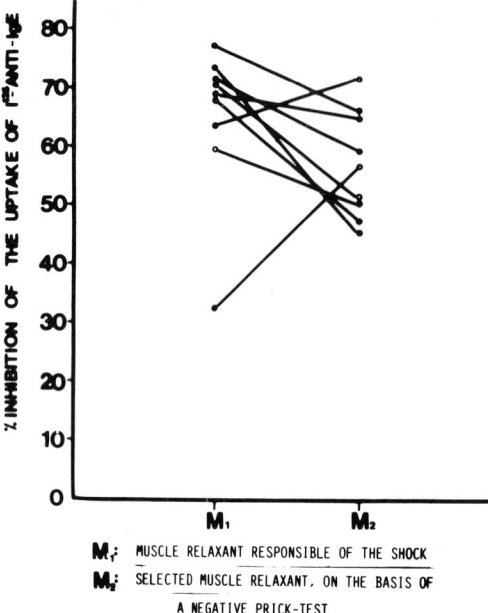

M₁: MUSCLE RELAXANT RESPONSIBLE OF THE SHOCK
M₂: SELECTED MUSCLE RELAXANT, ON THE BASIS OF
A NEGATIVE PRICK-TEST

Figure 2. Inhibition of QAS-RIA by M_1 and M_2.

latent hypersensitivity in all the subjects who are going to receive injections of muscle relaxants. Indeed, there is ample evidence for anaphylactic shocks occurring during the first use of muscle relaxants. This suggests a sensitization to other substances such as cosmetics, industrial products, and drugs containing quaternary ammonium ions [1].

Since 1986, these prick test have been performed in Nancy and have identified a subject who had latent sensitization to alcuronium. This detection was later confirmed by IDR, QAS-RIA, and LHR.

The *problem of cross anaphylaxis* appears in publications dealing with successive shocks induced by different muscle relaxants [9, 10]. On the other hand, it has been observed that the injection of a first muscle relaxant induces an anaphylaxis, even though the immediate injection of another one is well tolerated [26]. Conversely, a muscle relaxant may be injected without incident, and the use of another one, some minutes later, elicits a shock [20].

This shows how useful it would be to predict the risk of cross anaphylaxis and the harmlessness of a muscle relaxant that could be used later. The crossreactivity (CR) is well demonstrated by RIA inhibition: All muscle relaxants give an inhibition curve that is related to the

affinity for the antibodies studied [9–14]. The highest inhibition is obtained with the drug implicated in the shock in about 70% of the cases (Figure 2). Crossreactivity studied by IDR is present in 84% of individuals, but only 10% show crossreactivity to all muscle relaxants [22]. In a comparative study of both techniques, involving 34 patients with an allergy to suxamethonium or alcuronium, CR by IDR was lower than CR studied by RIA [24]. This is because factors other than the affinity of antibodies play a part in allowing the bridging of IgE antibodies, the prelude to the release of chemical mediators. Tests for bridging, like skin tests and LHR, seem well suited to predict the innocuousness of a muscle relaxant. In a study of 13 cases of hypersensitivity to muscle relaxants, a chosen muscle relaxant on the basis of negative prick tests gives a negative ID test 10 times and LHR 12 times (Figure 2). The chosen muscle relaxant also gives a lower inhibition than the incriminated drug in 10 cases (Figure 3). Vecuronium and pancuronium are most often concerned. Three patients subsequently had an operation without the slightest problem with these muscle relaxants.

Patients	ID tests		LHR	
	M1 (10^{-6} ->10^{-2})	M2 (10^{-1})	M1 (%)	M2 (%)
1	+ 10^{-2}	-	-	-
2	+ 10^{-3}	+	-	-
3	+ 10^{-4}	-	nd	- *
4	+ 10^{-3}	-	+ (47)	-
5	+ 10^{-6}	-	+ (69)	+ (59)
6	+ 10^{-2}	-	-	-
7	+ 10^{-3}	-	+ (56)	- *
8	+ 10^{-3}	-	+ (35)	-
9	+ 10^{-3}	+	+ (27)	-
10	+ 10^{-2}	-	-	- *
11	+ 10^{-2}	-	+ (23)	-
12	+ 10^{-3}	-	+ (57)	-
13	+ 10^{-3}	+	+ (15)	-

*M_2 was used subsequently without accident.

Figure 3. Comparison of the intradermal tests and leucocyte histamine release to the incriminated, and selected muscle relaxants, as selected by prick tests.

Prevention of cross anaphylaxis by monovalent hapten should be envisaged, like with penicillin and dextrans. The principle is that a monovalent molecule, when used in sufficient excess, inhibits the interaction between drugs with the same epitopes, and antibodies. It thus prevents the bridging of specific IgE (penicillin) or the forming of IgE immune complexes (dextrans). The monovalent hapten of penicillin gave rise to 5–10% anaphylactic reactions and had to be abandoned, though better results have been obtained with dextrans [5].

The choice of a substance depends on certain preconditions:

— The presence of a quarternary ammonium ion and the absence of tertiary nitrogen in the molecule.

— Substance readily available in the form of an injectable drug.

— Free of negative pharmacological effects. This eliminates ganglioplegics.

— No interference with the pharmacological effect of muscle relaxants.

— Having induced no anaphylactic reaction of any sort (information obtained from the pharmaceutical laboratory and the central data bank for pharmacology).

The reactivity of the substance, and the verification that it behaves like a monovalent hapten, have to be ascertained by four tests:

— inhibition of positive QAS-RIA

— negativity of LHR

— negativity of IDR with undiluted solution

— competitive inhibition of skin tests and LHR by the muscle relaxant.

A third phase is the in vivo study in three stages:

— verification of the cardiovascular tolerance of high doses of the substance in patients who have to undergo a G.A.;

— study of tolerance of intravenous injections in patients who are allergic to muscle relaxants;

— study of changes in skin-reactivity threshold and planimetry of IDR with the muscle relaxant, before and 15 minutes after IV injection of the monovalent hapten.

It may be hoped that these studies would allow us subsequently to propose the systematic injection of a monovalent hapten before the use of any muscle relaxant, and that in this way the seriousness and frequency of anaphylactic reactions to muscle relaxants would be considerably reduced.

References

1. Baldo, B. A., and M. Fisher. 1983. Substituted ammonium ions as allergenic determinants in drug allergy. Nature, 306: 262–264.
2. Baldo, B. A., and M. Fisher. 1983. Anaphylaxis to muscle relaxant drugs: Crossreactivity and molecular basis of binding of IgE antibodies detected by radio-immuno-assay. Molecular Immunol. 20: 1393–1400.
3. Boileau, S., M. Hummer-Sigiel, R. Moeller, and N. Drouet. 1985. Réévaluation des risques respectifs d'anaphylaxie et d'histaminolibération avec les substances anesthésiologiques. Ann. Fr. Anesth. Réanim. 4: 195–204.
4. Comroe, J. H., and R. D. Dripps. 1946. The histamine-like reaction of curare and tubocurarine injected intracutaneously and intraarterially in man. Anaesthesiology 7: 260–262.
5. De Weck, A. L., and Ch. Schneider. 1972. Specific inhibition of allergic reactions to penicillin by a monovalent hapten. Experimental immunologic and toxicologic studies. Int. Arch. Allergy 42: 782–797.
6. Didier, A., D. Cador, P. Bongrand, R. Furstoss, P. Fourneron, M. Senft, F. Philip-Joet, D. Charpin, J. Charpin, and D. Vervloet. 1987. Role of the quaternary ammonium ion determinants in allergy to muscle relaxants. J. Allergy Clin. Immunol. 79: 578–584.
7. Doenicke, A. 1980. Pseudo-allergic reactions due to histamine release during intravenous anaesthesia. Pseudo-allergic reactions: Involvement of drugs and chemicals. Karger, Basel, 7: 224–250.
8. Fisher, M. 1979. Intradermal testing in the diagnosis of acute anaphylaxis during anesthesia. Results of five years' experience. Anaesth. Intens. Care 7: 58–61.
9. Fisher, M. 1980. Anaphylaxis to muscle relaxants: Cross-sensitivity between relaxants. Anaesth. Intens. Care 8: 211–213.
10. Fisher, M., and M. C. Y. Chan. 1982. Anaphylaxis to both decamethonium and suxamethonium. Anaesth. Intens. Care 10: 153–155.
11. Galletly, D. C. 1986. Comparative cutaneous histamine release by neuromuscular blocking agents. Anaesth. Intens. Care 14: 365–369.
12. Gueant, J. L., L. Khamel, D. A. Moneret-Vautrin, S. Widmer, M. C. Laxenaire, and J. P. Nicolas. 1986. Méthode radio-immune de détection des IgE spécifiques à l'alcuronium. Ann. Fr. Anesth. Réanim. 5: 570–573.
13. Gueant, J. L., E. Mata, B. Monin, P. Gerard, M. C. Laxenaire, D. A. Moneret-Vautrin, and J. P. Nicolas. 1988. Biological and clinical evaluation of a radio immune assay for detection of specific anti-muscle relaxant IgE. In: Biologie prospective. G. Siest, ed. London: J. Libbey, in press.

14. Harle, D. G., B. A. Baldo, and M. Fisher. 1985. Assays for and cross-reactivities of IgE antibodies to the muscle relaxants Gallamine, Decamethonium and Succinylcholine. J. Immunol. Meth. 78: 293–305.

15. INSERM. 1983. Enquête épidémiologique sur les anesthésies. Premiers résultats. Ann. Fr. Anesth. Réanim. 2: 331–385.

16. Jerums, G., S. Whittingham, and P. Wilson. 1967. Anaphylaxis to suxamethonium. Brit. J. Anaesth. 39: 73–76.

17. Laxenaire, M. C., D. A. Moneret-Vautrin, and D. Vervloet. 1985. The French experience of anaphylactoid reactions. In: Anaphylactoid reactions in anesthesia. D. J. Sage, ed. Boston, pp. 145–160.

18. Levine, B. B., and A. P. Redmond. 1968. The nature of the antigen antibody complexes initiating the specific wheal and flare reaction in sensitized man. J. Clin. Invest. 47: 555–567.

19. Leynadier, F., M. Sansanicq, J. D. Didier, and J. Dry. 1987. Prick-tests in the diagnosis of anaphylaxis to general anesthetics. Br. J. Anaesth. 59: 683–689.

20. Mishima, S., and T. Yamasura. 1984. Anaphylactoid reaction to pancuronium. Anesth. Analg. 63: 865–866.

21. Moneret-Vautrin, D. A., M. C. Laxenaire, and R. Moeller. 1981. Anaphylaxis due to succinylcholine. Immuno-allergological studies in thirteen cases. Clin. Allergy 11: 175–183.

22. Moneret-Vautrin, D. A., and C. Mouton. 1985. Anaphylaxie aux myorelaxants. Valeur prédictive des intradermoréactions et recherche de l'anaphylaxie croisée. Ann. Fr. Anesth. Réanim. 4: 186–191.

23. Moneret-Vautrin, D. A., M. C. Laxenaire, S. Widmer, and M. Hummer. 1987. Intérêt des prick-tests dans le dépistage de l'anaphylaxie aux myorelaxants. Ann. Fr. Anesth. Réanim. 6: 352–355.

24. Moneret-Vautrin, D. A., L, Kamel, J. L. Gueant, M. C. Laxenaure, S. el Kholty, and J. P. Nicolas. 1988. Anaphylaxis to muscle relaxants: Cross sensitivity studied by radio-immunoassays compared to intradermal tests, in 34 cases. J. Allergy Clin. Immunol., in press.

25. Paton, W. 1957. Histamine release by compounds of simple chemical structure. Pharmacol. Review 9: 269–328.

26. Stirton-Hopkins, C. 1988. Life-threatening reaction to atracurium. Brit. J. Anaesth. 60: 597–598.

27. Tetzlaff, J. E., and Gellman, M. D. 1986. Anaphylactoid reaction to atracurium. Can. Anaesth. Soc. J. 33: 647–650.

28. Vervloet, D., A. Arnaud, P. Vellieux, S. Kaplaski, and J. Charpin. 1979. Anaphylactic reactions to muscle relaxants under general anaesthesia. J. Allergy Clin. Immunol. 63: 348–353.

29. Vervloet, D., E. Nizankowska, A. Arnaud, M. Senft, and J. Charpin. 1983. Adverse reactions to suxamethonium and other muscle relaxants under general anaesthesia. J. Allergy Clin. Immunol. 71: 552–563.

30. Vervloet, D., M. Benzarti, A. Arnaud, and J. Charpin. 1985. Reproducibilité des tests cutanés aux myorelaxants. Ann. Fr. Anesth. Réanim. 4: 184–185.

31. Withington, D. E., K. B. P. Leung, L. Bromley, G. K. Scadding, and F. L. Pearce. 1987. Basophil histamine release. A study in allergy to suxamethonium. Anaesthesia 42: 850–854.

Drug-Induced Lyell's Syndrome (Toxic Epidermal Necrolysis)

*Johannes Ring**

In 1956, A. Lyell first named the syndrome of "Toxic epidermal necrolysis" (TEN) in four patients with the dramatic clinical characteristics of "scalded skin" due to different causes [12]; there are earlier reports in the literature on similar skin conditions (see [2, 7, 18]). In a retrospective 1967, Lyell classified 4 subgroups of TEN [13], namely, the drug-induced, the staphylococcal, a group of "miscellanea" (bacterial sepsis, viral infection, vaccination, graft versus host reaction) as well as an idiopathic form.

Clinical Symptoms and Histology

Today, two forms of Lyell's syndrome can be clearly distinguished: The staphylococcal Lyell's syndrome (also called "staphylococcal scalded skin syndrome" = SSSS) [6, 14] mostly occurring in children with little mucosal involvement and subcorneal blister formation (Figure 1). The new definition of TEN comprises only those conditions in which the whole epidermis is located in the blister roof showing necrotic keratinocytes (Figure 2) and very little inflammation ("empty corium")—this in contrary to cases of fixed drug eruption or erythema multiforme [25].

The blister formation is subepidermal with destruction of basal cells similar to epidermolysis bullosa iunctionalis. The basal membrane can be demonstrated almost unchanged at the bottom of the blister in the electronmicroscope (Figure 3).

The experiences presented here are based on existing monographs, [2, 7], a literature research for the years 1975–1985 as well as the own experience with 26 cases of the Munich Department of Dermatology, making up a total of 308 cases evaluated in addition to the above-mentioned monographs and the recently published series of Créteil [16a].

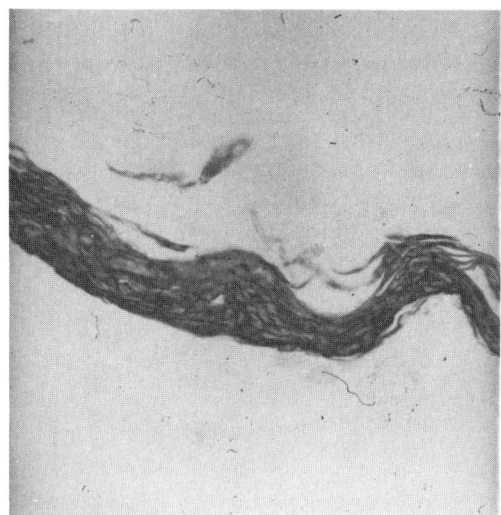

Figure 1. Histology of a blister roof in staphylococcal Lyell's syndrome: Subcorneal blister formation.

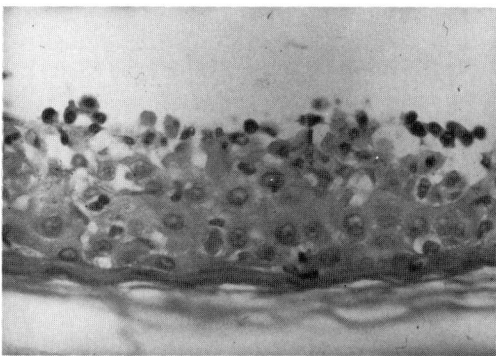

Figure 2. Histology of blister roof in toxic epidermal necrolysis: Subepidermal blister formation with necrotic keratinocytes.

Clinical symptoms comprise a prodromal phase with fever, blepharitis, conjunctivitis, and malaise (often interpreted as viral infection); an erythematous exanthem appears which is confluating and blistering leading to large areas of epidermolysis. The typical clinical symptom is a positive Nikolski sign on an erythematous lesion (Figure 4). The patient seems to be "swimming in his own skin" (Fig-

---

*   Dermatologische Klinik und Poliklinik der Ludwig-Maximilians-Universität, 8000 München, West-Germany.

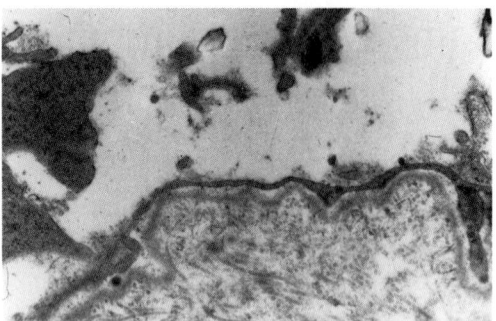

Figure 3. Electronmicroscopy of the blister bottom in toxic epidermal necrolysis: The basal lamina stays intact at the bottom of the blister (with friendly permission of C. Luderschmidt [18]).

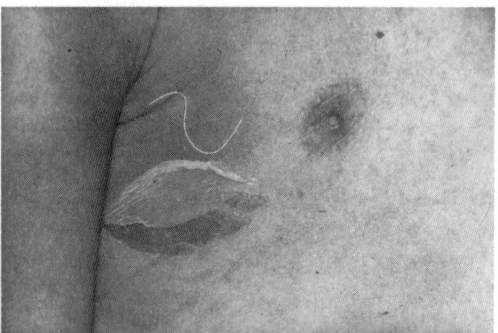

Figure 4. Positive Nikolski sign in toxic epidermal necrolysis.

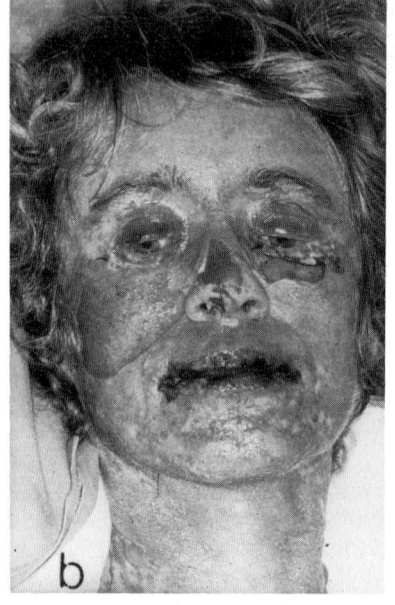

Figure 5. Large areas of epidermolysis in a patient with drug-induced Lyell's syndrome.

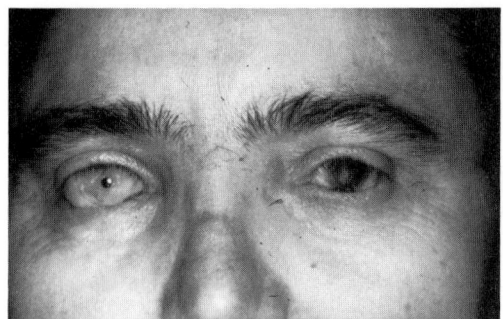

Figure 6. Late sequels of cicatricial conjunctival changes after drug-induced Lyell's syndrome.

ure 5). The mucosal surfaces are regularly involved. Diffuse alopecia is common as well as involvement of the nails. The skin lesions go always along with severe disease (e.g., high fever), the fluid loss leading to hypovolemia, sometimes shock. There is often involvement of internal organs (toxic dystrophy of the liver, tubular necrosis of the kidney, interstitial nephritis, endo-myocarditis) as well as the central nervous system (brain edema). Superinfections like pneumonia or gastrointestinal bleeding can complicate the disease [2, 7, 16a].

Factors of ill prognosis include old age, too late hospitalization, extent of blister formation, early incidence of leukopenia, initial renal insufficiency (high blood urea levels) as well as increased blood sugar concentrations [2, 7, 18, 23]. After successful therapy, the skin lesions heal within two to four weeks with desquamation of the epidermal compartment. Quite commonly finger and toe nails are lost. Postinflammatory hyper- as well as hypopigmentation is common. The mucosal membrane changes tend to heal slower. Especially conjunctival involvement may lead to synechia formation and loss of visus by vascularisation of the cornea (Figure 6).

Epidemiology

Drug-induced Lyell's syndrome is more common among elderly individuals and possibly in patients with HIV infection; there is a female to male ratio of 2:1. There are little exact data on the incidence of Lyell's syndrome in the literature. According to Schöpf et al. [in preparation], who performed a large-scale epidemiological trial in Germany, the risk of a drug-induced Lyell's syndrome in the West-German population is 0.7 per million inhabitants.

There seems to be a certain genetic susceptibility with a significant increase of HLA-B 12 in TEN generally. With regard to the eliciting drugs, sulfonamide-related cases seem to be linked to HLA-A 29, B 12 and DR 7, whereas NSAID-related cases show a linkage to A 2 and B 12 [20].

Etiologic Agents

In many textbooks, lists of drugs are presented that have been discussed in connection with Lyell's syndrome. Upon closer examination, the causal relationship between certain drugs and TEN seems often arbitrary. In our experience patients mostly took several different medications in the relevant time period (for new drugs one to three weeks prior to onset of symptoms, 24–48 hours for re-applications). In a kind of "tautology" from a comparison with the literature, the "culprit" drug is selected among possible ten or more others which are as suspect from a theoretical point of view!

In a detailed analysis of the 308 above-mentioned cases, it was only possible in 67 cases to find a "culprit" drug, when the criterium was that this drug was either the *only drug* the patient was taking, the *only newly introduced drug*, or that the causal relationship was *proven by reexposition* (which has been done by mistake, neglect or in controlled provocation) (Table 1). In this analysis nonsteroidal anti-inflammatory drugs (NSAID), antimicrobial chemotherapeutics, central nervous system-active drugs, allopurinol, and others were found. It should be stressed that there are clear-cut cases of TEN without any drug involved. We observed one case of TEN seemingly after intake of a herbal tea ("Teufelskrallen-Tee") [18]; cases of TEN have been described after tonic water, aetheric oils, eye drops, and isoproterenol powder [3, 7, 18].

Table 1. TEN: Culprit drugs (67 of 306 cases) ("single," "only new," or "reexposition").

NSAID	26
(pyrazolones	11)
Antimicrobials	22
(sulfonamides	8)
Allopurinol	5
Others	2

The epidemiological analysis is further complicated by clear deficits in dermatologic description of the lesions in many reports. Unclear terms as "shedding," "desquamation," "erythema multiforme," etc., make it impossible to clearly differentiate Lyell's syndrome from other entities.

The missing information on the total number of applications of the respective drug furthermore often prevents the real estimation of the exact incidence of this life-threatening side effect.

Pathophysiology

The pathophysiology of drug-induced Lyell's syndrome is largely unknown. There are, however, a variety of hypotheses that favor either immunological or nonimmunological reactions (Table 2). Analogies to graft-versus-host reaction seem attractive on the basis of animal experimental models [1, 15].

Table 2. TEN: Pathophysiological concepts.

Immune reactions
➤Allergy (type II): Ab or CTL against keratinocytes?
➤Allergy (type III): Ig and C deposits?
➤Allergy (type IV): Patch test and LTT results?
➤GVH: "Altered self"?
➤Monocyte-mediated cytotoxicity?
➤Combination of infection plus drug?

Non-immunological mechanisms
➤Pharmacotoxicity and underlying enzyme defect?
➤Enzyme activity?
➤Active oxygen species?
➤Microbial toxins?
➤(Prodromi already by toxin or cytokine?)
➤Combined UV + drug?

We would like to discuss three rather new aspects as possible working hypotheses for future research in this area:

Cytokines from Epidermal Cells

It seems possible that substances from macrophages, which have been found in the epidermis [19], keratinocytes, or other epidermal cells, play a pathogenic role (e.g., interleukin 1 which produces fever and affects many other organs, interleukin 2 which lead to exanthematous eruptions, etc.). The so-called "prodromal phase" could be seen as the first stage of the disease produced by effects of cytokines.

Microbial Toxins

The "toxic shock syndrome" (TSS) reported in 1978 by Todd et al. [24] is defined by fever, exanthem (diffuse and sometimes erythrodermic as well as blistering), mucosal membrane involvement, hypotension, multiorgan involvement and exclusion of other infectious diseases [4]. Many of the cases of TSS have very similar clinical characteristics reminding one of drug-induced Lyell's syndrome [8, 18]; the majority of TSS cases, however, does not show large-scale epidermolysis, but rather desquamative dermatitis especially in the palmo-plantar area after 8 to 10 days (similar to scarlet fever).

The staphylococcal toxin of TSS (TSST-1) has been isolated and can be distinguished in animal experiments from exfoliatin producing SSSS: Exfoliatin cleaves the epidermis within the stratum granulosum without cell destruction [4, 6], while TSST-1 induces a blister beneath the stratum granulosum together with keratincyte necrosis [9]. One might speculate about a new at present unknown toxin inducing at least some of the symptoms of TEN (Table 3).

Photosensitization

Looking at the list of "culprit" drugs (Table 1), it is striking that most of them are well known photosensitizers [3, 7, 18]. In an analysis of the seasonal variation in toxic epidermic necrolysis, we found a trend toward a higher prevalence in Spring and Summer, especially when NSAID-induced cases were taken into consideration [18].

It also seems interesting that in many cases the first symptoms start in the face and in the extremities [18]. We observed one case of drug-induced Lyell's syndrome occurring after a heavy sunburn (Figure 7). So one could speculate about an additional affect of UV light in the pathogenesis of this disease. Figure 8 summarizes the various possible pathophysiological factors that either alone or in combination may lead to the development of TEN.

Diagnosis and Therapy

Table 4 lists diagnostic measures that should be taken, if possible. There are reports about positive skin and lymphocyte transformation tests [11, 17, 21, 22]. According to our experience, there is no proof that a generalized TEN may be provoked by skin tests (patch tests, prick tests)

Some authors have performed oral provocation [10]. The indication to this has to be carefully thought of as well as the test dose (1:1000 and lower) and the test condition (in the hospi-

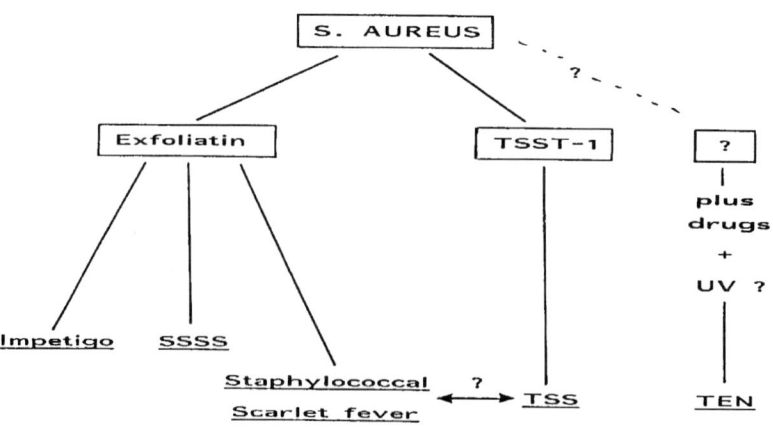

Table 3. Hypothetical concepts of microbial toxins possibly involved in TEN.

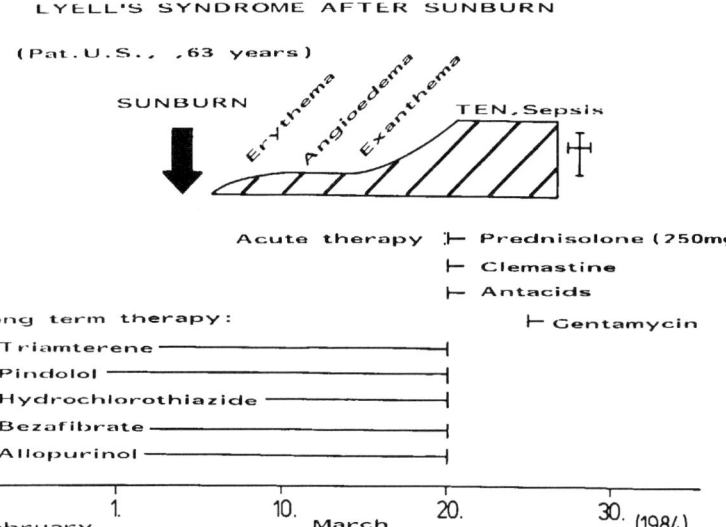

LYELL'S SYNDROME AFTER SUNBURN

(Pat.U.S., ,63 years)

SUNBURN   Erythema Angioedema Exanthema   TEN, Sepsis

Acute therapy ├ Prednisolone (250mg)
              ├ Clemastine
              ├ Antacids
                  ├ Gentamycin

Long term therapy:
– Triamterene
– Pindolol
– Hydrochlorothiazide
– Bezafibrate
– Allopurinol

1.   10.   20.   30. (1984)
February   March

Figure 7. Case of a 63-year-old patient suffering from Lyell's syndrome starting after a sunburn.

Table 4. TEN: Diagnosis.

➤Dermatologic examination
➤Blister roof histology (cryo section)
➤Biopsy for dermatopathology
➤Bacteriology (skin, mucous membranes, maybe foci)
➤In vitro diagnosis (e.g., lymphocyte transformation)
➤Skin test (after 8–12 weeks)
— epicutaneous
— prick, i.d. (dilution! 1 substance/die only!)

tal under emergency conditions, one substance a day). The treatment of drug-induced Lyell's syndrome comprises general measures, local and systemic therapy (Table 5). Local treatment has to include an early ophthalmologic intervention with contact lenses and frequent application of eye drops in order to prevent synechia formation. Certain "caveats" should be taken into consideration (Figure 9). Glucocorticosteroids should, if at all, only be given in the early phase of the exanthem prior to large scale necrolysis (e.g., four days of methylprednisolone: 1000–500–250–50 mg).

In the stage of wide-scale blistering, glucocorticosteroids rather seem to exert a negative effect promoting septic complications [16, 16a, 18, 23]. Some authors recommend, on the basis of pathophysiological considerations, an early and prophylactic antibiotic treatment with unsuspect drugs. In spite of modern medical and intensive care, the lethality of drug-induced Lyell's syndrome still ranges around an alarming 30% [2, 7].

Table 5.

TEN: Local treatment
➤Balneotherapy
➤Metalline foil
➤Take of necrotic epidermis
➤Antiseptics (e.g., AgNO$_3$, pyoktanin, chlorhexidin, povidoneiodine)
➤Antibiotic gauze (e.g., furantoin; *cave: sulfonamides!*)
➤Covering (polyurethane foam, gel, etc.)
➤Mucous membrane care (oral, genital)
➤Eye prophylaxis (contact lenses, artificial tears)
➤*No bandaid!*

TEN: Systemic therapy
➤Glucocorticosteroids in early phase (e.g., 1000-250-100-20 mg prednisolone, day 1–4). Not for long-term therapy!
➤Antibiotics when signs of sepsis or leukopenia (prophylactically?). Select least suspected substances.
➤Heparin (thrombosis prophylaxis)
➤Central analgesics

TEN: Therapy (General)
➤Hospital → single room → intensive care unit
➤Withdraw all suspected drugs
➤Warmth
➤Special bed (e.g., airstream), turn every 3 h
➤Fluid, electrolytes, colloids
➤Gastric tube

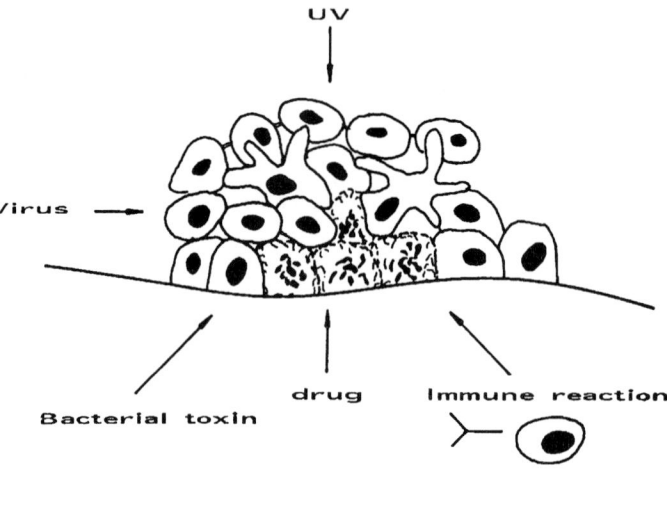

Figure 8. Pathophysiological synopsis of different possible etiologic factors in toxic epidermal necrolysis.

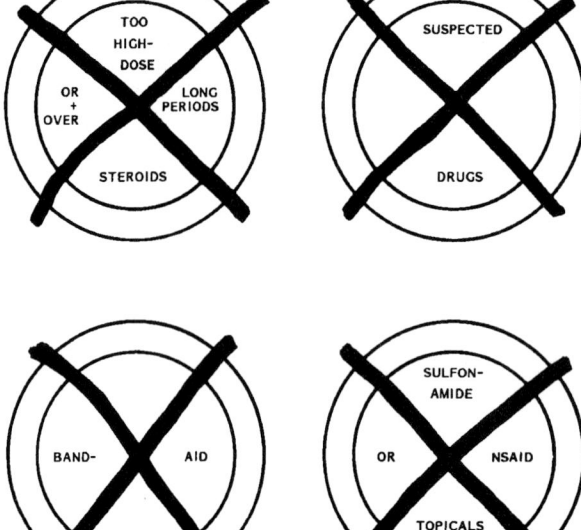

Figure 9. Caveats in the treatment of toxic epidermal necrolysis.

References

1. Billingham, R. E., and J. W. Streilein. 1968. Toxic epidermal necrolysis and homologous disease in hamsters. Arch. Der. 98: 528.
2. Braun-Falco, O., and H. J. Bandmann (Eds.). 1970. Das Lyell-Syndrom. Das Syndrom der verbrühten Haut. Huber: Bern.
3. Bouletreau, P., M. J. Ray, M. Bret, G. Carret, and J. P. Flandrois. 1984. Le syndrome de choc toxique staphylococcique. Ann. Fr. Anesth. Rean. 3: 309–311.
4. Davis, J. P., P. J. Chesney, P. J. Wand, and M. LaVenture. 1980. Toxic-shock syndrome: Epidemiologic features, recurrence, risk factors and prevention. New Engl. J. Med. 303: 1429–1435.
5. Dimond, R. J., and K. D. Wuepper. 1976. Purification and characterization of a staphylococcal epidermolytic toxin. Infect. and Immun. 13: 627–623.
6. Elias, P. M., P. Fritsch, and E. H. Epstein jr. 1977. Staphylococcal scalded skin syndrome. Arch. Derm 113: 207–219.
7. Goerz, G., and Ruzicka, T. 1978. Lyell-Syndrom. Grosse: Berlin.
7a. Guillaume, J. C., J. C. Roujeau, J. Revuz, D.

Penso, and R. Touraine. 1987. The culprit drugs in 87 cases of toxic epidermal necrolysis (Lyell's syndrome). Arch. Dermatol. 123: 1166–1170.

8. Hurwitz, M, H. P. Rivera, M. H. Gooch, T. G. Slama, A. Handt, and J. Weiss. 1982. Toxic shock syndrome or toxic epidermal necrolysis? J. Amer. Acad. Derm. 7: 246–254.

9. Kapral, F. A. 1982. Epidermal toxin production by staphylococcus aureus strains from patients with toxic shock syndrome. Ann. intern. Med. 96, Part 2: 972–974.

10. Kleinhans, D., and Th. Fuchs. 1984. Orale Provokation bei einem durch Barbitursäure verursachten Lyell-Syndrom. Akt. Derm. 10: 122–124.

11. Luderschmidt, Chr., O. Linderkamp, and J. Ring. 1985. Drug-induced toxic epidermal necrolysis (Lyell's syndrome) in a 4-year-old girl. Europ. J. Pediat. 14: 91–93.

12. Lyell, A. 1956. Toxic epidermal necrolysis: an eruption resembling scalding of the skin. Brit. J. Derm. 68: 355–361.

13. Lyell, A. 1967. A review of toxic epidermal necrolysis in Britain. Brit. J. Derm. 79: 662–671.

14. Melish, M. E., L. A. Glasgow, and M. D. Turner. 1972. Staphylococcal scalded skin syndrome: Isolation and partial characterization of the exfoliative toxin. J. infect. Dis. 125: 129–140.

15. Merot, Y., and J. H. Saurat. 1985. Clues to pathogenesis of toxic epidermal necrolysis. Int. J. Derm. 24: 165–168.

16. Parsons, J. M. 1985. Management of toxic epidermal necrolysis. Cutis 36: 305–311.

16a. Revuz, J., D. Penso, J. C. Roujeau, J. C. Guillaume, C. R. Payne, J. Wechsler, and R. Touraine. 1987. Toxic epidermal necrolysis. Clinical findings and prognosis in 87 patients.

Arch. Dermatol. 123: 1160–1165.

17. Ring, J. 1987. Diagnostik von Arzneimittel-bedingten Unverträglichkeitsreaktionen. Hautarzt 38: 16–22.

18. Ring, J, G. Wimschneider, and Chr. Luderschmidt. 1987. Arzneimittel-induziertes Lyell-Syndrom. In: Fortschritte prakt. Dermatol. Venerol., Bd. XI. O. Braun-Falco and W. B. Schill, eds. Springer-Verlag: Berlin, pp. 252–264.

19. Roujeau, J. C., L. Dubertret, S. Moritz, J. Jouault, M. Heslan, J. Revuz, and R. Touraine. 1985. Involvement of macrophages in the pathology of toxic epidermal necrolysis. Brit. J. Derm. 113: 425–430.

20. Roujeau, J. C., T. H. Huynh, J. C. Guillaume, C. Braq, J. Revuz, and R. Touraine. 1987. Genetic susceptibility to toxic epidermal necrolysis. Arch. Dermatol. 123: 1171–1173.

21. Schöpf, E., K. H. Schulz, R. Kessler, M. Taugner, and W. Braun. 1975. Allergologische Untersuchungen beim Lyell-Syndrom. Z. Hautkr. 50: 865–873.

22. Schulz, K. H. 1972. Lymphocytentransformationstest bei Arzneimittelallergie. Arch. Derm. Forsch. 244: 309–312.

23. Steigleder, G. K. 1985. Behandlung der toxischen epidermalen Nekrolyse. Z. Hautkr. 60: 763–765.

24. Todd, J., M. Fishaut, F. Kapral, and T. Welch. 1978. Toxic-shock syndrome associated with phage-group-I staphylococci. Lancet ii: 1116–1118.

25. Wolff, H. H., R. L. Dimond, and O. Braun-Falco. 1978. Das staphylogene Lyell-Syndrom. In: Pädiatrische Dermatologie. J. J. Herzberg, ed. Schattauer: Stuttgart, pp. 191–197.

Cross-Reactivity Between Aspirin and Other Drugs/Dietary Chemicals. A Critical Review

Donald D. Stevenson*

ASA and NSAIDs cross-react routinely in ASA-sensitive asthmatic and urticaria patients. By contrast, less potent analgesics, such as salsalate and acetaminophen, which in contrast to NSAIDs barely inhibit cyclooxygenase enzyme, cross-react with ASA infrequently and only with high concentrations of the drugs. A number of drugs, preservatives, and dyes that do not block cyclooxygenase have been reported to cross-react in ASA sensitive patients. However, evidence for this is inconclusive, and repeat studies have not confirmed cross-sensitivity for tartrazine, azo dyes, hydrocortisone succinate dextropropoxyphene, sulfites, and MSG.

Aspirin (ASA) sensitivity refers to a condition found in patients who have either chronic rhinitis, sinusitis, nasal polyps, and/asthma or chronic uritcaria with or without angioedema. Such patients are identified as being ASA-sensitive only after they have experienced either a respiratory or cutaneous reaction to ASA or non-steroidal anti-inflammatory drugs (NSAID). Except for sensitivity reactions, these patients are indistinguishable from other asthmatic or chronic urticaria patients. *ASA disease* is the underlying respiratory or cutaneous inflammation, which persists in the absence of ASA and precedes or follows ASA sensitivity [1–4]. Approximately 10–20% of asthmatics and 20–30% chronic urticaria patients are afflicted with these sensitivity reactions [1, 2].

In view of the close association between reactions to ASA and NSAIDs, two lines of investigation have dominated this field for the past 20 years. First, attempts to discover the mechanisms of ASA sensitivity have focused upon how ASA and NSAIDs—despite great dissimilarity of molecular sizes and shapes—can initiate such reactions [3]. Second, extending these observations about cross-reactivity between ASA and NSAIDs, investigators have attempted to prove cross-reactivity to other drugs, chemicals and dyes [3, 5].

In 1977, Szczeklik and his associates conducted a series of in vitro experiments that demonstrated that ASA and NSAID share an important pharmacologic effect on arachodanic acid metabolism, namely, inhibition of the gateway enzyme cyclooxygenase [6]. Furthermore, during oral challenges of known ASA-sensitive asthmatics, these authors showed that NSAIDs that inhibited cyclooxygenase in vitro with the least concentration of drug were the most potent NSAIDs in cross-reactions with ASA. Interestingly, drugs, such as dextropropoxyphene that do not block cyclooxygenase did not induce respiratory reactions in known ASA-sensitive asthmatic subjects.

Although the shared in vitro pharmacologic effect was predicative of the presence and even the degree of cross-sensitivity, support for the theory that ASA blockade of cyclooxygenase in any cell system in some manner produces the ASA/NSAID reactions has never materialized [7], and more recent data show that ASA appears to have other effects, namely, release of a leukotriene (LTC4) and histamine into nasal secretions during ASA induced reactions [8]. As this investigation unfolds, it would not be surprising to conclude that ASA/NSAID block cyclooxygenase, eliminating the generation of cycloprostaglandin products, an event not related to the pathogenesis of the ASA/NSAID reactions, and at the same time a genetically susceptible or virus-altered cell(s)—perhaps respiratory mast cells, eosinophils, or platelets—react directly with ASA/NSAID to release leukotrienes, histamine, and perhaps other inflammatory mediators.

With respect to cross-reactivity, all NSAIDs except benoxyprofen (an NSAID that does not block cyclooxygenase) cross-react with ASA 100% of the time, if large enough dosages of the cross-reacting drugs are used [1, 6, 9]. Furthermore, cross-desensitization between ASA and

* Scripps Clinic and Research Foundation, La Jolla, CA, USA.
 Supported by NIH Grants RR-00833 and IA-10386.

NSAIDs occurs routinely, strongly suggesting that similar mechanisms for both initiating and inhibiting sensitivity reactions are operative [10, 11]. From a practical standpoint, any ASA-sensitive asthmatic patient, after ASA desensitization, can substitute any NSAID for ASA without adverse respiratory reaction [1, 11].

Cross-reactivity to weak inhibitors of cyclooxygenase in vitro has been more difficult to prove. Current evidence supports the earlier assumption of Szczeklik et al. [6] that poor inhibitors of cyclooxygenase are likely to cross-react poorly—if at all. With respect to acetaminophen, those studies which reported a low to absent incidence of cross-reactivity between ASA and acetaminophen, challenged with dosages of acetaminophen at or below 650 mg (5, 12–14). By contrast, Delaney [15] challenged ASA-sensitive asthmatics with 600 mg acetaminophen, without inducing reactions, and then increased the dosage to 1000 mg, with 28% of the same patients now experiencing a respiratory reaction.

At the Scripps Clinic and Research Foundation, we recently had the opportunity to study three ASA-sensitive asthmatics who gave an associated history of wheezing episodes 2 h after ingesting one or two Extra Strength Tylenol® (500 mg acetaminophen capsule). All three patients had ASA respiratory sensitivity, proven during oral ASA challenges with provoking dosage of ASA 60 mg. All experienced asthmatic reactions to acetaminophen during controlled oral challenges with acetaminophen 1000 mg, but not with 500 mg. Attempts to desensitize two patients to 1000 mg and 1500 mg of acetaminophen were successful though only temporary, and attempts to desensitize to 2000 mg were not successful. Cross-desensitization, after inducing tolerance to ASA [11] was also successful in two patients who were able to ingest 1000 mg of acetaminophen without adverse effect while in the ASA desensitized state. Therefore, the study suggested that acetaminophen behaves like ASA/NSAIDs with respect to hypersensitivity reactions of the respiratory tract, except that large doses of the drug are needed to initiate mild respiratory tract reactions, and in only a subpopulation of ASA sensitive asthmatics.

Another weak prostaglandin cyclooxygenase inhibitor is salsalate (disalcylic acid). In a recent study at our institution, 2 of 10 known ASA sensitivity asthmatics cross-reacted to Salsalate but only when the provoking dose reached 2 grams. Furthermore, after ASA desensitization, both asthmatics could then ingest Disalcid 2 g without any adverse effect, again demonstrating cross-desensitization. In summary, the same principle appears: weak cyclooxygenase inhibitors, requiring large doses of drug to produce mild respiratory reactions in only a subpopulation of potentially susceptible ASA sensitive asthmatics.

The third area of discussion involves a variety of drugs, dyes, and food additives which have *not* been shown to block cyclooxygenase and yet have been reported to cross-react in ASA sensitive asthmatics [3, 5, 16, 21]. The major compounds that have been reported to cross-react are tartrazine [3, 5, 16, 21], other azo and non-azo dyes [3], hydrocortisone succinate [19], dextropropoxyphene [20], sulfites [21], and MSG [18]. For those who reported such cross-sensitivity, an attractive theory to explain on-going urticaria or asthma and rhinitis with polyp formation, in the absence of exposure to ASA, is the daily ingestion of dyes, preservatives, and flavor enhancers. Yet, despite the listed reports and this attractive theory, there are serious questions about whether or not such cross-sensitivity even exists [22].

A major obstacle in conducting challenges is to reproduce a specific effect from a challenge substance without injury to the patient or observing a spontaneous fluctuation of the natural underlying disease and inappropriately assigning cause to a challenge substance [23]. If bronchial airways are irritable, carrying out forced expiratory volume spirometry maneuvers can decrease FEV1 values by >20% and induce wheezing episodes which are entirely spontaneous and occur after ingesting placebo capsules [23, 24]. Likewise, chronic idiopathic urticaria waxes and wanes as a natural consequence of the disease. This area of research is particularly vexing because systemic corticosteroids for asthma and antihistamines for urticaria are frequently required to counter primary disease activity by suppressing hyperactive airways in the bronchial tree or suppressing urticaria. Critics argue that subsequent negative challenges, using any challenge substance, are only negative because medications had been taken by the study subjects and were blocking reactions that would otherwise appear. The dilemma is that withholding corticosteroids or antihistamines allows spontaneous bronchial airway irritability or urticaria to return, coincidental to challenge with a study capsule, providing a report in the literature which is incorrect.

With these considerations in mind, we will briefly examine the six challenge substance listed earlier, attempting to show why it is our contention that cross-sensitivity between these substances and ASA is neither expected nor occurs [22]. Tartrazine cross-sensitivity has been championed by a number of authors [3, 5, 16, 17], and this subject has been reviewed extensively [24, 25]. Gerber et al. [26] have shown that tartrazine does not block cyclooxygenase enzyme in vitro and therefore would not be expected to cross-react with ASA/NSAIDs. There are 5 studies in the literature that do not confirm the presence of ASA and tartrazine cross-sensitivity [25, 27–30]. In the largest study, Stevenson et al. [25] challenged 150 ASA sensitive asthmatics with tartrazine 25 mg and 50 mg, and 6 (4%) experienced decline in FEV1 values suggesting a cause-and-effect asthmatic response. However, when these same patients were rechallenged at a later date, using one-day placebo challenges to establish baseline bronchial stability and double-blind placebo-controlled challenges with tartrazine in similar dosages, repeat challenges were all negative [25]. In the same paper, 5 ASA sensitive urticaria patients were challenged with tartrazine, and none reacted to tartrazine. Yet, in the same admission to the GCRC all 5 reacted to ASA despite taking antihistamines during the challenge period. By contrast, one ASA-tolerant urticaria patient developed urticaria 1 hour after ingesting tartrazine 25 mg during 2 double-blind placebo-controlled oral challenges.

This study is instructive for several reasons. First of all, in the asthma challenge studies, if we had accepted the screening challenge results as final, a characteristic of all prior studies reporting tartrazine cross-sensitivity, we also would have reported false positive reactions as if a true cross-sensitivity existed in 4% of the patients. Second, the large size of our ASA-sensitive asthmatic population of 150 patients makes it unlikely that small percentages of cross-reactivity would not be uncovered. Third, all patients experienced large and sustained reactions to ASA while taking the same anti-asthmatic medications used during the tartrazine challenges, suggesting that true respiratory reactions could occur if tartrazine was capable of generating them.

With respect to urticaria induced by tartrazine, the same observations apply. First, tartrazine did not induce urticaria in a small number of ASA-sensitive urticaria patients, a finding entirely different from the NSAIDs, which routinely induce urticaria flares upon first exposure to the drug. Second, the doses of tartrazine used in this study, 25 mg, followed by 50 mg (cumulative doses of 75 mg) far exceed dietary or pharmaceutical exposure, making it impractical to argue that sufficient exposure to tartrazine was not carried out. Third, since one of our urticaria patients did react with urticaria to 25 mg of tartrazine, our challenge methods must have been adequate to demonstrate urticaria when tartrazine could induce this type of reaction. Finally, since this reaction occurred in a patient who, at another time, did not react to ASA, the mechanism of tartrazine induced urticaria is likely to be unrelated to the pathogenic sequences suspected for true cross-sensitive between ASA and the NSAIDs.

Azo and non Azo dyes are available in most diets, and therefore some physicians have suggested that their continued ingestion is responsible for chronic asthma or urticaria [17]. Despite routine challenges with these dyes, we have never been able to identify cross-sensitivity in any of our known ASA-sensitive asthmatics or urticaria patients [22]. This is consistent with an excellent study by Weber et al. [27], in which known ASA-sensitive asthmatics failed to react to these dyes. Likewise, despite the report of hydrocortisone-associated asthma [19], we have been unable to document its occurrence in 15 consecutive known ASA-sensitive asthmatics. Dextropropoxyphene sensitivity has not been adequately studied. Dr. Szczeklik's and our groups have never encountered an ASA sensitive patient who could not take this analgesic. Sulfite sensitivity in asthma is well documented. However, we have challenged 32 consecutive ASA-sensitive asthmatics with up to 200 mg sulfites, without adverse effect. MSG sensitivity in asthma has been reported to occur in suspected ASA sensitivity asthmatics [18, 21]. We have never documented MSG sensitivity in an ASA-sensitive asthmatic. Therefore, it is difficult to burden ASA-sensitive patients with the additional responsibility of avoiding a variety of dietary substances that probably do not cross-react. A much more likely probability is that each of the substances listed above can cause unique and specific reactions in susceptible patients. However, any occurrence of such a "reaction" in an ASA-sensitive asthmatic or urticaria patient might be purely coincidental. In fact, since none of these chemicals inhibit cyclooxygenase in vitro, there is no predictive reason to suspect cross-sensitivity. Indeed, most "reactions" reported in the literature are probably measurements of the primary ASA disease fluctuations, while withholding essential medications and assigning cause and effect responsibility to innocent bystander challenge substances.

References

1. Stevenson, D. D. 1984. Diagnosis, prevention and treatment of adverse reactions to aspirin and nonsteroidal anti-inflammatory drugs. J. Allergy Clin. Immunol. 74: 617.
2. Stevenson, D. D., and R. A. Simon 1988. Aspirin sensitivity: Respiratory and cutaneous manifestations. In: Allergy: Principles and Practice. E. Middleton, C. E. Reed, and E. F. Ellis, eds. St. Louis: C.V. Mosby, p. 1537.
3. Samter, M., and R. F. Beers. 1968. Intolerance to aspirin: Clinical studies and consideration to pathogenesis. Ann. Intern. Med. 68: 975.
4. Lumry, W. R., J. G. Curd, and D. D. Stevenson. 1984. Aspirin-sensitive asthma and rhinosinusitis: Current concepts and recent advances. Ear, Nose and Throat Journal. Feb.: 102.
5. Spector, S. L., C. H. Wangaard, and R. S. Farr. 1979. Aspirin and concomitant idiosyncracies in adult asthmatic patients. J. Allergy Clin. Immunol. 64: 500.
6. Szczeklik, A., R. J. Gryglewski, and G. Czernigwska-Mysik. 1977. Clinical patterns of hypersensitivity to nonsteroidal anti-inflammatory drugs and their pathogenesis. J. Allergy Clin. Immunol. 60: 276.
7. Stevenson, D. D., and R. Lewis. 1987. Proposed mechanisms of aspirin sensitivity reactions, Editorial. J. Allergy Clin. Immunol. 80: 788.
8. Ferreri, N. R., W. C. Howland, D. D. Stevenson, and H. L. Spiegelberg. 1988. Release of leukotrienes, prostaglandins, and histamine into nasal secretions of aspirin-sensitive asthmatics during reaction to aspirin. Am. Rev. Resp. Dis. 137: 847.
9. Mathison, D. A., and D. D. Stevenson. 1979. Hypersensitivity to nonsteroidal anti-inflammatory drugs; Indications and methods for oral challenge. J. Allergy and. Immunol. 64: 669–674.
10. Lumry, W. R., J. G. Curd, R. S. Zeiger, and D. D. Stevenson. 1983. Aspirin sensitive rhinosinusitis: The clinical syndrome and effects of aspirin administration. J. Allergy and Clin. Immunol. 71: 580.
11. Pleskow, W. W., D. D. Stevenson, R. A. Simon, D. A. Mathison, M. Schatz, and R. S. Zieger. 1982. Aspirin desensitization in aspirin sensitive asthmatic patients: Clinical manifestations and characterization of the refractory period. J. Allergy and Clin. Immunol. 69: 11.
12. Falliers, C. J. 1983. Acetaminophen and aspirin challenges in subgroups of asthmatics. J. Asthma 20(s): 39.
13. Szczeklik, A., and R. J. Gryglewski. 1983. Asthma and anti-inflammatory drugs: Mechanisms and clinical patterns. Drugs 25: 533.
14. Henochowicz, S. 1986. Acetaminophen-induced asthma in a patient with aspirin idiosyncrasy. Immunol. Allergy Pract. 60: 43.
15. Delaney, J. C. 1976. The diagnosis of aspirin idiosyncrasy by analgesic challenge. Clin. Allergy 6: 177.
16. Freedman, B. J. 1977. Asthma induced by sulfur dioxide, benzoate and tartrazine contained in orange drinks. Clin. Allergy. 7: 407.
17. Juhlin, L., G. Michaelsson, and O. Zetterstrom. 1972. Urticaria and asthma induced by food and drug additives in patients with aspirin sensitivity. J. Allergy Clin. Immunol. 50: 92.
18. Allen, D. H., J. Delohery, and G. Baker. 1987. Monosodium L-glutamate-induced asthma. J. Allergy Clin. Immunol. 80: 530.
19. Partridge, M. R., and G. J. Gibson. 1978. Adverse bronchial reactions to intravenous hydrocortisone in 2 aspirin sensitive patients. Br. Med. J. 1: 1521.
20. Smith, A. P. 1971. Response of aspirin allergic patients to challenge by some analgesics in common use. Br. Med. J. 1: 494.
21. Baker, G. J., P. Collette, and D. H. Allen. 1981. Bronchospasm induced by metabisulfite-containing foods and drugs. Med. J. Aust. 2: 614.
22. Simon, R. A. 1984. Adverse reactions to drug additives. J. Allergy Clin. Immunol. 74: 623.
23. Stevenson, D. D. 1988. Oral challenges to detect Aspirin and sulfite sensitivity in asthma. NE and Regional Allergy Proceedings 9: 135.
24. Mathison, D. A., D. D. Stevenson, and R. A. Simon. 1985. Precipitating factors in Asthma: Aspirin, sulfites and other drugs and chemicals. Chest 67S: 50.
25. Stevenson, D. D., R. A. Simon, W. R. Lumry, and D. A. Mathison. 1986. Adverse reactions to tartrazine. J. Allergy and Clin. Immunol. 78: 182.
26. Gerber, J. G. et al. 1979. Tartrazine and the prostaglandin system. J. Allergy Clin. Immunol. 63: 289.
27. Weber, R. W., M. Hoffman, D. A. Raine, and H.

S. Nelson. 1979. Incidence of bronchoconstriction due to aspirin, azo dyes, non-azo dyes and preservatives in a population of perennial asthmatics. J. Allergy and Clin. Immunol. 64: 32.

28. Vedantham, P., M. M. Menon, T. D. Bell, and D. Bergin. 1977. Aspirin and tartrazine oral challenge: Incidence of adverse response in chronic childhood asthma. J. Allergy and Clin. Immunol. 60:8.

29. Tarlo, S. M., and I. Broder. 1982. Tartrazine and benzoate challenge and dietary avoidance in chronic asthma. Clin. Allergy 12: 303.

30. Haripparsad, D., N. Wilson, C. Dixon, and M. Silverman. 1984. Oral tartrazine challenge in childhood asthma: Effect on bronchial reactivity. Clin. Allergy 14: 81.

Adverse Reaction to Food and Drug Additives

*Ronald A. Simon**

The list of additives used by the food and pharmaceutical industries is extensive and includes thousands of antioxidants, flavors, colors, preservatives, sweeteners, thickeners, and many others. Yet, most of the agents used have not been implicated in hypersensitivity reactions. In addition, many of the reports of adverse reactions to additives were made by investigators not experienced in hypersensitivity reactions, were anecdotal, or not rigorously controlled. Table 1 identifies the most common additives and those that have been implicated in causing adverse reactions.

Table 1. Additives most commonly associated with adverse reactions.

FD&C dyes
— Tartrazine (FD&C yellow #5)
Parabens
— Parahydroxy benzoic acid
— Methyl, ethyl, butyl parabens
— Sodium benzoate
Butylated hydroxyanisole (BHA)
Butylated hydroxytoluene (BHT)
Nitrates
Nitrites
Monosodium glutamate (MSG)
Sulfites
Sulfur dioxide
Sodium sulfite
Potassium bisulfite
Metabisulfite
Aspartame (Nutrasweet)

The food dye and coloring act (FD&C) approved dyes are coal tar derivatives. These agents are known to provoke contact hypersensitivity. The best known dye is tartrazine (FD&C yellow #5). In addition to tartrazine, there is a group of AZO dyes that include ponceau (FD&C red #4) and sunset yellow (FD&C #6). Amaranth (FD&C red #5) was banned from use in the United States in 1975 because of claims of carcinogenicity. Non-AZO dyes include brilliant blue (FD&C blue #1), erythrosine (FD&C red #3), and indigotin (FD&C blue #2).

Use of FD&C-approved dyes is so ubiquitous in foods and drugs that isolated reactions, in otherwise normal individuals, are not reported as such. Rather, these dyes have been reported to provoke chronic urticaria or asthma. However, the prevalence of reactions to any food or drug additives (including tartrazine and the other dyes) in patients with chronic urticaria and angioedema is unknown. This is not because of inadequate numbers of studies, but arises rather from the lack of properly and vigorously controlled studies and inherent problems in challenging patients with chronic urticaria. There are advantages and disadvantages in studying patients while their disease is active or inactive, on medications or off medications. In addition, most studies suffer from lack of a period of evaluation during straight placebo challenges to determine baseline levels of symptomatology. Finally, most studies simply report the appearance or increase in hives, no attempt being made at quantitation. Even with these problems in study design; selecting populations with a history suggesting reactions to tartrazine or other dyes or having had a response to an additive free diet; studies indicate that less than 10% of such individuals are sensitive to tartrazine (and in fact other additives). In our studies at Scripps Clinic, utilizing double-blind placebo-controlled challenges after a period of baseline observation with symptom scores to quantify objective changes in the subjects' skin, we found that only 1 of 25 subjects with chronic idiopathic urticaria/angioedema reacts to tartrazine.

Tartrazine is also the most frequently implicated additive from provoking asthmatic reactions. However, critical review of the medical literature would suggest that sensitivity to tartrazine in asthmatic subjects is, at best, extremely unusual. In the best double-blind placebo control studies Weber et al. in adults and Vedanthan et al. in children found no tartrazine-sensitive subjects among groups of approximately 50 in each report having chronic

* Department of Clinical Research, Scripps Clinic and Research Foundation, La Jolla, California, USA.

467

asthma, most times steroid dependent. If tartrazine sensitivity exists at all in asthma, it is likely to be in the aspirin-sensitive group. Yet, for more than the last 15 years, we have been performing double-blind placebo-controlled challenges with tartrazine in aspirin-sensitive asthmatics at Scripps Clinic, and in over 165 such challenges, we have yet to find a single positive response. There is only one positive challenge in a double-blind, placebo-controlled report of tartrazine provoked asthma in the medical literature. Interestingly, this patient was not aspirin-sensitive and also did not experience amelioration of asthma symptoms while on a tartrazine-free diet.

Since reactions to AZO dyes other than tartrazine and non-AZO dyes are far less commonly reported than those to tartrazine, these agents will not be discussed further.

Parabens are aliphatic esters of parahydroxybenzoic acid and include methyl, ethyl, propyl, and butyl parabens. Sodium benzoate is a closely related substance and is usually reported to cross react with other parabens. These agents are widely used as preservatives in foods and drugs and are clearly recognized as causes of severe contact dermatitis (PABA-containing sunscreens). In three well-documented reports, parabens have been associated with immediate hypersensitivity reactions resulting in diffuse urticaria and angioedema. These reports involved parabens used as preservatives in drugs (local anesthetics and corticosteroids), not in foods. The three subjects reported were otherwise normal and able to ingest parabens without an apparent difficulty. Keeping in mind the problems discussed earlier with studies of tartrazine in urticaria, parabens have also been reported to exacerbate chronic urticaria in less than 10% of subjects challenged. There is only one double-blind placebo-controlled report of benzoate-provoked asthma in the medical literature. Interestingly, this patient was not aspirin-sensitive and also did not experience amelioration of asthma symptoms while on a benzoate-free diet.

BHA (butylated hydroxyanisole) and BHT (butylated hydroxytoluene) are antioxidants that are commonly used in breakfast cereals and other grain products to maintain crispness and prevent rancidity. There have been no well-documented reports of hypersensitivity to these agents when consumed in the amounts normally ingested in foods. However, toxic reactions (usually neuropsychiatric) have been noted when BHT is taken in pharmacologic doses (100–1000 mg per day) as an anti-aging, anti-cancer, or anti-herpes agent (lay book and "health food" store remedies).

Nitrates and nitrites are widely used as preservatives in processed meats (frankfurters, salamies, etc.). However, their popularity stems from their flavoring and coloring attributes. These agents have not, in review of the literature, been associated with hypersensitivity reactions, but can provoke vascular headache. Furthermore, their metabolic products (nitrosamines) are known carcinogens.

Monosodium glutamate (MSG) is a non-essential dicarboxylic amino acid that forms about 20% of our normal dietary protein. MSG is added to food as a flavor enhancer particularly in oriental food and has been commonly reported to produce a variety of symptoms including headache, myalgias, backache, neck pain, nausea, diaphoresis, and chest heaviness (dubbed the "Chinese Restaurant Syndrome"). MSG has not been implicated in producing urticaria. MSG has been associated with asthma in reports by Allen et al. from Australia. The initial report described asthma occurring 10–12 hours after a Chinese meal. Subsequent reports by the same authors noted additional patients with more immediate (1–2 hour) reactions. Recently, a single patient has been reported with MSG-provoked asthma confirmed by multiple double-blind, placebo-controlled challenges. This patient was also reported as sulfite sensitive. A recent letter to the *Lancet* describes a subject with angioedema occurring 16 hours after monosodium glutamate ingestion. A single-blind, placebo-controlled ingestion challenge supported this association.

Aspartame (Nutrasweet®), a dipeptide of aspartic acid and phenylalanine, has been reported to provoke urticaria in one double-blind, placebo-controlled study in two individuals. Reports of Nutrasweet®-provoked headaches have been variable with both positive and negative findings depending upon study design.

Sulfiting agents have been widely used for centuries to freshen and prevent oxidative discoloration (browning) of foods. Sulfiting agents include sulfur dioxide and sodium potassium sulfite, bisulfite and metabisulfite. Sulfites are also used to sanitize and inhibit the growth of non-desirable micro organisms in the fermentation industry. Extreme levels of sulfites were found on fresh foods and vegetables (such as salad bars). In August of 1986, the FDA banned the use of sulfites on any foods served as fresh in restaurants. Currently, the highest levels can be found in dry fruits (such as apricots), potatoes, wine, and some seafoods. Processed foods with more than trace amounts of sulfites (10 ppm SO_2) must have sulfite-containing labels on package materials. Wine bottled after January 1988 must also bear a label with sulfite inscription. FDA regulation concerning sulfite use on potatoes remains pending.

Sulfiting agents have clearly been shown by a number of double-blind controlled reports from several investigators in several different countries to be the cause of life-threatening asthmatic reactions. In fact, prior to their ban from fresh fruits and vegetables, more than 12 deaths were reported to be likely related to sulfite sensitivity. While the number of sulfite-sensitive asthmatics remains unknown, reports from three different groups indicate that approximately 5% of the asthmatic population can experience anything from mild wheezing to severe life-threatening, asthmatic episodes following ingestion of sulfite-containing foods and beverages. Although the mechanism of sulfite sensitivity is unknown, it is likely—in the overwhelming majority of asthmatics—to involve the inhalation of sulfur dioxide generated from sulfite solutions in warm acidic environments. There are only two reports (three patients total) of sulfite-sensitive asthmatics with positive skin tests to sulfites suggesting an IgE-mediated mechanism. Our studies also indicate that some asthmatics with severe reaction to sulfites have low levels of the enzyme sulfite oxidase which is necessary to oxidase sulfite into the inactive sulfate form. These asthmatics, like the skin-test-positive asthmatics, respond to sulfite ingested in capsule form. Other asthmatics, with less mild history, react only to sulfite containing solutions (generating sulfur dioxide).

There are isolated case reports of non-asthmatic reactions to sulfites. These generally involve urticaria and angioedema. Unfortunately, rigorously controlled double-blind, placebo-controlled challenges have either not been performed or have not provoked the reactions noted by their history in these individuals. In challenges with 25 subjects with chronic idiopathic urticaria and angioedema at the Scripps Clinic, we have not seen reactions to metabisulfite. Two cases of anaphylaxis related to sulfite ingestion with positive skin test have been reported. Three reports looked at sulfite sensitivity in subjects with idiopathic anaphylaxis. Only one subject among 130 subjects challenged was found to be sulfite sensitive in one of the studies. In another, none of the 25 subjects with idiopathic anaphylaxis were found to be sulfite sensitive. However, one other subject experienced a systemic reaction following a sulfite skin test. The third study found no subjects sensitive to sulfite among 12 individuals with idiopathic anaphylaxis.

More than a decade ago, Feingold wrote that a significant percentage of hyperactivity in children could be traced to additives. Since then, some uncontrolled studies have purported to show that a diet free of salicylates and additives results in a marked improvement in the behavior of hyperactive children. However, well-controlled studies have failed to support this hypothesis.

Suggested Reading

1. Simon, R. A. 1986. Adverse reactions to food additives, N. Engl. Reg. Allergy Proc. 7: 533.

2. Simon, R. A. 1984. Adverse reactions to drug additives. J. Allergy Clin. Immunol. 74: 623–630.

3. Simon R. A., and D. D. Stevenson. 1988. Sulfite-sensitivity. In: Allergy principles and practices. Middleton, Reed, Ellis, eds. St. Louis: C.V. Mosby Co.

4. Lipton, M. A., and J. P. Mayo. 1983. Diet and hyperkenisis—An update. J. Am. Dietetic Assoc. 83: 132–134.

5. Ortolani, C., E. Pastorello, A. Fontana, S. Gerosa, M. Ispano, V. Pravettoni, F. Rotondo, C. Mirone, and Zanussi, 1988. Chemicals and drugs as triggers of food associated disorder. Ann. of Allergy 60: 358–366.

6. Stevenson, D. D., R. A. Simon, W. Lumry, and D. A. Mathison. 1986. Adverse reactions to tartrazine. J. Allergy Clin. Immunol. 78: 182.

7. Stevenson, D. D., and R. A. Simon. 1981. Sensitivity to ingested metabisulfites in asthmatic subjects. J. Allergy Clin. Immunol. 68: 26–32.

8. Hannuksela, M., and A. Lahti. 1986. Peroral challenge tests with food additives in urticaria and atopic dermatitis. Int. J. Derm. 25: 179.

9. Allen, D. H., J. Delohery, G. J. Baker, and R. Wood. 1983. Monosodium glutamate induced asthma. J. Allergy Clin. Immunol. 71: 98.

10. Kulcycki, A. Jr. 1986. Aspartame-induced urticaria. Ann. Int. Med. 104: 207.

11. Schiffman, S., C. E. Buckley, H. A. Sampson, E. W. Massey, J. N. Baraniuk, J. V. Follett, and Z. S. Warwick. 1987. Aspartame and susceptibility to headache. N. Engl. J. Med. 317: 1181–1185.

12. Koehler, S. M., and A. Glaros. 1988. The effect of aspartame on migraine headache. 28: 10.

Changing Habits in Food and Drug Additives (Europe)

*Philippe C. Frei**

The habits concerning food and drug additives can be those of the manufacturers, the population (consumers), and the few patients who occasionally suffer from adverse reactions to these chemicals, mainly asthma, urticaria, and polypous rhinitis.

The habits of the manufacturers have changed slightly in Europe as a consequence of regulations limiting the addition of chemicals. Progress has been made in the labeling of products, enabling a selection by subjects hypersensitive to additives, without depriving the others of the advantages of such substances, for example, preservatives.

It is difficult to estimate a possible change in the habits of the population at large. A trend toward eating more fresh products is appearing, however, sometimes even to excess, even among persons not at all reactive to additives.

Patients change their habits more or less correctly according to the quality of the medical information received. The crucial problem is still determination of the extent of the role of additives in the individual case. The diagnosis is difficult and relies on the effect of an additive-free diet and/or oral provocation tests, which have several pitfalls. The place of certain additives in this pathology is still controversial.

First, the habits of the *manufacturers* might have changed, either as a consequence of changes in the chemicals added to food or drugs, or because they improved the labeling of packages. Manufacturers might have taken these measures either as a compliance to new regulations, or following their own decision. Second, a change might also be observed in the habits of the *consumers* in general, concerning either their consumption of food or that of pharmaceuticals. Finally, we have to consider the more specific habits of the few *patients* who experience adverse reactions to food and drug additives.

We can also ask ourselves whether there is any justification for changing the habits, that is, for promotion among manufacturers, consumers, or patients avoidance of the use or consumption of certain food chemicals? In other words, what evidence is there that additives actually trigger adverse reactions? Doesn't this controversial subject [1] consist more of anecdotes than of proven facts? If the evidence that such reactions do exist is really given, is the size of the hypersensitive population large enough or the reactions severe enough to impose measures on the whole population? For instance, is it reasonable to deprive the whole population the advantage of

Figure 1.

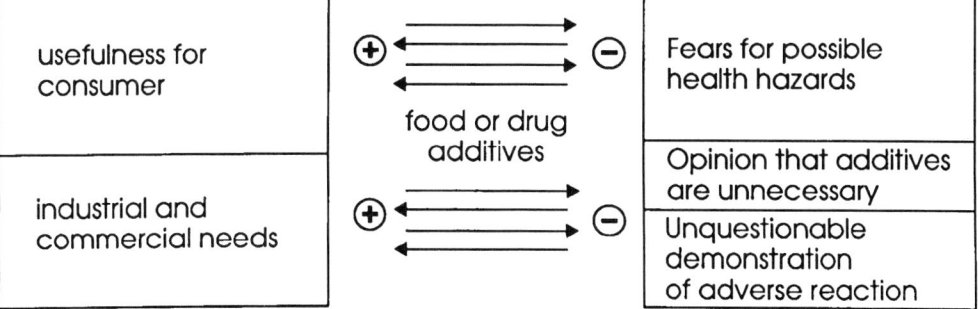

---

* Division of Immunology and Allergy, Centre Hospitalier Universitaire Vaudois (CHUV), CH-1011 Lausanne, Switzerland.

471

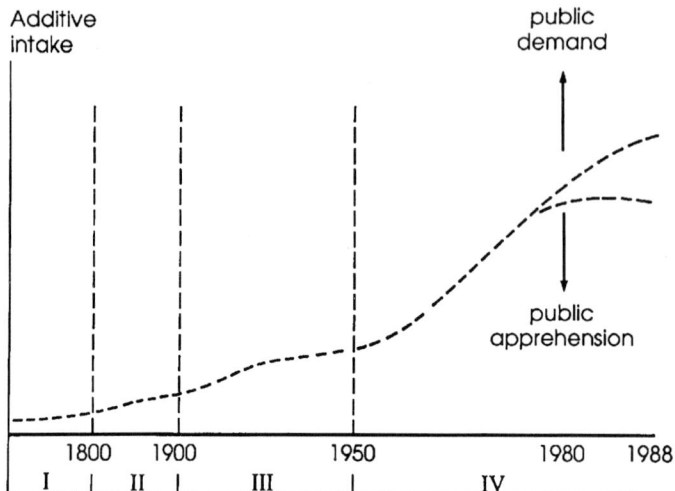

Figure 2.

useful antioxidants and preservatives that allow one to prepare meals rapidly? Shouldn't we rather avoid any conflict between general social welfare on the one hand and rare pathological conditions on the other? Indeed, in recent years, food and drug additives happened to be kept in the middle of many different kinds of contrary forces (Figure 1).

Habits have also changed differently according to the phase of additive history considered [1]. In phase I (Figure 1), food additives consisted mainly of sulfiting agents, which had been added to wine even in ancient times [2]. The first increase in additive intake occurred in the 19th century (phase II). The more marked increase during the 20th century has been related to canned food (phase III), with a very rapid increase since the 1950s (phase IV), arising from the fast-food restaurants and the increasing need to eat rapidly. Figure 2 shows how apprehension among consumers [1] in recent years has tended to counterbalance the increase resulting from public demand.

Symptoms

These can be summarized by viewing the three main kinds of adverse reactions known to the allergist: asthma, polypous rhinitis, and urticaria. Two or three of these manifestations often occur simultaneously. In adults, the association of asthma and urticaria is fairly typical of reactions to additives, since food constituents may provoke urticaria but hardly asthma.

One, two, or all three of these conditions may occur as acute episodes after meals, more often after restaurant meals [3], and mainly among patients over 40. They are frequently accompanied by blood eosinophilia or a history of drug reactions [4].

That other manifestations like headache, anaphylaxis, digestive or behavioral problems might result from additive intolerance is much less proven, or for the most part rare [3, 4, 5, 6, 7].

Reactions to additives occur frequently in patients suffering also from IgE-mediated asthma or rhinitis. We recently found [8] a high incidence of IgE-mediated reactions in patients otherwise reactive to additives, as shown by oral provocation tests (OPT). A group of 34 patients suspected of having asthma or urticaria to additives were orally challenged. Of the 24 with positive OPTs, 13 (54%) were considered "allergic" according to history, skin tests, RAST, and total IgE. Among the 10 with negative OPTs, 40% were found to be "allergic."

Patients experiencing asthma or acute sneezing after additive ingestion are also not infrequently those who suffer as well from exercise-induced asthma.

Some physiological and clinical similarities were noted between the reactions described here and reactions arising from different other triggers like those listed in Table 1. This observation led in 1980 to the concept of "pseudoallergic reactions" (PAR) [9, 10], this concept and term now not infrequently in use in Europe.

Table 1. Pseudoallergic reactions (PAR) [9, 10].

Non-immunological reactions mimicking allergy, following the intake of:
— aspirin + NSAI
— food and drug additives
— morphine and morphine-like substances
— radiographic contrast media
— local anesthetics
— intravenous immunoglobulins
— dextrans and gelatin
— oligopeptidic hormones
— several others

Chemicals Responsible for Eliciting Pseudoallergic Reactions

There is more or less a kind of hierarchy between the different compounds suspected to elicit such reactions. The most frequently recognized as able to do so are listed in Table 2. For those mentioned at the top of the list, the evidence that they trigger reactions is fairly well documented. For the others, such documentation is poor, and for some the reactions are certainly very rare or anecdotal. Tartrazine is still the best studied of the coloring agents. Among the antioxidants and/or preservatives, the groups of the various sulfites has been best studied during recent years [2, 11]. At least six deaths, related to sulfite intake after a restaurant meal, have been reported in the United States, all in asthmatics [12, 13]. Reports on reactions to BHT (butylated hydroxytoluene) are rarer [14]. Nitrites, mostly added to preserve pork meat, have been suspected to induce PARs, in particular headaches. It is also possible that they provoke headaches because of their pharmacologic action as vasodilators [15, 16].

Apart from the severity of the reactions and the likelihood that they trigger the reaction, the chemicals can also be ranked according to the difficulty for consumers to avoid them in the course of daily food intake. For instance, tartrazine, which can be readily identified, is much more easily avoided than the sulfites, which cannot be detected by the consumer and are more broadly distributed, for instance, in restaurant salads, in beverages, wine [17], etc.

Table 2 mentions also the E numbers (or European numbers) that have been given to additives by the European Community. They can be used by the manufacturers as codes for labeling.

Table 3 lists the different groups of chemicals added to food and drug formulations, as well as some active drug components that often trigger the same kind of reactions. Coloring agents and preservatives are by far the additives most commonly used in food and drug preparations. The role of other types of chemicals is very limited. Among flavoring agents, aspartame has been suspected of inducing urticaria [18] and other adverse reactions [19]. The flavor en-

Table 2. Additives responsible for eliciting pseudoallergic reactions.

Dyes	Preservatives
tartrazine = yellow 5 = E102	Na-, K-metabisulfite = E223–224
erythrosine = red 3 = E127	Na-, K-disulfite = E221–222
amaranth = red 2 = E 123	Sulphur dioxide (SO_2) = E220
sunset yellow = yellow 6 = E110	Na-, K-, benzoate = E211–212
ponceau = red 4 = E 124	Na, K-, Ca-sorbates = E201–202, –203
	Na-nitrite = E250
caramel = E150	Na-nitrate = E251

Table 3. Substances eliciting pseudoallergic reactions.

NSAI	Additives to		Drug formulations
	Food		
aspirin	coloring agents		coloring agents
indomethacin	preservatives		preservatives
aminopyrine			
phenylbutazone	antioxidants (BHA, BHT)		
mefenamic acid	emulsifiers		
ibuprofen	gelifiers and		
	thickening substances		
many others	flavoring agents		
	acidifiers (asa)		
	flavor enhancers		
	(Na-, K-, NH_2-glutamates)		
	others		

hancers include the glutamates, which have been made responsible for the so-called Chinese restaurant syndrome, consisting of numbness of the face or chest, burning, warmth, tightness, weakness, and chest pain [20]. Glutamate asthma [21] or angioedema/urticaria were described later [8, 22]. These reactions have been overdiagnosed. They are certainly very rare.

Diagnosis

The role of such chemicals in asthma and urticaria cannot be demonstrated by skin test nor by any in vitro assay. Their role can be strongly suggested by a careful patient's history. For instance, repeated reactions after drinking wine [17], colored drinks, or after restaurant meals [3] are suggestive. A written list of the ingestants taken during the few hours preceding the attacks can be helpful. Physicians and patients should be aware of the local regulations on food additives in order to more correctly suspect what additive could be contained in each food. The physicians should also be informed on what additives are added to pharmaceuticals.

The possible role of additives can best be shown through an improvement of the clinical conditions after an additive-free diet of about two weeks, prescribed first as a diagnostic measure [8, 23]. Finally, oral provocation tests (OPTs) can contribute to the diagnosis [4, 8]. OPTs consists of oral intake of various food additives given in progressive doses to a fasting subject, after some 14 days of an additive-free diet. Results are considered as positive (1) in the case of asthma, if a decrease in the peak flow rate of at least 20% is measured, (2) in the case of urticaria, if skin lesions clearly appear, and (3) in any case, if lacrimation, sneezing, cough, or diarrhea appear.

Thanks to OPTs, a causative role of additives was shown by several authors, for instance, with sulfites [17, 24, 25], tartrazine [26, 27], several additives in asthma [8, 28] or in urticaria [29, 30, 31].

OPTs are unfortunately time-consuming, since chemicals must be tested cautiously, in progressive doses, and with a sufficient time interval between two different additives. In urticaria, OPTs are also of limited value, because of the lack of any quantitative estimation of the skin reactions. But the most important drawback of OPTs is that they are often hardly repeatable. This could result from the fact that starting with small doses, before reaching the eliciting ones, might induce a kind of rush desensitization. It is also possible that the amount of an additive—however equivalent to what was taken during a meal—does not induce a response because of the lack of association with other additives or other kinds of stimulations occurring during meals [32]. An additional difficulty is related to the sulfites, in that some patients react to their inhalation rather than to their ingestion. In this respect, OPTs should be performed by administered the substance dissolved in water, rather than as capsules. But this, unfortunately, increases the difficulty of administering the substance blind.

Prevalence of Reactions to Food Additives

Which part of the population is, in fact, concerned by the possibility of a change in their habits. Figures are difficult to establish, because most studies were performed on selected groups of persons. The prevalence has been calculated to be some 0.1% of the whole population [23, 33, 34]. In a study performed with sulfites in asthmatics, the prevalence of reactions to those substances was of 3.9% [24]. It was about 10–20% in asthmatics studied with dyes and preservatives [35, 36]. The prevalence has been found to be significantly higher (30%) in asthmatics older than 45 years, or in asthmatics without any IgE-mediated reactions demonstrable. A prevalence of 30–50% was found in cases of chronic urticaria [37, 38]. About 5–10% of the aspirin-sensitive patients react to additives as well.

Regulations on Food Additives

Total interdiction has been obtained for tartrazine or azo dyes in some areas, for instance, in Sweden [30] and in France. For other additives—or in other countries—a limitation in quantity is often prescribed. For the sulfites, for instance, some regulations limit their quantity to 10 mg/kg (as SO_2), but allow an exception for different kinds of food, such as dried fruits, which may contain up to 2000 mg/kg. Finally, the regulations may limit the number of foods to which the addition of one given additive is permitted. In several European countries, sulfites, azo dyes, and benzoates are, for instance, permitted to be added to about 20 foodstuffs [39, 40].

The question is now: What do manufacturers actually add? In fact, many of them rather stay on the safe side of the regulations. They also try to substitute seminatural substances.

Unfortunately, this satisfying and heartening trend has not yet gone that far for drug additives. We recently made a survey on the additive content of the 1500 formulations most frequently used in Switzerland [41]. Seven percent of the tablets were shown to contain tartrazine and 11% erythrosine. Twenty-six percent of the effervescent tablets contained sunset yellow, this dye being found in 18% of the powders and 10% of the syrups. Eight percent of the syrups also contained benzoate, which was found in 50% of the various oral solutions. Sorbates were present in 23% of the nebulizers and pressurized aerosols prescribed to asthmatics. A comparison between formulations sold in 1982 and in 1986 showed no change, except for a decrease in the addition of tartrazine, which was present in 10% of the tablets in 1982 and 6% in 1986. Coloring agents and preservatives are still added today to some formulas specially sold to allergic patients. For instance, 8 of 10 antihistamine syrups were found to contain benzoate, 2 sorbates, and 2 sunset yellow.

Labeling

The policy most recommended today should consist of better information for the few hypersensitive subjects rather than constrictions imposed on the population at large. Labeling is the best way to offer broad and sufficient protection and to enable the offending agent to be avoided.

The regulations on the specific labeling of food of food and drug additives differ from one country to another. The European Community Scientific Committee for food set out regulations in 1982 and established the "E

numbers," which mean "approved by the European Community" [29, 42]. In the U.K., according to the "Labelling in Food Regulation, 1984," all additives had to be listed by name or code by July 1986 [23, 32]. In the Federal Republic of Germany, labeling is mandatory for food additives. For instance, sulfites must be labeled when over 50 mg/kg (SO_2) for all foodstuffs, but not for wine. In Switzerland, labeling has been mandatory for food additives since 1984 and for drug additives since 1986, by name or by EC codes.

Finally, it is interesting to look at what the manufacturers actually mention on packages, leaflets, or boxes. The labeling by category names, such as "coloring agents" is useless, since it does not permit any selection by the patient. The nominative declaration of all additives "recognized" as capable of eliciting reactions is already a better step. However, it does not permit the recognition of a reaction to a substance, which would only exceptionally be a trigger. The full labeling of all additives offers in the end the best safety to the patient and might also in the future allow the possible recognition of reactions to substances not yet implicated in pseudoallergic reactions [43].

How does the *population at large* behave regarding additives? What is its perception of the problem? Food additives have received a bad press in recent years. A tendency to eat less canned food seems to have appeared in Europe. The E numbers may have started to offer a disincentive to purchasing [32]. In some countries, there is a trend toward a decrease in the use of food additives, mainly of the coloring agents, because it is what the consumer sees and what is less necessary. Just a "cover-up" is indeed not very acceptable.

In particular the use of dyes in sweet beverages or in pastries is tending to decrease slightly. The suppression of any coloring agents is sometimes used in advertising: "no artificial coloring." There are also differences between European countries. In some Mediterranean countries, with better possibilities of obtaining fresh fruits or with a stronger tradition of fresh vegetables, the acceptability of non-colored foodstuffs is better.

However, there is probably no tendency toward a drop in sulfite intake, because of the content of sulfite in wine and soft drinks. At the level of the whole population, the habits have, in fact, not changed much, as information

Table 4. Daily alimentary intake of sulfites (after 40).

Country	SO₂/person/day (mg) mean	max	With/without alcoholic drinks	Method
Netherlands	3	13	with	total alimentation analyses
Switzerland	4.2	25	without	sulfite analyses and
	27.5		with	consumption statistics
Belgium	5.3	23	without	mean consumption
	8–10	23	with	and sulfite analysis
		144	with 350 ml wine	
Germany (FRG)	20		with	
	9–10		without	estimation
		144	with	mean drink consumption in wine drinkers
	12.2		without	mean consumption
	24.8		with	in whole population

is often poor. Some consumers even avoid fresh fruits because they believe that the main problem lies in the surface treatment. Examples of daily alimentary intake of sulfites are given in Table 4. The table shows how different the level of sulfite ingestion can be, depending on whether or not alcoholic beverages are considered [40].

How to the few *patients* experiencing additive reactions behave regarding avoidance of food additives? They often do not identify their possible role as well as that of food constituents. They cannot see the role of preservatives as well as that of dyes. Their habits depend much on the medical information they receive, but sometimes—even if well informed—they are not ready to recognize an additive, because they do not like to avoid the foodstuff containing that particular additive (e.g., sulfite in wine!).

Fear of chemicals in the cooking pot is increasing somewhat in Europe. The role of additives sometimes tends to be exaggerated [32, 42], perhaps as a consequence of the dismissal of responsibility to others, because of exaggerated ecological principles, or because one does not tolerate that possible risks be imposed by the food or drug companies. Many of us have observed cases of obsessiveness in additive-free diet. But even if the role of additives is limited, the addition of conservants and colors—intended to increase profits by attracting more consumers—should be reduced and its use avoided in giving only a factitious appearance.

References

1. Fennema, O. M. 1987. Food additives—An unending controversy. Am. J. Nutr. 46: 201.
2. Bush, R. K., S. L. Taylor, and W. Busse. 1986. A critical evaluation of clinical trials in reactions to sulfites. J. Allergy Clin. Immunol. 78: 191.
3. Settipane, G. A. 1987. The restaurant syndrome. New Engl. and Reg. Allergy. Proc. 8: 39.
4. Hannuksela, M., and T. Haahtela. 1987. Hypersensitivity reactions to food additives. Allergy 42: 561.
5. Crayton, J. W. 1986. Adverse reactions to food: Relevance to psychiatric disorders. J. Allergy. Clin. Immunol. 78: 243.
6. Mattes, J. A., and R. Gittelman-Klein. 1978. A crossover study of artificial food coloring in the hyperkinetic child. Am. J. Psychiatry 5: 987.
7. Ribon, A., and S. Joshi. 1982. Is there any relationship between food additives and hyperkinesis? Ann. Allergy 48: 275.
8. Genton, C., P. C. Frei, and A. Pécoud. 1985. Value of oral provocation tests to aspirin and food additives in the routine investigation of asthma and chronic urticaria. J. Allergy Clin. Immunol. 76: 40.
9. Dukor, P., P. Kallos, H. D. Schlumberger, and G. P. West. 1980. Pseudoallergic reactions–PAR. Vol. 1 to 4. Basel: Karger.
10. Kallos, P., and H. D. Schlumberger. 1987. Pseudoallergic reaction–PAR. Int. Arch. Allergy. Appl. Immunol. 82: 1.
11. Pryzbilla, B., and J. Ring. 1987. Sulfit-Überempfindlichkeit. Hautarzt 38: 445.
12. Jacobson, M. F. 1985. Food technology. N. Engl. J. Med. 313: 413.
13. Subcommittee on Oversight and Investigations, Hearings of the House Committee on Energy

and Commerce, March 27, 1985.

14. Moneret-Vautrin, D. A., G. Faure, and M. C. Bene. 1986. Chewing-gum preservative induced toxidermic vasculitis. Allergy 41: 546.

15. Moneret-Vautrin, D. A., C. Einhorn, and J. Tisserand. 1980. Le rôle du nitrite de sodium dans les urticaires histaminiques d'origine alimentaire. Ann. nutr. aliment. 34: 1125.

16. Henderson, W. R., and N. H. Raskin. 1972. "Hotdog" headache: Individual susceptibility to nitrite. Lancet ii: 1162.

17. Dahl, R., J. M. Henriksen, and H. Harving. 1986. Red wine asthma: A controlled challenge study. J. Allergy Clin. Immunol. 78: 1126.

18. Bradstock, M. K., M. K. Serdula, J. S. Marks, R. J. Bernard, N. T. Crane, P. L. Remington, and F. T. Trowbridge. 1986. Evaluation of reactions to food additives: The aspartame experience. Amer. J. Clin. Nutr. 43: 464.

19. Maher, T. 1987. Natural food constituents and food additives: The pharmacologic connection. J. Allergy Clin. Immunol. 79: 413.

20. Kennedy, R. A. 1986. The Chinese restaurant syndrome. An anecdote revisited. Food chem. toxic. 24: 301.

21. Allen, D. H., and G. H. Baker. 1981. Chinese restaurant asthma. N. Engl. J. Med. 305: 1154.

22. Squire, E. N. 1987. Angio-oedema and monosodium glutamate. Lancet i: 988.

23. Young, E., S. Patel, R. Stoneham, R. Rona, and J. D. Wilkinson. 1987. The prevalence of reaction to food additives in a survey population. J. Royal Coll. Physicians (London) 21: 241.

24. Bush, R. K., S. L. Taylor, K. Helden, J. A. Nordlee, and W. W. Busse. 1986. Prevalence of sensitivity to sulfiting agents in asthmatic patients. Am. J. Med. 81: 816.

25. Stevenson, D. D., and R. A. Simon. 1981. Sensitivity to ingested metabisulfites in asthmatic subjects. J. Allergy Clin. Immunol. 68: 26.

26. David, T. J. 1987. Reactions to dietary tartrazine. Arch. Dis. Child. 62: 119.

27. Stevenson, D. D., R. A. Simon, W. R. Lumry, and D. A. Mathison. 1986. Adverse reactions to tartrazine. J. Allergy Clin. Immunol. 78: 182.

28. Ortolani, C., E. Pastorello, M. T. Luraghi, F. Della Torre, M. Bellani, and C. Zanussi. 1984. Diagnosis of intolerance to food additives. Ann. Allergy 53: 588.

29. Supramaniam, G., and J. O. Warner. 1986. Artificial food additive intolerance in patients with angio-oedema and urticaria. Lancet ii: 907.

30. Juhlin, L. 1987. Additives and chronic urticaria. Ann. Allergy. 59: 119.

31. Thune, P., and A. Granholt. 1975. Provocation tests with antiphlogistica and food additives in recurrent urticaria. Dermatologica 151: 360.

32. Lessof, M. H. 1987. Adverse reactions to food additives. J. Royal Coll. Physicians (London) 21: 237.

33. Poulsen, E. 1980. Danish report on allergy and intolerance to food ingredients and food additives. Toxicology Forum, Aspen, Colorado.

34. Commission of the Europ. Communities. Brussels. 1981. Report of a working group on adverse reactions to ingested additives. 111: 556.

35. Weber, R. W., M. Hofmann, A. R. Dudley, and H. S. Nelson. 1979. Incidence of bronchoconstriction due to aspirin, azo dyes and preservatives in a population of perennial asthmatics. J. Allergy Clin. Immunol. 64: 32.

36. Moneret-Vautrin, D. A. 1986. Food antigens and additives. J. Allergy Clin. Immunol. 78: 1307.

37. Juhlin, L. 1981. Recurrent urticaria and angio-oedema: Clinical investigation of 330 patients. Br. J. Dermatol. 104: 369.

38. Michaëlsson, G., and L. Juhlin. 1973. Urticaria induced by preservatives and dye additives in food and drugs. Br. J. Dermatol. 88: 525.

39. Ordonnance sur les additifs admis dans les denrées alimentaires (Switzerland). 1.10.1986/4.11.1987. Département de l'Intérieur/Chancellerie d'Etat.

40. Wever, J. 1986. Sulfit in Lebensmitteln—ein Gesundheitsrisiko? Z. Ernährungswiss. 25: 146.

41. Kolly, M., A. Pécoud, and P. C. Frei. 1989. Additives contained in drug formulations most frequently prescribed in Switzerland. Ann. Allergy, in press.

42. E numbers, doctors and patients: Food for thought. 1984. Drug. Ther. Bull. 22: 41.

43. Lück, E. 1987. Lebensmittelzusatzstoffe aus der Sicht des Lebensmittelchemikers. Z. Hautkr. 62: 36.

Advances in Vaccination

G. J. V. Nossal*

Vaccines remain history's most cost-effective public health tools, and therefore it is very appropriate that a Congress of Allergology and Clinical Immunology should receive an overview of what is happening in the field of vaccination worldwide. Before discussing the vaccines of the future, it is worth recalling that the current expanded program of immunization being coordinated by the WHO, UNICEF, and other agencies represents one of the few shining beacons in an otherwise very troubled world public health scene. In March of 1988, the world's leading experts on maternal and child health met and set an ambitious agenda for the 1990s. This conference ("Bellagio III") had a curiously optimistic flavour; its ambitious but achievable goals included:

— the global eradication of poliomyelitis by the end of the 20th century;

— the reduction of measles deaths by 95%;

— the virtual elimination of neonatal tetanus;

— a 70% decrease in deaths from diarrhoeal diseases; and

— a 50% reduction in maternal mortality.

The capacity to take such a positive stance arises from the spectacular success of the global immunization program, which is already reaching over 50% of the world's children, a vast improvement from the situation 10 years ago. The reason for bringing the issue up in a scholarly treatise such as this is to stress the immensity of the stakes for which we are playing. If, by the close of the century, an infrastructure exists for the delivery of the current childhood vaccines to 90% or more of the world's children, the new and improved vaccines arising from research over this period can be grafted onto the existing efforts, a process that should appeal enormously to third-world nations as they at first hand see the child and maternal health benefits derivable from vac-

cines. This prospect should encourage the research community in the efforts with which this lecture deals.

The new biology has made an enormous contribution to the search for new and improved vaccines. Essentially, the mass synthesis of any peptide or protein that would be desired in a molecular vaccine is now a matter of technology alone. The fundamental principles of molecular biology and protein chemistry have been solved. However, the largest underlying and unsolved problem in modern vaccinology is immunopotentiation, that is, how to make the new generation of molecular vaccines sufficiently immunogenic. This huge issue is relevant to the whole spectrum of diseases we might wish to control, even though the types of immune response required for disease control will vary from case to case. Rather than listing the many types of vaccine that are in the research pipeline, this contribution concentrates on the major approaches to immunopotentiation under very active research at the moment.

New and Improved Molecular Vaccines

Traditionally, vaccines have fallen into three major headings, namely, live attenuated vaccines, killed microorganisms, or molecular vaccines (albeit somewhat crude ones) such as tetanus toxoid or diphtheria toxoid. In the search for new and improved vaccines, this basic pattern has been continued but refined. For live, attenuated organisms, highly sophisticated genetic manipulations are producing bacterial and viral variants with known properties, and furthermore avirulent organisms are being used as carriers of foreign genes which, following expression, could act as vaccines for some completely different microorganism from the attenuated strain in question. This is basically

* The Walter and Eliza Hall Institute of Medical Research, P.O. Royal Melbourne Hospital, Victoria 3050, Australia. This work was supported by the National Health and Medical Research Council, Canberra, Australia; by Grant AI-03958 from the National Institute of Allergy and Infectious Diseases, United States Public Health Service; and by the generosity of a number of private donors to The Walter and Eliza Hall Institute.

a recombinant attenuated organism. For the newer killed vaccines, biotechnology has so far not made a substantial contribution. However, for molecular vaccines, where there is a lot of active research, several different approaches are jostling for priority. There are proponents of the chemical synthesis route, who argue that pure peptides, perhaps attached to some defined carrier, will prove effective, thus obviating the need for any recombinant DNA technology, or for purification from potentially toxic bacterial products. On the other hand, there are a greater number of proponents of the genetic engineering approach, using biological synthesis in bacterial, yeast, or mammalian cells after appropriate genetic engineering. Finally, a still different approach is that of anti-idiotypic antibodies, which under appropriate circumstances can act as an "internal image" of the original immunogen, and thus evoke an immune response.

All molecular vaccines rest on a set of five assumptions, which require validation in each particular situation. First, there is the assumption that a subset of epitopes will be sufficient to produce protective immunity. By comparison with either a live attenuated vaccine or a killed vaccine comprising the whole microorganism, each molecular vaccine presents only a minor proportion of the antigenic universe of the whole organism. This is certainly a limitation, but there are also situations in which it might be a signal benefit, such as in diseases like malaria, where it seems highly likely that part of the "strategy" of the organism is to direct the majority of the immune attack against certain tandemly repeated epitopes of molecules, the immune response to which is not at all protective. If, in a situation like that, one can be intelligent enough to isolate only those antigens or portions of antigens, the immune response to which is essential for host protection, then the exclusion of irrelevant epitopes is a positive benefit. Secondly, the new biotechnologies—be they synthetic or recombinant DNA—will have to overcome the many production problems, again particular for each case. It must be remembered that, for most of its history, vaccinology has been a kind of "cottage industry," the technology for the bacterial vaccines being relatively straightforward—and even that for the viral vaccines now being well standardised. A substantial learning curve will be necessary as we enter the new era.

The third assumption is that the correct immune effector mechanism will be identified by the vaccine developer. There is not much point in developing a vaccine that will cause excellent antibody production, when what is needed for host protection is strong T cell immunity. Citing the case of malaria once again, the tide has certainly turned here recently, with T cell immunity appearing to be far more prominent than previously imagined [1].

The fourth assumption is that adjuvants or other immunopotentiating agents of sufficient efficacy and safety for human use will become available. This point represents a significant roadblock at the present time.

Finally, and related to the first assumption, it is to be hoped that safety will be assured through the exclusion of undesirable contaminants and of epitopes that may in fact be helpful to the microorganism rather than the host.

Some vaccines have recently entered clinical trial that could already be defined as molecular vaccines. These include bacterial polysaccharides such as the polyvalent pneumococcal vaccines; the hepatitis B vaccine, which is essentially pure polymerised hepatitis B surface antigen; the putative birth control vaccine, consisting of all or portion of the b chain of human chorionic gonadotrophin conjugated to a toxoid; and the putative anti-sporozoite vaccine for falciparum malaria, consisting of three repeats of the tetrapeptide of the circumsporozoite antigen conjugated to toxoid. For the latter cases, the results of clinical trials are eagerly awaited.

Principles for Increasing Immunogenicity

A large range of procedures to enhance immunogenicity have evolved over several decades through measures that retain a considerable empirical element. The most potent methods, e.g., Freund's complete adjuvant, certainly combine a number of the separate principles listed below. We shall deal only briefly with the chief principles involved.

Slowing the Absorption of the Immunogen

Large, sudden pulses of pure protein antigens risk activating the suppressor limb of immune responses, particularly if the intravenous route is used. Slow absorption from a subcutaneous depot site permits extensive access to the widely scattered dendritic cells and macrophages, and also ensures that antigen will still be available after the initial burst of clonal proliferation, thus permitting some facets of a secondary response. Slow absorption is favoured by adsorbing antigens onto aluminium hydroxide ("alum precipitation"), placing antigens into water-in-oil emulsions, incorporating antigens into liposomes, and other similar manipulations. This method is conceptually close to the next one.

Rendering the Antigen Particulate

Particles are more attractive to macrophages and tilt the balance in favour of immunity rather than suppression. This can vary from a simple heat-induced aggregation to sophisticated polymerisation strategies, including the self-aggregation characteristic of antigens such as the soluble antigen of hepatitis B virus. In the case of liposomes or oily droplets, there is a combined effect of particulateness and slow absorption, as there is with alum precipitation.

Co-Exhibition of the Antigen with a Highly Immunogenic Agent

If one particular vaccine is highly immunogenic, the adjuvant effect of that vaccine—and also the characteristics it may possess for guiding the response toward a particular immunological pathway—may "spill over" into a response to an antigen co-administered with it. For example, killed H. pertussis or C. parvum bacteria are powerfully immunogenic; if a pure protein is given in the same injection, the response to it is enhanced. Certain immunogens (for reasons that are unclear) guide the response in particular directions, e.g., extracts of a parasite such as Nippostrongylus brasiliensis elicit powerful IgE responses. Pure proteins co-administered will also evoke an IgE response. Presumably this is somehow tied up with the spectrum of lymphokines evoked by particular agents, which guide isotype switch patterns. The polyclonal activating characteristics of lymphokines may also underlie the enhancement of immune responses in general.

Chemical Immunopotentiation

A long history of research underlies a search for a pure, safe, effective, non-toxic, small organic molecule that mimics the potentiation of the whole immune response that can be achieved with killed M. tuberculosis or other toxic microbial extracts such as E. coli lipopolysaccharide. A review of this area is outside the scope of this paper. Suffice it to say that no uniformly satisfactory agent has been approved for human use, and a dissociation between toxicity and efficacy has been difficult to achieve. Covalent coupling of the immunoactive agent and the immunogen of interest is one approach worth following.

Attachment to a Suitable Carrier Protein

This has already been mentioned, but the nature of the carrier requires definition. It is important that the antigen in question activate helper T lymphocytes, not only because T cells are essential for protection in many situations, but also because the T helper cell is required for antibody production, affinity maturation, and isotype switch, all of which are necessary in many protective situations. It is now clear that many proteins possess only one or, at best, very few T cell epitopes, that is, linear sequences of amino acids capable of fitting into the putative antigen-binding cleft of the major histocompatibility complex (MHC) molecule [2]. In practice, most whole microorganisms contain antigens possessed of such epitopes, though it is of interest that some humans are genetically poor responders to highly relevant antigens such as hepatitis B or schistosomal antigens [3]. However, in any given polypeptide vaccine, the number of such epitopes may be small or even zero; hence the requirement to link the polypeptide to a highly immunogenic carrier. The definition of a suitable carrier for human vaccines is not an easy matter. There is merit in considering a useful carrier such as diphtheria or tetanus toxoid, yet the possibility remains that pre-existent immunity to the carrier may have unpredictable effects on the immunogenicity of the polypeptide of interest. The use of a randomly chosen, highly immunogenic carrier such as keyhole limpet haemocyanin also poses ethical and regulatory problems, not the least being an assurance of freedom from endotoxin. There is sufficient work currently going on related to the properties required in a T cell epitope to make one optimistic concerning future tailor-made carrier proteins, though care will need to be taken to avoid immune response gene effects, perhaps by maintaining some heterogeneity in the carrier.

Genetically Engineered Microorganisms as Carriers of Genes for Important Antigens

This notion was pioneered by Paoletti [4] and Moss [5], who engineered the vaccinia virus also to include genes coding for important host-protective antigens of various pathogens. The general idea is by no means confined to vaccinia virus. For example, adenoviruses may turn out to represent more acceptable viral carriers of antigen genes. Moreover, an extensive body of work supports the notion that *Salmonella* bacteria can be engineered to carry a wide variety of antigens, the approach, of course, being most germane to enteric infections such as cholera or bacillary dysentery, though by no means confined to them. These recombinant attenuated living vaccines have many attractions. It must be remembered that vaccinia viruses and, even more so, BCG have enjoyed wide usage in human populations, and though side effects of a serious nature are not unknown, they are rare. The case becomes even more persuasive when one considers the relatively slow development of adjuvants suitable for human use. Moreover, many experimental, veterinary, and medical examples attest to the fact that live, attenuated vaccines are very potent, conferring immunity that may be lifelong. An interesting variant was introduced by Langford et al. [6]. Arguing that cell surface-associated antigens were more likely to evoke a strong T-cell response than secreted antigens, they added coding information for the transmembrane domain of an immunoglobulin heavy chain to the gene for the soluble S antigen of *P. falciparum*, and inserted the hybrid gene into vaccinia. The construct was found to lead to greatly enhanced immunogenicity. Of course, there is no reason that this basic idea should be confined to just a single gene. In fact, in our laboratory there are now several constructs that could be referred to as "super-

genes" in which a variety of coding regions for quite different antigens are stacked end to end in the one vaccinia virus construct.

A further elaboration of this idea is to insert genes for various interleukins into engineered vaccinia viruses already carrying genes for important antigens. For example, the response to vaccinia itself can be markedly enhanced by the insertion of the IL-2 gene into the virus, permitting immunodeficient mice to recover from an otherwise fatal infection. However, it is becoming apparent that the early hopes for a marked enhancement of the immune response in normal animals by this stratagem are unlikely to come to fruition, at least with IL-2. Nevertheless, the approach is certainly worthy of continued exploration.

Examples of Early Vaccine Research from The Walter and Eliza Hall Institute

Apart from the malaria vaccine research already mentioned, and extensively summarised elsewhere, recent research from The Walter and Eliza Hall Institute can illustrate some of the fascinating problems of a scientific nature that confront the search for new and improved vaccines. For example, the group of Dr. Graham F. Mitchell [7] has uncovered a potential vaccine candidate molecule in schistosomiasis through the use of detective work involving an animal model. It was noted that, in the mouse, there was a marked genetic element in the worm burden resulting from a particular challenge inoculum. Antibody preparations from infected mice of each of the two strains were prepared in order to pose the question of whether there was some antigen or antigens recognised by the resistant strain but not recognised by the susceptible strain. Two-dimensional gel electrophoresis of extracts of adult worms revealed one particular protein that was consistently identified by the sera of infected resistant mice, but not by the susceptible strain. This material was prepared in sufficient amounts for N-terminal amino acid analysis, construction of an oligonucleotide probe, and search in a cDNA library revealed the corresponding clone. Sequence data information obtained by this strategy was submitted to computer search, and it turned out that the molecule of interest was highly homologous to glutathione-S-transferase. Enough of this enzyme was prepared as a fusion protein to permit an immunisation trial in mice. Encouraging results have been obtained, and while it is unlikely that the enzyme alone will be enough to constitute a useful human vaccine, this may represent the first occasion on which an important parasite enzyme has been shown to have some host-protective immunogenic activity.

The leishmaniases constitute another group of parasitic diseases collectively of considerable public health importance. Dr. Emanuela Handman and her colleagues have been investigating possible vaccine approaches and have identified a *Leishmania* lipophosphoglycan derived from the parasite which they believe might make an interesting vaccine candidate [8]. It is furthermore believed that this molecule is involved in the attachment of the single-celled parasite to the membrane of the macrophage it must penetrate in order to multiply. It is important to remember that some host-protective pathogen-derived antigens are carbohydrate in nature rather than protein, and of course here neither recombinant DNA technology nor peptide synthesis will provide the answers to production. However, in the case of the *Leishmania* lipophosphoglycan, it appears likely that conventional culture techniques followed by chemical isolation will suffice to provide sufficient material for suitable vaccine trials.

Conclusions

What is particularly exciting about progress in vaccinology at the moment is the new spirit within the academic community. Until about a decade ago, academic research in immunology and practical progress in vaccinology were poles apart. The vast bulk of the energy of the academic community was devoted either to fundamental aspects, or to diseases principally of relevance to the industrialised nations, such as cancer, autoimmune diseases, allergy, and the problems of organ transplantation. This meant that progress in practical immunisation depended on disciples of other disciplines, such as virology and bacteriology. Now, however, the academic community has realised its responsibilities to the Pasteurian legacy. Well before the AIDS virus made its appearance on

the scene, an increasing number of leading researchers had turned their attention to the health problems of the tropical developing countries, and particularly to immunoparasitology. It goes without saying that the intense desire for an AIDS vaccine has accelerated the trend. The decade that we have passed through has had its sobering component. Much progress has been made on many fronts, but formidable problems such as antigenic variation, the need for a T cell epitope, and the lack of a suitable human adjuvant have made progress slower than one might have hoped. Still, one key achievement is the fact that the academic community and the practically oriented vaccine developer are now in active dialogue across many fronts.

Some formidable roadblocks remain for the would-be vaccine inventor. There is really little incentive for the pharmaceutical industry to invest heavily, because in the last analysis vaccines are not particularly profitable. High research costs, high quality control problems, governments as purchasers in many instances, and infrequent usage all make vaccines less profitable than drugs. An even greater factor is the product liability issue, which deters numerous companies from even entering the race. On the other hand, within the academic community there is relatively little glamour attached to vaccine development. Although there are many fascinating problems of the host-pathogen relationship that obviously need to be explored, much of vaccine research in this modern era boils down to questions such as –Which antigen? Which carrier? Which adjuvant? What dose? How many doses at what spacing?"—and these are not questions of the highest intellectual interest. Finally, university-based groups are clearly not efficient at developmental research, scale-up or meeting the maze of regulatory requirements. All of this being so, we should perhaps be encouraged by the progress that has been made. What is most heartening of all is that truly productive consortia have been formed between leading academic groups and leading pharmaceutical companies. I am happy to say that in the latter case, humanitarian motives have been high on the agenda in some instances. We must persist in these endeavours, because in many countries vaccines represent essentially the only hope for lowering childhood mortality and morbidity to acceptable levels.

References

1. Weiss, W. R., M. Sedegah, R. L. Beaudoin, L. Miller, and M. F. Good. 1988. CD8+ T cells (cytotoxic/suppressors) are required for protection in mice immunized with malaria sporozoites. Proc. Natl. Acad. Sci. USA. 85: 573–576.

2. Good, M. F., D. Pombo, I. A. Quakyi, E. M. Riley, R. A. Houghten, A. Menon, D. W. Alling, J. A. Berzofsky, and L. H. Miller. 1988. Human T-cell recognition of the circumsporozoite protein of *Plasmodium falciparum*: Immunodominant T-cell domains map to the polymorphic regions of the molecule. Proc. Natl. Acad. Sci. USA. 85: 1199–1203.

3. Sasazuki, T., and S. Matsushita. 1987. MHC-Linked immune suppression genes determine the phenotype of immune response to some natural antigens in humans. J. Immunogenet. 14: 99–101.

4. Panicali, D., and E. Paoletti. 1982. Construction of posviruses as cloning vectors: Insertion of the thymidine kinase gene from herpes simplex virus into the DNA of infectious vaccinia virus. Proc. Natl. Acad. Sci. USA. 79: 4927–4931.

5. Smith, G. L., M. Mackett, and B. Moss. 1983. Infectious vaccinia virus recombinants that express hepatitis B virus surface antigen. Nature, 302: 490–495.

6. Langford, C. J., S. J. Edwards, G. L. Smith, G. F. Mitchell, B. Moss, D. J. Kemp, and R. F. Anders. 1986. Anchoring a secreted plasmodial antigen on the surface of recombinant vaccinia virus infected cells increases its immunogenicity. Mol. Cell. Biol. 6: 3191–3199.

7. Mitchell, G. F., K. M. Davern, W. U. Tiu, M. D. Wright, K. L. Henkle, and M. V. Rogers. 1988. Resistance to infection with *Schistosoma japonicum* and *S. mansoni* in 129 mice: Speculation on the contribution of immune responses to schistosome glutathione s-transferases. Parasitol. Today, in press.

8. Mitchell, G. F., and E. Handman. 1987. Heterologous protection in murine cutaneous leishmaniasis. Immunol. Cell. Biol. 65: 387–392.

Analysis of Distinct Human T Cell Subsets Expressing a γ/δ Antigen Receptor

Alessandro Moretta*, Cristina Bottino**, Ermanno Ciccone**, Giuseppe Tambussi*, Silvano Ferrini**, Paola Varese**, Nicola Migone***, Maria Cristina Mingari**/****, Lorenzo Moretta**/****

The TCR gamma/delta+ cell subset differs from conventional T cells in a number of phenotypic and functional characteristics. The simultaneous lack of both CD4 and CD8 antigens allows to greatly enrich for TCR gamma/delta+ cells (by monoclonal antibodies and complement). Cloning of CD4⁻/CD8⁻ peripheral blood lymphocytes, under limiting dilution conditions, revealed that they are homogeneously composed of cytolytic cells that, in most instances, lyse tumor target cells.

The use of different monoclonal antibodies specific for TCR gamma/delta molecules allowed identification of two distinct subsets which bound BB3 and delta-TCSs-1 mAbs, respectively. The BB3-reactive TCR molecules were represented by Cγ1-encoded disulphide-linked heterodimers, whereas delta-TCS-1 reacted with Cγ2-encoded non-disulphide-linked molecules. Both BB3 and delta-TCS-1 mAb induced activation of cloned cells expressing the corresponding antigenic determinants. Analysis of the unfrequent delta-TCS-1⁺ clones which express surface CD8 molecules revealed that the "heavy" 55 kD form of (Cγ2-encoded) gamma-chain is selectively expressed by this cell type. Analysis of the distribution of subsets expressing different TCR gamma/delta isotypes showed that the Cγ1-encoded, BB3-reactive form is prevalent in the peripheral blood, but virtually absent in the thymus. In contrast, cells expressing the Cγ2-encoded, delta-TCS-1 reactive form are relatively unfrequent in peripheral blood, but represent the majority of TCR gamma/delta⁺ thymocytes.

Finally, "rare" (<5%) BB3⁻, delta-TCS-1⁻ clones were derived from peripheral blood WT31⁻ lymphcytes. These cells expressed in all instances a Cγ2 encoded non-disulphide-linked form of TCR indistinguishable from that recognized by delta-TCS-1 mAb.

The Two Major Subsets of TCR γ/δ+ Human Lymphocytes

A minor subset of human peripheral T lymphocytes express CD3-associated receptor for antigen (TCR) composed of gamma and delta chains. A remarkable phenotypic feature of most of these cells is the lack of surface expression of both CD4 and CD8 surface markers, which normally define the two major subsets of TCR alpha/beta⁺. Indeed, in a first series of experiments, we derived TCR gamma/delta⁺ clones from T cell populations depleted of CD4⁺ and CD8⁺ cells by treatment with mAb⁺ complement. These clones were analyzed for the reactivity with different mAbs directed to TCR gamma/delta. We found that the majority (i.e., about 70%) of clones derived from CD8⁻ Cd4⁻ peripheral blood T cells reacted with the mAb termed BB3, recently isolated in our laboratory [2]. Most of the remaining clones reacted with the delta-TCS-1 mAb but not with BB3 mAb; indeed, in no instances could we isolate clones expressing both the antigenic determinants recognized by the two mAbs [3]. Thus, BB3 and delta-TCS-1 mAbs react with distinct TCR gamma/delta⁺ cell subsets. More interestingly, these two cell subsets appear to express different molecular forms of the receptor. Indeed, all clones reacting with BB3 mAb displayed the Cγ1-encoded, disulphide-linked form of the receptor, whereas delta-TCS-1 mAb identified non-disulphide-linked molecules encoded by the Cγ2 gene segment [3]. In both forms of TCR gamma/delta, the gamma gene

---

*   Istituto di Istologia ed Embriologia Generale, Genova, Italy
**   Istituto Nazionale per la Ricerca sul Cancro, Genova, Italy
***   Dipartimento di Genetica, Biologia e Chimica Medica, Universita' di Torino, Torino, Italy
**** Istituto di Oncologia Clinica e Sperimentale, Genova, Italy.
      This work was supported in part by grants awarded by the Italian CNR P.F. Oncologia to A. Moretta, L. Moretta, and M. C. Mingari, and by the Associazione Italiana per la Ricerca sul Cancro (AIRC).

product displayed a molecular weight ranging between 41 and 44 kD; thus among such CD4⁻CD8⁻TCR gamma/delta⁺ clones (over 50 clones analyzed) we could not detect the high molecular form (55 kD) of the gamma chain that has been previously reported by others [1].

More recently, we have been able to derive TCR gamma/delta⁺ clones from purified TCR alpha/beta⁻ fractions of peripheral blood E-rosetting cells. Such cell populations, which were obtained after sorting WT31⁻ cells, contained variable proportions of CD3⁺ cells (ranging between 40% and 80%). Out of >10 TCR gamma/delta⁺ clones analyzed, about 70% reacted with BB3 mAb, whereas most of the remaining clones were delta-TCS-1⁺.

CD8⁺ TCRγ/δ⁺ Lymphocytes

It is well established that a remarkable feature of TCR gamma/delta bearing cells is the lack of expression of both CD4 and CD8 differentiation antigens. However, previous studies have indicated that a small fraction of these cells may express CD8 antigen [1]. Since in this set of experiments we selected WT31⁻ (TCR alpha/beta negative) cells (and not CD4⁻CD8⁻ cells as in the first set of experiments) the clones obtained should be representative of the whole TCR gamma/delta⁺ population and thus contain also CD8⁺ clones. Indeed, among all the clones analyzed, a small fraction (about 1:60) was found to express surface CD8 as detected by indirect immunofluorescence and cytofluorographic analysis. These CD8+ TCR gamma/delta⁺ clones reacted with delta-TCS-1

mAb, thus suggesting that they expressed the non-disulphide linked form of TCR gamma/delta (Figure 1). Indeed, cell surface iodination followed by immunoprecipitation with anti-CD3 mAb under conditions which preserve the CD3/TCR association (digitonin 1%) showed that all CD8⁺ clones analyzed expressed the non disulphide-linked form of TCR gamma/delta (Figure 2). However, the molecular

Figure 2. SDS-PAGE analysis of CD3-associated TCR molecules immunoprecipitated from the three major types of TCR gamma/delta⁻bearing human T lymphocytes. Ten cloned cells were surface labeled and then lysed in buffer containing digitonin. Cells lysates were immunoprecipitated by using anti-Leu4 (anti-CD3) mAb, lane a: clone D1.12 (CD8+, delta-TCS-1+), lane b: clone D5.100 (CD8-, delta-TCS-1+), lance c: clone GA17 (CD8-, BB3+).

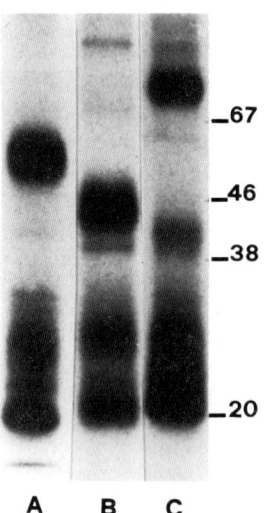

A   B   C

Figure 1. Cytofluorometric analysis of representative CD8⁺ and CD8⁻TCR gamma/delta+ clones. Note that all CD8⁺ clones were of the delta-TCS-1⁺ phenotype.

CD8⁺ AND CD8⁻ CLONES BEARING THE NON - DISULPHIDE LINKED FORM OF TCR γ/δ

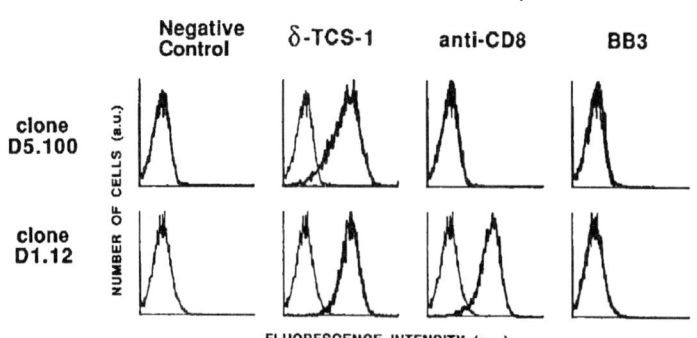

weight of the CD3-associated gamma-chains was considerably higher (55–60 kD) than that previously demonstrated on CD8$^-$TCR gamma/delta$^+$ clones (40–44 kD) isolated from the same donor [4].

The reactivity with a polyclonal anti-gamma chain rabbit antiserum indicated that the 55–60 kD and the 40–44 kD bands expressed by the two types (CD8$^+$ or CD8$^-$) of delta-TCS-1$^+$ clones represented the molecular product of the gamma chain genes. Similar 55–60 kD bands have been immunoprecipitated from all three CD8+ delta-TCS-1$^+$ clones isolated from peripheral blood. Interestingly, a similar band was precipitated also from a delta-TCS-1$^+$ clone derived from WT31$^-$ thymocyte populations. Although only 4 CD8$^+$ delta-TCS-1$^+$ clones could be analyzed (due to their low frequency and also to major difficulties in their in vitro expansion), it should be stressed that all the 25 CD8-delta-TCS-1$^+$ clones analyzed so far expressed the low molecular size (40–44 kD), non-disulphide-linked form of TCR gamma/delta. Therefore, in the panel of clones analyzed, expression—or lack thereof—of CD8 surface antigens appears to correlate with two different molecular sizes of non-disulphide-linked TCR gamma/delta [4]. It is noteworthy that Brenner et al. described a similar type of TCR gamma/delta molecules in immunoprecipitates from the IDP2 polyclonal cell line derived from an immunodeficiency patient. Approximately 50% of IDP2 cells were found to express CD8 surface antigens by FACS analysis [1].

In order to better characterize the TCR gamma/delta molecules expressed by CD8 clones, we further performed 2D-PAGE of CD3-associated molecules immunoprecipitated after lysis of surface iodinated cells in digitonin-containing buffer. It is of note that, by this type of analysis, no substantial differences in charge mobility could be detected among different CD8$^+$ clones (not shown). Indeed, the spots corresponding to the 55 kD gamma-chain expressed in CD8$^+$ clones resulted in slightly more acidic ones than those corresponding to the 40–44 kD gamma chains expressed in either BB3$^+$ or CD8-delta-TCS-1$^+$ clones. The charge mobility of the delta-chain expressed in CD8$^+$ clones could not be compared to that of the other two forms of TCR due to the poor labeling of this chain under the experimental conditions used. Similar prob-

lems of labeling of the 38 kD delta-chain are usually encountered in CD8$^-$delta-TCS-1$^+$ clones, whereas the very basic 44 kD delta-chain expressed in BB3$^+$ clones is normally strongly labeled [3].

Analysis of the DNA configuration at the TCR-gamma loci by means of a probe that can detect both the J1 and J2 regions was performed in three of these CD8$^+$TCR-gamma/delta$^+$ clones [4]. This analysis demonstrated that these 3 clones had rearranged both chromosomes. Thus, the absence of the germ line J1 and J2 containing segments together with the lack of hybridization to JP1 and JP2 specific probes clearly indicated that both the productive and non-productive V-J recombination had involved the most 3' J segments, i.e., J2. It follows that the constant portion of the expressed gamma-chains in the three clones should correspond to the Cγ2 gene segments, since the Cγ1 gene segments mapping upstream to J2 have been deleted.

In contrast to the Cγ1 locus, which codes for a constant region made up of three exons, the Cγ2 locus is polymorphic in size. At least two major alleles have been identified by gene cloning; one contains a duplication, the other a triplication of the second exon [5]. The 55 kD gamma-chain expressed by PEER leukemia cell line has been shown to be coded by a Cγ2 triplicated second exon [5]. Southern analysis by means of an exon 2-specific probe indicated that at least one copy of the triplication allele is present in all three clones (not shown).

Activation Characteristics of CD8$^+$, TCR Gamma/Delta$^+$ Clones

Mabs directed to CD3 or TCR complex (either alpha/beta or gamma/delta) have been shown to trigger the lytic machinery of cytolytic T cells expressing the corresponding receptor molecules [3]. We investigated whether anti-CD3 or anti-TCR gamma/delta (delta-TCS-1) mAb could induce activation of delta-TCS-1$^+$ CD8$^+$ clones. To this end, clones were tested for their ability to kill appropriate target cells represented by the Fcγ receptor-bearing P815 murine cell line. As shown in Table 1, the addition of soluble anti-CD3 mAb efficiently triggered delta-TCS-1$^+$ CD8$^+$ clones as well as delta-TCS-1$^+$ CD8$^-$ or BB3$^+$CD8$^-$ to lyse P815 target cells. On the other hand, delta-TCS-1 mAb activated

Table 1. Anti-TCR-/CD3 mAb-triggered activation of the lytic machinery in different TCR γ/δ+ clones.

Clone	Surface phenotype	mAb added to the cytolytic test*			
		none	anti-CD3	δ-TCS1	BB3
MV28	CD8+δTCS1+	7+	86	18	5
MV120	"	2	65	10	2
D1.12	"	9	71	23	6
T65	"	8	66	17	6
GA17	CD8-BB3+	14	95	12	89
G5.50	"	11	88	14	96
GB8	CD8-δ-TSC1+	3	72	68	4
M50B	"	8	83	89	6

*The various mAbs were added at the onset of the 4 h 51Cr release assay containing the Fc-receptor positive P815 cells.
+Data are expressed as a % specific 51Cr release at an approximate effector:target ratio of 1:1.

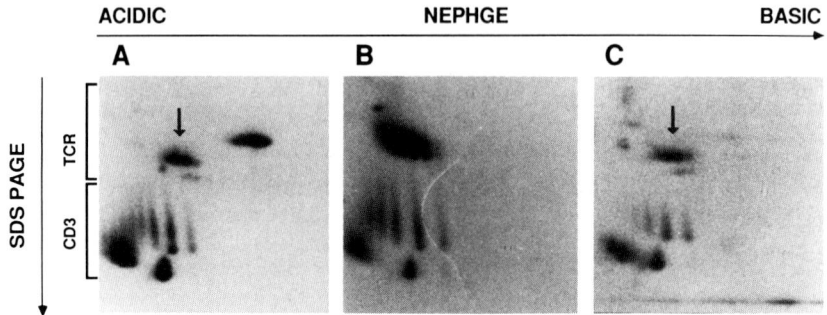

Figure 3. CD3-associated TCR molecules in TCR gamma/delta⁺, BB3⁻, delta TCS-1⁻ clones (Panel B) and in BB3-, Ti A⁺, delta-TCS-1+ clones (Panel C). These two types of "rare" clones are compared with a "conventional" BB3+, Ti A+, delta-TCS-1-clone (Panel A). Arrows indicate the similar gamma-chains that are detected in BB3-TiγA⁺ and in BB3⁺ TiγA⁺ clones.

CD8⁻delta-TCS-1⁺ clones but had only a marginal effect on CD8⁺ delta-TCS-1⁺ clones. Similar figures were obtained with anti-TCR gamma/delta-1, a mAb which appears to react with all forms of TCR gamma/delta (not shown).

It may be possible that the relative inefficiency of anti-TCR gamma-delta mAbs to induce activation of CD8⁺ delta-TCS-1⁺ clones may reflect a partial inability of this TCR type to transduce activation signals. On the other hand, since optimal activation could be induced by anti-CD3 mAbs, the defect would be inherent to the TCR itself or to an inefficient association with CD3 molecules. In addition, one may speculate that CD8 molecules, in cells carrying this particular form of TCR, may be needed in order to facilitate the binding of TCR to its natural ligand (MHC class I?) and/or the signal transduction.

Rare Phenotypes among TCR Gamma/Delta⁺ Cells

Analysis of large numbers of clones led to the isolation of a limited number of exceptions which could be classified in two major groups. In the first group, clones expressed the surface determinant recognized by the anti-TCR gamma/delta-1 mAb (which reacts with all known forms of TCR gamma/delta), but did not react with BB3 nor delta-TCS-1 mAb. These clones represent about 1:80 clones expressing TCR gamma/delta. In all instances the molecular characterization of TCR (Figure 2, Panel B) demonstrated that such clones express a Cγ2-encoded non-disulphide-linked form of receptor, either similar to that found in conventional delta-TCS-1⁺ clones or homologous to that of

CD8$^+$, delta-TCS-1$^+$ clones (in these cases such "double negative" clones expressed surface CD8). In the second group BB3$^-$, delta-TCS-1$^+$ clones reacted with the TiγA mAb which recognizes surface determinants related to the usage of Vγ9 gene segment [6].

While this phenotype is not unusual in TCR gamma/delta$^+$ thymocytes, in peripheral blood those cells that react with BB3 mAb are usually also reacting with TiγA mAb, indicating that most (>95%) of peripheral TiγA$^+$ cells utilize Cγ1 together with V9 (V9-JP rearrangement). However, in clones expressing the BB3-TiγA$^+$, delta-TCS-1$^+$ surface phenotype, Vγ9 is rearranged with J segments located upstream Cγ2. Indeed, the TCR immunoprecipitated from these cells is composed of non disulphide-linked chains. It is of note (Figure 2) that the mol. weight and the charge mobility of gamma-chains expressed in BB3$^+$ TiγA$^+$ clones (Panel A) and in BB3$^-$TiγA$^+$ clones (Panel C) are comparable; the most remarkable difference between these two types of TCR is the absence of the basic 45 kD delta-chain in BB3$^-$ TiγA$^+$ clones.

References

1. Brenner, M. B., J. McLean, D. P. B. Dyalynas, J. L. Strominger, J. A. Smith, F. L. Owen, J. G. Seidman, S. Ip, F. Rosen, and M. S. Krangel. 1986. Identification of a putative second T cell receptor. Nature (Lond.) 322: 145.

2. Ciccone, E., S. Ferrini, C. Bottino, O. Viale, I. Prigione, G. Pantaleo, G. Tambussi, A. Moretta, and L. Moretta. 1988. A monoclonal antibody specific for a common determinant of the human T cell receptor γ/δ directly activates CD3$^+$WT31$^-$lymphocytes to express their functional program(s). J. Exp. Med. 168: 1.

3. Bottino, C., G. Tambussi, S. Ferrini, E. Ciccone, P. Varese, M. C. Mingari, L. Moretta, and A. Moretta. 1988. Two subsets of human T lymphocytes expressing γ/δ antigen receptor are identifiable by monoclonal antibodies directed to two distinct molecular forms of the receptor. J. Exp. Med. 168: 491–505.

4. Moretta, A., C. Bottino, E. Ciccone, G. Tambussi, M. C. Mingari, S. Ferrini, G. S. Casorato, P. Varese, O. Viale, N. Migone, and L. Moretta. 1988. Human peripheral blood lymphocytes bearing T cell receptor γ/δ Expression of CD8 differentiation antigen correlates with the expression of the 55 kD Cγ2-encoded, γ-chain. J. Exp. Med., in press.

5. Pellicci, P.-G., M. Subar, A. Weiss, R. Dalla-Favery, and D. R. Littman. 1987. Molecular diversity of the human T-gamma constant region genes. Science 237: 1051.

6. Triebel, F., F. Faure, M. Graziani, S. Jitsukawa, M. P. Lefranc, and T. H. Hercend. 1988. A unique V-J-C-rearranged gene encodes a γ-protein expressed on the majority of CD3+ T cell receptor γ/δ-circulating lymphocytes. J. Exp. Med. 167: 694.

Differentiation and Regulation of Immunocompetent Cells: Interleukin 6 in Immune Regulation

*Tetsuya Taga, Katsuhiko Yamasaki, Tadashi Matsuda, Sachiko Suematsu,
Bo Tang, Toshio Hirano, Tadamitsu Kishimoto**

B cell differentiation factor (BSF2) has been molecularly cloned, and the studies with recombinant molecules demonstrated that the function of BSF2, which is now called IL-6, is not restricted to B cells, but rather shows a wide variety of biological functions on various tissues and cells. Among others, the most important functions of IL-6 are the induction of antibody response and acute phase reaction. Therefore, IL-6 may play a central role in the host defence mechanism against infection, inflammation, and tissue injuries. IL-6 also functions as myeloma/plasmacytoma growth factor, and the results with human myeloma cells demonstrated that IL-6 is an autocrine growth factor for myeloma cells. The findings in the transgenic mice with the Eμ-IL-6 gene proved that abnormal expression of the IL-6 gene in the B lineage cells is responsible for the generation of plasmacytomas. In addition to the essential role of IL-6 under normal homeostatic conditions, deregulation of the IL-6 expression leads to the generation of plasmacytomas and possibly to certain autoimmune diseases. Future studies on the regulation of the IL-6 gene expression and on the mechanism of the signal transduction through the IL-6 receptor will provide the necessary information for the molecular manipulation of the immune system.

Recent advances in molecular biology have allowed the cloning of the cDNAs of factors involved in the regulation of growth and differentiation of lymphocytes [1]. Three factors, IL-4 (BSF1), IL-5 (BCGFII), and IL-6 (BSF2), which are involved in B cell regulation, have been molecularly cloned [2–4], and the studies with recombinant molecules have confirmed that (i) IL-4 activates resting B cells, (ii) IL-5 induces growth and differentiation of activated B cells, and (iii) IL-6 induces the final maturation of B cells into antibody-producing cells.

However, the studies with recombinant molecules demonstrated that the functions of these molecules are not restricted to the B lineage cells, but show a wide variety of biological functions on various tissues and cells. For instance, the function of IL-4 include (i) activation of resting B cells, (ii) induction of isotype switching into IgG1 or IgE production, (iii) induction of mast cell growth, (iv) unregulation of Fcε receptor II expression on B cells and macrophages, and (v) induction of T cell growth [5]. Sincel IL-4 is involved in IgE production, FcεRII induction and mast cell growth, deregulation of IL-4 production may contribute to atopic diseases (Table 1).

The most typical example of a pleiotropic factor is IL-6 [1]. In this paper, we summarize the molecular genetics and biology of IL-6 and its receptor.

Table 1. IL-4 and immediate type hypersensitivity.

1) Induction of Isotype switching into IgE production
2) Inhibition of parasite-induced IgE production by anti-IL-4 antibody
3) Induction of mast cell growth
4) Induction of FcεRII expression on B cells and monocytes
5) Induction of IL-4 in anti-IgE-stimulated mast cells

IL-6 in B Cell Regulation

IL-6 was originally identified as a T cell-derived lymphokine which induced antibody production in B cells [6], and its cDNA was isolated [4]. Recombinant IL-6 could augment in vitro as well as in vivo antibody production

*   Institute for Molecular and Cellular Biology, Osaka University, 1-3, Yamada-Oka, Suita, Osaka 565, Japan.
    This study was supported in part by grants from the Ministry of Education, Science and Culture, Japan.

490

A Human PBL, in vitro

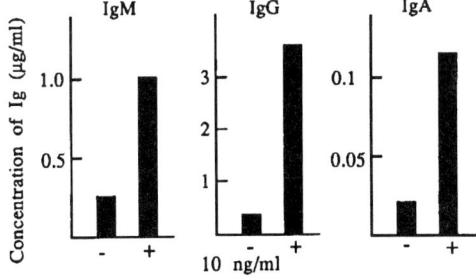

B Murine anti-SRBC response, in vivo

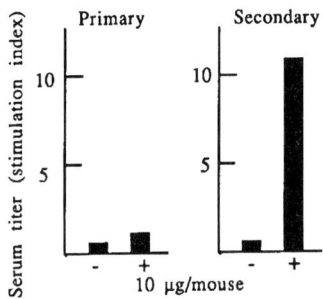

Figure 1. (A) Effects of IL-6 on PWM-induced immunoglobulin production in peripheral blood mononuclear cells. Human PBL were cultured in the absence (–) or in the presence (+) of 10 ng/ml of recombinant IL-6 for 8 days. Amounts of IgM, IgG, and IgA in the culture supernatant were determined by ELISA. (B) C3H/Hej mice were immunized with SRBC (1×10^8/mouse) and daily injected with rIL-6 (10 µg/mouse) (+) or human albumin (10 µg/mouse) (–). The serum anti-SRBC titer was examined by hemagglutination assay at day 7 (primary response). For secondary response, mice were immunized with SRBC (1×10^6/mouse) at an interval of 25 days, then treated with IL-6 and assayed in the same way as primary response.

[7, 8]; as shown in Figure 1, IL-6 augments Igs-production in PWM (pokeweed mitogen)-stimulated human PBL, and the administration of rIL-6 into SRBC-primed mice augments the in vivo anti-SRBC antibody response more than 10-fold [8].

Studies with anti-IL-6 antibody demonstrated that IL-6 is one of the essential factors for B cells to produce immunoglobulins (Igs); PWM-induced Ig-production in human PBL was almost completely inhibited by anti-IL-6 antibody [7]. In contrast, IL-6 did not inhibit mito-

gen- induced proliferation of B cells, indicating that IL-6 is required for antibody production, but not for B cell proliferation.

Pleiotropic Activities of IL-6

Following the molecular cloning of IL-6 (BSF2), it was revealed that other factors identified as IFNβ2 [9], 26 Kd protein [10], plasmacytoma growth factor [11], and hepatocyte stimulating factor [12, 13] were all identical to IL-6 (BSF2). These findings suggested that this molecule may have a wide variety of biological functions on various tissues and cells. And indeed, the studies carried out by several investigators utilizing recombinant IL-6 show the activity of IL-6 on various cells. Briefly, IL-6

– induces Ig-production in B cells (BSF2) [7];

– induces growth of plasmacytomas (plasmacytoma growth factor);

– induces acute phase proteins in hepatocytes (HSF) [12, 13];

– activates hematopoietic stem cells (multi-CSF) [14];

– induces growth of mitogen-stimulated T cells [15];

– induces cytotoxic T cells together with IL-2 (KHF) [16, 17];

– neural differentiation of rat pheocromocytoma, PC12 [18];

– induces differentiation of a myeloid leukemia cell line (M1) into macrophages [19];

– induces growth of glomerular mesangium cells [Horii et al., submitted].

The activities are summarized in Figure 2.

IL-6 Receptor

As expected from its pleiotropic function, the IL-6 receptor is expressed on a wide variety of cells as shown in Table 2 [20]. The number of the receptor molecules is in the range between 10^2 and 10^3, which is 100-fold lower than those for other growth factor receptors such as insulin and EGF. The paucity of the receptor molecules has made it extremely difficult to prepare monoclonal antibody or to purify their receptor molecules.

491

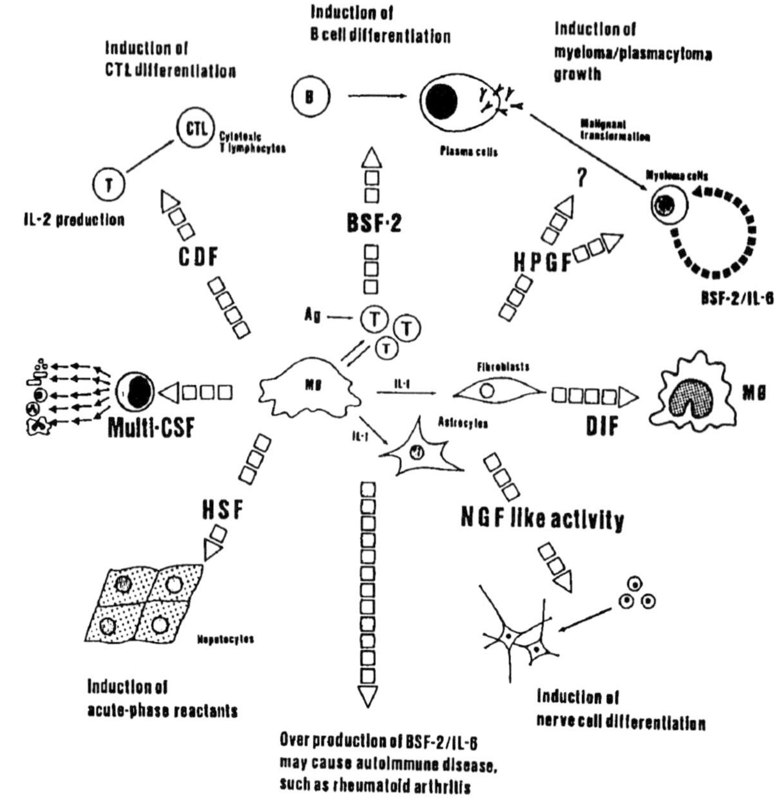

Figure 2. Pleiotropic functions of IL-6.

IL-6 provides multiple signals on different cells, such as growth-stimulatory, growth-inhibitory, and differentiation-inducing. In order to elucidate how a single ligand can provide multiple signals, the structure of the receptor must be determined. We employed a high- efficiency COS7 cell expression system with the CDM8 vector for the molecular cloning of the IL-6 receptor. The expressed receptors were detected with biotinated recombinant IL-6 and fluorescein-conjugated avidin. Cells expressing

the IL-6R were obtained with a fluorescence-activated cell sorter, resulting in the identification of a candidate plasmid clone, PBSF2R.236 [21]. The transfection of the cDNA into a human T cell line, JURKAT, would induce the expression of both high (Kd 17 pM) and low (710 pM) affinity receptors as observed in a human myeloma cell line, U266. The nucleotide sequence and the deduced amino acid sequence demonstrated that the IL-6R consists of 468 amino acids, including a signal peptide of 19 amino acids and a domain of ~90 amino acids that is similar to a domain in the immunoglobulin superfamily. The cytoplasmic domain of ~82 amino acids lacks a tyrosine/kinase domain, unlike other growth factor receptors. The structure of IL-6R is schematically described in Figure 3. The mechanism of its signal transduction could be mediated through an unknown biochemical pathway.

Table 2. Distribution of IL-6 receptor.

Cells	No. of receptors/cell
EBV-transformed B cell lines	200–3,000
Barkitt's lymphoma cell lines	not detectable
myeloma cells and cell lines	100–20,000
hepatoma cell lines	2,000–3,000
myeloid leukemia cell lines	2,000–3,000
rat pheochromocytoma cell line, PC12	ca. 1,200
resting B cells	not detectable
activated B cells	ca. 500
resting T cells	ca. 300

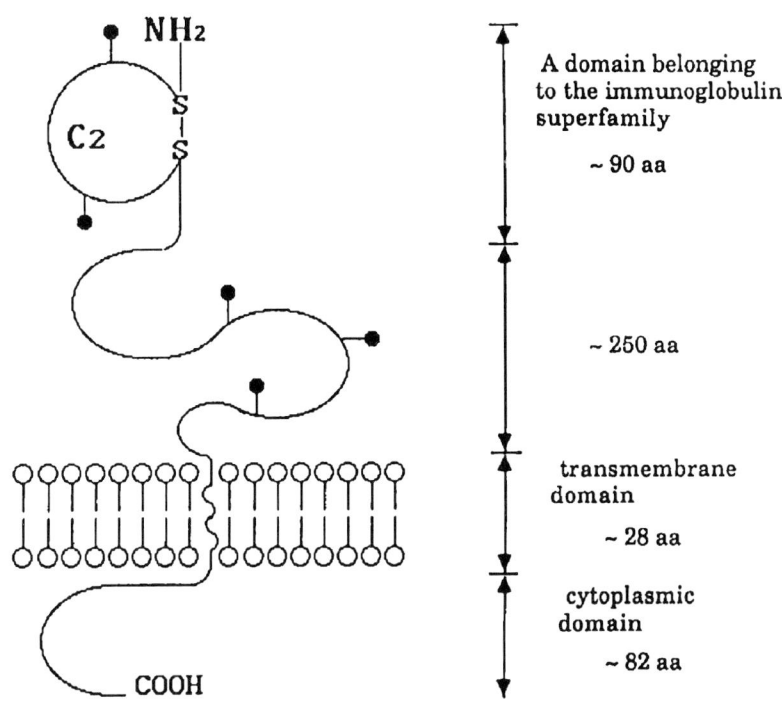

NH₂

C2

COOH

A domain belonging to the immunoglobulin superfamily

~ 90 aa

~ 250 aa

transmembrane domain

~ 28 aa

cytoplasmic domain

~ 82 aa

Figure 3. Schematic model of IL-6 receptor.

IL-6 and Myeloma/Plasmacytoma Generation

More than 20 years ago, M. Potter and his colleagues succeeded in the generation of plasmacytomas in mice by intrapeintoneal injection of mineral oil [22]. Subsequently, it was shown that mineral oil-induced granuloma produced large amounts of plasmacytoma growth factor. The purification and the molecular cloning of plasmacytoma growth factor demonstrated that it is identical with IL-6 [23]. In fact, IL-6 shows a potent growth activity on a murine plasmacytoma cell line. The concentration of IL-6 required for the induction of 50% maximum proliferation was only 0.002 ng/ml, which is 100-fold less than that for Ig-induction in B cells. The result suggests to us that deregulation of IL-6 production in the B lineage cells may be responsible for the oncogenesis of human multiple myelomas.

In order to examine this possibility, we isolated myeloma cells from 26 cases of myeloma patients and asked whether IL-6 can augment proliferation of myeloma cells, and whether myeloma cells produce IL-6. The result showed that myeloma cells in all 26 cases expressed

mRNA for IL-6, and their culture supernatants included IL-6 activity. In 12 out of 26 cases, recombinant IL-6 could augment the in vitro growth of myeloma cells. Interestingly, anti-IL-6 could inhibit the growth of myeloma cells. All of these results indicated that IL-6 is an autocrine growth factor for human myeloma cells and is essential for their growth [22].

The results obtained with human myeloma cells strongly suggest that deregulation of IL-6 expression in the B lineage cells may be involved in the development of myeloma/plasmacytoma. In order to prove it, we prepared transgenic mice with the IL-6 gene conjugated to the human Ig heavy chain enhancer gene (Eμ). Three mice in which the Eμ-IL-6 gene was integrated were obtained, and typical plasmacytomas were generated in these mice. The infiltration of typical plasmacytoma cells into spleen, lymph node, thymus, liver, and kidney was histologically confirmed. Their serum showed an increase in the level of IgG₁ with peaks of 1 g/ml. The results observed with the transgenic mice demonstrate that the abnormal expression of IL-6 in the B lineage cells is responsible for the generation of plasmacytomas.

References

1. Kishimoto, T., and T. Hirano. 1988. Molecular regulation of B lymphocyte response. Ann. Rev. Immunol. 6: 485–512.
2. Noma, Y., T. Sideras, T., Naito, A. Bergstedt-Lindqvist, C. Azuma, E. Severinson, T. Tanabe, T. Kinashi, F. Matsuda, Y. Yaoita, and T. Honjo. 1986. Cloning of cDNA encoding the murine IgG1 induction factor by a novel strategy using SP6 promotor. Nature 319: 640–646.
3. Kinashi, T., N. Harada, E. Severinson, R. Tanabe, P. Sideras, M. Konishi, C. Azuma, A. Tominaga, S. Bergstedt-Lindqvist, M. Takahashi, F. Matsuda, Y. Yaoita, K. Takatsu, and T. Honjo. 1986. Cloning of complementary DNA encoding T-cell replacing factor and identity with B-cell growth factor II. Nature 324: 70–73.
4. Hirano, T., K. Yasukawa, H. Harada, T. Taga, Y. Watanabe, T., Matsuda, S. Kashiwamura, K. Nakajima, K. Koyama, A. Iwamatsu, S. Tsunasawa, F. Sakiyama, H. Matsui, Y. Takahara, T. Taniguchi, and T. Kishimoto. 1986. Complementary DNA for a novel human interleukin (BSF- 2) that induces B lymphocytes to produce immunoglobulin. Nature 324: 73–76.
5. Lee, L., T. Yokota, T. Otsuka, P. Meyerson, D. Villaret, R. Coffman, T. Mosmann, D. Rennick, N. Roeham, C. Smith, A. Zlotnick, and K. Arai. 1986. Isolation and characterization of a mouse interleukin cDNA clone that expresses B-cell stimulatory factor 1 activities and T-cell and mast-cell-stimulating activities. Proc. Natl. Acad. Sci. USA 83: 2061–2065.
6. Hirano, T., T. Taga, N. Nakano, K. Yasukawa, S. Kashiwamura, K. Shimizu, K. Nakajima, K. H. Pyun, and T. Kishimoto. 1985. Purification to homogeneity and characterization of human B cell differentiation factor (BCDF or BSFp-2). Proc. Natl. Acad. Sci. USA 82: 5490–5494.
7. Muraguchi, A., T. Hirano, B. Tang, T. Matsuda, Y. Horii, K. Nakajima, and T. Kishimoto. 1988. The essential role of B cell stimulatory factor 2 (BSF-2/IL-6) for the terminal differentiation of B cells. J. Exp. Med. 167: 332–344.
8. Takatsuki, F., A. Okana, C. Suzuki, R. Chieda, Y. Takahara, T. Hirano, T. Kishimoto, J. Hamuro, and Y. Akiyama. Human recombinant interleukin 6/B cell stimulatory factor 2 (IL-6/BSF-2) augments murine antigen specific antibody responses in vitro and in vivo. J. Immunol., in press.
9. Zilberstein, A., R. Ruggieri, J. H. Korn, and M. Revel. 1986. Structure and expression of cDNA and genes for human interferon- β2, a distinct species inducible by growth-stimulatory cytokines. EMBO. J. 5: 2529–2537.
10. Haegeman, G., J. Content, G. Volckaert, R. Derynck, J. Tavernier, and W. Fiers. 1986. Structural analysis of the sequence coding for an inducible 25-kDa protein in human fibroblasts. Eur. J. Biochem. 159: 625632.
11. Van Snick, J., S. Cayphas, A. Vink, C. Uyttenhove, P. G. Coulie, M. R. Rubira, and R. J. Simpson. 1986. Purification and NH2- terminal amino acid sequence of a T-cell-derived lymphokine with growth factor activity for B-cell hybridomas. Proc. Natl. Acad. Sci. USA 83: 9679–9683.
12. Gauldie, J., C. Richards, D. Harnish, P. Lansdorp, and H. Baumann. 1987. Interferon β2-BSF-2 shares identity with monocyte derived hepatocyte stimulating factor (HSF) and regulates the major acute phase protein response in liver cells. Proc. Natl. Acad. Sci. USA 84: 72517255.
13. Andus, T., T. Geiger, T. Hirano, H. Northoff, U. Ganger, J. Bauer, T. Kishimoto, and P. C. Heinrich. 1987. Recombinant human B cell stimulatory factor 2 (BSF2/IFN-β2) regulates β-fibrinogen and albumin mRNA levels in Fao-9 cells. FEBS Lett. 15: 249–253.
14. Ikebuchi, K., G. G. Wong, S. C. Clark, J. N. Ihle, Y. Hirai, and M. Ogawa. Interleukin-6 enhancement of interleukin-3- dependent proliferation of multipotential hemopoietic progenitors. Proc. Natl. Acad. Sci. USA 84: 9035–9039.
15. Lots, M., F. Jirik, R. Kabouridis, C. Tsoukas, T. Hirano, T. Kishimoto, and D. A. Carson. 1988. BSF-2/IL-6 is a costimulant for human thymocytes and T lymphocytes. J. Exp. Med. 167: 1253–1258.
16. Takai, Y., G. G. Wong, S. C. Clark, S. J. Burakoff, and S. H. Herrmann. B cell stimulatory factor-2 is involved in the differentiation of cytotoxic T lymphocytes. J. Immunol. 140: 508–512.
17. Okada, M., M. Kitahara, S. Kishimoto, T. Matsuda, T. Hirano, and T. Kishimoto. IL-6/BSF-2 functions as a killer helper factor in the in vitro induction of cytotoxic T cells. J. Immunol., in press.
18. Satoh, T., S. Nakamura, T. Taga, T. Matsuda, T. Hirano, T. Kishimoto, and Y. Kaziro. Induction of neuronal differentiation in PC12 cells by B-cell stimulatory factor 2/interleukin 6. Mol. Cell. Biol., in press.
19. Miyaura, C., K. Onozaki, Y. Akiyama, T. Taniyama, T. Hirano, T. Kishimoto, and T. Suda. 1988. Recombinant human interleukin 6 (B-cell stimulatory factor 2) is a potent inducer of differentiation of mouse myeloid leukemia cells (M1). FEBS Letters 234: 17–21.
20. Taga, T., Y. Kawanishi, R. R. Hardy, T. Hirano, and T. Kishimoto. 1987. Receptors for B cell stimulatory factor 2 (BSF2): Quantitation, specificity, distribution and regulation of the expression. J. Exp. Med. 166: 967–981.
21. Yamasaki, K., T. Taga, Y. Hirata, H. Yawata, Y. Kawanishi, B. Seed, T. Taniguchi, T. Hirano, and

T. Kishimoto. 1988. Cloning and expression of human interleukin 6 (BSF-2/IFNβ2) receptor. Science 241: 825–828.

22. Potter, M., and C. Boyce. 1962. Induction of plasma cell neoplasms in strain Balb/c mice with mineral oil and mineral oil adjuvants. Nature 193: 1086–1087.

23. Van Snick, J., S. Cayphas, J.-P., Szikora, J.-C. Renauld, E. Van Roost, T. Boon, and R. J. Simp-son. 1988. cDNA cloning of murine interleukin-HP: Homology with human interleukin 6. Eur. J. Immunol 18: 193–197.

24. Kawano, M., T. Hirano, T. Matsuda, T. Taga, Y. Horii, K. Iwato, H. Asaoku, B. Tang, O. Tanabe, H. Tanaka, A. Kuramoto, and T. Kishimoto. 1988. Autocrine generation and essential requirement of BSF-2/IL-6 for human multiple myelomas. Nature 332: 83–85.

Chronic Inflammatory Joint Diseases: Role of Interleukin-1 and Interleukin-1 Inhibitor

Jean-Michel Dayer*

Interleukin-1 (IL-1) and tumor necrosis factor α (TNFα) may induce both catabolic and anabolic functions during the inflammatory process. The catabolic functions are illustrated by the stimulation of collagenase and prostaglandin production or by the decrease of proteoglycan synthesis, anabolic functions by the induction of fibroblast proliferation or the modulation of collagen and fibronectin synthesis. During inflammation cytokines increase at the local or systemic level but are possibly counteracted by so-called "anti-cytokines". We found that an IL-1 inhibitor blocks (1) PGE_2/collagenase production by human synovial cells and dermal fibroblasts, (2) production of IL-2 by lymphocytes exposed to IL-1, (3) proliferation of fibroblasts, and (4) binding of ^{125}I-IL-1α to lymphocytes. The IL-1 inhibitor binds to the IL-1 receptor and is distinct from IL-1. This molecule (mol. wt. 20–25 kD, pI 4.5–4.7) is heat- and protease-sensitive. The inhibitor does not affect functions induced by TNFα and has been found in high amounts in patients with juvenile rheumatoid arthritis. Since both IL-1 and TNFα are mediators of many similar functions, we examined the urine of febrile patients for the presence of a TNFα inhibitor. Using the TNFα-induced cytotoxicity test (L929 cells), we found a TNFα inhibitor of 30–35 kD with a pI of 5.5–6.1. The TNFα inhibitor blocks PGE_2 production induced by TNFα, but does not affect IL-1 binding to target cells. These results provide evidence that the bioactivity of IL-1 and TNFα may be altered by other substances interfering with the ligand.

Introduction

The significance of monocyte-macrophage products in connective tissue destruction was first recognized more than 10 years ago in the course of studies on the cell/cell interactions in chronic inflammation as exemplified by rheumatoid arthritis [1]. A monocyte product, termed mononuclear cell factor (MCF) was found to affect human rheumatoid synovial functions. MCF was defined by its effect on stimulation of the production of collagenase and prostaglandin E_2 (PGE_2) by adherent synovial fibroblasts [2, 3]. Both products are important in the process of tissue destruction and bone resorption. Monocytes were the primary source of MCF [4]. It was further demonstrated that MCF shared biochemical properties with lymphocyte-activating factor (LAF), subsequently termed interleukin-1 (IL-1) [5]. Further studies by numerous laboratories have shown that similar effects on the stimulation of collagenase and prostaglandin production could be observed with IL-1, using dermal fibroblasts, articular chondrocytes, or trabecular bone cells as target cells. Finally, both forms of human recombinant interleukin-1α and β (hrIL- 1α and β) have been shown to have MCF/IL-1 activity [6, 7, 8]. Other studies have shown that IL-1 plays a role not only in tissue destruction, but also in stimulating new matrix synthesis [9, 33]. IL-1 is a cytokine with multiple pleomorphic amplifying effects on immunological and inflammatory reactions [10–12]. It is a genetically unrestricted, immunologically nonspecific factor that is active at picomolar concentrations. The monocyte-macrophage seems to be the major source of IL-1, but numerous other cells can also synthesize this polypeptide. Both IL-1 molecules bind to the same cell surface receptor which has just been cloned [13].

* Division of Immunology and Allergy, Department of Medicine, Hôpital cantonal universitaire, CH-1211 Geneva 4, Switzerland.
This work was supported in part by the Fonds national suisse de la recherche scientifique (grant Nos. 3.449.0.83 and 3.400.0.86) and by "Subvention fédérale suisse pour la lutte contre les maladies rhumatismales".

Table 1. Role of IL-1 in connective tissue.

Destruction	Remodelling (repair, fibrosis)
Protease production	Fibroblast proliferation
Prostaglandin production	Synthesis of collagen and fibronectin
Direct bone resorption	Proteoglycan synthesis
Lymphocyte adhesion, migration, and proliferation	
Synovial cell sensitization to PGE$_2$	
endothelial damage	

Factors Modulating the Production and the Effects of IL-1 in the Context of Chronic Inflammation and Tissue Destruction

Considering the marked effect of IL-1 on collagenase and PGE$_2$ production, the factors modulating its production have to be examined in order to understand the mechanisms of inflammation and tissue destruction in joint diseases. The role of IL-1 in connective tissue destruction and remodeling is summarized in Table 1. Numerous interactions between cellular, humoral factors, and elements of the matrix regulate the production of IL-1.

Cellular Interactions

Although a variety of factors influences the secretion of IL-1 by monocyte-macrophages in several pathological states, T lymphocytes (T$_L$) are among the most important regulators of monocyte functions, so that co-culture of T lymphocytes with human peripheral blood monocyte-macrophages results in a marked increase of IL-1 production [4]. The precise role of T lymphocytes has been elucidated by Amento et al. [14], who utilized the human monocyte cell U937 and cloned T lymphocytes. The U937 cells do not produce IL-1 spontaneously, but only when stimulated with lectin, antigen-activated peripheral blood T lymphocytes, or similarly activated T lymphocyte clones [14]. Cell contact is not essential for this induction, since conditioned medium from activated T lymphocytes can also induce IL-1 production by the U937 cells. Clones consisting of either helper/inducer (T$_4$) or suppressor/cytotoxic (T$_8$) populations stimulate IL-1 production. In contrast to 1,25-dihydroxyvitamin D$_3$, αIFN, γIFN, and interleukin-2 failed to induce IL-1 production by U937 cells [15]. 1,25-dihydroxyvitamin D$_3$ increases IL-1 production in U937 if the monokine is stimulated with the T lymphokine(s) [16]. This potentiation is also found with γIFN instead of vitamin D$_3$ [17]. More recently, tumor necrosis factor (TNFα) has been found to stimulate IL-1 production [18] as well as LTB$_4$ when added to alveolar macrophages [19]. In contrast, PGE$_2$ appears to decrease IL-1 production by monocytes.

Humoral Interactions

Monocyte-macrophages can be stimulated directly to release IL-1 by endotoxin, aggregated immunoglobulins, or the Fc portion of immunoglobulin [20]. Self-associating IgG rheumatoid factor (RF) can also stimulate PGE$_2$ synthesis by monocyte-macrophages as well as IL-1 release [21]. Immune complexes (IC), consisting of the self-associating rheumatoid factors and found in serum as well as in synovial fluid from patients with rheumatoid arthritis, would provide further mechanisms whereby humoral factors may modulate cellular immune reactions in the inflammatory synovium.

Matrix Interactions

There has been considerable interest in the potential role of the extracellular matrix in regulating cell functions, regarding, for example, adherence, spreading, replication, and specific phenotypic expression [22]. There is also evidence that patients with rheumatoid arthritis have an altered cellular immune response to several different collagens [23]. We found, after culturing peripheral blood mononuclear cells on various purified collagen substrates, that collagen types II and III stimulate IL-1 production [24]. More recently, collagen type IX, a minor but important collagen type of the cartilage, has been found to markedly stimulate

IL-1 as well as PGE$_2$ production by human monocytes [25]. The inorganic phase of the bone (i.e., hydroxylapatite and calcium pyrophosphate dehydrate crystals) may also contribute to tissue destruction by stimulating IL-1, collagenase, and PGE$_2$ production [26].

Other Interactions and Drug Effects

Changes in the cellular morphology of the synovial cells appear also to be related to levels of PGE$_2$ in culture. The stellate aspect reflects the high level of PGE$_2$ to which the cells are exposed [27]. In this in vitro system, PGE$_2$ alone does not stimulate collagenase production by synovial cells, but may modify its response to IL-1. Certain synovial cell cultures that have been stimulated by IL-1 in the presence of high concentrations (10 μM) of indomethacin show a decrease of collagenase production. Collagenase production is restored in these cells by addition of low concentrations of PGE$_2$. Exogenously added PGE$_2$ or dibutyryl cAMP can overcome the indomethacin inhibition, suggesting that PGE$_2$ modulates collagenase expression through cAMP [27]. On the other hand, even at low concentrations (0.1 μM) of indomethacin, which still markedly inhibit PGE$_2$ synthesis, no change is observed in collagenase levels. In contrast, low concentrations (10 nM) of glucocorticosteroid block the production by synovial cells of both collagenase and PGE$_2$ [28, 29]. These results suggest that nonsteroidal anti-inflammatory drugs are poor or indirect inhibitors of collagenase production and by themselves may not be sufficient to stop collagen degradation in the RA patient. Another aspect of IL-1 is that it induces increased synovial cell sensitivity to PGE$_2$ as determined by PGE$_2$-induced cAMP response. This indicates that, within the synovium, IL-1 may upregulate the synovial cell and prepare it for a greater hormone (PGE$_2$) response, thus enhancing the PGE$_2$ effect in inflammation. Such changes in hormone sensitivity (induced by IL-1) do not occur only for PGE$_2$ but for other hormones involved in bone resorption, for example, the parathyroid hormone [30, 31].

Factors Modulating Production and Effects of IL-1 in the Context of Tissue Remodeling and Fibrosis

Cell Proliferation

IL-1 not only stimulates collagenase and PGE$_2$ production in cultured synovial cells, but also affects other cellular functions, depending sometimes directly on endogenous PGE$_2$ levels produced by the synovial cells and acting as an autocrine hormone. Thus, PGE$_2$ produced endogenously or added exogenously inhibits cell replication. However, when PGE$_2$ production by synovial cells is blocked by a cyclooxygenase inhibitor, a mitogenic effect of IL-1 is observed [31]. In cell cultures that produce little or no PGE$_2$, even in response to IL-1, the mitogenic effect of IL-1 is evident. In this regard IL-1 can be considered one of the cytokines involved in tissue repair and fibroblast proliferation.

Collagens, Fibronectin and Proteoglycan Synthesis

Concomitant with cartilage and bone destruction that develops throughout rheumatoid arthritis, attempts at tissue repair can be observed. Although it has been proved that proteoglycans are newly synthesized, there is no supporting evidence of newly synthesized collagen retaining its physiological function. Nearly all of the newly synthesized collagen becomes scar tissue (fibrosis) [32]. In synovial cells, IL-1 increases synthesis of types I and III collagen and fibronectin, and to a greater extent when PGE$_2$ production is inhibited by cyclooxygenase inhibitor [9]. However, the role of IL-1 as stimulator of collagen synthesis appears to be much less important than that of TGFβ. HrIL-1β can markedly stimulate proteoglycan synthesis by fibroblast synovial cells. This stimulation is not mediated by PGE$_2$ since addition of indomethacin did not prevent stimulation [33].

In a more general context, polypeptides produced from monocyte-macrophages (monokines) may be divided into two categories: (1) the "proinflammatory" monokines such IL-1α and β, TNFα and β, and (2) the "profibrotic" monokines such as insulin growth factors I and II (IGF-I and II), platelet-derived growth factors (PDGF), transforming growth factor β (TGFβ), interferon β (IFN-β). In contrast, IFN-γ is a strong inhibitor of collagen synthesis.

Inhibition of IL-1 Activity

Although the mechanisms by which the pleiotropic effects of IL-1 may be regulated in vivo are obscure, there is clear evidence for the presence of natural inhibitors. Inhibitors directed against IL-1 may act at different levels, by inhibiting monocyte-macrophage stimulation, synthesis and release of IL-1, or by inactivating IL-1 by proteolytic cleavage, aggregation, binding to a carrier, or competing at the IL-1 receptors. As is the case with many other polypeptide hormones, IL-1 activity is mediated via interaction with a plasma membrane receptor [13].

We observed that urine from febrile patients is inhibitory for both IL-1-dependent murine thymocyte proliferation and PGE_2/collagenase production by human synovial cells and dermal fibroblasts [34, 35]. Purification of this urine inhibitor involved ultrafiltration, ammonium-sulfate fractionation, ion-exchange chromatography, hydroxylapatite chromatography and Ultrogel AcA54 filtration. Inhibitory fractions eluted with an apparent molecular weight of 20–25 kD. At this stage of purification, the material was inhibitory for all IL-1 bioactivities tested, which include LAF/IL-1 and MCF/IL-1 activities as well as TNFα-induced IL-2 production [36]. The inhibitor thus appears to regulate IL-1-dependent activities of T and non-T target cells, implying that immune and non-immune responses may be controlled by the same molecule. More recently, we found that the inhibitor of IL-1 bioactivity blocked the specific binding of radioiodinated hrIL-1α to its receptor in dose-dependent fashion [37]. The inhibitor was distinct from IL-1 as determined by physical parameters (size, antigenicity) and receptor binding characteristics (apparent affinity, dissociation rate) [38]. The characteristics of the IL-1 INH are summarized in Table 2I.

TNFα, another monokine, found in high quantity in inflammatory fluids, also stimulates collagenase and PGE_2 production by dermal fibroblasts and synovial cells [39]. When

Table 2. IL-1 inhibitor.

Biochemical characteristics:
➤ ca. 20–25 kD; pI 4.5–4.7
➤ Heat label (100 °C, 30 min)
➤ Pronase-sensitive (37 °C, 24 h)
➤ Does not bind to ConA-sepharose
Functions and mechanism of action:
➤ Blocks IL-1α and IL-1β biologic activities
➤ Does not affect TNF biologic activities
➤ Reversal of IL-1-induced cytotoxicity
➤ Exerts competitive inhibition at the IL-1 receptor level (binds to IL-1 receptor)
Sources:
➤ Urine from patients with monocytic leukemia
➤ Urine from certain febrile patients
➤ Synovial and alveolar macrophages

investigating the urine of febrile patients for TNFα-inhibitory activity we found indeed another distinct inhibitor, specifically directed against tumor necrosis factor a [38]. This urine-derived TNFα INH has a mol. wt. of ~40–60 kD and a pI ranging from 5.5–6.1. It does not interfere with biological activities induced by IL-1. Similarly, the IL-1 INH is unable to block TNFα-induced cytotoxicity. Since TNFα is found in biologic fluids, it would be worthwhile to study this TNFα INH at the local site of the inflammation.

Conclusion

In chronic inflammation IL-1, defined as mononuclear cell factor (MCF), stimulates various types of cells to produce prostaglandin E_2, collagenase and neutral proteases that reflect mechanisms of tissue destruction. The same factor can also affect tissue remodeling and fibrosis. IL-1 has been found in various biological fluids (synovial fluids, serum, and urine). However, the control of IL-1 activities and their regulation in vivo is poorly understood. Inhibitors of LAF/IL-1 have been revealed in urine, serum, and cell-culture supernatant, but no in vivo inhibitory activity to MCF/IL-1 has been reported previously. Initially, we observed an MCF/IL-1 inhibitor (~25 kD) in urine from patients with monocytic leukemia, but the inhibitor is also present in other pathological conditions, such as in urine and serum from patients with juvenile rheumatoid arthritis [41] and in cultured mononuclear cells from inflammatory synovial fluid [12]. These findings may be sig-

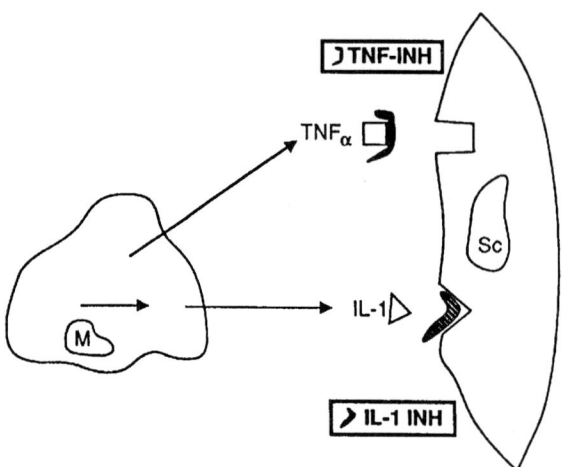

Figure 1. Monocyte-macrophage maturation: IL-1 and IL-1 INH production.

nificant insofar as the two distinct inhibitors to IL-1 and TNFα, respectively, could counteract the stimulation of collagenase and PGE_2 and thus be considered important natural molecules for modulating connective tissue destruction and remodeling. The mechanisms of inhibition for these inhibitors appear to differ. IL-1 INH binds to the receptor, and TNFα INH to the ligand (Figure 1). By means of this in vitro human cell culture model we were able to study cellular interaction between lymphocytes, monocyte-macrophages and synovial cells. Drugs or natural inhibitors may interrupt the chain of events at various levels and their study may lead to new therapeutic approaches in vivo.

References

1. Dayer, J.-M., and S. M. Krane. 1978. Clin. Rheum. Dis. 4: 517.
2. Dayer, J.-M., R. G. G. Russell, and S. M. Krane. 1977. Science 195: 181.
3. Dayer, J.-M., D. R. Robinson, and S. M. Krane. 1977. J. exp. Med. 145: 1399.
4. Dayer, J.-M., J. Bréard, L. Chess, and S. M. Krane. 1979. J. Clin. Invest. 64: 1386.
5. Mizel, S.B., J.-M. Dayer, S. M. Krane, and S. E. Mergenhagen. 1981. Proc. Natl. Acad. Sci. USA 78: 2474.
6. Dayer, J.-M., B. de Rochemonteix, B. Burrus, S. Demczuk, and C. A. Dinarello. 1986. J. Clin. Invest. 77: 645.
7. Wingfield, P., M. Payton, J. F Tavernier, M. Barnes, A. R. Shaw, K. Rose, G. Simona, S. Demczuk, K. Williamson, and J.-M. Dayer. 1986. Eur. J. Biochem. 160: 491.
8. Wingfield, P., M. Payton, P. Graber, K. Rose, J.-M. Dayer, A. R. Shaw, and U. Schmeissner. 1987. Eur. J. Biochem. 165: 537.
9. Krane, S.M., J.-M. Dayer, L.S. Simon, and M.S. Byrne. 1985. Collagen Rel. Res. 5:99.
10. Gery, I., R.K. Gershon, and B. H. Waksman. 1972. J. exp. Med. 136: 128.
11. Oppenheim, J. J., and I. Gery. 1986. Immunol. Today 7: 45.
12. Dinarello, C. A. 1986. The Year in Immunol. 2: 69.
13. Sims, J. E., C. J. March, D. Cosman, M.B. Widmer, H. R. MacDonald, C. J. McMahan, C. E. Grubin, J. M. Wignall, J. L. Jackson, S. M. Call, D. Friend, A. R. Alpert, S. Gillis, D. L. Urdal, and S. K. Dower. 1988. Science 241: 585.
14. Amento, E. P., J. T. Kurnick, A. Epstein, and S. M. Krane. 1982. Proc. Natl. Sci. USA 79: 5307.
15. Amento, E. P., J. T. Kurnick, and S. M. Krane. 1985. J. Immunol. 134: 350.
16. Amento, E. P., A. K. Bhalla, J. T. Kurnick, R. L. Kradin, T. L. Clemens, S. A. Holick, M. F. Holick, and S. M. Krane. 1984. J. Clin. Invest. 73: 731.
17. Roux-Lombard, P., A. Cruchaud, and J.-M. Dayer. 1986. Cell. Immunol. 97: 286.
18. Dinarello, C. A., J. G. Cannon, S. M. Wolff, H. A. Bernheim, B. Beutler, A. Cerami, I. S. Figari, M. A. Palladino Jr., and J. V. O'Connor. 1986. J. exp. Med. 163: 1433.
19. Polla, B., B. de Rochemonteix, A. F. Junod, and J.-M. Dayer. 1985. Biochem. Biophys. Res. Commun. 199:560.
20. Dayer, J.-M., J. H. Passwell, E. E. Schneeberger, and S. M. Krane. 1980. J. Immunol. 124: 1712.
21. Nardella, F. A., J.-M. Dayer, M. Roelke, S. M. Krane, and M. Mannik. 1983. Rheumatol. Int. 3: 183.
22. Kleinman, H. K., R. J. Klebe, and G. R. Martin. 1981. J. Cell. Biol. 88: 473.
23. Trentham, D. E., R. A. Dynesius, and J. R. David. 1978. N. Engl. J. Med. 299: 327.

24. Dayer, J.-M., D. E. Trentham, and S. M. Krane. 1982. Collagen Rel. Res. 2: 523.
25. Dayer, J.-M., S. Ricard-Blum, M.-T. Kaufmann, and D. Herbage. 1986. FEBS Lett. 198: 208.
26. Dayer, J.-M., V. Evêquoz, C. Zavadil-Grob, M. D. Grynpas, P. T. Cheng, J. Schnyder, U. Trechsel, and H. Fleisch. 1987. Arthr. Rheum. 30: 1372.
27. Baker, D. G., J.-M. Dayer, M. Roelke, H. R. Schumacher, and S. M. Krane. 1983. Arthr. Rheum. 26: 8.
28. Dayer, J.-M., S. M. Krane, R. G. G. Russell, and D. R. Robinson. 1976. Proc. Natl. Acad. Sci. USA 73: 945.
29. Dayer, J.-M., M. S. Roelke, and S. M. Krane. 1984. Biochem. Pharmacol. 33: 2893.
30. Goldring, S. R., J. M. Dayer, and S. M. Krane. 1984. Inflammation 8: 107.
31. Dayer, J.-M., S. R. Goldring, D. R. Robinson, and S. M. Krane. 1979. Biochim. Biophys. Acta 586: 87.
32. Krane, S. M., S. R. Goldring, and J.-M. Dayer. 1982. Lymphokines 7: 75.
33. Yaron, I., F. A. Meyer, J. M. Dayer, and M. Yaron. 1987. Arthr. Rheum. 30: 424.
34. Balavoine, J.-F., B. de Rochemonteix, A. Cruchaud, and J.- M. Dayer. 1984. Lymphokine Res. 3: 233A.
35. Balavoine, J.-F., B. de Rochemonteix, K. Williamson, P. Seckinger, A. Cruchaud, and J.-M. Dayer. 1986. J. Clin. Invest. 78: 1120.
36. Seckinger, P., K. Williamson, J.-F. Balavoine, B. Mach, G. Mazzei, A. Shaw, and J.-M. Dayer. 1987. J. Immunol. 139: 1541.
37. Seckinger, P., J. W. Lowenthal, K. Williamson, J.-M. Dayer, and H. R. MacDonald. 1987. J. Immunol. 139: 1546.
38. Dayer, J.-M., and P. Seckinger. 1988. In: The Control of Tissue Damage. A.M. Glauert, ed. Amsterdam: Elsevier, p. 151.
39. Dayer, J.-M., B. Beutler, and A. Cerami. 1985. J. exp. Med. 162: 2163.
40. Seckinger, P., S. Isaaz, and J.-M. Dayer. 1988. J. exp. Med. 167: 1511.
41. Prieur, A.-M., M.-T. Kaufmann, C. Griscelli, and J.-M. Dayer. 1987. Lancet II: 1240.
42. Roux-Lombard, P., C. Modoux, and J.-M. Dayer. 1988. Calc. Tissue Int. 42 (suppl.): A47.

Macrophages in Inflammation: Regulation of Tumor Necrosis Factor-α Synthesis by Prostaglandin E2 and Granulocyte-Macrophage Colony-Stimulating Factor

Harald Renz, Stefan Heidenreich, Jiang-Hong Gong, Jürgen Beck, Marianne Nain, Diethard Gemsa*

Tumor necrosis factor-α (TNF-α), a monokine of activated macrophages, participates in inflammation, stimulation of leukocytes and antitumor immunity. In this study, we report a dual effect of prostaglandin E2 (PGE2) which stimulated TNF-α synthesis at low and suppressed TNF-α synthesis at high concentrations. Enhanced TNF-α synthesis was associated with an intracellular increase of cyclic GMP, whereas suppression was mediated by an elevation of cyclic AMP. The important role of cyclic GMP was further substantiated by experiments showing that cyclic GMP, either exogenously added or endogenously generated by sodium nitroprusside, was efficiently stimulating TNF-α production. Although granulocyte-macrophage colony stimulating factor (GM-CSF) alone failed to stimulate TNF-α synthesis, it was capable of priming macrophages, initially for TNF-α release and subsequently for enhanced PGE2 production. The later-produced PGE2 may represent a negative feed-back inhibitor which down-regulates GM-CSF-induced TNF-α synthesis of activated macrophages.

Recently, it has been shown that TNF-α represents one of the most biologically active products of macrophages [1, 2]. Less TNF-α's antitumor effects but more its other biological activities such as induction of inflammation, cooperation with other cytokines during leukocyte stimulation, mediation of cachexia and shock symptoms have recently attracted an increased attention (key papers listed in [3, 4]).

The following study was designed to examine in detail the regulation of TNF-α synthesis in macrophages in response to two mediators, PGE2 and GM-CSF. Both compounds were selected since one, PGE2, has usually been associated with suppressive and the other, GM-CSF, with stimulatory effects on macrophages.

Results and Discussion

When TNF-α synthesis was stimulated by LPS in resident peritoneal macrophages from Lewis rats, PGE2 was suppressive if added at 5 ng/ml or higher concentrations (data not shown). This finding was in line with previous observations, since it supported the general concept that PGE2 is an inhibitor of leukocyte functions [5, 6]. Unexpectedly, in the absence of LPS stimulation, low concentrations of PGE2 (0.1 to 10 ng/ml) were capable of inducing a massive TNF-α synthesis (Figure 1). Based on these data, PGE2 exerted a dual activity on TNF-α production, a stimulation at low and a suppression at higher concentrations.

A further analysis revealed that PGE2-stimulated TNF-α synthesis correlated with an increase of intracellular cyclic GMP levels which, particular to PGE2 and no other prostanoid, were preferentially raised by low PGE2 doses (Figure 1). With higher PGE2 concentrations, an increase of cyclic AMP became apparent which, as expected, abolished TNF-α synthesis. This finding suggested that cyclic GMP may represent an intracellular signal to turn on TNF-α production. This assumption was verified by the experiments depicted in Table 1.

* Institute of Immunology, Philipps University, Robert-Koch-Str. 17, D-3550 Marburg, West Germany.
This work was supported by the Deutsche Forschungsgemeinschaft (Ge 354/5-2, Ge 354/7-1, He 1490/1-1).
Acknowledgements: We thank the following colleagues and corporations for donations of reagents: Dr. J. E. Pike, Upjohn Co., for PGE2; Dr. G. R. Adolf, Ernst-Boehringer-Institute, Vienna, for murine TNF-α; Dr. E. Schlick, BASF/Knoll, Ludwigshafen, for human TNF-α; Dr. F. Seiler and Dr. D. Krumwieh, Behringwerke, Marburg, for GM-CSF.

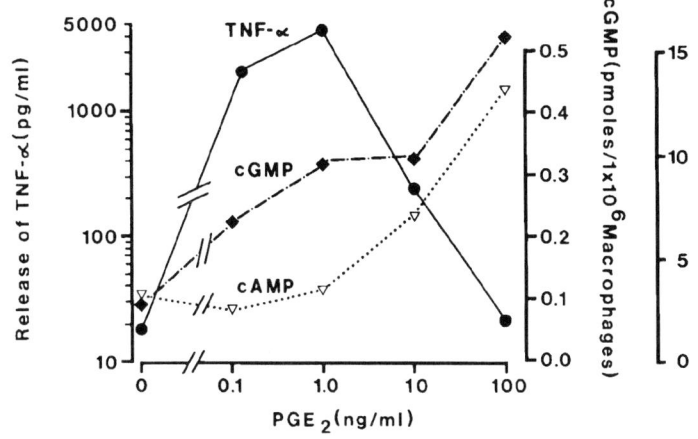

Figure 1. Release of TNF-α (●) from PGE₂-stimulated macrophages and correlation with intracellular levels of cyclic GMP (◆) and cyclic AMP (▽). Rat macrophages (1×10^6/ml) were incubated with indicated concentrations of PGE₂ and cyclic nucleotide concentrations were determined after 15 min by RIA. TNF-α release was measured by bioassay on L929 fibroblasts after 20 h of incubation (reprinted with permission of the *Journal of Immunology*).

Table 1. Effect of cyclic nucleotides on TNF-α release from macrophages.

Macrophage treatment*	Release of TNF-α (pg/ml)	
	–LPS	+LPS
None	28 ± 7**	2464 ±375
Cyclic GMP, 10^{-3} M	2160 ± 23	>3500
Sodium nitroprusside, 10^{-3} M	>3500	>3500
Cyclic AMP, 10^{-3} M	6 ± 2	53 ± 10
Theophylline, 10^{-3} M	8 ± 2	178 ± 37
Isoproterenol, 10^{-3} M	35 ± 8	1440 ± 221

*Resident peritoneal macrophages from Lewis rats (0.5×10^6/ml) were incubated for 20 h with indicated compounds in the presence or absence of LPS (1 µg/ml). Release of TNF-α in the culture supernatant was determined by bioassay on L929 fibroblasts.
**Mean ± S.D. on four identical cultures.

Addition of exogenous cyclic GMP as well as selective stimulation of guanylate cyclase by sodium nitroprusside were both efficient inducers of TNF-α synthesis, whereas exogenous cyclic AMP or agents raising intracellular cyclic AMP such as theophylline or isoproterenol were inefficient and, furthermore, counteracted LPS-induced TNF-α synthesis. Further evidence (not presented here) clearly indicated that low PGE₂ concentrations and cyclic GMP acted at the transcriptional level by enhancing TNF-α gene expression.

PGE₂- and cyclic GMP-induced TNF-α synthesis was also found in freshly harvested human monocytes, but not in rat macrophages that were intraperitoneally elicited by casein or activated by *C. parvum*. Thus, it appears that a certain pre-stimulation or activation stage precludes PGE₂-mediated TNF-α production. It would be interesting to study whether unstimulated mononuclear phagocytes may always display an enhanced responsiveness to those agents that raise cyclic GMP, which would indicate a preparedness for up-regulating signals. In contrast, already stimulated/activated cells may preferentially respond to cyclic AMP-elevating agents which cause a down-regulation of a variety of functions.

The apparent dualistic role of PGE₂, namely, low dose stimulation and high dose inhibition of TNF-α synthesis, argues for a modulation of the previous concept that solely attributes to PGE₂ the role of a negative feed-back inhibitor [5–7]. Based on our results, it is entirely feasible that low PGE₂ concentrations, which may be generated locally during microbial and other inflammatory processes, may aid in enhancing the functions of resident macrophages by releasing TNF-α which has previously been shown to be a co-factor of macrophage activation [3]. Only when macrophages have reached a sufficiently high level of stimulation/activation can their concomitantly produced PGE₂ act as an autocrine factor to down-regulate the initially induced macrophage activation.

In contrast to PGE₂, GM-CSF has usually been regarded as a factor that not only pro-

Table 2. GM-CSF-activated macrophages: Suppression of TNF-α synthesis by release of PGE_2.

	Release of	
Macrophage treatment*	TNF-α (ng/ml)	PGE_2 (ng/ml)
None	1.1 ± 0.3**	25.2 ± 3.2
GM-CSF	0.2 ± 0.1	57.0 ± 4.2
Indomethacin	0.6 ± 0.3	0.4 ± 0.3
GM-CSF + indomethacin	4.1 ± 0.3	0.2 ± 0.1

*Peritoneal macrophages from DBA/2 mice (1×10^6) were preincubated for 20 h with GM-CSF (300 U/ml), indomethacin (0.5 µg/ml), or a combination therof. Thereafter, LPS (1 µg/ml) was added, and after 18 h, release of TNF-α and PGE_2 was determined.
**Mean ± S.D. of four identical cultures.

motes proliferation and differentiation of macrophage precursor cells, but additionally activates already fully mature macrophages [8–10]. When considering macrophages, on the one hand, as particularly responsive cells to activating signals and, on the other hand, as potentially deleterious to surrounding tissue, it appears likely that activating factors such as GM-CSF may require a counteracting signal that, typical for macrophages, may be produced as an autocrine factor.

To analyze the effect of GM-CSF on TNF-α synthesis, murine peritoneal macrophages were incubated for different time periods with this cytokine. Although GM-CSF alone was incapable of stimulating TNF-α release from macrophages, it displayed the typical properties of a priming factor. Initially, within the first 8 h of incubation, it primed for enhanced TNF-α synthesis when macrophages were tested by a triggering stimulus such as LPS

(data not shown). However, this priming effect entirely disappeared upon further incubation with GM-CSF and was completely superseded by a suppressive effect on TNF-α synthesis after 20 h (Table 2). Despite suppressed TNF-α release, GM-CSF was found to have potently induced TNF-α gene transcription by 20 h of treatment (data not shown), which suggested that after prolonged GM-CSF treatment, a factor must have concomitantly been generated that interfered with efficient translation of TNF-α mRNA into the protein product. Table 2 demonstrates that treatment of GM-CSF-primed macrophages with the cyclooxygenase blocker indomethacin entirely reverted GM-CSF's suppressive effect on TNF-α synthesis and fully restored its priming properties. The responsible arachidonic acid metabolite was most likely PGE_2, since (1) enhanced amounts of PGE_2 were produced upon longer incubation with GM-CSF and (2) indomethacin-restored macrophages were again suppressed when exogenous PGE_2 was added back in amounts produced by GM-CSF-primed macrophages.

It was particularly important that PGE_2's inhibitory effect became evident only when macrophages were treated with GM-CSF for a prolonged time period. This finding indicates that GM-CSF acts on macrophages in a dual, but temporally delayed fashion: first by priming for enhanced TNF-α synthesis and only later by priming for an inhibitor of TNF-α produc-

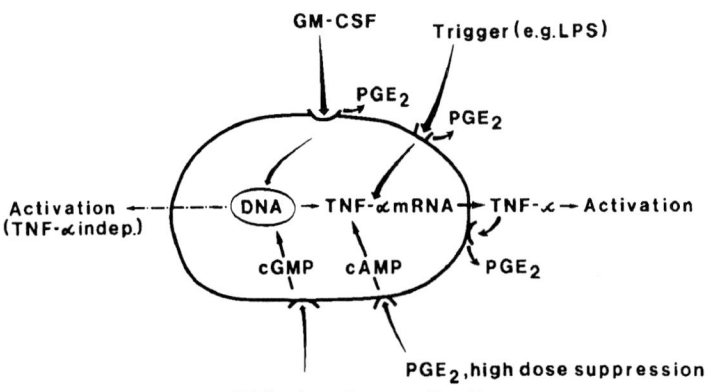

Figure 2. Autoregulatory circuit in macrophages responding to GM-CSF, TNF-α and PGE_2.

tion, PGE_2, which was produced by macrophages in an autocrine manner.

Although during an inflammatory response a variety of mediators may be called into action, it appears that the macrophage products TNF-α and PGE_2 occupy a prominent position [1, 2, 5, 6]. Both factors are not acting independently, rather, as shown here, mutual interactions take place which either up- or down-regulate macrophage activation. Within the framework of cytokine interactions, we also postulate that GM-CSF is a contributing factor that conditions macrophages for an enhanced secretory activity.

Our current working hypothesis with regard to interdependence of GM-CSF, TNF-α and PGE_2 is outlined in Figure 2. Based on the available evidence, GM-CSF appears to act at the transcriptional level by enhancing TNF-α gene expression. This leads to an accumulation of TNF-α mRNA which may readily be translated into the biologically active TNF-α protein by exogenous stimuli such as LPS. In this scenario, GM-CSF as well as LPS and TNF-α are also potent stimulators of the arachidonic acid metabolism which results in release of PGE_2. Initially, when low PGE_2 amounts are produced, a preferential effect on intracellular cyclic GMP generation has been shown which, in turn, acts at the transcriptional/translational level to produce more TNF-α. However, more TNF-α may induce higher PGE_2 concentrations which are capable of generating intracellular cyclic AMP that is inhibitory and blocks TNF-α mRNA translation into TNF-α protein. This autoregulatory circuit may serve as an example how a cytokine/mediator network may adapt macrophage activation to a well-balanced inflammatory response. Pathogenic effects may occur when substantial parts of such a network are deranged and factors such as TNF-α are continuously produced in high amounts, flood the organism and cause undesirable side effects such as shock or cachexia.

References

1. Old,L. J. 1985. Tumor necrosis factor (TNF). Science 230: 630.
2. Sherry,B., and A.Cerami. 1988. Cachectin/tumor necrosis factor exerts endocrine, paracrine, and autocrine control of inflammatory responses. J. Cell Biol. 107: 1269.
3. Heidenreich, S., M. Weyers, J.-H. Gong, H. Sprenger, M. Nain, and D. Gemsa. 1988. Potentiation of lymphokine-induced macrophage activation by tumor necrosis factor-α. J. Immunol. 140: 1511.
4. Renz, H., J.-H. Gong, A. Schmidt, M. Nain, and D. Gemsa. 1988. Release of tumor necrosis factor-α from macrophages. Enhancement and suppression are dose-dependently regulated by prostaglandin E2 and cyclic nucleotides. J. Immunol., 141: 2388.
5. Goodwin, J. S., and D. R. Webb. 1980. Regulation of the immune response by prostaglandins. Clin. Immunol. Immunopathol. 15: 106.
6. Gemsa, D. 1981. Stimulation of prostaglandin E release from macrophages and possible role in the immune response. In Lymphokines, Vol. 4. E. Pick, ed. Academic Press, New York, p. 335.
7. Schultz, R. M., N. A. Pavlidis, W. A. Stylos, and M. A. Chirigos. 1978. Regulation of macrophage tumoricidal function: A role of prostaglandins of the E series. Science 202: 320.
8. Grabstein, K. H., D. C. Urdal, R. J. Tushinski, D. Y. Mochizuki, V. L. Price, M. A. Cantrell, S. Gillis, and P. J. Conlon. 1986. Induction of macrophage tumoricidal activity by granulocyte-macrophage colony-stimulating factor. Science 232: 506.
9. Weiser, W. Y., A. van Niel, S. C. Clark, J. R. David, and H. G. Remold. 1987. Recombinant human granulocyte/macrophage colony-stimulating factor activates intracellular killing of Leishmania donovani by human monocyte-derived macrophages. J. Exp. Med. 166: 1436.
10. Dahinden, C. A., J. Zingg, F. E. Maly, and A. de Weck. 1988. Leukotriene production in human neutrophils primed by recombinant human granulocyte/macrophage colony-stimulating factor and stimulated with the complement component C5a and FMLP as second signals. J. Exp. Med. 167: 1281.

Cytokines in the Regulation of MHC-Restricted T-Cell Functions: A Human Graft versus Host Disease Model

*Dietger Niederwieser and Christoph Huber**

The observation that nominal antigens are recognized in context with MHC-antigens represents one of the most intriguing key-findings about the mechanisms of T-cell mediated immune recognition [1]. As a consequence, the inability of an antigen-specific T-cell to be stimulated by or to lyse an antigen-bearing cell target can be caused by either of the two not mutually exclusive mechanisms: first, by an inappropriate expression and/or presentation of the nominal antigen and/or second, by an inappropriate expression of the restricting MHC element. Although consensus exists about the limited and tissue- specific expression of class II MHC-antigens, much controversy exists about the amount of class I MHC antigens in different tissues. While most of us have been taught that class I MHC antigens are abundantly expressed on almost every nucleated cell, detailed analyses have demonstrated that the majority of non-hemopoetic tissues have very little if any of these surface structures [2, 3]. It has also been shown that cytokines such as the interferons and TNFs profoundly influence biosynthesis and surface expression of MHC antigens [4, 5]. On the basis of these findings one might expect that constitutive expression of MHC antigens and modification by endogenous cytokines crucially determines T-cell mediated tissue damage. In this article we provide evidence in a human graft versus host disease (GvH-D) model for the validity of this assumption.

Material and Methods

Patients

Patients transplanted with allogeneic bone-marrow from their HLA- identical and MLC- negative siblings for treatment of hemopoetic malignancy were investigated. The conditioning regimen consisted of ultra-high chemotherapy with cyclophosphamide followed by hyperfractionated total body irradiation. Prophylactic immunosuppression consisted of Cyclosporin A. Skin biopsies were obtained prior to transplantation from recipients and their donors to establish long-term keratinocyte cultures. Peripheral blood mononuclear cells (PMNC) were also harvested and cryopreserved before transplantation. Recipient peripheral blood mononuclear cells were collected after transplantation at the time of hemopoetic reconstitution, when total mononuclear blood cell counts exceeded 1000 cells/μl.

Establishment of GvH-D Lines

IL-2 dependent GvH-D lines were established from post-transplant recipient T-cells restimulated with PMNC and supplemented with IL-2. A commercially available preparation of T-cell supernatant enriched for IL-2 and depleted of contaminating lectins and other major impurities was utilized (Lymphokult, Biotest, Frankfurt). Cultures were established in Costar macrowells until cluster formation was visible. They were than transferred to tissue culture flasks, expanded by twice weekly restimulation with the original stimulator cell and maintained with IL-2 containing media.

Maximum time for expansion did not exceed three weeks. Lines were characterized by phenotypical analysis using a panel of monoclonal antibodies directed against the various T-cell associated surface structures. They were

* Div. Clinical Immunobiology, Dept. Internal Medicine, Univ. Hospital, Anichstr. 35, A-6020 Innsbruck, Austria. This work was financially supported by the Austria Research Grants "Zur Förderung der wissenschaftlichen Forschung," Project no. 6526, and by funds of the Ernst Boehringer/Institut für Arzneimittelforschung in Vienna. *Acknowledgements:* We are indebted to Mrs. A. M. Födinger for skillful technical assistance, Dr. J. Tratkiewicz for editing, and Mrs. M. Price-Placzek for secretarial assistance.

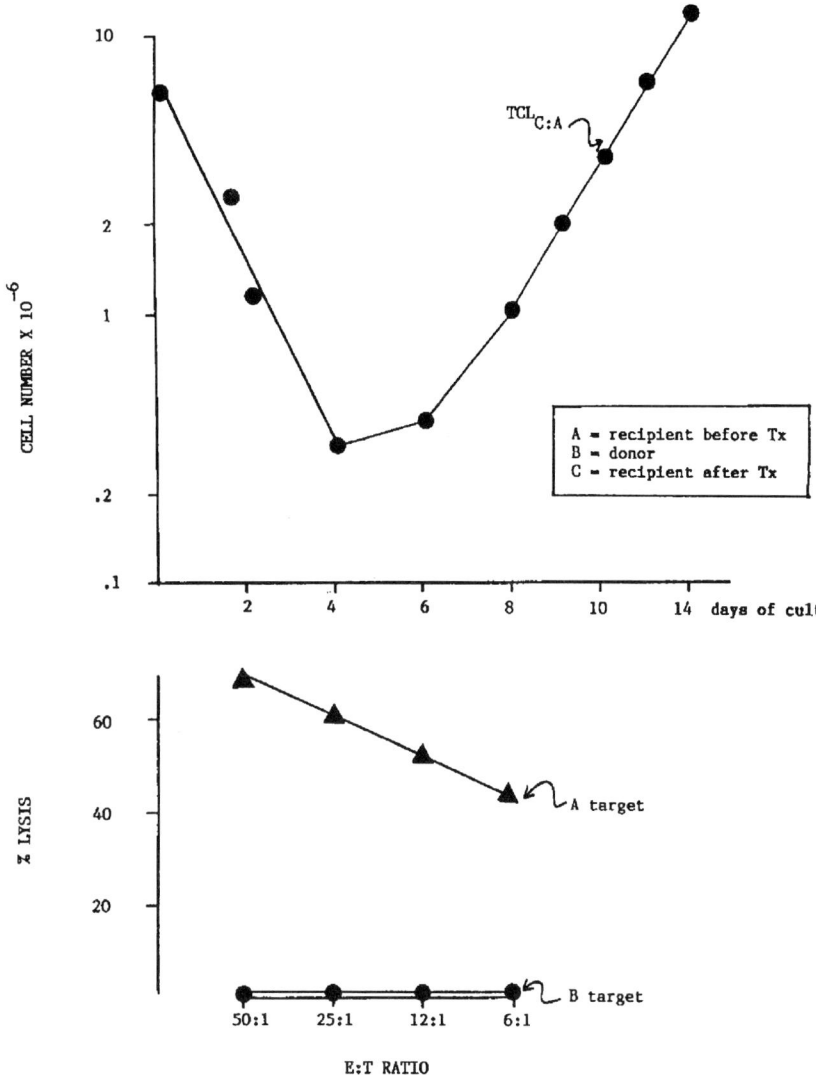

Figure 1. Growth properties and cytotoxic capacity of a GvH-D line.

also characterized for their functional capacities to recognize, in a proliferative assay, or to destroy recipients pretransplant hemopoetic or epidermal cells. PMNC and keratinocytes of donor origin served as controls. In addition, GvH-D T-cell lines were also used to study the segregation patterns of the nominal and the restricting MHC antigens involved in the patients families. MLC and CML assays were performed as previous described [6].

Results

Establishment and Characterization of GvH-D Lines

T-cells, harvested from the peripheral blood of patients subsequent to allogeneic bone-marrow transplantation, were restimulated with the patients' own pretransplant PMNC cells. In

507

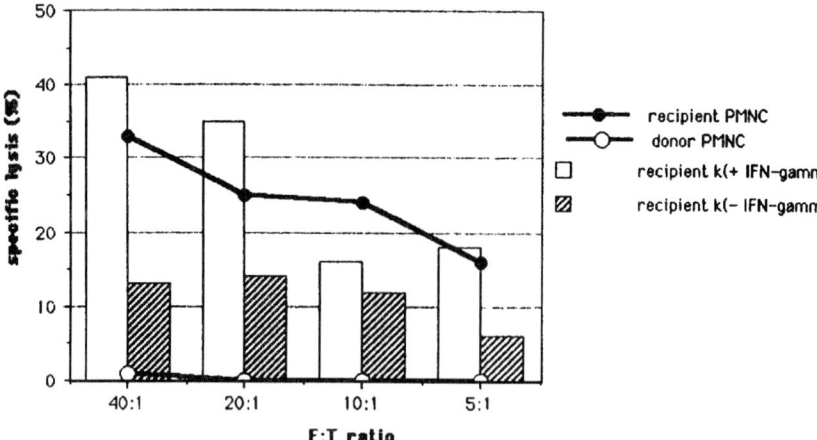

Figure 2. Susceptibility of recipient PMNC, untreated or IFN-γ treated recipient keratinocytes (k) and donor PMNC to lysis by a GvH-D line.

Table 1. Means of normalized IFN-γ serum levels before and after GvH-D (n=5).

Days before and after	−6	−4	−2	0	2	4	6
IFN-γ % (mean±SD)	16±11	47±0	55±38	100±0	64.7±91	83.2±28	56±42

the presence of IL-2-containing T-cells supernatants, lines with exquisite specificity for pretransplant PMNC were recovered from all patients exhibiting acute or chronic GvH-D. We failed, however, to establish such lines with discriminatory capacity in the presence of recombinant or highly purified natural IL-2. An example of the growth properties and the cytotoxic capacity of such a GvH-D line is shown in Figure 1. Lines exhibiting specificity for the recipients own pretransplant PMNC were further tested in family studies.

These investigations are in agreement with others, as we obtained clear evidence for the restricted recognition of the putative minor histocompatibility (HA) antigen(s) by class I MHC antigens [7]. Thus, it appears that in GvH-D patients, T-cells with minor HA specificity restricted by class-I MHC antigens can be regularly recovered from the blood stream.

Differential Reactivity of GvH-D Lines

GvH-D lines were tested against recipients pretransplant PMNC and keratinocytes. Target cells were untreated or preincubated with various concentrations of rIFN-alpha or rIFN-γ for 72 hours. These cells were either used as targets in CML-assay or were analyzed for MHC-antigen expression after staining with the appropriate monoclonal antibodies and FACS-ana-

lyses. The results of such an experiment are demonstrated in Figure 2. As indicated, mononuclear blood cells bearing the appropriate minor HA were readily lysed, whereas keratinocytes of the same derivation were resistant. Pretreatment of resistant keratinocyte targets with rIFN-γ increased both their class I MHC-antigen expression and susceptibility to lysis. Thus, it appears that only tissues with a high constitutive expression of class I MHC antigens are susceptible to lysis by minor HA specific, and class I MHC antigens are susceptible to lysis by minor HA specific and class I MHC restricted cytolytic T-cells. Moreover, the tolerance state observed in the case of keratinocytes, which have a low constitutive expression of class I MHC antigens, can be readily reversed by IFN- induced enhancement of the restricting MHC-elements.

Elevated levels of Endogenous IFN-γ Precede Clinical Presentation of GvH-D

As discussed in the previous paragraph IFN-γ plays a key-role in the in vitro control of a peculiar immune-tolerance state caused by an inappropriate expression of the restricting MHC- element of an antigen-specific T-cell response. If this also applies to the in vivo situation, GvH-D-associated tissue damage to the epidermis should be exclusively seen in the presence of endogenous levels of IFN-γ. We monitored endogenous IFN-gamma levels in patients at various days before and after transplantation. The results summarized in Table 1 indicate that GvH-D is associated with increased levels of this cytokine, and that this increase precedes clinical disease manifestation by several days.

Discussion

The aim of our studies was to further elucidate the role of differential expression of MHC-antigens in manifestation of T-cell- mediated tissue damage, using a human GvH-D model. The use of minor HA-specific and MHC-restricted cytolytic T-cells in the above model demonstrated that the susceptibility of different target tissues related to their constitutive expression of class I MHC. High expression on hemopoetic cells was associated with detectable lysis, whereas low expression on non-hemopoetic cells such as on keratinocytes was associated with resistance. Although the data do not allow one to discriminate between differential expression of the minor HA on these targets or differential expression of their restricting MHC- elements, our previous studies with MHC-specific T-cells would favor the view of the MHC-antigen as the crucial control element [7]. The use of class I MHC specific CTL revealed essentially the same hierarchy in the lysis of hemopoetic versus non-hemopoetic target cells. A further observation supporting the view of MHC-expression being critical in determining the extent of tissue injury is derived from our observation of the impact of cytokines on both lysis in CML and the expression of class-I MHC. When keratinocyte targets were exposed to α- or γ-IFN and further used as targets in a CML-assay or assessed for their class I MHC-antigen density by FACS-analysis, a distinct pattern was obtained. Whereas α-IFN, even at very high concentrations, only slightly increased class I MHC antigen expression and only minimally affected lysis in CML, a significant increase in surface antigen expression and almost identical lysis as that observed on hemopoetic targets was also seen with keratinocytes. It thus appears that MHC-restricted antigen- specific T-cells can discriminate between different organs on the basis of their differential constitutive MHC-expression. If this is the case, and if IFNs can readily break

such peripheral tolerance states in tissues with low constitutive class I MHC expression, a clear-cut correlation should exist between demonstration of endogenous IFN-γ levels and clinical manifestation of tissue injury. In the human GvH-D model, such an association is in fact readily demonstrable. No clinical presentation of GvH-D is seen in the absence of increased levels of endogenous IFN-γ, furthermore, increasing levels of the cytokine can be detected prior to clinical manifestation of disease.

From these studies it seems likely that T-cell-mediated tissue damage of organs with low constitutive MHC expression is greatly influenced by cytokine-inducing agents. IFN biosynthesis is known to be induced by virus infection. In fact, triggering of both GvH-D and of certain autoimmune states by virus infection has been frequently reported. Mechanisms such as the one discussed might explain this relationship.

References

1. Doherty, P. C., and R. M. Zinkernagel. 1975. A biological role for the major histocompatibility antigens. Lancet 2: 1406.
2. Skoskiewicz, M. J., R. B. Colvin, E. E. Schneeberger, and P. R. Russel. 1985. Widespread and selective induction of major histocompatibility complex-determined antigens in vivo by gamma- interferon. J. Exp. Med. 162: 1645.
3. Daar, A. S., S. V. Fuggle, J. W. Fabre, A. Ting, and P. J. Morris. 1984.The detailed distribution of HLA-A,B,C antigens in normal human organs. Transplantation 38: 287.
4. Steeg, P. S., R. N. Moore, H. M. Johnson, and J. J. Oppenheim. 1982. Regulation of murine macrophage IA antigen expression by lymphokine with immune interferon activity. J. Exp. Med. 156: 1780
5. Lindahl, P., I. Gresser, P. Leary, and M. Tovey. 1976. Interferon treatment of mice: Enhanced expression of histocompatibility antigens on lymphoid cells. Proc. Natl. Acad. Sci. USA 73: 1284.
6. Niederwieser, D., J. Auböck, J. Troppmair, M. Herold, G. Schuler, G. Boeck, J. Lotz, P. Fritsch, and Ch. Huber. 1988. IFN-mediated induction of MHC antigen expression on keratinocytes and its influence on in vitro alloimmune responses. J. Immunol. 140: 2556.
7. Goulmy, E., J. W. Gratama, E. Blokland, F. E. Zwaan, and J. J. Van Rood. 1983. A minor transplantation antigen detected by MHC restricted cytotoxic T-lymphocytes during graft-versus-host-disease. Nature 302: 159.

HLA-B27 and Enteric Bacteria in the Pathogenesis of Ankylosing Spondylitis

Andrew F. Geczy*, John S. Sullivan*, John K. Prendergast**,Carmel M. Edwards*

The importance of the association between the human histocompatibility antigen HLA-B27 and ankylosing spondylitis (AS) is undisputed, but the biological significance of this association remains unresolved. Our group has demonstrated cross-reactivity between a range of enteric bacteria and a specific determinant found only on the cells of HLA-B27-positive individuals with ankylosing spondylitis. We have proposed that the genetic element coding for this cross-reactive determinant is freely transmissible, and that its acquisition by B27-positive cells in vivo represents an important step in the pathogenesis of AS.

Ankylosing spondylitis (AS) is a relatively uncommon inflammatory arthropathy of the axial skeleton which frequently also involves the large peripheral joints [1]. Some early genetic studies of AS demonstrated a tendency for familial aggregation [2]; however, research on possible pathogenic mechanisms underlying the development of this disease did not really commence until 1973 when Brewerton et al. [3] and Schlosstein et al. [4] reported an intimate association between AS and HLA-B27. In most ethnic groups studied, about 90% of individuals who develop AS are positive for HLA-B27, but less than 1 in 50 HLA- B27-positive individuals develop the disease [5, 6]. The limited distribution of AS in the general HLA-B27-positive population, together with its discordant occurrence in some identical twins, as well as its close relationship to arthropathies of known infectious aetiology, indicates that additional factors might also play a role in the triggering of AS.

It was largely on this basis, and particularly in the light of a preliminary report suggesting cross-reactivity between HLA-B27 and some *Klebsiella* organisms [7], that we originally embarked on studies on the possible relevance of *Klebsiella* and HLA-B27 to AS. The concept that cross-reactive determinants might be involved in the pathogenesis of As was extended by Ebringer and his associates, who showed that sera from a rabbit immunized with HLA-B27-positive lymphocytes had increased binding activity against *Klebsiella* antigens [8].

These, and more recent immunochemical studies suggesting that structural similarity between some bacterial antigens and HLA-B27 may be relevant to the pathogenesis of AS, have been claimed to support the molecular mimicry hypothesis on the one-gene theory [9]. According to this theory, environmental agents (e.g., viruses or bacteria) and self-antigens share antigenic determinants, and this sharing may result in the failure of the immune system to recognize as foreign certain determinants on the environmental organism. One consequence of shared determinants between self and foreign antigens is the production against foreign antigens of humoral or cell-mediated effector mechanisms, which may attack certain target cells expressing self-antigens and thereby initiate an inflammatory reaction. Support for this theory has come from two recent studies which demonstrated specific cross-reactivity between HLA-B27 and the nitrogenase enzyme from *Klebsiella pneumoniae* [10] as well as between HLA-B27 and a surface membrane protein from a certain strain of *Yersinia* [11].

By contrast, our observations and their interpretation are basically different from the molecular mimicry hypothesis promoted by several other groups [8–12]. Our findings suggest that the cells of HLA-B27-positive patients with ankylosing spondylitis (B27+AS+), but not those of HLA-B27-positive normal individuals (B27+AS–), express on their surface an antigenic complex that is cross-reactive with a broad spectrum of enteric bacteria [13]. Since this cell-surface structure is not detectable serologically on the cells of HLA-B27-negative AS

---

* New South Wales Red Cross Blood Transfusion Service, 153 Clarence Street, Sydney, 2000 N.S.W. Australia.
** Department of Biochemistry and Molecular Biology, Harvard University, Cambridge, MA 02138, U.S.A.
This work was supported in part by grants from the National Health and Medical Research Council of Australia.

patients or those of normal individuals, it is reasonable to assume that HLA-B27 either forms part of a "cross-reactive complex" or is involved in its expression [14]. Subsequent work has shown that the majority of organisms isolated from the bowel flora of B27+AS+ individuals display a cross-reactive marker [15], i.e., a marker, antisera to which specifically recognize B27+AS+ cells; and that these organisms persist in these individuals for periods of up to 2 years [15, L.E. McGuigan, unpublished observations]. Such "cross-reactive" bacteria are rarely found in the bowel flora of HLA-B27-positive or -negative healthy individuals [15].

Collectively, these data suggest that the apparently unique presence and persistence of cross-reactive bacteria in the bowel flora of B27+AS+ individuals might be relevant to the pathogenesis of AS.

An extension to these studies has shown that the cells of B27+AS– clinically normal individuals can be rendered susceptible to lysis by antisera to certain cross-reactive enteric bacteria, following their incubation in the culture medium obtained from the appropriate bacterial isolate. The molecule responsible for this modification has been termed modifying factor [16]. This factor, which has a predominantly outer-membrane location, has a molecular weight of approximately 30,000 and an isoelectric point of 5.5 [17, 18]. An immunochemically similar factor has been isolated from the culture supernatants of B27+AS+. lymphoblastoid cell lines (LCL) [19] and an antiserum raised to the affinity-purified B27+AS+ LCL-derived factor displays similar specificity to antisera produced against cross-reactive bacteria [20]. Although in vitro "modified" B27+AS– cells may provide a useful model for studying the in vivo situation with respect to cells from B27+AS+ individuals, there are two important differences between in vitro "modified" and "in vivo" cells:

1. The in vitro modification of B27+AS– cells is a transient phenomenon, and when "modified" cells are cultured without exogenous MF, the serologically detectable marker is lost in 8 to 12 hours [14].

2. B27+AS+ cell lines constitutively express the cross-reactive determinant in the absence of exogenously added modifying factor, even after repeated subculturing [21].

Hence, the essential difference between the in vitro "modified" B27+AS– cells and the B27+AS+ cells is that the former represent simply a transient modification, the latter a permanent modification. We have proposed that the B27+AS+ cells has acquired the gene necessary for the constitutive expression of modifying factor, while the in vitro "modified" B27+AS+ cell has merely bound the product of this putative gene. Thus, when it is cultured in modifying factor-free medium, it loses this "modified" determinant [22]. The suggestion that eukaryotic cells acquire prokaryotic genetic material represents a novel pathogenetic mechanism which is somewhat controversial, but which is nevertheless consistent with our findings. In earlier studies it was shown that caesium chloride-purified plasmid preparations from "cross-reactive" bacteria can transform "non-cross-reactive" bacteria (e.g., E. coli C600) in such a way that these transformed organisms permanently acquire the genetic element coding for modifying factor (unpublished results). More recently, plasmid preparations from a clinical isolate (Salmonella typhimurium BTS 111) and from a cross-reactive transformant (E. coli C600-pBB1) have been shown to hybridize with Southern blots of Pst 1-treated digests of genomic DNA from 7 out of 10 B27+AS+ patients: no hybridization was detected with genomic DNA from either B27-positive or -negative normal individuals (unpublished results).

At this stage, no definite link has been established between the HLA-B27-associated modifying factor on B27+AS+ cells and the aetiopathogenesis of AS, but at least one reasonable hypothesis can be formulated. Since B27+AS+ cells express a type of altered self-determinant, it is possible that some kind of an immunological process, involving specific cytolytic cells (e.g., T-lymphocytes) against B27-associated structures, might lead to the destruction of target tissue displaying "modified" HLA-B27. Assuming that tissues in the axial and peripheral parts of the skeleton express B27-associated determinants, it remains to be explained why in AS, the sacroiliac region is affected more frequently than the peripheral joints. However, there are several ways in which cytotoxic mechanisms may be involved in the pathogenesis of AS. Firstly, cells in the sacroiliac region may present cytotoxic effector cells a more "recognizable" structure than cells in the vicinity of the peripheral joints. Secondly, the activity or concentration of CTL, or both, may be greater in the sacroiliac region. Ultimately, the inflammatory consequences of tissue injury at these sites as a result of CTL activity may be more pronounced than in other parts of the skeleton. Support for at least some of these suggestions has come from our more recent studies, which provide persuasive evidence that certain CTL can recognize modifying factor in the context of HLA-B27 [23]. We have shown that CTL can be induced either by stimulating the peripheral blood mononuclear cells (PBMC) of an HLA-B27-negative individual with the PBMC of an HLA-identical sibling suffering from AS or by immunizing in vitro, B27+AS– PBMC with autologous PBMC modified by "cross-reactive" bacterial antigens [23]. These CTL specifically lyse B27+AS+ PBMC, but not PBMC from B27-positive or -negative normal controls or from B27-negative AS patients. In vivo, one of the consequences of CTL activity might be the destruction of target tissue bearing B27-associated determinants, followed by an inflammatory episode, possibly during the early stages of the disease. Perhaps even more relevant to disease pathogenesis is the finding [J.S. Sullivan and A.F. Geczy, unpublished data] that neutrophils and monocytes from B27+AS+ but not from B27+AS– individuals can function as targets for HLA-B27-restricted CTL. These preliminary observations raise the intriguing possibility that these cells might participate in the inflammatory reactions that appear to be a prominent feature of AS.

Concluding Remarks

The remarkable association between HLA-B27 and AS, first described in 1973, promised to elucidate many aspects of the pathogenesis of this disease, but more than a decade after this initial report we are left with many more questions than answers. Despite rapid progress in our understanding of the structure and function of the HLA system, we are still unable to identify the unique features of the HLA-B27 gene or its product that renders an individual susceptible to AS. The continuing and often confused debate about the putative environmental agent which may trigger AS emphasizes how little we really understand about the pathogenesis of this MHC-linked disease. Nevertheless, the combined immunochemical and molecular, biological approaches adopted by our group during the past eight years should continue to yield new insights and thus make the study of As a little less forbidding that it has been in the past.

References

1. Hart, F. D. 1980. Clinical features and complications. In Ankylosing spondylitis. J. M. H. Moll, ed. Churchill Livingstone, London, p. 52.
2. Emery, E. A., and J. S. Lawrence. 1967. Genetics of ankylosing spondylitis. J. Med. Genet 4: 239.
3. Brewerton, D. A., M. Caffrey, F. D. Hart, D. C. O. James, A. Nicholls, and R. D. Sturrock. 1973. Ankylosing spondylitis and HL-A27. Lancet 1: 904.
4. Schlosstein, L., P. I. Terasaki, R. Bluestone, and C. M. Pearson. 1973. High association of HLA antigen W27 with ankylosing spondylitis. N. Engl. J. Med. 288: 704.
5. Tiwari, J. L., and P. I. Terasaki. 1985. HLA and disease associations. Springer-Verlag, N.Y.
6. Hickling, P., and V. Wright. 1983. Seronegative arthritides. In Oxford textbook of medicine. D. J. Weatherell, J. G. G. Ledingham, and D. A. Warrell, eds. Oxford University Press, Oxford, p. 22.
7. Ebringer, P., P. Cowling, N. Ngwa-Suh, D. C. O. James, and R. W. Ebringer. 1976. Cross-reactivity between Klebsiella aerogenes species and B27 lymphocyte antigens as an aetiological factor in ankylosing spondylitis. In HLA and disease. J. Dausset and A. Svejgaard, eds. INSERM, Paris, p. 27.
8. Ebringer, A. 1983. The cross-tolerance hypothesis, HLA-B27 and ankylosing spondylitis. Br. J. Rheumatol. 22: 53.
9. Ebringer, A., M. Baines, and T. Ptaszynska. 1985. Spondyloarthritis, uveitis, HLA-B27 and Klebsiella. Immunol. Rev. 86: 101.
10. Schwimmbec, P. L., D. T. Y. Yu, and M. B. A. Oldstone. 1987. Autoantibodies to HLA-B27 in the sera of HLA-B27 patients with ankylosing spondylitis and Reiter's syndrome. J. Exp. Med. 166: 173.
11. Chen, J. H., D. H. Kono, Z. Yong, M. S. Park, M. B. A. Oldstone, and D. T Y. Yu. 1987. A Yersinia pseudotuberculosis protein which cross-reacts with HLA-B27. J. Immunol. 139: 3003.
12. Ogasawara, M., D. H. Kono, and D. T. Y. Yu. 1986. Miomicry of human histocompatibility HLA-B27 antigens by Klebsiella. Infect. Immun. 51: 901.
13. Prendergast, J. K., J. S. Sullivan, A. Geczy, L. I. Upfold, J. P. Edmonds, H. V. Bashir, and E.

Reiss-Levy. 1983. Possible role of enteric organisms in the pathogenesis of ankylosing spondylitis and other seronegative arthropathies. Infect. Immun. 41: 935.

14. Geczy, A. F., K. Alexander, H. V. Bashir, J. P. Edmonds, L. Upfold, and J. Sullivan. 1983. HLA-B27, *Klebsiella* and ankylosing spondylitis: Biological and chemical studies. Immunol. Rev. 70: 23.

15. Mcguigan, L. E., J. K. Prendergast, A. F. Geczy, J. Edmonds, and H. V. Bashir. 1986. Significance of non-pathogenic cross-reactive bowel flora in patients with ankylosing spondylitis. Ann. Rheum. Dis. 45: 566.

16. Geczy, A. F., K. Alexander, H. V. Bashir, and J. Edmonds. 1980. A factor(s) in *Klebsiella* culture filtrates specifically modifies an HLA-B27-associated cell-surface component. 283: 782.

17. Sullivan, J., L. Upfold, A. F. Geczy, H. V. Bashir, and J. P. Edmonds. 1982. Immunochemical characterization of *Klebsiella* antigens which specifically modify and HLA-B27-associated cell-surface component. Hum. Immunol. 5: 295.

18. Upfold, L. I., J. S. Sullivan, and A. F. Geczy. 1986. Biochemical studies on a factor isolated from *Klebsiella* K43 BTS 1 that cross-reacts with cells from HLA-B27-positive patients with ankylos-

ing spondylitis. Hum. Immunol. 17: 224.

19. Orban, P., J. S. Sullivan, A. F. Geczy, L. I. Upfold, N. Coulits, and H. V. Bashir. 1983. A factor shed by lymphoblastoid cell lines of HLA-B27-positive patients with ankylosing spondylitis, specifically modifies the cells of HLA-B27-positive normal individuals. Clin. Exp. Immunol. 53: 10.

20. Sullivan, J. S., and A. F. Geczy. 1987. An antiserum to a disease-associated factor from the cells of an HLA-B27-positive patient with ankylosing spondylitis specifically recognizes an HLA-B27 associated determinant. Arth. Rheum. 30: 439.

21. Alexander, K., C. Edwards, I. S. Misko, A. F. Geczy, H. V. Bashir, and J. P. Edmonds. 1981. The distribution of a specific HLA-B27-associated component on the tissues of patients with ankylosing spondylitis. Clin. Exp. Immunol. 45: 158.

22. Sullivan, J. S., J. Prendergast, and A. F. Geczy. 1983. The aetiology of ankylosing spondylitis: Does a plasmid trigger the disease in genetically susceptible individuals? Hum. Immunol. 6: 185.

23. Geczy, A. F., L. E. McGuigan, J. S. Sullivan, and J. P. Edmonds. 1986. Cytotoxic T lymphocytes against disease-associated determinant(s) in ankylosing spondylitis. J. Exp. Med. 164: 932.

Autoreactive T Cells in Rheumatic Disease

Hans H. Peter, Michael Schlesier*, Ari E. Hinkkanen**, Viktor Steimle**,
Arlette Urlacher***, Gaby Haas*, Andreas Neumann*, Inga Melchers*,
Jörg T. Epplen*** *

Rheumatic joints contain an elevated number of activated T cells [1, 2], the stimulating antigens of which are currently subject of intense research in many laboratories. While evidence has been provided that locally persisting antigen may stimulate T cells in Lyme arthritis [3], molecular mimikry between *Klebsiella pneumoniae* nitrogenase and an HLA-B-27 epitope has been postulated to perpetuate chronic inflammatory joint disease in ankylosing spondylitis [4]. For rheumatoid arthritis (RA), animal models propose collagen type II [5] and proteoglycans [6] as potential candidates for triggering a local autoreactive T cell response. Although attractive, these hypotheses do not rule out the possibility that an essential part of the immune reaction in rheumatic joints is directed against self-MHC determinants which show an increased local expression or may be associated with different autologous peptides to which tolerance has not been induced during ontogeny. Autoreactive T cells with specificity for MHC class II determinants have been isolated from normal donors after immunization with foreign antigens [7]; they are therefore by no means specific for autoimmune diseases. However, in RA the number of autoreactive T cells may be altered and their regulatory control may be disturbed.

We have been investigating the role of autoreactive T cells in rheumatic diseases over the last four years and asked the following specific questions:

1. Are autoreactive T cells readily detectable in rheumatic diseases?

2. Is the frequency of autoreactive T cells elevated in rheumatic diseases?

3. To which antigens do autoreactive T cells from rheumatic patients react?

4. Are *Borrelia burgdorferi* (B.b.)-specific T cells increased in frequency in patients with Lyme arthritis?

By summarizing the results of our recent investigations we will try to give answers to some aspects of these questions.

Are Autoreactive T Cells Readily Detectable in Rheumatic Diseases?

Originally we started out with bulk cultures of peripheral blood (PBL) and synovial fluid lymphocytes (SFL) in the presence of 5% autologous serum plus lectin-free or recombinant interleukin 2 (rIL-2) [8]. The aim was to expand in vivo activated T cells. Under these conditions, normal PBL could not be expanded, and SFL from RA patients grew better than PBL, suggesting high suppressive activity in bulk cultures. After 14 days growing cultures were cloned by limiting dilution (LD) with 1 or 5 cells/well in the presence of irradiated autologous feeder cells. 5% autologous serum and 0.1 µg/ml PHA. Growing clones were expanded and tested for proliferative responses against autologous and allogeneic stimulator cells. In one thoroughly analyzed RA patient autoreactive T cell clones/lines were clearly demonstrable. To our surprise most of these clones reacted also against allogeneic stimulator cells suggesting either polyclonality, antigen-specific reactivity (alloreactivity may be viewed as reactivity against self-MHC plus an unknown antigen X) or a broad unspecific reactivity of the established clones. Phenotypically 11 out of 16 clones were CD8$^+$/CD4$^-$, 5 CD4$^+$/CD8$^-$ and 1 CD4$^+$/CD8$^+$. Attempts to demonstrate anti-bacterial or anti-mycoplasma specificity of the clones were unsuccessful. Interestingly, in the same study we failed to gen-

* Abteilung für Rheumatologie und Klinische Immunologie, Med. Univ. Klinik Freiburg, FRG.
** Max-Planck-Institut für Psychiatrie, Planett/Martinsried bei München, FRG.
*** Centre de Transfusion Sanguine, Strasbourg, France.
    Supported by BMFT Grant No. 01 VM 8605 and DFG Ep7/3-2.

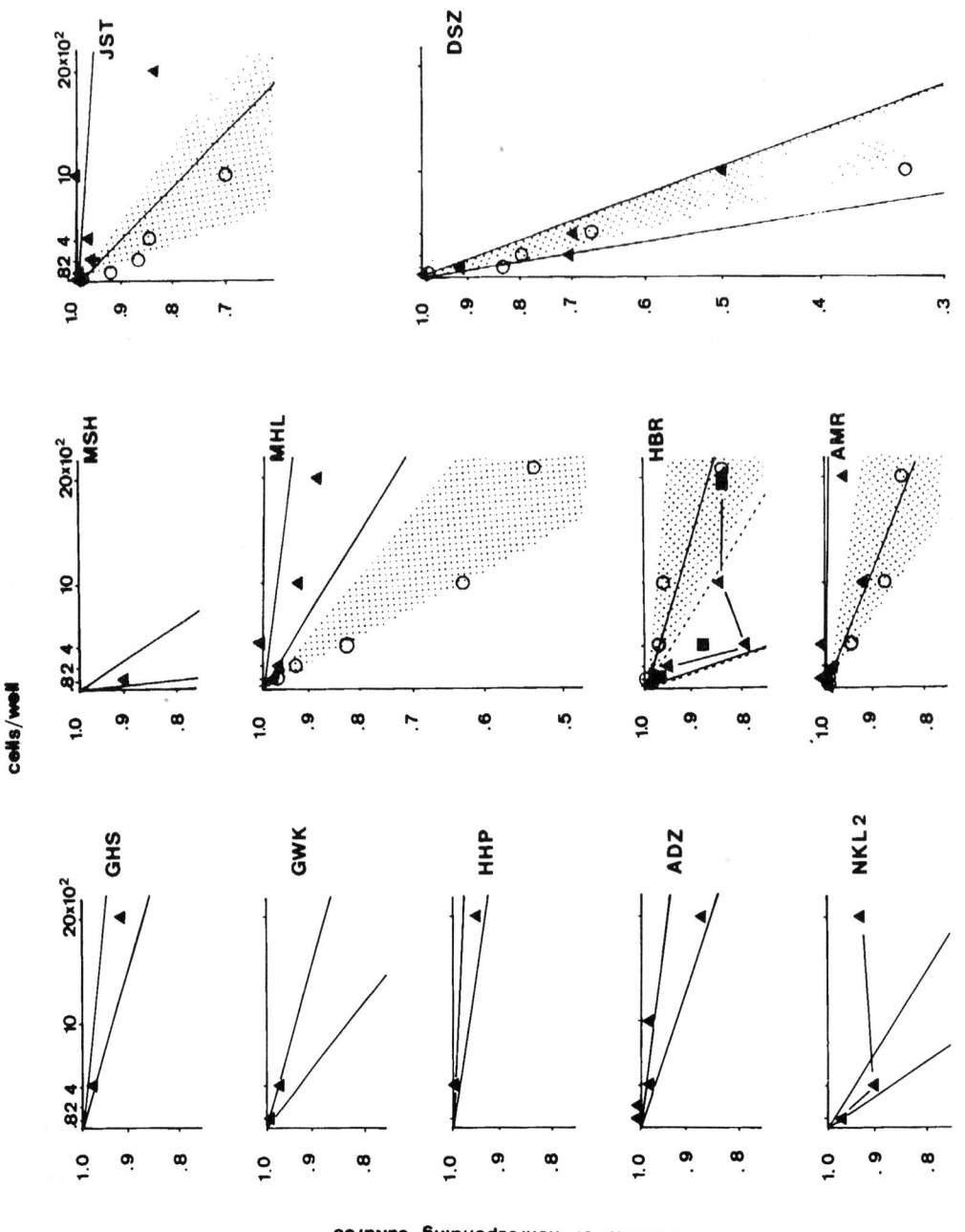

Figure 1: Frequencies of autoreactive T cells from PBL (▲) of controls (left column) and from PBL (▲) and SFL (-o-) of patients with RA and Lyme arthritis (middle and right column). Patient HBR was tested before gold therapy (PBL ■) and during gold therapy (PBL ▲, SFL -o-). 95% confidence intervals are indicated by straight lines for PBL and by shaded areas for SFL.

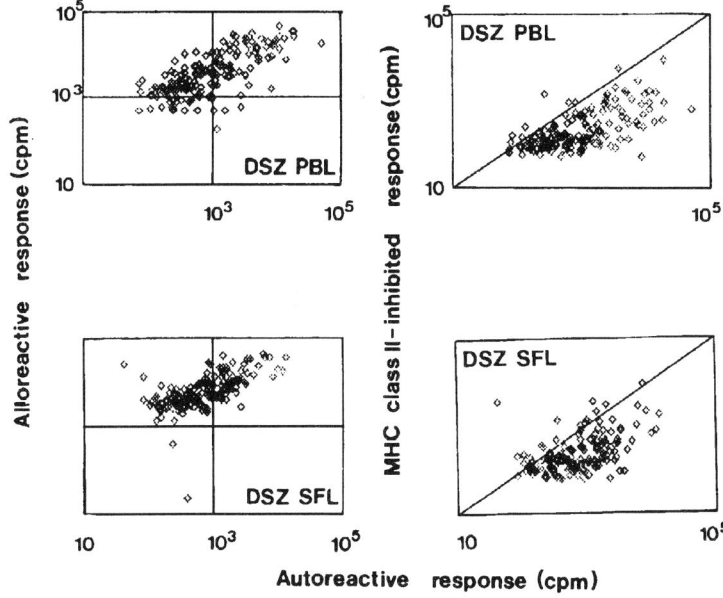

Figure 2: Auto- and alloreactivity of LD-derived T cell lines from PBL and SFL of a 36-year-old patient (DSZ) with Lyme arthritis (left column). The proliferative responses are distributed in 4 rectangles: *Lower left:* background proliferation; *upper left:* alloreactive lines only; *upper right:* auto- and alloreactive lines; *lower right:* strictly autoreactive lines. The two graphs of the right column show the inhibition of the autoreactive SFL and PBL responses by monoclonal anti-DR/DP antibody (shift into the lower triangle).

erate autoreactive T cell clones/lines from allogeneic mixed lymphocyte cultures (MLC), while we had no difficulties to establish allospecific clones.

Is the Frequency of Autoreactive T Cells Elevated in Rheumatic Diseases?

In a second series of experiments we estimated frequencies of in vivo activated autoreactive T cells in LD cultures (20 to 2000 cells/well) again using strictly autologous culture conditions and rIL-2 as the only stimulant [9]. Autoreactive T cells were readily detectable in every control person and rheumatic patient tested. The mean frequencies of growing and autoreactive T cells (measured by proliferation against autologous PBL) were 10-fold higher in patients with RA or Lyme arthritis than in controls (Figure 1). Again the great majority of the established clones/lines (we considered only cultures which according to Poisson statistics had a >80% chance to be monoclonal) reacted broadly against autologous and allogeneic stimulator cells. The reactivity of most clones was inhibited by a monoclonal anti-DR/DP (Tü35) antibody (Figure 2). Interestingly, there was no increase of autoreactive T cells in synovia as compared to blood. In analogy to published studies on the alloreactivity of antigen-

specific T cell clones [10], we interpreted alloreactivity of the in vivo primed and in vitro with rIL-2 expanded T cells as reactivity against self-MHC + X. Alternatively, T cells with broad specificity, reacting against the novel HLA-DY determinants [11] may also be taken into consideration. An interesting observation relates to the cell range of the LD cultures at which autoreactive T cells may be preferentially detected. Thus low cell counts between 1 and 400 cells/well are particularly suitable to unravel auto-reactive T cells; at higher cell inputs (>400 cells/well) they often fail to grow possibly due to suppressive mechanisms.

To which Antigens Do Autoreactive T Cells from Rheumatic Patients React?

The specificity of strictly autoreactive and crossreactive T cell clones was studied in detail in a 21-year-old patient (U.A.) with HLA-B27+ reactive arthritis and a homozygous DRw11 serotype (Table 1). From this patient's blood and synovial fluid, 135 T cell lines were established, and 33 with high probability of clonality (6 from blood, 27 from synovial) were further analyzed for phenotype, function, and specificity [12]. The majority of the clones expressed CD4+/CD8- (26/33), a minority CD8+/CD4- (3/33) or CD4-/CD8- (4/33). Only two clones

517

Table 1. Specificity of the autoreactive T cell clone UA-S2.

Stimulator	HLA haplotype*	Response (cpm)**
Medium		180
U.A. (patient)	a,c	27260
H.A. (mother)	a,b	26800
G.A. (father)	c,d	1900
A.A. (brother)	b,d	900
I.R. (sister)	a,c	11922
J.H. (aunt)	a,b	11015
J.A. (daughter)	n.t.	347
UA-LBL (EBV)	a,c	498
UA-S24 (Tc clone)	a,c	280

*Haplotypes: (a) A2 or 32, B27, Cw1, DRw11, (b) A2 or 32, B7, Cw7, DR2, (c) A2 or 32, B51, C–, DRw11, (d) A2 or 32, B57, Cw6, DR7
**Proliferative response measured as 3H-TdR uptake.

ular cloning from genomic and cDNA libraries of UA-S2 DNA, a novel DRw11 variant was found (DRw11.3), the β1-chain of which differs at positions 71 and 86 from the known DRw11.1 variant and at positions 67 and 164 from DRw11.2 [13]. The gene encoding for the DRβ1 chain of the second DRw11 variant (probably DRw11.1) present in patient U.A. is currently searched for in the patient's and his father's genome. Whether UA-S2 recognizes an autologous MHC determinant alone or in conjunction with a hitherto unidentified peptide remains to be seen by transfection experiments of the different DRβ1 genes into L cells or B-cell lines (B-LCL) followed by stimulation experiments with UA-S2. Circumstantial evidence points to a peptide specificity of UA-S2, since the clone only proliferates to irradiated PBL but not to an autologous B-LCL (Table 1) or to other DRw11⁺, autologous T cell lines. It is feasible that certain PBL carry an autologous

Table 2. Autoreactive T cell clones from A HLA-B27+ reactive arthritis.

T cell clone	Origin	Phenotype	Target antigen	Cβ usage	Rearrangement of	
					Vβ 6.7 or 6.1	Va element of UA-S2
UA-S2	synovia	CD4⁺/8⁻	auto*	Cβ2	+	+
UA-S24	synovia	CD4⁺/8⁻	auto/allo	Cβ2	+	***
UA-86	synovia	CD4⁻/8⁻	auto/allo	?**	-	-
UA-S97	synovia	CD4⁻/8⁻	auto/allo	Cβ1	-	-
UA-B34	blood	CD4⁻/8⁺	auto/allo	?**	-	-

*Autoreactivity is defined as proliferative response to autologous irradiated BPL (DRw11.3+), alloreactivity as response to two unrelated BPL donors (DRw11-).
**Not Cβ2, ***Va of UA-S2 deleted

failed to proliferate in response to either autologous or allogeneic stimulator cells; 30 clones/lines reacted broadly with autologous and allogeneic stimulator cells and only one synovia-derived CD4⁺ helper T cell clone (UA-S2) exhibited a strictly autoreactive reaction pattern restricted to the maternal DRw11+ haplotype (Table 1). Since by serological means the patient was homozygous for DRw11, but the paternal DRw11⁺ haplotype failed to stimulate UA-S2, a microheterogeneity between father and mother was assumed in the DRβ1-chain gene encoding for the DRw11 specificity. This hypothesis could be confirmed by primed lymphocyte typing (PLT) with a reagent specific for a DRw11 subtype (most likely DRw11.1) that recognizes the paternal but not the maternal haplotype [12]. By molec-

peptide, e.g., a cell-type-specific antigen [14] which is recognized by UA-S2 in a MHC-restricted manner similar to the Mls gene products in mice [15]. The autologous B-LCL may lack or have lost this peptide during culture, or less likely, it may not adequately express the relevant DRw11 haplotype which is needed as restriction element for UA-S2.

The T cell receptor (TCR) α and β chains or UA-S2 have meanwhile been sequenced [16] and revealed a novel Va element rearranged to a known Ja segment; the expressed Vβ6.7 element has been described before, in UA-S2 it is rearranged to Dβ2.1—Jβ2.3—Cβ2. Most interestingly, one other clone (UA-S24) from the same patient uses also the Vβ6.7 element which is rearranged to the Jβ2 cluster (Table 2). Thus, UA-S2 appears to be unique in that it recog-

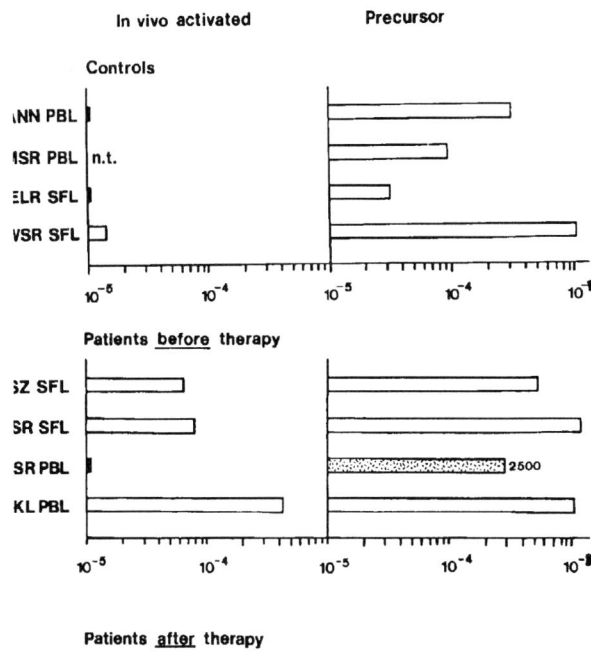

Figure 3: Frequencies of in vivo activated *Borrelia burgdorferi*-specific T cell lines from normal controls and patients with Lyme arthritis (left column). The T cell precursor frequencies are shown on the right column. Shaded bars indicate non-linear LD-curves suggesting suppression of B.b.-specific T cell proliferation.

nizes an autologous DRw11.3 epitope alone or in conjunction with an autologous peptide whereas clone UA-S24 which is stimulated by autologous and allogeneic stimulator cells most likely recognizes self-MHC plus a foreign peptide. This difference in specificity may be explained by different Va elements and/or differences in the N nucleotide composition of the Vβ—Dβ—Jβ junctions.

Are *Borrelia burgdorferi* (B.b.)-Specific T Cells Increased in Frequency in Patients with Lyme Arthritis?

To this end we performed autologous LD cultures (156 to 20,000 cells/well) as described in section 2 either with or without addition of *Borrelia burgdorferi* (B.b.) sonicates. Established T cell clones/lines were then tested for their proliferative response to B.b. antigens presented by autologous irradiated PBL [17]. This protocol provides three sets of information:

1. It allows to test for precursor frequencies of B.b. specific T cells (LD in the presence of B.b., followed by testing of clones on B.b.-presenting PBL);

2. It allows to test for frequencies of in vivo activated B.b. specific T cells (LD in the absence of B.b. followed by testing of clones on B.b.-presenting PBL);

3. It allows to test for B.b.-induced autoreactive T cells (LD in the presence of B.b. followed by testing of clones against autologous stimulators).

Some preliminary results are presented in Figure 3. Healthy individuals had only very few in vivo-activated B.b.-specific T cells in their peripheral blood (<1/60,000), but showed similar precursor frequencies (1/800 to 1/30,000) as patients with Lyme arthritis (1/800 to 1/8000). Conversely, in vivo-activated B.b.-specific T cells were readily detectable in blood and synovial fluid of patients with Lyme arthritis (1/1300 to 1/15,000). Interestingly, following successful antibiotic treatment of Lyme arthritis, non-linear LD curves at higher cell numbers were observed, indicating suppression of B.b.-specific T cell growth.

Conclusions

Provided appropriate LD culture conditions (autologous serum, autologous feeder cells, and rIL-2) are employed, in vivo-activated autoreactive T cells are readily detectable in blood and synovial fluid of rheumatic patients. The frequency of autoreactive T cells is elevated in patients with rheumatic diseases, and most of the established lines/clones show a broad proliferative response to autologous and allogeneic stimulator cells. Only few clones exhibited strict autoreactivity; in one patient the functional difference of a strictly autoreactive clone (UA-S2) versus an auto- and alloreactive clone (UA-S24) from the same synovial LD culture could be traced down to subtle differences in the TCRβ-chain gene structure or to the use of a different Va element, respectively. The MHC product recognized by UA-S2 turned out to be a DRβ1 chain variant of DRw11 which may serve as restriction element for a hitherto unknown autologous peptide. Finally, in patients with Lyme arthritis, we proved that our LD culture system is capable of estimating frequencies for B.b.-specific, in vivo-activated T cells as well as for their precursor cells in blood and synovial fluid. The tools for analyzing autoreactive T cells described here may greatly enhance our understanding of the role of T cells during induction and perpetuation of RA and other MHC-linked autoimmune diseases.

References

1. Burmester, G. R., D. T. Y. Yu, A. M. Irani, H. G. Kunkel, and R. J. Winchester. 1981. Ia[+] T cells in synovial fluid and tissues of patients with rheumatoid arthritis. Arthr. Rheum. 24: 1370.

2. Knobloch, C., M. Schlesier, R. Dräger, M. Gärtner, and H. H. Peter. 1985. Quantitative absorption of interleukin 2 by peripheral blood and synovial fluid lymphocytes from patients with rheumatoid arthritis. Rheumatol. Int. 5: 133.

3. Steer, A. C., P. H. Duray, and E. C. Butcher. 1988. Spirochetal antigens and lymphoid cell surface markers in Lyme synovitis. Arthr. Rheum. 31: 487.

4. Schwimmbeck, P. L., D. T. Y. Yu, and M. B. A. Oldstone. 1987. Auto-antibodies to HLA B27 in the sera of HLA B27 patients with ankylosing spondylitis and Reiter's syndrome. Molecular mimikry with *Klebsiella pneumoniae* as potential mechanism of autoimmune disease. J. Exp. Med. 166: 173.

5. Trentham, D. E. 1985. Immune response to collagen. In: Immunology of rheumatic diseases. S. Gupta and N. Talal, eds. Plenum, pp. 301–323.

6. van Eden, W., J. E. R. Thole, R. van der Zee, A. Noordzij, J. D. A van Embden, E. J. Hensen, I. and R. Cohen. 1988. Cloning of the mycobacterial epitope recognized by T lymphocytes in adjuvant arthritis. Nature 331: 171.

7. Tilkin, A. F., J. Michon, D. Juy, M. Kayabanda, Y. Henin, G. Sterkers, H. Betuel, and J. P. Levy. 1987. Autoreactive T cell clones of MHC class II specificities are produced during responses against foreign antigens in man. J. Immunol. 138: 674.

8. Schlesier, M., C. Ramb-Lindauer, M. Gärtner, and H. H. Peter. 1984. Analysis T cell cultures and clones from a patient with classic rheumatoid arthritis. Evidence for the existence of autoreactive T cell clones in blood and synovial fluid. Rheumatol. Int. 4 (Suppl.): 1.

9. Schlesier, M., G. Haas, G. Wolff-Vorbeck, I. Melchers, and H. H. Peter. 1988. Autoreactive T cells in rheumatic disease. I. Analysis of growth frequencies and autoreactivity of T cells from patients with rheumatoid arthritis and Lyme disease. J. Autoimmunity, in press.

10. Ashwell, J. D., C. Chen, and R. H. Schwartz. 1986. High frequency and nonrandom distribution of alloreactivity in T cell clones selected for recognition of foreign antigen in association with self class II molecules. J. Immunol. 136: 389.

11. Pawelec, G., N. Fernandez, Th. Brocker, E. M. Schneider, H. Festenstein, and P. Wernet. 1988. DY determinants, possibly associated with novel class II molecules, stimulate autoreactive CD4[+] T cells with suppressive activity. J. Exp. Med. 167: 243.

12. Schlesier, M., C. Ramb-Lindauer, R. Dräger, A. Urlacher, M. Robin-Winn, and H. H. Peter. 1988. Autoreactive T cells in rheumatic disease. II. Function and specificity of an autoreactive T helper cell clone established from a HLA-B27[+] reactive arthritis. Immunobiology, in press.

13. Steimle, V., A. Hinkkanen, M. Schlesier, and J. T. Epplen. 1988. A novel HLA-DRβ1 sequence from the DRw11 haplotype. Immunogenet. 28: 208.

14. Marrack, P., and J. Kappler. 1988. T cells can distinguish between allogeneic major histocompatibility complex products on different cell types. Nature. 332: 840.

15. Janeway, C. A., K. Fischer-Lindahl, and U. Hämmerling. 1988. The Mls locus: New clues to a lingering mystery. Immunology Today. 9: 125.

16. Hinkkanen, A. E., V. Steimle, M. Schlesier, H. H. Peter, and J. T. Epplen. 1988. The antigen receptor of an autoreactive T cell clone from human rheumatic synovia. Immunogenet., in press.

17. Neumann, A., M. Schlesier, A. Vogt, I. Melchers, and H. H. Peter. 1988. Borrelia burgdorferi reactive T cells in lyme arthritis (LA). Immunobiology 178: 146 (Abstract).

Disturbed Immune-Endocrine Communication in Autoimmune Disease

Georg Wick and Hans-Peter Brezinschek*

Immunizations with exogenous antigens results in a surge of the serum glucocorticoid hormone levels concomitant with the immune response in rodents and normal chickens. The same effect can be obtained by injections of the supernatant of mitogen-stimulated spleen cells (conditioned medium). These increased glucocorticoid levels are believed to suppress the immune response against a second, different antigen (antigenic competition). As shown by other authors interleukin 1 (IL-1) released by macrophages in the course of an immune response seems to be the main mediator of glucocorticoid release via stimulation of the hypothalamic-pituitary-adrenal axis. In the present communication we show for the first time that this immune-endocrine feedback loop is malfunctioning in an animal model for an organ specific autoimmune disease, the Obese strain (OS) of chicken with spontaneous autoimmune thyroiditis. We localized the defect to the hypothalamic-pituitary portion of feedback loop and in part clarified its molecular nature. Elucidation of these pathophysiological changes may open new ways for a more selective therapy of autoimmune diseases.

Immuno-neuro-endocrinology has evolved as a relatively young interdisciplinary field of research from the notion that interactions between the three major communication systems of the body are common. The recent availability of appropriate animal models, of various mediators produced in pure form via DNA recombinant technology in addition to the already known classical hormones, the access to monoclonal antibodies as specific and sensitive investigative tools, the molecular characterization of hormone receptors, and the use of new, sophisticated tissue-culture techniques have confirmed that the interrelationship between the nervous, the immune, and the endocrine systems are extremely complex. On the other hand, the unravelling of these interactions by interdisciplinary efforts is not only important for the understanding of physiological and pathological processes, but may also provide insight into biochemical pathways that can be manipulated therapeutically with relative ease. The best example for such a therapeutic intervention is perhaps the use of glucocorticoids as inflammatory and immuno- suppressive drugs. The present contribution concentrates on one single facet of the interaction between the immune and the endocrine system: the immunoregulatory role of endogenously produced glucocorticoids and the pathological alteration of this regulatory principle in autoimmune disease.

Interaction Between the Immune and Glucocorticoid Systems

Antigenic challenge leads to a surge of glucocorticoid levels in the serum of normal mice, rats, and chickens with a peak at 3 to 6 days, i.e., coincident with the serum antibody peak [1, 2, 3]. The mechanism leading to this increase is based on the release of one (or several) mediator(s) from cells of the immune system, the so-called glucocorticoid increasing factor(s) (GIF) [4]. The main component of GIF has been identified as interleukin 1 (IL-1) [5], but additional glucocorticoid increasing components should also be considered. Recombinant murine IL-1 and human IL-1 can induce the release of corticotropin releasing factor (CRF) by the hypothalamus, which in turn induces the production of adrenocorticotropic hormone (ACTH) in the pituitary and thus entails stimulation of the adrenal cortex and the production of glucocorticoids, i.e., corticosterone (CN) [6]. Another possibility, discussed by different

*   Institute for General and Experimental Pathology, School of Medicine, University of Innsbruck, and Immunoendocrinology Research Unit of the Austrian Academy of Sciences, Innsbruck, Austria.
    This work was supported by the Austrian Research Council (Grant No. S-41/05) and the Jubiläumsfonds of the Austrian National Bank (Grant No. 2784). We acknowledge the collaboration and discussion with Drs. G. Krömer, R. Fässler, K. Hála and H. Dietrich. Dr. K. N. Traill kindly improved the English language of our manuscript.

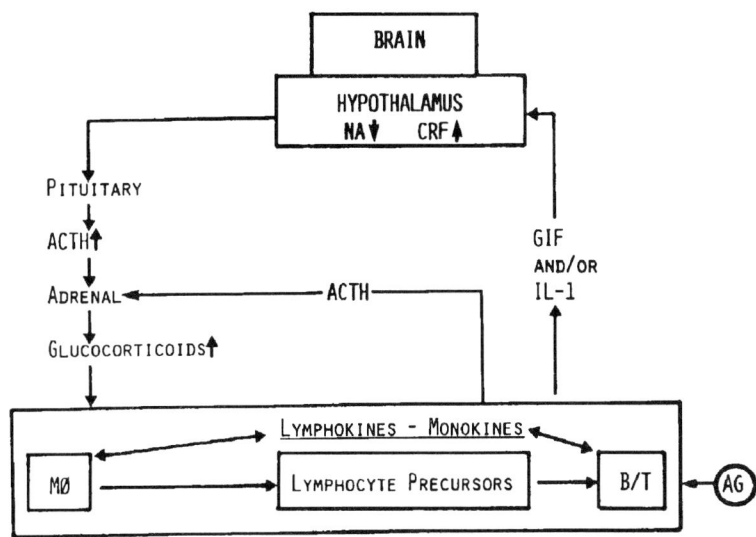

Figure 1. Immunoendocrine feedback loop: Two possible pathways resulting in corticosterone elevation have been suggested, i.e., an indirect stimulation via the hypothalamohypophysealaxis and a direct effect via an ACTH-like substance, produced by the stimulated immune system. No evidence for the latter pathway was found in the present experiments.

groups [2] could be the production of ACTH by cells of the immune system, which then would stimulate the adrenals directly (Figure 1).

Besedovsky et al. [7] have shown that injection of a second antigen into an animal at the time of the glucocorticoid peak induced by the first antigen elicits no, or only a minor, immune response ("antigenic competition"). This may be explained by the fact that glucocorticoids exert their immunosuppressive effect primarily during the phase of induction of the immune response and not during the growth-factor-dependent differentiation phase. Induction of clones potentially reactive to the second antigen will therefore be suppressed by the high-glucocorticoid concentration, but the reaction to the first antigen will not be affected.

Since autoimmune diseases are characterized by a hyperreactivity against different autoantigens, it was deemed of interest to investigate whether functional alterations of the above-mentioned feedback loop may contribute to this abnormal immunological reactivity. For these studies we have chosen an animal model that develops a spontaneous autoimmune thyroiditis (SAT) that closely resembles human Hashimoto thyroiditis in all clinical, serological, pathohistological, and endocrinological aspects. This is the Obese strain (OS) of chickens, most probably the best studied animal model for a spontaneous organ specific autoimmune disease [8, 9, 10].

Before embarking on these studies, we confirmed that the above-mentioned mechanisms of antigen-induced glucocorticoid secretion are also operative in an avian species. In addition, we also showed that—similar to the situation in rodents—the injection of supernatants from concanavalin A (ConA) stimulated chicken spleen cell cultures into normal White Leghorn (NWL) chickens also induced a surge in CN serum levels [11]. The administration of dexamethasone, a glucocorticoid superagonist, was able to inhibit this effect via suppression of ACTH production. This observation also showed that in our system no ACTH production by cells of the immune system, and thus direct stimulation of the adrenals, did occur. Finally, inhibition of prostaglandin synthesis by indomethacin also had no influence on GIF activity in vivo [17].

Further attempts to elucidate the nature of GIF in the chicken provided the following data: GIF activity seems to be phylogenetically conserved because ConA supernatants of mouse spleen cell cultures were also effective in increasing CN in chickens: Interleukin 2 (IL-2) was excluded as a possible mediator of GIF activity, because IL-2 receptor bearing chicken lymphoblasts were not able to absorb the activity. Molecular chromotography and HPLC separation showed that the active fraction had a molecular weight of about 15 to 16 KD, and this fraction also reacted with polyclonal and monoclonal antibodies against human IL-1a.

We therefore concluded that also in the chicken, IL-1 is the principal active component of GIF [H.P. Brezinschek et al., in preparation]. In this context it is important to note that in previous experiments chicken IL-1 has been found to be active in co-stimulation assays on mouse cells, in contrast to IL-2 and gamma-interferon, which did not show biological interspecies cross-reactivity (12).

Disturbed Immune Endocrine Feedback Loop in OS Chickens with Spontaneous Autoimmune Thyroiditis

When the above-mentioned experiments were repeated with OS chickens, it was first shown that animals of this strain gave similar primary immune responses to heterologous antigens, e.g., sheep blood cells, but showed significantly decreased CN serum levels as compared to age and sex matched NWL controls [11].

When OS and NWL chickens were injected with ConA supernatants from NWL spleen cultures, a significantly higher, dose-dependant CN response was again observed in NWL as compared to OS birds [11]. A defect in GIF production by OS spleen cells was, however, excluded because ConA supernatants of OS spleen cell cultures were as effective in normal birds as supernatants from NWL cultures at inducing a normal CN response. A suppression of the pituitary ACTH production by dexamethasone could be overcome in both strains by injection of the ACTH analogue Synacthen®, thus speaking for a normal responsiveness of the adrenals in the OS. This observation is also emphasized by the fact, that baseline CN values, i.e., before immunization or injection of conditioned medium, is the same in OS and NWL chickens. We conclude from the data obtained so far that the defect of immune-endocrine communication in the OS is situated within the hypothalamic-pituitary axis within the above-described feedback loop.

Genetic analysis of the altered responsiveness to GIF was done by cross-breeding OS birds with the inbred normal CB strain, back crossing the F1 generation with both OS and CB birds, and also producing F2 chickens. Data of these experiments have been published in detail elsewhere [13, 14] and can be summarized as follows: GIF hyperresponsiveness of OS chickens is controlled by one autosomal dominant gene that is not associated with the major histocompatibility complex (MHC). Abnormal GIF responsiveness is not always associated with thyroiditis, i.e., the disease sometimes occurs in animals showing a normal GIF response. Since the development of SAT is a multigenic process and the role of glucocorticoids can only be conceived as being involved in the fine tuning of the immune system, these latter observations do not argue against them being one of the modulatory factors involved in the pathogenesis of the disease.

The functional relevance of the observed phenomena could be demonstrated by injecting conditioned medium into OS and NWL chickens and concomitantly monitoring the development of the CN serum profile and T-cell mitogen responsiveness of peripheral blood lymphocytes. It could be clearly shown that mitogen responsiveness decreased in parallel with the increase of CN and that OS responses remained significantly higher than those of NWL chickens [11].

Finally, we recently identified a new endogenous virus (ev 22) in Southern blots of OS chicken DNA restriction enzyme digests hybridized with a Rous sarcoma virus-specific probe that contains the whole avian endogenous virus information [9, 10, 15]. This ev 22 occurs only in the OS and was not found in any other strain. Interestingly, its presence correlates significantly with the abnormal immune-endocrine interaction in this strain [13]. Current attempts of our group are aimed at further elucidating the possible role of this correlation by cloning of the new ev and its flanking regions.

In addition to the diminished response of the neuroendocrine system to signals of the immune system, a further unrelated defect has been found in the OS, namely, a decreased basal glucocorticoid tonus [16]. The glucocorticoid tonus is defined as the balance between free, hormonally active glucocorticoid hormone and the fraction bound to corticosteroid binding globulin (CBG). OS chickens show significantly elevated CBG serum levels. This genetically determined alteration segregates independently of the described abnormal immune-endocrine interaction [13] but may aggravate the effects of the latter.

Therapeutic Considerations

Based on these results and our previous experience which showed the OS to be an apt model for the assessment of immunomodulatory drugs, OS chickens were treated from the day of hatching until the third week of age with hydrocortisone; this regimen led to complete prevention or significant improvement of SAT in a dose-dependent manner [16].

In summary, we have for the first time provided evidence that an altered immune-endocrine dialogue may be one of the factors involved in the development of an autoimmune disease [17]. Based on these data new concepts for the elucidation of the multifactorial pathogenesis of autoimmune diseases can be devised and the rationale for more selective therapies conceived, e.g., the use of synthetic steroid analogues that still possess immunosuppressive potential without undesired endocrine side effects.

References

1. Besedovsky, H. O., A. del Rey, and E. Sorkin. 1983. What do the immune system and the brain know about each other? Immunol. Today 4: 342.
2. Blalock, J. E., and E. M. Smith. 1985. The immune system: our mobile brain? Immunol. Today 6: 115.
3. Payan, D. G., J. P. McGillis, and E. J. Goetzl. 1987. Neuroimmunology. Adv. Immunol. 39: 299.
4. Besedovsky, H. O., A. del Rey, E. Sorkin, W. Lotz, and U. Schwulera. 1985. Lymphoid cells produce an immunoregulatory glucocorticoid increasing factor (GIF) acting through the pituitary gland. Clin. exp. Immunol. 59: 622.
5. Besedovsky, H. O., A. del Rey, E. Sorkin, and C. A. Dinarello. 1986. Immunoregulatory feedback between interleukin-1 and glucocorticoid hormones. Science 233: 652.
6. Sapolsky, R., C. Rivier, G. Yamamoto, P. Plotsky, and W. Vale. 1987. Interleukin-1 stimulates the secretion of hypothalamic corticotropin-releasing factor. Science 238: 522–524.
7. Besedovsky, H., A. del Rey, and E. Sorkin. 1979. Antigenic competition between horse and sheep red blood cells as a hormone-dependent phenomenon. Clin. exp. Immunol. 37: 106.
8. Cole, R.K., J. H. Kite, and E. Witebsky. 1968. Hereditary autoimmune thyroiditis in the fowl. Science 160: 1357.
9. Wick, G., J. Möst, K. Schauenstein, G. Krömer, H. Dietrich, A. Ziemiecki, R. Fässler, S. Schwarz, N. Neu, and K. Hála. 1985. Spontaneous autoimmune thyroiditis—a bird's eye view. Immunol. Today 6: 359.
10. Wick, G., K. Hála, H. Wolf, A. Ziemiecki, R. S. Sundick, M. StöfflerMeilicke, and M. DeBeats. 1986. The role of genetically determined primary alteration of the target organ in the development of spontaneous autoimmune thyroiditis in obese strain (OS) chickens. Immunol. Rev. 94: 113.
11. Schauenstein, K., R. Fässler, H. Dietrich, S. Schwarz, G. Krömer, and G. Wick. 1987. Disturbed immuneendocrine communication in autoimmune disease: Lack of corticosterone response to immune signals in obese strain chickens with spontaneous autoimmune thyroiditis. J. Immunol. 139: 1830.
12. Hayari, Y., K. Schauenstein, A. Globerson. 1982. Avian lymphokines. II. Interleukin1 activity in supernatants of mitogen-stimulated chicken spleen cells. Dev. Comp. Immunol. 6:785.
13. Krömer, G., R. Fässler, K. Hála, G. Boeck, K. Schauenstein, H. P. Brezinschek, N. Neu, H. Dietrich, R. Jakober, and G. Wick. 1988. Genetic analysis of extrathyroidal features of Obese strain (OS) chickens with spontaneous autoimmune thyroiditis. Eur. J. Immunol., in press.
14. Krömer, G., N. Neu, T. Kuehr, H. Dietrich, R. Fässler, K. Hála, and G. Wick. 1988. Immunogenetic analysis of spontaneous autoimmune thyroiditis of Obese strain (OS) chickens. Submitted for publication.
15. Ziemieki, A., G. Krömer, R. G. Müller, K. Hála, and G. Wick. 1988. Ev 22, a new endogenous avian leukosis virus locus found in chickens with spontaneous autoimmune thyroiditis. Arch. Virol. 100: 267.
16. Fässler, R., H. Dietrich, G. Krömer, S. Schwarz, H. P. Brezinschek, and G. Wick. 1988. Diminished glucocorticoid tonus in Obese strain (OS) chickens with spontaneous autoimmune thyroiditis: Increased plasma levels of physicochemically unaltered corticosteroid binding globulin but normal total corticosterone plasma concentration and normal glucocorticoid receptor contents in lymphoid tissue. J. steroid. Biochem. 30: 375.
17. Krömer, G., H. P. Brezinschek, R. Fässler, K. Schauenstein, and G. Wick. 1988. Physiology and pathology of an immunoendocrine feedback loop. Immunol. Today 9: 163.

Monitoring the Progress of Immune Complex Disease: Assays for Complement Activation Fragments

*Shaun Ruddy**

Nonspecific tests for the measurement of plasma levels of immune complexes are subject to a variety of extraneous influences, resulting in remarkable amounts of variation in results from day to day and from laboratory to laboratory. Serial studies generally are more informative. Added to this variance is the remarkable heterogeneity of the diseases such as systemic lupus erythematosus, rheumatoid arthritis, and systemic vasculitis in which measurements of immune complexes are performed. Although immune complex assays have been valuable for informing investigators about the pathogenesis of disease, they have proved less useful for following the progress of a particular disease in an individual patient. For the latter, measurements of complement levels are more reliable and more informative. Immunoassays employing monoclonal antibodies that are specific for fragments produced during complement activation of this system increase the sensitivity and specificity of complement assays in monitoring the progress of immune complex disease.

The notion that immune complexes cause disease is supported by a large body of both experimental and clinical evidence. Both animal models such as acute or chronic serum sickness induced by antigen injection with the formation of an immune response and clinical investigations in diseases such as systemic lupus erythematosus and rheumatoid arthritis have provided a firm basis for associating tissue damage with immune complexes. In human disease, the data include immunofluorescent observations of deposits of immunoglobulins and complement in damaged tissues. Complexes of DNA with anti-DNA have been found in kidneys from patients with systemic lupus, of IgG with anti-IgG in synovial tissues from patients with rheumatoid arthritis, and of hepatitis antigen and antibody in the vessels of patients with vasculitis. Supporting information includes the demonstration of hypercatabolism of complement proteins with resulting falls in plasma or synovial fluid levels in many of these diseases. Although other pathogenetic mechanisms, including disorders of the cellular lim of the immune response may be responsible for some of the tissue damage observed, there is widespread agreement of the importance of immune complexes as cause of disease.

More than 40 different methods for detecting immune complexes have been described. McDougal et al. [1] examined the performance characteristics of the five most widely performed assays and found a remarkable degree of variability both within laboratories for different assays and between laboratories. In an attempt to eliminate some of this variation, Nydegger [2] has proposed an international reference preparation of synthetic immune complexes. In an extensive review, Moxley [personal communication] has examined the clinical utility of the various competing immune complex assays. He found that they did distinguish inflammatory rheumatic disease, including systemic lupus erythematosus, rheumatoid arthritis, or vasculitis from noninflammatory disease, but that they did not differentiate between subsets of inflammatory rheumatic diseases. With the exception of the solid-phase C1q binding assay for systemic lupus erythematosus, the immune complexes assays were of less use than other commonly available (and less expensive) laboratory tests in correlating with and predicting disease activity.

*   Division of Rheumatology, Allergy and Immunology, Department of Internal Medicine, Medical College of Virginia, Virginia Commonwealth University, Richmond, Virginia, U.S.A.
    This is Publication No. 255 from the Charles W. Thomas Fund.

526

Measurement of Complement Components

As a consequence of their participation in an immune reaction during a disease, the complement proteins become altered and are rapidly cleared from the plasma space. When this acceleration catabolism exceeds any compensatory increases in synthesis, a fall in plasma level results. Concentrations of complement proteins are measured by immunoassays with antibody specific for the protein in question. Although the results of measurements of most of the complement proteins in a large number of disease states have been described, the components most frequently used in clinical situations are C3 and C4. Although it is still unacceptably high and a source of confusion, the coefficient of variation of complement measurements is much less than that for immune complex assays, either day to day or between laboratories. The range of normal for complement proteins is quite broad, often of the order of 50% of the normal mean [3]. In the case of C4, the high frequency of null alleles coding for non- synthesis and inherited partial deficiency is partly responsible for the broad normal range. Thus, serial changes in levels for a given patient over a period of time are often more informative than comparison with an absolute range of normal. C3 and C4 concentrations are widely used as an index of disease activity in systemic lupus erythematosus. Falls in levels of C4 often presage the development of lupus nephritis; reduced levels of C3 usually indicate the *presence* of nephritis. With the exception of disease that has become extra-articular, complement measurements are not informative in rheumatoid arthritis or, for that matter, most other rheumatic disease.

By no means all patients with active systemic lupus erythematosus will have subnormal levels of C3 and C4. In an attempt to increase the sensitivity of complement measurements, assays for split products or cleavage fragments produced during complement activation have been devised. The anaphylatoxin fragment, C3a, cleaved from C3 by either the classical or alternative pathway convertases, is not normally detectable in serum. Differential precipitation of native C3 from the peptide C3a by exposure of the sample to acid conditions allows the subsequent measurement of C3a by a radioimmunoassay using competition for binding to antibody by [125-I]C3a. Using this assay, Abramson et al. [4] have found elevations in the plasma of patients with SLE. We have found elevations in synovial fluid from patients with rheumatoid arthritis when compared to synovial fluids from patients with degenerative or traumatic arthritis [5]. In a prospective study of plasma specimens, levels of C3a were found to correlate with the activity of rheumatoid arthritis as assessed by a joint index or disease activity index [6]. The correlation values were similar to those for serum C-reactive protein and for the Westergren erythrocyte sedimentation rate. In correlations of the disease indices with combinations of laboratory tests, any pair of laboratory tests correlated more strongly than did any one test.

We have used an enzyme-linked immunoassay for Bb, the fragment of factor B produced when Factor D cleaves it during alternative pathway activation, to examine synovial fluids. The assay was developed by Cytotech Corp., San Diego, CA. Preliminary results, shown in Figure 1, indicate that this assay discriminates successfully between rheumatoid arthritis and degenerative joint disease. The results are at least as good as those for C3a. Buyon and co-workers [7] used this Bb assay in parallel with an assay for the Ba fragment of Factor B in

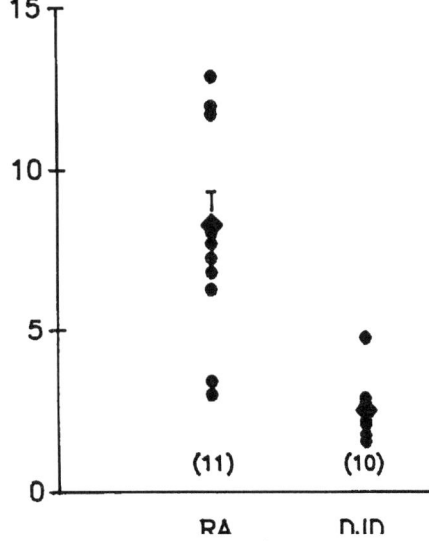

Figure 1. Concentrations of Bb fragment in synovial fluids from patients with rheumatoid arthritis (RA) or degenerative joint disease (DJD). The sample size is given in the parenthesis below each set of points.

systemic lupus erythematosus. They found that elevated levels of Ba/Bb more accurately reflected disease severity than did the total hemolytic complement, which was often depressed in patients with only moderately active or inactive SLE. Elevations of Ba/Bb were also better predictors of flares in disease than was the total hemolytic complement or levels of C4 or C3.

References

1. McDougal, J. S., M. Hubbard, P. L. Strobel, and F. C. McDuffie. 1982. Comparison of five assays for immune complexes in the rheumatic diseases: Performance characteristics of the assays. J. Lab. Clin. Med. 100: 705.

2. Nydegger, U. E., and S. E. Svehag. 1984. Improved standardization in the quantitative estimation of soluble immune complexes making use of an international reference preparation. Results of a collaborative multicentre study. Clin. Exp. Immunol. 58: 502.

3. Ruddy, S. 1985. Plasma protein effectors of inflammation: Complement. In: Textbook of rheumatology (2nd ed.). W. N. Kelley, E. D. Harris, S. Ruddy and C. B. Sledge, eds. Philadelphia: W. B. Saunders, p. 83.

4. Belmont, H. M., P. Hopkins, H. S. Edelson, H. B. Kaplan, R. Ludewig, G. Weissman, and S. Abramson. 1986. Complement activation during systemic lupus erythematosus: C3a and C5a anaphylatoxins circulate during exacerbations of disease. Arthritis Rheum. 29: 1085.

5. Moxley, G., and S. Ruddy. 1985. Elevated C3 anaphylatoxin levels in synovial fluids from patients with rheumatoid arthritis. Arthritis Rheum. 28: 1089.

6. Moxley, G., and S. Ruddy. 1987. Elevated plasma C3a anaphylatoxin levels in rheumatoid arthritis patients. Arthritis Rheum. 30: 1097.

7. Buyon, J., Tamerius, J., Kolb, W., Morrow, P., Winchester, R., Weissman, G., and S. Abramson. 1988. Determination of plasma complement split products (CSP) in lupus is the most sensitive predictor of disease activity. Arthritis Rheum., in the press.

The Use of Lymphokines in Therapy

Michael T. Lotze and Steven A. Rosenberg*

The use of a variety of different recombinant cytokines alone or in conjunction with other biologic reagents have now been identified as therapeutically effective approaches in murine models and more recently in patients with cancer. In addition, monoclonal antibodies directed against human tumors as well as adoptive therapy with cellular reagents alone or in conjunction with cytokines represent promising new approaches. The availability of recombinant cytokines has allowed substantial progress to be made and the development of biologic therapy as a fourth modality of cancer treatment has now joined surgery, chemotherapy, and radiotherapy by providing convincing evidence of therapeutic efficacy. Evaluation of the clinical effects of these cytokines when administered at physiologic and pharmacologic doses provides insight into the molecular mechanisms associated with several human diseases.

It is estimated that there are approximately 30–100,000 genes contained within the human genome. Each of these genes encode protein products important for embryogenesis, physiologic responses to the environment, and reproduction. The advent of molecular biologic techniques suggests that each of the products of these genes is potentially accessible for use as pharmacologic reagents as they exist in nature or as modified subsequently for use. The prior development of medical therapeutics progressed on the basis of chance observations regarding physiologic effects of various substances when introduced into man and more recently through understanding of the basic biochemistry of these processes. The availability of techniques to produce the very molecules which have evolved to subserve biologic functions represents an important and revolutionary advance. This has perhaps most clearly been demonstrated in the rapid progress in the cloning and expression of recombinant cytokines. Over 15 different recombinant proteins have now been administered to humans. Many

of them represent hormones produced within the endocrine or immune systems. The availability of recombinant lymphokines and monokines has made possible the elucidation of many additional activities of these otherwise scarce molecules. Further, the administration of these reagents is associated with many systemic effects reminiscent of previously poorly explained syndromes, including myocardial depression, cholestasis and jaundice, fever and cancer cachexia. Indeed, it may be that the release of these individual factors is central to the development of these syndromes.

Our own experience with the use of recombinant cytokines began with studies of human Interleukin-2 (IL-2), which serve as the basis for many of the immunotherapies that we have developed for patients with cancer [1, 2]. Subsequently, evaluation of other cytokines, including tumor necrosis factor (TNF), alpha interferon, granulocyte-macrophage colony stimulating factor (GM-CSF), have been carried out by our group. It is not possible here to summarize all of the preclinical data as well as the biologic basis for their clinical use; this information is available from many of the references. The recombinant cytokines with possible clinical use that are currently available are listed in Table 1. Below, we will highlight what is known about the clinical effects of these cytokines.

Alpha Interferon

Alpha or leucocyte interferon and beta-1 interferon, which is derived from fibroblasts, share a common receptor and have very similar effects in vitro. Most clinical trials to date have been done with recombinant alpha interferon [35–37], and it appears in those studies done with beta interferon [38, 39] that similar effects are noted. The mechanism by which interferon mediates anti-tumor effects is unclear, but postulated mechanisms include direct anti-

*   Tumor Immunology Section, Surgery Branch, National Cancer Institute, Building 10, Room 2B47, Bethesda, MD 20892.
    Acknowledgement: We appreciate the careful preparation of this manuscript by Ms. Mary Ann Bodnar.

Table 1. Recombinant cytokines with possible clinical uses.

Name	Human Trials	Molecular Weight	Relevant Bio-logic Effects	Toxicity	Ref. No.
IL-1	-	15–17,000	Hematopoietic growth factor, stimulatory for NK activity, endogenous pyrogen lympho-cyte activating factor. Protect bone marrow from radiation toxicity, decrease IL-2 induced vascular leak	Fever	3-5
IL-2	+	15,000	T cell growth factor, induces lytic activity (LAK) for fresh tumor, alters traffic of lymphoid cells	Fever, chills, leaky capillary syndrome, cholestatic jaundice, de-creased systemic vascular resistance	6-13
IL-3	-	25,000	Pluripotent erythroid and myeloid CSF synergizes with other CSFs, including GM-CSF growth factor for B cells and T cells	None in primates at 5– 50 µg/kg/d; increase acute phase reactants	14, 15
IL-4	+	21,500	Inhibits some IL-2 driven re-sponses and proliferation; B cell and T cell growth and differentiation factor	None described in ro-dents; primate and human testing in progress	16-18
IL-5	-	45–60,000	Differentiation of eosinophils; T cell replacing factor; in-crease IgA secretion	Unknown	19, 20
IL-6	-	19–30,000	Interferion, B cell differentia-tion factor, hepatocyte stimu-lating factor, increase hepatic acute phase reactants	None described in rodents	21, 22
GM-CSF	+	14–34,000	Neutrophil (PMN) monocyte and eosinophil growth factor; increase PMN phagocytes, chemotaxis	Bone pain, fever, myalgia, anorexia, weight gain, edema, rash, hypo-tension, respiratory distress	23-27
G-CSF	+	19,600	Neutrophil and erytroid colonies stim..lated; activates PMN for oxidative metabolism and ADCC	Bone pain	28
M-CSF	-	45,000	Monocyte stimulation to release monokines (IL-1, TNF)	None reported in rodents	29, 30
TNF-	+	17–60,000	Tumor necrosis synergy with IL-2 antitumor effect	Fever, chills, hypo-tension, GI hemorrhage	31-34
Alpha interferon	+	17.5–21,000	Antiviral agent, differ-entiating agent, anti-pro-liferative	Fever, chills, myalgia, cardiac arrhythmias, fatigue, mild hepatopathy	35-37
Beta interferon	+	18,500	Anti-viral agent, differ-entiating agent, anti-pro-liferative	Fever, chills, myalgia, malaise, nausea, vomit-ing, mild hepatopathy	38, 39
Gamma interferon	+	40–60,000	Antiviral, differen-tiative, anti-proliferative	Fever, chills, myalgia, nausea, vomiting, head-ache, increased SGOT	40-42
Erythro-poietin	+	18–34,000	Erythropoiesis	Hypertension, hyper-kalemia	43

IL = interleukin, NK = natural killer, CSF = colony-stimulating factor, GM = granulocyte-macrophage, PMN = polymorphonuclear leucocyte, ADCC = antibody-dependent cellular cytotoxicity, GI = gastrointestinal proliferative effects on tumor as well as possible effects on host immune effector mechanisms. Efficacy in hematologic malignancies including chronic myelogenous leukemia, hairy cell leukemia, epidemic Kaposi's sarcoma associated with the acquired immunodeficiency syndrome, as well as cutaneous T-cell and non-Hodgkin's lymphomas have been found. Responses in 25–80% of cases have been noted. Melanoma and renal cell carcinoma have responded in approximately 20% of patients. Recombinant interferon alpha is now licensed for use by the U.S. Food and Drug Administration in the treatment of hairy cell leukemia.

The major toxicities associated with alpha interferon include profound malaise at high doses as well as fever, mild transaminase elevations and a neuropsychiatric syndrome including confusion. Its use in combination with IL-2 in murine metastasis models has been more effective than either alone with demonstrable synergy. Clinical trials with alpha interferon and IL-2 have been initiated at the NCI and suggest enhanced efficacy when compared to IL-2 alone especially in patients with renal cell carcinoma.

Interleukin-2

Interleukin-2 has been demonstrated to have marked efficacy in the treatment of patients with melanoma and renal cell carcinoma in conjunction with the adoptive transfer of lymphokine-activated killer cells as well as with the adoptive therapy with tumor-infiltrating lymphocytes [6–13, 44]. The rationale for the use of IL-2 in vivo were based on its central role following antigenic or mitogenic stimulation. Decreased ability to produce IL-2 is associated with pathologic states, and the laboratory abnormalities in these conditions can be corrected by addition of IL-2 in in vitro cultures. Further, immune reactivity can be demonstrated to be inhibited by antibodies to IL-2 and IL-2 receptor-bearing cells both in vivo and in vitro. Immune response can be blocked by antibodies to the IL-2 receptor. For example, one can prolong cardiac allografts survival by using antibodies to the IL-2 receptor.

Toxicities related to IL-2 administration include problems related to a vascular leak syndrome characterized by requirement for exogenous fluid and on occasion vasopressor administration to maintain adequate organ profusion. A mild and reversible myocardial depression can be demonstrated as well as a reversible profound cholestatic jaundice and prerenal azotemia in most patients. An example of the effects of low doses of IL-2 on hepatobiliary excretion of technicium coupled disida, a hepatobiliary scanning agent, demonstrating profound cholestasis, is shown in Figure 1. This and other side effects of IL-2 are readily reversible, and although treatment-related morbidity occurs in virtually every patient, there is only a 1–2% overall mortality in now well over 700 patients treated on IL-2-based therapies.

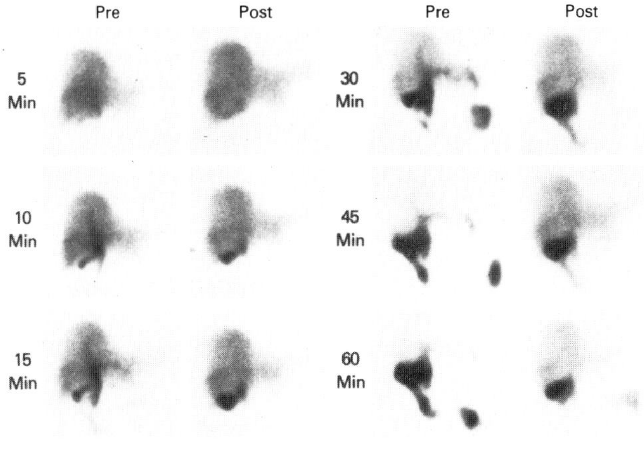

Figure 1. Delayed excretion of Tc-99m-Disida in a patient receiving 20,000 units/kg of IL-2 three times a day. A hepatobiliary scan was obtained prior to IL-2 treatment with prompt visualization of the liver at 5 minutes and almost complete clearing of the liver by 45 minutes with virtually all activity in the biliary tree or gut by 60 minutes. Conversely, in the same patient, delayed excretion into the biliary tree and more prominent retention in the liver are noted for as long as 60 minutes. This represents one of the many clinical findings associated with IL-2 administration in humans. (From B. Fisher et al.: Interleukin-2 induces profound reversible cholestasis: A detailed analysis in treated patients. Submitted for publication.)

We performed a prospective randomized trial of high-dose IL-2 alone or given with lymphokine-activated killer cells for the treatment of patients with advanced cancer. The adoptive transfer of LAK cells increases the incidence of complete but not overall responses in treated patients. Others have reported similar responses when giving IL-2 by alternative schedules. We have recently demonstrated that the addition of IL-2 to treatment with monoclonal antibodies increases the apparent whole body retention of the antibody consistent with the capillary leak syndrome, and we have demonstrated in murine models that combinations of IL-2 and anti-tumor monoclonal antibodies to the B16 melanoma are more effective than either one alone. Based on these studies, we have initiated combination protocols recently with the monoclonal antibodies 17.1A, L6, and B72.3, all antibodies to colorectal carcinomas. Total doses of 600 mg/m^2 to 6 g/m^2 are planned in conjunction with both high- and low-dose IL-2.

Gamma Interferon and Tumor Necrosis Factor

Tumor necrosis factor (TNF) was initially identified with two distinct biologic activities. Specifically, these included the induction of hemorrhagic necrosis in tumors, especially those implanted subcutaneously in mice and as a factor causing the wasting diathesis known as cachexia in animals with chronic infections. This was associated with a reduction in lipoprotein lipase activity [31]. We have evaluated the role of tumor necrosis factor in murine [32, 33] models and have been able to demonstrate that tumor necrosis factor has greater toxicity in tumor-bearing as compared to non-tumor-bearing animals, and that single doses are capable of causing necrosis and reduction in size in murine tumors transplanted under the skin as well as in the liver. Long-term antitumor responses correlated with the immunogenicity of the tumors. TNF is synergistic with IL-2 in murine studies, but when used alone in cumulative doses up to 1 mg/m^2, little efficacy has been noted in clinical trials [34]. Similarly, in our clinical studies combining doses of up to 300 μg/m^2 TNF administered as a single intravenous dose once a day for three days followed by IL-2 administration, no additional efficacy compared to IL-2 alone has been noted. Toxicity associated with TNF treatment include fever and chills, hypotension, and at the highest doses mild to moderate renal insufficiency. A mild hepatopathy manifested by increases in transaminase levels was noted in our studies.

Gamma interferon has been given as an intravenous, intraperitoneal, or intramuscular treatment regimen [40–42]. Immunologic activity in-

Figure 2. Synergistic effect of interferon and TNF and increasing MHC molecules on cultured tumor lines. Tumor 444 is a cultured renal cell carcinoma which was stained with antibodies to both class I and class II determinants. Markedly enhanced expression of class II molecules was noted with treatment. Interestingly, K562, which expressed neither molecule well prior to treatment, only had class I molecules induced. This ability to modify cell surface determinants may be of importance in biologic therapy. (From E. A. Wiebke et al.: Cytokines alter target cell susceptibility to lysis, I: Evaluation of non-MHC restricted effectors reveals differential effects on natural and lymphokine-activated killing. Submitted for publication.)

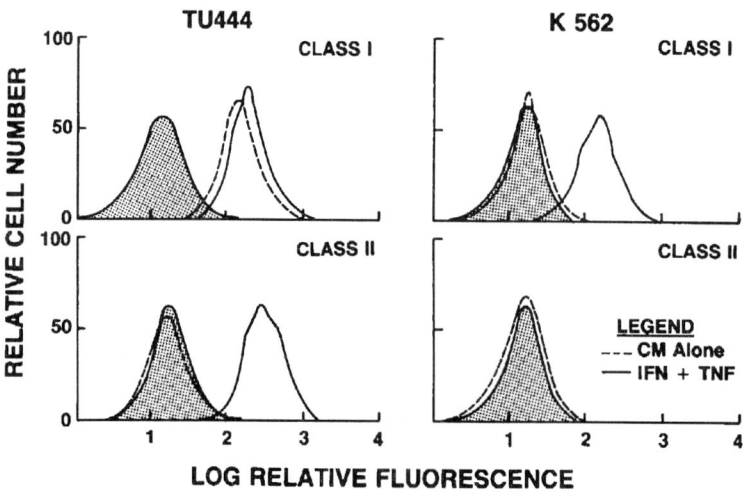

cludes enhanced hydrogen peroxide production by monocytes as well as increased Fc receptor expression. Toxicity has included chills, fever, headache, myalgias, fatigue, nausea, and vomiting. Doses up to 0.25 mg/m^2 intramuscularly and 0.4 mg/m^2 intraperitoneally or intravenously can be tolerated without major toxicity. Little substantive activity has been noted in a variety of different non-hematologic neoplasms. For this reason, combinations of gamma interferon with other agents should be considered given their profound biologic effects. In laboratory studies that we have performed, gamma interferon and tumor necrosis factor are markedly synergistic in upregulating major histocompatibility complex antigens, as is shown in Figure 2. Further, these agents have been very effective in increasing the susceptibility of cultured tumor targets to autologous specific tumor-infiltrating lymphocytes which have been expanded in IL-2. Such combinations alone, with IL-2, or with the adoptive transfer of tumor-infiltrating lymphocytes, are intriguing possibilities.

Interleukin-4

IL-4 was initially identified as a B-cell stimulatory factor which caused proliferation of B-cells following treatment with antibody to immunoglobulin-M as an activation signal [16]. In addition, IL-4 increased the expression of class II molecules on resting B-cells and enhanced the secretion of both IgG1 and IgE. We have been interested in its use as a T-cell growth factor and have been able to demonstrate that IL-4 enhances the growth of tumor specific infiltrating lymphocytes from human melanomas when used with IL-2 from human melanoma [17]. Based on these studies, we have initiated phase I clinical trials of IL-4 alone with plans to combine it with IL-2 in patients with cancer based on this study as well as ones done in mice [18]. Doses of 1 µg/m^2 given daily for up to a week have been well tolerated in three patients.

Colony-Stimulating Factors

The first colony-stimulating factor administered to humans was the granulocyte-macrophage CSF (GM-CSF), which has now been administered in the setting of the neutropenia associated with AIDS, myelodysplastic syndromes, and cancer [23–27]. Patients receiving recombinant GM-CSF after high-dose chemotherapy and autologous bone-marrow transplantation also had accelerated myeloid recovery. In our studies administering up to 100 µg/kg/day of GM-CSF intravenously, no anti-tumor effects were noted, and marked malaise, fever, and dyspnea requiring discontinuance after 12–18 days was noted. Marked increases (Figure 3) in white cell number have been noted. Granulocyte CSF has been administered to patients with urothelial tumors [28]. A dose-dependent increase in neutrophil

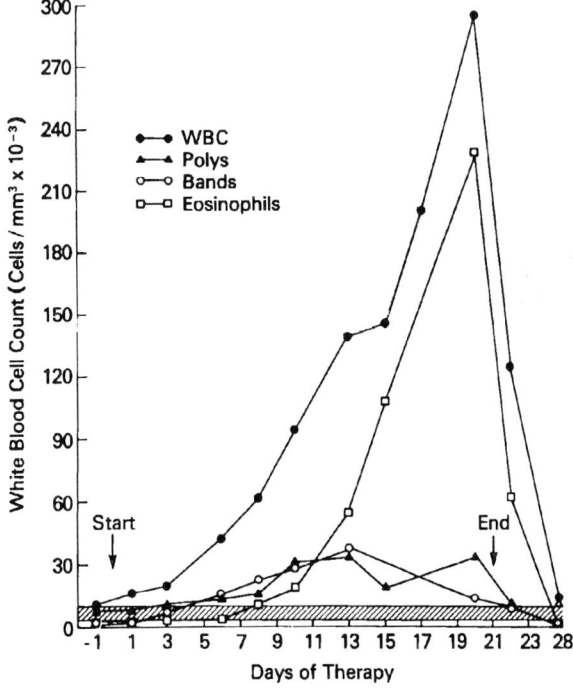

Figure 3. Continuous infusion of recombinant GM-CSF in humans is associated with marked elevations in peripheral white blood cell counts. In this patient, GM-CSF was administered at 30 µg/kg/day with marked increases in the number of white cells which were predominantly eosinophils, but also increased number of mature granulocytes and immature band forms. Following conclusion of treatment, prompt decrease in granulocyte numbers is noted.

counts as well as decreased number of days in which patients had decreased neutrophil counts associated with the administration of chemotherapy was noted. Interestingly, a decrease in the severity and incidence of mucositis as well as in the incidence of febrile neutropenia was noted. Monocyte CSF has not yet been administered to patients, but may have a role in cancer treatment in view of its ability to activate monocytes to mediate tumor killing, as well as in infectious diseases [29, 30].

Future Prospects

Much of our current enthusiasm for the use of lymphokines in therapy was predicted on the early but limited success of recombinant alpha interferon and IL-2 in hematologic malignancies as well as in melanoma and renal cell carcinoma. In addition to their demonstrable clinical utility, these trials have taught us much about the biology of these reagents and has allowed us to ask more penetrating questions regarding their biologic role. The evolution of adoptive immunotherapy using cellular reagents, monoclonal antibodies, and now an increasing list of recombinant cytokines makes the opportunities for impacting on cancer even greater. Substantial attention in the future will be attended to the use of these agents alone and in combination as probes of biologic action as well as therapeutic agents capable of disturbing the homeostatic balance maintained between the host and the tumor.

References

1. Lotze, M. T., and S. A. Rosenberg. 1986. Protocol design for lymphokine testing in clinical studies of human cancer. Lymphokine Research 5: S177–S181.
2. Lotze, M. T., and S. A. Rosenberg. 1988. The immunologic treatment of cancer. CA—A Cancer Journal for Clinicians 38: 68–94.
3. Neta, R., and J. J. Oppenheim. 1988. Why should internists be interested in interleukin-1? Ann. Int. Med. 109: 1–3.
4. Dinarello, C. A. 1988. Biology of interleukin-1. FASEB J. 2: 108–115.
5. Neta, R., M. B. Sztein, J. J. Oppenheim, S. Gillis, and S. D. Douches. 1987. The in vivo effects of interleukin-1. I. Bone marrow cells are induced to cycle after administration of interleukin-1. J. Immunol. 139: 1861–1966.
6. Lotze, M. T., and S. A. Rosenberg. 1988. Interleukin-2 as a pharmalogic reagent. In Interleukin-2, Vol. 1. E. K. Smith, ed. Academic Press, Orlando, FL, p. 237–294.
7. Rosenberg, S. A. 1988. Cancer therapy with interleukin-2: Immunologic manipulations can mediate the regression of cancer in humans. J. Clin. Oncol. 6: 403–406.
8. Rosenberg, S. A., M. T. Lotze, and J. J. Mule. 1988. New approaches to the immunotherapy of cancer using interleukin-2. Ann. Int. Med. 109: 853–864.
9. Denicoff, K. D., D. R. Rubinow, M. Z. Papa, C. Simpson, C. A. Seipp, M. T. Lotze, A. E. Chang, D. Rosenstein, and S. A. Rosenberg. 1987. The neuropsychiatric effects of treatment with interleukin-2 and lymphokine-activated killer cells. Ann. Int. Med. 107: 293–300.
10. Wiebke, E. A., S. A. Rosenberg, and M. T. Lotze. 1988. Acute immunologic effects of interleukin-2 therapy in cancer patients: Decreased delayed type hypersensitivity response and decreased proliferative response to soluble antigens. J. Clin. Oncol. 6: 1440–1449.
11. Cotran, R. S., J. S. Pober, M. A. Gimbrone J., T. A. Springer, E. A. Wiebke, A. A. Gaspari, S. A. Rosenberg, and M. T. Lotze. 1987. Endothelial activation during interleukin-2 immunotherapy. A possible mechanism for the vascular leak syndrome. J. Immunol. 139: 1883–1888.
12. Rosenberg, S. A., M. T. Lotze, L. M. Muul, A. E. Chang, F. P. Avis, S. Leitman, W. M. Linehan, C. N. Robertson, R. E. Lee, J. T. Rubin, C. A. Seipp, C. G. Simpson, and D. E. White. 1987. A progress report on the treatment of 157 patients with advanced cancer using lymphokine-activated killer cells and interleukin-2 or high-dose interleukin-2 alone. N. Engl. J. Med. 316: 889–897.
13. Sosman, J. A., P. C. Kohler, J. Hank, K. H. Moore, R. Bechhofer, B. Storer, and P. M. Sondel. 1988. Repetitive weekly cycles of recombinant human interleukin-2: Responses of renal carcinoma with acceptable toxicity. JNCI 80: 60–63.
14. Donahue, R. E., J. Seehra, M. Metzger, D. Lefebvre, B. Rock, S. Carbone, D. G. Nathan, M. Garnick, P. K. Shegal, D. Laston, E. LaVallie, J. McCoy, Y.-C. Yang, and S. C. Clark. 1988. Human IL-3 and GM-CSF act synergistically in stimulating hematopoiesis in primates. Science 241: 1820–1822.
15. Kimoto, M., V. Kindler, M. Higaki, C. Ody, S. Izui, and P. Vassalli. 1988. Recombinant murine IL-3 fails to stimulate T or B lymphopoiesis in vivo, but enhances immune responses to T cell-dependent antigens. J. Immunol. 140: 1889–1894.
16. Miyajima, A., S. Miyatake, J. Schreurs, J. De Vries, N. Arai, T. Yokota, and K.-I. Arai. 1988.

Coordinate regulation of immune and inflammatory responses by T cell-derived lymphokines. FASEB J. 2: 2462–2473.

17. Kawakami, Y., S. A. Rosenberg, and M. T. Lotze. 1988. Interleukin-4 promotes the growth of tumor-infiltrating lymphocytes cytotoxic for human autologous melanoma. J. Exp. Med. In press.

18. Kern, D. E., D. J. Peace, J. P. Klarnet, M. A. Cheever, and P. D. Greenberg. 1988. IL-4 is an endogenous T cell growth factor during the immune response to a syngeneic retrovirus-induced tumor. J. Immunol. 141: 2824–2830.

19. Harriman, G. R., and W. Strober. 1987. Interleukin-5, a mucosal lymphokine. J. Immunol. 139: 3553–3555.

20. Lopez, A. F., C. J. Sanderson, J. R. Gamble, H. D. Campbell, I. G. Young, and M. A. Vadas. 1988. Recombinant human interleukin-5 is a selective activator of human eosinophil function. J. Exp. Med. 167: 219–224.

21. Jablons, D. M., J. J. Mule, J. K. McIntosh, P. B. Sehgal, L. T. May, C. M. Huang, S. A. Rosenberg, and M. T. Lotze. 1988. Interleukin-6/interferon-2 as a circulating hormone: Induction by cytokine administration in humans. J. Immunol. Submitted.

22. Gauldie, J., C. Richards, D. Harnish, P. Lansdorp, and H. Baumann. 1987. Interferon 2/B-cell stimulatory factor type 2 shares identity with monocyte-derived hepatocyte-stimulating factor and regulates the major acute phase protein response in liver cells. Proc. Natl. Acad. Sci. USA 84: 7251–7254.

23. Groopman, J. E., r. T. Mitsuyasu, M. J. DeLeo, D. H. Oette, and D. W. Golde. 1987. Effect of recombinant human granulocyte- macrophage colony-stimulating factor on myelopoiesis in the acquired immunodeficiency syndrome. N. Engl. J. Med. 317: 593–598.

24. Vadhan-Raj, S., M. Keating, A. LeMaistre, W. N. Hittelman, K. McCredie, J. M. Trujillo, H. E. Broxmeyer, C. Henney, and J. U. Gutterman. 1987. Effects of recombinant human granulocyte-macrophage colony-stimulating factor in patients with myelodysplastic syndromes. N. Engl. J. Med. 317: 1545–1552.

25. Kleinerman, E. S., R. D. Knowles, L. B. Lachman, and J. U. Gutterman. 1988. Effect of recombinant granulocyte/macrophage colony- stimulating factor on human monocyte activity in vitro and following intravenous administration. Cancer Res. 48: 2604–2609.

26. Baldwin, G. C., J. C. Gasson, S. G. Quan, J. Fleischmann, R. Weisbart, D. Oette, R. T. Mitsuyasu, and D. W. Golde. 1988. Granulocyte-macrophage colony-stimulating factor enhances neutrophil function in acquired immunodeficiency syndrome patients. Proc. Natl. Acad. Sci.

USA 85: 2763–2766.

27. Brandt, S. J., Peters, W. P., S. K., Atwater, J. Kurtzberg, M. J. Borowitz, R. B. Jones, E. J. Shpall, R. C. Bast Jr., C. J. Gilbert, and D. H. Oette. 1988. Effect of recombinant human granulocyte-macrophage colony-stimulating factor on hematopoietic reconstitution after high-dose chemotherapy and autologous bone marrow transplantation. N. Engl. J. Med. 318: 869–876.

28. Gabrilove, J. L., A. Jakubowski, H. Scher, C. Sternberg, G. Wong, J. Grous, A. Yagoda, K. Fain, M. A. S. Moore, B. Clarkson, H. F. Oettgen, K. Alton, K. Welte, and L. Souza. 1988. Effect of granulocyte colony-stimulating factor on neutropenia and associated morbidity due to chemotherapy for transitional-cell carcinoma of the urothelium. N. Engl. J. Med. 318: 1414–1422.

29. Broxmeyer, H. E., D. E. Williams. G. Hangoc, S. Cooper, S. Gillis, R. K. Shadduck, and D. C. Bicknell. 1987. Synergistic myelopoietic actions in vivo after administration to mice of combinations of purified natural murine colony-stimulating factor 1, recombinant murine interleukin-3, and recombinant murine granulocyte/macrophage colony-stimulating factor. Proc. Natl. Acad. Sci. USA 84: 3871–3875.

30. Broxmeyer, H. E., D. E. Williams, S. Cooper, A. Waheed, and R. K. Shadduck. 1987. The influence in vivo of murine purified colony- stimulating factor-1 on myeloid progenitor cells in mice recovering from sublethal dosages of cyclophosphamide. Blood 69: 913–918.

31. Beutler, B., and A. Cerami. 1987. Cachectin: More than a tumor necrosis factor. N. Engl. J. Med. 316: 379–385.

32. Asher, A., J. J. Mule, C. M. Reichert, E. Shiloni, and S. A. Rosenberg. 1987. Studies on the antitumor efficacy of systemically administered recombinant tumor necrosis factor against several murine tumors in vivo. J. Immunol. 138: 963–974.

33. McIntosh, J. K., J. J. Mule, M. J. Merino, and S. A. Rosenberg. 1988. Synergistic antitumor effects of immunotherapy with recombinant interleukin-2 and recombinant tumor necrosis factor-α. Cancer Res. 48: 4011–4017.

34. Blick, M., S. A. Sherwin, M. Rosenblum, and J. Gutterman. 1987. Phase I study of recombinant tumor necrosis factor in cancer patients. Cancer Res. 47: 2986–2986.

35. Merigan, T. C. 1988. Human interferon as a therapeutic agent. N. Engl. J. Med. 318: 1458–1460.

36. Gutterman, J. U., S. Fine, J. Quesada, S. J. Horning, J. F. Levine, R. Alexanian, L. Bernhardt, M. Kramer, H. Spiegel, W. Colburn, P. Trown, T. Merigan, and Z. Dziewanowski. 1982. Recombinant leukocyte A interferon: Pharmacokinetics, single-dose tolerance, and biologic effects in

cancer patients. Ann. Int. Med. 96: 549–556.

37. Quesada, J. R., J. Reuben, J. T. Manning, et al. 1984. Alpha interferon for induction of remission in hairy-cell leukemia. N. Engl. J. Med. 310: 15–18.

38. Rinehart, J. J., D. Young, J. Laforge, D. Colborn, and J. A. Neidhart. 1987. Phase I/II trial of interferon beta serine in patients with renal cell carcinoma: Immunological and biological effects. Cancer Res. 47: 2481–2487.

39. Sarna, G., M. Pertcheck, R. Figlin, and B. Ardalan. 1986. Phase I study of recombinant beta ser 17 interferon in the treatment of cancer. Cancer Treat. Rep. 70: 1365–1372.

40. Maluish, A. E., W. J. Urba, D. L. Longo, W. R. Overton, D. Coggin, E. R. Crisp, R. Williams, S. A. Sherwin, K. Gordon, and R. G. Steis. 1988. The determination of an immunologically active dose of interferon-gamma in patients with melanoma. J. Clin. Oncol. 6: 434–445.

41. D'Acquisto, R., M. Markman, T. Hakes, S. Rubin, W. Hoskins, and J. L. Lewis Jr. 1988. A phase I trial of intraperitoneal recombinant gamma-interferon in advanced ovarian carcinoma. J. Clin. Oncol. 6: 689–695.

42. Goldstein, D., J. Gockerman, R. Krishnan, J. Ritchie Jr., C. Y. Tso, L. E. Hood, E. Ellinwood, and J. Laszlo. 1987. Effects of gamma interferon on the endocrine system: Results from a phase I study. Cancer Res. 47: 6397–6401.

43. Eschbach, J. W., J. C. Egrie, M. R. Downing, et al. 1987. Correction of the anemia of end-stage renal disease with recombinant human erythropoietin: Results of a combined phase I and II clinical trial. N. Engl. J. Med. 316: 73–78.

44. Topalian, S. L., D. Soloman, F. P. Avis, A. E. Chang, D. L. Freerksen, W. M. Linehan, M. T. Lotze, C. N. Robertson, C. A. Seipp, P. Simon, C. G. Simpson, and S. A. Rosenberg. 1988. Immunotherapy of patients with advanced cancer using tumor-infiltrating lymphocytes and recombinant interleukin-2: A pilot study. J. Clin. Oncol. 6: 839–853.

Therapeutic/Prophylactic Effects of Thymopentin with Respect to Its Mechanisms of Action

*Kalman Bolla**

The influence of thymopentin on various target cell populations is discussed as the main aspect of its mechanisms of action. Experimental and clinical observations are presented and reviewed which suggest that the immunomodulatory, immune-reconstructive and antiinflammatory effects are three independent characteristics of this pentapeptide. The simultaneous activation of various mature T-cells is shown as a basic mechanism of immunomodulation. For better predictability of the functional effects, it is proposed to distinguish between silent, preventive, and regulative forms of immunomodulation. The influence of thymopentin on immature or deficient T-cells and on monocytes/macrophages is suggested as an explanation for its immune-reconstructive and antiinflammatory effects, respectively. Finally, experiments are reported which support the general statement that therapeutic approaches able to modify the functional stage and/or proportion of the target cells may result in interactions with any immunomodulator.

Thymopentin is the synthetic pentapeptide segment 32–36 of the thymic hormone thymopoietin [1–2]. The natural hormone and/or thymopentin have been shown to be able to influence the maturation and/or function of various cell types. Thus, they can induce differentiation of prothymocytes by increasing the intracellular cyclic AMP [2–4], accelerating the differentiation of immature granulocytes [5], and either inhibiting or stimulating the induction of surface antigens characteristic for B cell lines [2, 6]. Changes in the function of various T-cells [7–9] monocytes/macrophages [10–12] and neutrophils [10] have also been reported in the presence of thymopentin or after treatment with this pentapeptide. Together with reports on the variability of effects on the target cells, several observations have been published on promising clinical results with thymopentin treatment in a wide range of indications: primary immunodeficiencies [13], frequently recurring herpes infection [14–15], therapy-resistant leprosy [16], condyloma [17], and *Trichophyton rubrum* infection [18] as well as rheumatoid arthritis [19, 20], atopic dermatitis [21], chronic inflammatory processes [22], prevention of infections in elderly [23], etc.

In order to elaborate rational therapeutic approaches with thymopentin, it seemed necessary to reduce the events to be considered. In this sense, the immunomodulatory, immunoreconstructive, and the antiinflammatory effects of thymopentin have been identified and investigated in some detail.

Immunomodulation with Thymopentin

The term *immunomodulation* is used in the literature without a generally accepted definition. Based on targeted experiments and theoretical considerations [24, 25], we interpret it as a common name for those biological processes that can temporarily increase the functional capacity of one or more immune competent cell populations. As long as the functions of such cells are not triggered by an appropriate stimulus, the increase in the functional capacity remains physiologically silent. The possible increase in the functional capacity of a cell population necessarily depends on the availability of the cells involved. Since it can be different in a resting or reacting immune system, we proposed to use the terms preventive and regulative immunomodulation, respectively [24].

In the case of thymopentin, the simultaneous activation of different T-cells has been shown (in vitro and in vivo) as a potential basic mech-

* CILAG International Research Center, Hochstr. 201/209, CH-8201 Schaffhausen, Switzerland.
Acknowledgements: The author thanks Dr. R. Cappel (Inst. Pasteur, Bruxelles), Prof. J. Duchateau (Hop. Univ. Saint-Pierre, Bruxelles), Dr. E. Faist (Ludwig-Maximilians-Univ., München), Prof. W. Glinz and P. Grob (Universitätsspital, Zürich), Dr. T. Michalak (Memorial Univ. Newfoundland), and Prof. W. Mohr (Universität Ulm) for their contribution.

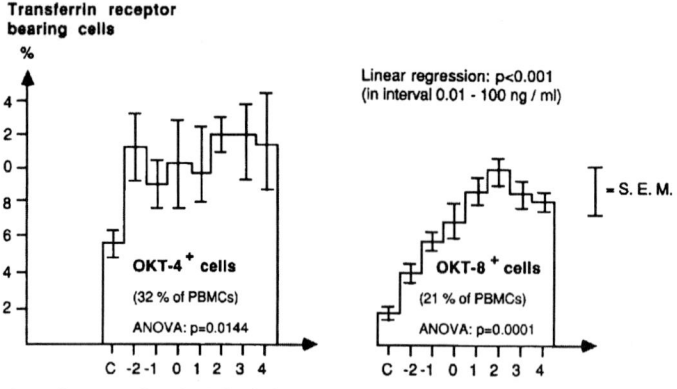

Figure 1. Effect of thymopentin on the induction of transferrin receptor-bearing cells in various populations of peripheral blood mononuclear cells (PBMCs) of healthy blood donors; n = 8 [25].

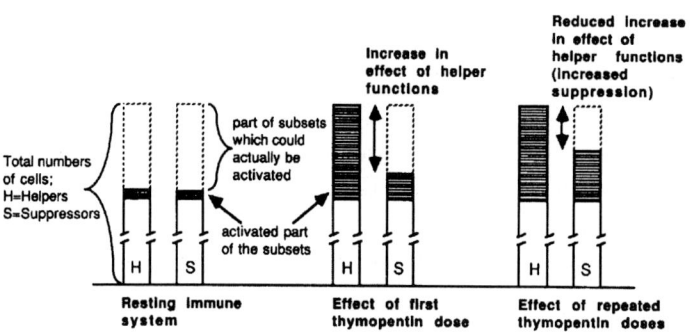

Figure 2. Simplified model for explanation of the effect of repeated doses of thymopentin on helper and suppressor functions [26].

anism of immunomodulation [25]. In the in vitro part of this study, the increase in the percentage of transferrin-receptor-bearing cells was used as a marker for activation. Thymopentin simultaneously—but to a different degree—activated the OKT-4 and OKT-8 positive cells. While the lowest concentration of thymopentin already induced maximal activation in the OKT-4 positive cell population, a concentration-dependent increase was observed in the OKT-8 positive cell population (Figure 1).

The thymopentin-induced increase in the functional capacity of various T-cell populations was also demonstrated in the in vivo experiments [25]. In addition, the results of these experiments strongly suggest that the duration of the activated stage is different in the various cell types. This possibility may be important with regard to the frequency of drug application.

The simultaneous but quantitatively different activation of various T-cells may explain some characteristic aspects of thymopentin's immunomodulatory effects. The different affinity of the various cell types to thymopentin would explain the influence of dose, while the presence of cell types that can be activated at all and their actual proportions would reflect the crucial importance of the immune status of the subject treated. Assuming that only a certain percentage of cells in a subset can be in an activated state, subsets containing activated cells would either entirely or partially escape additional activation. In this case, a simplified model (Figure 2) which takes into account only the activation of T helper and suppressor cells could explain why, for instance, the primary antibody response is stimulated by a single dose of thymopentin rather than by multiple doses [24]; after maximal activation of the helper subset, thymopentin can activate only other cell types, i.e., suppressor cells in this case. Consequently, repeated daily doses of thymopentin will result in reduced stimulation or even inhibition of the immune response. Similar reasoning can hold true for the difference observed in the immune response when

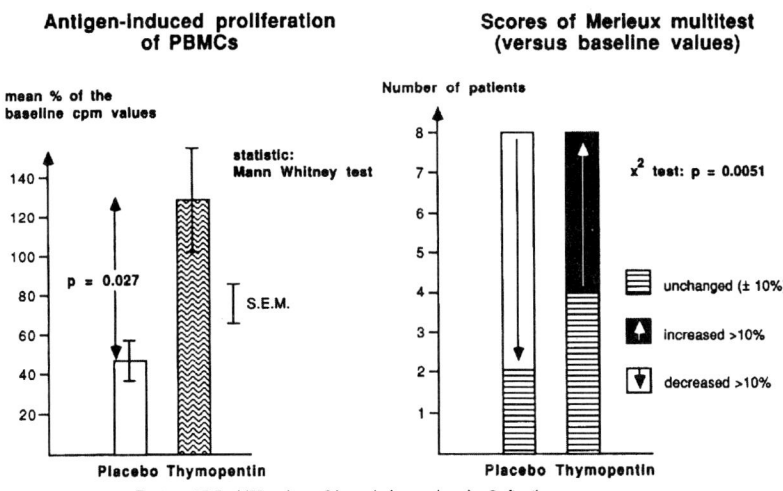

Antigen-induced proliferation of PBMCs

mean % of the baseline cpm values

Scores of Merieux multitest (versus baseline values)

Number of patients

statistic: Mann Whitney test

p = 0.027

S.E.M.

x^2 test: p = 0.0051

unchanged (± 10%)

increased >10%

decreased >10%

Placebo Thymopentin

Placebo Thymopentin

Treatment 0.5 ml (50 mg) s. c. 2 hours before and on day 2 after the surgery

Figure 3. Changes in immune parameters in surgical patients. Assessments before and seven days after the surgery. Treatment either with 0.5 ml placebo or thymopentin (50 mg) s. c. 2 hours before and on day 2 after heart surgery; n = 8/group [26].

identical single doses of thymopentin were administered either before or after the HSV-2 infection [24]. In this case, the pretreatment would induce higher activation in the helper than in the suppressor cell populations at the time of infection, thus stimulating the immune response. On the other hand, when thymopentin was administered just after the infection, only the suppressor and not the helper cells, which are already involved in the ongoing immune response, can additionally be activated.

The Effects of Thymopentin on Temporary Immune Depression

Considering observations showing that appropriate treatment with thymopentin can increase the functional capacity of the helper mechanism, transitory immune depression, i.e., prevention of opportunistic infections in such situations, represents a potential indication for immunomodulatory therapy with this drug. To assess this possibility, a series of experiments and clinical studies were performed [26].

In the first step, a mice model was established. After infection with LD-10 of herpes simplex virus (HSV-2), immune depression with a duration of about 2 weeks can be demonstrated. One week after the challenge with HSV-2, the mice were infected with 10^4 TCID-50 of Coxsackie virus (CV). This dose cannot induce any mortality in healthy mice, but resulted in a mortality rate of over 90% in the immune-depressed animals. A single dose of thymopentin given on day 4 after the infection with HSV-2 strongly reduced the grade of HSV-2-induced immune depression and the sensitivity of the mice against the secondary (CV) infection (mortality rate: 45%, p < 0.001).

In subsequent clinicopharmacological studies we were able to demonstrate that temporary immune depression following surgical trauma can also be prevented with thymopentin [27, 28]. For monitoring the immune-depression antigen-induced proliferation of peripheral blood, mononuclear cells (PBMCs) and the Mérieux multitest were used. Thymopentin 50 mg given s.c. two hours before the surgery and on the second postoperative day corrected both parameters by the end of the first postoperative week (Figure 3).

Correction of immune parameters in surgical patients does not necessarily result in the prevention of opportunistic infections. The first evidence suggesting this potential benefit has been gathered in cooperation with Zurich University (W. Glinz and P. Grob). Patients with severe polytrauma (injury severity score -ISS-

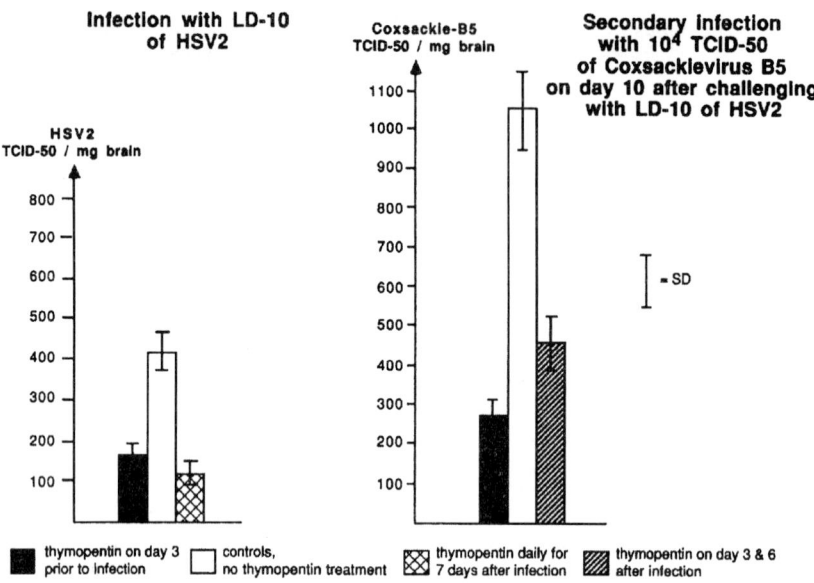

Figure 4. Effect of thymopentin (100 ng/kg, i. p.) on virus spreading in mice (n = 6/group) assessed on day 7 after infection (collaboration with R. Cappel).

over 16) were enrolled into an open (partly randomized) clinical study. In the first part of the study, the patients were treated with a single dose of thymopentin 50 mg s.c. either on the day of the trauma or on one of the subsequent days up to day 4. The randomly selected controls were not treated with thymopentin. After entering 18 patients into this study, we had the impression [26] that the first injection should be given as early as possible and at least a second dose should also be administered. Based on this impression and on the observations gathered in the animal experiments, days 1 and 4 were selected for thymopentin treatment. This treatment regimen has been applied in 29 such patients up till now, and only five of them developed opportunistic infections. These observations require confirmation in a double-blind setting; nevertheless, this low infection rate suggests the therapeutic application of thymopentin-induced immunomodulation in this indication. This suggestion is also supported by the fact that the overall infection rate in such polytraumatized patients is around 50% in this department [29], and this figure was even higher in the control group during the current study period.

The Effects of Thymopentin on Acute/Subacute Viral Infections

Enhancing of the functional capacity of the helper mechanisms may provide a rationale for immunomodulatory therapy in acute infections. The beneficial effects of thymopentin in experimental HSV-2 infection, especially its preventive effect in lethal infections [24, 30] and its influence on interferon response [31], pointed to investigating the virus spreading/elimination in animals treated with thymopentin.

In a series of experiments, mice were infected with LD-10 of HSV-2 and treated with either 100 ng or 1 mg/kg dose/s of thymopentin. Six-six mice per group were sacrificed on different days after the infection, and virus titration was performed from brain tissue in each. In a second series, mice infected with LD-10 of HSV-2 were challenged with 10^4 TCID-50 of Coxsackie virus (CV) ten days after the infection with HSV-2. In this experiment, thymopentin was administered either on day 3 before or on days 3 and 6 after the secondary infection. Again 6-6 mice per group were sacrificed on different days, but only after the secondary infection. The Coxsackie titer was assessed in brain tissue. The results are shown in

Figure 4. The thymopentin treatment significantly reduced the titer of both viruses (collaboration with R. Cappel).

Since the inhibitory effect of thymopentin on the virus spreading is not virus-specific (observed in DNA and RNA virus infection), a therapeutic trial was set up for checking this effect in a hepatitis B virus infection model. Seventeen woodchucks were infected with woodchuck hepatitis virus (WHV) and after randomization treated daily either with thymopentin 1 mg/kg or placebo s.c. After the infection, blood was taken from the animals at weekly intervals for assessing the WH_sAg titer in the serum. The treatment started after the first positive value had been achieved, and continued until two subsequent samples were negative for this parameter. In addition to the serological assessments, histological evaluation was performed. Thymopentin treatment significantly improved the serological parameters (Figure 5), and according to the preliminary evaluation also reduced the severity of the histological alterations (collaboration with T. Michalak).

Both indication fields discussed above represent substantial potential for the clinical use of thymopentin, though further studies are necessary for elaboration of optimized treatment regimens. This statement is particularly valid for therapeutic objectives which aim at increasing the functional capacity of suppressor mechanisms.

Immune reconstruction with Thymopentin

The influence of thymopentin on the activation of mature T-cells cannot explain clinical findings such as the long-lasting beneficial effect of thymopentin on patients with frequently relapsing HSV infection [14, 15]. Since the duration of thymopentin-induced activation of mature T-cells is not that long, it can be anticipated that additional mechanisms are also influenced.

A defect of cellular immunity has been considered as one of the most important factors in the pathophysiology of frequently recurring herpes simplex infections [32]. Considering the role of thymic hormones in T-cell differentiation, *an immunoreconstructive effect of thymopentin* would represent a possible explanation for the long-lasting effect observed in our patients. Newly matured T-cells, or completion of the functional maturation of morphologically mature T-cells, would maintain the beneficial therapeutic effect as long as these cells survive.

Thymopentin has been shown to induce T-cell maturation in vitro [2, 33, 34] as well as in vivo [2]. Thymopentin has also been reported to be able to improve or even correct age-related or thymectomy-induced immune deficiencies [35, 36]. A long-lasting corrective effect was also observed in the cellular immunity of elderly volunteers after thymopentin treatment for one month when it was administered as in our study, i.e., 50 mg s.c. thrice a week [23]. In that setting, the long-lasting therapeutic outcome of the immune reconstruction was reflected by the significantly reduced number of upper respiratory tract infections.

To explore whether immunomodulation and immunoreconstruction could concomitantly be induced by thymopentin, we compared the drug's effect on the primary complement-de-

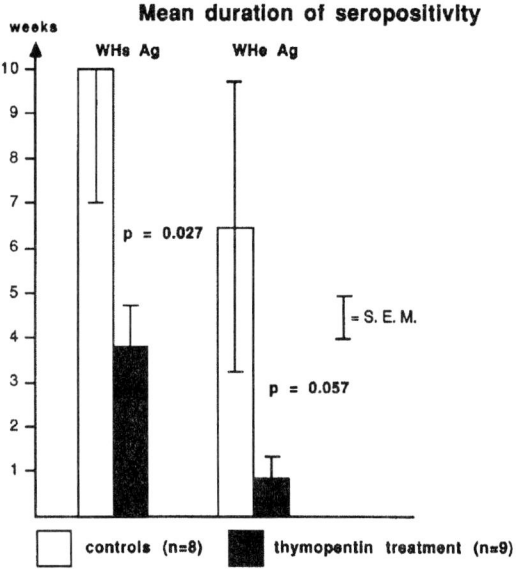

Figure 5. Serological observations after daily treatment with thymopentin (1 mg/kg, s. c.) or placebo in woodchuck hepatitis (collaboration with T. Michalak).

541

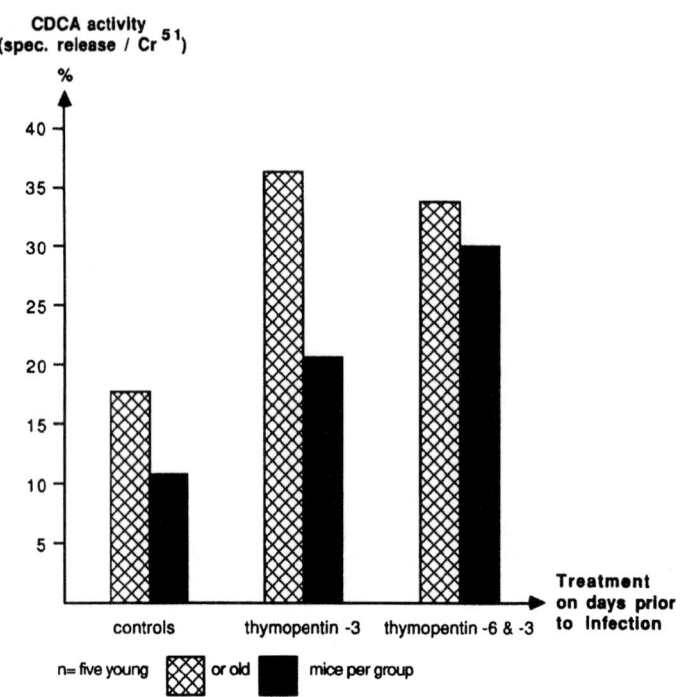

CDCA activity
(spec. release / Cr^{51})
%

Figure 6. Effect of thymopentin (100 ng/kg, i. p.) on primary complement dependent cytotoxic antibody (CDCA) response in young and old mice infected with LD-10 of HSV 2. Assessment from pooled sera of 5 mice per group on day 7 after the infection (collaboration with R. Cappel).

pendent cytotoxic antibody (CDCA) response of old (>12 months) and young (6-week-old) mice infected with LD-10 of HSV-2. The result of this explorative experiment (collaboration with R. Cappel) is summarized in Figure 6. As expected, the CDCA response in the old controls was weaker than in the young ones. When treated with thymopentin 3 days prior to infection, both groups experienced antibody response enhancement by about 100%. However, if the mice received thymopentin on days 6 and 3 prior to viral inoculation, only the group of old mice showed further increase in this antibody response. We may assume that the first injection of thymopentin (on day −6) not only activated the mature T-cells, but also increased the availability of these cells for further activation in the immunodeficient old mice. Both maturation of additional helper cells and correction of a possible functional defect in the mature T-cells could result in such increased availability. These mechanisms could probably not be triggered in healthy young mice.

The different target cell populations and the difference in the duration of the functional effects strongly suggest that *immunomodulation and immunoreconstruction are two substantially*

different effects of thymopentin. The primary targets of the first are mature T-cells, while immature or functionally deficient T-cells could represent the substrate for the second effect.

Both immunoreconstruction and immunomodulation may result in modified immune responses. Nevertheless, it seems reasonable to distinguish between these two processes at least as a working hypothesis. Considering immune reconstruction as a separate entity investigation into this field could offer a new approach for clinical management of various chronic diseases.

Thymopentin's Antiinflammatory Effect

Rheumatoid arthritis was one of the first clinical indications in which thymopentin was investigated. Regarding this indication, promising clinical results which have been proved also in double-blind settings [20, 37] were first reported after its administration in form of short i.v. infusion. This treatment regimen was proposed after a clinicopharmacological study showed that s.c. treatment with thymopentin

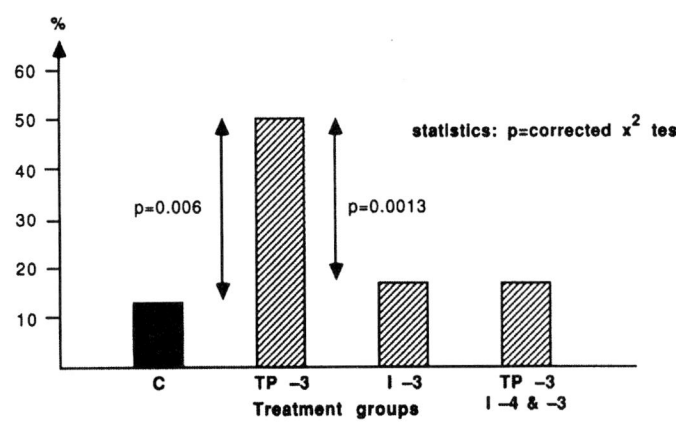

Figure 7. Interaction between thymopentin and indomethacin. Surviving rate registered in groups of 30 mice treated i. p. with thymopentin (100 ng/kg) and/or indomethacin (1 mg/kg) before infection with LD-90 of HSV 2 (collaboration with R. Cappel).

C = infected controls without treatment
TP = thymopentin treatment on day "x" related to the infection
I = indomethacin treatment on day/days "x" related to the infection

stimulated the antibody response, while i.v. dosing inhibited it [38]. Unfortunately, concomitant therapy with fixed dose of NSAID and/or a low dose of steroids was allowed in all the clinical studies performed in this indication.

Putting the target cells and their reactions into the focus of a rational therapeutic approach with immune modulatory/reconstructive drugs led us to reanalyze the results gathered in rheumatoid arthritis patients. According to this concept, interaction can be expected between an immunomodulator and whatever therapeutic approach that may influence the proportion and/or function of the target cells.

Thymopentin has been shown to modulate the pokeweed mitogen (PWM)-induced IgG production in peripheral blood mononuclear cell (PBMCs) cultures [39]. In this model 3 ×10^7 mol indomethacin completely abolished the concentration-dependent modulatory ef-

Figure 8. Influence of daily treatment either with thymopentin (2 mg/kg, s. c.) or indomethacin (1 mg/kg, s. c.) on the progression of adjuvant arthritis in rats (collaboration with W. Mohr).

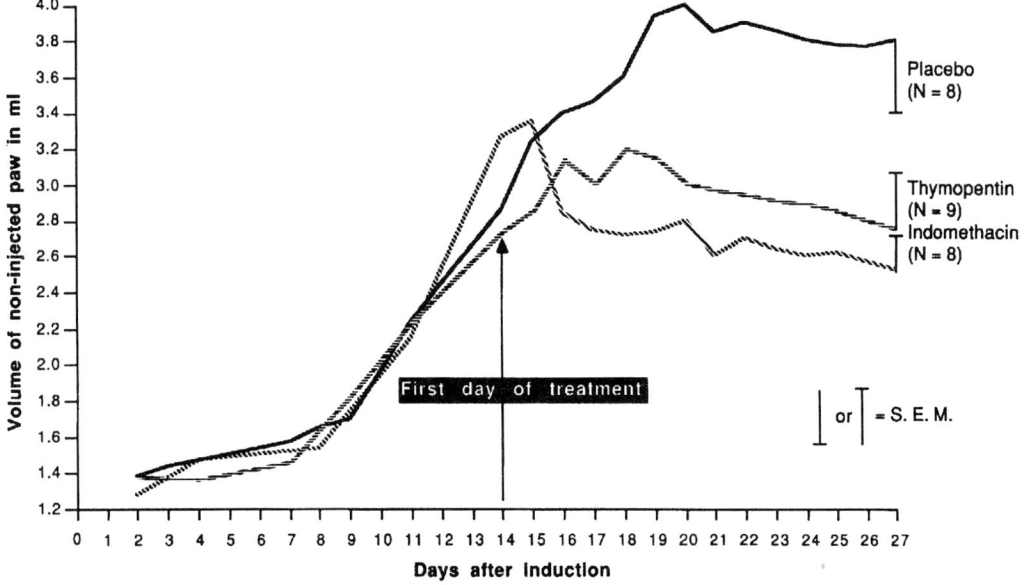

fect of thymopentin [12]. An interaction could also be observed in vivo when HSV-2-infected mice were treated with thymopentin and indomethacin (Figure 7). In this experiment, indomethacin abolished the preventive effect of thymopentin which had been demonstrated in the animals infected with LD-90 of HSV-2 (collaboration with R. Cappel).

In view of the interaction between thymopentin and indomethacin, the immunomodulatory effect of the pentapeptide seemed insufficient to explain its beneficial effect in rheumatoid arthritis. Since first of all inflammatory parameters were significantly improved with thymopentin treatment, we postulated that this substance also possesses an antiinflammatory effect. This assumption was also supported by observations showing that thymopentin can influence the function of monocytes/macrophages and neutrophils [10–12], and ensure a significant improvement in patients with gonarthrosis and tendovaginitis after local application [22]. Experiments on adjuvant arthritis models (collaboration with W. Mohr) have provided further evidence for this hypothesis. Figure 8 shows that daily treatment with thymopentin or indomethacin ensured similar effects in this model. Both treated groups showed significant improvement compared to the controls.

Retrospectively, the beneficial effect of thymopentin in rheumatoid arthritis may be due to its antiinflammatory effect rather than the immunomodulatory one. The antiinflammatory effect of thymopentin and the possible

interaction with other NSAIDs would indicate its use as monotherapy in this indication. The real potential of thymopentin in the therapy of rheumatoid arthritis can only be judged after such clinical trials.

Conclusion

As a contribution to the elaboration of rational therapeutic approaches with thymopentin, its target cells and the consequences of their reactions were put into the focus of consideration. Thymopentin simultaneously, but to a different degree, influences various cell types. Its clinical effect is always the net result of interactions between the various cell types in-

volved. The availability of the target cells for thymopentin can be different in various diseases and could be modified by concomitant therapy as well. Both the reactions of the different target cells and their availability have to be considered when elaborating specific treatment regimens with thymopentin.

References

1. Schlesinger, D. H. and G. Goldstein. 1975. The amino acid sequence of thymopoietin II. Cell 5: 361.
2. Goldstein, G., M. P. Scheid, E. A. Boyse, D. H. Schlesinger and J. Van Wauwe. 1979. A synthetic pentapeptide with biological activity characteristic of the thymic hormone thymopoietin. Science 204: 1309.
3. Scheid, M. P., G. Goldstein, and E. A. Boyse. 1978. The generation and regulation of lymphocyte populations. Evidence from differentiative induction system in vitro. J. exp. Med. 147: 1727.
4. Audhya, T. K., M. P. Scheid, and G. Goldstein. 1984. Contrasting biological activities of thymopoietin and splenin, two closely related polypeptide products of thymus and spleen. Proc. Natl. Acad. Sci. USA 81: 2847.
5. Kagan, W. A., G. J. O'Neill, G. Goldstein, and R. A. Good. 1977. Induction of human granulocyte differentiation in vitro by ubiquitin and thymopoietin. Blood 50: 275.
6. Abbott, J., and K. Ngiam. 1981. Sequential expression of B lymphocytes surface antigens in vitro. Eur. J. Immunol. 11: 411.
7. Sunshine, G. H., R. S. Basch, R. G. Coffey, K. W. Kohen, G. Goldstein, and J. Hadden. 1978. Thymopoietin enhances the allogenic response and cyclic GMP levels of mouse peripheral, thymus-derived lymphocytes. J. Immunol. 120: 1594.
8. Audhya, T., G. A. Heavner, D. J. Kroon, and G. Goldstein. 1984. Regulatory Peptides 9: 155.
9. Heavner, G. A., T. Audhya, D. Kroon, and G. Goldstein. 1985. Structural requirements for the biological activity of thymopentin analogs. Arch. Biochem. Biophys. 242: 248.
10. Waymack, J. P., S. J. Gonce, P. Miskell, and J. W. Alexander. 1985. Mechanisms of action of two new immunomodulators. Arch. Surg. 120: 43.
11. Waymack, J. P., J. Metz, D. Garnet, H. Sax, and J. W. Alexander. 1985. Effect of immunomodulators on macrophage function in burned animals. Surg. Forum 36: 10.
12. Duchateau, J., and K. Bolla. 1988. Immunomodulation with thymopentin. In vitro studies. Oncology, in press.
13. Aiuti, F., L. Businco, M. Fiorilli, E. Galli, I. Quinti, S. Le Moli, R. Seminara, and G.

Goldstein. 1983. Birth defects: Original Article Series 19: 267.

14. Bolla, K., D. Djawari, E. M. Kokoschka, J. Petres, S. Liden, R., Gonseth, P. Amblard, M. G. Bernengo, J. J. Bonerandi, A. Claudy, H. Degreef, J. DeMaubeuge, J. Meynadier, J. H. Seurat, E. Schöpf, W. Höbel, and E. Sundal. 1985. Prevention of recurrences in frequently relapsing herpes labialils with thympoentin. A randomized double-blind placebo-controlled multicenter study. Surv. Immunol. Res. 4(1): 37.

15. Bolla, K., J. DeMaubeuge, S. Liden, J. Bonerandi, and E. Sundal. 1988. Treatment of genital herpes simplex infections with thymopentin. A double-blind placebo-controlled study. Int. J. Immunotherapy, in press.

16. Castells, A., J. Terencio, A. Ramirez, E. Sundal, and K. Bolla. 1985. Thymopentin treatment in patients with chemotherapy-resistant lepromatous leprosy. Surv. Immunol Res. 4(1): 63.

17. Fransen, L., J. Anthoons, G. Hoogewijs, and K. Bolla. 1988. Thymopentin treatment in genital warts of long duration. Cancer Detection and Prevention, in press.

18. Molin, L., and K. Bolla. 1985. Thymopentin in chronic Trichophyton rubrum infection. Surv. Immunol. Res. 4(1): 135.

19. Franchimont, P., C. Hauwert, and K. Bolla. 1985. Thymopentin in active chronic rheumatoid arthritis. An open, monitored study in 16 patients. Surv. Immunol. Res. 4(1): 81.

20. Malaise, M. G., C. Hauwert, P. Franchimont, B. Danneskiold-Samsoe, R. Bach-Andersen, D. Gross, H. Gerber, H. Gerschpacher, H. Stocker, and K. Bolla. 1985. Treatment of active rheumatoid arthritis with slow intravenous injections of thymopentin. Lancet 832.

21. Kang, K., K. D. Cooper, and J. M. Hanifin. 1983. Thymopoietin pentapeptide (TP-5) improves clinical parameters in lymphocyte subpopulation abnormalities in atopic dermatitis. J. Am. Acad. Dermatol. 8: 372.

22. Pipino, F., and D. Vittore. 1988. Experience with thymopentin in the treatment of periarthritis humeroscapularis, tendinitis and gonarthrosis by local infiltration. Arzneim.-Forsch. 38: 116.

23. Di Perri, T., and Gruppo Italiano di Studio sugli Ormoni Timici. 1987. Efficacia e tollerabilita della Timopentina in pazienti a rischio di infezioni. Recenti Progressi in Medicina 78: 1.

24. Bolla, K., J. Duchateau, and R. Cappel. 1987. Strategical aspects of immunomodulation based on the influence of thymopentin on immune responses. In Immune Regulation by Characterized Polypeptides. G. Goldstein, J. F. Bach, and H. Wigzkell, eds. New York: Alan R. Liss, Inc., p. 61.

25. Bolla, K., R. Cappel, and J. Duchateau. 1987. Activation of peripheral blood lymphocytes as a potential basic mechanism of immunomodulation. Int. J. Immunotherapy III: 71.

26. Bolla, K., R. Cappel, J. Duchateau, and E. Faist. 1988. Immunomodulation as a potential therapeutic approach in immunodeficiencies. In Immune Consequences of Trauma, Shock and Sepsis. E. Faist, ed. Springer-Verlag, Heidelberg, in press.

27. Faist, E., A. Riedel, and K. Bolla. 1987. Influence of thymopentin on postsurgical immune deficiency: A clinical pilot study. Int. J. Pharm. Res. VII: 83.

28. Faist, E., W. Ertzel, B., Salmen, A. Weiler, C. Ressel, K. Bolla, and G. Hebera. 1988. The immune enhancing effect of perioperative thymopentin administration in elderly patients undergoing major surgery. Arch. Surg., in press.

29. Grob, P., M. Holch, W. Fierz, W. Glinz, and S. Geroulanos. 1988. Pediatr. Infect. Dis. J. 7: 37.

30. Cappel, R., F. DeCuyper, K. DeNeef, W. Höbel, and K. Bolla. 1985. Effect of thympopentin on the mortality and immune response after an experimental herpes simplex infection in mice. Surv. Immunol. Res. 4(1): 48.

31. Cappel, R., K. DeNef, F. DeCuyper, and K. Bolla. 1987. Effect of thymopentin treatment and HSV 2 infection on the interferon production in BALB/c mice. In Immune Regulation by Characterized Polypeptides. G. Goldstein, J. F. Bach, and H. Wigzell, eds. New York: Alan R. Liss, Inc., p. 75.

32. Liden, S. 1985. Herpes simplex. Clinical and pathogenic aspects. Surv. Immunol. Res. 4(1): 24.

33. Verhaegen, H., W. DeCock, J. De Cree, and G. Goldstein. 1980. Comparison of the in vitro effects of thymopoietin pentapeptide and levamisole on peripheral E-rosette forming cells. Thymus 1: 195.

34. Nash, L., R. Good, A. Hatzfeld, G. Goldstein, and G. Incefy. 1981. In vitro differentiation of two surface markers for immature T cells by the synthetic pentapeptide, thymopoietin 32-36. J. Immunology 126: 150.

35. Weksler, M. E., J. B. Innes, and G. Goldstein. 1978. Immunological studies of aging IV. The contribution of thymic involution to the immune deficiencies of aging mice and reversal with thymopoietin 32-36. J. exp. Med. 148: 996.

36. Goldberg, E. H., G. Goldstein, E. A. Boyse, and M. P. Scheid. 1981. Effect of the TP-5 analogue of thymopoietin on the rejection of male skin by aged and thymectomized female mice. Immunogenetics 13: 201.

37. Lemmel, E. M., G. L. Bach, W. Bolten, D. Brackers, Z. Fahmy, H. Mattern, I. Stroehmann, and A. Wittenborg. 1988. Immunomodulierende Therapei der chronischen Polyarthritis mit Thymopentin. Dtsch. med. Wschr. 113: 172.

38. Duchateau, J., G. Delespesse, and K. Bolla. 1983. Phase variation in the modulation of the human immune response. Immunol. Today 4: 213.

39. Duchateau, J., H. Collet, and K. Bolla. 1987. Influence of thymopentin on candidin-induced proliferation and PWM-induced IgG production of human lymphocytes. In Immune Regulation by Characterized Polypeptides. G. Goldstein, J. F. Bach, and H. Wigzell, eds. New York: Alan R. Liss, Inc., p. 83.

Immunopathogenic Mechanisms of HIV Infection: Studies on the Induction of Virus Expression

*Anthony S. Fauci**

The slow progression of disease after initial infection with the human immunodeficiency virus (HIV) in the vast majority of affected individuals suggests that a latent, or low level, chronic infection occurs in vivo. We have established an in vitro model system for the study of latent or chronic infections with HIV and have used this system to delineate the possible mechanisms involved in the switch from restricted virus replication to high levels of virus production. In this regard, we have shown that specific cytokines can upregulate the expression of HIV from chronically infected cell lines, and that induction of HIV expression occurs via activation of the HIV promotor.

Much has been learned about the interaction between the human immunodeficiency virus (HIV) and host cells since the acquired immunodeficiency syndrome (AIDS) was first recognized in 1981. The two major cellular targets for HIV are T4 lymphocytes and cells of monocyte/macrophage origin, including dendritic cells, Langerhans cells, and astroglial cells (reviewed in [1]). These cells have in common the presence of the CD4 molecule on their surface. The CD4 molecule has been shown to be a high affinity receptor for the HIV envelope glycoprotein (gp120) [2, 3].

Infection with HIV in vivo results in a spectrum of clinical manifestations, ranging from asymptomatic disease to full-blown AIDS. During the asymptomatic phase, T4 cell numbers are normal; however, over time, T4 cell numbers begin to decline, ultimately resulting in immunosuppression and opportunistic diseases [4]. Since progression of disease occurs over an extended, variable period of time, it is postulated that HIV remains in a latent —integration without virus expression—or low-level, chronically expressed state until the virus is activated. Once activation occurs, viral replication and T4 cell death follow, resulting in the spread of infection to other cells.

Latent or Low-Level Chronic HIV Infection

HIV is rapidly cytolytic for T4 cells in vitro [5], with cell death likely occurring as a result of a massive explosion of virions from the cell surface [6]. However, certain cells survive that do not produce virus, but virus expression can be induced following exposure of infected cells to activating agents [7]. HIV has also been shown to infect cells of the monocyte/macrophage lineage in vitro [8–11]. In contrast to the rapid cytopathic effect of HIV on T4 cells, HIV-infected monocyte/macrophages are not readily killed by the virus. Consistent with this finding is the observation that, in monocyte/macrophages, HIV is produced predominantly intracellularly within cytoplasmic vesicles [12]. Thus, the fatal explosion of virus from the surface of T4 cells apparently does not occur in monocyte/macrophages.

Non-cytopathic infection of cells in vitro by HIV has also been recently demonstrated in human bone marrow cells [13]. By using a positive selection cell fractionation technique, pure myeloid progenitor cells were obtained and directly infected with HIV. From electron microscopic analysis of the infected bone marrow cultures, it was evident that HIV was replicating intracellularly. In fact, in some cells, entire areas of the cytoplasm were replaced with mature virions. The cell type in the bone marrow that became infected were progenitor cells of monocyte lineage. Like the mature monocyte/macrophage, progenitor bone marrow cells are apparently resistant to HIV-induced cytopathic effects and thus may function as reservoirs of HIV in the infected individual.

Regulation of HIV Expression

There are several unique features of HIV that allow it to regulate its own replication. Like

* National Institute of Allergy and Infectious Diseases, National Institutes of Health, Bethesda, MD 20892

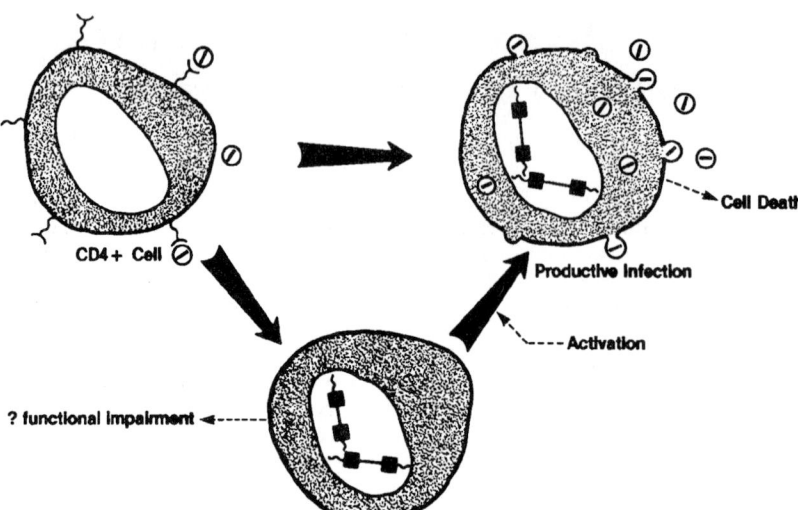

Figure 1. HIV Infection of CD4+ Lymphocytes. Infection of target cells by HIV can result in direct virus production and cell death. Alternatively, the HIV provirus can remain in a latent state, with little or no virus production. Activation signals can transform a latent or chronic infection into a productive one.

other retroviruses, the HIV genome consists of RNA sequences that code for the core proteins (*gag*), the envelope proteins (*env*), and the reverse transcriptase and integrase (*pol*) [14]. However, the genetic structure of HIV is far more complex than other retroviruses (reviewed in [1]). In addition to the flanking long terminal repeat (LTR) sequences that contain important regulatory regions for HIV replication, HIV has at least six additional genes (*tat, rev, vif, nef, vpr*, and *vpu*).

The *tat* gene encodes a protein that activates viral gene expression in trans and is essential for virus replication. *Rev* is an upregulator of expression of viral capsid and envelope proteins and is required for replication. *Vif*, while not absolutely necessary for virus replication, is essential to the efficient generation of infectious virions. The function of the gene product of *Vpr*, a protein that is immunogenic in HIV-infected individuals, is presently not known (reviewed in [1]). The newest gene to be identified is *Vpu* [15, 16]. Since infection of T lymphocytes with a *vpu* mutant HIV resulted in five- to ten-fold less progeny virus but more *gag, pol*, and *env* proteins, it has been postulated that *vpu* is required for efficient virus replication and may have a role in virion assembly or maturation [16].

In contrast to those regulatory genes whose principal function is to increase virus replication and infectivity, the role of *nef* is one of downregulation of virus production (reviewed

in [1]). In addition, it has recently been demonstrated that the *nef* gene product is a myristylated GTP-binding phosphoprotein that can downregulate the expression of CD4 in a T cell line [17].

Activation of Latent or Chronic HIV Infections

The consequence of the existence of multiple regulatory genes in HIV is that infection with this virus can result in a host of different outcomes, from true latency with a total absence of viral gene expression to low level, restricted viral replication, to a highly productive, lytic event (Figure 1). This spectrum of events is manifested in vivo in the long and variable clinical course of infection. Thus, in order to halt the progression of HIV-induced disease in infected individuals, it is of utmost importance to understand the factors that influence the various possible outcomes of infection with HIV and to delineate the mechanisms whereby a latent or restricted replicative state is converted into a productive infection.

It was shown early on that both untreated peripheral blood lymphocytes (PBL) and phytohemagglutinin (PHA)-exposed PBL could be infected with HIV, but that only the PHA-stimulated lymphocytes produced detectable reverse transcriptase (RT) activity indicative of a productive infection [18]. Similar experiments using antigen-induced activated PBL showed that the activated cells were 10 to 100 times more susceptible to virus replication than the untreated controls [19].

Because HIV-infected individuals can be coinfected with a variety of other pathogenic viruses, it was of interest to examine whether exposure to heterologous viruses had an effect on HIV expression. In cotransfection experiments, it was shown that heterologous viral genes can upregulate the expression of an indicator gene that is linked to HIV LTR sequences (reviewed in [20]). In addition, exposure of in vitro HIV-infected PBL to noninfectious HTLV-1 virions resulted in the production of large quantities of HIV [21].

Since HIV expression could be augmented by mitogens, antigens, and heterologous viruses, the next question to be addressed was whether normal physiologic cellular inductive signals could activate HIV. Thus, we established a model system for cytokine-induced upregulation of HIV that utilized a chronically HIV-infected clone, U1, derived from a promonocytic cell line, U937. U1 produced low levels of HIV, but after induction with 13-phorbol-12-myristate acetate (PMA), virus expression increased 20-fold [22]. In addition, virus expression in U1 cells was significantly increased following exposure to PHA-induced supernatants containing multiple cytokines and by recombinant granulocyte/macrophage colony-stimulating factor alone [23].

Induction of HIV Expression by TNF-alpha

The model system for the study of HIV expression was extended to include a chronically HIV-infected T cell clone, ACH-2, that was derived from HIV infection of A3.01 cells. Using these cells, we demonstrated that supernatants from elutriated human monocytes stimulated with lipopolysaccharide (LPS), and tumor necrosis factors-alpha and -beta can upregulate HIV expression [24; Folks, T. et al., manuscript in preparation, 27]. It has also been determined that tumor necrosis factor-alpha is the active component in the LPS-monocyte supernatant. The addition of antisera to TNF-alpha to the LPS-monocyte supernatants resulted in an inhibition of the induction of HIV [24].

In order to investigate the mechanisms of action of TNF-alpha, A3.01 cells were transfected with a plasmid containing the HIV LTR linked to the chloramphenicol acetyl transferase (CAT) indicator gene. Following exposure of the transfected cells to TNF-alpha, there was a significant increase in the level of CAT activity. This experiment demonstrates that the induction of HIV by TNF-alpha can be attributed to activation of the HIV promotor by a transactivating mechanism.

TNF-alpha is an immunoregulatory molecule that functions during normal immune responses [25] and is found in high levels in individuals with opportunistic infections [26]. Thus, it is possible that progression of HIV-induced disease could be the result of ordinary infections that stimulate TNF-alpha production. Once the T4 cell counts are depressed and opportunistic infections occur, further production of TNF-alpha would hasten the downward spiral of immune function.

References

1. Fauci, A. S. 1988. The human immunodeficiency virus: infectivity and mechanisms of pathogenesis. Science 239: 617.
2. Klatzmann, D., F. Barre-Sinoussi, M. T. Nugeyre, C. Dauguet, E. Vilmer, C. Griscelli, F. Vezinet-Brun, J. C. Gluckman, J.-C. Chermann, and L. Montagnier. 1984. Selective tropism of lymphadenopathy associated virus (LAV) for helper-inducer T lymphocytes. Science 225: 59.
3. Dalgleish, A. G., P. C. L. Beverley, P. R. Clapham, D. H. Crawford, M. F. Greaves, and R. A. Weiss. 1984. The CD4 (T4) antigen is an essential component of the receptor for the AIDS virus. Nature 312: 763.
4. Fauci, A. S. 1985. Immunological abnormalities in the acquired immunodeficiency syndrome (AIDS). Clin. Res. 32: 491.
5. Popovic, M., M. G. Sarngadharan, E. Read, and R. C. Gallo. 1984. Detection, isolation, and continuous production of cytopathic retroviruses (HTLV-III) from patients with AIDS and pre-AIDS. Science 224: 497.
6. Leonard, R., D. Zagury, I. Desportes, J. Bernard, J.-F. Zagury, and R. C. Gallo. 1988. Cytopathic effect of human immunodeficiency virus in T4 cells is linked to the last stage of virus infection. Proc. Natl. Acad. Sci. 85: 3570.
7. Folks, T., D. M. Powell, M. M. Lightfoote, S. Benn, M. A. Martin, and A. S. Fauci. 1986. Induction of HTLV-III/LAV from a nonvirus-producing T-cell line: implications for latency. Science 231: 600–602.

8. Levy, J. A., J. Shimabukuro, T. McHugh, C. Casavant, D. Stites, and L. Oshiro. 1985. AIDS-associated retroviruses (ARV) can productively infect other cells besides human T helper cells. Virology 147: 441.

9. Ho, D. D., T. R. Rota, and M. S. Hirsch. 1986. Infection of monocyte/macrophages by human T lymphotropic virus type III. J. Clin. Invest. 77: 1712.

10. Nicholson, J. K. A., G. D. Cross, C. S. Callaway, and S. J. McDougal. 1986. In vitro infection of human monocytes with human T lymphotropic virus type III/lymphadenopathy-associated virus (HTLV-III/LAV). J. Immunol. 137: 323.

11. Salahuddin, S. Z., R. M. Rose, J. E. Groopman, P. D. Markham, and R. C. Gallo. 1986. Human T lymphotropic virus type III infection of human alveolar macrophages. Blood 68: 281.

12. Orenstein, J. M., M. S. Meltzer, T. Phipps, and H. E. Gendelman. 1988. Cytoplasmic assembly and accumulation of human immunodeficiency virus types 1 and 2 in recombinant human colony-stimulating factor-1 treated human monocytes: An ultrastructural study. J. Virology 62: 2578.

13. Folks, T. M., S. W. Kessler, J. M. Orenstein, J. Justement, E. Jaffe, and A. S. Fauci. 1988. Infection and replication of human immunodeficiency virus-1 (HIV-1) in highly purified progenitor cells from normal human bone marrow. Science, in press.

14. Rabson, A. B., and M. A. Martin. 1985. Molecular organization of the AIDS retrovirus. Cell 40: 477.

15. Cohen, E. A., E. F. Terwilliger, J. G. Sodroski, and W. A. Haseltine. 1988. Identification of a protein encoded by the vpu gene of HIV-1. Nature 334: 532.

16. Strebel, K., T. Klimkait, and M. A. Martin. 1988. A novel gene of HIV-1, vpu, and its 16-kd product. Science 241: 1221.

17. Guy, B., M. P. Kieny, Y. Riviere, C. Le Peuch, K. Dott, M. Girard, L. Montagnier, and J.-P. Lecocq. 1987. HIV F/3′ orf encodes a phosphorylated GTP-binding protein resembling an oncogene product. Nature 330: 266.

18. Folks, T. M., J. Kelly, S. Benn, A. Kinter, J. Justement, J. Gold, R. Redfield, K. W. Sell, and A. S. Fauci. 1986. Susceptibility of normal human lymphocytes to infection with HTLV-III/LAV. J. Immunol. 136: 4049.

19. Margolick, J. B., D. J. Volkman, T. M. Folks, and A. S. Fauci. 1987. Amplification of HTLV-III/LAV infection by antigen-induced activation of T cells and direct suppression by virus of lymphocyte blastogenic responses. J. Immunol. 138: 1719.

20. Rosenberg, Z. F., and A. S. Fauci. 1988. Immunopathogenic mechanisms in human immunodeficiency virus (HIV) infections. Ann. N.Y. Acad. Sci., in press.

21. Zack, J. A., A. J. Cann, J. P. Lugo, and I. S. Y. Chen. 1988. HIV-1 production from infected peripheral blood T cells after HTLV-1 induced mitogenic stimulation. Science 240: 1026.

22. Folks, T. M., J. Justement, A. Kinter, S. Schnittman, J. Orenstein, G. Poli, and A. S. Fauci. 1988. Characterization of a promonocyte clone chronically infected with HIV and inducible by PMA. J. Immunol. 140: 1117.

23. Folks, T. M., J. Justement, A. Kinter, C. A. Dinarello, and A. S. Fauci. 1987. Cytokine-induced expression of HIV in a chronically infected promonocyte cell line. Science 238: 800.

24. Clouse, K. A., D. Powell, I. Washington, G. Poli, K.Strebel, W. Farrar, P. Barstad, J. Kovacs, A. S. Fauci, and T. M. Folks. Monokine regulation of human immunodeficiency virus-1 expression in a chronically infected human T cell clone. J. Immunol., in press.

25. Kehrl, J. H., M. Mon-Alvarez, G. A. Delsing, and A. S. Fauci. 1987. Lymphotoxin is an important cell derived growth factor for human B cells. Science 238: 1144.

26. Lahdevirta, J., C. P. J. Maury, A.-M. Teppo, and H. Repo. 1988. Elevated levels of circulating cachectin/tumor necrosis factor in patients with acquired immunodeficiency syndrome. Amer. J. Med. 85: 289.

27. Folks, T. M., K. A. Clouse, J. Justement, A. Rabson, E. Duh, J. H. Kehrl, and A. S. Fauci. Tumor necrosis factor-alpha induces the expression of the human immunodeficiency virus from a chronically infected T cell clone. In preparation.

Immune Response to HIV

Stephen G. Norley and Reinhard Kurth*

Defining which aspects of the immune response to HIV are capable of preventing infection, and which viral epitopes can stimulate these responses, is a major aspect of AIDS vaccine development. The potential roles of the various immune mechanisms in relation to vaccine design are reviewed and discussed.

Central to the theme of developing an AIDS vaccine is characterization of the immune response following infection and vaccination. This is essential because attempts to induce a protective immunity using "classical" vaccination strategies, based primarily on the elicitation of neutralizing antibody, have met with universal failure, and it is now clear that in order to design an effective immunoprophylaxis, we must know which immune mechanisms—or combinations thereof—are capable of preventing the initial infection from becoming established. The viral antigens/epitopes stimulating these immune mechanisms must then be identified and used as the basis for a putative vaccine. In this review we briefly discuss the present knowledge of different anti-HIV effector mechanisms and how this knowledge is being applied to vaccine development.

Neutralizing Antibody

The identification of HIV as the causative agent of AIDS stimulated immediately an intense effort world-wide to characterize the neutralizing antibody response to the virus. Once a variety of suitable test systems had been established, it was quickly shown that the majority of HIV-1 seropositive individuals harbor antibodies able to neutralize HIV-1 in vitro [1]. However, the titers of neutralizing antibody were generally low, and the reactivity was, at best, group specific [2]. HIV-2-infected patients, on the other hand, have recently been shown to possess a low level of antibody able to neutralize both HIV-1 and HIV-2 [3]. The demonstration of anti-HIV neutralizing antibodies was quickly followed up by the promising generation of neutralizing antibodies in ex-

perimental animals receiving inoculations of a variety of putative vaccine preparations, particularly purified envelope glycoprotein produced from recombinant systems [4]. These antibodies, however, were generally characterized by their relatively low titers and narrow type specificity. Furthermore, when chimpanzees possessing a "good" circulating neutralizing antibody response were challenged with a very low dose of the homologous virus, there was no significant effect on the course of the infection. In an effort to define the situation at the molecular level, many groups have worked to identify the precise epitopes eliciting and acting as targets for neutralizing antibody. Using synthetic peptide technology, point-mutation analysis, and monoclonal antibodies, it has been possible to map the major neutralizing epitopes on the envelope protein. Results from different laboratories are not completely in agreement, and it seems that there are a number of major neutralizing antibody-stimulating regions of the envelope glycoprotein. The major epitope apparently maps to the middle of the gp120 and appears to be reactive in a type-specific manner [5], whereas other regions of env, particularly the transmembrane gp41, exhibit a wider group specificity [6]. The latter seem to act by preventing penetration (rather than by blocking of initial binding) and should certainly be considered for inclusion in a putative vaccine. However, as other epitopes reside in regions of hypervariability their use in a broadly protective vaccine seem limited.

Complement Activating Antibodies

One possible mechanism by which antibodies can attack infected cells is by binding to cell surface viral proteins and stimulating complement. However, most studies, including our own, have found that antibodies able to initiate the complement cascade, and hence specific

---

*   Paul-Ehrlich-Institut, Frankfurt, West Germany.

lysis of infected cells, are rarely present in the sera of HIV infected patients [7]. By "fine-tuning" assay conditions, however, it is possible to demonstrate the limited lysis of HIV infected cells in the presence of specific antibody and complement [8], and it is quite feasible that the production of such antibodies could be stimulated by a vaccine presenting the correct epitopes in a suitable way.

Natural Killer Cells

Although primarily involved in immune surveillance against tumor cells, NK cells can, under the correct conditions, attack HIV-infected cells [9], and we have preliminary evidence indicating that the spread of virus in culture is reduced in the presence of these cells. It is possible that enhancement of NK activity by lymphokines released after suitable stimulation of T-cells and monocytes by a vaccine could help to control the initial infection, although the effect would be rather non-specific. Unfortunately, there is evidence that the overall lytic action of NK cells against target cells is dramatically decreased in patients with AIDS [10].

Antibody-Dependent Cellular Cytotoxicity

The potential role for ADCC in the control of HIV infection has received an increasing amount of attention over the last two years, primarily because this is one antibody-directed effector mechanism that has a proven ability to attack HIV infected cells [11, 12]. The envelope glycoprotein appears to present the major target for ADCC attack [13], and the epitopes that seem to serve as the major target for ADCC reside in the more conserved regions near the carboxy terminal of the gp120 or in the gp41 region itself.

Consequently, other groups have shown a measure of group specificity in the reaction [14]. Our laboratory has developed a sensitive ADCC system and has found that, without exception, antibodies from HIV-1 seropositive patients have the ability to initiate lysis of cells infected with a variety of different HIV-1 strains. Furthermore, we have demonstrated the presence in a number of individuals of anti-

bodies able to promote lysis of cells infected with HIV-1 and those infected with HIV-2. This represents the first incidence of a functional immune mechanism able to mount a lytic attack of cells infected with either group of viruses and has clear potential as the basis for a broad-spectrum vaccine. By use of cold-target competition assays, we have shown that the epitope(s) recognized by these cross-reactive sera are present on both HIV-1- and HIV-2-infected cells, and it seems possible, therefore, that some isolates of HIV may possess or express epitopes that stimulate the production of antibodies able to initiate ADCC attack of cells infected with any strain of HIV-1 or HIV-2. Furthermore, we have shown that the presence of an active ADCC system in cell culture can limit the spread of HIV after addition of infected cells. These results have clear implications for the development of a broad spectrum anti-HIV vaccine.

Cytotoxic T-Lymphocytes

Perhaps the greatest potential for a vaccine lies in the stimulation of a cytotoxic T-lymphocyte (CTL) response. These specifically stimulated cytotoxic cells often represent the major antiviral immune mechanism [15] and have been shown in a number of systems to be wholly responsible for eliminating disease [16]. Stimulation of HIV-specific CTLs by a vaccine should present a formidable barrier to infection. A number of groups have demonstrated the presence of specific CTLs in HIV infected patients [17–19], but work in this field is hampered by the fact that a CTL will only recognize its target antigen on the surface of the cell if it is associated with the appropriate class I MHC molecule, which usually necessitates the use of infectible autologous cells or cell lines from each individual. CTLs usually recognize antigens processed and expressed by cellular mechanisms, and the available target antigens are therefore not limited to the external glycoproteins [20]. Indeed, using vaccinia vectors expressing a variety of HIV genes, different groups have shown the presence of CTLs specific for envelope (env), core (gag), and even polymerase (pol) proteins [19, 21, 22]. As the latter two are relatively well conserved between strains, they may form the basis for a putative vaccine. Design of a vaccine to stimulate a CTL response has to overcome the fact that a good CTL response is difficult to achieve with non-replicating antigen. Even with the identification of the epitopes responsible for CTL stimulation, injection of purified proteins or synthetic peptides may be ineffective [15]. This is the reason why the development of a live virus vaccine, probably based upon the expression of the required epitopes in a harmless virus vector, is so important. Indeed, in a unique set of trials, one group [23] has recently described the successful stimulation in humans of a HIV-specific CTL response following infection with a live vaccinia virus expressing the HIV envelope gene, although, for various reasons, this vector would not be suitable for general use. It may be possible, however, to overcome the requirement for a replicating viral vaccine to stimulate the CTL response if the sequence and structure of the epitopes recognized by the CTL precursor can be mimicked to such an extent that the need for processing and expression are circumvented.

In summary, although the initial "crude" vaccine preparations failed to elicit a protective immune response in the animal model, the ongoing detailed analysis of potentially effective immune mechanisms and the viral epitopes which stimulate them should allow the design of a protective vaccine. Such a vaccine will almost certainly need to stimulate the cellular immune system in addition to the humoral, and will probably take the form, at least initially, of a live genetically engineered virus.

References

1. Robert-Guroff, M., M. Brown, and R. C. Gallo. 1985. HTLV-III-neutralizing antibodies in patients with AIDS and AIDS-related complex. Nature. 316: 72.
2. Weiss, R. A., P. R. Clapham, J. N. Weber, A. G. Dalgleish, L. A. Lasky, and P. W. Berman. 1986. Variable and conserved neutralisation antigens of human immunodeficiency virus. Nature. 324: 572.
3. Weiss, R. A., P. R. Clapham, J. N. Weber, D. Whitby, R. S. Tedder, T. O'Connor, S. Chamaret, and L. Montagneir. 1988. HIV-2 antisera cross-neutralize HIV-1. AIDS. 2: 95.
4. Robey, W. G., L. O. Arthur, T. J. Matthews, A. Langlois, T. D. Copeland, N. W. Lerche, S. Oroszlan, D. P. Bolognesi, R. V. Gilden, and P. J. Fischinger. 1986. Prospect for prevention of human immunodeficiency virus infection: Purified 120-kDa envelope glycoprotein induces neutralizing antibody. Proc. Natl. Acad. Sci. USA 83: 7023.
5. Palker, T. J., M. E. Clark, A. J. Langlois, T. J. Matthews, K. J. Weinhold, R. R. Randall, D. P. Bolognesi, and B. F. Haynes. 1988. Type-specific neutralization of the human immunodeficiency virus with antibodies to env-encoded synthetic peptides. Proc. Natl. Acad. Sci. USA 85: 1932.
6. Ho, D. D., M. G. Sarngadharan, M. S. Hirsch, R. T. Schooley, T. R. Rota, R. C. Kennedy, T. C. Chanh, and V. L. Sato. 1987. Human immunodeficiency virus neutralizing antibodies recognize several conserved domains of the envelope glycoproteins. J. Virol. 61: 2024.
7. Nara, P. L., W. G. Robey, M. A. Gonda, S. G. Carter, and P. J. Fischinger. 1987. Absence of cytotoxic antibody to human immunodeficiency virus-infected cells in humans and its induction in animals after infection or immunization with purified envelope glycoprotein gp120. Proc. Natl. Acad. Sci. USA 84: 3793.
8. Toth, F.D., J. Kiss, B. Szabo, G. Füst, E. Ujhelyi, S. R. Hollan, and L. Vaczi. 1988. Complement-dependent cytotoxic antibodies to HIV-induced cell surface antigens in HIV seropositive haemophiliacs. IV Int. Conf. AIDS. Abst. 2177.
9. Ruscetti, F. W., J. A. Mikovits, V. S. Kalyanaraman, R. Overton, H. Stevenson, K. Stromberg, R. B. Herberman, W. L. Farrar, and J. R. Ortaldo. 1986. Analysis of effector mechanisms against HTLV-I and HTLV-III/LAV infected lymphoid cells. J. Immunol. 136: 3619.
10. Sirianni M. C., S. Soddus, W. Malorni, G. Arancia, and F. Aiuti. 1988. Mechanism of defective natural killer cell activity in patients with AIDS is associated with defective distribution of tubulin. J. Immunol. 140: 2565.
11. Rook, A. H., H. C. Lane, T. Folks, S. McCoy, H. Alter, and A. S. Fauci. 1987. Sera from HTLV-III/LAV antibody-positive individuals mediate antibody-dependent cellular cytotoxicity against HTLV-III/LAV-infected T cells. J. Immunol. 138: 1064.
12. Ljunggren, K., E.-M. Fenyö, G. Biberfeld, and M. Jondal. 1987. Detection of antibodies which mediated human immunodeficiency virus-specific cellular cytotoxicity (ADCC) in vitro. J. Immunol. Methods. 104: 7.
13. Shepp, D. H., S. Chakrabarti, B. Moss, and G. V. Quinnan, Jr. 1988. Antibody-dependent cellular cytotoxicity specific for the envelope antigens of human immunodeficiency virus. J. Infect. Dis. 157: 1260.
14. Lyerly, H. K., D. L. Reed, T. J. Matthews, A. J. Langlois, P. A. Ahearne, S. R. Petteway, Jr., and K. J. Weinhold. 1987. Anti-GP 120 antibodies from HIV seropositive individuals mediate

broadly reactive anti-HIV ADCC. AIDS Res. Hum. Retroviruses. 3: 409.

15. Rouse, B. T., S. G. Norley, and S. Martin. 1988. Antiviral cytotoxic T lymphocyte induction and vaccination. Rev. Infect. Dis. 10: 16.

16. Jonjic, S., M.-D. Val, G. M. Keil, M. J. Reddehase, and U. H. Koszinowski. 1988. A non-structural viral protein expressed by a recombinant vaccinia virus protects against lethal cytomegalovirus infection. J. Virol. 62: 1653.

17. Walker, C. M., D. J. Moodey, D. P. Stites, and J. A. Levy. 1986. CD8+ lymphocytes can control HIV infection in vitro by suppressing virus replication. Science. 234: 1563.

18. Plata, F., B. Autran, L. P. Martins, S. Wain-Hobson, M. Raphaël, C. Mayaud, M. Denis, J. M. Guillon, and P. Debré. 1987. AIDS virus-specific cytotoxic T lymphocytes in lung disorders. Nature. 328: 348.

19. Walker, B. D., C. Flexner, T. J. Paradis, T. C. Fuller, M. S. Hirsch, R. T. Schooley, and B. Moss. 1988. HIV-1 reverse transcriptase is a target for cytotoxic T-lymphocytes in infected individuals.

20. McMichael, A. J., C. A. Michie, F. M. Gotch, G. L. Smith, and B. Moss. 1986. Recognition of influenza A virus nucleoprotein by human cytotoxic T lymphocytes. J. gen. Virol. 67: 719.

21. Shepp, D. H., F. Daguillard, D. Mann, and G. V. Quinnan. 1988. Human class 1 MHC-restricted cytotoxic T-lymphocytes specific for human immunodeficiency virus envelope antigens. AIDS. 2: 113.

22. Walker, B. D., S. Chakrabarti, B. Moss, T. J. Paradis, T. Flynn, A. G. Durno, R. S. Blumberg, J. C. Kaplan, M. S. Hirsch, and R. T. Schooley. 1987. HIV-specific cytotoxic T lymphocytes in seropositive individuals. Nature. 328: 345.

23. Zagury, D., J. Bernhard, R. Cheynier, I. Desportes, R. Leonard, M. Fouchard, B. Reveil, D. Ittele, Z. Lurhuma, K. Mbayo, J. Wane, J.-J. Salaun, B. Goussard, L. Dechazal, A. Burny, P. Nara, and R. C. Gallo. 1988. A group specific anamnestic immune reaction against HIV-1 induced by a candidate vaccine against AIDS. Nature. 332: 728.

Science. 240: 64.

Results of Clinical Trials of Anti-Retrovirus Therapy in AIDS

*Michael H. Grieco**

Nucleoside analogues that inhibit HIV-1 RT appear to be a fruitful area for continued research. AZT, a pyrimidine nucleoside has clearly been shown to be clinically effective and to prolong life following PCP. Other promising nucleoside analogues include ddC, ddI, and d4T. Reduction of HIV-1 p24 antigenemia is a clear effect of AZT and ddC, and appears also to result from treatment with foscarnet and possibly from Ampligen, suggesting that other drugs may be able to inhibit viral replication and modify the clinical course of HIV-1 infection.

Multiple agents are under study that may modify infection by free virus. These include dextran sulfate, AL-721, soluble CD4, anti-Leu 3A monoclonal antibody, and castanospermine, which are in various phases of development as potential theraputic agents. The rapid development of AZT as a clinical effective agent has underscored the realistic potential for the control of HIV-1 infection with drugs acting synergistically to inhibit infection at multiple sites in the replication cycle.

Development of treatment for HIV-1, the etiologic agent for AIDS, is regarded as a necessary condition for the long-term control of infection with this retrovirus. An ideal drug would be orally effective, viricidial, relatively non-toxic, and would be able to access infected lymphocytes, monocytes, the central nervous system, and endothelial cells as well as any other cells that might be infected with HIV-1 in the host.

These will be difficult goals to achieve. However, the accomplishments thus far provide significant hope for the future in developing at least long-term effective inhibitory drug treatment.

The stages of HIV replication that may be target for theraputic intervention are summarized in Table 1 [1–3].

Zidovudine (Azidothymidine, AZT)

The 2',3'-dideoxynucleotides are nucleoside analogues in which modification of the 3'-hydroxy group prevents formation of phosphodiester linkage for nucleic acid chains. In 1964 Horwitz et al. [4] first synthesized AZT, which was subsequently shown to be active against Friend murine leukemia virus in 1974 and HIV-1 in 1985 [5] in vitro at concentrations of greater than 0.1 mM, while inhibition of proliferation of uninfected lymphocytes required greater than 1 mM. Infected cells of the monocyte-macrophage series are less sensitive than infected lymphocytes, probably because of reduced phosphorylation. The activity of producing AZT requires the actions of cellular thymidine kinases to convert to AZTMP, then to AZTDP and finally AZTTP. AZTTP inhibits HIV-1 RT about 100 times more effectively than cellular polymerase. AZT competetively inhibits thymidylate kinase and reduces levels of dTTP, while AZTTP is incorporated into proviral DNA strands and results in chain termination because of preferential binding to HIV-1 RT. Inhibition of the reverse transcriptase site of action has been fruitful and has led to identification of several other nucleoside analogues with marked in vitro activity (Table 1), but only AZT has been established as effective clinically.

After oral administration, AZT is rapidly absorbed with a mean half-life of approximatety one hour and mean peak and trough levels after a 250 mg dose of 0.62 and 0.16 µg/ml respectively. The drug does penetrate the CSF with levels of about 50% of the corresponding serum concentration.

After the results of a Phase I pilot study in 19 patients with AIDS and ARC were reported, a

* Chief, Division of Allergy, Clinical Immunology and Infectious Diseases, St. Luke's\Roosevelt Hospital Center, 428 West 59th Street, New York, NY 10019-1196; and Professor of Clinical Medicine, College of Physicians and Surgeons of Columbia University, New York, NY.
This work was supported by NIH Clinical Studies Group Grant AI 25901.

Table 1. Viral replication and possible sites of pharmacologic intervention.

Site	Candidate drug
I. Adherence of CD4 and 2nd step fusion	Castanospermine Dextran sulfate AL-721 Peptide T Soluble CD4 Anti-idiotype CD4 Anti-idiotype gp120
II. Entry into target cell and uncoating of RNA	None available
III. Reverse transcriptase	Zidovudine (AZT) 2',3'-dideoxycytidine 2',3'-dideoxyadenosine 2',3'-dideoxyinosine 2',3'-dideoxy-2',3'dideohydrocytidine (D4C) 2',3'-dideoxy-2',3'dideohydrothymidine (D4T) 3'-azido-2',3'-dideoxyuridine (CS-87) Foscarnet
IV. Viral RNase (III, IV, V endoded by *pol* gene)	RNase H inhibitors
V. Viral integrase	None available
VI. Transcriptase	None available specific for HIV-1—Ampligen may work here
VII. Translation	Inhibitors of TAT, REV, or VIF "Ante-sense" constructs Interferons, Ampligen, Ribavirin
VIII. Post-translational processing	Interferon, myristylation, glycosylation or protease inhibitors or modifers

Phase III model study was organized and 282 patients were enrolled from February to June 1986 in a clinical trial at 12 centers in the United States [7, 8], 145 receiving AZT orally, 250 mg every 4 hours and 137 placebo. Patients with AIDS were within 4 months of first attack of PCP and patients with ARC were advanced. By September 1986, the study was terminated because of significant reduction of mortality in the AZT arm. Subjects in the AZT arm continued on the drug while patients in the placebo arm were converted to AZT, 200 mg every 4 hours, which terminated further long-term placebo control evaluation. The AZT arm, for long-term comparison of mortality, must be evaluated with historical data from New York [9] and San Francisco [10]. The results concerning mortality from the original and extended studies are summarized in Table 2, and the New York and San Francisco mortality data for PCP infection alone are provided as well. The more favorable outcome noted in New York City in AZT-untreated subjects may be due to bias resulting from lack of follow-up [11]. At six months, 1 of the patients on AZT had died compared to 19 on placebo. The estimated mortality rate was 6.2% at 9 months, 10.3% at 12 months and 21.3% at 18 months. This contrasts with the historical control values following PCP of 54.6% in NYC and 70% in San Francisco at 12 months subsequent to diagnosis.

Other theraputic and adverse effects are listed in Tables 3 and 4. This includes the original and extended AZT trial, the compassionate-use trial in over 4800 patients enrolled from October 1986 to March 1987, and other reports in the literature. As a result of the original and extended trials, AZT was licensed in the United States in 1987 for use after diagnosis of PCP and for an absolute CD4 lymphocyte count of less than $200/mm^3$. Within three years of the demonstration of AZT's activity against HIV-1, this drug has been administered to over 20,000 individuals throughout the world. This is remarkable achievement and represents a model for future drug development.

A number of studies are now in progress to further evaluate the role of AZT in treatment. Viral synergy has been detected with AZT combined with acyclovir, ampligen, GMCSF, alpha interferon, and the glycosylatian inhibitor castanospermine [12]. Clinical studies of AZT and alpha interferon as well as AZT and

Table 2. Mortality in the original AZT double-blind, placebo-controlled trial and extended AZT administration.

Observation after start of therapy (months)	AZT arm (N=145)	Control arm (N=137)	Historical controls for PCP NYC (9)/ San Francisco (10)
6	1 (.7%)	19 (14%)	
9	9 (6.2%)	12 AIDS, 7 ARC	
12	10.3% (est)		54.6%/70%
18	31 (21.3%)		
24			75.0%/98%
36			79.6%/—
48			80.4%/—
60			83.3%/—

Table 3. Clinical results from double-blind, placebo-controlled trial of AZT, open extended trial, compassionate use trial, and other reports.

1. Decreased severity of opportunistic infection.
2. Decreased frequency of OI not clear.
3. Transient increase in CD4 cells.
4. Improved DTH.
5. Decrease of progressive weight loss.
6. HIV-1 p24 antigen is reduced.
7. PCP subjects enrolled within 3 months had improved responses.
8. Predictors of poor outcome:
    ➤initial Karnowsky score less than 90%
    ➤hemoglobin levels less than 11 g/dl
    ➤CD4 counts less than 100/cm^3
    ➤transfusion-induced infection
9. neurological benefits?
10. HIV-associated thrombocytophen?
11. psoriasis?
12. lymphocytic interstitial pneumonia?

Table 4. Toxicity reported from double-blind, placebo-controlled trial of AZT, open extended trial, compassionate use trial, and other reports [12].

1. Macrocytic anemia
2. Neutropenia
3. Headaches
4. Nausea
5. Myalgia
6. Insomnia
7. Rarely hypocellular marrow
8. Fever
9. Rash
10. Nail pigmentation [13]
11. Reversible confusion
12. Necrotizing myopathy [14, 15]

acyclovir, AZT plus GMCSF and AZT plus interleukin-2 are in place or are being planned.

Many of these studies are being planned to be carried out by the NIH, NIAID-sponsored AIDS Clinical Trials Program, which consists of 35 research centers throughout the United States. Several active AZT trials are itemized in Table 5 and provide a view of current efforts to extend the knowledge base to expand the clinical use of AZT.

Acyclovir, another nucleoside analog, can potentiate the anti-HIV activity of AZT in all cultures without potentiating its toxicity [16]. One pilot study in 8 patients indicated tolerance of AZT 100 mg and acyclovir 800 mg every 4 hours [17]. Improved clinical efficacy remains to be established. Desciclovir (DCV) is the 6-deoxy congener of acyclovir. It is a prodrug that is well absorbed and extensively converted to acyclovir by host xanthine oxidase. The oral dosing of this drug yields levels of acyclovir comparable to intravenous acyclovir dosing and may be useful if clinical AZT-acyclovir synergy is demonstrated.

Other Nucleosides

Another pyrimidine, 2′,3′-dideoxycytidine, is even more potent than AZT on a molar basis. This is the most potent inhibitor in the ATH8 system. Inactive inhibition of HIV is achieved at concentrations of 0.5 mM at high viral doses and 10 mM concentrations at low viral doses. This drug is relatively resistant to cytidine deaminase, is well absorbed when administered orally in animals, cleared by the kidneys, and had produced relatively few toxic effects

Table 5. Elective AZT trials with AZT alone.

I. AZT alone:
ACTG 001: AIDS-associated KS
ACTG 005: AIDS dementia and CNS infection
ACTG 017: HIV+ asymptomatic hemophilia
ACTG 016: Early ARC
ACTG 019: HIV+ and/or PGL
ACTG 003: Pediatric AIDS or PGL
ACTG 049: Infants with perinatal exposure
ACTG 043: Pediatric HIV+ symptomatic
ACTG 052: Pediatric symptomatic HIV infection
Burroughs Wellcome: HIV AbNeg HCW,
Occupational exposure (800-448-7845)
ACTG 061: AIDS dementia complex
ACTG 062: HIV+ with hepatic disease
ACTG TX302: Accidental massive exposure to HIV
In planning: Treatment of infected pregnant
women
AZT crossing of placenta in mice has been
demonstrated by blockade of Cas-Br-E
neurotropic type C retrovirus.

Table 6. AZT in combination with other drugs.

a. Alpha interferon and beta interferon
   ACTG 013 and 014: AIDS-associated KS
   ACTG 068: AIDS/ARC
   Triton Biosciences: KS, AIDS, ARC
b. Alpha interferon plus GM-CSF
   Schering: AIDS-associated KS
c. Acetaminophen
   ACTG 032: ARC/AIDS
d. Acyclovir
   ACTG 010: ARC/PGL
   European Multicenter: AIDS/ARC/HIV+ symptomatic
   ACTG 063: AIDS post first episode PCP
   ACTG 070: AIDS with retinitis
e. Chemotherapy
   ACTG 008: AIDS, systemic B-cell lymphoma
   ACTG 009: AIDS primary CNS lymphoma
f. Desciclovir, a 6-deoxycongener of acyclovir that
   is converted to acyclovir by xanthine oxidase
   ACTU 007: AIDS/ARS
g. Dideoxycytidine, alternating with AZT
   ACTG 047 and 050: AIDS/ARC open label dose
   ranging
   using doses of AZT 200 mg and ddC 0.01 and
   0.03 mg/kg q4h
h. Foscarnet
   ACTG 053: AIDS/ARC on AZT
i. GM-CSF
   NIH: AIDS/ARC, alternating therapy trial
   ACTU 065: AIDS/ARC dose ranging trial
j. Gamma interferon
   ACTU 072: AIDS
k. Gamma globulin
   Burroughs Wellcome: Pediatric HIV infection
   ACTG 051: Pediatric symptomatic HIV infection
l. Interleukin-2
   ACTU 042: HIV+ asymptomatic
   ACTU 024: PGL
   ACTU 067: AIDS/ARC
m. Others
   Probenecid/Quinine, TMP/SMX, Vitamin B12,
   rEro

in laboratory animals. A Phase I study [18] examined 5 dosage regimens of ddC—0.03 mg/kg/8h, 0.03 mg/kg/4h, 0.06 mg/kg/4h, 0.09 mg/kg/4h, 0.25 mg/kg/8h—in 20 patients. The drug crossed the blood-brain barrier, decreased p24 values by week 2, and increased CD4 levels. Unfortunately, a painful peripheral neuropathy developed in 10 patients after 6–14 weeks of treatment. Sixty-one AIDS/ARC patients were enrolled in an open study by Skowron et al. [19] and randomized to 0.06, 0.03, 0.01, or 0.005 mg/kg orally every 4 h for 12 or 24 weeks. Fifty-one of 61 ddC treated patients developed neuropathy [14] at 0.06 mg, 15 at 0.03 mg, 10 at 0.01 mg, and 12 at 0.005 mg. Antigen p24 reduction was noted even with the lower doses of 0.03, 0.01, and 0.005. In addition to neuropathy, fever, rash and stomatitis were reported in each dose group. ACTG 050 is studying the use of alternating AZT and ddC to minimize the hematologic toxicity of the former and the neurotoxicity of the latter. Since this is a second drug shown to decrease p24 antigen in serum, every effort is being made to evaluate this drug in a manner that affords acceptable toxicity.

The 2′,3′-dideoxy, 2′,3′-didehydro derivatives of the pyrimidines, cystidine (d4C) and thymidine (d4T), have potent in vitro anti-HIV-1 activity, although d4T appears to be less toxic for H9 cells as does 3′-azido-2′,3′ dideoxyuridine (CS-87), a synthenized pyrimidine nucleoside analog of AZT Phase I trials are in the development stage.

2′,3′-dideoxy analogs of purine bases, adenosine (ddA) and inosine (ddI) have also shown strong in vitro inhibition of HIV-1 proliferation, again by acting as chain terminators. The ddA concentration required for maximal anti-HIV activity in a 7-day assay is some 20-fold higher than ddC but ddA becomes cytolytic to ATH8 cells only at levels 40-fold higher. ddA is a prodrug and is countered by serum adenosine deaminase to ddI which is subsequently converted intracellularly to ddA. Since ddA causes renal toxicity in dogs and rats after cleavage in the stomach to release adenine, there has been substantial concern that oral administration of ddA might be nephrotoxic in humans. The equally potent ddI is cleared in the stomach to hypoxanthine and is not expected to be nephrotoxic. ddA has been given to 8 patients in a pilot study but further trials are not contemplated.

ddI acts as a precursor to ddATP and is thought to exert antiviral activity through this enzyme. Athough ddI is about 10 times less potent than AZT, it is 100-fold less toxic than either AZT or ddC in vitro. Preliminary observations from the previous ddA study suggests that ddI may have a short half-life in serum but a larger half-life intracellularly. A phase I study is being conducted at the NIH and an ACTG trial, 064, is planned for phase I dose ranging.

There continues to be a great deal of interest in developing other patent nucleoside inhibitors since a member of this group, AZT, has been shown to be clinically effective and may be a beacon to more potent and effective drugs.

Interference with CD4 Binding or Viral-Cell Fusion

a) *Castanospermine:* Castanospermine (CAS) is a plant alkaloid, isolated from seeds of the Australian chestnut tree *Castanospermine australe*, that has shown to be a potent inhibitor of the endoplasmic reticulum enzyme, alpha-glucosidase I. By inhibiting glucosidase I, castanospermine prevents the removal of glucose residues during the normal processing of glycoproteins. The resultant proteins contain incompletely processed carbohydrate chains, an alteration that has profound effects on cell surface expression and the function of some glycoproteins. Castanospermine inhibits replication of HIV and dramatically inhibits syncytium formation in a transfected CD4+ cell line expressing the HIV envelope gene. Syncytium inhibition appears to occur through alteration of the envelope glycoprotein and not by alteration of the CD4 molecule. CD4 receptor-gp120 glycoprotein binding is not altered by CAS, but processing from gp160 to gp120 is decreased by this compound (suggesting that this is the mechanism of inhibition of syncytium formation). Antiviral effects of CAS ap-

pear to result from decreased virion infectivity due to interference with post-CD4-binding steps in the process of virus entry, as well as a decrease in cell-to-cell virus transmission secondary to syncytium inhibition. Studies in humans have not been performed.

b) *Dextran Sulfate:* This compound is a polysaccharide with a molecular weight of 7000–8000 and a sulfate content of 17–20% that appears to block HIV-1 entry into cells and to inhibit cell to cell infection and syncytia formation [20, 21]. Thirty-four patients have been enrolled in a Phase I dose finding study [22], 900 mg escalating to 5400 mg. Only 10 patients were p24 antigen-positive prior to therapy, and no significant change was noted. Related toxicity included diarrhea, CNS symptoms, and dysphonia. An ACTG Phase I trial is underway to extend dose finding in a larger cohort of p24 antigen-positive subjects. Wide community use in the United States has preceeded any evidence of laboratory or clinical efficacy.

c) *AL-721:* AL-721 is a lipid compound composed of neutral lipids, phosphatidylcholine and phosphatidylethanolamine in a 7:2:1 ratio. The objective of this open study reported by Grieco et al. [23] was to evaluate the effects of AL-721 in vivo in an 8-week open trial in which 10 g twice daily was administered on a low fat diet to 8 HIV-infected subjects with lymphadenopathy syndrome (LAS).

Serial lymphocyte cocultivation studies in 7 patients with initial culture positivity appeared to demonstrate reduction of reverse transcriptase peak counts in 5, with the trough noted in 4 at 8 weeks, and in 1 at 4 weeks following termination of therapy. The mean values for all 7 patients revealed a baseline value of 73419 with decrease to a low of 27418 at 8 weeks.

Mean levels of total lymphocytes, T-4, T-8, and T-11 cells were not altered, but lymphoproliferative responses to concanavalin A and pokeweed mitogens appeared to be augmented in 4 of the 8 subjects in association with AL-721 treatment. No side effects were noted.

In a subsequent follow-up study using a normal diet in the same subjects, lymphocyte cocultivation and mitogen-induced rsponses were less consistently affected when 15 g twice daily AL-721 was readministered. In addition, serum HIV p24 and CD4 levels were not altered during both the 8-week open and the subsequent AL-721 readministration. Four of the 8 patients have progressed to AIDS over the subsequent 14 months. The results of this study do not support the broad presumption of efficacy held by some members of the community infected with HIV-1.

d) *Anti-Leu-3A:* Anti-Leu-3A is a murine monoclonal antibody preparation which is an anti-idiotype to a monoclonal antibody to CD4 antigen. This antibody with anti-idiotype determinants may imitate CD4 antigen and bind to HIV gp160. Four patients have been treated with this drug, 1 mg intramuscularly, for over 3 weeks.

e) *Recombinant Soluble CD4:* rsT4 molecules are soluble, secreted forms of CD4 antigen that have been recombinantly produced by stable transfection of mammalian (CHO, myeloma) or insect cell lines (SF9) with vectors encoding versions of CD4 that lack its transmembrane and cytoplasmic portions. rsT4 has been shown to have the in vitro ability to inhibit HIV-1 infectivity, replication, and virus-induced cell fusion (syncytium formation). It is believed to achieve such inhibition by acting as a soluble virus receptor which interferes with the binding of HIV gp120 to intact CD4 antigen present on the surface of CD4+ cells, an essential step in HIV infection of such cells. Smith et al. [24] have produced two soluble CD4 analogs possessing an affinity and specificity for gp120 comparable to intact CD4 and which are capable of neutralizing the infectivity of HIV-1. Both forms of rsT4 virtually abolished growth of HIV-1 in CD4+ H9 cells.

In a dose-escalating IV study of rsT4.1 (Biogen) in 2 primates, a short half-life of approximately 30 minutes was determined with no observable toxicities. A theoretical concern about the clinical utility of rsT4 is its potential to interfere with normal immunologic function at in vivo concentrations necessary to inhibit HIV infectivity. Thus, HIV-1 may bind to a CD4 epitope necessarily conserved for the normal role this antigen plays in the immune system—thought to be T helper cell interaction with class II major histocompatibility complex (MHC) antigens on antigen presenting cells. If this is the case, rsT4 may itself be immunosuppressive. Phase I trials are in progress.

Foscarnet

Trisodium phosphonoformate is a pyrophosphate analog. This drug has in vitro anti-viral activity against all human herpes viruses. Its mode of action is by selective inhibition of viral DNA-polymerases at concentrations not affecting cellular DNA-polymerases. The human herpes viruses are inhibited by 30 µg/ml of foscarnet but different primary isolates of HSV and CMV differ in their sensitivities to foscarnet. A number of retroviruses are sensitive to foscarnet, including HIV, apparently by inhibition of RT.

Bergdahl et al. [25] enrolled 21 ARC patients in an open label controlled trial of foscarnet (PFA) or no treatment in Sweden. Eleven of 21 patients received foscarnet 50 mg/kg IV every 8 h for 28 days with a 2-month follow-up. Of the 10 patients who were p24 positive at entry, all 6 patients treated with PFA had a decrease in p24 after 4 weeks of treatment as compared to none of 4 in the control group. 0/11 treated patients progressed to AIDS as compared to 2/10 control patients who developed PCP during the initial 1 month treatment and 2 month follow-up period.

Jacobson et al. [26] studied 11 AIDS patients with CMV retinitis administered PFA 60 mg/kg IV every 8h for 14 days at UC San Francisco. 7/11 had detectable p24 prior to treatment. After the 14 days, 7/7 had a decrease in p24 between 4%–89% with a mean reduction of 58% overall. Three patients had p24 antigen levels increase to 54%–91% of their baseline values while on a maintenance dose of PFA 60mg/Kg (5 × week). Dose modifications were dependent on creatinine clearance. No significant change in CD4+ cell counts were noted.

In the Swedish study, all 19 treated patients noted increased thirst, 13/19 had headaches, nausea and anorexia, and 9/19 had pain in the costovertebral region. Other co-workers in France did not observe renal impairment in AIDS patients for CMV retinitis with foscarnet 200 mg/kg/day, when patients were over-hydrated with 2 liters isotonic saline solution prior to administration of foscarnet.

ACTU trials, 015 and 028, are active for CMV retinitis and ARC/PGL respectively. Since foscarnet must be administered continuosly and intravenously, its role for treatment of HIV-1 infection is limited. However, it may become a useful anti-CMV agent with a side benefit of inhibition of HIV replication. This is a third drug with substantial ability to reduce circulating p24 levels.

Ribavirin

Ribavirin is a synthetic nucleoside derivitive of the antibiotic pyrazomycin. It shows broad spectrum antiviral activity against DNA and RNA viruses, and is licensed by the FDA for its use in aerosol form for the treatment of respiratory syncytial viral (RSV) infections. This drug inhibits inosine monophosphate dehydrogenase (IMP), which converts IMP via xanthosine monophosphate to guanosine monophosphate. Competition of various enzymes for the resulting decreased pool of guanosine triphosphate (GTP) may account, at least in part, for the antiviral effect. Ribavirin resembles guanosine chemically and its antiviral action can be reversed by adding guanosine to treated cultures. Ribavirin further interferes with the guanylation step for 5′capping of viral mRNA and inhibits viral RNA polymerases, which are responsible for mRNA priming and elongation.

Multiple studies have been reported and have been equivocal with 600–800 mg oral daily doses [27]. An effect on p24 antigen has not been noted [28]. Additional studies are underway evaluating the effect of ribavirin at higher doses of up to 2400 mg/day in HIV-infected individuals including ATCG 034, a Phase I dose ranging trial. Treatment with this drug has been associated with mild anemia elevated bilirubin, insomnia, headache, and irritability. It should be reemphaszed that ribavirin antagonizes the effect of AZT on HIV replecation in vitro, a finding that might have clinical relevance [29].

Ampligen

Ampligen is a mismatched, double-stranded RNA molecule. It is a polynucleotide derivative of poly I-poly C with occasional uracil residues in the polypyrimidine strand to provide RNA-ase cleavage sites. This drug has the potential ability to augment cellular immunity as well as having antiviral properties. Ampligen has shown strong anti-HIV activity both in vitro and in vivo. In addition, ampligen crosses the blood-brain barrier. Ampligen has been shown to afford protection from HIV infection to the HIV-permissive T-cell line C-3 or the T-lymphoblastoid cell line CEM when incubated in growth media supplemented with ampligen at 10–50 µg/ml prior to virus challenge [30]. Ampligen may have a dual mechanism of action: direct antiviral action (including activation of dsRNA-dependent intercellular enzymes, such as RNA-ase L) and various indirect (immunomodulatory) actions.

Mitchell et al. [31] studied the in vitro effects of ampligen (25 µg/ml) and ampligen combined with AZT. HIV RNA was assayed in both C3 and H9 cells after repeated viral challenge in the presence of ampligen alone and ampligen combined with AZT. Virtually no HIV RNA was detected in cultures treated with ampligen, while the combination resulted in complete inhibition of HIV RNA. Pellegrino et al. [31] found that the inhibition of HIV RNA accumulation from ampligen occurs rapidly and early in the HIV life-cycle.

Strayer and co-workers [32] reported the effect of ampligen therapy on patients with HIV-related immune dysfunction. Forty (35 ARC/HIV+ and 5 AIDS) patients were treated with Ampligen 100–250 mg IV infusion twice weekly for 6–16 months. 83% ARC/HIV+ symtomatic and 75% AIDS patients who were tested demonstrated improvement in delayed-type hypersensitivity (DHR) within 12 weeks of treatment. A decrease in p24 antigen was noted in 13/14 patients treated with 200–250 mg who were initially p24 positive at baseline (mean p24 decrease of 39% from 776 ng/ml pre-treatment to 472 ng/ml in these 13 patients after 2–8 months on study). Median T4 cell count at time of entry was 238 cells/mm^3. T4 cell count increased 4.3% (30 patiients) after 4 months, 8% (10 patients) after 8 months, and 17% (6 patients) after 12 months. ARC patients reported a symptomatic improvement in the following: diarrhea, night sweats, and fatigue. In 11/15 ARC patients, a decrease in lymphadenopathy was noted. Four KS patients had progressive disease between 2–5 months into treatment. Five ARC patients progressed to AIDS (1 KS, 3 AIDS) while on treatment, and 1 ARC patient developed KS after discontinuing ampligen for 8 weeks.

This appears to be another drug which may influence p24 antigen levels although the effect does not appear to be as pronounced as with AZT, ddC, and foscarnet. A pharmaceutical-firm-sponsored study is in progress as a double-blind placebo-controlled trial in ARC subjects using 200 mg of ampligen administered intraveniously twice weekly.

The ACTG has Phase I drug ranging trials 038 and 054 for seropositive and AIDS/ARC subjects.

Conclusion

Thus far, two nucleoside analogues, AZT and ddC, foscarnet and possibly ampligen, appear to suppress p24 antigen. Of these, only AZT has been established as having a clinically significant benefit. It is likely that multiple agents to control HIV infection will become available over the next few years.

Further and updated information regarding HIV chemotherapy is available in the AIDS/HIV Experimental Treatment Directory compiled and published by the American Foundation for AIDS Research. This publication benefits from technical assistance from the Professional Outreach Program of the National Institute of Allergy and Infectious Diseases.

References

1. Hirsch, M. S. 1985. Prospects of therapy for infections with human T-lymphotropic virus, type III. Ann. Int. Med. 103: 750–754.
2. Yarchoan, R., and S. Broder. 1987. Development of antiretroviral therapy for the acquired immunodeficiency syndrome and related disorders. New. Engl. J. Med. 316: 557–564.
3. DeClercq, E. 1986. Chemotherapeutic approaches to the treatment of the acquired immunodeficiency snydrome (AIDS). J. Med. Chem. 29: 1561–1569.
4. Horowitz, J. P., J. Chua, and M. Noel. 1964. The monomesylates of 1-(2'-deoxy-beta-D-lyxofuranosyl) thymidine. J. Organ. Chem. 29: 2076–2078.
5. Mitsuya, H., K. J. Weenhold, and P. A. Furman. 1985. 3'-azido-3'-deoxythymidine (BWA509U): An antiviral agent that inhibits the infectivity and cytopathic effect of human T-lymphotrypec virus type III/lymphadenopathy-associated virus in vitro. Proc. Natl. Acad. Sci. USA 87: 7096–7100.
6. Richman, D. D., R. S. Kornbluth, and D. A. Carson. 1987. Failure of dideoxynucleosides to inhibit human immunodeficiency virus replication in cultured human macrophages. J. Exp. Med. 166: 1144–1149.
7. Richman, D. D., M. A. Fischl, M. H. Grieco, M. S. Gottlieb, P. A. Volberding, O. L. Laskin, J. M. Leedom, J. E. Groupman, D. Mildvan, M. S. Hirsch, G. G. Jackson, D. T. Durach, S. Nusinoff-Lehrman, and the AZT Collaborative Working Group. 1987. The toxicity of AZT in the treatment of patients with AIDS and ARC. A double-blind, placebo-controlled trial. New Engl. J. Med. 317: 192–197.
8. Fischl, M. A., D. D. Richman, M. H. Grieco, M. S. Gottlieb, P. A. Volberding, O. L. Laskin, J. M. Leedom, J. E. Groupman, D. Mildvan, R. T. Schooley, G. G. Jackson, D. T. Durach, D. King, and the AZT Collaborative Group. 1987. The efficacy of AZT in the treatment of patients with AIDS and ARC. A double-blind placebo-controlled trial. New Engl. J. Med. 317: 185–191.
9. Rothenberg, R. M., R. Woelfel, J. Stoneburner, J. Miller R. Parker, and B. Truman. 1987. Survival with AIDS. Experience with 5833 cases in New York City. New Engl. J. Med. 317: 1297–1302.
10. Bacchette, P., D. Osmond, R. E. Chaisson, S. Dritz, G. W. Rutherford, L. Swig, and A. R. Moss. 1988. Survival patterns of the first 500 patients with AIDS in San Francisco. J. Infect. Dis. 157: 1044–1047
11. Bacchette, P., D. Osmond, R. E. Chaisson, and A. R. Moss. 1988. Survival with AIDS in New York. New Engl. J. Med. 318: 1464–1465.
12. Hirsch, M. S. 1988. Azidothymidine. J. Infec. Dis. 157: 427–431.
13. Furth, P. A., and A. M. Kazakis. 1987. Nail pigmentation changes with azidothymidine (zidovidine). Ann. Int. Med. 107: 350.
14. Bessen, L. J., J. B. Greene, E. Louie, P. Seitzman, and H. Weinberg. 1988. Severe polymyositis-like syndrome associated with zidovidine therapy of AIDS and ARC. New Engl. J. Med. 318: 708.
15. Gorard, D. A., K. Henry, and R. J. Guiloff. 1988. Necrotizing myopathy and zidovidine. Lancet 1: 1050.
16. Mitsuya, H., and S. Broder. 1987. Strategies for antiviral therapy in AIDS. Nature 325: 773–778.
17. Surbone, A., R. Yarchoan, N. McAtee, R. Blum, M. Maha, J.-P. Allain, R. V. Thomas, H. Mitsuya, M. Leuther, S. Nusinoff-Lehrman, J. M. Pluda, F. K. Jacobsen, H. A. Kessler, C. E. Myers, and S. Broder. 1988. Treatment of AIDS and ARC with a regimen of AZT and acyclovir. Ann. Int. Med. 108: 534–540.
18. Yarchoan, R., C. F. Perno, R. V. Thomas, R. W. Klecker, J.-P. Allain, R. J. Wills, N. McAtee, M. A. Fischl, R. Dubinsky, M. C. McNeeley, H. Mitsuyu, J. M. Pluda, T. J. Lawley, M. Leuther, B. Safai, J. M. Collins, C. E. Myers, and S. Broder. 1988. Phase I Studies of 2',3'-dideoxy-cytidine in severe human immunodeficiency virus infection as a single agent and alternating with AZT. Lancet 1: 76–80.
19. Skowron, G., T. C. Merigan, S. Bonzette, D. Richman, R. Utlamchandani, M. Fischl, R. Schooley, M. Hirsch, W. J. Soo, C. Pettinelli, and the ddC

Study Group of the AIDS Clinical Trials Group. 1988. Abstract #3015, IV Int. Conf. AIDS, page 223.

20. Ueno, R., and S.Kuno. 1987 Dextran sulfate, a potent anti-HIV agent in vitro having synergism with AZT. Lancet 1: 1379.

21. Mitsuyu, H. 1988. Dextran sulfate suppression of viruses in the HIV family: Inhibitors of virion binding to CD4+ cells. Science 240: 646–649.

22. Abrams, D. I., S. Kuno, R. Wong, K. Jeffords, J. Molaghan, M. Nash, R. Wong, and R. Ueno. 1988 A phase I trial of oral UA 001 (Dextran Sulfate) in patients with AIDS and ARC. 1988. IV Int. Conf. AIDS Abstract #3580, p. 161.

23. Grieco, M. H., M. Lange, E. Buimovici-Klein, M. M. Reddy, A. England, G. F. McKinley, K. Ong, and C. Metroka 1988 Open study of AL-721 treatment of HIV infected subjects with generalized lymphadenopathy syndrome: An eight-week open trial and follow-up. Antiviral Research 9: 177–190.

24. Smith, D. H., R. A. Byrn, and S. A. Marsters. 1987. Blocking of HIV-1 infectivity by a soluble secreted form of the CD4 antigen. Science 238: 1704–1707.

25. Bergdahl, S., A. Sonnersberg, J. Albert, J. Sjovall, A. Larsson, M. Halvarsson, A. Aust-Kettes, B. Jakobsson, and O. Strannegard. 1988. Antiviral effects against HIV in patients with AIDS-related complex given intermittent IV foscarnet. Abstract #3588, IV Int. Conf. AIDS, page 163.

26. Jacobson, M. A., S. Crowe, J. Levy, F. Aweeka, J. Gambertoglio, N. McManus, and J. Mills. 1988. Beneficial effect of intermittent intravenous fos-

carnet on HIV infection in patients with AIDS, Abstract #3586, IV Int. Conf. AIDS, page 163.

27. Crumpacker, C., W. Heagy, G. Bubley, J. E. Monroe, R. Finberg, S. Hussey, L. Schnipper, D. Lucey, T. H. Lee, M. F. McLane, M. Essex, and C. Mulder. 1987 Ribavirin treatment of AIDS and ARC. Ann. Int. Med. 107: 664–674.

28. Vernon, A., R. S. Schulof, and the Ribavirin Study Group. 1987. Serum HIV core antigen in asymptomatic ARC patients taking oral ribavirin or placebo. Abstract T.8.b. IIIrd Int. Conf. AIDS, page 58.

29. Vogt, M. W., K. L. Hartshorn, P. A. Furman, T.-C. Chou, J. A. Fyfe, L. A. Coleman, C. Crumpacker, R. T. Schooley, and M. S. Hirsch. 1987. Ribavirin antagonizes the effect of AZT on HIV replication. Science 235: 1376–1379.

30. Montefiore, D. C. 1987. Antiviral activity of a mismatched double-strand of RNA (ampligen) against HIV in vitro. Proc. Natl. Acad. Sci. USA 84: 2985–2989.

31. Mitchell, W. M., D. C. Montefiore, W. E. Robinson, M. G. Pellegrino, and D. H. Gillespie. 1988. Inhibition of HIV-1 RNA accumulation by mismatched double-stranded RNA (ampligen) and zidovudine. Abstract #3613, IV Int. Conf. AIDS, page 170.

32. Strayer, D. B., I. Brodsky, L. Einck, S. M. Miller, P. Mansell, H. F. Henreques, D. M. Parente, R. S. Schulof, G. L. Simon, H. Paxton, W. H. Meyer, D. Paul, A. G. Grillo-Lopez, and W. A. Carter. 1988. Ampligen therapy in ARC/Pre-ARC. Abstract #3046, IV Int. Conf. AIDS, page 23.

The Interferons: Results of Clinical Trials of Anti-Alpha-Interferon (IFN) in AIDS

*Joseph A. Bellanti, Stephen M. Peters, Barbara Zeligs, Simon V. Skurkovich**

Based upon the hypothesis that acid labile alpha-IFN may downregulate the immune system, a study was performed to evaluate the safety and clinical efficacy of anti-alpha-IFN in patients with AIDS. Four patients with CDC-defined AIDS who had recovered from *P. carinii* pneumonia received daily intramuscular injections of sheep anti-alpha-IFN immunoglobulin (1.5 to 9×10^6 IU/day) for either 6 days (patients #1, #2), 11 days (patient #3) or 14 days (patient #4), during which time and subsequently thereafter clinical and laboratory parameters were evaluated at monthly intervals. Following treatment all 4 patients reported a subjective increase in sense of well-being and a clearance of facial erythroderma. After 14 days of treatment, patient #1 experienced an 8 lb weight gain and patient #4 a 4 lb weight gain. Prior to treatment all patients had detectable levels of alpha-IFN which was either partially (3/4) or totally (1/4) acid-labile. During the treatment period, no pH stable or acid-labile aberrant alpha-IFN could be detected in the blood of the subjects. Although no serious adverse or toxic effects were observed following treatment, 3 or 4 patients experienced either localized or a mild generalized maculopapular exanthem on the 9th to 10th day, which disappeared within a week.

Following treatment all subjects displayed a leukocytosis with neutrophilia either during the first 7-day period (patients #1 and #2) or within 14 days (patients #3 and #4); no significant changes in lymphocyte counts or in CD4/CD8 populations were observed. The results of these studies thus far suggest that there is a good correlation between the patients' acid-labile alpha-IFN levels and clinical status and that clinical improvement was seen following neutralization of the acid-labile IFN. The approach is feasible with negligible side effects and suggests that continuous removal of acid-labile IFN correlates with clinical improvement. However, the long-term efficacy of anti-alpha-IFN in the treatment of AIDS will require further studies of dosage and frequency of administration. At the present time an extracorporeal approach in which serum alpha-IFN will be removed using immunoadsorbent columns is being investigated.

Although originally described as a family of anti-viral proteins [1], it is now clear that the interferons (IFNs) comprise a heterogeneous collection of proteins and glycoproteins with a wide variety of biologic functions including cellular regulation, cellular differentiation [2], and intracellular communication; particularly significant are the immunoregulatory activities of the IFNs in humoral and cell-mediated immunity [3–6].

There are three known types of human IFNs differing in antigenic, chemical, and biological properties: alpha or leukocyte, beta or fibroblast, and gamma or immune IFN. Normal natural IFN alpha is pH stable. It is synthesized in the host as a family of at least 15 subtypes [7–8], which consist predominantly of pH-stable and some acid-labile subtypes [9]. It is possible that under normal conditions all these subtypes are produced in the same balanced proportions. Patients with certain immunologically mediated disorders, e.g., rheumatoid arthritis, systemic lupus erythematosus, and most recently the acquired immune deficiency syndrome (AIDS), have IFN alpha in the blood that is acid-labile, i.e., loses activity when treated with acid at pH 2. We have postulated [10, 11] that this increase in the amount of acid-labile alpha-IFN (due either to the production of new pH-labile alpha-IFN or other types of defective IFNs or to the decrease in the production of the pH stable types of IFN alpha) exerts a negative immunoregulatory effect. The purpose of the present studies was to treat 4 patients with AIDS with an anti-alpha-IFN immunoglobulin and to determine the reactogenicity and clinical efficacy of this treatment.

---

* Departments of Pediatrics and Microbiology and International Center for Interdisciplinary Studies of Immunology, Georgetown University School of Medicine, Washington, DC, and Advanced Biotherapy Concepts, Inc., Columbia, MD, USA.

Materials and Methods

Subjects

Four patients with CDC-defined AIDS who had recovered from *P. carinii* pneumonia were recruited into the study. The clinical characteristics and presentations are shown in Table 1.

Preparation and Source of Anti-Alpha-IFN Antibody

An anti-human alpha-IFN antibody was prepared by hyperimmunization of sheep with multiple injections of human alpha-IFN emulsified in complete Freund's adjuvant. Serial bleedings of the sheep were performed to establish maximal titers of anti-alpha IFN antibody and large bleedings were performed at appropriate intervals to obtain batch quantities of antiserum.

Purified sheep gamma globulin was prepared by ammonium sulfate fractionation followed by absorption with human serum albumin, chicken ovalbumin, and human leukocyte membrane extracts in normal human serum to remove cross-reacting antibodies. The final preparation was sterile filtered through a 0.22 μ filter and bottled in sterile pyrogen-free bottles.

Assays for Serum Alpha-IFN and Anti-Alpha-IFN

Serum interferon titers were measured by a modified bioassay using MDBK cells (Maria Darby bovine kidney cell line: American Type Culture Collection, Rockville, MD) as targets, and vesicular stomatitis virus (Indiana strain) VSV as a challenge [12]. The interferon titers were expressed as the reciprocal of the dilution at which 50% protection from VSV-induced cytopathogenicity occurred. Interferon standards were included with every assay and serial endpoint dilutions of serum were adjusted according to the results of standards and were expressed as IU/ml. Serum samples which were assayed for acid-labile alpha-IFN were diluted with 0.1 M HCl in RPMI to a pH 2.0 and incubated at 4°C for 24 h after which they were adjusted to pH 7.2 with 0.1 M NaOH. Control specimens were treated in a similar fashion but diluted with RPMI alone.

Serum alpha-IFN antibody assays were performed by incubating appropriate two-fold dilutions of antiserum with 8–10 reference units of human alpha-IFN for 1 h at 37°C followed by the assay of serum alpha-IFN as described above. Control anti-alpha-IFN standards were tested with each assay and the antiserum titers were reported as a mean titer for ml for 50% neutralization of 8–10 reference units of human alpha-IFN.

Table 1. Clinical characteristics prior to treatment.

				Initial presentation						Initial serum α-IFN (IU/ml)	
Pt #	Age/sex (yr) (M/F)	HIV Ab	P. carinii	CMV culture	Candidiasis	Lympha-denopathy	Weight loss	Fatigue	Others	Total activity	Activity after acid treatment
1	38/M	+	+	−	+	+ (cervical)	+	+	Facial erythroderma	125	0
2	43/M	+	+	+	+	+ (cervical)	−	−	Facial erythroderma	125	25
3	31/M	+	+	+	+	−	−	+	Acneform eruptions, diarrhea, pneumonia (MAI)	125	25
4	35/M	+	+	+	+	−	+	+	Facial erythroderma, diarrhea	125	25

Entrance Criteria and Immunization Schedule

After informed consent was obtained each subject had a complete history and physical examination performed. Entrance criteria consisted of the following:

1) all subjects were in category 4 of the AIDS Classification System of the CDC,

2) no AZT or other immune modulator treatment for at least one month prior to treatment,

3) patients with Kaposi's sarcoma were excluded,

4) all subjects had negative histories of allergy to animal protein and were also skin tested to sheep protein prior to treatment.

Patients received daily intramuscular injections of sheep anti-alpha-IFN immunoglobulin (1.5 to 9×10^6 IU/day) for either 6 days (patients #1 and #2), 11 days (patient #3), or 14 days (patient #4), during which time and subsequently thereafter at monthly intervals clinical laboratory (hematologic, biochemical, and immunologic) parameters were evaluated.

Results

Clinical Characteristics and Results of Treatment

The clinical characteristics of the four patients prior to treatment are summarized in Table 1. All of the patients were white male homosexuals ranging in age from 31 to 43 years. All had detectable HIV antibody, and all had recovered from *P. carinii* pneumonia 1–2 years previously. Three patients (#2, #3, #4) had positive CMV isolates from the urine, and all four had evidence of oral candidiasis. Patients #1 and #2 had evidence of cervical lymphadenopathy; patients #1 and #4 had significant weight loss, and patients #1, #3 and #4 fatigue. Of interest was the finding of facial erythroderma in three of the four patients and an acneform eruption in patient #3. All patients had detectable serum alpha-IFN, most of which was acid-labile.

The results of treatment are summarized in Table 2. Two of the four patients (#1 and #4) had significant weight gain (patient #1 +8 lb, patient #4 +4 lb) and an increase in energy level was seen in three of the patients (#1, #3, #4) with an increase in appetite in patient #1. The erythroderma or skin manifestations cleared in all patients following treatment; three of the four (patients #1, #3, #4) within 1-week period and within 1-month period (patient #2).

Table 2. Results of treatment*.

Pt #	Subjective changes					Skin manifestations			
	Weight gain (lb)	Energy level**	Appetite**	Erythro-derma	Other	Localized (site of inj.)	Generalized	Pain	Itching
1	+8	+++	++	improved		P	O	P	P
2	N.C.	N.C.	N.C.	N.C.		P	P	O	P
3	N.C.	++	N.C.		Improved acne		O	O	OO
4	+4	+	N.C.	Improved markedly		P	O	P	P

*Treatment 2–4 × 10^8 units anti-α-IFN/day
Patients 1 & 2 treated 6 days, patients 3 & 4 treated 11–14 days
**Degree of improvment:
N.C. = no change
+ = 25%
++ = 50%
+++ = 75%
++++ = 100%
***P = present, O = absent

No major adverse manifestations were seen following treatment. Mild swelling and tenderness were seen at the site of injection in three of four patients (patients #1, #3, #4) and a generalized rash in patient #2 which cleared within one week. No evidence of serum sickness was observed in any of the patients or any other major immediate hypersensitivity reactions.

Laboratory Studies

A variety of changes were seen in the peripheral leukocyte counts. Patients #1 and #2, who were treated for 6-day periods, demonstrated a rise in total leukocytes and in polymorphonuclear leukocytes within the first days of treatment. A compensatory decrease in lymphocytes was also observed during this period, which then reversed over a 14-day period. Patients #3 and #4, who were treated for longer periods, showed a more protracted increase in white cells and polymorphonuclear leukocytes but no significant change in lymphocytes. No significant changes in CD4 (T4) or CD8 (T8) or CD-2 (T11) populations were seen in any of the patients following treatment. More significant were the changes in lymphocyte mitogenic responses to PHA, PWM, and ConA. Patient #1 showed minor increases in PHA by 35 days. A more significant rise in PHA and PWM was observed in patient #2 by 60 days. Patient #3 showed a mild increase in PHA by the 21st day; no significant changes were observed in patient #4.

Current Clinical Status

Shown in Table 3 is a summary of the more recent findings seen in longer term follow-up of these patients. Patient #1, who had shown initial improvement on this treatment, later began an alternative anti-viral chemotherapy. He developed severe bone marrow suppression and leukopenia, and soon expired. His blood showed a very high level of acid-labile alpha-IFN. Acid-labile interferon was not detected in patient #2 since his treatment, and he has remained clinically well. Patient #3 improved after his initial treatment, and no acid-labile IFN was found in his blood. Five months later his condition deteriorated and the levels of acid-labile IFN were found elevated. He was then retreated for a 12-day period and his acid-labile IFN decreased and his clinical condition improved (enhanced energy, appetite, disappearance of rash). Based upon the data of this retreated patient, we were strongly encouraged that repeated removal of the acid-labile alpha-IFN was achieving a therapeutic effect. Although he improved for a 5-month period, he developed a systemic coccidiomycosis infection at this time, deteriorated rapidly, and expired in June 1988 before any opportunity for retreatment. The clinical condition of patient #4 improved initially but subsequently deteriorated with a recurrence of *P. carinii* pneumonia. Although it was planned to retreat this patient, he deteriorated before a second course of antibody could be administered and expired on 7/15/88.

Table 3. Results of anti-α-IFN treatment in patients with AIDS.

| Patient | Dates | Treatment | | Serum α-IFN (IU/ml) | | Total ab α-IFN | |
		Duration (days)	Pre	During	Post (2–12 mos.)	Clinical course
1*	10/14/86–10/19/86	6	125/125	<5/<5	625/500	Died 7/6/87
2	1/9/87–1/14/87	6	125/100	<5/<5	<5/<5	Clinically well
3*	4/21/87–5/4/87	14	125/100	<5/<5	125/<5	Initial improvement, followed by subjective deterioration
	10/7/87–10/19/87	12	625/625	<5/<5	<5/<5	Improvement; died 6/88
4*	4/22/87–5/1/87	11	125/100	<5/<5	25/25	Deterioration; died 7/15/88

*patients expired

Discussion

The results of these studies thus far suggest that there is a good correlation between the patients' acid-labile alpha-IFN levels and clinical status, and that clinical improvement was seen following neutralization of the acid-labile IFN. Thus, these preliminary studies have supported our original hypothesis and have encouraged us to proceed further with this approach.

The approach is based upon the hypothesis that disturbances in the synthesis of interferon, i.e., alpha-IFN, accompanied by sharp increases in the production of an aberrant acid-labile type of alpha-IFN represents a major factor in the continuous dysregulation and immunosuppression seen in patients in varying stages of human immunodeficiency virus (HIV) infection, e.g., AIDS. It has been found that the serum of patients with frank AIDS or ARC has elevated levels of aberrant alpha interferon. This interferon abnormality is hypothesized to represent a "fault" in the normal immune cascade, related to the HIV infection which initially disturbed interferon synthesis and, subsequently, the immune system [11]. It is hypothesized that the level of aberrant alpha interferon reflects viral replication. Anti-interferon immunoglobulin administered to such patients presumably binds to the hyperproduced aberrant alpha interferon and neutralizes it.

Recent evidence has provided a possible mechanism for this postulated action of acid-labile IFN and the manner in which the continuous presence of alpha-IFN may be responsible for the clinical deterioration of patients with AIDS. Recent studies [13–15] have demonstrated that lymphocytes incubated with alpha-IFN in vitro or lymphocytes taken from patients treated with alpha-IFN in vivo show a loss of alpha-IFN receptors on a variety of target cells including specific subpopulations of lymphocytes. These observations lend further support for an abnormal modulation of lymphocyte responsiveness by the continuous presence of this acid-labile interferon. In future studies we shall be directing our efforts to the continual removal of acid-labile interferon from the blood of these patients using an extracorporeal device. The advantages of this approach are that it should be more efficient, should allow more frequent treatment, and would have the added advantage of reducing potential allergic reactions by eliminating the need for administration of a foreign antiserum to patients.

References

1. Isaacs, A., and Lindenmann, J. 1957. Virus interference. I. Interferon. Proc. R. Soc. London Ser. B 145: 258.
2. Rossi, G. B. 1985. In: Interferon 6, I. Gresser, ed. Orlando, FL: Academic Press, p. 31.
3. Skurkovich, S. V., E. G. Klinovy, I. M. Aleksandrovskaya, N. V. Levina, N. A. Arkhipova, and T. I. Bulycheva. 1973. Stimulation of transplantation immunity and plasma cell reaction by interferon in mice. Immunology 25: 317.
4. Skurkovich, S. V., A. S. Skorikova, and E. I. Eremkina. 1978. Enhancement by interferon of lymphocyte cytotoxicity in normal individuals to cells of human lymphoblastoid lines. J. Immunol. 121: 1173.
5. Sonnenfeld, G. A., and T. Merigan. 1979. A regulatory role for interferon in immunity. Ann. N.Y. Acad. Sci. 332: 345.
6. Stewart, W. E., II. 1981. The interferon system. New York: Springer-Verlag.
7. Owerbach, D., W. J. Rutter, T. B. Shows, P. Gray, D. V. Goeddel, and R. M. Lawn. 1981. Leukocyte and fibroblast interferon genes are located on human chromosome 9. Proc. Natl. Acad. Sci. 78: 3123.
8. Vilcek, J., A. E. Friedman-Kien, D. Henriksen-DeStefano, J. A. Sonnabend, O. T. Preble, and R. M. Friedman. 1984. In: The epidemic of Kaposi's sarcoma and opportunistic infections. A. E. Friedman-Kien and L. J. Laubenstein, eds. New York: Masson, p. 193.
9. Landgraf, S., and D. C. Chadha. 1983. IFN Scie. Mem. 1, Sept.
10. Skurkovich, S., and E. I. Eremkina. 1975. The probable role of interferon in allergy. Ann. Allergy 35: 356.
11. Skurkovich, S., B. Skurkovich, and J. A. Bellanti. 1987. A unifying model of the immunoregulatory role of the interferon system: Can interferon produce disease in humans? Clin. Immunol. Immunopath. 43: 362.
12. Familetti, P. C., S. Rubinstein, and S. Pestka. 1981. A convenient and rapid cytopathic effect inhibition assay for interferon. In: Methods of enzymology, Vol. 78. Interferons. S. Pestka, ed. New York, London, Toronto, Sydney, San Francisco: Academic Press, p. 387.
13. Faltynek, C. R., G. L. Princler, and J. R. Ortaldo. 1986. Expression of IFN-α and IFN-α receptors on normal human small resting T lymphocytes and large granular lymphocytes. J. Immunol. 136: 4134.

14. Lau, A. S., G. E. Hannigan, M. H. Freedman, and B. R. G. Williams. 1986. Regulation of interferon receptor expression in human blood lymphocytes in vitro and during interferon therapy. J. Clin. Invest. 77: 1632.

15. Faltynek, C. R., and G. L. Princler. 1986. Modulation of interferon-α and interferon-α receptor expression during T-lymphocyte activation and proliferation. J. Interferon Research 6: 639.

Immunological Strategies for Therapeutic Destruction of HIV and HIV-Infected Cells in Asymptomatic Patients

Alec H. Sehon*

It is proposed that the immunological armamentarium developed for the in vivo destruction of tumor cells by the use of "magic bullets" may be adapted for the annihilation of HIV and HIV-infected cells. It is suggested that for this purpose anti-HIV antibodies be labelled with radionuclides, anti-viral drugs, or toxins. To overcome the inherent immunogenicity of these immunotoxins (IT), which would undermine their effectiveness, it is recommended that the patients be rendered tolerant to IT by pre-administration of immunosuppressive conjugates of IT with monomethoxypolyethylene glycol (mPEG). The rationale for this tolerogenic regimen is based on results obtained in the author's laboratory demonstrating that mPEG conjugates of xenogeneic immunoglobulins (xIg) may induce tolerance to xIg. It is anticipated that this therapeutic modality would at least prolong the asymptomatic phase of HIV-infected individuals and slow down, if not prevent altogether, the development of full-blown AIDS.

Working Hypothesis

There is increasing recognition of the overwhelming difficulties in producing in the foreseeable future an effective anti-HIV vaccine [1] and of the danger of inducing instead anti-HIV antibodies that may actually *enhance* the infectivity of the virus by promoting its attachment to and penetration into cells possessing Fc receptors [2]. Hence, in this paper, I propose an alternative therapeutic strategy involving the use of *passively administered, modified anti-HIV antibodies* for the protection of asymptomatic HIV carriers.

Viral epitopes of HIV have been shown to be accessible—albeit in vitro—on HIV-infected cells to xenogeneic monoclonal and polyclonal anti-HIV antibodies [3, 4]. By analogy, with methods developed for the destruction of tumor cells in cancer patients, by the use of immunotoxins (IT) [5, 6] it is postulated that infected T(CD4) cells bearing HIV epitopes as well as HIV virions released from these and other infected cells could be destroyed and/or inactivated in vivo by "magic bullets" consisting of conjugates of anti-HIV monoclonal antibodies (MAbs) with appropriate toxins, radionuclides, or anti-viral agents; for the sake of brevity, all these potentially viricidal anti-HIV conjugates will be referred to as IT. Although there are many more cells (monocytes/macrophages, dendritic, Langerhans, and glial cells) containing the HIV genome in a cryptic, latent form than cells expressing HIV epitopes, the strategy proposed in this paper for *arresting the progression of HIV infection to full-blown AIDS* rests on the hypothesis that

1. conserved HIV epitopes, such as those of the gp120 viral envelope [7], are accessible in vivo to the corresponding anti-HIV MAbs not only on free HIV but also on some of the infected cells, and

2. under the protective umbrella of the appropriate anti-HIV IT, any virus released from or appearing on infected cells (as well as these cells) would be captured and destroyed by the IT in circulation before having the chance of infecting new cells.

It may also be envisaged that direct administration of anti-HIV IT into the cerebrospinal fluid may arrest the neurological effects of HIV, as apparently successfully achieved by

*   MRC Group for Allergy Research, Department of Immunology, The University of Manitoba, Winnipeg, MB, Canada, R3E 0W3.
Acknowledgements: This study was supported by grants from the Medical Research Council of Canada and the N.I.A.I.D., National Institutes of Health, Bethesda, MD. The secretarial assistance of Gail Falkenberg and Shamina Singh is acknowledged.

intrathecal targeting of radiolabelled MAbs to tumor antigens in patients with neurological malignancies [8]. These strategies, in common with passive immunization in other diseases, would be expected to reduce the patient's viral burden and the spread of the virus in and from healthy seropositive individuals. The development in recent years in many laboratories of increasing numbers of murine MAbs, goat and monkey antibodies to a variety of HIV envelope epitopes [3, 4, 7] renders the hypothesis testable.

Possible Induction of Immunological Tolerance in HIV-Carriers to Xenogeneic Anti-HIV MAbs and IT by the Corresponding Conjugates with Monomethoxy-polyethylene Glycol (mPEG)

The obvious possible complications due to the injection of anti-HIV MAbs or of the corresponding IT into asymptomatic patients—who for all intents and purposes still possess a functional immune system—is the inherent immunogenicity of these immunological bullets in humans. It is to be also noted that toxins are even more immunogenic than xenogeneic immunoglobulins [9]. Therefore, it is to be anticipated that these patients will produce antibodies to these immunological reagents, and that—in addition to undermining the effectiveness of the immunotherapy—the resulting immune complexes may lead to diverse pathophysiological effects, e.g., serum sickness, anaphylactic symptoms, and hepatotoxicity [5, 10]. To overcome these complications, it is suggested that the proposed use of "magic bullets" be combined with *a method developed in this laboratory for conversion of diverse antigens [11]—including xenogeneic immunoglobulins (xIg) [12]—to nonimmunogenic and tolerogenic derivatives which suppress specifically the host's immune response to the antigens in question.* This conversion involves the coupling of an appropriate number of mPEG molecules (mol. wt. of about 3000 or 6000) onto the antigen molecule; the resulting conjugates were shown in mice to be particularly suppressogenic if administered prior to injection of the unmodified antigen [11, 13].

The tolerance induced by mPEG conjugates was demonstrated to be due to suppressor T (Ts) cells which also produced soluble factors (TsFs) capable of suppressing specifically the immune response. Moreover, these TsFs were shown to be protease-sensitive, but resistant to treatment with RNase or DNase [14]. It is also to be noted that, in very recent experiments [15], it was shown that TsFs could be isolated from the extract of these Ts cells by an immunosorbent synthesized by immobilizing murine B16G MAbs produced to an unrelated TsF [16]. Interestingly, the eluted TsFs had also the ability to bind to the specific antigen that had been incorporated into the mPEG conjugates used for induction of the tolerance and for generation of Ts cells. Thus, the TsFS induced by tolerogenic mPEG conjugates appear to consist of two domains, i.e., one antigen-specific domain and the other domain sharing an antigenic epitope(s) with other TsFs. Since in all likelihood TsFs are proteins, they would be amenable to synthesis by recombinant DNA (rDNA) methodology, and one may visualize that the synthetic products could be used in lieu of tolerogenic mPEG conjugates of the corresponding IT.

Despite the recent elegant synthesis of tailormade chimeric [17] and "humanized" antibodies [18] by genetic engineering, it is likely that—even if these antibodies were nonimmunogenic in man—because of the high immunogenicity of toxins the effectiveness of the corresponding IT, just as that of xenogeneic MAbs, would be counteracted by the immune response of the recipient. Therefore, studies were recently undertaken in this laboratory for the synthesis of tolerogenic mPEG conjugates of xIg, in the expectation that injection of these tolerogens prior to initiation of the treatment with nonpegylated xIg would induce specific immunosuppression, and that, consequently, it would be possible to administer subsequently the xIg without engendering anti-xIg antibodies [12, 13].

In the absence of the resources required to test the validity of this premise with mouse MAbs in nonhuman primates, the model developed consisted of inbred strains of adult mice, human monoclonal (myeloma) immunoglobulins (HIgG) as a source of xIg, and heat aggregated HIgG (i.e., haHIgG) as the immunizing antigen in absence of adjuvant; the HIgG was aggregated by heating at 63°C for

571

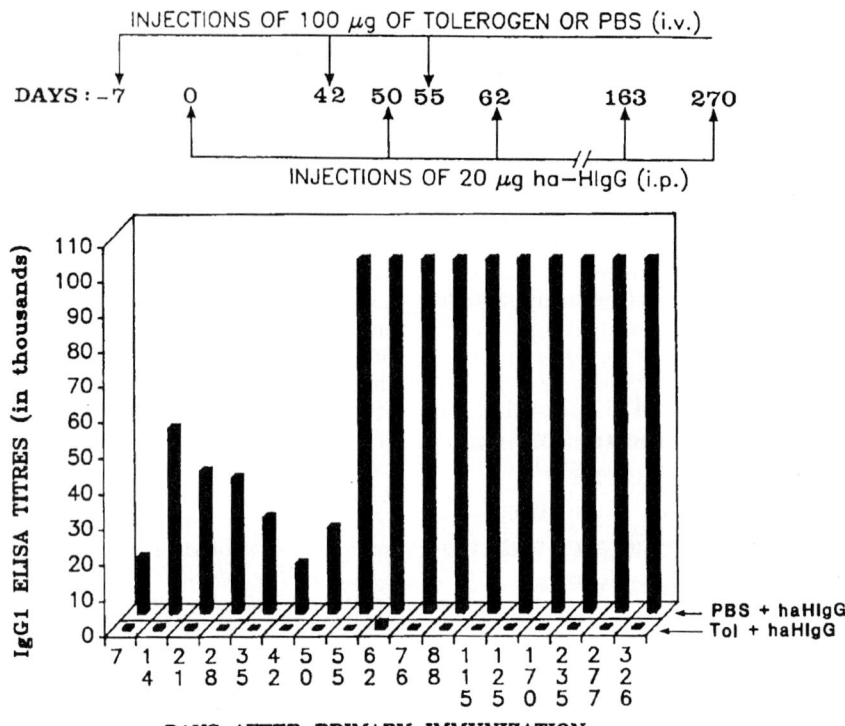

Figure 1. Induction of tolerance to HIgG by the treatment of mice with HIgG(mPEG)$_{22}$. The control group received PBS and the test group three injections of 100µg of HIgG(mPEG)$_{22}$ on days –7, 42, and 55. Both groups were immunized five times with 20µg of haHIgG on days 0, 50, 62, 163 and 270. (The days are to be read vertically.)

25 min in order to increase its immunogenicity without the use of adjuvants. By using a diversity of protocols, differing in the number of doses of a given conjugate and of intermittent injections of haHIgG, it was shown that a long-lasting state of tolerance to HIgG (in excess of 300 days) was established in mice by pre-administration of the corresponding HIgG (mPEG)$_n$ conjugates [13]. Moreover, the suppression encompassed multiple IgG subclasses, i.e., IgG1, IgG2a and IgG2b anti-HIgG antibodies.

The typical results of the experiment illustrated in Figure 1 demonstrate that injection of the HIgG(mPEG)$_{22}$ on days –7, 42, and 55 resulted in suppression of the IgG1 anti-HIgG antibody response in excess of 95% in animals that received 5 doses of the antigen over a period of 270 days. In an other experiment designed to test the specificity of the immunosuppressive effect of HIgG(mPEG)$_{22}$ (data not given here), it was demonstrated that injection of an unrelated antigen, i.e., OA, on day 146

into mice immunosuppressed to HIgG, induced an IgG1 anti-OA antibody response that was essentially identical to that induced in mice which had not been treated with HIgG (mPEG)$_{22}$.

Since "pegylation" of anti-HIV MAbs or of their IT would result in a marked reduction or total loss of their antigen binding capacity due to conformational changes and/or masking of their antigen binding sites, treatment with tolerogenic mPEG conjugates of IT by themselves may not prove too effective. Therefore, to ensure the efficacy of the treatment, the therapeutic regimen would consist of two steps: The first, *immunosuppressive phase* would involve a series of injections of tolerogenic mPEG conjugates of MAbs, or of mPEG conjugates of the corresponding IT, for induction of tolerance in the host to the epitopes of MAbs and/or IT; and the second, *effector phase* would involve injections of the nonpegylated MAbs or IT, and intermittent injections of the corresponding mPEG conjugates. The crucial issue which still remains to be clarified is whether or not mPEG conjugates are capable of suppressing the immune response also to the idiotypic determinants of cell-bound MAbs [23, 24].

As a further refinement of the treatment, the *efficacy of targeting the immunological bullets* onto HIV epitopes could be increased by the depletion of free HIV, autologous anti-HIV antibodies, and of possible immune complexes thereof from the circulation of asymptomatic HIV carriers. This depletion could be achieved by prior plasmapheresis utilizing two immunosorbent cartridges in series, one consisting of immobilized anti-HIV antibodies and the other of immobilized HIV epitopes. Clearly, this therapy could be supplemented by anti-viral agents; some of the highly potent anti-viral drugs—which cannot be administered systemically because of their toxicity—could be actually coupled to anti-HIV IT for their selective delivery onto HIV or onto infected cells with HIV on their surface.

The Possible Supplementary Therapeutic Use of mPEG Conjugates of CD4 or CD4-Tx

In view of the increasing interest in using synthetic CD4 for blocking the infectivity of HIV [19–21], one may also visualize the use of CD4-Tx conjugates which would be expected not only to bind to HIV, but also to inactivate the virus. However, the concern has been expressed [22] that an influx of synthetic CD4 may induce anti-CD4 auto-antibodies that would sabotage the immune system—as does HIV—by reaction with cells carrying the CD4 marker. Clearly, this concern would be even more justified for the probably immunogenic CD4-Tx. Therefore, as for the above proposed therapeutic strategies involving xenogeneic anti-HIV antibodies or their toxin derivatives, it is recommended that treatment with CD4 or CD4-Tx be preceded by immunosuppression of the recipient to the respective epitopes with tolerogenic mPEG conjugates of CD4 or CD4-Tx.

Anticipated Results

The proposed therapeutic regimens are expected to be effective mainly in the early stage after infection and prior to conversion from the asymptomatic phase to full-blown AIDS. These strategies are predicated on the assumption that

1. not all of the patient's cells having CD4 receptors would have been infected prior to the beginning of the treatment, and

2. newly differentiated cells would be spared infection by the virus which would be sequestered or destroyed by the passively administered antibodies or IT.

Clearly, this passive immunization therapy would be expected to prolong the asymptomatic phase of HIV-infected individuals by reduction of their viral burden [25]. Thus, one may gain the time needed for preventing the development of full-blown AIDS by

1. induction of a vigorous autologous anti-HIV immune response by an effective vaccine whenever this becomes available [26], and

2. supportive therapies with new agents, such as synthetic CD4, CD4-Tx conjugates, or appropriate anti-viral drugs.

Finally, in support of using mPEG conjugates in humans, it ought to be pointed out that administration of mPEG conjugates of immunogenic proteins, such as allergens and xenogeneic enzymes, has proven a safe therapeutic procedure in patients suffering from common allergies [27], adenosine deaminase deficiency [28], and cancer [29].

References

1. Ada, G. L. 1988. Plenary lecture: Prospects for HIV vaccines. IV Int. Conf. on AIDS, Stockholm, June 16.
2. Matsuda, S., M. Gidlynd, K. Nillsson, A. Nygren, E. M. Feny, and H. Wigzell. 1988. Enhancement of HIV replication in human monocytes by low titers of anti-HIV antibodies in vitro. Abstract 2070, IV Int. Conf. on AIDS, Stockholm, June 12–16.
3. Fung, M. S. C., C. Sun, and N.-C. Sun. 1987. Monoclonal antibodies that neutralize HIV-1 virions and inhibit syncytium formation by infected cells. Biotechnol. 5: 940–946.
4. Lyerly, H. K., T. J. Matthews, A. J. Langlois et al. 1987. Human T-cell lymphotropic virus IIIb glycoprotein (gp120) bound to CD4 determinants on normal lymphocytes and expressed by infected cells serves as target for immune attack. Proc. Natl. Acad. Sci. 84: 4601–4605.

5. Dillman, R.O. 1985. Monoclonal antibodies in the treatment of cancer. C.R.C. Crit. Rev. Oncol. Hematol. 1: 357.

6. Frankel, A. E. 1988. Immunotoxins. Boston: Kluwer Academic Publishers.

7. Ho, D. D., J. C. Kaplan, I. E. Rackauskas, and M. E. Gurney. 1988. Second conserved domain of gp120 is important for HIV infectivity and antibody neutralization. Science 239: 1021–1023.

8. Lashford, L. S., A. G. Davies, R. B. Richardson, S. P. Bourne, J. A. Bullimore, H. Eckert, J. T. Kemshead, and H. B. Coakham. 1988. A pilot study of ^{131}I monoclonal antibodies in the therapy of leptomeningeal tumors. Cancer 61: 857–868.

9. Mischak, R., C. Foxall, K. Knebel, L. Spitler, V. Byers, L. Currant, and R. W. Baldwin. 1988. Human antibody responses to murine monoclonal antibody-ricin A chain immunotoxins. 3rd Intl. Conf. on Monoclonal Immunoconjugates for Cancer, San Diego, California (Abstract No. 27).

10. Zimmer, A. M., R. E. Goldman-Lieken, and J. M. Kazikiew. 1987. Radioimmunotherapy retreatment of cutaneous T cell lymphoma: Effect of plasmapheresis on human antimurine antibody titers. J. Nucl. Med. 28: 603 (Abstract No. 193).

11. Sehon, A. H. 1982. Suppression of IgE antibody responses with tolerogenic conjugates of allergens and haptens. Prog. Allergy 32: 161–202.

12. Wilkinson, I., C.-J. C. Jackson, G. M. Lang, V. Holford-Strevens, and A. H. Sehon. 1987. Tolerance induction in mice by conjugates of monoclonal immunoglobulins and monomethoxypolyethylene glycol. Transfer of tolerance by T cells and by T cell extracts. J. Immunol. 139: 326–331.

13. Maiti, P. K., G. M. Lang, and A. H. Sehon. 1988. Tolerogenic conjugates of xenogeneic monoclonal antibodies with monomethoxypolyethylene glycol: I. Induction of long-lasting tolerance to xenogeneic monoclonal antibodies. V. Int. Congr. on Advances in the Applications of Monoclonal Antibodies in Clinical Oncology. London, U.K., May 25–27, Int. J. Cancer (in press).

14. Wilkinson, I. 1988. Ph.D. Dissertation, The University of Manitoba, March.

15. Athota, R., and A. H. Sehon. unpublished data.

16. Steele, J. K., A. T. Stammers, A. Chan, and J. Levy. 1986. Characterization of an anti-idiotypic T cell hybridoma involved in the regulation of the immune response to the P815 mastocytoma. J. Immunol. 137: 3550–3556.

17. Brüggemann, M., G. T. Williams, C. I. Bindon, M. R. Clark, M. R. Walker, R. Jefferis, H. Waldmann, and M. S. Neuberger. 1987. Comparison of the effector functions of human immunoglobulins using a matched set of chimeric antibodies. J. Exp. Med. 166: 1351–1361.

18. Riechmann, L., M. Clark, H. Waldmann, and G. Winter. 1988. Reshaping human antibodies for therapy. Nature (London). 332: 323–327.

19. Clapham, P. R., D. Whitby, A. G. Dalgleish, P. Maddon, R. Axel, R. Sweet, and R. A. Weiss. 1988. Soluble CD4 neutralizes infectivity and syncytia of HIV-1, HIV-2 and SIV. IV Int. Conf. on AIDS, Stockholm, June 16.

20. Fisher, R., J. Bertonis, B. Chao, D. Costopoulos, T. Liu, J. Maraganore, W. Meier, R. Flavell, V. Johnson, B. Walker, and R. Schooley. 1988. Development of recombinant soluble CD4 as a novel HIV antiviral. IV Int. Conf. on AIDS, Stockholm, June 16.

21. Byrn, R., D. Capon, T. Gregory, S. Chamow, and J. Groopman. 1988. In vitro inhibition of HIV-1 infection with purified soluble recombinant CD4. IV Int. Conf. on AIDS, Stockholm, June 16.

22. Haseltine, W. A. 1988. Plenary Lecture: Replication and pathogenesis of AIDS virus. IV Int. Conf. on AIDS, Stockholm, June 14.

23. Benjamin, R. K., S. P. Cobbold, M. R. Clark, and H. Waldmann. 1986. Tolerance to rat monoclonal antibodies. J. Exp. Med. 163: 1539–1552.

24. Jonker, M., and J. H. A. M. Den Brok. 1987. Idiotype switching of CD4-specific monoclonal antibodies can prolong the therapeutic effectiveness in spite of host anti-mouse IgG antibodies. Eur. J. Immunol. 17: 1547–1553.

25. Salk, J. 1987. Prospects for the control of AIDS by immunizing seropositive individuals. Nature 327: 473–476.

26. Levine, A. M., B. E. Henderson, R. Dworsky, M. S. Ascher, H. W. Sheppard, L. C. Cullman, D. R. Hicks, C. Munson, D. J. Carlo, J. Ambrahamson, and R. Salk. 1988. Response of HIV infected individuals with ARC to inoculation of gamma-irradiated HIV. Abstract 6567, IV Int. Conf. on AIDS, Stockholm, June 12–16.

27. Dreborg, S., and E. Akerblom. Immunotherapy with polyethylene glycol modified allergens. In: Crit. Rev. Therapeutic Drug Carrier Systems. S. Bruck, ed. Boca Raton, FL: CRC Press, Inc., in press.

28. Hershfield, M. S., R. H. Buckley, M. L. Greenberg, A. L. Melton, R. Schiff, C. Hatem, J. Kurtzberg, M. L. Markert, R. H. Kobayashi, and A. Abuchowski. 1987. Treatment of adenosine deaminase deficiency with polyethylene glycol-modified adenosine deaminase. N. Eng. J. Med. 316: 589–596.

29. Abuchowski, A., G. M. Kazo, C. R. Verhoest, T. Van Es, D. Kafke Witz, M. L. Nucci, A. T. Viau, and F. F. Davis. 1984. Cancer therapy with chemically modified enzymes. I. Anti-tumor properties of polyethylene glycol-asparaginase conjugates. Cancer Biochem. Biophy. 7: 175–186.

SUBJECT INDEX*

---

*   This index has been prepared on the basis of the *key words* supplied by the authors. The page number(s) refer(s) to
     the first page(s) of the respective article(s).